VOLUME ONE

Textbook of Plastic, Maxillofacial and Reconstructive Surgery

SECOND EDITION

VOLUME ONE

Textbook of Plastic, Maxillofacial and Reconstructive Surgery

SECOND EDITION

EDITORS

Gregory S. Georgiade, M.D., F.A.C.S.

Associate Professor, General Surgery and
Plastic, Maxillofacial and Reconstructive Surgery
Duke University Medical Center
Durham, North Carolina

Nicholas G. Georgiade, D.D.S., M.D., F.A.C.S.

Professor Emeritus and Former Chief
Division of Plastic, Maxillofacial, Reconstructive and Oral Surgery
Duke University Medical Center
Durham, North Carolina

Ronald Riefkohl, M.D., F.A.C.S.

Clinical Associate Professor
Plastic, Maxillofacial and Reconstructive Surgery
Duke University Medical Center
Durham, North Carolina

William J. Barwick, M.D.

Assistant Professor
Plastic, Maxillofacial and Reconstructive Surgery
Duke University Medical Center
Durham, North Carolina

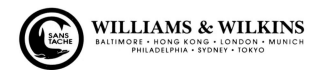

WILLIAMS & WILKINS
BALTIMORE · HONG KONG · LONDON · MUNICH
PHILADELPHIA · SYDNEY · TOKYO

Editor: Timothy H. Grayson
Managing Editor: Victoria M. Vaughn
Copy Editor: Megan Westerfeld
Designer: Norman W. Och
Illustration Planner: Ray Lowman
Production Coordinator: Raymond E. Reter
Cover Designer: Norman W. Och

Copyright © 1992
Williams & Wilkins
428 East Preston Street
Baltimore, Maryland 21202, USA

Accurate indications, adverse reactions, and dosage schedules for drugs are provided in this book, but it is possible that they may change. The reader is urged to review the package information data of the manufacturers of the medications mentioned.

Printed in the United States of America

First Edition 1987

Library of Congress Cataloging in Publication Data

Textbook of plastic, maxillofacial, and restructive surgery / editors.
  Gregory S. Georgiade . . . [et al.].—2nd ed.
      p.   cm.
  Rev. ed. of Essentials of plastic, maxillofacial, and
reconstructive surgery.   c1987.
  Includes bibliographical references and index.
  ISBN 0-683-03454-5
  1. Surgery, Plastic.   I. Georgiade, Nicholas G., 1918–
  [DNLM: 1. Surgery, Plastic.   WO 600 T355]
RD118.E87   1992
617.9′5—dc20
DNLM/DLC
for Library of Congress   90-13151
                                                  CIP

                              92 93 94 95 96
                      1 2 3 4 5 6 7 8 9 10

To
RUTH GEORGIADE
Associate in the Department of Surgery
for her continued dedication and penchant for accuracy
and details in the final preparations
of these many manuscripts and bibliographies.

Foreword

When the first edition of this outstanding text was written, it was a pleasure to write a strong Foreword in view of the eminence of the contributors and the high quality of its content. It is now a privilege to recognize that it has been a very successful effort and is widely read. For these reasons, the publishers requested a second edition under the editorship of Dr. Gregory S. Georgiade, Associate Professor of Surgery and Plastic Surgery at the Duke University Medical Center. Once again a text of exceptional significance has been produced and can be highly recommended.

Emphasis should be placed upon the fact that Dr. Nicholas G. Georgiade, formerly Professor and Chairman of the Division of Plastic and Maxillofacial Surgery at Duke University Medical Center, was the first Editor, and provided a sound basis for the text. He developed a work of high caliber and relevance, and these features have been maintained and expanded in the present edition. Of particular significance are the quality of the illustrations and the fact that they have been carefully selected to illustrate pertinent points. This feature has particular significance in the field of plastic and maxillofacial surgery since the clinical results and final appearance are of significance both to the patient and to a host of observers. It is important to emphasize that the text includes chapters covering such topics as speech pathology and psychological aspects of plastic surgical patients, with appropriate attention given the subject of medicolegal professional liability.

In this edition a number of changes have been made. Twenty chapters are now authored by new contributors, placing emphasis on the fact that an orderly rotation of participants is essential to maintain updated presentations of the wide number of topics included in this work. Like its predecessor, it can be predicted that this edition of *Textbook of Plastic, Maxillofacial and Reconstructive Surgery* will continue to exert a major impact upon this field.

David C. Sabiston, Jr., M.D.
James B. Duke Professor of Surgery
Department of Surgery
Chairman Department of Surgery
Duke University Medical Center
Durham, North Carolina

Preface

The extremely popular and successful first edition was so well received that the editors determined that a timely second edition encompassing an even greater base of information in this expanding specialty should be published. The editors' objectives were to update the information in original chapters and to also introduce new and additional chapters yielding a new "state-of-the-art" textbook. This new revised text now has over 100 chapters and has been divided into nine sections: Basic Principles; Skin and Soft Tissues; Head and Neck; Aesthetic Surgery; Breast and Chest; Genitalia; Microsurgery; Hand; Trunk and Lower Extremity; and Practical Concepts of the Plastic Surgery Practice. This text continues to be as comprehensive as possible, including the many illustrations and complete updated bibliographies as well as recommended readings that are an important contribution to each of the chapters.

Acknowledgments

We would like to thank all the contributing authors who so willingly contributed their knowledge, time, and expense to the production of this new second edition.

The office staff, namely, Judy Hall, Nancy Sipes, Lena Carver, and Jackie Howard, are complimented for the computerization of these manuscripts. The always helpful staff at Williams and Wilkins, including Ms. Vicki Vaughn, Mr. Tim Grayson, Mr. Raymond Reter, and many others, are to be commended for their assistance.

Contributors

Hassein S. Abul-Hassan, M.D.
Division of Plastic & Reconstructive Surgery, University of Louisville School of Medicine, Louisville, Kentucky

Bernard S. Alpert, M.D., F.A.C.S.
Assistant Clinical Professor of Surgery, University of California at San Francisco, and Chief, Department of Plastic Surgery, San Francisco Institute of Plastic Surgery, Davies Medical Center, San Francisco, California

Mark A. Anton, M.D.
Newport Beach, California

David P. Apfelberg, M.D., F.A.C.S.
Director, Comprehensive Laser Center, Palo Alto Medical Foundation, Palo Alto, California; and Assistant Clinical Professor of Plastic Surgery, Stanford University Medical Center, Stanford, California

Louis C. Argenta, M.D., F.A.C.S.
Professor of Surgery and Chairman, Department of Plastic & Reconstructive Surgery, Bowman Gray School of Medicine, Wake Forest University, Winston-Salem, North Carolina

Sherrell J. Aston, M.D., F.A.C.S.
Clinical Associate Professor, Plastic Surgery, New York University School of Medicine, and Surgeon Director, Department of Plastic Surgery, Manhattan Eye, Ear & Throat Hospital, New York, New York

Joseph Banis, Jr., M.D., F.A.C.S.
Associate Professor, Division of Plastic & Reconstructive Surgery, University of Louisville, Louisville, Kentucky

Fritz E. Barton, Jr., M.D., F.A.C.S.
Professor & Chairman, Division of Plastic Surgery, University of Texas Southwestern Medical School, Dallas, Texas

William J. Barwick, M.D.
Assistant Professor, Division of Plastic & Reconstructive Surgery, Duke University Medical Center, Durham, North Carolina

Bruce S. Bauer, M.D., F.A.C.S., F.A.A.P.
Associate Professor of Surgery, Northwestern University Medical School, and Chief, Division of Plastic Surgery, The Children's Medical Hospital, Chicago, Illinois

Ellen Beatty, M.D.
Associate, Florida Orthopaedic Institute, Tampa, Florida

Patricia Bitter, M.D.
General Surgery Resident, Hennepin County Medical Center, Minneapolis, Minnesota

Scott A. Brenman, M.D.
Clinical Assistant Professor, Division of Plastic Surgery, Pennsylvania Hospital of the University of Pennsylvania, Philadelphia, Pennsylvania

Jean Trimble Bried, P.A.
Atlanta, Georgia

Gregory M. Buncke, M.D.
Assistant Clinical Professor in Surgery, University of California at San Francisco, San Francisco, California

Harry J. Buncke, M.D., F.A.C.S.
Clinical Professor of Plastic Surgery, University of California at San Francisco, and Director, Microsurgical Replantation, Transplantation Service, Davies Medical Center, San Francisco, California

A. Jay Burns, M.D.
Assistant Professor, Division of Plastic Surgery, University of Texas Southwestern Medical School, Dallas, Texas

H. Hollis Caffee, M.D., F.A.C.S.
Professor of Surgery, Division of Plastic Surgery, University of Florida College of Medicine, Gainesville, Florida

James H. Carraway, M.D., F.A.C.S.
Chairman, Department of Plastic Surgery, Eastern Virginia Medical School, Norfolk, Virginia

Thomas J. Carrico, M.D., F.A.C.S.
Richmond Plastic Surgeons, Inc., Richmond, Virginia

Culley C. Carson, III, M.D., F.A.C.S.
Professor of Urology, Division of Urology, Duke University Medical Center, Durham, North Carolina

John Cassel, M.D., F.A.C.S.
Clinical Associate Professor of Plastic Surgery, University of Miami School of Medicine, Miami, Florida

K. Ning Chang, M.D., F.A.C.S.
Assistant Clinical Professor of Surgery, University of California at San Francisco, and Attending, Plastic & Reconstructive Surgery, Pacific Presbyterian Medical Center, San Francisco, California

Robert A. Chase, M.D., F.A.C.S.
Emile Holman Professor of Surgery, Stanford University, Stanford, California

Norman M. Cole, M.D., F.A.C.S.
Associate Clinical Professor of Plastic Surgery, University of Louisville, Louisville, Kentucky; and Assistant Clinical Professor of Plastic Surgery, University of Kentucky, Lexington, Kentucky

Eugene H. Courtiss, M.D., F.A.C.S.
Associate Clinical Professor of Surgery, Harvard Medical School, and Consultant in Plastic Surgery, Massachusetts General Hospital, Boston, Massachusetts

Edwin Cox, M.D.
Assistant Consulting Professor, Division of Hematology & Oncology, Duke University Medical Center, Durham, North Carolina

Court B. Cutting, M.D.
Assistant Professor of Surgery (Plastic Surgery), and Director of the Cleft Palate Clinic, Institute of Reconstructive Plastic Surgery, New York University Medical Center, New York, New York

Anthony J. DeFranzo, M.D., F.A.C.S.
Associate Professor of Surgery, Department of Plastic and Reconstructive Surgery, Bowman Gray School of Medicine, Winston-Salem, North Carolina

A. Lee Dellon, M.D., F.A.C.S.
Associate Professor of Plastic Surgery, and Associate Professor of Neurologic Surgery, The Johns Hopkins University School of Medicine, Baltimore, Maryland

Donald M. Ditmars, Jr., M.D., F.A.C.S.
Head, Division of Plastic Surgery, Department of Surgery, Henry Ford Hospital, and Clinical Assistant Professor of Surgery, University of Michigan, Detroit, Michigan

Marek K. Dobke, M.D.
Division of Plastic Surgery, University of California Medical Center, San Diego, California

G. Stephenson Drew, M.D.
Assistant Professor, Division of Plastic Surgery, Medical College of Georgia, Augusta, GA

Edward Eades, M.D.
Adobe Plastic Surgery, P.C., Tucson, Arizona

Milton Edgerton, Jr., M.D., F.A.C.S.
Alumni Professor of Plastic & Maxillofacial Surgery, Department of Plastic Surgery, University of Virginia Health Science Center, Charlottesville, Virginia

Richard Ellenbogen, M.D.
Ellenbogen Plastic Surgical Institute, Los Angeles, California

Ray A. Elliott, Jr., M.D., F.A.C.S.
Clinical Professor of Surgery (Plastic), and Associate Clinical Professor of Orthopaedics (Hand), Albany Medical College, Albany, New York

Jack Fisher, M.D., F.A.C.S.
Assistant Clinical Professor, Department of Plastic & Reconstructive Surgery, Vanderbilt University, Nashville, Tennessee

Jack C. Fisher, M.D., F.A.C.S.
Professor of Surgery and Head, Division of Plastic Surgery, University of California Medical Center, San Diego, California

David H. Frank, M.D., F.A.C.S.
Associate Professor, University of California Medical Center, University Hospital, San Diego, California

William S. Garrett, Jr., M.D., F.A.C.S.
Clinical Assistant Professor of Plastic Surgery, University of Pittsburgh, Pittsburgh, Pennsylvania

David Gault, F.R.C.S.
Senior Registrar in Plastic Surgery, The Hospital for Sick Children, London, England

Gregory S. Georgiade, M.D., F.A.C.S.
Associate Professor of Surgery, and Associate Professor of Plastic, Maxillofacial and Reconstructive Surgery, Duke University Medical Center, Durham, North Carolina

Nicholas G. Georgiade, D.D.S., M.D., F.A.C.S.
Professor Emeritus of Plastic, Maxillofacial and Reconstructive Surgery, Division of Plastic, Maxillofacial, and Reconstructive Surgery, Duke University Medical Center, Durham, North Carolina

David Gilbert, M.D.
Stanford, California

Kenna S. Given, M.D., F.A.C.S.
Professor and Chief, Division of Plastic Surgery, Medical College of Georgia, Augusta, Georgia

John M. Goin, M.D., F.A.C.S.
Los Angeles, California

Marcia Kraft Goin, M.D., Ph.D.
Los Angeles, California

J. Leonard Goldner, M.D.
Professor Emeritus of Orthopaedic Surgery, Duke University Medical Center, Durham, North Carolina

Richard D. Goldner, M.D.
Assistant Professor of Orthopaedic Surgery, Duke University Medical Center, Durham, North Carolina

Mark S. Granick, M.D., F.A.C.S.
Associate Professor of Surgery (Plastic), Medical College of Pennsylvania, and Clinical Associate Professor of Surgery (Plastic), Hahnemann University, and Attending Surgeon, Division of Plastic and Reconstructive Surgery, Presbyterian Cancer Center, Philadelphia, Pennsylvania

Richard O. Gregory, M.D., F.A.C.S.
Orlando, Florida

Jeffrey P. Groner, M.D.
Assistant Professor of Surgery, Division of Plastic & Reconstructive Surgery, Washington University School of Medicine, St. Louis, Missouri

James C. Grotting, M.D., F.A.C.S.
Associate Professor, Division of Plastic Surgery, The University of Alabama at Birmingham, Birmingham, Alabama

Dwight C. Hanna, M.D., F.A.C.S.
Clinical Professor of Surgery, University of Pittsburgh School of Medicine, Pittsburgh, Pennsylvania

John M. Harrelson, M.D.
Associate Professor of Orthopaedic Surgery, and Assistant Professor of Pathology, Chief, Musculoskeletal Oncology Section, Duke University Medical Center, Durham, North Carolina

Thomas Benedict Harter, M.D.
Louisville, Kentucky

Carl R. Hartrampf, Jr., M.D., F.A.C.S.
Clinical Professor, Department of Surgery, Division of Plastic Surgery, Emory University School of Medicine, Atlanta, Georgia

Paul A. Hatcher, M.D.
Assistant Professor, Department of Urology, University of Tennessee Medical Center, Knoxville, Tennessee

Gregory P. Hetter, M.D., F.A.C.S.
Las Vegas, Nevada

David H. Hildreth, M.D.
Assistant Professor, Orthopaedics, Hand and Reconstructive Microsurgery, University of Texas Health Science Center, Houston, Texas

James G. Hoehn, M.D., F.A.C.S.
Professor and Chief, Albany Medical College, Albany, New York

Andrew T. Huang, M.D.
Professor of Hematology & Oncology, Duke University Medical Center, Durham, North Carolina

Norman Hugo, M.D., F.A.C.S.
Professor and Chairman, Division of Plastic & Reconstructive Surgery, Columbia Presbyterian Medical Center, New York, New York

Dennis Hurwitz, M.D., F.A.C.S.
Clinical Associate Professor of Surgery (Plastic), and Attending Physician at the Montefiore-University Hospital and Children's Hospital of Pittsburgh, Pittsburgh, Pennsylvania

Ian T. Jackson, M.D., F.R.C.S., F.A.C.S., F.R.A.C.S. (Hon)
Director, Institute for Craniofacial and Reconstructive Surgery, Southfield, Michigan

Jonathan S. Jacobs, D.M.D., M.D., F.A.C.S.
Associate Professor of Plastic Surgery, Eastern Virginia Medical School, Norfolk, Virginia

Saulius Jankauskas, M.D.
Los Angeles, California

Arthur Jensen, M.D.
Division of Plastic and Reconstructive Surgery, School of Medicine, University of California at Los Angeles, Los Angeles, California

M. J. Jurkiewicz, D.D.S., M.D., F.A.C.S.
Professor of Surgery, Emory University School of Medicine, Atlanta, Georgia

Morton L. Kasdan, M.D., F.A.C.S.
Clinical Professor of Plastic Surgery, University of Louisville School of Medicine, Louisville, Kentucky; and Associate Clinical Professor, Occupational Medicine, Albert B. Chandler Medical Center, University of Kentucky, Lexington, Kentucky

Bernard L. Kaye, M.D., F.A.C.S.
Jacksonville, Florida

John G. Kenney, M.D., F.A.C.S.
Plastic & Reconstructive Surgery of Charlottesville, Charlottesville, Virginia

Lowell R. King, M.D., F.A.C.S.
Professor of Urology, Duke University Medical Center, Durham, North Carolina

Harold E. Kleinert, M.D., F.A.C.S.
Clinical Professor of Surgery, University of Louisville School of Medicine, Louisville, Kentucky; and Clinical Professor of Surgery, Indiana University–Purdue University School of Medicine, Indianapolis, Indiana

Thomas J. Krizek, M.D., F.A.C.S.
Professor and Chief, Department of Surgery, University of Chicago Medical Center, Chicago, Illinois

Don La Rossa, M.D., F.A.C.S.
Professor of Surgery (Plastic), University of Pennsylvania School of Medicine, Philadelphia, Pennsylvania

Margaretha Willemina Langman, P.S., DRA
Louisville, Kentucky

Donald R. Laub, M.D., F.A.C.S.
Clinical Associate Professor of Surgery, Stanford University Medical School, Palo Alto, California

Donald R. Laub, Jr., M.D.
Resident in Surgery, University of Oregon Medical School, Tigord, Oregon

David C. Leber, M.D., F.A.C.S.
Harrisburg, Pennsylvania

James A. Lehman, Jr., M.D., F.A.C.S.
Akron, Ohio

Kenneth A. Leopold, M.D.
Assistant Professor, Department of Radiation Oncology, Duke University Medical Center, Durham, North Carolina

Scott Levin, M.D.
Assistant Professor, Plastic and Reconstructive Surgery, Division of Plastic & Reconstructive Surgery, Duke University Medical Center, Durham, North Carolina

John R. Lewis, Jr., M.D., D.A.B., F.A.C.S., F.I.C.S.
The Institute of Aesthetic Plastic Surgery, Atlanta, Georgia

William Lineaweaver, M.D.
Associate, Microsurgical Replantation Transplantation Department, Davies Medical Center, San Francisco, California

Ralph T. Manktelow, M.D., F.R.C.S.(C.)
Professor & Chairman, Division of Plastic Surgery, Department of Surgery, Toronto General Hospital & the Hospital for Sick Children, Toronto, Canada

Paul N. Manson, M.D., F.A.C.S.
Professor and Chief of Plastic Surgery, The Johns Hopkins Medical Institutions, and Director of Plastic Surgery, The Maryland Institute for Emergency Medical Services Systems, Baltimore, Maryland

Carl H. Manstein, M.D., F.A.C.S.
Chief of Plastic Surgery, Jean's Hospital in Philadelphia, and Chief of Plastic Surgery, The Hospital of the Geriatric Center, and Attending in Plastic Surgery, Albert Einstein Medical Center, and Associate in Plastic Surgery, Temple University, Philadelphia, Pennsylvania

Mark E. Manstein, M.D.
Assistant Surgeon to Pennsylvania Hospital, and Clinical Associate at University of Pennsylvania Hospital, and Attending in Plastic Surgery, Albert Einstein Medical Center, Philadelphia, Pennsylvania; and Attending in Plastic Surgery, Holy Redeemer Hospital, Meadowbrook, Pennsylvania

Malcolm W. Marks, M.D., F.A.C.S.
Associate Professor of Surgery, Department of Plastic & Reconstructive Surgery, Bowman Gray School of Medicine, Wake Forest University, Winston-Salem, North Carolina

Robert M. Mason, Ph.D., D.M.D.
Professor of Orthodontics, Duke University Medical Center, Durham, North Carolina

Stephen J. Mathes, M.D., F.A.C.S.
Professor of Surgery, Head, Division of Plastic & Reconstructive Surgery, University of California at San Francisco, San Francisco, California

G. Patrick Maxwell, M.D., F.A.C.S.
Assistant Clinical Professor, Nashville Plastic Surgery Clinic, Nashville, Tennessee

Alex McArthur, M.D.
Newport News, Virginia

Joseph G. McCarthy, M.D., F.A.C.S.
Lawrence D. Bell Professor of Plastic Surgery, and Director of the Institute of Reconstructive Plastic Surgery, New York University School of Medicine, New York, New York

Kenneth S. McCarty, Jr., M.D., Ph.D.
Associate Professor, Department of Pathology & Medicine, Duke University Medical Center, Durham, North Carolina

Robert McFarlane, M.D., M.Sc., F.R.C.S.(C), F.A.C.S.
Professor and Chairman, Division of Plastic Surgery, The University of Western Ontario, London, Ontario, Canada

Mary H. McGrath, M.D., F.A.C.S.
Professor of Surgery, and Chief, Division of Plastic & Reconstructive Surgery, George Washington University Medical Center, Washington, D.C.

Peter J. McKenna, M.D.
Fellow in Plastic Surgery, University of Pittsburgh, Pittsburgh, Pennsylvania

Timothy A. Miller, M.D., F.A.C.S.
Professor of Surgery, University of California School of Medicine, and Chief of Plastic Surgery, Wadsworth Veterans Hospital, Los Angeles, California

Professor Dr. Hanno Millesi
Department of Plastic and Reconstructive Surgery, I. Chirurgische Universitätsklinik, Allgemeines Krankenhaus, Vienna, Austria

Penny L. Mirrett, M.A.
Center for Speech & Hearing Disorders, Duke University Medical Center, Durham, North Carolina

Richard A. Mladick, M.D., F.A.C.S.
Plastic Surgery Center, Inc., Virginia Beach, Virginia

Joseph A. Moylan, M.D., F.A.C.S.
Professor of Surgery, Department of Surgery, Duke University Medical Center, Durham, North Carolina

Ross H. Musgrave, M.D., F.A.C.S.
Pittsburgh, Pennsylvania

David T. Netscher, M.D.
Assistant Professor, Division of Plastic Surgery, Baylor College of Medicine, Houston, Texas

E. Douglas Newton, M.D., F.A.C.S.
Pittsburgh, Pennsylvania

Joel M. Noe, M.D., F.A.C.S.
Clinical Assistant Professor of Surgery (Plastic), Harvard Medical School, Boston, Massachusetts

James A. Nunley, II, M.D., F.A.C.S.
Associate Professor, Division of Orthopaedic Surgery, Duke University Medical Center, Durham, North Carolina

Suzanne M. Olbricht, M.D.
Instructor, Dermatology, Harvard Medical School, and Director, Dermatosurgery Unit, Beth Israel Hospital, Boston, Massachusetts

Timothy J. Panella, M.D.
Associate Professor, Division of Hematology & Oncology, Department of Medicine, Duke University Medical Center, Durham, North Carolina

Earle E. Peacock, Jr., M.D., F.A.C.S.
Chapel Hill, North Carolina

Robert M. Pearl, M.D., F.A.C.S.
Assistant Physician-in-Chief, The Permanente Medical Gropu, Inc., Santa Clara, California

George C. Peck, M.D., F.A.C.S.
Chief, Department of Plastic & Reconstructive Surgery, Beth Israel Hospital, Passaic, New Jersey

George C. Peck, Jr., M.D.
Attending Plastic Surgeon, Department of Plastic and Reconstructive Surgery, Beth Israel Hospital, Passaic, New Jersey; and St. Barnabas Hospital, Livingston, New Jersey; and Clara Maass Hospital, Belleville, New Jersey

William Christopher Pederson, M.D.
Clinical Associate Professor and Head of Division of Plastic and Reconstructive Surgery, University of Texas Health Sciences Center, San Antonio, Texas

Joel Pessa, M.D.
Assistant Professor of Plastic and Reconstructive Surgery, Dartmouth-Hitchcock Medical Center, Lebanon, New Hampshire

Robert Peterson, M.D.
Division of Plastic Surgery, Baylor College of Medicine, Houston, Texas

Joseph Michael Pober, M.D., F.A.C.S.
St. Luke's-Roosevelt Hospital Center, Columbia University College of Physicians & Surgeons, and Clinical Instructor in the Department of Surgery (Plastic), College of Medicine, State University of New York Health Science Center, and Department of Surgery (Plastic), Cabrini Medical Center, The New York Medical College, New York, New York

Leonard R. Prosnitz, M.D.
Professor and Chief of Division of Radiation Oncology, Duke University Medical Center, Durham, North Carolina

Charles L. Puckett, M.D., F.A.C.S.
Professor and Head, Division of Plastic Surgery, University of Missouri Health Science Center, Columbia, Missouri

Peter Randall, M.D., F.A.C.S.
Professor Emeritus of Plastic Surgery, Hospital of the University of Pennsylvania, Philadelphia, Pennsylvania

Ronald Riefkohl, M.D., F.A.C.S.
Clinical Associate Professor of Plastic & Reconstructive Surgery, Division of Plastic & Reconstructive Surgery, Duke University Medical Center, Durham, North Carolina

John E. Riski, Ph.D.
Assistant Clinical Professor, Center for Speech & Hearing Disorders, Duke University Medical Center, Durham, North Carolina

Richard P. Rizzuti, M.D.
Assistant Professor of Plastic Surgery and Chief of Division of Plastic Surgery, East Carolina University School of Medicine, Greenville, North Carolina

Martin C. Robson, M.D., F.A.C.S.
Chief, Division of Plastic Surgery, The University of Texas Medical Branch at Galveston, Galveston, Texas

Ross Rudolph, M.D., F.A.C.S.
Head, Division of Plastic & Reconstructive Surgery, Scripps Clinic and Research Foundation, La Jolla, California; and Associate Clinical Professor of Plastic Surgery, University of California, San Diego, California

Robert C. Russell, M.D., F.R.A.C.S., F.A.C.S.
Associate Professor, and Director, Microsurgery Research Unit, Southern Illinois University School of Medicine, Springfield, Illinois

Renato Saltz, M.D.
Clinical Instructor, Division of Plastic Surgery, and Instructor, Biomedical Engineering, School of Engineering, University of Alabama at Birmingham, Birmingham, Alabama

Richard Carlton Schultz, M.D., F.A.C.S.
Clinical Professor of Surgery (Plastic), Division of Plastic Surgery, University of Illinois, Chicago, Illinois

Hillard F. Seigler, M.D., F.A.C.S.
Professor of Surgery and Professor of Immunology, Duke University Medical Center, Durham, North Carolina

Donald Serafin, M.D., F.A.C.S.
Professor and Chief, Division of Plastic & Reconstructive Surgery, Duke University Medical Center, Durham, North Carolina

Donald Silver, M.D., F.A.C.S.
Professor and Chairman, Department of Surgery, University of Missouri-Columbia, Columbia, Missouri

Paul J. Smith, F.R.C.S.
Consultant Plastic & Hand Surgeon and Honorary Senior Lecturer in Child Health, The Hospital for Sick Children, London, England

Mark P. Solomon, M.D., F.A.C.S.
Chief, Division of Plastic Surgery, and Associate Professor of Surgery (Plastic), The Medical College of Pennsylvania, and Clinical Associate Professor of Surgery (Plastic), Hahnemann University, and Attending Surgeon, Division of Plastic and Reconstructive Surgery, Presbyterian Cancer Center, Philadelphia, Pennsylvania

Melvin Spira, M.D., F.A.C.S.
Professor and Chairman, Division of Plastic Surgery, Baylor College of Medicine, Houston, Texas

Samuel Stal, M.D., F.A.C.S.
Associate Professor of Plastic Surgery, Baylor College of Medicine, Houston, Texas

Alexander C. Stratoudakis, M.D., F.A.C.S.
Athens, Greece

Daniel C. Sullivan, M.D.
Associate Professor, Department of Radiology, Duke University Medical Center, Durham, North Carolina

John Taras, M.D.
Division of Orthopaedic Surgery, Duke University Medical Center, Durham, North Carolina

Charles P. Vallis, M.D., F.A.C.S.
Lynn, Massachusetts

Allen L. Van Beek, M.D., F.A.C.S.
Clinical Assistant Professor, Department of Surgery, University of Minnesota, Minneapolis, Minnesota

Nancy Van Laeken, M.D., F.R.C.S.(C.)
Associate Clinical Professor, Division of Plastic Surgery, Department of Surgery, University of British Columbia, Vancouver, British Columbia, Canada

Luis O. Vasconez, M.D., F.A.C.S.
Professor and Chief, Division of Plastic Surgery, University of Alabama at Birmingham, Birmingham, Alabama

Frank A. Vicari, M.D., M.S.
Attending Plastic Surgeon, The Children's Memorial Hospital, and Clinical Assistant Professor of Surgery, Northwestern University Medical School, and Division of Plastic Surgery, The Children's Medical Hospital, Chicago, Illinois

Michael P. Vincent, M.D., F.A.C.S.
Chief, Plastic Surgery, Bethesda Naval Hospital, and Assistant Professor of Surgery, Uniformed Services, University Health Services, Bethesda, Maryland

Vincent Voci, M.D.
Charlotte, North Carolina

Robin T. Vollmer, M.D.
Assistant Clinical Professor, Department of Pathology, Duke University Medical Center, and Director of Anatomic Pathology, VA Medical Center, Durham, North Carolina

Paul M. Weeks, M.D., F.A.C.S.
Professor & Chairman, Division of Plastic Surgery, Washington University School of Medicine, St. Louis, Missouri

Margaret E. Williford, M.D.
Assistant Clinical Professor, Department of Radiology, Duke University Medical Center, Durham, North Carolina

Jeffrey L. Wisnicki, M.D., F.A.C.S.
Chairman, Department of Surgery, Palms West Hospital, and Chief of Plastic Surgery, John F. Kennedy Memorial Hospital, West Palm Beach, Florida

S. Anthony Wolfe, M.D., F.A.C.S.
Clinical Professor of Plastic & Reconstructive Surgery, University of Miami School of Medicine, Miami, Florida

Lawrence S. Zachary, M.D.
Chief Resident, Plastic & Reconstructive Surgery, Wayne State University, Detroit, Michigan

Vincent N. Zubowicz, M.D., F.A.C.S.
Clinical Professor of Plastic Surgery, Emory University Affiliated Hospitals, and Chief, Division of Plastic Surgery, Georgia Baptist Medical Center, Atlanta, Georgia

Contents

VOLUME ONE

ONE: Basic Principles

TWO: Skin and Soft Tissues

THREE: Head and Neck

VOLUME TWO

FOUR: Aesthetic Surgery

FIVE: Breast and Chest

SIX: Genitalia

SEVEN: Microsurgery

EIGHT: Hand

NINE: Trunk and Lower Extremity

ONE

Basic Principles

1

Biology of Tissue Injury and Repair

Thomas J. Krizek, M.D., F.A.C.S.

Introduction

The organism is said to be the interface at which chemical reactions between life and the environment take place. When tissue disruption occurs, a complex coordinated series of events are set in motion to repair the wound. Certain lower forms of life enjoy the ideal end result of complete anatomical, physiological, and functional restitution of the tissues to the normal condition. However, organisms that are more evolutionarily complex have lost this ability for regeneration. In its place, the less desirable process of healing is substituted and, with it, the "scar."

In a review of current concepts of wound healing, Howes and Hoopes (1) commented on the

groping, frequently illogical and meandering methods of dealing with healing problems. Wounds have been boiled, frozen, dried, wetted, stressed, strained, torn, minced, burned, cooled, stained, assayed, and treated with a wide variety of topical agents and dressing techniques. In spite of man's strong desire to aid healing, he has gained little control, if any, over either the rate or the quality of healing.

Because the study of wounds and wound healing is basic to the art of surgery, comprehension of these processes is fundamental to surgical practice. This chapter will therefore review the complex yet fascinating biology of tissue injury and repair.

Basic Anatomical Concepts

Although a detailed review of anatomical features of various tissues is beyond the scope of this review, wound management cannot be approached thoughtfully nor accomplished meaningfully in the absence of these considerations.

SKIN

The skin has two layers that constitute its basic anatomy, each playing a significant role in wound management.

EPIDERMIS

The outer epidermis is our protective waterproofing layer and the part of us that the world sees. Its color, texture, and in particular any deformity or scar are manifest here. The germinal or basal layer is constantly replenishing itself and pushing dying cells and keratin to the surface. Any superficial injury, such as an abrasion or burn, may destroy this outermost waterproofing layer and allow both weeping of tissue fluids from within and the absorption of medications or the invasion of bacteria from without. Because the germinal layer is intact in superficial wounds such as scrapes and superficial burns, healing usually occurs without scarring. Inasmuch as the melanocytes are also in the germinal layer, discoloration may occur (lighter after some superficial burns, darker as tanning after sunburns). Because the naked nerve fibers end in the germinal layer, superficial injuries are irritating to large numbers of nerve endings and are particularly painful. Because the epidermis has no collagen fibers, it has little inherent tensile strength. When a wound is carefully coapted, epithelial cells migrate quickly and will often seal a wound within a few hours (and thus waterproof it).

DERMIS

Collagen in the dermis is a fibrous protein deposited by fibroblasts that, through its intrinsic fiber strength and by its complex cross-linkages (weave), holds us together. The epidermis rests on the collagenous dermis in an irregular surface interface (papillary ridges) that makes them mechanically difficult to separate. In a coapted wound, the epidermis rapidly seals the wound, but it is the collagen in the dermis that must be laid down across the wound to give it strength. The dermis contains the epithelial-lined skin appendages that include the eccrine or sweat glands and the sebaceous oil glands. Each empties into a hair follicle. The major blood supply to the skin is through vessels in the dermis; there are none in the epidermis.

Wound Healing

When the continuity of the skin has been violated by scraping off the epidermis (abrasion or burn), crushing (contusion), or cutting or tearing (laceration), the steps in the reparative process are remarkably economical and effective defense processes.

INFLAMMATORY PHASE

Traditionally, wound healing has been divided artificially into phases. There is some disagreement about the exact events that occur within each phase and there is overlap; however, their use emphasizes chronological landmarks that characterize the healing process. The initial step is acute inflammation to establish hemostasis and mobilize components of the immune system in response to chemical, bacterial, or mechanical injury.

Vascular Response

The initial vascular response to bleeding is one of vasoconstriction, which lasts 5–10 min. Injury activates the coagulation cascade so that platelet adhesion and aggregation lead to the formation of a clot. Platelets also release several intracellular substances into the extracellular space that affect other processes in wound repair. Among these are: prostaglandins, which affect leukocytes; thromboxane, which produces potent vasoconstriction; chemotactic factors, which attract granulocytes; biogenic amines which enhance vascular tone and permeability; fibroblasts, which produce proliferative factors and collagenase with its inhibitor.

After vasoconstriction there is a period of active vasodilation and increased permeability of the smaller blood vessels (2). Some active substances, such as histamine from tissue mast cells and serotonin, directly increase the permeability of the microcirculation and cause dilation of venules. The process is enhanced by enzymes that destroy norepinephrine, which maintains the vessel tone. Proteolytic enzymes attack the endothelium and also activate kallikrein, which, in turn, activates the kinins. These then markedly increase vascular permeability, increasing the amount of protein and cells within the wound. These events, in addition to mechanical injury to the microcirculation, continue to increase vascular permeability for about 72 hr. Thus, the origins of signs of inflammation can be seen—erythema and warmth from the vasodilation, edema from the increase in cells and plasma, and pain from the increased tissue pressures.

Cellular Response

Within the inflammatory phase, cellular response begins shortly after vascular changes are first observed. A few hours after wounding, leukocytes (granulocytes) migrate by diapedesis across the walls of vessels into the injured areas and are stimulated by chemotactic factors. In the absence of infection or a foreign body, the granulocytes decrease rapidly in the wound, spilling out their hydrolytic enzymes to assist further in breakdown of bacteria and debris. Conversely, bacteria or foreign material

will perpetuate the inflammatory process. Although inflammation is not in itself a scar, it precedes scar formation. The duration and intensity of the inflammatory reaction help determine the extent of scar formation. There is little collagen deposited across an inflamed wound. Because it is collagen that ultimately provides strength, there can be no real gain in strength until inflammation ends and collagen deposition begins. Only when successful closure of the wound occurs can the next stage begin.

For many years, materials released by the neutrophils were postulated to provide a stimulus for subsequent fibroplasia. Carrel (3) first suggested that "minimal trauma" was essential for wound repair, but excessive trauma with marked inflammation may delay healing. When the inflammation phase is prolonged by increasing amounts of invasive bacteria and devitalized tissue, the physiological response may be above and beyond that caused by the initial injury.

Mononuclear phagocytizing cells and transformed macrophages soon appear in the wound. These cells may be the pivotal ones in wound healing. They release a number of chemotactic and growth factors that activate and stimulate the division of fibroblasts and new blood vessels. Macrophages soon become the dominant cell type within 3–4 days after injury.

Mast cells make their appearance simultaneously with the round cells, lymphocytes, macrophages, and monocytes. They are believed to release polysaccharides and enzymes, including heparin, histamine, and their hydrolytic enzymes. The precise role of mast cells is not known, but they may be involved in the breakdown of debris and removal of collagen.

LAG PHASE OR SUBSTRATE PHASE

When Howes and others (4) studied the small gains in tensile strength of the healing wound during the first 3–5 days, this period was labeled the "lag phase." During this time, the wound debris must be removed, and capillary fibroblasts and endothelial cells must migrate. Dunphy and Udupa (5) suggested that this period of active preparation should be more aptly named the "substrate phase." During the time of acute inflammation, fibroblasts appear at the edges of the wound in the first 24 hr and peak at 3–5 days.

The mucopolysaccharide ground substance is believed to provide an environment for the subsequent deposit of collagen and may even be involved in later maturation of the collagen fibers during the maturation phase (6). Whatever their eventual function, there is no evidence that the glycoproteins, mucopolysaccharides, or other elements of the ground substance make any contribution to the tensile strength of the wound during the substrate phase. Indeed, the principal contributor to this feature of the healing wound in the earliest stage is the fibrin clot, noted during the discussion of the inflammatory response. Within the first 24 hr, the wound has a measurable amount of tensile strength that results from the fibrin clot as well as from epithelization.

PROLIFERATIVE PHASE (EPITHELIAL REGENERATION, CONTRACTION, AND FIBROPLASIA)

The second phase of wound repair takes place from day 5 until the third week after wounding. During this period, epithelial and connective tissue proliferate. Epithelial regeneration plays an essential part in the restoration of the tissue by providing an efficient barrier against invasive bacteria. The process includes mobilization or loosening of the basal cells from their dermal attachments and migration to the place of defect with proliferation and replacement by mitosis of preexisting cells. Finally, by differentiation, cell function is restored. The epithelial cell movement across a denuded area is predictable and relentless. It continues as long as the wound is denuded of epithelial cells. The fundamental process that initiates division and migration has not been elucidated, but the process continues until the epithelial cell comes into contact with another epithelial cell. In the past, it was thought that dedifferentiation and migration of cells played the major role, but it is now believed that mitosis involving basal cell layers is also important.

In wounds closed by first intention, in which margins are coapted, the process of epithelialization may be complete in 24–48 hr. Wounds that close by secondary intention have a more involved process. At the donor site for a split-thickness skin graft, little early mitotic activity exists. By 36–48 hr, there is increased mitotic activity with thickening of the epithelial layer. The proliferation arises from the margins as well as from epidermal appendages in the dermis (the rete or papillary ridges). In the full-thickness wound, there is little migratory effort for 3–5 days until an adequate granulation bed exists. The migration of epithelial cells follows in close relation to the granulation bed. Proliferation starts on either side and follows along the cut edge of the dermis across the granulation bed until the edges meet. The deep epithelial surface gradually thickens with ultimate junction in the line of repair. Thickness may increase in some as much as 1 mm/day (7).

The second major event in the proliferative phase is wound contraction or "intussusceptive growth," by which large wounds close without scarring. This phenomenon is a form of tissue remodeling and may represent the vestige of a function now lost. Because a wound must be *closed* before it can begin the remainder of the healing phase, the body attempts to accomplish this by epithelialization and contraction. Epithelial cells, by multiplying and migrating across the surface of an open wound, will help to cover the open wound. Wound shrinking at the edges also serves the attempt at closure. All wounds contract, and they do so from end to end, not from side to side. If an excised wound is 2 cm long when it is closed, it may be 1.8 cm long when it has finished healing. If the wound is a curve or a circle, the tissue within the curve may be bunched up as contraction occurs (the "trapdoor"). If the wound is allowed to remain open for a long time and inflammation is severe, the contraction processes may become far advanced. It is further aggravated

by stress on the wound. Therefore, an inflamed chronic wound running across a joint may be so shortened when healed as to limit motion. This is called a contracture. Contraction is normal; contracture is the joint-limiting, pathological end result of excess contraction.

One of the more recent significant findings in the study of wound healing has been the discovery of a cell that has both fibroblast and smooth muscle characteristics. In 1971, Gabbiani et al. (8) first postulated the presence of myofibroblast cells in a contracting wound. Further studies by Rudolph et al. (9) demonstrated that the rate of wound contraction partially depended on the number of myofibroblasts within the wound. Additional work (10) indicated that the myofibroblasts are distributed throughout the wound, not just at the margins. Thus, the entire granulation surface serves as a contractile organ whereby the myofibroblasts shorten the wound, followed by collagen deposition and cross-linking to maintain the degree of contraction. Through such a lock-step mechanism, the bed of the contracting wound shortens in progressive fashion.

The third major development in the proliferative phase is the production of substances of connective tissue repair. Early histologists were impressed by the increase in fibroblasts and collagen during healing and suggested that a correlation might exist between the number of fibroblasts, the quantity of collagen, and the tensile strength of the scar (11). Indeed, scar tissue would seem to develop from the production of collagen molecules by fibroblasts. These molecules aggregate to form fibers, followed by a weaving of the fibers and fibrils into a purposefully ordered pattern. The molecule in the appropriate environment of the ground substance is formed into a larger, more stable collagen by intra- and intermolecular bonds. Basically, the protein from fibroblasts (procollagen) has a high proline content. Collagen that forms the fibers and fibrils is an extracellular substance. To become extracellular requires a special hydroxylation step from the peptide proline to the unique collagen amino acid hydroxyproline. With the hydroxylation of proline and lysine, final assembly can take place.

The solubility of collagen and the nature of its polymerization have been extensively studied. Tropocollagen is composed of three chains, each with a molecular weight of about 95,000. In native proteins, the individual chains are arranged as a left-handed helix, producing a rope-like structural molecule. Intramolecular and intermolecular cross-linking by aldehyde groups develops early during fibroplasia. The secondary gain in tensile strength during the period of remodeling is more related to the intermolecular bonds.

Fibroblasts also produce glycosaminoglycans (mucopolysaccharides) once they have migrated into the wound. The precise role of the mucopolysaccharides in wound healing is not fully understood. Most of the glycoprotein in the wound during the first few days appears to be derived from serum glycoproteins. The production of new polysaccharides in the wound is closely related to the period of collagen formation and fibroplasia. Bentley (12) demonstrated that chondroitin sulfate appears early in the wound at about days 4–6, and its concentration increases concomitantly following the progressive curve of collagen formation. Simultaneously, there is a reduction in the concentration of hyaluronic acid, which rises again at the end of fibroplasia.

The glycosaminoglycans are repeating disaccharide units attached to the protein core. As they are secreted by fibroblasts, these substances are hydrated to contribute to the "ground substance, an amorphous gel that may play a role in subsequent aggregation of collagen fibers" (13).

At the end of the inflammatory stage (about 5–7 days in clean, primarily closed wounds) the wound has about 10% of its ultimate tensile strength. After 15–20 days, the wound can resist normal stress. Much more collagen is formed than is ultimately needed, and wound tensile strength continues to increase for several weeks. By 3 weeks, the synthesis of wound collagen remains high, but the net collagen accumulated is matched by collagen degradation. At 6 weeks the wound has reached about 60% of strength, and it reaches its maximum in 3–6 months. However, healed wounds rarely regain more than 70–80% of the intact skin strength.

MATURATION OR REMODELING PHASE

Although a wound probably never becomes as strong as intact skin, the scar matures over time and the collagen fibers (laid down in disarray in the fibroplasia phase— they are like steel wool, potentially strong but poorly organized) begin to be rewoven in response to stress. The fibers are lined up (like weaving steel wool into a cable) along stress lines, and the more stretch on the wound the more cable-like the scar will be. Big scars may seem to be stronger. In actuality, because strength is dependent on weave rather than amount of collagen, a fine hairline scar may be stronger than a thick scar.

During this phase, which may last a year or longer, the scar will flatten, the redness will fade, and the pruritus will disappear. When this happens, one can expect that the wound has reached its maximum healing and time will contribute no more. The fibroblasts appear to be responsible for reabsorption and production of new collagen. The zone of activity in which this chemical process takes place is localized in an area approximately 0.75 mm on either side of the wound edge (14). If tension is placed on the wound, it is noted that the random collagen fibers appear to line up parallel to the forces of tension. Within 3 months, the scar becomes flatter, softer, and lighter in color. The collagen becomes thicker and denser, and the blood vessels constrict and disappear.

It should be obvious that a fresh wound that is ill-placed or poorly aligned can be no more than an ill-placed or poorly aligned mature scar a year later. Although vitamins and a nutritious diet may be prudent for healthy living, there is no evidence that the addition or supplementation of vitamins (C, E, etc.) or additional nutritious food will make a difference in the healing of the usual wound in an otherwise healthy person.

Once again, emphasis must be placed upon the ideal milieu and stimuli for wound healing to progress in an orderly fashion with minimal connective tissue formation.

Factors Affecting the Wound Healing Process

Although the phenomenon of wound healing is relatively fixed in an orderly progression of events, the rate of wound healing in any of the phases can be regulated by many factors. That a healing wound does not develop separately from the organism or its environment is evident.

For years mankind has hoped to accelerate wound healing favorably, but we have painfully learned that very little can be done therapeutically to hasten repair beyond the normal. A variety of substances have been purported to hasten tissue repair, including scarlet red, gentian violet, balsam of Peru, powdered cartilage and bone, zinc oxide, and oxygen. Most of these agents probably restore healing to a more optimal level rather than accelerate the process.

NUTRITION

All else being equal, wounds in the young heal more rapidly than those in the elderly whether this be by increased fibroplasia, decreased susceptibility to infection, increased general cell proliferation, or just improved nutrition. Protein deficiency is believed to retard vascularization and lymphatic formation, to lower resistance to infection, and to inhibit several phases of wound healing. In such an environment, there is a delay in both fibroplasia and the development of tensile strength. In 1949, Localio and his associates (15) reported that the feeding of d,l-methionine to protein-depleted animals restored the substrate period to its normal length and increased the rate of fibroplasia. This suggests that this single amino acid is necessary for synthesis by fibroblasts of both mucopolysaccharides and collagen. Although administration of methionine does appear to restore the healing process to a normal rate, the reversal of protein starvation requires time. Protein deficiency states should be corrected before the operation.

Trauma abruptly alters the metabolic status quo. The postinjury state is marked by increased heat production; gluconeogenesis; negative nitrogen, potassium, sulfur, and phosphorus balance; early hyperglycemia; and modification in carbohydrate utilization. Also occurring are elevated serum concentrations of free fatty acids with ketosis; sodium, chloride, and water retention; potential depletion of ascorbic acid, thiamine, riboflavin, nicotinamide, and vitamin A; and possible deficiencies of trace metals such as zinc, copper, and iron. Coupled with these events are potentially great caloric requirements associated with multiple injuries, burns, and sepsis. When postoperative nutritional problems are superimposed on possible preexisting nutritional problems (e.g., malignancy, increased age, diabetes, or gastrointestinal

[GI] disorders such as Crohn's disease or cirrhosis), the potential for nutritional disaster exists. If malnutrition does occur, such patients exhibit a potential for weakness, greater susceptibility to anesthetics and shock, impaired liver and GI tract function, retarded wound healing, serious infections, prolonged hospitalization, and death. It should also be noted that a given wound will heal slower in an individual with another significant injury (e.g., a burn with a concomitant long bone fracture).

VITAMINS

Vitamin C

The importance of vitamin C as a cofactor necessary for collagen synthesis has been recognized since the development and prevention of scurvy in sailors during previous centuries. Man cannot synthesize vitamin C and normally has storage for only 4 or 5 months. Ascorbic acid is an active reducing agent involved in the production of superoxide radicals, an important intermediary in respiration and in the synthesis of an antibacterial substance from leukocytes. In addition, vitamin C (or rather its ester equivalent, ascorbate) is required for the hydroxylation of proline and lysine. In the scorbutic individual, collagen lysis outstrips synthesis, causing a weakening of collagen, increased capillary permeability, fragility, and rupture and hemorrhage of vessels. It has not been established whether the increased requirement for vitamin C reflects an accumulation of ascorbic acid at the wound site or an increased rate of vitamin C metabolism. Excessive doses of vitamin C do not further accelerate wound healing.

Vitamin A

Vitamin A is important in vision, reproduction, epithelium maintenance and multiplication, synthesis of proteoglycans, stabilization of lysosomal membranes, and the enhancement of cellular immunity. Experiments have shown vitamin A accelerates healing of skin lesions, whereas deficiencies retard epithelialization, wound closure, collagen synthesis rates, and cross-linking of new collagen. In addition, vitamin A deficiency causes depletion of vitamin C reserves. Moreover, vitamin E seems to enhance absorption, storage, and utilization of vitamin A. Importantly, vitamin A offsets the inhibitory effects of adrenal steroids on wound repair, even when applied locally. Large stores are maintained in the liver, and supplementation is not required with routine surgical procedures. In the malnourished patient, 25,000 IU/day is adequate for normal wound repair.

Vitamin E

The role of vitamin E in wound healing is unknown. Ehrlich et al. (16) observed that vitamin E inhibited wound healing by decreasing tensile strength and accumulation of collagen. It had no effect on glucocorticoid inhibition of wound healing, and its actions were reversed by vitamin A. It is believed that vitamin E may exert its activity by its membrane stabilizing effects.

OXYGEN

Oxygen is considered an essential substrate for effective wound healing. During healing, the wound consumes a greater amount of oxygen than normal tissues (17, 18). The partial pressure of oxygen (pO_2) within tissue is dependent upon several physical properties, including distance from the nearest capillary, intercapillary distance, rate of oxygen consumption, and a diffusion coefficient specific for that tissue. When a wound occurs, local capillaries are injured, reducing the availability of oxygen. Thus, the oxygen requirement for repair is greatest when the local circulation is least able to satisfy the need. Although the tissue pO_2 in the healed wound is measured at 30–50 mm Hg, the minimal pO_2 necessary for healing is not known. Hunt and Pai (19) clearly observed that fibroblast replication was potentiated at partial pressures of 30–40 mm Hg. However, collagen synthesis required higher oxygen partial pressures.

Recent studies (20) indicate that the rate of epithelial cell proliferation in wounds is directly proportional to the arterial oxygen tension at the wound site. Oxygen increases the efficiency of collagen formation. Collagen cannot escape from the fibroblast unless a specific portion of the proline and lysine has been hydroxylated. Other studies (21) indicate that reduced oxygen may result in the formation of underhydroxylated collagen, causing a weakening of the tensile strength in wounds.

MICROENVIRONMENT, HOST RESISTANCE, AND INFECTION (22–24)

The humoral and cellular defense mechanisms of the body are usually sufficient to control infection and promote wound healing. However, they cannot function efficiently in an environment of debris, necrotic tissue, hematoma, and virulent and numerous bacteria. In all these instances, bacteria may compete effectively with phagocytes, fibroblasts, endothelial cells, and epithelium, leading to infection and delayed wound healing. Patients susceptible to infection because of impaired host defenses include those mentioned previously (e.g., elderly with serious diseases, diabetics, cancer patients, and patients who have sustained major trauma or surgery).

Prostaglandins

Inflammatory reactions in skin are due to many different processes. Prostaglandins and their metabolites have been implicated in the inflammatory and immunological responses that the body employs to facilitate wound healing. Although prostaglandins may be directly involved by influencing the metabolism and activity of other inflammatory cells (lymphocytes, macrophages, neutrophils) or by interacting themselves with other components of inflammation (bradykinin and histamine), their primary role in these responses is not yet established.

Epidermal reparative processes involve a complex interaction among essential fatty acids, prostaglandins, epidermoid proliferation, epidermal maturation, and keratinization. Of all the prostaglandins, PGE_2 has the most maturation and keratinization. It also has the most clearly defined relationship to epidermal maturation and keratinization.

Conclusions

The goal of management of soft tissue injuries is the successful closure of the wound. Only when the wound is closed can inflammation end, fibroplasia begin, and remodeling result in a stable scar. Although regulation of wound healing may be possible in the future, the surgeon of today must understand the biology of tissue injury and its repair to provide the optimal conditions for wound healing.

References

1. Howes RM, Hoopes JE: Current concepts of wound healing. *Clin Plast Surg* 4:173, 1977.
2. Peacock EE, VanWinkle W: In: *Surgery and Biology of Wound Repair*. Philadelphia, WB Saunders Co, 1970.
3. Carrel A: The treatment of wounds. *JAMA* 55:2148, 1910.
4. Howes EL, Sooy JW, Harvey SC: The healing of wounds as determined by their tensile strength. *JAMA* 92:42, 1929.
5. Dunphy JE, Udupa KN: Chemical and histochemical sequences in the normal healing wounds. *N Engl J Med* 253:847, 1955.
6. VanWinkle W Jr: The tensile strength of wounds and factors that influence it. *Surg Gynecol Obstet* 129:819, 1969.
7. Dingman RO: Factors of clinical significance affecting wound healing. *Laryngoscope* 83:1540, 1973.
8. Gabbiani G, Hirschel BJ, Ryan GB, et al: Granulation tissue as a contractile organ: A study of structure and function. *J Exp Med* 135:719, 1972.
9. Rudolph R, Guber S, Suzuki M, et al: The life-cycle of the myofibroblast. *Surg Gynecol Obstet* 145:389, 1977.
10. Rudolph R: Location of the force of wound contraction. *Surg Gynecol Obstet* 148:547, 1979.
11. Madden JW, Peacock EE: Studies on the biology of collagen during wound healing: I. Rate of collagen synthesis and deposition in cutaneous wounds of the rat. *Surgery* 64.288, 1968.
12. Bentley JP: Rate of chondroitin sulfate formation in wound healing. *Ann Surg* 165:186, 1967.
13. Bryant WM: Wound healing. *Ciba Found Symp* 29:2, 1977.
14. Adamsons RJ, Musco F, Enquist IF: The chemical dimensions of a healing incision. *Surg Gynecol Obstet* 123:515, 1966.
15. Localio SA, Gillette L, Hinton JW: Biological chemistry of wound healing; effect of dl-methionine on healing surface wounds. *Surg Gynecol Obstet* 89:69, 1949.
16. Ehrlich P, Tarver H, Hunt TK: Inhibitory effects of vitamin E on collagen synthesis and wound repair. *Ann Surg* 175:235, 1972.
17. Hunt TK, Zederfeldt B, Goldstick TK: Oxygen and healing. *Am J Surg* 118:521, 1969.
18. Hunt TK, Twomey P, Zederfeldt B, et al: Respiratory gas tensions and pH in healing wounds. *Am J Surg* 114:302, 1967.
19. Hunt TK, Pai MP: The effect of varying ambient oxygen tensions on wound metabolism and collagen synthesis. *Surg Gynecol Obstet* 135:561, 1972.
20. Silver IA: Oxygen tension and epithelialization. In Maibach HI, Rovee DT (eds): *Epidermal Wound Healing*. Chicago, Year Book Medical Publishers, 1972, pp 291–305.
21. Uitto J, Prockop DJ: Synthesis and secretion of under hydroxylated procollagen at various temperatures by cells subject to temporary anoxia. *Biochem Biophys Res Commun* 60:414, 1974.
22. Bierens de Haan B, Ellis H, Wilks M: The role of infection on wound healing. *Surg Gynecol Obstet* 138:693, 1974.
23. Burke JF, Morris PJ, Bondoc CC: The effect of bacterial inflammation on wound healing. In Dunphy JE, VanWinkle W (eds): *Repair and Regeneration*. New York, McGraw-Hill, 1969, pp 19–30.
24. Krizek TJ, Robson MC: Evolution of quantitative bacteriology in wound management. *Am J Surg* 130:579, 1975.

2

Normal and Pathological Wound Healing

Thomas J. Carrico, M.D.

Introduction

All surgeons must understand the complex biological and biochemical series of events termed wound healing in order to manipulate them to the best advantage of their patients. The purpose of this chapter is to describe the major components of the normal as well as the pathological wound healing processes. Intervention with pharmacological or mechanical means will also be discussed.

"Normal" Wound Healing

Wounding is immediately followed by coagulation, altered vascularity, and inflammation, all of which modulate healing.

Coagulation is mediated by platelets, and during thrombus formation, platelet factors are released. Platelet-derived growth factor is a polypeptide that is known to be a potent mitogen for fibroblasts and is chemotactic for human skin fibroblasts (1–4).

Inflammation soon follows as small blood vessels dilate and capillary permeability increases, allowing circulating neutrophils, followed by monocytes, to migrate into the wound. Inflammatory cells were once though to control bacterial proliferation and remove debris. However, macrophages also play a role in the induction of fibroblast migration and proliferation and subsequent collagen synthesis (5). Depletion of wound macrophages significantly decreases deposition of wound collagen. Several studies suggest a significant role of prostaglandins in this process (6), supporting the possible use of prostaglandin inhibitors such as ibuprofen to control inflammation.

The surgeon has often viewed inflammation as a foe, but an adequate inflammatory response is indeed vital to normal wound healing. In fact, recent fetal rabbit studies by Krummel et al. (7) show a complete lack of a classic inflammatory stimulus. This results in failure of wound contraction and, therefore, healing by secondary intention in punch or unsutured wounds. These studies restate the need for inflammation in order to achieve "normal" wound healing.

Wound breaking strength has been enhanced in rats by synthetic growth hormones (8). This dosage was effective when given within 24 hr of wounding, indicating a synergistic effect on the inflammatory phase of wound repair. Clinical use of hormones and specific growth factors may open a new era of pharmacological manipulation of the healing wound.

Strength and integrity of all tissue repairs rely on the synthesis, cross-linking, and deposition of collagen. Ribosomal hydroxylation of proline and lysine is required for the synthesis of the nascent collagen chain. This hydroxylation requires specific enzymes—lysyl and prolyl hydroxylase—both of which require oxygen, alpha-ketoglutarate, ascorbate, and iron as cofactors. Corticosteroids inhibit these hydroxylating enzymes, but the steroid effect on the enzymes is counteracted by vitamin A. Therefore, the physician should recognize that hypoxia, ascorbate, or iron deficiencies, as well as exogenous corticosteroids, can inhibit wound strength and integrity.

Collagen is secreted from the cell in a triple-helical configuration with terminal peptide fragments attached to each end of the molecule. These terminal peptide fragments are normally cleaved from the collagen molecule before cross-linking by two specific proteases. Failure of cleavage causes a specific type of Ehlers-Danlos syndrome.

Collagen cross-linking is what actually gives strength to and maintains the integrity of the healed wound. "Cross-links" are covalent bonds between adjacent collagen molecules, resulting in a three-dimensional triple helix molecule (9). A number of compounds can inhibit the formation of collagen cross-links in animals. The potent lathyrogen beta-aminopropionitrile (BAPN) causes bone deformation, aortic aneurysms, and joint dislocations when fed to growing animals. All reflect an inhibition of collagen cross-linking (10). This may have exciting potential as a pharmacological agent to control scarring in humans.

Collagen degradation mediated by the enzyme collagenase is equally important as collagen synthesis in the process of wound healing. After wounding, the rates of both collagen synthesis and degradation rise and fall in an ordered and sequential fashion (11–13) so that enough collagen is synthesized, cross-linked, deposited, and removed to provide wound strength and integrity without excessive scarring. The mechanisms that normally regulate the delicate balance between collagen synthesis and degradation are currently being defined.

There are at least seven genetically distinct types of human collagen. Types I and III are the major components of skin. Recent data reveal that, within hours after wounding, types IV and V collagen are present in the wound, followed shortly thereafter by the appearance of type III. The early collagens may provide a matrix or scaffolding for the subsequent events of repair.

All of the processes described so far occur in the

wound that is closed primarily, either immediately or delayed. For a wound to close by secondary intention, contraction and epithelialization must occur.

Although the mechanism of contraction was the subject of controversy for many years, it is now generally thought that the myofibroblast (a fibroblast-like cell with smooth muscle components) is the responsible contractile cell. Myofibroblasts were first described by Majno et al. (14) and have been found subsequently in many animal and human contracting tissues. How contraction leads to contracture remains unclear. It is hypothesized that myofibroblasts are the responsible contractile cells and that it is collagen that holds the newly contracted tissues in position. Although studies by Peacock and associates (15, 16) suggest that pharmacological inhibition of smooth muscle contraction will prevent contracture, there is no satisfactory clinical method to implement these findings.

Epithelialization is also the major healing phenomenon of the partial-thickness wound. Mitosis and migration occur to restore integrity to the partial loss of skin. Various types of dressings and pharmacological agents that purport to enhance this process have been marketed. However, the only firm evidence to date suggests that epithelialization is more rapid with a hydrophobic rather than a hydrophilic dressing.

Epidermal growth factor (EGF), a small polypeptide, is a potent growth factor for human fibroblasts and has been shown to significantly enhance epithelialization when applied topically to skin defects in mice (18) and to burn wounds in pigs (19).

Transforming growth factor-beta (TGF-B) is another polypeptide that has been shown to accelerate wound repair experimentally (20, 21). This appears to be a combination of increasing influx of monocytes and fibroblasts as well as an increase in collagen deposition.

The potential for these growth factors to enhance "normal" wound healing and treat defects in "pathological" wound healing excites the imagination of every physician dealing with problem wounds.

Congenital Alterations in Wound Healing

Any of the steps in the complex process of wound healing may be disrupted by congenital inborn errors in metabolism that are manifested by production of abnormal collagen and/or pathological wound healing. Evident disorders resulting from genetic defects in collagen metabolism include several types of Ehlers-Danlos syndrome, osteogenesis imperfecta, cutis laxa, and the spondyloepiphyseal dysplasia (22).

A number of enzyme deficiencies are recognized, including those of lysyl hydroxylase, lysyl oxidase, and procollagen protease (22). In addition, immunogenetic factors may be significant in the production of a number of disorders, such as rheumatoid arthritis (23).

Diabetes is an inherited disorder with multifaceted defects in wound healing. There are mechanical impairments and metabolic defects in patients with this condition. Diabetic wound hypoxia occurs secondary to both microangiopathy and major arterial occlusion from accelerated atherosclerosis. Impaired sensation of diabetic neuropathy results in repeated mechanical trauma and also impedes healing.

Insulin deficiency significantly decreases collagen synthesis in animals (24, 25). Goodson and Hunt (26) have demonstrated that insulin is more important in the early phases of healing, corresponding to the inflammatory response. This coincides with known defective leukocyte functions (specifically, decreased chemotaxis, phagocytosis, and intracellular killing). These defects are manifested clinically by the increased incidence of wound infection in diabetics (27).

Supplemental vitamin A may improve healing in diabetes. Seifter et al. (28) showed a stimulation of the early inflammatory response in wounded, nondiabetic rats. These authors also found that supplemental vitamin A could improve wound healing in diabetics in the absence of insulin (29).

In managing diabetic wounds, the effects of neuropathy and microangiopathy cannot be altered. However, large vessel disease should be corrected when appropriate, and areas of sensory loss must be protected. Adequate control of hyperglycemia is of great importance, especially in the perioperative period. Optimization of arterial pO_2, local perfusion pressure, and minimization of wound contamination are mandatory. Supplemental vitamin A in doses of 25,000 units/day appears beneficial (30).

Another category of congenital pathological wound healing occurs in patients who exhibit "surface overhealing." Keloid formation and hypertrophic scars, including burn scars, are in this group. All are manifested by overabundant deposition of collagen. Peacock et al. (31) described the clinical differences between keloid and hypertrophic scar. Keloid extends beyond the boundaries of the original skin wound, invades surrounding tissue, and often recurs after surgical removal. In contrast, hypertrophic scar, although raised, remains within the normal line of incision or injury and tends to regress gradually. There is a clear familial and racial predilection for keloid that may follow an autosomal dominant pattern. They may occur on any area of the body and, with the exception of newborns, have been reported in all age groups (32).

Histologically, keloids are characterized by overabundant deposition of dermal collagen (33). It has been clearly demonstrated that collagen synthesis is significantly greater in keloids than in hypertrophic scars, normal scars, or in normal skin (33–35). Collagen degradation also appears to be abnormal in keloid. Although high levels of collagenase activity are found in keloid tissue culture abstracts (36, 37), this activity is probably inhibited in vivo by the presence of alpha$_2$-macroglobulin, a potent collagenase inhibitor (38, 39).

An immune component to keloid formation is suggested (40) but still poorly defined. Antibody-antigen interactions could stimulate a chronic inflammatory response that enhances fibroblast proliferation and collagen deposition as described earlier. Keloid tissue immunoglobulin G (IgG) levels are significantly greater than those

NORMAL AND PATHOLOGICAL WOUND HEALING—*Chapter 2*   **11**

in normal skin or scar controls, suggesting that a local immune response is, indeed, involved in keloid formation (41).

Hypertrophic burn scars are similar in appearance to both keloid and hypertrophic scars. These scars are commonly found at the border of skin grafts and in deep second- and third-degree burns that heal by secondary intention. Areas that heal slowly contain high concentrations of inflammatory cells and are probably sites of increased collagen synthesis. A second important unique characteristic of hypertrophic burn scars is that they do not form until patients are healthy. That collagen antibodies have been found in burn patient serum (42), and that there is increased IgG deposited in burn skin (43) and in the serum recovered from burn patients (44) imply that the immune response is involved in the pathogenesis of the hypertrophic burn scar.

The clinician has few methods for controlling overabundant collagen deposition in patients who demonstrate "overhealing." These methods to control surface scar fall into three general categories: (a) regulation of collagen metabolism; (b) use of pharmacological agents; and (c) mechanical measures.

First is the regulation of collagen metabolism. The intralesional use of the corticosteroid triamcinolone (9-alpha-fluoroacetonide) produces keloid regression (45, 46). Steroids have multiple effects, which could explain this phenomenon. Corticosteroids may inhibit fibroblast migration, decrease collagen synthesis, increase collagenase activity, and decrease alpha-globulin deposition. The dose of triamcinolone (40 mg/ml) never exceeds 80 mg every 6 weeks. Pregnancy and peptic ulcer disease are contraindications to this therapy.

Radiation therapy has been used to treat keloid and hypertrophic scars, but we believe the risks of radiation-induced tissue damage and carcinoma, however small, outweigh the benefit of using this method to treat benign lesions.

Several pharmacological agents may prove efficacious in treatment. These include colchicine, which retards fibroblast collagen secretion (47), enhances collagenase activity (48), and inhibits wound contraction (49). BAPN irreversibly inhibits lysyl oxidase, preventing subsequent collagen cross-linking (50), and high doses of D-penicillamine produce the same effect by chelating copper (51). Although systemic use of these agents may improve pharmacological control of excess collagen deposition, they do have effects on systemic collagen metabolism. Therefore, we believe the use of topical BAPN fumarate holds the greatest promise in treatment of cutaneous lesions characterized by overabundant collagen deposition.

The last category of control methods are mechanical measures. These include surgical excision, which leads usually to recurrence unless adjunctive corticosteroid injections are used postoperatively. Data to support the use of pressure devices and splints do not exist, although anecdotal successes with them have been noted. Z-plasty or W-plasty scar revisions only serve to convert a linear problem to a "Z"- or "W"-shaped one, which becomes even more unsightly.

Acquired Pathological Wound Healing

Surgeons are increasingly confronted with problems of healing in immunosuppressed patients. Corticosteroids as well as other anti-inflammatory agents are widely used in control of many systemic diseases as well as to control the rejection of transplanted organs. These agents are definitely "two-edged swords" with many documented side-effects, including significant alterations in healing. Anti-inflammatory steroids decrease the tensile strength of closed wounds (52), slow the rate of epithelialization (53) and neovascularization (54), and severely inhibit contraction (55).

The mechanism for these defects is twofold. First, steroids diminish prolyl hydroxylase and lysyl oxidase activity (56, 57). Steroids may also increase collagenase activity. The poor healing and relatively fragile skin noted in these patients are probably related to inadequate deposition of cross-linked collagen. The second mechanism involves the direct action of steroids on the inflammatory process. Sandberg (58) showed reduced tensile strength of closed wounds only if steroids were given within 3 days after wounding, a time corresponding to the full development of the inflammatory response. Similarly, Ehrlich and Hunt (59) noted that fibroblast migration into the wound could only be inhibited if the animals were treated with corticosteroid before wounding.

Vitamin A given concurrently with steroids can reverse the inhibitory effects of glucocorticoids on repair as measured by tensile strength (59, 60). This is secondary to reversal of corticoid inhibition of inflammation (61). Wound contraction, however, is not completely reversed (62).

The effect of vitamin A on the immunosuppressive action of steroids is a controversial issue because vitamin A has been reported both to have no effect (63, 64) and to have a significant effect on those properties (65, 66). Haick et al. (67) demonstrated that cell-mediated immunity and humoral antibody production were similar in two groups of animals receiving steroids alone or in combination with vitamin A.

Vitamin A, in doses of 25,000 units/day, is recommended for improvement in wound healing in patients receiving steroids (30). Cautious use of this modality in transplant patients is warranted because some authors have noted a diminished immunosuppressive effect of steroids with the use of vitamin A (65, 66).

Another group rapidly growing in numbers consists of patients receiving chemotherapy. The effect of chemotherapeutic agents on wound healing has been well summarized by Ferguson (68). These agents have effects in several areas.

One is overall marrow suppression with resultant decreases in circulating blood elements. It has been shown, however, that leukopenia at the time of wounding and during the inflammatory phase has no effect on wound débridement, fibroblast proliferation, or connective tissue formation (69, 70). Macrophages are sufficient for normal phagocytosis of cellular debris as well as stimulation of fibroblast proliferation and neovascularization (71). However, the absence of polymorphonuclear leukocytes during the inflammatory phase can predispose to wound infection, which prolongs the inflammatory phase and retards wound healing.

Profound cell depletion, however, does impair wound breaking strength and wound collagen deposition, as demonstrated by Peterson (72).

Other wound-healing effects are peculiar to specific agents. Certain agents (e.g., cyclophosphamide) have been found to inhibit the early vasodilatory phase of inflammation, again prolonging healing (73–75). Most cytotoxic agents exert their antineoplastic effects by interfering with DNA replication, RNA production, protein synthesis, or cell division. These effects influence the healing wound by inhibiting fibroblast proliferation or by directly decreasing collagen formation.

Inasmuch as there is no evidence to date that perioperative administration of antineoplastic agents decrease rates of tumor recurrence or mortality over delayed postoperative chemotherapy, it seems wise to delay treatment after major operations until the early phase of wound repair has been completed.

Possibly the most vexing of wound-healing problems is in radiation-injured tissues. Despite recent improvements in radiotherapy techniques, significant injury to the tissues still occurs. Although the biochemical and structural changes have not been defined, most investigators believe that the fundamental wound-healing problem is tissue hypoxia secondary to an obliterative endarteritis. However, Rudolph et al. (76) suggest that radiation injury is not associated with obliterative endarteritis. Current management of chronic radiation ulcers is excision with new, well-vascularized tissues being transplanted to the area in the form of pedicled or "free" musculocutaneous flaps (77, 78). This concept is valid for any organ or tissue. Basic characterization of the biochemical alterations in radiated tissues is one of the most important goals in wound-healing research. Surprisingly, very little work has been done in this important area.

Physiological Parameters Influencing Wound Healing

Certain physiological variables encountered clinically have major impact on the success or failure of the healing wound. Recent contributions to the understanding of nutrition, tissue oxygenation, and circulating volume as significant influences on wound healing are now discussed.

Although centuries of clinical observation suggest that poorly nourished patients have impaired wound healing, specific deficiencies are just beginning to be defined. Recent advances in the metabolic response to injury have led to clinical intervention in the form of enteral or parenteral hyperalimentation to assist the malnourished patient to abate infection and wound-healing problems. Nevertheless, it is unclear as to what, why, and how these modalities alter wound healing if, indeed, they alter it at all.

First, in animal studies (79), there are significant changes in wound healing that occur in the presence of a severe degree of malnutrition, when weight loss exceeds one third of the normal body weight. Severe malnutrition results in a profound reduction in the strength of abdominal and skin wounds, but strength changes of colonic anastomoses are less pronounced. These different tissue responses have been noted by other authors, and appear to affect the collagen of skin or parietal tissues for the most part (80, 81). These and other studies (82, 83) support the use of short-term hyperalimentation for the severely malnourished patient before elective surgery.

The normally nourished patient who sustains a large injury has a complex endocrine and metabolic response. Briefly, the patient is abruptly hypermetabolic with negative balances of nitrogen, potassium, sulfur, and phosphate. Gluconeogenesis increases, carbohydrate utilization is altered, and there are increased free fatty acids in the serum with ketosis. Requirements of vitamin A, ascorbic acid, thiamine, riboflavin, and nicotinamide are increased. Intravenous hyperalimentation with amino acids, high concentrations of carbohydrate, and fat emulsion in this setting is well supported in the literature (84).

Kinney (85) has shown that, in patients undergoing elective abdominal operations without complications, there is a relatively small change in the metabolic rate. Nutritional support beyond normal caloric requirements in this setting seems unwarranted.

Collagen synthesis is critically dependent on the availability of molecular oxygen to form the hydroxyprolyl and hydroxylysyl residues. Uitto and Prockop (86) have shown that even temporary anoxia may result in fibers of low mechanical strength. The rate of wound healing is now known to be a function of arterial pO_2, over a certain physiological range. Niinikoski (87) has shown in animals that the net collagen accumulation in the dead space of wounds decreased with hypoxia and increased with hyperoxia with a peak at 70% O_2. This has been confirmed by Hunt and Pai (88).

Wounds in ischemic tissues become infected more frequently than wounds in well-vascularized tissues. Hunt and colleagues (89) found that infection could be diminished by increasing wound oxygen supply. They concluded that the effectiveness of the phagocytic defense system varies with change in the oxygen environment. It is possible that bacteria, fibroblasts, and phagocytes compete for what little oxygen is available in the wound. Infection results when sufficient bacteria are present to overwhelm the phagocytic response or to diminish the oxygen supply to a point where intracellular destruction becomes impaired.

The nutritional status and oxygen tension of the wound all depend on the delivery of their components to the local area by the microcirculation. This, in turn, is a function of the circulating volume. Sandblom (90) found decreased breaking strength in wounds of rabbits made anemic by bleeding. The animals were often dehydrated and hypovolemic. He also showed that dehydration alone can decrease wound strength. Sandberg and Zederfelt (91) replaced lost blood volume with dextran and restored healing toward normal. Chang et al. (92) reported that, even with normal arterial pO_2, tissue oxygenation will be low if blood volume is low. Therefore, wound healing can be markedly impaired with a decreased circulating volume. The surgeon must be aware that cardiac output and blood volume must be maintained at normal levels to promote normal healing.

Conclusion

In conclusion, wound healing is a complex interaction of mechanical, physiological, and biochemical events. An alteration in any facet of this intricate process will inevitably lead to prolonged or abnormal healing, often with devastating effects. The use of growth factors to enhance or modulate repair is a vital area of current wound healing research and holds great promise for the future.

References

1. Graham MF, Diegelmann RF, Cohen IK, et al: Effects of inflammation on wound healing: In vitro and in vivo studies. In Hunt TK (ed): *Soft and Hard Tissue Repair: Biological and Clinical Aspects.* New York, Praeger Scientific, 1984, p 361.
2. Rutherford RB, Ross R: Platelet factors stimulate fibroblasts and smooth muscle cells quiescent in plasma serum to proliferate. *J Cell Biol* 69:196, 1976.
3. Seppa H, Grotendorst GR, Seppa S, et al: Platelet derived growth factor is chemotactic for fibroblasts. *J Cell Biol* 92:584, 1982.
4. Lawrence WT, Solomon G, Link GW, et al: Mitogenic activity in excisional wounds in rats and its stimulation by PDGF. *Surg Forum* 39:637, 1988.
5. Leibovich SJ, Ross R: A macrophage dependent factor that stimulates the proliferation of fibroblasts in vitro. *Am J Pathol* 84:501, 1976.
6. Lord JT, Ziboh VA, Cagle WD, et al: Prostaglandins in wound healing: possible regulation of granulation. In Samuelsson B, Ramwell PW, Paolette R (eds): *Advances in Prostaglandin and Thromboxane Research,* Vol VII. New York, Raven Press, 1980, p 865.
7. Krummel TK, Nelson JM, Diegelmann RF, et al: Fetal responses to injury in the rabbit. *J Pediatr Surg* 22:640, 1987.
8. Hollander DM, Devereux DF, Marafino BJ, et al: Increased wound breaking strength in rats following treatment with synthetic human growth hormone. *Surg Forum* 35:612, 1984.
9. Tanzer ML: Crosslinking of collagen. *Science* 180:561, 1973.
10. Barrow MV, Simpson CF, Miller EJ: Lathyrism: A review. *Q Rev Biol* 49:101, 1974.
11. Cohen IK, Moore CD, Diegelmann RF: Onset and localization of collagen synthesis in open rat skin wounds. *Proc Soc Exp Biol Med* 160:458, 1979.
12. Enquist IF, Adamson RJ: Collagen synthesis and lysis in healing wounds. *Minn Med* 48:1695, 1965.
13. Grillo HK, Gross J: Collagenolytic activity during mammalian wound repair. *Dev Biol* 15:300, 1967.
14. Majno G, Gabbiani G, Hirshcel BJ, et al: Contraction of granulation tissue in vitro: Similarity to smooth muscle. *Science* 173:548, 1971.
15. Morton D Jr, Steinbronn K, Lato M, et al: Effect of colchicine on wound healing in rats. *Surg Forum* 25:47, 1974.
16. Peacock EE Jr, Madden JW: Administration of beta-aminopropionitrile to human beings with urethral strictures: A preliminary report. *Am J Surg* 136:600, 1978.
17. Rovee RT, Kurowky LA, Labun J: Effect of local wound environment of epidermal healing. In Maibach HI, Rovee DT (eds): *Epidermal Wound Healing.* Chicago, Year Book Medical Publishers, 1972, pp 159–181.
18. Niall M, Ryan GB, O'Brien BM: The effect of epidermal growth factor on wound healing in mice. *J Surg Res* 33:164, 1982.
19. Brown GL, Curtsinge LJ, Brightwell JR, et al: Human epidermal growth factor accelerates epithelialization of partial-thickness burns. Abstract—Presented at the Association for Academic Surgery 19th Annual Meeting, 1985, p 67.
20. Lawrence WT, Norton JA, Sporn MB, et al: The reversal of an Adriamycin-induced healing impairment with chemo attractants and growth factors. *Ann Surg* 203:142, 1986.
21. Mustoe TA, Pierce GF, Thomason A, et al: Accelerated healing of incisional wounds in rats induced by transforming growth factor Beta. *Science* 237:1333, 1988.
22. McKusick VA: *Heritable Disorders of Connective Tissues.* St. Louis, CV Mosby Co, 1972.
23. Harris ED Jr, Faulkner CS, Brown FE: Collagenolytic systems in rheumatoid arthritis. *Clin Orthop* 110:303, 1975.
24. Arquilla ER, Wringer EJ, Nakajo M: Wound healing: A model for the study of diabetic microangiopathy. *Diabetes* (Suppl) 25:811, 1976.
25. Goodson WH, Hunt TK: Studies of wound healing in experimental diabetes mellitus. *J Surg Res* 22:221, 1977.
26. Goodson WH, Hunt TK: Wound healing in experimental diabetes mellitus: Importance of early insulin therapy. *Surg Forum* 29:95, 1978.
27. Cruse PJE, Foord R: A five year prospective study of 23,649 surgical wounds. *Arch Surg* 107:206, 1973.
28. Seifter E, Crowley LV, Rettura G, et al: Influence of vitamin A on wound healing in rats with femoral fracture. *Ann Surg* 181:836, 1975.
29. Seifter E, Rettura G, Padawer J, et al: Impaired wound healing in streptozotocin diabetes: Prevention by supplemental Vitamin A. *Ann Surg* 194:42, 1981.
30. Levenson SM, Seifter E, VanWinckle W Jr: Nutrition. In Hunt TK, Dunphy JE (eds): *Fundamentals of Wound Management.* New York, Appleton-Century-Crofts, 1979, p 325.
31. Peacock EE Jr, Madden JW, Trier WC: Biologic basis for the treatment of keloids and hypertrophic scars. *South Med J* 63:755, 1970.
32. Cohen IK, McCoy BJ: The biology and control of surface overhealing. *World J Surg* 4:289, 1980.
33. Cohen IK, Keiser HR, Sjoerdsma A: Collagen synthesis in human keloids and hypertrophic scar. *Surg Forum* 22:488, 1971.
34. Cohen IK, Diegelmann RD, Johnson ML: Effects of corticosteroids on collagen synthesis. *Surgery* 82:15, 1977.
35. Craig RDP, Schofield JD, Jackson SS: Collagen biosynthesis in normal human skin, normal and hypertrophic scar and keloid. *Eur J Clin Invest* 5:69, 1975.
36. Cohen IK, Diegelmann RL, Keiser HR: Collagen metabolism in keloid and hypertrophic scar. In Longacre JJ (ed): *The Ultrastructure of Collagen.* Springfield, IL, Charles C Thomas, 1976, p 199.
37. Milsom JP, Craig RDP: Collagen degradation in cultured keloid and hypertrophic scar tissue. *Br J Dermatol* 89:635, 1973.
38. Diegelmann RF, Bryant CP, Cohen IK: Tissue alpha-globulins in keloid formation. *Plast Reconstr Surg* 59:418, 1977.
39. Eisen AZ, Bauer EA, Jeffrey JJ: Human skin collagenase: The role of serum alpha globulins in the control of activity in vivo and in vitro. *Proc Natl Acad Sci USA* 68:248, 1971.
40. Chytikova H, Kulhanek V, Horn V: Experimental production of keloids after immunization with autologous skin. *Acta Chir Plast* (Praha) 1:72, 1959.
41. Cohen IK, McCoy BJ, Mohanakumar T, et al: Immunoglobulin, complement and histocompatibility antigen studies in keloid patients. *Plast Reconstr Surg* 63:689, 1979.
42. Dobke M, Danowska A, Kondrat W: Antinuclear, antimitochondrial and anti-smooth muscles auto-antibodies following thermal trauma. *Burns* 5:195, 1979.
43. Daniels JC, Fukushima M, Larson DL, et al: Tissue levels of various globulins in burned patients. *J Trauma* 11:699, 1971.
44. Daniels JC, Larson DL, Abston S, et al: Serum protein profiles in thermal burns. *J Trauma* 14:137, 1974.
45. Griffith H: The treatment of keloids with triamcinolone acetonide. *Plast Reconstr Surg* 38:202, 1966.
46. Ketchum LD, Smith J, Robinson DW, et al: The treatment of hypertrophic scar, keloid, and scar contracture by triamcinolone acetonide. *Plast Reconstr Surg* 38:209, 1966.
47. Diegelmann RF, Peterkofsky B: Inhibition of collagen secretion from bone and cultured fibroblasts by microtubular disruptive drugs. *Proc Natl Acad Sci USA* 69:892, 1972.

48. Harris ED, Krane SM: Effects of colchicine on collagenase in cultures in rheumatoid synovium. *Arthritis Rheum* 14:669, 1971.

49. Ehrlich HP, Grislis G, Hunt TK: Evidence for the involvement of microtubules in wound contraction. *Am J Surg* 133:706, 1977.

50. Peacock EE Jr, Madden JW: Some studies on the effects of BAP in patients with injured flexor tendons. *Surgery* 66:215, 1969.

51. Albergoni V, Cassini A, Favero N, et al: Effect of penicillamine on some metals and metalloproteins in the rat. *Biochem Pharmacol* 24:1131, 1975.

52. Ehrlich HP, Hunt TK: The effect of cortisone and anabolic steroids on the tensile strength of healing wounds. *Ann Surg* 170:203, 1969.

53. Baker BL, Whitaker WL: Interference with wound healing by the local action of adrenocortical steroids. *Endocrinology* 46:544, 1950.

54. Howes EL, Plotz CM, Blunt JW, et al: Retardation of wound healing by cortisone. *Surgery* 28:177, 1950.

55. Stephens FO, Dunphy JE, Hunt TK: Effect of delayed administration of corticosteroids on wound contraction. *Ann Surg* 173:214, 1971.

56. Benson SC, Luvalle PA: Inhibition of lysyl oxidase and prolyl hydroxylase activity in glucocorticoid treated rats. *Biochem Biophys Res Commun* 99:557, 1981.

57. Cutreneo KR, Costello D, Fuller GC: Alteration of proline hydroxylase activity by glucocorticoids. *Biochem Pharmacol* 20:2797, 1971.

58. Sandberg N: Time relationship between administration of cortisone and wound healing in rats. *Acta Chir Scand* 127:446, 1964.

59. Ehrlich HP, Hunt TK: Effects of cortisone and vitamin A on wound healing. *Ann Surg* 167:324, 1968.

60. Hermann JB, Woodward SC: Stimulation of fibroplasia by vitamin A. *Surg Forum* 20:500, 1969.

61. Ehrlich HP, Tarver H, Hunt TK: Effects of vitamin A and glucocorticoids upon inflammation and collagen synthesis. *Ann Surg* 177:222, 1973.

62. Hunt TK, Ehrlich HP, Garcia JA, et al: Effect of vitamin A on reversing the inhibitory effect of cortisone on healing of open wounds in animals and man. *Ann Surg* 170:633, 1969.

63. Brazenor G, Stephens FU: The effect of vitamin A on the immunosuppressive action of cortisone of skin homografts in mice. *Aust NZ J Surg* 42:314, 1973.

64. Neifeld JP, Lee HM, Hutcher NC: Lack of effect of vitamin A on corticosteroid induced immunosuppression. *J Surg Res* 19:225, 1975.

65. Cohen BE, Cohen IK: Vitamin A: Adjuvant and steroid antagonist in the immune response. *J Immunol* 111:1376, 1973.

66. Jurin M, Tannok IF: Influence of vitamin A on immunologic response: *Immunology* 23:283, 1972.

67. Haick A, Johnson D, Raju S: Vitamin A does not alter immunosuppressive properties of simultaneously administered steroids. *Am Surg* 47:533, 1981.

68. Ferguson MK: The effect of anti-neoplastic agents on wound healing. *Surg Gynecol Obstet* 154:421, 1982.

69. Simpson DM, Ross R: The neutrophilic leukocyte in wound repair. A study with antineutrophil serum. *J Clin Invest* 51:2009, 1972.

70. Wahl SM, Arend WP, Ross R: The effect of complement depletion on wound healing. *Am J Pathol* 74:73, 1974.

71. Leibovich SJ, Ross R: The role of the macrophage in wound repair: A study with hydrocortisone and antimacrophage serum. *Am J Pathol* 78:71, 1975.

72. Peterson JM, Barbul A, Breslin RJ, et al: Significance of T-lymphocytes in wound healing. *Surgery* 102:300, 1987.

73. Desprez JD, Kiehn CL: The effects of cytotoxan (cyclophosphamide) on wound healing. *Plast Reconstr Surg* 26:301, 1960.

74. Karppinen V, Myllarniemi H: Vascular reaction in the healing laparotomy wound under cytostatic treatment. *Acta Chir Scand* 136:675, 1970.

75. Myllarniemi H, Peltokallio P: The effect of high dose cyclophosphamide therapy in the abdominal cavity of the rat: Adhesions and their vascular pattern. *Ann Chir Gynecol Fenn* 63:238, 1974.

76. Rudolph R, Arganese T, Woodward M: The ultra-structure and etiology of chronic radiotherapy damage in human skin. *Ann Plast Surg* 9:282, 1982.

77. Rudolph R: Complications of surgery for radiotherapy skin damage. *Plast Reconstr Surg* 70:179, 1982.

78. Tessmer CF: Radiation effects in skin. In Berdjis CC (ed): *Pathology of Irradiation*. Baltimore, Williams & Wilkins, 1971, pp 146–170.

79. Irvin TT: Effects of malnutrition and hyperalimentation on wound healing. *Surg Gynecol Obstet* 146:33, 1978.

80. Caback V, Dickerson JWT, Widdowson EM: Response of young rats to deprivation of protein or of calories. *Br J Nutr* 17:601, 1963.

81. Harkness M, Harkness RD, James DW: The effect of a protein-free diet on the collagen content of mice. *J Physiol* 144:307, 1958.

82. Bozzetti F, Terno G, Longoni C: Parenteral hyperalimentation and wound healing. *Surg Gynecol Obstet* 141:712, 1975.

83. Steiger E, Allen TR, Daly JM, et al: Beneficial effects of immediate postoperative total parenteral nutrition. *Surg Forum* 22:89, 1971.

84. Levenson MS, Seifter E: Dysnutrition, wound healing and resistance to infection. *Clin Plast Surg* 4:375, 1977.

85. Kinney JM: Energy requirements of the surgical patient. In Ballinger WF, et al (eds): *Manual of Surgical Nutrition*. Philadelphia, WB Saunders Co, 1975, pp 223–235.

86. Uitto J, Prockop DJ: Synthesis and secretion of underhydroxylated procollagen at various temperatures by cells subject to temporary anoxia. *Biochem Biophys Res Commun* 60:414, 1974.

87. Niinikoski J: Oxygen and wound healing. *Clin Plast Surg* 4:361, 1977.

88. Hunt TK, Pai MP: The effect of varying ambient oxygen tensions on wound metabolism and collagen synthesis. *Surg Gynecol Obstet* 135:561, 1972.

89. Hunt TK, Linsey M, Grislis G, et al: The effect of differing ambient oxygen tensions on wound infection. *Ann Surg* 181:35, 1975.

90. Sandblom P: The tensile strength of healing wounds. *Acta Chir Scand* 89 (suppl), 1944.

91. Sandbert N, Zederfelt B: Influence of acute hemorrhage on wound healing in the rabbit. *Acta Chir Scand* 118:367, 1960.

92. Chang N, Goodson WH, Gottrup F, et al: Direct measurement of wound and tissue oxygen tension in postoperative patients. *Ann Surg* 197:470, 1983.

3

Basic Principles of Surgical Techniques

Robert M. Pearl, M.D., F.A.C.S. and Robert A. Chase, M.D., F.A.C.S.

As surgeons, our greatest contribution to wound care is to take every action to assure an optimal setting for the wound to heal without interference. The biological processes—vascular, cellular, humoral, and biochemical—that together constitute inflammation, are essential occurrences in repair. To eliminate inflammation would be to deter the necessary accumulation of building blocks or substrates for the repair process to progress. Mechanical and chemical impediments to the natural progression and speed of healing include: motion at the wound interface; microbial invasion, which diverts the healing process to one of defense; interference with blood circulation, which transports cellular and chemical elements to the wound and removes by-products of absorptive débridement; and the repair process itself.

For thousands of years, surgeons have recognized that the final outcome of a procedure is dependent on precise surgical technique. In the 13th and 14th centuries, débridement of wounds and accurate apposition of their edges were stressed (1). In the 16th century, Paré noted the consequences of poor technique (2). In the 19th century, Pasteur and Lister emphasized asepsis (3–5). Finally, in the 20th century, Halsted outlined the basic tenets of surgical technique (6).

Although these principles are still relevant, the explosion in plastic and reconstructive surgery and maxillofacial surgery over the last decade has expanded the meaning of these concepts. Microsurgery and craniofacial techniques, including rigid fixation, are now essential parts of the surgeon's armamentarium. The expected results today often equal the exceptional outcome of the past. In this chapter, we will examine the basic principles of surgical technique; the details of their specific applications will be left for the individual sections.

Halsted's basic tenets of surgical technique stressed (a) asepsis, (b) hemostasis, (c) obliteration of dead space, (d) preservation of blood supply, (e) gentleness, and (f) no tissue tension at the suture line. When preoperative preparation, operative exposure, and rigid fixation are added, the foundation for both per primum healing and stable, long-term results is complete.

Preoperative Preparation

As surgical procedures become more complex, so must the preoperative planning and evaluation become more exact. Symmetry, balance, and absence of disfigurement are the goals. To achieve these, the reconstructive surgeon must assess facial form and function, including vascular supply, soft tissue cover, bony stability, passive and active motion, and innervation. A detailed anatomical exam is required, not only of the bone, muscle, and nerves, but also of the vascular supply and fascia. Physiological function must be assessed, including such problems as temporomandibular joint dysfunction, nasal airway obstruction, diplopia, and the tendency to dry eye syndrome. Adequate photography, dental study models, and computed tomography scans allow the surgeon to define the problem in three dimensions.

The incision must be planned not only to be the least conspicuous, but also to allow for future procedures. As an example, damage to the temporal artery at a first operation should be avoided if later a temporalis fascial flap or microvascular transfer might be needed.

In the operating room, appropriate instrumentation, adequate lighting, including a comfortable headlight, and magnification, including loupes and microscope, must be available. Intubation with a right-angle connector secured over a pad on the forehead allows access to the neck, mandible, maxilla, and orbits. Similarly, an oral tube wired to the teeth and secured to the chest provides access to the maxilla, orbits, and skull.

Asepsis

PREPARATION OF INTACT SKIN

Preparation of intact skin for surgical assault, whether by incision, abrasion, or puncture, consists of mechanical cleansing and bacteriocidal flooding. Detritus, or matter on the skin surface including naturally sloughing keratin, is removed. Inasmuch as intact skin is a waterproof protective barrier, it is possible to use antiseptics and various antimicrobial agents without fear of damaging unprotected and vulnerable tissues beneath the skin surface. There are numerous solutions that combine detergent or soap and antibacterial substances. Each commercial product has its advocates. So long as the solution contains these general ingredients, the intact skin will be optimally "prepped." Careful washing with the solution on the night preceding surgery may help cleanse and sterilize the skin at the site of proposed surgery.

The presence of hair at the proposed wound site or close to it is a nuisance and a potential threat to asepsis. Conservative hair removal over the area to be incised or prepared is best done just before surgery and skin preparation. Once hair is removed, the skin can be more readily prepared. Hair left at the incision site may get cut during the incision, and free hairs become irritating foreign bodies within the wound.

Although asepsis is the goal, this is rarely possible in the maxillofacial region. The intact skin of the entire face should be cleansed with a bacteriocidal solution to permit intraoperative comparison of the local site with the contralateral normal side. The preparation should extend onto the scalp. Hair in the incision line itself should be trimmed to minimize foreign body in the wound. However, full head shaving is rarely required because there is no evidence that the intraoperative shaving of hair is helpful in preventing infection. Furthermore, there is evidence that shaving the night before is detrimental.

In procedures where the mouth, pharnyx, sinuses, or nose are entered, bacterial contamination is inevitable. Under these circumstances, the surgeon should maximize the patient's defenses by the use of systemic antibiotics, preservation of vascular supply, avoidance of dead space, provision of adequate soft tissue cover, and selection of autologous rather than alloplastic materials.

PREPARATION—THE OPEN WOUND

Any chemical strong enough to be antiseptic is also injurious to exposed and vulnerable tissues unprotected by skin. Thus, the open wound itself is best prepared by gentle irrigation and washing with noninjurious fluids such as normal saline or balanced salt solution. Foreign materials not floated free by such washing are best removed by surgical débridement with sterile instruments. The intact skin around the open wound may be prepared as outlined for intact skin, but prep solutions must not be allowed to flow into the open wound.

Hemostasis

A hematoma provides a nidus for infection, compromises the overlying skin flaps, delays revascularization, and induces scar formation. The surgeon must use care to coagulate or ligate vessels and to drain areas where this is not possible, such as at osteotomy sites. Blood collections should be evacuated when they occur. Bipolar coagulation should be utilized in areas adjacent to the cornea, facial nerve, or brain.

Adequate Operative Exposure

Adequate exposure is required to facilitate extensive reconstructive procedures. Repair through small local incisions and wounds often leads to incomplete correction. Incisions should be placed so as to be inconspicuous (i.e., bicoronial or intraoral) or to produce minimal scars (i.e., extended lateral canthotomy or transcolumella). Incisions are placed in optimal locations such as the relaxed skin tension lines or along the lower ciliary margins. The incision itself should be perpendicular to the skin surface

or beveled in the region of hair follicles. Subperiosteal elevation avoids damage to the overlying motor nerves. In addition, by maintaining the fascial integrity, one prevents herniation of fat or other soft tissues into the operative fields. Flap elevation and undermining must be performed in anatomical planes.

The elasticity or compliance of skin and its mobility over underlying deep fascia, bone, or muscle allow it to drape over the underlying body architecture. At the same time, it hugs to the walls of concavities such as the axilla, submental neck, and palm of the hand, rather than webbing or tenting across such concavities. The skin adapts to the need to stretch and contract and to wrinkle regularly, forming predictable creases over areas of motion. Surgery or trauma may disrupt these normal characteristics by altering an area that is normally elastic, by creating a scar, or by changing the nature of the attachment of skin to underlying structures.

The fibrous tissue in scar is nonelastic and thus resists the stretching where it is essential for normal range of anatomical movement. A scar subjected to repeated efforts to stretch may react by becoming hypertrophic and rope-like.

Geometric reorientation of scars and movement of skin and soft tissue to fill a void are the primary objectives of such procedures as Z-plasty, V-Y advancement, adjacent tissue shifts, and interpolated flaps. It behooves the surgeon to understand the geometry of such maneuvers so that there is advanced knowledge of the exact site of scars after geometric repositioning.

The Z-plasty is a fundamental strategy with endless applications in wound geometry. Cleft lip repairs, other than simple straight line closure, are all modifications of the Z-plasty principle. If the reconstructive need is to alter the direction of a linear wound or scar, the surgeon should know precisely the new wound configuration as it would be after Z-plasty. The principle of the classical Z-plasty for a linear wound or scar is to draw parallel lines one on each side of the wound at about 60° to it and with dimensions that will allow interchange of the two flaps. If one wishes the new transverse arm of the new configuration to fall along a crease or predictable line, the two parallel lines should start at a point along the desired line.

Obliteration of Dead Space

This tenet classically refers to gaps in the soft tissues that can result in hematoma or seroma formation, serve as a locus for infection, and produce soft tissue contracture. However, these sequelae can also follow failure to reconstruct the bony framework. Failure to anatomically reposition the facial skeleton and bone graft the residual defects following fracture can produce bony relapse, contracture of the soft tissue envelope, and permanent disfiguration. Similarly, the failure to replace bone loss from the facial or cranial skeleton leads to local hematoma, poor healing, delayed union with subsequent motion, and an unsatisfactory functional and aesthetic outcome.

Preservation of Blood Supply

Throughout the preoperative planning and intraoperative procedure, the surgeon must be cognizant of every opportunity to increase the vascular supply to the reconstructive area. The Doppler probe allows the surgeon to identify and preserve axial vessels of the head and neck. Magnification and gentle technique are essential to avoid inadvertently damaging the vascular pedicle.

Axial flaps are more likely to survive and combat contamination than random pattern ones (7). Myocutaneous flaps can augment the local circulation and oxygen supply in vascularly compromised areas (8). Following trauma or frontal facial advancement, when one needs to separate the brain from a contaminated area such as the nose, a vascularized pericranial flap is superior to a nonvascularized graft. Similarly, in contradistinction to a nonvascularized fat or dermal graft, a vascularized transfer of soft tissue will survive in toto, remain soft, and maintain its volume.

Gentleness

Gentleness in the handling of tissue maintains the viability of each of the living cells, be they in the skin, soft tissues, or bone. Skin edges should never be pinched; instead, they should be elevated with skin hooks. Sharp dissection following anatomical planes provides a relatively bloodless field. Constant irrigation of desiccated soft tissues and bone increases cellular survival. Sufficiently large incisions will minimize traction on the wound margins. Gentle identification of nerves will avoid neuropraxia, and subperiosteal elevation of muscles will obviate transection, shortening, and fibrosis of these functional units.

Skin closure should strive to be exact; edges should be everted, and sutures should be placed at identical levels on each side. Small caliber sutures, loosely tied and removed early, will improve the ultimate scar.

Avoidance of Tissue Tension at the Suture Line

The avoidance of tissue tension allows primary healing and decreases the body's fibroblastic response. In the skin, excess tension on the suture line leads to hypertrophic or wide scars. When the forces are excessive on a fracture site or osteotomy, distraction and delayed or fibrous union results. Excess tension on vascular repairs induces thrombogenesis, and excess tension is the main cause of failed nerve repair. Undermining, primary tissue expansion, and skin grafts and flaps can help to minimize tension at the skin wound edges. Similarly, bone, vein, or nerve grafts can accomplish the same goals in the deeper tissues.

Rigid Fixation

By avoiding motion at fracture sites, one can promote more rapid healing, avoid displacement, permit early mobilization, and minimize the chances of infection. Immobilization is the sine qua non of both fracture union and successful bone grafts. Although wire fixation can be adequate, rigid plate or screw fixation is more commonly required. Plates must be of adequate length with a minimum of two screws on each side of the repair site. Full fracture reduction must be assured prior to plate application. Plate type and size, screw length, and site of application must be appropriate to counterbalance the forces at the fractures sites.

When surgical procedures were limited to the skin and soft tissues, avoidance of infection and the production of a well-coapted skin edge were the signs of sound surgical technique. Today's surgical procedures aim to achieve restoration of both form and function. To reach this goal, the surgeon needs to preserve and expand the vascular supply, restore and augment the bony skeleton, resuture and reposition muscles, and repair and transfer nerves. Each of these requires that the surgeon adhere to the basic tenets that have evolved over centuries. Ultimately, genetic engineering will eliminate the congenital problems, and transplantation will correct the acquired ones. However, until that era dawns, the surgeon who has mastered the basic principles of surgical technique will be the one who routinely obtains the best results.

References

1. Theodoric: Chirurgia in Guy de Chauliac, *Ars chirurgica* (n.41), fol. 140. recto.
2. Paré A: *The Workes of that Famous Chirurgion Ambrose Parey,* trans. Thomas Johnson (London, 1634) pp 324, 429, 457–464. Johnson's translation was from the 1582 Latin edition of Paré's 1579 collected works, the second French edition.
3. Lister J: On a case illustrating the present aspect of the antiseptic system of treatment in surgery. *Br Med J* 1:31, 1871.
4. Lister J: On a new method of treating compound fracture, abscess, etc. *Lancet* 1:326–329, 357–359, 387–389, 507–509; 2:95–96, 1867.
5. Pasteur L, Joubert JF, Chamberland CE: La Theorie des germes et ses applications a la médecine et a la chirurgie. *CR Acad Sci* 86:1037, 1878.
6. Halsted WS: In Burket WC (ed): *Surgical Papers.* Baltimore, The Johns Hopkins Press, 1924, pp 311–586.
7. Pearl R, Arnstein D: A vascular approach to the prevention of infection. *Ann Plast Surg* 14:443, 1985.
8. Chang N, Mathes SJ: Comparison of the effect of bacterial innoculation in musculocutaneous and random pattern flaps. *Plast Reconstr Surg* 70:1, 1982.

4

Skin Grafting

Jack C. Fisher, M.D., F.A.C.S. and Marek K. Dobke, M.D.

When the history of 20th century plastic surgery is written, ample reference will be made to microsurgery, myocutaneous flaps, tissue expansion, perhaps even pharmacological control of graft rejection, if current research frontiers are pursued. Nevertheless, we propose that skin grafting will stand as this century's most important clinical advance in reconstructive surgery.

Biological transfer of skin, both allogeneic and autologous, was initially described during the 19th century. Historical precedent is generally credited to Reverdin (1), a surgical resident working in Paris, whose achievement was reported in 1870. George David Pollock, a British surgeon, applied the first successful autograft to a burn wound in England. Just a few months later, probably without knowledge of Reverdin's work, he then turned to skin sources from other than the patient, first from an unspecified donor and eventually from himself (2). Pollock's description of the result probably represents the earliest account of immunological skin rejection; however, it is unlikely that he understood what was going on at the time.

Clinical use of grafted skin awaited 20th century refinements. Prior to World War I, only very thin (Thiersch) or full-thickness (Wolff) grafts were used. Halsted applied large full-thickness grafts to his mastectomy wounds; they were known as "Davis" grafts in America. Blair and Brown first reported their clinical use of split skin grafting in 1929 (3), and many believe that their work constitutes the landmark plastic surgery achievement of this century. Widespread acceptance of split skin grafting was later assured by invention of the dermatome by Earl Padgett and George Hood (4). Meanwhile, Blair remained partial to a knife for graft harvest.

When American plastic surgery units crossed the Atlantic during World War II, they discovered that skin grafting was uncommonly practiced; the tubed flap dominated reconstructive surgery. Sir Harold Gillies was the reigning master of local flap transfer for repair of most traumatic deformities. John Converse recalls teaching conferences with Sir Harold early in the war; opinions would be sought for the best way to close a certain defect. Gillies on one occasion turned to Converse and said, "Now if you say you're going to use a graft, I will send you back to America!" (5).

Sir Archibald McIndoe was one British plastic surgeon who used split skin grafts on a large scale, applying the method for rapid closure of extensive burn injuries. Skin grafting was not commonly used by German or French surgeons until after World War II, when the dermatome and improvements on Blair's knife became available to all European nations.

Wounds That Require Skin Grafts

Two kinds of wounds confront the plastic surgeon: those without skin loss, and those with a skin deficit. Simple lacerations, partial abrasions, and surgical incisions can be closed either primarily by suture or, if infected, secondarily at a later time. Leg ulcers, full-thickness burns, avulsions, and pressure sores are all examples of wounds with skin loss. Closure of these defects depends on two natural mechanisms, epithelial migration and wound contraction, or upon surgical intervention with tissue delivery, for example, as a skin graft or flap.

Before the introduction of skin grafting, surgeons had no choice but to wait for contraction and epithelial migration. Contraction is the expected consequence of granulation tissue formation in a wound defect. Epithelium seeks to cover a surface wound from the margins by advancing over the highly vascular collagen-rich surface. Both are painstakingly slow processes; they can be depended upon in areas in which the skin is mobile and easily drawn together, such as the abdomen or buttocks, but they are never reliable for scalp or extremity defects, where the skin is already drawn tight.

Contraction is, in part, dependent on the action of contractile fibroblasts (myofibroblasts), which are cells rich in actin fibers that display many of the physiological properties of smooth muscle (6). Myofibroblasts are present during the phases of wound healing when contraction takes place. They are identifiable by electron microscopy. They disappear after contraction stops and wound closure is complete (7).

The inherent force of wound contraction becomes apparent when surface defects on joint surfaces are permitted to close spontaneously. No amount of splinting can halt the contraction process. The resulting deformity is called a contracture.

Epithelium that migrates from the margins of a wound is fragile and exists without the rete pegs that normally assure union between the epidermis and dermis. Migratory epithelium is therefore avulsed easily by shearing forces. Migrating epithelium is clinically recognizable as a blue-gray border encircling the granulating wound. Mi-

FIGURE 4.1. Diagram demonstrates schematically the histology of normal skin, emphasizing the skin appendages (hair follicles and sweat glands) that yield new epithelium following split graft harvest. On the left, skin grafts of varying thicknesses are depicted. (From Rudolph R, Fisher JC, Ninnemann JL: *Skin Grafting.* Boston, Little Brown, 1980.)

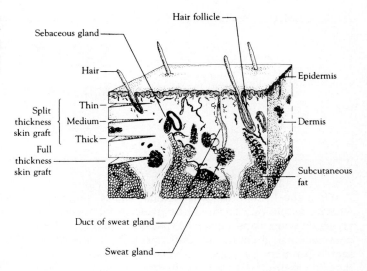

croscopically, the advancing epithelium assumes a neoplastic appearance, especially after the chronic presence of the wound. Long-standing epithelial migration can lead to carcinogenesis after many years of unresolved healing (8).

Today, surgeons intervene with skin grafts or skin flaps rather than depend on the natural healing processes. There is good reason to graft well in advance of active contraction in order to limit deformity and disability. Partial-thickness (split) skin grafts will slow the rate of contraction in a wound but not eliminate it altogether. Full-thickness grafts and skin flaps can stop contraction if applied early to surface defects (Fig. 4.1).

Preparing Wounds for Skin Grafting

Skin grafts require a living regenerative surface for successful neovascularization. Grafting means tissue transfer without preservation of blood supply. Therefore, vascular union must develop quickly in order for the graft to survive transfer.

Cortical bone denuded of its periosteum cannot accept a skin graft; neither are tendons, nerves, or cartilage without their respective investing connective tissue suitable surfaces for grafting. Most other tissues, including muscle, fat, fascia, and even dura and periosteum, readily accept skin grafts if certain criteria are met:

1. *Viability:* The wound surface must be viable. It must have a blood supply and must be débrided of all non-living tissue. Acutely injured tissue must be protected with a biological or synthetic membrane. Following débridement, chronic wound surfaces must be protected, or else further necrosis will take place.
2. *Hemostasis:* Following débridement, all bleeding must be controlled, or a graft cannot be expected to live. More skin grafts fail because of a hematoma than most surgeons recognize or admit.
3. *Bacterial Equilibrium:* Most granulating surfaces contain bacteria. However, quantitative microbiological studies show that wounds with bacterial densities less

than 10^5/g organisms will accept grafts more readily than wounds with higher levels of contamination (9). Quantitative (biopsy) culture of the wound surface is a useful diagnostic aid prior to skin grafting. The traditional swab culture is unreliable and does not tell the surgeon anything about bacterial density within the wound.

4. *Systemic Equilibrium:* Patients with certain illnesses are not good candidates for grafting. For example, those who receive steroid medication do not vascularize grafts as well. Venous stasis can be as disabling to graft viability as is arterial insufficiency. Diabetes, hematological disorders, and prior radiation produce their own handicaps to graft acceptance. Some of these preconditions can be treated and stabilized prior to grafting; others cannot.

The following question is often asked by the inexperienced skin grafter: What should be placed on the wound surface to make it ready for a graft? No applied substance can substitute for blood supply or meticulous débridement. Commonly used solutions like the organic iodines (povidone) are probably without biological advantage. Also, they contain inflammatory ingredients like detergents and are so deeply pigmented that they obscure the surgeon's ability to examine the wound surface.

A physiological salt solution is quite adequate. However, we prefer to use a very dilute solution of sodium hypochlorite (10% in saline). Known historically as Dakin's solution following its introduction during World War I, it can be prepared easily by diluting laundry bleach 1:10. Dakin's solution releases free chlorine and oxygen and dissolves thin residual layers of fibrin. It can also neutralize the foul odor that often accompanies a chronic wound. We believe that benefits from its strong antimicrobial potential exceed by far some cellular damage due to its local toxicity. Dressings for a wound surface should be moistened at the time of application and again at the time of removal. The traditional wet-to-dry dressing is unnecessarily painful as well as damaging to migrating epithelium.

Selecting the Appropriate Donor Site(s)

Choice of a suitable donor site must take into account the type of graft needed: full- or split-thickness skin, thick split or thin, small area or large, etc.

SPLIT-THICKNESS SKIN

For the smallest requirements, such as a fingertip, a postage stamp-sized split graft from the upper inner arm is ideal. For moderate needs, begin with the lateral buttock. This area is less painful when the patient is supine and is easily hidden by swimwear or summer clothing. When a greater need must be met, extend to the posterior buttock, then onto the more visible thigh. For very extensive burns, the additional choices in order of preference are abdomen, back, scalp, anterior chest wall, arms, and lastly the lower leg. Lower extremity donor sites may not heal well.

Visible areas should be avoided for small grafting needs because men, women, and children alike sense embarrassment whenever evidence of prior skin grafting is unnecessarily emblazoned on their thighs.

The buttock and thigh areas are ideal when thick split skin is needed for durability. Avoid the groin and antecubital regions; here only the very thinnest grafts can be harvested without risking exposure of subcutaneous fat.

Facial grafting requires special attention to color matching (Fig. 4.2). Leg skin assumes a darker, brownish hue on the face long after grafting, even though pigments may look the same initially. This principle applies equally to patients of all ethnic origins. Scalp skin is an excellent donor site for facial defect grafting if partial-thickness skin flaps are used to avoid transferring hair follicles. Unfortunately, scalp skin is too hyperpigmented for use in pale-skinned individuals if skin from a blush zone is required. This leaves no ideal choice. We have replaced deeply pigmented facial grafts with shoulder skin and achieved an acceptable color match.

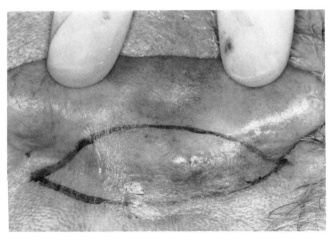

FIGURE 4.3. Postauricular graft donor site.

FULL-THICKNESS SKIN

Only limited grafting needs can be served by a full-thickness skin graft. The resulting defect must be sutured. The thinnest skin is the eyelid, followed by postauricular (Figs. 4.3 and 4.4), preauricular, supraclavicular, antecubital, and groin skin.

Skin Harvest

Plastic surgeons have adopted the agricultural term "harvest" when they refer to cutting skin grafts. A variety of instruments are used, depending on the quantity and thickness of the graft required.

Full-thickness grafts may be excised by dissection. Experienced surgeons carefully separate the skin from the underlying fat. Whenever fat is excised in continuity with skin, it must be carefully removed (defatted) *prior to* application (Fig. 4.5). Donor defects are closed in two layers—a deeper closure with absorbable suture, and a run-

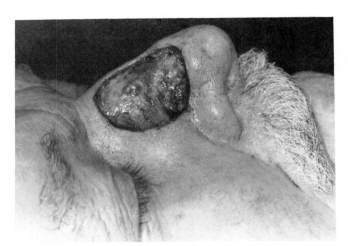

FIGURE 4.2. Nasal skin defect following excision of basal cell carcinoma.

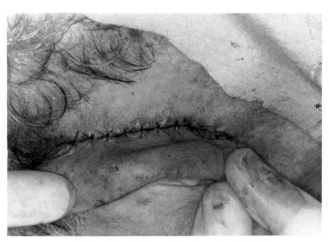

FIGURE 4.4. Donor site closed primarily.

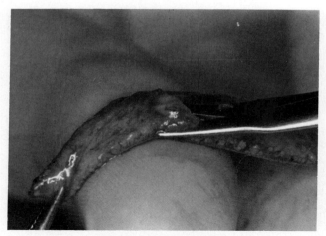

FIGURE 4.5. Full-thickness graft defatted with fine scissors.

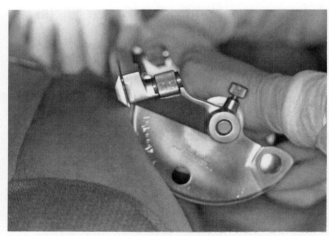

FIGURE 4.7. Reese drum dermatome: split graft taken across buttock.

ning pull-out suture for the skin. The fat should never be scraped off; this will *injure* the dermis unnecessarily.

The invention of the dermatome by Padgett and Hood contributed to the popularity of split skin grafting during and after World War II. Skin grafting technique is often learned today using the Brown electric or air-powered dermatome (Fig. 4.6). We prefer the air drive model because of its faster blade. Split grafts are cut between 0.012- and 0.018-inch thickness. Application of very thin grafts may close the wound but will not halt contraction. Thicker grafts are more durable and contract less, but they must be taken from sites where the skin is of sufficient thickness (buttock, thigh, back).

Power dermatomes are best used on surfaces with underlying muscle padding. Skin is more effectively removed from the abdomen or chest wall using a drum dermatome (Fig. 4.7). Drum dermatomes rely on the principle that adhesive surfaces, direct or removable, will bind to the skin sufficiently for a manually operated blade to cut a split graft (Fig. 4.8). Errors in the use of a drum

dermatome are usually related to inadequate preparation. Always use a fat-dissolving solvent (e.g., ether, acetone, or alcohol) before applying the dermatome. Drum dermatomes should not be used on the scalp; hair shafts are too dense for the adhesive to stick. The donor scalp should be infiltrated with saline. This allows the power dermatome to function against a padded surface. Drum dermatomes are favored for the most precise harvest of skin grafts of predictable thickness. Surgeons favor the Reese or the Padgett models based on personal experience. Both operate on the same principle.

Not to be forgotten is the fine art of free cutting skin grafts. Many of our British colleagues maintain facile skills with the Humby, Ferris Smith, or similar grafting knives. Whether or not you choose to develop skill with a long-bladed knife, you should achieve skill with small knives like the Goulian (made by Weck), a very useful instrument for taking small split grafts of consistent thickness.

The trick with free cutting skin is (*a*) concentration to

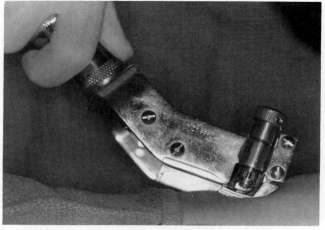

FIGURE 4.6. Brown dermatome (air-driven): correct angle for taking split grafts.

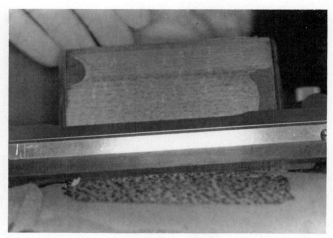

FIGURE 4.8. Split graft adherent to drum adhesive as blade cuts at selected skin thickness.

maintain blade angle and graft thickness and (*b*) remembering to slice (like roast beef) rather than to push.

Pinch grafting, an old technique, ought to be discarded completely. Surgeons used to pierce the skin with a needle, draw the skin to a point and slice with the scalpel blade. The resulting graft contained full-thickness skin in the middle and partial-thickness skin at the borders and was unsatisfactory. Pinch grafts do not take well, and the donor sites will often heal with hypertrophic scars.

Skin Graft Storage

Both skin autografts and allografts can be stored at 4°C for a limited period of time. This technique is useful if the graft is to be used within a few days after harvesting. The graft should be spread on moist cotton gauze. The addition of tissue culture medium may enhance viability, and antibiotics may help to prevent microbial growth.

Storage for up to 2 weeks is an acceptable clinical practice. For longer periods of time, skin banking conditions must be developed, and grafts should be stored in a frozen or lyophilized state.

Delayed Graft Application

Occasionally, after lesion excision and skin graft harvesting, completion of hemostasis and wound-bed infection can be a problem. When this occurs, the harvested graft may be stored, either on the donor site or at 4°C for several days, and then applied as a delayed graft. This grafting can be easily performed at the bedside. It is our usual practice to delay skin grafting of free muscle flap surfaces for 2–3 days and to cover them once it becomes apparent that there are no problems with flap circulation (10).

There is experimental evidence that a graft applied to a wound surface within the 48-hr delay period will meet early granulation with angiogenic proliferation of the wound bed, thus promoting graft survival.

Donor Site Care

Split-thickness skin graft donor sites can be expected to heal in stages like any wound. They represent partial abrasions. Following bleeding and hemostasis, an inflammatory reaction develops. A protective fibrin shield forms over the wound surface. After 2 or 3 days, active epithelial proliferation can be observed. Epidermis regenerates by growth and migration of epithelial cells from the hair follicles and skin appendages. The dermis should be covered by new epithelium in 5–10 days, depending on the thickness of graft taken.

As soon as the graft is taken, apply to the donor site a wrung out sheet of lubricated gauze followed by a lap pad. Do not remove the first layer as new bleeding will occur. After securing the skin graft, return to the donor site, remove the lap pad, express accumulated clot from beneath the gauze, apply a layer of Telfa or Xeroform, and wrap with gauze. On the following day, remove all but the first layer, leaving the lubricated gauze to come off spontaneously just as a scab does. Exposing a donor site decreases surface temperature from 98°F to 91°F, thereby decreasing the potential for bacterial growth.

Conversion of a donor site to a full-thickness wound requiring its own graft is a complication of grafting, caused either by cutting to an excessive depth or by inattention to postoperative wound care. If subcutaneous fat is observed during the harvest of a graft, that graft should be immediately sutured back down and a new graft obtained elsewhere. These inadvertent avulsions usually revascularize quickly, albeit with a scar that must later be explained to the patient.

The differences between lubricated gauzes are subtle. Do not apply any of the currently available synthetic skin substitutes. None offers any advantage over traditional methods for donor site care. Some will stick to the donor site. Biobrane, an extremely effective temporary skin substitute for wound surfaces, is expensive and inhibits both wound contraction and epithelial migration, which is not desirable in a donor site.

Graft Immobilization

If a graft is not held immobile long enough to receive its new blood supply, then it cannot succeed. The problem of an unsuccessful graft is easily explained, but its cause, and therefore its solution, can elude us. The failure of a graft is often attributed to infection, but the failing graft is often also the graft that was inadequately secured.

Grafts may be sutured, stapled, or taped to the wound margin or to each other (Fig. 4.9). Grafts are fragile; shearing forces will tear them if they are affixed under tension. For prevention of those troublesome shearing forces, we prefer two extremes: no dressing at all, or else a tie-over dressing.

Leaving a graft open to view sounds more daring than it is; however, it requires a cooperative patient as well as nursing staff willing to observe and take action when serum or clot accumulation is discovered or when subtle graft movement is seen. This is not a suitable technique

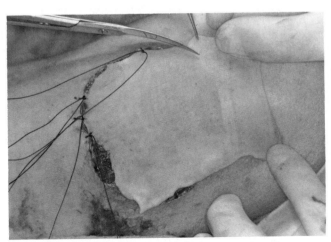

FIGURE 4.9. Split graft applied to wound surface.

for a child, an uncooperative adult, certain body regions, or an intimidated nursing staff.

A tie-over dressing, inaccurately called a stent, may be the best insurance for graft immobilization (Fig. 4.10). Conventional dressings seem to loosen with time, no matter how expertly applied. Some will say that a tie-over dressing takes too long, but they will waste more time grafting a second time after the initial attempt fails. Furthermore, a tie-over dressing ought to be done quickly. Do not fuss over tiny sutures. Use 4-0 silk and large needles for faster handling, quickly tie the ends long, and go onto the next stitch (Figs. 4.11 and 4.12). If the scrub nurse can stay ahead of you, then you are probably not suturing fast enough.

Other bad habits to avoid include:

1. Placing the wrong side down (inverted grafts will not grow).
2. Leaving clots beneath the graft before applying a dressing.
3. "Pie-crusting": making multiple small holes in the graft, presumably for drainage. It is far better to take more time for hemostasis.

How Grafts Heal

If a graft is successfully held immobile on its wound bed, it will gradually regain the pink color it lost at the time of harvest. This return of color begins within a few hours as passive absorption of red cells takes place from the wound into the preexistent but vacated vascular channels of the graft.

The graft in this tentative status is also nourished by a plasma exchange of nutrients (plasmatic imbibition). Fluid is passively absorbed by the graft, and this leads to edema within 2 or 3 days. Finally, the proliferating capillary tufts of the granulating bed unite with the vascular spaces of the graft; the result is revascularization (take).

Grafts slowly gain durability and lose their edema. This marks the maturing phase of healing, which is characterized by changes in dimension, pigmentation, and sensibility.

We speak in error of a graft contracting. Contraction is a characteristic of the wound surface, not of the graft. Nevertheless, skin grafts will themselves "shrink" if they have been drawn too tightly across a defect. Grafts should therefore cover a defect easily and without tension. A wound will contract to some degree following grafting; barely a trace occurs following a full-thickness graft, but as much as 30–35% may occur after a split-thickness graft application.

Pigment cells of the skin are extraordinarily sensitive to injury during skin transfer. Therefore, most grafts undergo an initial loss of pigmentation, followed by hyper-pigmentation, and finally by gradual return to normal. Donor sites will pass through a similar pigment transition. For some patients, the distance between donor and recipient site can produce problems with respect to color match. The tawny (in whites) and dark (in blacks) hue of the leg does not look good on the face or neck.

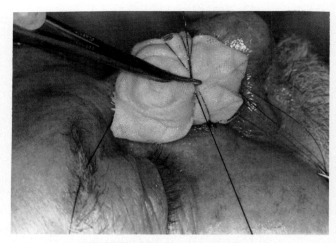

FIGURE 4.10. Tie-over dressing.

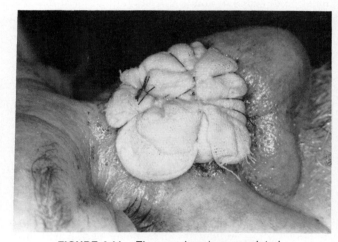

FIGURE 4.11. Tie-over dressing completed.

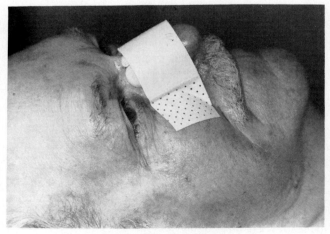

FIGURE 4.12. Simple dressing.

Re-innervation is incomplete in most grafts, yet it is better in split grafts than in full-thickness grafts or in flaps. Pontén (11) has determined by two-point discrimination testing that skin grafts can, at best, assume sensibility characteristics of the recipient wound, not of the original donor site.

Even under ideal vascularization and maturation conditions, certain unwanted sequelae may result (e.g., scaling because the graft cannot yet lubricate itself or milia due to obstructed or buried sweat glands). Scaly skin should be lubricated daily with a lanolin-containing moisturizing lotion. Milia should be opened and drained.

Special Techniques

MESH GRAFTING

A mechanical device can multiply pierce a graft, allowing it to be expanded into a mesh of varying size. The longer the slits, the greater the expansion ratio. Certain wounds lend themselves to meshing (e.g., an irregular, concave surface in which exudate puddles or an enormous burn wound with scarcity of donor sites).

Readers who are now aware of wound contraction and epithelization will immediately recognize the disadvantage of meshing: it leaves an incompletely covered surface that must contract further to achieve closure.

Those who make a habit of meshing every graft do not understand the principles of wound coverage. The quality of a healed surface is dependent on the thickness and integrity of the graft applied. Avoid applying meshed grafts to a face, a hand, or any flexor surface (neck, knee, etc.)

CHINESE METHOD OF SKIN GRAFTING

The so-called Chinese concept of treating extensive third-degree burns involves staged excision and intermingled transplantation of auto- and allogeneic skin. This method of treatment was developed in the 1960s by Chinese surgeons (12).

In this procedure, small segments of available split-thickness autografts are inserted into windows on the healing allograft sheets. As allogeneic epidermis is rejected, autogeneic epidermis migrates from the autologous islands, epithelializing allogeneic dermis.

The long-term fate of allogeneic dermis is presently under investigation. It appears that the time difference between the rejection of auto- and allogeneic epidermis is the basis for the success of the Chinese method. Autogeneic epidermis grows over allogeneic dermis, which gradually is replaced by autologous elements. However, cytogenetic investigations demonstrate that viable allogeneic cells may survive for several months (13; Fig. 4.13).

DERMAL-FAT GRAFTING

For padding, composite grafts of dermis and fat have been successfully used. Following removal of epidermis, these grafts can be buried. Their limitation is that much of

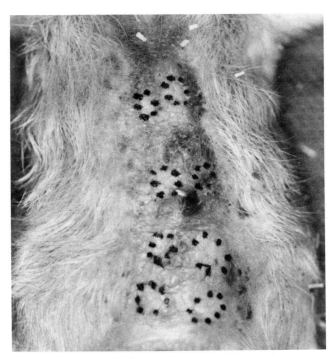

FIGURE 4.13. Intermingled graft 5 weeks posttransplantation (experimental rat model).

the fat will resorb. Surgeons who continue to use this old technique tend to rely only upon grafted dermis, not the fat.

MUCOSAL GRAFTING

Skin does not fare well inside the mouth. Like all grafts, skin retains its original characteristics. Whenever a secretory surface is required (e.g., conjunctiva, nasal lining, buccal mucosa), a mucosal graft is appropriate.

Grafts of mucosal membrane may be transferred as either full-thickness or split-thickness grafts. A special dermatome (Castroviejo) is available for harvesting small split mucosal grafts. Full-thickness mucosa contracts after harvest; therefore, a larger graft than the anticipated need should be harvested.

The best sources for mucosal grafts are the buccal surface, nasal septum, and conjunctiva. The conjunctiva is thinnest; the septum is thickest.

COMPOSITE GRAFTING

A composite graft includes more than one kind of tissue. For example, a wedge of ear, including skin and cartilage, is ideal for reconstructing alar defects. A graft of nasal septum and overlying mucosa can be used for eyelid reconstruction.

Composite grafts are necessarily limited in dimension because they must derive blood supply from the recipient wound. Furthermore, the donor site must be closed primarily. Great care must be taken with composite tissue transfers: recipient wound preparation, suture immobilization, and graft handling must be flawless, or vascularization will not take place.

HAIR TRANSPLANTS

Hair-bearing grafts are a composite tissue; they include skin and enough subcutaneous tissue to protect intact hair follicles. Either plugs or strips are taken from hair-bearing areas and transferred carefully to balding zones. Shafts subsequently fall out of the follicles, but new hair will grow if the entire graft has been vascularized.

CULTURED SKIN GRAFTS

As techniques for tissue culture improved during the 1970s, attempts were made to create cultured skin substitutes that might help permanently heal large defects. Whenever autologous skin is in short supply, as for the treatment of extensive third-degree burns or giant hairy nevi, cultured skin grafting techniques may be another alternative for the coverage of large deficiencies.

In vitro cultivation and serial culturing of keratinocytes make production of viable epithelial sheets possible. Cultured epithelium alone, however, does not provide mechanically and aesthetically satisfactory long-term coverage. Various modifications in composite grafts, using a combination of cultured epidermal cells and allogeneic dermis or collagen appear to be superior to epithelial sheets alone (Figs. 4.14 and 4.15).

As in the Chinese method of skin grafting, low dermal immunogenicity allows for healing of allogeneic dermis. In composite auto/allogeneic skin grafts, allogeneic dermis may function as a dermis and support the cultured autologous epidermal component (14; Figs. 14.16 and 14.17).

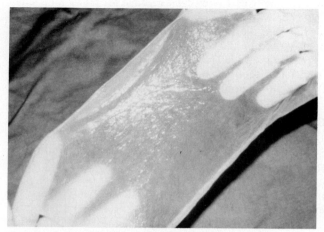

FIGURE 4.14. Porous and resorbable collagen-glycosaminoglycan membrane as a dermal substitute for composite cultured skin equivalent.

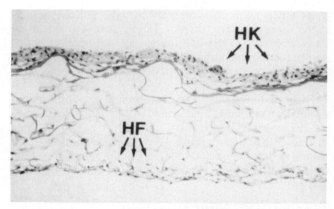

FIGURE 4.15. Composite culture skin equivalent: autologous human keratinocytes (HK) attached to nonporous surface of collagen-glycosaminoglycan substitute; autologous human fibroblasts (HF) are populated within internal pores.

Why Skin Grafts Fail

Given the choice, we would all prefer a perfect graft take every time, but our best hopes are not always realized. The occasional skin grafter can expect at best a partial graft take. We have overheard surgeons claim that a graft was a success when no more than half of that graft remained viable.

Clinical success requires that all of the graft becomes revascularized. In order to achieve success routinely, establish a high standard and consider anything less than 100% revascularization to be a failure, then seek an explanation for that failure. Do not shift the blame to anyone but yourself.

By the time a graft has clearly failed, decomposing skin may have already stimulated the formation of pus. Therefore, infection is often blamed for the failure of the graft, the implication being that the graft loss was beyond the surgeon's control.

The most common reason for graft loss is hematoma, followed closely by inadequate immobilization of the graft. Each of these factors is within the surgeon's control. Extra moments taken to achieve complete hemostasis will save many hours of a surgeon's time and days of hospitalization for regrafting. The difference between a firmly held graft and a dressing that permits graft movement is the life of that graft!

Misjudgment of the wound, its vascularity, and its inherent bacterial density can lead to failure due to bacterial contamination. Biopsy culture before scheduled grafting can help to avoid this cause of failure.

A less common error is the application of the graft epidermal side down. Always place the dermal (shiny) surface down. Vascularization requires union between a granulating surface and the graft dermis.

Grafted skin cannot maintain its neovasculature if held in a dependent position. Lower extremity wounds must be elevated for 2 weeks after graft application. Afterward, external elastic compression is needed whenever

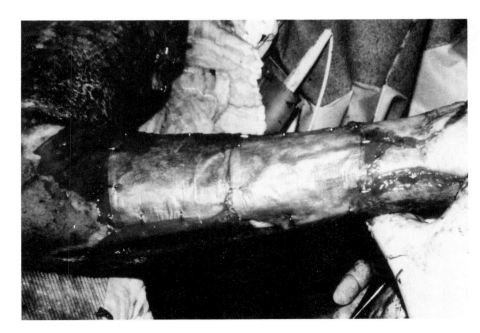

FIGURE 4.16. Two 8.5 × 8.5-cm composite cultured skin equivalents placed on right forearm wound after fascial excision of full-thickness burn wound.

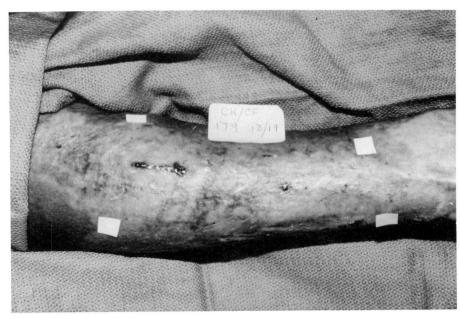

FIGURE 4.17. The same wound 16 days later: good healing of composite cultured skin equivalent.

the leg is in a dependent position. Small blisters on a newly grafted surface indicate excessive hydrostatic pressure.

Summary

Develop your biological understanding of the grafting process. Perfect your skin grafting skills. Free transfers of tissue are likely to remain this century's most significant gift to reconstructive surgery. For a more detailed understanding of skin grafting principles and methods, consult a comprehensive monograph on the subject (15).

ACKNOWLEDGMENTS

Photographs 14 through 17 are courtesy of Matthew Cooper, M.D. and John F. Hansbrough, M.D., Department of Surgery, UCSD Medical Center, San Diego, CA.

References

1. Klasen HJ: *History of Free Skin Grafting*. Heidelberg, Springer-Verlag, 1981.
2. Freshwater FM, Krizek TJ: Skin grafting of burns: A centennial. *J Trauma* 11:862, 1971.
3. Blair VP, Brown JB: The use and uses of large split skin grafts of intermediate thickness. *Surg Gynecol Obstet* 49:82, 1929.

4. Padgett EC: Skin grafting in severe burns. *Am J Surg* 43:626, 1939.

5. Converse JM: Introduction to plastic surgery. In Converse JM (ed): *Reconstructive Plastic Surgery,* Vol 1. Philadelphia, Saunders, 1977.

6. Gabbiani G, Hirschel BJ, Ryan GB, Statkov PR, Majno G: Granulation tissue as a contractile organism. *J Exp Med* 135:719, 1972.

7. Rudolph R, Guber S, Suzuki M, Woodward M: The life cycle of the myofibroblast. *Surg Gynecol Obstet* 145:389, 1977.

8. Peacock EE: *Wound Repair,* 3rd edition, Philadelphia, Saunders, pp 187–191.

9. Robson MC, Krizek TJ: Predicting skin graft survival. *J Trauma* 13:213, 1973.

10. James MI, McGrouther DA: Delayed exposed skin grafting: A 10-year experience of the technique. *Br J Plast Surg* 38:124, 1985.

11. Pontén B: Grafted skin—observations on innervation and other qualities. *Acta Chir Scand (Suppl)* 257:1, 1960.

12. Yangl CC, Shih TS, Xu WS: A Chinese concept of treatment of extensive third degree burns. *Plast Reconstr Surg* 70:238, 1982.

13. Kistler D, Hafemann B, Hettich R: Cytogenetic investigations of the allodermis after intermingled skin grafting. *Burns* 15:82, 1989.

14. Cuono CB, Langdon R, Birchall N, Barttlebort S, McGuire J. Composite autologous-allogeneic skin replacement: Development and clinical application. *Plast Reconstr Surg* 80:626, 1987.

15. Rudolph R, Fisher JC, Ninnemann JL: *Skin Grafting.* Boston, Little, Brown, 1979.

5

Basic Principles of Skin Flaps

Jack Fisher, M.D., F.A.C.S.

Introduction

In the past, a discussion on skin flaps in reconstructive plastic surgery would have devoted considerable space to the random pattern flap, the tubed pedicle flap, waltzing of tissue to distance sites, and the delay phenomenon. However, with our present understanding of blood supply to tissues (specifically, skin) and the clinical development of musculocutaneous, muscle, and fasciocutaneous flaps, there is less need for use of random tissue and less dependency on the delay phenomenon. Free tissue transfer has further decreased the need for the concept of waltzing tissue over multiple stages to distant sites. Nevertheless, knowledge of the anatomy and physiology of skin and skin flaps is essential.

The design and execution of a well-planned skin flap procedure, often randomly based in such areas as the head and neck, remain important. In other areas of the body, many new flaps with defined vascular anatomy have been described. This has been especially true with the advent of free tissue transfer because there is increasing interest in identifying specific sites from which skin can be raised with a known dominant vascular pedicle.

This chapter will present topics important for a basic understanding of skin flaps, including the vascular anatomy of skin. Our present understanding of blood supply of the skin in association with the underlying muscle and fascia has produced a fundamental change in the practice of plastic and reconstructive surgery. Advances in knowledge have led to the development of musculocutaneous and fasciocutaneous flaps. It has also provided the basis for development of the field of microvascular free tissue transfer (1). Although newer techniques have superseded many of the skin flap procedures, pathogenesis of skin flap necrosis, the delay phenomenon, and revascularization of skin remain important topics. Much research has been devoted to the pharmacological manipulation of skin flaps in order to improve survival. Methods of monitoring skin flap viability remain of great interest to both researchers and clinicians. Each of these important issues will be reviewed.

Skin Flap Classification According to Vascular Anatomy

Understanding the vascular anatomy of skin flaps requires a basic knowledge of the blood supply throughout the body. The subdermal vascular plexus and its relationship to skin perfusion must be considered in the content of the blood supply to the underlying muscle and fascia and of the body as a whole (Fig. 5.1). Accurate knowledge of vascular anatomy is an important prerequisite to successful skin flap transfer. Numerous methods for directly or indirectly manipulating and augmenting the blood flow to an area of skin have been described. However, these manipulations can do little to salvage a flap poorly designed with respect to vascular anatomy.

A simplified scheme of the blood supply to skin has been described, consisting of three major components. First is the segmental vasculature, which consists of branches of the aorta (e.g., femoral, intercostal vessels). Second is the perforating vessels, which are supplied by the segmental vessels and connect to the third group, the cutaneous vasculature. There are two major subgroups within the cutaneous vasculature: the musculocutaneous perforators, which are the blood supply to most of the skin of the body, and the direct cutaneous vessels, which supply a limited number of anatomical sites. The direct cutaneous vessels form the axial pattern or arterial flaps, which will be discussed below.

The main blood supply to the skin comes from the musculocutaneous perforators, a fact that has gained great clinical importance in the last decade. These musculocutaneous vessels are arranged perpendicularly and supply a limited territory of overlying skin. This is in contrast to the direct cutaneous vessels that run parallel to the skin at a limited number of anatomical sites. Thus, one method of classification of skin flaps is logically based on their vascular anatomy.

RANDOM PATTERN (CUTANEOUS) FLAP

The random pattern flap has no specific arterial-venous system (2). This flap has significant limitations that were determined previously by length/width ratios. However, experimental work has shown that it is the blood supply of the flap, and not the width of it, that determines the length that the surviving piece can be (1, 3). The concept of the musculocutaneous perforator not only allowed for development of the musculocutaneous flap, but it also provided an understanding of the blood supply to the skin of the random pattern flap. Perfusion by musculocutaneous perforators in the base of the flap provides perfusion of the dermal-subdermal plexus of the flap (Fig. 5.2).

FIGURE 5.1. A simplified representation of skin blood supply with both random and axial pattern distributions is shown.

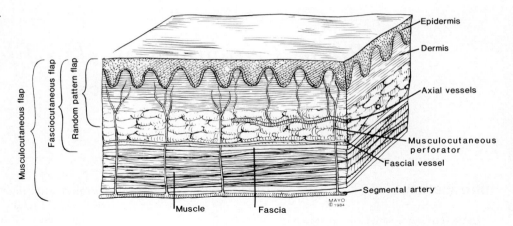

AXIAL PATTERN (ARTERIAL) FLAP

The axial pattern flap is a skin flap with a defined anatomical arterial-venous system (2). It includes a specific direct cutaneous artery in its longitudinal axis (1). This vessel runs superficial to the muscle within the subcutaneous tissue (Fig. 5.3). The axial pattern flap may be raised to at least the length of the arterial-venous system that runs within it and can be even longer (2). This is because a portion of the flap distal to the vessels survives as random skin. The axial pattern flap includes the underlying subcutaneous tissue that contains the direct cutaneous vessel, and there is significant variation of flap thickness depending upon the amount of surface fat of the individual. An axial pattern flap in which the skin bridge base has been divided and is only attached by its vascular pedicle is referred to as an "island flap" (Fig. 5.4). The axial pattern island flap has evolved into the model for potential free tissue transfer by microvascular techniques (4).

Two of the early axial pattern flaps used clinically were the deltopectoral flap popularized by Bakamjian and the groin flap described by McGregor and Jackson (5). However, there are many axial pattern flaps that have been described and used clinically (Table 5.1).

Skin Flap Classification According to Mobilization

A simple classification of skin flaps into local or distant has been developed and is well known (6).

LOCAL FLAPS

Local flaps can be divided into two groups: those that rotate about a point to reach the defect, and those that advance into the defect.

Flaps That Move Around a Fixed Point

Rotation Flap

The movement is in an arc around a fixed point and primarily in one plane. This is a semicircular flap (Fig. 5.5).

Transposition Flap

This rectangular flap rotates on a pivot point. The more it is rotated, the shorter the flap effectively becomes (Fig.

FIGURE 5.2. A random pattern (cutaneous) flap is shown. The intact musculocutaneous perforators in the base of the flap perfuse the dermal-subdermal plexus of the elevated portion of the flap.

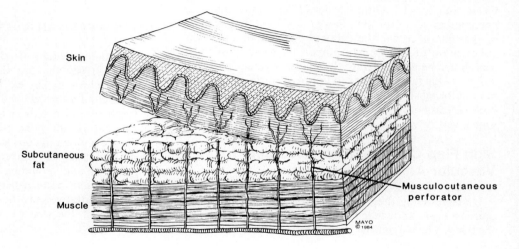

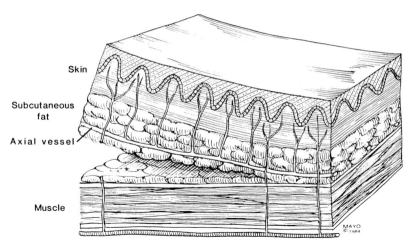

FIGURE 5.3. An axial pattern (arterial) flap is shown. The axial vessel is elevated with the flap. As depicted, there may be an overlap between territories of direct cutaneous vessels and musculocutaneous perforators.

Skin

Subcutaneous fat

Axial vessel

Muscle

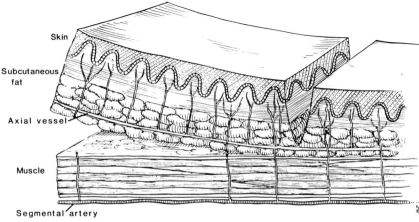

FIGURE 5.4. An island flap is shown. The axial vessel is elevated with the flap, and the skin bridge at the base is divided, isolating the flap only on its vascular pedicle.

Skin

Subcutaneous fat

Axial vessel

Muscle

Segmental artery

FIGURE 5.5. A rotation flap is shown. Movement is in an arc around a fixed point.

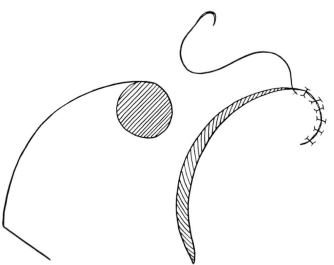

Table 5.1.
Axial Pattern Flaps

Flap	Blood Supply
Median forehead	Supratrochlear vessels
Nasolabial	External nasal angular vessels
Deltopectoral	Internal mammary perforators
Groin	Superficial circumflex iliac artery
Dorsalis pedis	Dorsalis pedis artery

5.6). An example of the transposition flap is the rhomboid (Limberg) flap (Fig. 5.7).

Interpolated Flap

The donor site is separated from the recipient site, and the pedicle of the flap must pass over or under the tissue to reach the recipient area (Fig. 5.8). An example is a nasolabial flap for reconstruction of the nose.

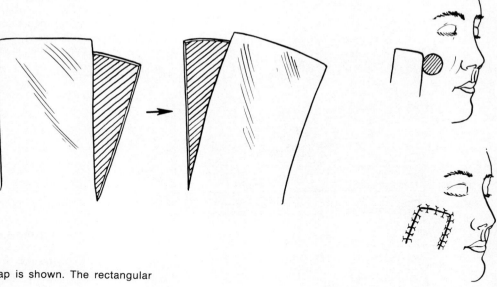

FIGURE 5.6. A transposition flap is shown. The rectangular flap is rotated on a pivot point.

Advancement Flaps

The primary motion is in a straight line from donor site to recipient site without rotation or lateral movement. Advancement flaps include the following.

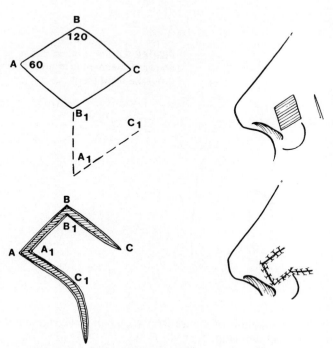

FIGURE 5.7. A Limberg's flap (rhomboid flap) is shown. This is used for closure of rhomboid defects with angles at 60° and 120° and sides of equal length. The short diagonal of the rhomboid is extended equal to its own length (B_1 to A_1) and then back-cut at 60° (A_1 to C_1). The base of the flap is parallel to the lines of maximal extensibility, and the secondary effect is closed by a shift of tissue.

Single-Pedicle Advancement Flap

A rectangle of skin is moved forward primarily on the basis of the elastic properties of skin (Fig. 5.9).

Bipedicle Advancement Flap

An incision is made parallel to the defect and the flap is undermined and advanced. Often, this type of advancement requires skin grafting to close the donor site (Fig. 5.10).

V-Y Advancement Flap

A V-shaped incision in the skin is closed by advancing the sides of the "V" and closing it in the shape of a "Y" (Fig. 5.11). This technique is commonly used to repair defects resulting from fingertip injuries.

DISTANT FLAPS

As with local flaps, distant flaps can be based on blood supply of either a random or an axial pattern. Distant flaps are those that are separated from the defect. They can be based on a pedicle and transferred directly to the defect, such as a groin flap used to cover a defect of the hand (Fig. 5.12) or the deltopectoral flap for head and neck reconstruction. The method of microvascular free tissue transfer has essentially replaced the indirect flap transfer today.

Delay Phenomenon

"Delay" is defined as a method of augmenting the surviving length of a flap (7). With the development of axial

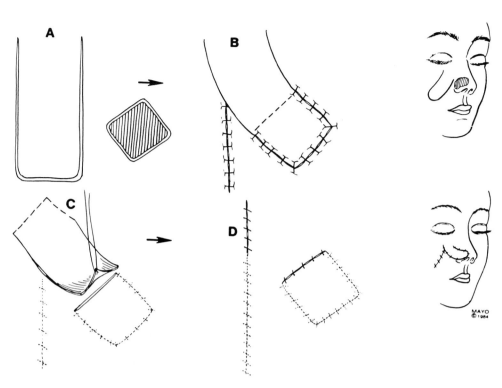

FIGURE 5.8. An interpolated flap is shown. **A,** The flap is outlined and elevated. **B,** The donor site is closed, and flap is inset into the defect. **C,** Once the flap is revascularized, its pedicle is divided. **D,** Insetting is completed.

pattern, musculocutaneous, fasciocutaneous, and microvascular free flaps in recent years, the importance of the delay phenomenon has been dramatically reduced. Although there is less clinical dependence on the delay phenomenon now, it remains an important topic relating to the mechanisms of tissue perfusion and viability.

MECHANISM

It has long been known that, if a skin flap is raised in several stages, a greater length will survive than if the flap is transferred in a single stage. It has been thought that partial interruption of the blood supply to a skin flap be-

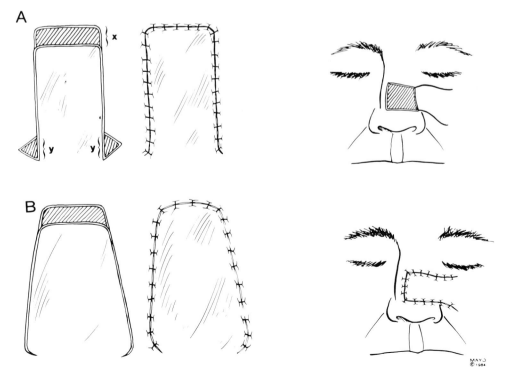

FIGURE 5.9. An advancement flap is shown. **A,** In the advancement flap, triangles (y) (Burrow's triangle) of skin have been removed lateral to the base equal to the distance of the advancement ($x = y$). **B,** Incisions are made into the base of flap to assist in advancement.

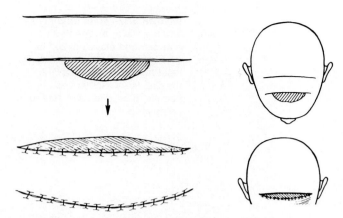

FIGURE 5.10. A bipedicle advancement flap is shown with incisions parallel to the defect.

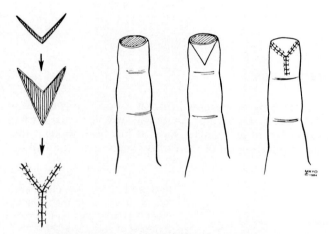

FIGURE 5.11. A V-Y advancement flap is shown.

fore its complete elevation and transfer either enhances its blood supply or increases its tolerance to ischemia. Although there has been considerable clinical success with its application, confusion remains as to the exact mechanism of the delay phenomenon.

Because of its importance in reconstructive surgery, the delay phenomenon has attracted a great deal of research. The findings have been contradictory or nonreproducible, and this has further confused the issue. Early work in this field attributed the benefits seen in delay to increased vessel size, reorientation of vessels along the axis of the flap, increased vessel number, and improved blood flow (8, 9). Other research has shown only a temporary increase in number of vessels during delay (10). It has also been stated that delay conditions the flap to survive in a state of relative hypoxia (10). This is in contrast to the concept that delay works by improving vascularity in the flap (11).

Ischemia appears to be an important factor in the delay phenomenon (12). It has been shown that increased pCO_2 levels are associated with increased flap survival. The assumption is that an increased pCO_2 reflects greater ischemia. Ischemia also appears to be an important factor in skin flap revascularization.

Another important concept with conflicting experimental results is that of arteriovenous shunting. In one series of experiments, blood flow was demonstrated in areas of skin flaps destined to become necrotic (13). In this work, angiography showed filling of blood vessels in areas that did not fluoresce after injection of fluorescein dye into the vascular system. The assumption made was that, because of open arteriovenous shunts, nutrient blood flow did not reach the distal skin even though the area was perfused. On the basis of this model, the delay phenomenon was attributed to fewer patent arteriovenous shunts after delay, compared to acutely elevated flaps.

Further research in the area of arteriovenous shunting and the delay phenomenon has given varying results (14). Although further investigations have questioned the validity of the arteriovenous shunt concept as a major factor

FIGURE 5.12. A groin flap can be used as a distant pedicle flap to cover the defects of the hand. The pedicle is divided after adequate revascularization by the recipient bed of the hand.

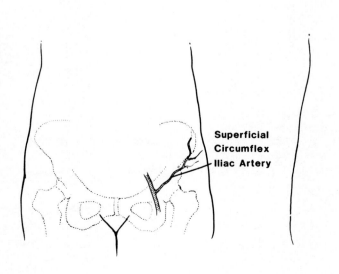

Superficial Circumflex Iliac Artery

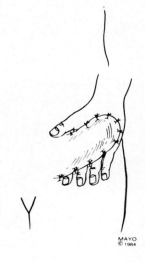

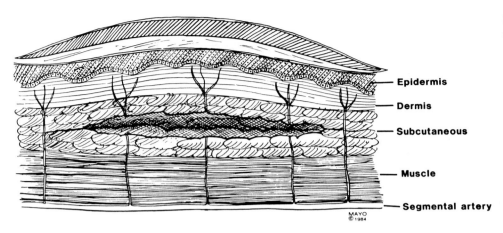

in the delay phenomenon and in the pathogenesis of skin flap failure, there is some evidence that arteriovenous shunting does occur at least in the proximal portion of the flap (15). Whether the delay phenomenon is due to a decrease in arteriovenous shunting, the stimulus of hypoxia, or reorientation of blood supply, delay does increase blood flow to skin flaps (16).

It is known that arteriovenous shunts are under sympathetic control, and there is the possibility of closing these shunts to enhance nutrient blood flow to the distal flap by appropriate pharmacological agents (13). Whatever the mechanism of the delay phenomenon, if one were able to mimic it pharmacologically, multiple surgical steps might be avoided. Arteriovenous shunting is discussed further in the sections on Pathogenesis of Skin Flap Failure and Improving Skin Flap Survival.

TIMING OF DELAY

Data concerning the timing of delay procedures are inconsistent. Recommendations varying from 10 days to 3–4 weeks (17, 18). Experimental data indicate that the increase in blood flow reaches a maximum as early as 1 week after the delay procedure (19).

SURGICAL TECHNIQUE

The method of generating a surgical delay varies with the blood supply of the skin to be elevated. In those areas

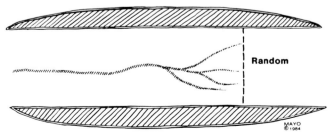

FIGURE 5.14. Surgical delay of an axial pattern flap requires division of the skin parallel to and beyond the direct cutaneous vasculature. Undermining may be less important in this setting.

with significant musculocutaneous perforators, just cutting the skin on each side of a potential flap will accomplish little. In such an area, it is necessary to undermine the flap in order to decrease blood flow significantly and to initiate the delay phenomenon (Fig. 5.13). Where there are direct cutaneous vessels or there are few deep perforators, undermining may not be critical because blood flow is primarily in an axial pattern and dividing the skin parallel to the blood supply may be adequate (Fig. 5.14). Thus, the type of flap and its relationship to perforating or axial vessels must be taken into consideration when performing a delay procedure.

Pathogenesis of Skin Flap Failure

In spite of improved understanding of skin blood supply and advances in reconstructive techniques, skin flap failure is still a significant problem. Potential factors contributing to unsuccessful outcomes are both intrinsic and extrinsic (15). Extrinsic factors, more obvious and potentially controllable, include wound infection, systemic hypotension, and compression or tension of the flap. With appropriate intervention, these factors may be altered, thereby decreasing flap necrosis.

However, the major cause of skin flap failure, and the most difficult to manipulate, is inadequate blood supply (15, 20), an intrinsic factor.

Initially, it was thought that flap necrosis was primarily due to poor venous drainage. It was also thought that the length/width ratio was the critical factor in flap survival. This clinical rule was adhered to until research proved otherwise: in animal models, similar flaps of different widths survived essentially to the same lengths (1, 3). If a large artery and a large vein run through a flap, *the surviving length of the flap* is limited only by the length of the axial blood supply (3). Thus, current evidence points primarily to insufficient arterial inflow as the primary cause of skin flap failure (15).

Because it is believed that flap necrosis is secondary to arterial insufficiency, any arteriovenous shunting that occurs within a flap is likely to impede perfusion and contribute to necrosis (21). A marked increase in erythrocyte volume in the distal region of pedicle flaps has been found and suggests that, due to open vascular shunts, the blood has bypassed the nutrient vessels of the skin (22). Other work that has shown increased hematocrit values in the poorly supplied distal areas of skin flaps has been interpreted as demonstrating a stasis phenomenon in ischemic tissue, not arteriovenous shunting (23). It is safe to say that arteriovenous shunting plays some role in skin flap necrosis but arterial insufficiency is the primary intrinsic cause.

One of the extrinsic factors associated with skin flap necrosis is hematoma. The pressure of an underlying hematoma has been thought to compromise the dermal-subdermal circulation and thus lead to necrosis. Although pressure from an extensive hematoma may be a factor, it appears that a direct toxic effect within the blood contributes to skin flap necrosis (24). This toxic effect is not related to bacterial contamination, and if the hematoma is removed within 24 hours, the flap can be salvaged. Also, a delay procedure protected these experimental flaps from hematoma-associated necrosis. Further studies have demonstrated a substance in whole blood that acts on vascular smooth muscle to influence blood flow to skin (25). The hematoma itself is not toxic to cells of the skin, but some substance in it causes vasoconstriction of the microcirculation (25).

Tension has also been implicated in skin flap necrosis. However, skin with a good blood supply can withstand high tension without necrosis (20). Tension is more likely to contribute to necrosis in flaps with a marginal blood supply. Other factors such as gravity, edema, abnormal clotting, and vascular spasm probably play minor, if any, roles in skin flap necrosis (20).

Another potentially significant external factor in the pathogenesis of skin flap necrosis is cigarette smoking because it may act on blood supply. Tobacco smoke contains numerous constituents, including nicotine, particulate matter, and gaseous components such as carbon monoxide, carbon dioxide, and nitrous oxide (26). It has been known for many years that cigarette smoking causes diminished blood flow (27), and this effect on the circulation has been attributed primarily to the effects of nicotine directly on the vasculature (28, 29). It may also be due to stimulation of the sympathetic ganglia and the adrenal medulla (30) by nicotine causing increased levels of circulating epinephrine and norepinephrine (31).

The carbon monoxide in cigarette smoke (3–6% of the smoke) is bound by hemoglobin to produce carboxyhemoglobin, which can limit the oxygen-carrying capacity of blood (32). Increased carboxyhemoglobin concentration and smoking are also associated with endothelial changes in the vasculature (33) and increased platelet adhesiveness (34, 35).

The acute effects of smoking on the cutaneous microcirculation in elevated skin flaps have been investigated experimentally (26). Blood vessel diameter and erythrocyte velocity during smoking were studied, and both decreased. These effects of cigarette smoking disappeared in 10 min after cessation of smoking. Although there is evidence that smoking decreases blood flow, the important question is whether or not it also decreases skin flap survival. Experiments using nicotine revealed no effect on skin flap survival (36), but others using cigarette smoke have shown a significant decrease in survival of skin flaps (32, 37). Based on the available data, it is not unreasonable to implicate cigarette smoking in skin flap failure.

Revascularization of Skin Flaps

There are three important questions concerning the revascularization of flaps: (*a*) When is the flap adequately vascularized from its recipient bed to tolerate division of its base or pedicle? (*b*) Where in the recipient bed does the revascularization originate? (*c*) What is the stimulus that initiates this revascularization? Each of these factors is important in planning the division of a pedicle skin flap.

RATE OF REVASCULARIZATION

What is the rate at which revascularization occurs and becomes adequate to sustain a flap independent of its original blood supply? Experimental data do not always correlate with clinical experience. Surgeons traditionally wait 2–3 weeks before dividing the pedicle, but much of the experimental data indicates that adequate revascularization occurs sooner. There is also considerable variation among the experimental results, with revascularization to sustain skin flaps in various animal models varying 5–10 days (22, 38).

Data from experimental work on free flaps give useful information relating to pedicle skin flaps. In these models, revascularization adequate to sustain the tissue occurred in 5–6 days (39, 40). This research in animals such as pigs, rats, and rabbits may not correlate with the human clinical situation, especially that in smaller animals, in which revascularization occurs in just a few days.

Recent clinical experience with free tissue transfers has given further insight into the rate of revascularization. Several clinical cases have been reported in which microvascular free skin flaps lost their vascular pedicle within days of transfer, with varying degrees of survival. In one case, a free deltopectoral flap lost its vascular pedicle at 14 days and 75% of the flap survived (41). In another report, loss of the pedicle at 10 days resulted in 30% survival of the flap (39). Based on clinical judgment, most surgeons wait at least 2–3 weeks before dividing the pedicle of a skin flap.

SOURCE OF REVASCULARIZATION

Animal research has evaluated the relative contributions of the wound edges and the wound bed in the revascularization process (38). It appears that both are important. Because of the source of the blood supply, an axial pattern flap may have a different route of revascularization than a random pattern flap. The quality of the recipient bed is also important in flap revascularization. Irradiated or scarred recipient areas are likely to contribute less to revascularization compared to a healthy bed.

STIMULUS OF REVASCULARIZATION

It appears that ischemia is the critical factor in initiating this process (42). It has been shown experimentally that revascularization of skin flaps occurs first in the region of slowest isotope clearance, suggesting that the stimulus for revascularization is greater in the more hypoxic, distal area of the flap (22). An initial increase in uptake of intravenously injected dye has also been demonstrated in the relatively ischemic distal portion of the pedicle flap until 7–10 days. Then the entire flap stains with dye. Revascularization between the flap and its recipient bed begins in 3 or 4 days after the operation, and it begins at the most hypoxic distal portion of the flap. Other research has shown that ischemia results in an increase in both size and density of the vessels associated with skin flap revascularization (43).

BENEFITS OF STAGED DIVISION OF PEDICLE FLAP

There is microangiographical evidence that, when the flap pedicle is divided in stages, there is an increase in the number and size of vessels compared to cases in which flaps are divided acutely (43). Once the pedicle of a flap is divided, the flap is completely dependent on the recipient bed for its blood supply; thus, the purpose of staged division of the pedicle is increased flap survival, which has been confirmed both clinically and experimentally. In addition to making the division safer, staged division of the pedicle may allow division to be done earlier by causing a relative ischemia and stimulating the revascularization process. However, it is possible that the well-vascularized flap in an ischemic bed may undergo less revascularization because of the lack of stimulation for vessel growth (44).

Improving Skin Flap Survival

The volume of research in skin flap survival is impressive, but many of the results have been inconsistent, nonreproducible, or poorly documented. Recent work looking at the McFarlane dorsal rat flap model may explain the contradictory results of many flap physiology studies (44). It appears that a significant portion of the McFarlane dorsal rat flap survives independent of nutrient blood flow and behaves as a full-thickness skin graft (45). There is little direct evidence that any of the agents tried has actually improved survival of a flap in which there was a compromised circulation (46). Due to the lack of clinical application of experimental flap research, there is limited justification for the use of any of these agents in the clinical setting. With improvements in flap design and the current understanding of blood supply, techniques designed to salvage the failing flap may have less clinical significance. Once skin necrosis develops in a flap, there is little control over the final outcome.

Work in this field has taken two basic directions. There have been attempts to improve the blood flow to the flap or attempts to improve the flap's ability to tolerate ischemic insult (47). There are also noxious substances that may have a negative influence on skin flap survival, and these factors need to be identified.

IMPROVING SKIN FLAP BLOOD FLOW PHARMACOLOGICALLY

Agents to improve skin flap blood flow generally have a complex mode of action, and it is difficult to isolate their effects. Results have been inconsistent from one species to another with the same drug, and extrapolating pharmacological effects from animal to man is even more difficult. Further, some of the theories on which drug use is based may be incorrect. Therefore, the agents used may not be logical choices if the thesis of flap failure is incorrect.

Sympatholytic agents such as phenoxybenzamine, reserpine, 6-hydroxydopa, propranolol, and guanethidine have been tried with varying degrees of success, failure, and inconsistency. The results of studies using these agents have been reviewed elsewhere (47), and the success of these drugs depends on the accuracy of the theories of flap necrosis. If arteriovenous shuntings plays a major role in skin flap necrosis, then an agent that can close these channels should result in improved nutrient circulation (13). However, if one assumes that arterial insufficiency alone is the problem and that arteriovenous shunting plays little role, then an alpha-adrenergic receptor blocking agent is needed to cause increased blood flow (47).

Other attempts at improving blood flow to skin flaps have been directed toward inducing vasodilation. Isoxsuprine has received particular attention; some reports show increased skin flap survival, and others do not (25, 47–52). One problem with drug treatment research is that animals have a panniculus carnosus. In animals such as the rat, the panniculus is an integral part of the skin's blood supply, and what is thought to be a skin flap may be a musculocutaneous flap. In the pig, the skin is not as dependent on the blood supply of the panniculus (1). Pigs pretreated with isoxsuprine had improved muscle flap survival but no improvement in skin flap survival (51). That isoxsuprine has a greater effect on skeletal muscle blood supply than on the blood supply of skin is the most likely explanation of this finding (51). Other work has shown increased skin flap survival in the rat with hematoma-induced necrosis when treated with isoxsuprine (25); however, the flap was most likely musculocutaneous, and the isoxsuprine may have been working primarily on the underlying muscle and indirectly affecting the overlying skin.

Other agents that appear to act as vasodilators include histamine, hydralazine, and prostaglandin inhibitors (47). Skin can produce prostaglandins, which can cause vasoconstriction, and during skin flap elevation, the prostaglandins may be released. Thus, treatment with prostaglandin inhibitors might increase flap survival (52). However, because of conflicting data, it is not certain if vasodilators truly contribute to skin flap survival.

CHANGING THE RHEOLOGICAL PROPERTIES OF BLOOD

Another approach to improving skin flap blood flow is based on the flow mechanics of liquids—attempts have been made to alter characteristics of blood components or solution viscosity. Chemical agents have been added to the blood, or the concentration of one or more components has been decreased. Drugs used both experimentally and clinically include pentoxifylline, heparin, and dextran. Pentoxifylline has several modes of action, including altering deformability of erythrocytes, decreasing platelet aggregation, and lowering blood viscosity (53). It is believed that its main value in increasing flap survival is its ability to increase erythrocyte deformability and flexibility (53). Although it was shown experimentally to increase flap survival, its success in clinical application is less certain. Heparin has been shown to increase flap survival experimentally (54). Results with low-molecular-weight dextran have been less favorable (55).

Changing the viscosity of blood consists of protein depletion, lowering hematocrit levels, and perfusion with solutions of varying viscosities. Although anemia potentially decreases the amount of oxygen carried to the tissues, there is experimental evidence that the associated decreased viscosity improves skin flap survival (56). In a similar fashion, protein depletion lowers serum viscosity and enhances experimental skin flap survival (57). As with other approaches to increased flap survival, results are variable, and it is unlikely that making patients anemic or hypoproteinemic will have clinical acceptance.

ENHANCING TOLERANCE TO ISCHEMIA

Methods to improve the flap's ability to tolerate ischemic insult have included hyperbaric oxygen, hypothermia, moist environment, and systemic corticosteroid therapy. Another approach is using drugs that alter cellular metabolism and protect against ischemia (58). This last approach originates from research in organ storage and preservation and may hold some promise. Hyperbaric oxygen (59), hypothermia (60), and moist dressings (61, 62) have all produced improved survival of experimental skin flaps. Systemic administration of steroids has been shown to increase the survival of skin flaps in animals (58, 63). Steroids are known to stabilize cell membranes, cause vasodilation with presumed improved oxygen consumption, and have complex action of enzyme biosynthesis. The specific mode of action of steroids on the microcirculation is unknown.

MONITORING SKIN FLAP VIABILITY

Skin flap failure is a significant clinical problem, and objective methods of assessing flap viability would be useful. Pedicle skin flaps traditionally have problems in their distal portion. In order to salvage this portion of the flap, one must either quickly change external factors such as kinking or hematoma or institute early pharmacological treatment to be effective. With greater accuracy in predicting the survival length of flaps, complications could be reduced. Subjective methods such as assessment of flap viability by color, capillary refill, and dermal bleeding require significant clinical experience. Variables such as oxygen content of blood, dilation of the capillaries, blood flow, and skin pigmentation can affect these subjective evaluations (23).

At present, in addition to clinical assessment, fluorescein dye is commonly used to assess viability. As traditionally used, this method gives only intermittent data within a period of time and is subject to error, depending on the impressions of the observer.

The ideal test of skin flap viability should be safe for both the patient and the flap. It should be an accurate, reliable method that provides results rapidly and can be repeated (64). Methods for assessing blood flow and viability in skin flaps can be divided into four categories—clinical tests, chemical tests, radioisotope methods, and instrument-based methods (65).

Of the chemical tests, intravenous injection of the vital dye fluorescein is the most commonly used. Fluorescein diffuses out of the capillaries and into the interstitial fluid, producing a yellow-green color in the skin exposed to ultraviolet light (66). It is important to remember that one is observing extracellular fluorescein, and this is not a reflection of the blood flow. Fluorescein is considered a safe substance, and complications have been infrequent, considering its widespread use. The problems most often consist of vomiting and nausea, although pruritus and urticaria have been reported (67). Close monitoring of patients during bolus administrations of fluorescein has shown a significant incidence of hypotension (68). Whether this is a vasovagal reaction, a direct vasospastic effect of the dye, or an anaphylactoid reaction is unknown. Although there is a component of subjective clinical judgment in the traditional use of fluorescein, it appears to be a relatively reliable reflection of the limits of the functional microcirculation (66).

An attempt has been made to reduce the subjective component of the fluorescein method by using fiberoptic dermofluorometry (69). This technique allows for more frequent examinations with smaller volumes of fluorescein. It may provide objective data by which tissue fluorescence can be quantified.

Radioisotopes can give a measurement of blood flow limited to a particular point in time. Although this technique is useful experimentally, it does not meet the need for continuous efficient monitoring in a clinical case.

The possibilities of monitoring skin flap viability with sophisticated instrumentation have been based on temperature, transcutaneous gas (pO_2 or pCO_2), tissue pH, photoplethysmography, Doppler shift flow metering, electromagnetic flow metering, and interstitial fluid pressure measurements (23, 65, 69–71). Results with these techniques have been variable. At present, clinical assessment and intravenous fluorescein dye are the most commonly used methods of assessing skin flap viability.

References

1. Daniel RK, Williams HB: The free transfer of skin flaps by microvascular anastomoses: An experimental study and reappraisal. *Plast Reconstr Surg* 52:16, 1973.
2. McGregor IA, Morgan G: Axial and random pattern flaps. *Br J Plast Surg* 26:202, 1973.
3. Milton SH: Pedicled skin-flaps: The fallacy of the length : width ratio. *Br J Surg* 57:502, 1970.
4. Daniel RK, Taylor GI: Distant transfer of an island flap by microvascular anastomoses. *Plast Reconstr Surg* 52:111, 1973.
5. Jackson IT: Flaps design and management. In Calnan J (ed): *Recent Advances in Plastic Surgery.* NewYork, Churchill-Livingstone, 1976, pp 153–172.
6. Grabb WC: Classification of skin flaps. In Myers MB, Grabb WC (eds): *Skin Flaps.* Boston, Little, Brown & Co, 1975, pp 145–154.
7. Blair VP: *Surgery and Diseases of the Mouth and Jaws: A Practical Treatise on the Surgery and Diseases of the Mouth and Allied Structures.* St. Louis, CV Mosby Co, 1912.
8. German W, Finesilver EM, Davis JS: Establishment of circulation in tubed skin flaps: An experimental study. *Arch Surg* 26:27, 1933.
9. Bardach J, Kurnatowski A: Blood supply of a Filatov's skin flap. *Acta Chir Plast* 3:290, 1961.
10. McFarlane RM, Heagy FC, Radin S, et al: A study of the delay phenomenon in experimental pedicle flaps. *Plast Reconstr Surg* 35:245, 1965.
11. Myers MB: Attempts to augment survival in skin flaps—mechanism of the delay phenomenon. In Grabb WC, Myers MB (eds): *Skin Flaps.* Boston, Little, Brown & Co, 1975, pp 65–79.
12. Myers MB, Cherry G, Milton S: Tissue gas levels as an index of the adequacy of circulation: The relation between ischemia and the development of collateral circulation (delay phenomenon). *Surgery* 71:15, 1972.
13. Reinisch JF: The pathophysiology of skin flap circulation (the delay phenomena). *Plast Reconstr Surg* 54:585, 1974.
14. Prather A, Blackburn JP, Williams TR, et al: Evaluation of tests for predicting the viability of axial pattern skin flaps in the pig. *Plast Reconstr Surg* 63:250, 1979.
15. Kerrigan CL: Skin flap failure: Pathophysiology. *Plast Reconstr Surg* 72:766, 1983.
16. Guba AM: Study of the delay phenomenon in axial pattern flaps in pigs. *Plast Reconstr Surg* 63:550, 1979.
17. Gillies HD, Millard DR: *The Principles and Art of Plastic Surgery.* Boston, Little, Brown & Co, 1957.
18. Myers MB, Cherry G: Differences in the delay phenomenon in the rabbit, rat and pig. *Plast Reconstr Surg* 47:73, 1971.
19. Guba AM, Callahan J: Nutrient blood flow in delayed axial pattern skin flaps in the pig. *Plast Reconstr Surg* 64:372, 1979.
20. Myers MB: Investigations of skin flap necrosis. In Grabb WC, Myers MB (eds): *Skin Flaps.* Boston, Little, Brown & Co, 1975, pp 3–10.
21. Reinisch JF: Discussion. *Plast Reconstr Surg* 72:775, 1983.
22. Young CMA: The revascularization of pedicle skin flaps in pigs. A functional and morphologic study. *Plast Reconstr Surg* 70:445, 1982.
23. Kerrigan CL, Daniel RK: Monitoring acute skin-flap failure. *Plast Reconstr Surg* 71:519, 1983.
24. Mulliken JB, Healey NA: Pathogenesis of skin flap necrosis from an underlying hematoma. *Plast Reconstr Surg* 63:540, 1979.
25. Hillelson RL, Glowacki J, Healey NA, et al: A microangiographic study of hematoma-associated flap necrosis and salvage with isoxsuprine. *Plast Reconstr Surg* 66:528, 1980.
26. Reus WF, Robson MC, Zachary L, et al: Acute effects of tobacco smoking on blood flow in the cutaneous micro-circulation. *Br J Plast Surg* 37:213, 1984.
27. Franke FE, Hertzman AB: Effects of cigarette smoking on the skin circulation (abstract). *Am J Physiol* 129:357, 1940.
28. Sarin CL, Austin JC, Nickel WO: Effects of smoking on digital blood-flow velocity. *JAMA* 229:1327, 1974.
29. Roth GM, McDonald JB, Sheard C: The effect of smoking cigarettes and of intravenous administration of nicotine on the electrocardiogram, basal metabolic rate, cutaneous temperature, blood pressure and pulse rate of normal persons. *JAMA* 125:761, 1944.
30. Gebber GL: Neurogenic basis for the rise in blood pressure evoked by nicotine in the cat. *J Pharmacol Exp Ther* 166:255, 1969.
31. Cryer PE, Haymond MW, Santiago JV, et al: Norepinephrine and epinephrine release and adrenergic mediation of smoking-associated hemodynamic and metabolic events. *N Engl J Med* 295:573, 1976.
32. Lawrence WT, Murphy RC, Robson MC, et al: The detrimental effect of cigarette smoking on flap survival: An experimental study in the rat. *Br J Plast Surg* 37:216, 1984.
33. Astrup P, Kjeldsen K: Carbon monoxide, smoking, and atherosclerosis. *Med Clin North Am* 58:323, 1974.
34. Birnstingl MA, Brinson K, Chakrabarti BK: The effect of short-term exposure of carbon monoxide on platelet stickiness. *Br J Surg* 58:837, 1971.
35. Davis JW, Davis RF: Acute effect of tobacco cigarette smoking on the platelet aggregate ratio. *Am J Med Sci* 278:139, 1979.
36. Falcone RE, Ruberg RL: Pharmacologic manipulation of skin flaps: Lack of effect of barbiturates or nicotine. *Plast Reconstr Surg* 66:102, 1980.
37. Schultz RC, Nolan JT, Jenkins R, et al: Acute effects of cigarette smoke exposure on experimental skin flaps. Presented at the meeting of the American Association of Plastic Surgeons, Chicago, IL, May 6–9, 1984.
38. Tsur H, Daniller A, Strauch B: Neovascularization of skin flaps: Route and timing. *Plast Reconstr Surg* 66:85, 1980.
39. Serafin D, Shearin JC, Georgiade NG: The vascularization of free flaps: A clinical and experimental correlation. *Plast Reconstr Surg* 60:233, 1977.
40. Strauch B, Sharzer L, Glaser B, et al: Neovascularization: What is the relationship between contact surface area and volume of tissue? *Plast Surg Forum* 2:225, 1979.
41. Gilbert A, Beres J: Une complication inhabituelle d'un lambeau libre. *Ann Chir Plast Esthet* 21:151, 1976.
42. Myers MB, Cherry G: Blood supply of healing wounds: Functional and angiographic. *Arch Surg* 102:49, 1971.
43. Cohen BE: Beneficial effect of staged division of pedicle in experimental axial-pattern flaps. *Plast Reconstr Surg* 64:366, 1979.
44. Fisher J, Wood MB: Late necrosis of a latissimus dorsi free flap. *Plast Reconstr Surg* 74:274, 1984.
45. Hammond DC, Brooksher RD: An isolated dorsal skin flap model in the rat. Department of General Surgery, Blodgett/St. Mary's Hospitals, Grand Rapids, MI (in press).
46. Cherry GW: Discussion. *Plast Reconstr Surg* 70:549, 1982.
47. Kerrigan CL, Daniel RK: Pharmacologic treatment of the failing skin flap. *Plast Reconstr Surg* 70:541, 1982.
48. Kinseth F, Adelberg MG: Prevention of skin flap necrosis by a course of treatment with vasodilator drugs. *Plast Reconstr Surg* 61:738, 1978.
49. Finseth F, Adelberg MG: Experimental work with Isoxsuprine for prevention of skin necrosis and for the treatment of failing flap. *Plast Reconstr Surg* 63:94, 1979.
50. Finseth F: Clinical salvage of three failing skin flaps by treatment with a vasodilator drug. *Plast Reconstr Surg* 63:304, 1979.
51. Cherry GW: The differing effects of Isoxsuprine on muscle flap and skin flap survival in the pig. *Plast Reconstr Surg* 64:670, 1979.
52. Sasaki A, Harii K: Lack of effect of Isoxsuprine on experimental random flaps in the rat. *Plast Reconstr Surg* 66:105, 1980.
53. Takayanagi S, Ogawa Y: Effects of pentoxifylline on flap survival. *Plast Reconstr Surg* 65:763, 1980.
54. Sawhney CP: The role of heparin in restoring the blood supply in ischemic skin flaps: An experimental study in rabbits. *Br J Plast Surg* 33:430, 1980.
55. Myers MB, Cherry G: Design of skin flaps to study vascular insufficiency: Failure of Dextran 40 to improve tissue survival in devascularized skin. *J Surg Res* 7:399, 1967.
56. Earle AS, Fratianne RB, Nunez FD: The relationship of hemat-

ocrit levels of skin flap survival in the dog. *Plast Reconstr Surg* 54:341, 1974.

57. Ruberg RL, Falcone RE: Effect of protein depletion on the surviving length in experimental skin flaps. *Plast Reconstr Surg* 61:581, 1978.

58. Mes LGB: Improving flap survival by sustaining cell metabolism within ischemic cells: A study using rabbits. *Plast Reconstr Surg* 65:56, 1980.

59. Arturson G, Khanna NN: The effects of hyperbaric oxygen dimethyl sulfoxide and complamin on survival of experimental skin flaps. *Scand J Plast Reconstr Surg* 4:8, 1970.

60. Kiehn CL, DesPrez JD: Effects of local hypothermia on pedicle flap tissue. I: Enhancement of survival of experimental pedicles. *Plast Reconstr Surg* 25:349, 1960.

61. Sasaki A, Fukuda O, Soeda S: Attempts to increase the surviving length in skin flaps by moist environment. *Plast Reconstr Surg* 64:526, 1979.

62. McGrath MH: How topical dressings salvage "questionable" flaps: Experimental study. *Plast Reconstr Surg* 67:653, 1981.

63. Mendelson BC, Woods JE: Effect of corticosteroids on the surviving length of skin flaps in pigs. *Br J Plast Surg* 31:293, 1978.

64. Creech BJ, Miller SH: Evaluation of circulation in skin flaps. In Grabb WC, Myers MB (eds): *Skin Flaps*. Boston, Little, Brown & Co, 1975, pp 21–38.

65. Jones BM: Monitors for the cutaneous microcirculation. *Plast Reconstr Surg* 73:843, 1984.

66. McGraw JB, Myers B, Shanklin KD: The value of fluorescein in predicting the viability of arterialized flaps. *Plast Reconstr Surg* 60:710, 1977.

67. Stein MR, Parker CW: Reactions following intravenous fluorescein. *Am J Ophthalmol* 72:861, 1971.

68. Buchanan RT, Levine NS: Blood pressure drop as a result of fluorescein injection. *Plast Reconstr Surg* 70:363, 1982.

69. Silverman DG, LaRossa DD, Barlow CH, et al: Quantification of tissue fluorescein delivery and prediction of flap viability with the fiberoptic dermofluorometer. *Plast Reconstr Surg* 66:545, 1980.

70. Serafin D, Lesesne DB, Mullen RY, Georgiade NG: Transcutaneous pO$_2$ monitoring for assessing viability and predicting survival of skin flaps: Experimental and clinical correlations. *J Microsurg* 2:165, 1981.

71. Fisher JC, Parker PM, Shaw WW: Laser Doppler flowmeter measurements of skin perfusion changes associated with arterial and venous compromise in cutaneous island flaps. Microsurg 6:238, 1985.

6

Muscle and Musculocutaneous Flaps

Stephen J. Mathes, M.D., F.A.C.S. and K. Ning Chang, M.D., F.A.C.S.

Muscle and musculocutaneous flaps are now well established tools for the reconstruction of many complex wounds. These wounds are difficult to manage because of (a) exposed vital structures such as bones, tendons, vessels, and mediastinal wounds; (b) compromised ability to heal because of such factors as prior irradiation; (c) extensive loss of skin, subcutaneous tissue, and mucosal lining; and (d) exposed prosthetic materials and grafts. Examples of these types of wounds include infected median sternotomy wound, lower extremity trauma, head and neck cancer defect, chronic osteomyelitis, and osteoradionecrosis. In fact, muscle and musculocutaneous flaps have been important applications in many surgical specialties, including general surgery, cardiothoracic surgery, orthopaedic surgery, urology, gynecological surgery, and neurosurgery (1–13).

Muscle and musculocutaneous flaps offer several important advantages. The flaps can provide a large amount of skin and bulk. They have constant vascular anatomy that allows safe elevation and prediction of the arc of rotation. The flaps are less susceptible to infection and more likely to achieve wound healing compared to commonly used skin flaps. A large muscle flap can often be transposed while leaving minimal external contour defect.

Vascular Anatomy of Muscles (14–17)

Muscle blood supply is based on one or more vascular pedicles that enter the muscle belly between its origin and insertion. The artery enters the muscle, ramifies, and gives off musculocutaneous perforators to the skin. The musculocutaneous perforators arborize in the dermal-subdermal plexus and supply the cutaneous territory overlying the muscle (Fig. 6.1). The dominant pedicle is defined on the basis of (a) anatomical study using angiography technique, and (b) clinical observation of the ability to sustain muscle circulation after surgical manipulation of the muscle for use as a flap. Division of the dominant vascular pedicle of the muscle generally results in avascular necrosis of the muscle. The minor pedicle represents smaller vascular attachments to the muscle. When divided, the muscle circulation is sustained by the larger dominant vascular pedicles.

While there is great variability in the size, shape, and function of muscles in the human body, five patterns of vascular anatomy are recognized in muscles (17; Fig. 6.2).

Muscles of Type I pattern contain a single vascular pedicle. An example is the tensor fascia lata, which is supplied by the transverse branch of the lateral circumflex femoral artery.

The Type II pattern contains both dominant and minor vascular pedicles. The larger dominant vascular pedicle will sustain circulation in the muscle after division of the minor pedicles. This is the most common pattern of circulation observed in human muscle. An example is the gracilis, which is supplied by the medial circumflex femoral artery (the dominant pedicle) and branches from superficial femoral arteries (the minor pedicles).

A Type III pattern has two major pedicles. These pedicles either have separate regional sources of circulation or are located on opposite sides of the muscle. An example is the gluteus maximus, which is supplied by inferior and superior gluteal arteries.

Type IV pattern muscles are supplied by multiple vascular pedicles. Each pedicle provides circulation to a portion of the muscle. Division of more than two or three of these pedicles during elevation results in distal muscle necrosis. The sartorius, for example, receives multiple branches from the superficial femoral artery.

A Type V pattern consists of one major vascular pedicle and several secondary segmental vascular pedicles. Both types of pedicles provide significant sources of circulation to the muscles. A selected list of the vascular anatomy of the more commonly used muscles is provided in Table 6.1.

Arc of Rotation

The extent of elevation of the muscle from its normal anatomical position without devascularization and its subsequent ability to reach an adjacent defect determine the arc of rotation. The point of rotation is determined by the site of entrance of the dominant pedicle into the muscle. Only muscles distal to the point of rotation are actually useful as a transposition flap. The points of rotation for muscles of Types I, II, III, and V are located at one end or the proximal one third of the muscle. Muscles of Type IV, with a segmented vascular pattern, have a very limited arc of rotation. Type V muscles have two arcs of rotation. The latissimus dorsi can be elevated around the thoracodorsal artery to cover a large defect in the anterior chest. Posteriorly, it can be elevated and rotated based on paramedian vessels to cover a midline defect (Fig. 6.3A and B).

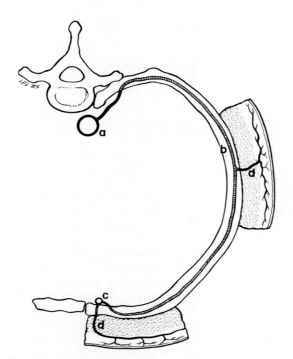

FIGURE 6.1. Cross-section of the body showing (**a**) aorta, (**b**) intercostal artery, (**c**) internal mammary artery, and (**d**) musculocutaneous perforators.

Table 6.1.
Classification of Vascular Anatomy of Muscles

Type I pattern	Gastrocnemius (medial head)
	Gastrocnemius (lateral head)
	Rectus femoris
	Tensor fascia lata
Type II pattern	Biceps femoris
	Gracilis
	Peroneus brevis
	Peroneus longus
	Platysma
	Semimembranosus
	Semitendinosus
	Soleus
	Sternocleidomastoid
	Trapezius
	Vastus lateralis
	Vastus medialis
Type III pattern	Gluteus maximus
	Rectus abdominis
	Temporalis
Type IV pattern	Extensor digitorum longus
	Extensor hallucis longus
	Flexor digitorum longus
	Flexor hallucis longus
	Sartorius
	Tibialis anterior
Type V pattern	Latissimus dorsi
	Pectoralis major

In addition to rotational movement, the muscle can be used as a turnover flap. The best example is the reconstruction of a median sternotomy wound using pectoralis major muscle based on musculocutaneous perforators from the internal mammary artery.

Musculocutaneous flaps can also be used as advancement flaps. Examples are V-Y advancement of a gluteus maximus musculocutaneous flap for reconstruction of a sacral defect or V-Y advancement of a hamstring musculocutaneous flap for an ischial defect (18, 19).

Functional Preservation in the Use of Muscle and Musculocutaneous Flaps

If the muscle origin or insertion or the motor nerve is divided during flap elevation, the muscle will no longer serve its original function. This may result in functional disability or alteration of form and contour. Several techniques can be used to minimize the detrimental effects by (*a*) choosing a muscle from a group of synergistic muscles, and (*b*) using only a portion of the muscle as needed. Gracilis, for example, is expendable because the remaining and more powerful adductor muscles will preserve the function. Muscles of the extremities, such as tibialis anterior, flexor digitorum longus, or extensor digitorum longus, have long tendons. For coverage of a small defect, careful dissection of part of the muscle from the tendon allows transposition without disruption of the muscle-tendon unit. In flat, broad muscles of the trunk (e.g., latissimus dorsi, pectoralis major, trapezius), only part of the muscle may have to be transposed, leaving the motor nerve and a major portion of the origin and insertion intact.

Motor Innervation

The motor nerve generally enters the proximal muscle close to the origin. The motor nerve is often closely associated with the dominant vascular pedicle to the muscle. Muscle denervation noted on preoperative evaluation may indicate an associated injury to the vascular pedicle. Location and preservation of the motor nerve are essential in free functional muscle transplantation. Specific effort to divide the motor nerve will not always significantly reduce muscle bulk in the denervated muscle. Required proximal dissection subjects the vascular pedicle to risk of injury.

Specialized Tissue Flaps

MUSCLE AND SKIN GRAFT OR MUSCULOCUTANEOUS FLAP

Superficial muscle may be elevated as a muscle flap and skin grafted or elevated with overlying skin as a musculocutaneous flap. This depends on both the reconstructive need of a particular defect and the aesthetic and functional considerations of each method. In general, the use of muscle flap alone, without the overlying skin island, is

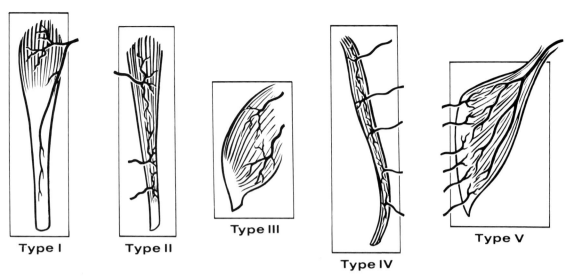

Type I   Type II   Type III   Type IV   Type V

FIGURE 6.2. Patterns of vascular anatomy of muscle are illustrated. See the text for description. (Reproduced with permission from Mathes SJ, Nahai F: Classification of the vascular anatomy of muscles: Experimental and clinical correlation. *Plast Reconstr Surg* 67:177, 1981.)

least likely to cause external contour deformity. The inclusion of skin island in the muscle flap may result in unacceptable donor site deformity in certain parts of the body. In these situations, muscle flap alone is preferred. Certain three-dimensional complex wounds can be filled better by using muscle alone. An example would be osteomyelitis cavities. Epimysium may be incised, and the muscle expanded when there is discrepancy between the flap and the reconstructive defect. Muscle flaps make

excellent recipient sites for skin graft. Skin-grafted muscle flaps can offer durable surfaces, as in reconstruction of plantar surface of the heel when the muscle flap is transferred and skin grafted (20). In some situations, the inclusion of overlying skin is either required or preferable. Examples include a postmastectomy chest wall deformity, pressure sores, and an extirpative defect around the head and neck region in which skin or mucosal replacement is required.

MUSCULOCUTANEOUS PERFORATORS AND MUSCULOCUTANEOUS FLAPS

The vascular supply of the skin comes from direct cutaneous arteries and musculocutaneous perforators (Fig. 6.4). Direct cutaneous vessels predominate in the head region and around the limb girdles, joints, digits, and genitalia. In the rest of the body, significant amounts of cutaneous circulation come from the underlying muscles (Fig. 6.5).

The location and size of the musculocutaneous perforators have been studied both through dye injection study of cadavers and through clinical experiences. Figure 6.6 illustrates the location of the larger musculocutaneous perforators in the anterior truncal region, which reach the skin from pectoralis major and rectus abdominis muscles.

The pattern of the blood supply to the underlying muscle must be taken into account when designing the overlying skin island. In general, the Type I blood supply will support all the overlying skin of the muscle unit. With Type II blood supply, the proximal area of skin or that area over the dominant pedicle is far more reliable than the skin territory over the distal pedicle. With Type III blood supply, each half of the muscle can be elevated separately with overlying skin. Muscles with Type IV blood supply have limited usefulness as musculocutaneous flaps because each of the segmented pedicles car-

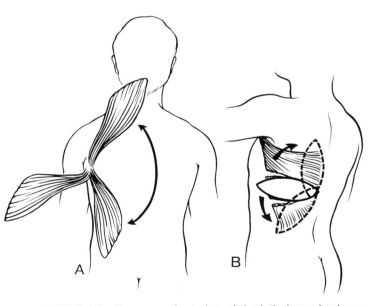

FIGURE 6.3. Two arcs of rotation of the latissimus dorsi are based on (**A**) the thoracodorsal artery, and (**B**) the posterior intercostal perforators. (Reproduced with permission from Mathes SJ, Nahai F: Classification of the vascular anatomy of muscles: Experimental and clinical correlation. *Plast Reconstr Surg* 67:177, 1981.)

FIGURE 6.4. Cross-section of the leg showing skin blood supply from (**A**) direct cutaneous artery, and (**B**) musculocutaneous arteries. Both types of vessels ramify to form (**C**) fascial plexus, which connects with (**D**) dermal-subdermal plexus.

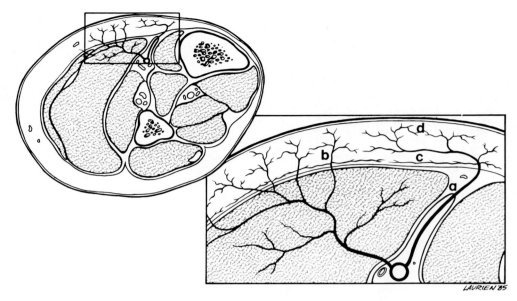

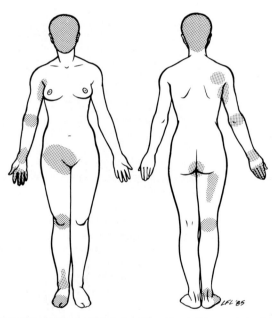

FIGURE 6.5. Blood supply of the skin is illustrated. *Shaded areas* are supplied predominantly through direct cutaneous vessels, and the *unshaded area* is supplied predominantly through musculocutaneous perforators. (From Mathes SJ, Nahai F: *Clinical Applications for Muscle and Musculocutaneous Flaps.* St. Louis, CV Mosby Company, 1982, p 97.)

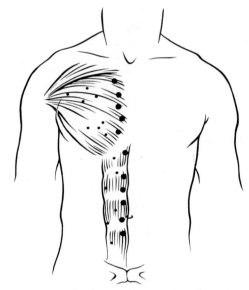

FIGURE 6.6. Musculocutaneous perforators through pectoralis major and rectus abdominis into skin of anterior trunk. The *dots* indicate the location of musculocutaneous perforators. (Modified from Mathes and Nahai [16], p 110.)

ries a segmental area of overlying skin. The Type IV blood supply is quite useful because skin islands can be based on both the major proximal supply or the secondary segmental blood supply to the muscle. In general, musculocutaneous perforators are found between muscle fibers and the overlying skin. There are no perforators between the tendon or fascia and the overlying skin. The tensor fascia lata and gastrocnemius are cases in point; these muscles carry the skin over the fascia lata and

Achilles tendons, respectively, through perforating vessels that enter the skin directly over the muscle fibers and not through the fascia lata or the Achilles tendon. Figure 6.7 illustrates the use of rectus abdominis as a muscle transposition flap for (*a*) an infected median sternotomy wound, and (*b*) for breast reconstruction.

The area of skin island that can be safely elevated beyond the muscle is variable. In addition to the all-important consideration regarding the vascular supply of the muscle, other determining factors include: (*a*) the size of the musculocutaneous perforators; (*b*) the distance they reach beyond the border of the muscle; and (*c*) the axial

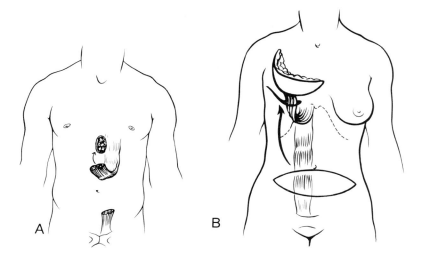

FIGURE 6.7. The use of rectus abdominis muscle as (**A**) a muscle flap, and (**B**) extended skin island musculocutaneous flap. (Modified from Mathes and Nahai [16], p 230.)

orientation of the vessels. In general, the broad, flat truncal muscles with large perforators are able to carry skin island several centimeters beyond the muscle; in breast reconstruction, large amounts of lower abdominal skin are carried by the rectus abdominis muscle. In contrast, skin over the distal aspect of long and narrow muscles such as gracilis can be unreliable. A useful maneuver to ensure maximal circulation to the skin island beyond the muscle is to take the fascia with the skin whenever the fascia is available; the fascia carries a vascular plexus that can augment the circulation to the skin (21, 22).

SPECIALIZED APPLICATION OF MUSCLE FLAP

Restoration of specialized body function can be achieved by the use of muscle flaps. When the muscular motor nerve is coapted to a suitable donor motor nerve at the recipient site during microsurgical transplantation of a muscle flap, the motor function can be restored. Serratus anterior, pectoralis minor, and other muscles have been used for reanimation of the paralyzed face. Gracilis muscles have been transplanted to the forearm to achieve finger flexion in Volkmann's ischemic contracture (23–25). A neurosensory flap can be designed by incorporating a cutaneous sensory nerve into a musculocutaneous flap. Such a flap has been used successfully for replacement of extensive plantar foot and heel defects (26).

Healing and Infection in Flaps

Heavy contamination, the presence of infection, and decreased vascularity are often encountered in a wound to be reconstructed. Successful outcomes often depend on the ability of the flap to bring in adequate blood supply. Musculocutaneous flaps and muscle flaps have been demonstrated to be effective in management of chronic and difficult wounds such as chronic osteomyelitis, osteoradionecrosis, and massive lower extremity injuries. Such clinical observation has been confirmed by animal experiments in which musculocutaneous flaps, random

pattern flaps, and fasciocutaneous flaps were subjected to bacterial inoculation in both the dermal portion and in the wound space underneath the flaps. Intradermal injection of staphylococci resulted in a most extensive degree of skin necrosis in random pattern flaps. The cutaneous portion of the musculocutaneous flap was the least affected. The musculocutaneous flap was most effective in containing bacterial proliferation in the wound space after bacterial inoculation, followed by the fasciocutaneous flap. Introduction of bacteria into the wound space underneath the random pattern flap led to frequent flap necrosis. The greatest amount of collagen was deposited in the wound space in musculocutaneous flaps (27, 28).

Several factors have been demonstrated to account for the difference observed in the various types of flaps, including dermal blood flow, tissue oxygen tension, and blood flow in the muscles. Tissue hypoxia has been shown to significantly impair bacteriocidal capability of leukocytes. It also leads to impaired collagen deposition (29). Successful management of a difficult wound with a flap depends on the proper selection of the flap as well as optimization of tissue oxygen tension and perfusion to the flap.

References

1. Mathes SJ, Feng L-J, Hunt TK: Coverage of the infected wound. *Ann Surg* 198:420, 1983.
2. Nahai F, Rand R, Hester TR, Bostwick J, Jurkiewicz MJ: Primary treatment of the infected sternotomy with muscle flaps: A review of 211 consecutive cases. *Plast Reconstr Surg* 84:434, 1989.
3. Ariyan S: The pectoralis major sternomastoid and other musculocutaneous flaps for head and neck reconstruction. *Clin Plast Surg* 7:89, 1980.
4. Mathes SJ, Alpert B, Chang N: Use of the muscle flap in chronic osteomyelitis: Experimental and clinical correlation. *Plast Reconstr Surg* 89:815, 1982.
5. Byrd HS, Cierny G, Tibbet JB: The management of open tibial fracture with associated soft tissue loss: External pin fixation with early flap coverage. *Plast Reconstr Surg* 68:73, 1981.
6. Godina M: Early microsurgical reconstruction of complex trauma of the extremity. *Plast Reconstr Surg* 78:285, 1986.

7. Lesavoy MA, Dubrow TJ, Wackym PA, Eckardt JJ: Muscle flap coverage of exposed endoprosthesis. *Plast Reconstr Surg* 83:90, 1989.

8. Greenberg B, LaRossa D, Lotke PA, Murphy JB, Noone RB: Salvage of jeopardized total-knee prosthesis: The role of the gastrocnemius muscle flap. *Plast Reconstr Surg* 83:85, 1989.

9. Mixter RC, Turnipseed WD, Smith DJ, Acher CW, Rao VK, Dibbell DG: Rotational muscle flaps: A new technique for covering infected vascular grafts. *J Vasc Surg* 9:472, 1989.

10. Kennedy NM, Breach JH, Shepherd JH, et al: The use of myocutaneous flap following radical excision of the external genitalia. *Br J Urol* 59:272, 1987.

11. McCraw JB, Massey FM, Shanklin KD, Horton CG: Vaginal reconstruction with gracilis myocutaneous flaps. *Plast Reconstr Surg* 58:176, 1976.

12. Tobin GR, Day TG: Vaginal and pelvic reconstruction with distally based rectus abdominis myocutaneous flap. *Plast Reconstr Surg* 81:62, 1988.

13. Ryan JA Jr, Gibbons RP, Correa RJ Jr: Urologic use of gracilis muscle flap for non-healing perineal wounds and fistulae. *Urology* 26:456, 1985.

14. McCraw JB, Dibbell DG, Carraway JH: Clinical definition of independent myocutaneous vascular territories. *Plast Reconstr Surg* 60:341, 1977.

15. Mathes SJ, Nahai F: *Clinical Atlas of Muscle and Musculocutaneous Flaps.* St. Louis, CV Mosby Company, 1979.

16. Mathes SJ, Nahai F: *Clinical Applications for Muscle and Musculocutaneous Flaps.* St. Louis, CV Mosby Company, 1982.

17. Mathes SJ, Nahai F: Classification of the vascular anatomy of muscles: Experimental and clinical correlations. *Plast Reconstr Surg* 67:177, 1981.

18. Fisher J, Arnold PG, Waldorf J, Woods JE: Gluteus maximus musculocutaneous V-Y advancement flap for large sacral defect. *Ann Plast Surg* 11:517, 1983.

19. Hurteau JE, Bostwick J, Nahai F, Hester R, Jurkiewicz MJ: V-Y advancement of hamstring musculocutaneous flap for coverage of ischial pressure sore. *Plast Reconstr Surg* 68:539, 1981.

20. May JW, Halls MJ, Simon SR: Free microvascular muscle flaps with skin graft reconstruction of extensive defects of the foot. *Plast Reconstr Surg* 75:627, 1985.

21. Tolhurst DE, Halseker B, Zeeman RJ: The development of fasciocutaneous flap and its clinical applications. *Plast Reconstr Surg* 7:597, 1983.

22. Carriquiry C, Costa MA, Vasconez LO: Anatomic study of septocutaneous vessels of the leg. *Plast Reconstr Surg* 76:354, 1985.

23. Terzis JK: Pectoralis minor: A unique muscle for correction of facial palsy. *Plast Reconstr Surg* 83:767, 1989.

24. Zuker R: Volkmann's ischemic contracture. *Clin Plast Surg* 16:537, 1989.

25. Zhu SX, Zhang BX, Yao JX, et al: Free musculocutaneous flap transfer of extensor digitorum brevis muscle by microvascular anastomosis for restoration of function of thenar and adductor pollicis muscles. *Ann Plast Surg* 15:481, 1985.

26. Chang KN, DeArmond SJ, Buncke HJ: Sensory reinnervation in microsurgical reconstruction of the heel. *Plast Reconstr Surg* 78:652, 1986.

27. Chang N, Mathes SJ: Comparison of the effect of bacterial inoculation in musculocutaneous and random pattern flaps. *Plast Reconstr Surg* 70:1, 1982.

28. Calderon W, Chang N, Mathes SJ: Comparison of the effect of bacterial inoculation in musculocutaneous and fasciocutaneous flaps. *Plast Reconstr Surg* 77:785, 1986.

29. Hunt TK, Halliday B, et al: Impairment of microbicidal function in wound: Correction with oxygenation. In Hunt TK, Heppenstal RB, Pin E, Rovee D (eds): *Soft and Hard Tissue Repair— Biological and Clinical Aspects.* New York, Praeger Scientific Publishing Company, 1984, p 455–468.

7

Composite Grafts

Ross H. Musgrave, M.D., F.A.C.S. and James A. Lehman, Jr., M.D., F.A.C.S.

The term "composite graft," indicates that the graft is derived from two or more germ layers and contains at least two layers of tissue; i.e., skin and cartilage, mucosa and cartilage, or skin and fat. König (1) is usually credited as the innovator of composite grafts, having described the procedure in 1887. In 1914, he reported a 50% survival rate in a series of 47 cases in which alar defects were repaired with composite grafts from the ear (2). Thereafter, little enthusiasm for such grafts was displayed as a result of the perceived risk of failure. In 1935, Limberg (3) reported 47 cases of free composite grafts with an 87% success rate (only six failed). However, interest was not rekindled until 1946 when Dupertuis (4) reported the successful transfer of 15 composite earlobe grafts in nasal reconstructions. His use of the earlobe as a source of material occurred before his knowledge of previous work in the field. Apparently, Zeno independently described the use of a composite earlobe graft (5) just before Dupertuis.

Since that time, numerous reports of success with composite grafts have been reported in the literature (6–23). A majority of the reports described free composite transplants of skin and fat (and cartilage, occasionally) from the ear to the nasal area. Variants of the composite graft have also been reported. Flanagin (21) described a successful free full-thickness graft, including muscle and mucous membranes, from the lower to the upper lip. In 1912, Joseph (22) reported the repair of a nostril defect with a graft from the opposite alar base. In 1959, Douglas (24) reported 17 successful digital replacements with composite grafts. The free nipple graft in mammaplasty, popularized by Adams (25) and Conway (26), is another variant of the composite graft and includes skin, ducts, erectile tissue, smooth muscle, and some fat. Composite grafts from one eyelid to another, including cartilage and mucous membranes, have been used to advantage (27). Nasal septal cartilage and mucosa have likewise been useful in reconstruction of the lower eyelid (28).

In microtic ears, Brent (29–31), Tanzer (32), Rueckert (33), Converse (34), and Hall and Stevenson (35) have each used segments of the opposite ear, including cartilage and skin, either to add a tragus or to reconstruct a semblance of conchal cupping.

Survival of these relatively massive free grafts suggests that they are actively vascularized within a short time, possibly a few hours, after transplantation. From our clinical experience, it appears that early establishment of circulation in the composite earlobe grafts depends on direct vessel anastomoses between the subdermal plexus of the recipient wound edge and the subdermal plexus of the graft. Vascular anastomosis logically must occur before actual capillary invasion of the graft from the wound edge can be accomplished. According to Goldmann's "plasmatic circulation" theory (36), it seems unlikely that the success of these bulky grafts can be accomplished by interchange of extracellular fluid. Both clinical and experimental evidence suggest a rapid hemic vascularization in composite grafts as well as in split- and whole-thickness skin grafts. The most plausible mechanism by which vascularization occurs within a few hours after transfer is that of direct vessel-to-vessel anastomosis between the graft and the recipient bed.

The anastomosis of vessels was suggested over a century ago by Bert (37) and Thiersch (38). Histologically, Davis and Traut (39) demonstrated anastomoses within 22 hours after the application of skin grafts in dogs. Further documentation of early vascularization via anastomosis is provided by the observations of Douglas (24), Converse and Rapaport (18), Calnan (40), McLaughlin (10), and Rees (6). McLaughlin carefully observed the life cycle of composite earlobe grafts and noted a pink blush within 6 hr after transfer and a positive digital pressure test in 24 hr. A similar pattern has been revealed in our clinical observations. In most instances, composite earlobe grafts that were filleted resulted in limited vascular anastomosis via their raw (fatty) *under*surface. This may be due to the relative paucity of vessels in the subcutaneous fat of both the recipient and the donor tissue, or to the absence of host vessels when the graft is of necessity placed directly on cartilage. For this reason, precise approximation of the skin and dermal edge is necessary. The temptation to wedge in an extra millimeter of graft must be resisted; the union of vessels actually seems to be enhanced when these grafts are under a little tension.

As described by McLaughlin (10), composite grafts go through four stages from application to "take." Initially, the graft is a pearly white color, followed by a period (6–10 hr) in which there is a pale pink tinge, and then rapidly by a mottled cyanosis in areas of the graft. The inset earlobe graft commonly progresses in rapid fashion from a pale pink color through a mottled dark purple discoloration. (This progression may be of concern to the inexperienced surgeon.) Then, over a period of 5–10 days, the successfully applied graft resolves in a pinkish color. Some of the dark mottling may persist and eventually peels off like a superficial eschar.

FIGURE 7.1. Wedge-shaped earlobe graft (*left*) can provide larger segment of posterior surface fat, dermis, and epithelium. The graft is filleted, and anterior skin discarded. Note the hexagonal configuration of recipient bed (even more important when area to be grafted is located on tip of nose). Small (1-mm) rubber drains shown in illustration on *right* are all removed by 36 hr.

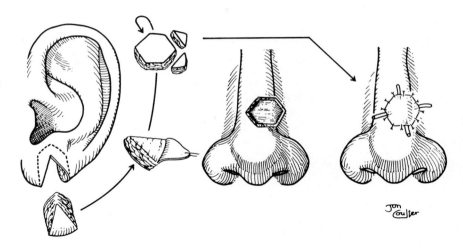

There have been some changes in technique since the work of Dupertuis in the 1940s, but the basic principles for this surgery remain the same. The defect to be reconstructed must be freshly constituted surgically and free of heavy scar and radiation changes. The graft must be handled with extreme care and should be harvested under local anesthesia without epinephrine if possible. Careful tissue handling of both the donor and the recipient area, as well as thorough hemostasis of the recipient bed are essential during the surgical procedure. To prevent pressure damage to the tissue, forceps should be avoided in favor of fine dural hooks or even the surgeon's fingers. Grafts to the nasal tip should not be placed on exposed alar cartilage, although this may sometimes be unavoidable. Frequently, some perichondrium or soft tissue can be sutured over an area of exposed cartilage with very fine catgut sutures.

Preparation of the nasal recipient bed requires careful dissection. If the cartilage has been excised and there is a small rent in the nasal lining, small absorbable sutures can be employed before placement of the composite graft. If nasal tip cartilage is involved in a neoplastic growth, it can be excised with the specimen and a composite graft placed on the raw surface of the nasal mucosa. A much larger graft segment can be obtained from the *posterior* surface of the earlobe than from the anterior (Fig. 7.1). The recipient bed is prepared using local anesthesia (xylocaine 0.5% with epinephrine 1 : 200,000).

One technical improvement is that of making the recipient graft site hexagonal or octagonal. Round or oval grafts tend to become biscuit-like or puckered with scar contracture and, therefore, should be avoided. After the earlobe donor segment is obtained, it is filleted, tailored, and fitted into place; the anterior portion is discarded in most instances (Fig. 7.1). In filleted earlobe grafts, the crease joining the posterior lobular skin to the anterior skin should also be avoided. This small ridge will usually persist postoperatively because it is almost impossible to unfold the free edge of the earlobe to produce a flat graft. If placed directly in the midline, the ridge is fairly well camouflaged.

As suggested by Conley and Vonfraenkel (41), cooling enhances the take of a composite graft, apparently by decreasing the biological demands of the graft. (Herein the authors differ: Dr. Lehman is of the opinion there is no experimental evidence to confirm this position; however, Dr. Musgrave routinely uses iced saline in the postoperative management of earlobe grafts to the nasal tip.) A swatch of gauze is held in place with a Logan bow and moistened frequently by medicine dropper with iced saline. Cooling by evaporation is the essential process. Lowering the metabolism of the graft in this manner seems to enhance the rate of survival.

The greatest single deterrent to the "take" of a filleted-out earlobe graft is stasis within and/or a hematoma beneath the graft. In the first 48 hr postoperatively, cotton swabs moistened in hydrogen peroxide are used to gently "roll" the graft toward its periphery, where old dark blood and serum is extruded (sometimes a surprising amount). Small 1-mm drains are used at four points around the periphery of the graft (Fig. 7.1). All are removed by 36–48 hr because they represent four minute areas where end-to-end anastomoses of the vessels cannot take place. By the fourth postoperative day, the fine silk or nylon sutures are removed individually, and any remaining exudate is extruded through a suture perforation.

The graft must *not* be trimmed even if the purple discoloration fails to return to a pink color and it appears not to be viable. (Apparent failures have, at times, resulted in an acceptably healed contour.) The eschar must be allowed to remain in place for weeks if necessary. A mild antibiotic-steroid ointment is applied with a bandage daily. Ingrowth of epithelium from the edges with some deep scar tissue frequently provides an amazingly good cosmetic result where the surgeon and the patient had thought "all was lost."

For those patients who are being treated on an outpatient basis, an alternate method of postoperative wound management must be considered. A simple tie-over dressing (similar to that of a standard skin graft) with nasal packing will give adequate splinting and immobili-

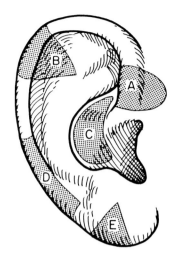

FIGURE 7.2. Donor areas from the ear provide numerous options, depending on the amount of cartilage desired. Areas **A** and **B** are the most frequently used sites for nostril rim reconstruction. Composite grafts, as in area **C,** provide convex curved cartilage and may include posterior skin when used for opposite-ear conchal reconstruction. Grafts from areas **D** and **E** do not, as a rule, contain cartilage.

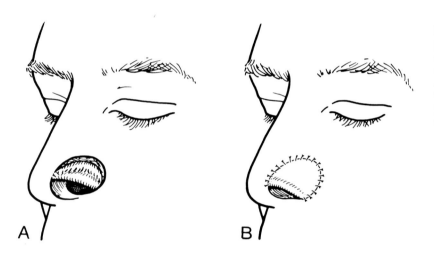

FIGURE 7.3. **A,** Turn-down of lining, which provides additional surface for apposition with composite graft. **B,** Graft in place with rolled edge of ear simulating nostril rim. Nasal lining (usually the anterior auricular surface) is sutured in place first. Petroleum jelly or greased packing, not shown, is part of splinting and dressing.

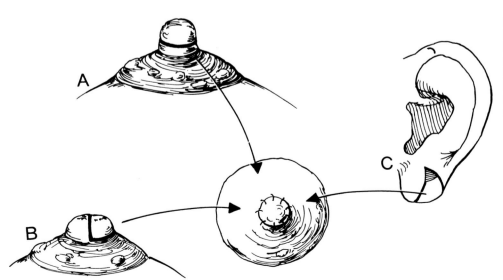

FIGURE 7.4. Nipple reconstruction using composite grafts is illustrated. For nipple reconstruction (**A**) the upper half of the opposite nipple, (**B**) the inferior half of the opposite nipple, and (**C**) the earlobe compose the graft.

zation. A small drain can be incorporated if it is believed necessary, and the patient can be discharged and follow-up performed in the office.

In avulsions of the nasal tip, if the missing portion can be obtained and is not too badly mangled, it can be cleansed and carefully sutured with a reasonable expectation of take in this richly vascularized area. When the missing portion cannot be used, composite grafts from the ear have been successfully employed as a primary procedure (42–44). Whether by surgery or by trauma, when the nostril rim defect involves lining and cartilage, the donor area should include both anterior and posterior auricle skin. This may be with or without cartilage, depending upon the requirements of the defect (Fig. 7.2). Filleting is not a part of this procedure. The edge of the graft will constitute the lining and should be tailored carefully and anchored in place first, using fine absorbable sutures (Fig. 7.3). By virtue of the donor area anatomy, the lining will usually be from the front of the ear and the exposed posterior auricular surface, which is usually larger. Ultimate color match of the graft is equally good whether anterior or posterior auricular skin is used.

Recently, composite grafts have been utilized for augmentation of the malar region (45) and nasal dorsum (46) with reasonable success, and this avoids the problems associated with alloplastic material. Composite grafts to fingertips (47) from the posterior surface of the earlobe employ principles similar to those for the nose. Splinting and immobilization require individualized improvisation.

In present-day reconstruction of breasts after thermal injury or ablative cancer surgery, reconstruction of the nipple is an integral part of restoring the breast form (48–51). The goal is to achieve a nipple that matches the color and projection size of the opposite nipple. The best tissue for such reconstructions is a composite graft from the opposite nipple. This offers the most realistic aesthetic result with only minimal donor site scarring.

Adequate nipple projection of the opposite, normal breast is the major factor influencing donor site selection (Fig. 7.4). If there is adequate projection, the opposite nipple offers a tissue graft of similar texture, size, and color. Approximately half of the normal nipple can be excised and transferred as a composite graft, using either the upper or lower half. A graft up to 7 mm will survive, and the donor site is allowed to reepithelialize. There have been no reported problems related to the nipple donor site.

References

1. König F: Eine neue Methode der Aufrichtung eingesunkener Nasen durch Bildung des Nasenruckens aus einem Haut-Periost, Knochenlappen der Stirn. *Arch Klin Chir* 34:165, 1887.
2. König F: Ueber Nasenplastik. *Beitr Klinisch Chir* 94:515, 1914.
3. Limberg AA: Rhinoplasty with free transplantation from auricle. *Soviet Phir* 9:70, 1935.
4. Dupertuis SM: Free earlobe grafts of skin and fat, their value in reconstruction about the nostrils. *Plast Reconstr Surg* 1:135, 1946.
5. Ivy RH: Lelio Zeno of Rosario and his contributions to plastic surgery (Editorial). *Plast Reconstr Surg* 42:587, 1968.
6. Rees TD: Transfer of free composite grafts of skin and fat. *Plast Reconstr Surg* 25:556, 1960.
7. Symonds FD, Crikelair GF: Auricular composite grafts in nasal reconstruction. *Plast Reconstr Surg* 37:433, 1966.
8. Crawford HH, Horton CE, Adamson JE: Composite earlobe grafts for one-stage reconstruction of facial defects. *Plast Reconstr Surg* 42:51, 1968.
9. Davenport G, Bernark FD: Improving the take of composite grafts. *Plast Reconstr Surg* 24:175, 1959.
10. McLaughlin CR: Composite ear grafts and their blood supply. *Br J Plast Surg* 7:274, 1954.
11. Lehman JA, Garrett WS, Musgrave RH: Earlobe composite grafts for the correction of nasal defects. *Plast Reconstr Surg* 47:12, 1971.
12. Sherlock EC: Use of composite grafts in reconstruction of the nasal rim. *South Med J* 62:1192, 1969.
13. Breach NM: Repair of a full-thickness nasal defect with an earlobe "sandwich" graft. *Br J Plast Surg* 32:94, 1979.
14. Smith RO, Dickinson JR, Cipcic JA: Composite grafts in facial reconstructive surgery. *Arch Otolaryngol* 95:252, 1972.
15. Gillies HD, Millard RD: *The Principles and the Art of Plastic Surgery,* Vol I. Boston, Little, Brown & Co, 1957, p 95.
16. Brown JB, Cannon B: Composite free grafts of two surfaces of skin and cartilage from the ear. *Ann Surg* 124:1101, 1946.
17. Szlazak J: Repair of nasal defects with free auricular grafts. *Br J Plast Surg* 1:176, 1948.
18. Converse JM, Rapaport FT: The vascularization of skin autografts and homografts: An experimental study in man. *Ann Surg* 143:306, 1956.
19. Davis WB, Thuss CH, Noble JH: Case report of unusual donor site of a composite graft. *Plast Reconstr Surg* 14:72, 1954.
20. Meade RJ: Composite ear grafts for construction of columella. *Plast Reconstr Surg* 23:134, 1959.
21. Flanagin WS: Free composite grafts from lower to upper lip. *Plast Reconstr Surg* 17:376, 1956.
22. Joseph J: *Handbuch der Speziellen Chirugie.* Berlin, Katz, Preysling, Blumenfield, 1912.
23. Avelar JM, Psillakis JM, Viterbo F: Use of large composite grafts in the reconstruction of deformities of the nose and ear. *Br J Plast Surg* 37:55, 1984.
24. Douglas B: Successful replacement of completely avulsed portions of fingers as composite grafts. *Plast Reconstr Surg* 23:213, 1959.
25. Adams WM: Free transplantation of the nipples and areolae. *Surgery* 15:186, 1944.
26. Conway H: Mannaplasty: Analysis of 110 consecutive cases with end results. *Plast Reconstr Surg* 10:303, 1944.
27. Robbins TH: Chondrodermal graft reconstruction of the lower eyelid. *Br J Plast Surg* 34:140, 1981.
28. Mustardé JC: *Repair and Reconstruction in the Orbital Region—A Practical Guide,* 2nd ed. London, Churchill Livingstone, 1980.
29. Brent B: The correction of microtia with autogenous cartilage grafts: I. The classic deformity. *Plast Reconstr Surg* 66:1, 1980.
30. Brent B: Reconstruction of the ear. In Grabb WC, Smith JW (eds): *Plastic Surgery,* 3rd ed. Boston, Little, Brown & Co, 1979, pp 299–320.
31. Brent B: The correction of microtia with autogenous cartilage grafts: II. Atypical and complex deformities. *Plast Reconstr Surg* 66:13, 1980.
32. Tanzer RC: Microtia—A long term follow-up of 44 reconstructed auricles. *Plast Reconstr Surg* 61:161, 1978.
33. Rueckert F: Reconstruction of the microtic ear. Presented at the International Symposium on Plastic Surgery, Beijing, China, June, 1984.
34. Converse JM: Construction of the auricle in unilateral congenital microtia. *Trans Am Acad Ophth Otolaryngol* 72:995, 1968.
35. Hall JD, Stevenson TR: Congenital ear deformity: Reconstruction using composite graft. *Ann Plast Surg* 21:145, 1988.
36. Goldmann E: Die kunstliche ueberhautung offener krebse durch haut-transplantationen nach Thiersch. *Zentralbl Allg Pathol* 1:505, 1890.
37. Bert P: Notes sur un cas de greffe animale. *C R Acad Sci* 61:587, 1865.
38. Thiersch K: Ueber die feineren anatomischen veranderungen

bei aufheilung von haut auf granulationen. *Arch Klin Chir* 17:318, 1874.

39. Davis JS, Traut HF: Origin and development of the blood supply of whole thickness skin grafts. *Ann Surg* 82:871, 1925.

40. Calnan J: Exposed delayed primary skin grafts: A clinical investigation. *Br J Plast Surg* 10:11, 1957.

41. Conley JJ, Vonfraenkel PH: The principle of cooling as applied to the composite graft in the nose. *Plast Reconstr Surg* 17:444, 1956.

42. Wynn S: Immediate composite graft to loss of nasal ala from dog bite. *Plast Reconstr Surg* 50:188, 1972.

43. Nagel F: Reconstruction of a partial auricular loss. *Plast Reconstr Surg* 49:340, 1972.

44. Maues MD, Yessenow RS: The use of composite auricular grafts in nasal reconstruction. *J Dermatol Surg Oncol* 14:994, 1988.

45. Sieman WR, Samiian MR: Malar augmentation using autogenous composite conchal cartilage and temporalis fascia. *Plast Reconstr Surg* 82:395, 1988.

46. Conley J: Intranasal composite grafts for dorsal support. *Arch Otolaryngol* 11:241, 1985.

47. Clarkson P: Composite ear grafts in repair of traumatic amputations of the fingertips. *Guys Hosp Gazette* 63:266, 1949.

48. Georgiade NG. Nipple-areola reconstruction. In Georgiade NG (ed): *Breast Reconstruction Following Mastectomy.* St. Louis, CV Mosby Co, 1979, pp 239–253.

49. Brent B, Bostwick J. Nipple-areola reconstruction with auricular tissues. *Plast Reconstr Surg* 60:353, 1977.

50. Bostwick J, Vasconez LO, Jurkiewicz MJ: Breast reconstruction after a radical mastectomy. *Plast Reconstr Surg* 61:682, 1978.

51. Cronin TD, Upton J, McDonough JM: Reconstruction of the breast after mastectomy. *Plast Reconstr Surg* 59:1, 1977.

8

Principles of Bone Transplantation

Alexander C. Stratoudakis, M.D., F.A.C.S.

The earliest attempt to transplant bone was published by Van Meek'ren in 1682 (1). Credit is generally given to Duhamel for the earliest scientific approach to osteogenesis. He placed silver wires subperiosteally and found, weeks later, that they were covered with bone. Duhamel believed this to be the result of the osteogenic properties of periosteum. This work was reported in 1742. On the other hand, Von Haller (1763) regarded the periosteum as being chiefly the support of blood vessels, which were agents for osteogenesis in the healing of fractures. He believed that osteogenesis was due to an exudation from arteries. Two sharply divided schools of thought arose, based on the views of these two men. Although Heine totally resected ribs subperiosteally and found that they grew back, the controversy was not settled until Flourens (1842) conclusively showed that periosteum is osteogenic and is the chief agent responsible for the healing of bone defects.

In 1867, Ollier reviewed the earlier literature and reported on his own experiment, concluding that the transplanted periosteum and bone remained alive and could, under proper circumstances, become osteogenic. He believed that viable bone with attached periosteum was the best form of graft to use; however, he also believed that the contents of the Haversian canals and the endosteum were important in bone regeneration.

On the other hand, Barth (1893–1898), a student of Marchand, claimed that all transplanted bone marrow and periosteum die and are replaced by surrounding tissue. He and Marchand were the first to use the term "creeping substitution" (*schleichender ersatz*) to describe the invasion of old bone by bud-like masses of new bone, without previous resorption of the old bone. They did not consider this to be the only method of replacement, admitting the occurrence of the usual method of resorption and apposition, but they felt that it was by far the most important process. The term creeping substitution has been frequently used, erroneously, to describe a process that is really resorption and apposition.

Axhausen (1907 and 1909) made a major contribution to the problem of osteogenesis and bone transplantation from his experiments, upon which he formulated his principles that periosteum has a high degree of survival and osteogenic activity in autografts, markedly less in homografts, and practically none in heterografts. He believed that all transplanted bone died, although most of the periosteum survived, to become a source of osteogenesis.

Later investigators concerned themselves with the problem of the contribution of the host bed to the regeneration of a graft, a subject that was complicated by the controversy between those who believed that bone can arise by metaplasia from surrounding connective tissue and those who believed it arises only from soft tissues associated with bone (2, 3).

Biology of Bone Transplantation

TERMINOLOGY

Autologous bone is the bone transplanted from one anatomical area to another. *Isograft* is a graft transplanted from one individual to another of the same inbred strain. The only clinical situation in which this could arise is in identical twins. *Homograft* is a graft transplanted from one individual to another of the same species. This type of graft is also referred to as *allogeneic* or *allograft*. *Heterograft* is a graft transplanted from an organism of one species to another. This type of graft is also referred to as a *xenograft*. Finally, nonviable bone processed by various methods and used for clinical or experimental applications, as well as synthetic or nonbiological materials used for the same purposes, will be referred to as *implants*, while the combination of autologous marrow with frozen or lyophylized banked bone is termed a *composite bone graft* (4).

BIOLOGY

Cell Survival

In the case of an autograft, there is little question that both the transplanted bone and the recipient tissues participate in the formation of new bone. The fact that osteogenic cells survive the transplantation of autogenous bone has been convincingly shown by various authors (5, 6). In fact, it has been shown that bone regeneration occurs from osteoprogenitor cells (preosteoblasts and osteoblasts) rather than from mature osteocytes, which degenerate by autolysis following transplantation, leaving empty lacunae. Preosteoclasts may also survive and initiate resorption of donor bone (7).

Stutzmann and Petrovic give a different account of bone cell histogenesis (8–12). According to them, the periosteum contains two cell types able to divide, the so-called skeletoblast and the preosteoblast. The skeletoblast, histologically a fibroblast-like cell, may divide up to 50 times, but its intermitotic interval is relatively long. The skeletoblast is the stem cell for either the preosteoblast or the secondary-type prechondroblast, or the preosteoclast. All these three cell varieties divide relatively frequently but never more than 10 times. When the preosteoblast matures into an osteoblast, it stops dividing. The so-called secondary-type prechondroblast is a cell present in the condylar cartilage of the mandible and also in the postfracture cartilaginous callus as well as in some varieties of bone sarcomas. When transformed into the secondary-type prechondroblast, the cell stops dividing. So, according to Stutzmann and Petrovic (8), and Petrovic, Stutzmann, and Oudet (9), bone regeneration occurs primarily from skeletoblast-derived cells, certainly not from osteoblasts and osteocytes. According to these authors, an "osteoprogenitor" cell *stricto sensu* does not exist. The only stem cell is the "skeletoblast." Finally, several authors (10–12) demonstrated that bone-resorbing cells are of extrinsic origin, originating from bone marrow and arriving through the blood as monocyte-type cells. In fact, what Trueta has described as cells originating from vessel walls are "blood monocyte-type" cells, which leave the blood stream and enter the tissues.

Osteoconduction

The process of growth of sprouting capillaries, perivascular tissue, and osteoprogenitor cells from the recipient bed into the three-dimensional structure of a bone graft or an implant is called *osteoconduction*. Osteoconduction occurs within a framework of nonbiological materials such as glass, ceramics, or plastics as well as within nonviable biological materials such as autoclaved bone, deproteinized bone, demineralized-trypsinized bone, and frozen or freeze-dried allogeneic bone (7).

Osteoinduction

The process of differentiation of fibroblast-like (skeletoblast, according to Stutzmann and Petrovic) migratory mesenchymal cells into osteoprogenitor cells on calcified tissue matrices that are either demineralized in the course of resorption or predemineralized in vitro is called *osteoinduction*. In other words, osteoinduction is the concept of a differentiated tissue such as transitional epithelium, cartilage, or bone having the capacity to induce cells of another tissue to differentiate into osteoblasts or chondroblasts and to form bone or cartilage (13). Once again, when dealing with bone transplantation, Stutzmann and Petrovic (8) and Petrovic, Stutzmann, and Oudet (9) consider that osteoinduction implies skeletoblasts and skeletoblast-derived cells but not "true" fibroblasts or any other cells. As for the cartilage, it is the secondary-type cartilage and not a primary-type (or articular type) cartilage.

The concept of osteogenic induction was first formulated by Levander in 1938 (14) and has been studied very extensively by Urist (7). Neither the mechanism nor the target site of this morphogenic phenomenon is known.

However, Urist has determined the critical components to be an insoluble noncollagenous bone morphogenetic protein (BMP), a proteolytic enzyme (BMPase), and a bone hydrophobic glycopeptide (HGP). Bone formation is regulated by the organic matrix; implants of inorganic or denatured bone or nonbiological substances do not produce bone when placed in a muscle pouch. In Stutzmann and Petrovic's view, it is because there are no skeletoblasts in the muscle pouch (A. Petrovic, personal communication, 1986).

The osteoinductive properties of bone are destroyed by autoclaving and by irradiation sterilization and are affected to various degrees by other manipulations in the processing of bone. Freeze-drying, for example, preserves enzymes that degrade constituents of bone matrix essential for the bone morphogenetic response. Sterilization with other chemical methods used in bone banks, such as β-propiolactone and hydrogen peroxide, destroy the BMP, whereas Thimerosal, which incidentally was used almost 25 years ago by Reynolds, inhibits BMPase without denaturation of BMP (7). Irradiation also reduces the breaking strength of bone in doses above 3 megarads; lower doses do not appear to have a significant effect on the mechanical properties of bone (15).

Burwell (13) had also addressed the subject of osteoinduction using a composite homograft-autograft model. He had arrived at conclusions similar to those of Urist— that the osteoinductive property of bone is contained in its organic matrix and that this capacity can be lowered by boiling, by immersion in Merthiolate solution, and most importantly, by removing its organic components before it is impregnated with marrow and implanted (13).

With respect to heterologous (xenogeneic) bone implants, calf bone had been used for a number of years in different forms such as *Kiel* bone (macerated with hydrogen peroxide), *Boplant* (extracted with detergent), and *"Os Purum"* (soaked in warm potassium hydroxide, acetone, and salt solution). The use of heterologous bone has by and large been discontinued, although Salama has reported the use of Kiel bone combined with autologous marrow in 110 operations (16). Urist states that there is currently no clinically acceptable xenoimplant. The fate of xenoimplants is sequestration or envelopment in a fibrous capsule. This has been shown both experimentally (17) and clinically (18).

Vascularization of Bone Grafts

Whether the initial revascularization of a bone autograft occurs by formation of anastomoses between vessels of the graft and those of the recipient bed, as occurs in split-thickness skin grafts, or by invasion of the graft by newly formed vessels is a matter of debate. Deleu and Trueta (19), having studied the phenomenon of bone revascularization in the anterior chamber of the eye of the guinea pig and the rat, concluded that such anastomoses do, indeed, occur. However, Albrektsson and Albrektsson (20) using an ingenious transparent chamber for direct in vivo observation of autograft revascularization in the rabbit, failed to observe any reutilization of preexisting graft vessels. Vascularization then must proceed by gradual penetration of the graft by host vessels while osteoclastic activity and apposition of new bone are taking place. The rate of vascularization depends on the species, on the size of the bone graft, and on the type of bone implant used (2). Cancellous grafts revascularize faster than cortical (19), and membranous bone revascularizes faster than mixed corticocancellous endochondral grafts (21).

Incorporation of the Bone Graft

The process of envelopment and interdigitation of the donor bone tissue with new bone deposited by the individual is termed *incorporation* (22). The quantity of donor bone resorbed is greater in cancellous than in cortical bone autografts and greater in autografts than in alloimplants. In all instances, the endpoint of incorporation generally falls short of complete replacement with living bone. When cortical bone is grafted in an adult, as much as 90% of the volume of the graft may be of donor origin. The donor tissue may remain unresorbed for as long as 13 years after the operation. In growing bones in children, tissue remodeling is so much more rapid than in adults that only microscopic quantities of the structure of the donor may be recognizable by the second year after transplantation (7). In dog experiments, Enneking (23) arrived at the following conclusions: (*a*) resorption of the necrotic bone transplant is independent of physiological skeletal metabolism; (*b*) appositional bone formation is influenced by the skeletal renewal rate; (*c*) torsional stress failure is correlated more with porosity than with microanatomical features; and (*d*) in autografts, at 48 weeks of healing, when physical resistance to torsional stress is nearly normal, only 60% of the transplant is resorbed and replaced by new bone. The same group of investigators studying cortical bone allografts in dogs concluded that the incidence of nonunion, fatigue fracture, increased porosity, increased cumulative new bone formation, decreased cross-sectional area, and decreased mechanical strength were significantly different when either fresh or freeze-dried allografts were compared to fresh autografts (24).

The list of donor site complications that are mentioned in the literature is impressive. However, with proper training, rigid adherence to the principles of bone harvesting, and correct choice of the donor site, the complication rate should be minimal.

Although autologous bone grafts are unquestionably superior to any other type of graft, the situation arises in which the use of grafts from a different source becomes necessary.

Antigenicity of Bone

Bone allografts elicit both humoral- and cell-mediated antigenicity (25, 26), proportional to the genetic disparity between host and donor. Bone allotransplantation is followed by a sequence of events that leads either to vascularization and eventual incorporation of the allograft or

alloimplant or to sequestration. The intensity of this reaction seems to depend on the genetic transplantation differences between donor and recipient, although in Muscolo's study (27), no clear relation could be established between the histocompatibility and the incorporation of the graft.

The sequence of events leading to incorporation of allografts proceeds at a much slower rate than in autografts (27), and they appear to be much more prone to infection, fracture, and nonunion (28). Antigenicity is reduced by various methods used to process and preserve the allograft, such as freezing or freeze-drying (29). Unfortunately, the above methods also have an adverse effect on the mechanical properties of bone, reducing the mechanical (torque) strength of bone (30). In the clinical use of processed allografts, antigenicity exerts only a limited effect on the outcome, and tissue typing has not been practiced in the reported clinical series. However, Mankin et al. (28) acknowledge that further studies are needed to better elucidate this point. Stevenson (25), in her experimental work, has detected antibodies in synovial fluid when no systemic antibodies could be detected, implying that matching for tissue antigens may reduce sensitization of the host. This would improve incorporation and reduce degenerative changes in the joint after implantation of an allograft.

Rejection becomes a much more serious problem in vascularized bone transfers, in which the musculoosseous grafts are rejected similarly to visceral organ grafts (31). The chronic immunosuppression that allows visceral organ transplantation carries an obligate morbidity. This morbidity is acceptable in the patient threatened by hepatic or renal failure, but it is unjustifiable in the patient requiring skeletal reconstruction of a nonvital body part (32). Efforts are continuing in the laboratory to elucidate the antigenic stimulus and to investigate methods of inducing tolerance by treatment of the graft as opposed to the patient. Transplantation immunity is inhibited by the development of serum blocking factors (enhancement), and eventually a stable state is reached between donor and recipient. The immune response to allografts or frozen bone alloimplants destroys the osteoinductive property (7).

AUTOGRAFT SUBSTITUTES

In the reconstruction of skeletal defects, autografts should be used whenever possible. Although allografting may be a less than optimal solution, it has become an important method in dealing with major skeletal loss when factors such as the size of the defect, donor site morbidity in patients already severely impaired by their disease and/or surgery, or the need to reconstruct an articular surface preclude the use of autografts (28). There are several reports of their use with high success rates (28, 33, 34).

Xenogeneic Bone

As noted earlier, the use of xenogeneic transplants has been abandoned by most surgeons, although sporadic reports of their use continues. The genetic transplantation differences between human tissue and that of other species (e.g., bovine), are such that the fate of such grafts is their eventual sequestration without any new bone formation.

Frozen Bone

Bone harvested under sterile conditions and kept frozen at −80°C does not undergo enzymatic destruction (35) and may be stored for long periods of time with seemingly little adverse effect on its function (36).

Freeze-Dried (Lyophylized) Bone

This is probably the most frequently used alloimplant. It is used mainly as a composite graft (i.e., in combination with marrow from the recipient). In orthopaedic surgery, it is used to fill defects resulting from the extirpation of bone tumors or cysts or as an adjunct in spinal fusions. It is also used extensively by periodontists to fill alveolar defects and by oral surgeons for reconstruction in the maxillofacial region. However, lyophylized bone has been shown to retain its antigenicity, and in applications where larger segments of bone are required with ability to withstand stress, the results have been very unfavorable, showing incomplete incorporation and decreased ability to withstand torsional stress (23). The bending strength was shown to be lowered to 55–90% of controls (37). Longitudinal cracks have also been observed when freeze-dried bone is rehydrated (38). It is suggested that freeze-dried bone be supplemented with generous amounts of autogenous iliac bone (7).

Deproteinized Bone

Such bone preparations lack osteoinductivity. Despite one report in which good results are claimed (39), experimental results indicate the failure to incorporate deproteinized bone into the host skeleton (14).

Demineralized Bone

In contrast to deproteinized bone, demineralized bone retains its osteoinductive properties and has been used by Mulliken et al. for reconstruction in the craniofacial region (40–42). It is acknowledged, however, that the use of radiation for sterilization diminishes osteoinductivity, and other ways to sterilize the implant are being investigated.

Chemosterilized Autolysed, Antigen-Extracted Allogeneic (AAA) Bone

This particular alloimplant has been described and is being used by Urist and Dawson (43). Cadaver bone is harvested as soon as possible after death and processed so that the BMP is preserved while nearly all the stain-

able intralacunar material is enzymatically digested. It is then freeze-dried. The breaking strength is claimed to be about one half that of whole, undemineralized wet bone. The highest success rates come from operations on young children with a high proliferative bone-growing capacity. Urist advises rigid immobilization of the recipient bone and on-laying rather than inlaying the graft in order to assure maximal contact with the host vascular bed. A series of spinal fusions utilizing this alloimplant has been published. The incidence of pseudarthrosis was slightly higher than that of a control series in which autogenous iliac bone was used, but the number of operations was too small to draw any conclusions (7, 43).

Inorganic, Nonbiological Implants

Use of such implants has been investigated as substitutes for autogenous grafts and allogeneic implants. Attempts were directed toward creating a porous material that would allow ingrowth of bone. Such an implant should possess the following properties: uniform pore distribution, optimal pore size, complete interconnection of pores, controlled pore-interconnection diameter, biocompatibility, sterilizability, and sufficient strength (44).

With the skeleton of the coral genus *Porites,* which has a skeleton analogous to osteon-evacuated bone, and using a process termed "replamineform" (indicating: replicated life form) for the fabrication of porous implant materials, several materials were tested by implantation in the femurs and tibias of dogs, in the form of cylinders 1.0 cm long and 0.5 cm in diameter. Among the materials tested, hydroxyapatite and calcium carbonate showed complete ingrowth at 8 weeks with "normal appearing and normally mineralizing osseous tissue." Furthermore, it was observed that in 1 year the calcium carbonate skeleton had been resorbed (44).

Hydroxyapatite implants fabricated by the above method were also tested by Holmes (45), who implanted them in the mandibles of dogs in which 2-cm defects were treated with implants placed in metal cast trays. At 2 months, bone extended into the implant for a distance of 3–5 mm. At 4 months, the entire length of the implant had been bridged in many of the porous channels. At 6 months, all the channels had been filled with lamellar bone with well-formed osteons. At 12 months, the architecture of the implant was notably diminished, and 88% of the implant area had been replaced by regenerated bone. It is noteworthy, however, that similar defects created in the mandibles of two dogs by the author and left *without* an implant were also completely bridged with regenerated bone at 6 months. In a more recent paper (46), Holmes tested experimentally the possibility of cranial reconstruction with porous hydroxyapatite. The final composition of the implant was 39.3% hydroxyapatite matrix, 17.2% bone ingrowth, and 43.5% soft tissue ingrowth. He concluded that a satisfactory contour can be obtained and the implant can function at least in part as a bone substitute. However, further understanding of the causes of nonunion, the extent of the predictable bone ingrowth, and the strength of the resultant implant-bone composition is required before the implant is used clinically for such critical applications, although its use in less critical applications has been the subject of several publications (47–49).

Calcium phosphate has also been tested (50) under the form of a ceramic biodegradable implant called "Synthos" (Miter Inc., Worthington, Ohio). This material can be carved into the desired shape and provides a uniform distribution of large interconnecting pores from 100 to 300 microns in size. Testing in the mandible, iliac crest, and inferior orbital rims of dogs was undertaken. Progressive invasion and replacement of the implant with bone were observed.

The above studies demonstrate the osteoconductive properties of the implants tested.

BONE AUTOGRAFTS

In 1972, an estimated 100,000 bone grafting operations were being performed in the United States annually (51). Since then, their increased application in all related surgical specialties has greatly increased this number, and Burchardt (22) in a more recent publication brings it up to 200,000. Autogenous bone is used in the vast majority of these cases. Fusion of joints, replacement of missing segments of bone, induction of healing in nonunited fractures, stabilization and retention of the facial skeleton in a displaced position (52), augmentation and normalization of facial contour, and creation of congenitally missing parts of the skeleton are clinical problems to which bone grafting provides the solution. The requirements of the bone graft vary greatly depending on the situation. Whereas one graft must be able to withstand torsional stress, a different graft will be chosen when early revascularization is the prime consideration. In a joint fusion, the contour of the graft may not be important, but in a craniofacial reconstruction, the shape is of particular relevance.

Donor Sites and Their Morbidity

A thorough working knowledge of each donor site with regard to the nature and properties of the bone it provides, as well as of the different possibilities in relation to the patient's age, is required if one is to utilize the transference of bone optimally and with the fewest possible sequellae. A description of the different donor sites follows.

The Cranium as a Source of Bone

This technique has become increasingly popular. Originally limited to a source of bone grafts for the cranial region during neurosurgical procedures, the cranium's use was extended to the reconstruction of the facial region by Tessier with excellent results (52). Calvarial bone is now being used with increasing frequency for congenital, traumatic, or surgically created deficits of the facial skeleton. Smith and Abramson (53) demonstrated in the

rabbit that membranous bone underwent less resorption than endochondral bone. The experimental work of Zins and Whitaker (54) has confirmed their findings and the clinical impression regarding the superiority of cranial bone for craniofacial reconstruction.

The technique of obtaining a cranial bone graft has been described in detail by Tessier (52).

In children, because of the tremendous regenerative capacity of the calvaria, cranial bone grafts are used almost exclusively in the reconstruction of the cranium and face. Defects created by the harvesting of cranial bone will be reconstituted, either totally or in part, up to the age of 3 or 4 years. In older children, when the calvaria is still too thin to split into inner and outer table, the donor defect should be covered either with autogenous graft from a different source or with an allogeneic implant. In adults, the cranial bone can easily be split into inner and outer tables. Generally, the outer table is used as the graft, and the inner table is returned to cover the donor site (52).

The location of the donor site is determined by the desired curvature. Generally, the parietal areas constitute the most appropriate donor sites. Small grafts may be obtained by burring the circumference of the outer table around the desired graft and carefully separating the outer from the inner table with a chisel at the level of the diploe. The harvesting of larger grafts requires a formal craniotomy.

Advantages of cranial bone grafts are: (a) the large quantity of bone available in children, in whom availability from other sources is limited; (b) less resorption as compared to endochondral bone grafts; (c) superior aesthetic results with proper selection of the curvature; (d) lack of significant postoperative pain; and (e) easy accessibility of the donor site, which either is part of the operative field in cranial or craniofacial procedures or can be draped out with the face when small grafts are needed during smaller procedures, such as the repair of an orbital floor defect. The disadvantages are few. Due to their rigidity, cranial bones do not conform to fill dead spaces and therefore may have to be combined with grafts from other sources such as the iliac crest or tibia (Tessier). The possibility of a dural tear or an epidural hematoma exists.

The Thorax as a Source of Autogenous Bone

The first rib graft was apparently performed as early as 1912 (55) with reconstruction of a mandible using autogenous rib strips.

The use of split rib grafts was popularized by Longacre, who performed a large number of reconstructions of defects of the cranium and facial skeleton. He noted that in children, those crania reconstructed with split ribs developed at a normal rate and that at 2 years new bone had formed large bony plates and only vestiges of the original ribs could be seen. He also commented on the rapid regeneration of ribs and on the fact that he had used the same, regenerated rib on occasion within 6 months to 1 year (56).

While split ribs are still used in craniofacial reconstruction, they have been replaced as the graft of choice by cranial bone. The regenerated rib in particular consists of dense cortical bone that Tessier (52) considers unsuitable for grafting. In harvesting autogenous ribs, an incision is made over the seventh rib. (A submammary incision is used in the female patient.) The dissection then proceeds under the latissimus dorsi muscle, splitting the fibers of the serratus as needed anteriorly. The ribs are harvested subperiosteally, with care to preserve the integrity of the pleura. Only alternate ribs are harvested. Following their removal, each rib bed is closed with a continuous absorbable suture. For small pleural tears, closure of the pleura under positive pressure is usually adequate. If a larger tear has occurred, temporary insertion of a thoracostomy tube should be carried out. Rib grafts should be avoided in children (52).

The Iliac Bone as a Source of Autogenous Grafts

The iliac bone is an excellent source of large quantities of cancellous and corticocancellous bone. The technique described by Tessier and published by Wolfe and Kawamoto (57) has yielded consistently good results with very little postoperative discomfort and minimal complications. With the hip elevated on a folded towel, the skin is retracted medially by an assistant. An incision is then carried out through skin and periosteum over the iliac crest, behind the anterior superior iliac spine. The iliac spine and the bone adjacent to it are left intact while the iliac crest is split sagittally, leaving the muscle attachments intact.

If a full-thickness bone graft is required, both medial and lateral halves of the iliac crest are reflected and retracted in continuity with the periosteum and muscle attachments. The graft is then taken in the desired shape and size. If only partial-thickness corticocancellous bone is needed, the medial portion of the crest is reflected, and the bone harvested. Additional quantities of cancellous bone can easily be harvested with a curette. The iliac crest is then reconstructed by direct wiring. A drain is generally not used. When properly carried out, this method allows the harvesting of a large quantity of bone without any aesthetic deficit. Young patients are usually able to ambulate on the day following the procedure with only a moderate amount of discomfort. This technique is not suitable for patients younger than 9 or 10 years of age because of incomplete ossification. Bone can be reharvested from the same area in 18–24 months (52).

In the younger child, the technique described by Crockford and Converse (58) may be used in the rare instance that an iliac bone graft will become necessary. The crest is left undisturbed, while the fascia lata and muscles are incised on the lateral surface down to bone and reflected. Bone is then harvested from the lateral surface, beneath the growth centers.

Published complications of iliac bone-graft harvesting include:

1. Herniation of abdominal contents through the scar (59, 60) is probably the result of disruption of the attachment of muscles on the iliac crest and harvesting of large full-thickness grafts. With preservation of the iliac crest and the periosteum, herniations should be totally preventable.
2. "Gluteus gait" is a persistent type of dragging limp caused by extensive stripping of the lateral surface of the ilium, with weakening of the attachments of the gluteal musculature and fascia lata. A "clicking" sound when the patient walks may be produced if the fascia lata slips suddenly over the greater trochanter instead of sliding smoothly over it. A strong repair of the fascia lata and accurate apposition of the edges of the periosteum should prevent any gait problems (55).
3. Meralgia paresthetica (neuropathy of the lateral femoral cutaneous nerve of the thigh is a complication that can be prevented by avoiding injury to the iliac spine and to the periosteum (61). The lateral femoral cutaneous nerve lies on the deep surface of the iliacus muscle. It leaves the pelvis just deep to the attachment of the inguinal ligament to the anterior superior iliac spine, but sometimes through the ligament or through the spine itself (62).
4. Fracture of the iliac crest occasionally occurs.
5. Hematoma formation is considered the most frequent complication, and most authors recommend leaving a drain in the wound. Tessier, however, feels that this is not necessary and closes the incisions without leaving a drain, claiming a very low incidence of hematoma formation (P. Tessier, personal communication.)

The Tibia as a Source of Autologous Bone

The importance of the tibia as a source of autologous bone has declined because primary bone grafts of clefts have by and large been abandoned and osteoperiosteal grafts are no longer in vogue. It is still useful, however, in providing a strip of cortical and some highly osteogenic cancellous bone. The technique of harvesting bone from the tibia was originally published by Breine and Johanson (64) and will be described here as currently performed by Tessier:

. . . an Esmarch bandage is applied to provide a *bloodless field*. Through a long curved incision, the skin and subcutaneous tissues are dissected from the anteromedial surface of the tibia, and the periosteum is incised medially, laterally, and distally, remaining attached only proximally from the level of the epiphysis to the mid-shaft of the tibia. With a very sharp osteotome, the periosteum with a thin layer of attached cortical bone is elevated in a distal-to-proximal direction, remaining attached as a proximally based osteoperiosteal flap. The underlying cortical bone of the medial surface of the tibia is then removed with the help of the osteotome, and the medullary cavity is entered. Cancellous bone is then curetted from the area of the proximal epiphysis, and the osteoperiosteal flap is sutured back in place. The skin is closed, and a snug dressing is applied. The harvested bone is generally used to supplement cranial grafts and to fill dead spaces, sparing the ilium for future use where multiple stages are planned. There is no deformity other than the surgical scar, and the patient experiences only a temporary difficulty in walking.

Other Autogenous Graft Donor Sites

For procedures involving the upper extremity, it is obviously advantageous to obtain the grafts from bones in the same surgical field. The *distal radius* and the *proximal ulna* have been used as a source of both cortical and cancellous bone with good results by McGrath and Watson (65). An oval-to-elliptical segment of cortical bone is removed by outlining the segment with multiple drill holes. Cancellous bone can then be curetted. When the ulna is used, the graft should be taken at least 2 inches below the olecranon to avoid weakness over the elbow joint. The radius is exposed between the first and second dorsal extensor compartments, and periosteum is reflected off its lateral aspect.

The *fibula* is the most suitable bone graft to bridge defects in the long bones that result either from traumatic losses or from the resection of tumors. Harvesting the fibula as a bone graft does not cause major functional deficits, provided the fibular head as well as the distal quarter of the fibula are not disturbed in order to maintain knee and ankle stability. Enneking (66) analyzed the results obtained in 40 patients who underwent such grafting operative procedures. Thirty-three patients had dual grafts, while seven had a single fibular graft. Dual grafts were used for major bones (humerus, femur, and tibia without fibula), while single grafts were used for the radius and for the tibia when the ipsilateral fibula was intact. In 25 patients, union was achieved in 12 months and in two in 20 months, while 12 patients required a supplementary cancellous graft at the site of nonunion to obtain stability. One patient required removal of an infected graft. Stress fractures of the grafts occurred in 18 of the 40 patients after union had occurred. The stress fractures healed in 15 of these patients; in six with no treatment, in seven with external immobilization, and in two after bone grafting of the ununited fracture. There were three persistent nonunions of stress fractures despite bone grafting, internal fixation, and electrical stimulation. *The length of the graft did not affect the incidence of nonunion, but it did affect the number of fatigue fractures.* The shorter grafts (7.5–12 cms) were associated with a 33% incidence of nonunion, while the longer grafts (12–25 cms) had a 32% rate of nonunion. *The incidence of fatigue fractures in the longer grafts (58%) was much greater than in the shorter grafts (17%).* The grafts decreased in density during the first 6 months but gradually regained their mass and were generally comparable to normal cortical bone at 2 years. As the patients became functional most (55%) of the grafts became more dense than normal. Some (34%) remained the same size, and a few (9%) atrophied (66).

Free Vascularized Bone Grafts

The first clinically successful free bone graft was reported by Taylor in 1975 (67). In selected patients, free vascularized bone grafts may offer considerable advantages over conventional bone grafting because large segments of bone transferred with their blood supply should heal to the recipient bone without the usual replacement by creeping substitution. The endosteal (nutrient) blood supply, however, must be preserved if predictable bone survival is to be achieved (68, 69).

It has been shown that epiphyseal growth is preserved following transfer of a vascularized bone segment (70, 71). When compound anterior rib segments were transferred with only their periosteal blood supply preserved, they showed no improved osteocyte survival or bone union as compared with conventional free grafts of the rib (72). More recently, Berggren et al. used bone grafts in dog mandibles and compared free vascularized bone grafts that had intact medullary and periosteal blood supply with grafts with only periosteal supply intact. They concluded that, in grafts with only periosteal blood supply, survival of the osteocytes and marrow is not as complete as in grafts with both medullary and periosteal blood supply. No difference in the ability to participate in healing to a recipient bone defect could be demonstrated (73). Moore et al. (74) compared vascularized and conventional rib grafts by biomechanical torsional testing and concluded that vascularized grafts were significantly stronger after 3 months of healing in the dog ulna model. These findings were also confirmed by Goldberg. In the clinical setting, however, the same complications reported by Enneking in his retrospective study of conventional bone grafts have also followed free vascularized bone grafts. Fatigue fracture, nonunion, and infection have been reported (75–77).

Pedicled Vascularized Bone Grafts

In the craniofacial region, vascularized calvarial bone may be transferred, retaining a vascular pedicle based on the temporalis muscle, either including the galea as recommended by McCarthy and Zide (78), or simply retaining periosteal continuity, which also preserves the blood supply as shown by Antonyshyn et al. (79). Such vascularized bone grafts (or more appropriately, flaps) have been shown to resorb less than free grafts (80) and to retain significant growth potential (81). If a suture is included in the flap, it also continues to grow, in contrast to a nonvascularized bone graft (82). However, if the blood supply to the transposed bone segment is interrupted, it resorbs to a greater degree than a nonvascularized bone graft, presumably because of the avascular sleeve of tissue that surrounds it (83). This method should probably be reserved for bone grafting in clinically unfavorable recipient sites (71).

Handling and Machining of Bone Grafts

It stands to reason that the least possible time should be allowed to lapse between the harvesting and the placement of the bone graft. During that period of time, the graft should not be allowed to dry out but should be kept in a liquid medium to ensure the viability of the maximum number of cells. In a comparative study of the various media for temporary storage of autografts, Marx et al. have determined that the best storage medium is either

D$_5$W or normal saline. The ability of the patient's serum to sustain cellular viability was extremely poor, and more elaborate tissue culture media offered no advantage over D$_5$W or normal saline (84).

Cortical and corticocancellous bone grafts are cut to the desired shape with a combination of bone-cutting forceps and electrical or air-powered saws and drills. It has been shown that the proper configuration of drill points and selection of appropriate drilling speeds are important in reducing the amount of mechanical and thermal damage to bone. Jacob et al. made the following recommendations: (a) bone drills must have an appreciable rake angle (cutting edge angle); (b) a point angle on the drill is desirable to prevent the drill from "walking" on the surface; (c) drilling should be done in the 750–1250 RPM range; (d) coolant in the form of saline should flood the entire drilling field (cold saline would possibly allow drilling at higher speeds); (e) the periosteum should be reflected away from the point where the drill will enter the bone to prevent the chips that are being ejected from the hole from being forced under this tissue and clogging the flutes of the drill; and (f) drill flutes should, for compact bone, be steep enough to remove chips at an even rate (85). Thompson (86) considers the optimal drilling speed to be about 500 RPM. He found that drilling at lower speeds causes fragmentation of the edges of the hole, while drilling at higher speeds increases the thermal changes in the bone. At 500 RPM, the temperature was about 43°C at 2.5 mm from the extraoral skeletal pin used for drilling in his experiments, while at 1000 RPM, the temperature was above 65.5°C (86). While the optimal drilling speed has not been universally agreed upon, the available studies indicate that it is in the vicinity of 500 to 1000 RPM and that the use of high-speed air-powered drills should be avoided.

References

1. Jobi a Meek'ren: *Observationes Medico Chirurgicae*. Ex officina Henrici et Theodori Boom, Amstelodami, 1682.
2. Chase SW, Herndon CH: The fate of autogenous and homogenous bone grafts. A historical review. *J Bone Joint Surg [Am]* 37:809, 1955.
3. Burchardt H, Enneking WF: Transplantation of bone. *Surg Clin North Am* 58:403, 1978.
4. Simmons DJ, Ellsasser JC, Cummins H, et al: The bone inductive potential of a composite bone allograft-marrow autograft in rabbits. *Clin Orthop* 97:237, 1973.
5. Ray RD: Vascularization of bone grafts and implants. *Clin Orthop Rel Res* 87:43, 1972.
6. Amsel S, Dell ES: Bone marrow repopulation of subcutaneously grafted mouse femurs. *Proc Soc Exp Biol Med* 138:550, 1971.
7. Urist M: Practical applications of basic research in bone graft physiology. *Instruc Course Lect* 25:1, 1976.
8. Stutzmann J, Petrovic A: Bone cell histogenesis: The skeletoblast as a stem cell for preosteoblasts and for secondary type prechondroblasts. *Progr Clin Biol Res* 101, 1982.
9. Petrovic A, Stutzmann J, Oudet C: Craniofacial growth research: In: *Cybernetics, Theory of Catastrophy*. Symposium on Skull Growth, Academic Medical Center of Amsterdam, 1985.
10. Lemoine C, Petrovic, A, Stutzmann J: Inflammatory process of the rat maxilla after molar autotransplantation. *J Dent Res* 49:1175, 1970.
11. Petrovic A: Cellules sanguines, plasma et coagulation. In Kayser C et al. (eds): *Traite de Physiologie*. Paris, Flammarion, 1970, pp 138–208.
12. Stutzmann J, Petrovic A, Shaye R: Analyse en culture organo-typique de la vitesse de formation-résorption de l'os alvéolaire humain prélève avant et pendant un traitement comprenant le déplacement des dents: nouvelle voie d'approche en recherche orthodontique. *L'Orthodontie Française* 50:399, 1979.
13. Burwell RG: Studies in the transplantation of bone. VIII. Composite homograft-autografts of cancellous bone: An analysis of inductive mechanisms in bone transplantation. *J Bone Joint Surg [Br]* 48:532, 1966.
14. Levander G: A study of bone regeneration. *Surg Gynecol Obstet* 67:705, 1938.
15. Pelker RR, Friedlaender GE: Biomechanical aspects of bone autografts and allografts. *Orthop Clin North Am* 18:235, 1987.
16. Salama R: Xenogeneic bone grafting in humans. *Clin Orthop Rel Res* 174:113, 1983.
17. Anderson KJ, Dingwal JA, Schmidt J, et al: The effect of particle size of the heterogenous bone transplant on the host tissue. *J Bone Joint Surg [Am]* 43:996, 1961.
18. Ramani PS, Kalbag RM, Gengupta RP: Cervical spinal interbody fusion with Kiel bone. *Br J Surg* 62:147, 1975.
19. Deleu J, Trueta J: Vascularization of bone grafts in the anterior chamber of the eye. *J Bone Joint Surg [Br]* 47:319, 1965.
20. Albrektsson T, Albrektsson B: Microcirculation in grafted bone; a chamber technique for vital microscopy of rabbit bone transplants. *Acta Orthop Scand* 49:1, 1978.
21. Kusiak JK, Zins JE, Ring E, et al: Early revascularization of membranous bone grafts. *Surg Forum* 32:567, 1981.
22. Burchardt H: Biology of bone transplantation. *Orthop Clin North Am* 18:187, 1987.
23. Enneking WF, Burchardt H, Puhl JJ, et al: Physical and biological aspects of repair in dog cortical bone transplants. *J Bone Joint Surg [Am]* 57:237, 1975.
24. Burchardt H, Jones H, Glowczewskie F, et al: Freeze-dried allogeneic segmental cortical bone grafts in dogs. *J Bone Joint Surg [Am]* 60:1082, 1978.
25. Stevenson S: The immune response to osteochondral allografts in dogs. *J Bone Joint Surg [Am]* 69:573, 1987.
26. Friedlander GE: Immune responses to osteochondral allografts. Current knowledge and future directions. *Clin Orthop* 174:58, 1983.
27. Muscolo DL, Caletti E, Schajowich F, Araujo ES, Marino A: Tissue-typing in human massive allografts of frozen bone. *J Bone Joint Surg [Am]* 69:583, 1987.
28. Mankin HJ, Gebhardt MC, Tomford WW: The use of frozen cadaveric allografts in the management of patients with bone tumors of the extremities. *Orthop Clin North Am* 18:275, 1987.
29. Friedlander GE, Strong DM, Sell KW: Studies on the antigenicity of bone. I. Freeze-dried and deep frozen allografts in rabbits. *J Bone Joint Surg [Am]* 58:854, 1976.
30. Pelker RR, Friedlander GE, Markham TC: Biomechanical properties of bone allografts. *Clin Orthop* 174:54, 1983.
31. Yaremchuk MJ, Nettlebad H, Randolph MA, Weiland AJ: Vascularized bone allograft transplantation in a genetically defined rat model. *Plast Reconstr Surg* 75:355, 1985.
32. Paskert JP, Yaremchuk MJ, Randolph MA, Weiland AJ: Prolonging survival in vascularized bone allograft transplantation. Developing specific immune unresponsiveness. *J Reconstr Microsurg* 3:253, 1987.
33. Jasty M, Harris WH: Total hip reconstruction using frozen femoral head allografts in patients with acetabular bone loss. *Orthop Clin North Am* 18:291, 1987.
34. Urbaniak JR, Aitken M: Clinical use of bone allografts in the elbow. *Orthop Clin North Am* 18:311, 1987.
35. Ehrlich MG, Lorenz J, Tomford WW, et al: Collagenase activity in banked bone. *Trans Orthop Res Soc* 8:166, 1983.
36. Mankin HJ, Doppelt SH, Sullivan TR, et al: Osteoarticular and intercalary allograft transplantation in the management of malignant tumors of bone. *Cancer* 50:613, 1982.
37. Triantafyllou N, Sotiropoulos E, Triantafyllou J: The mechanical properties of lyophylized and irradiated bone grafts. *Acta Orthop Belg* 41:35, 1975.

38. Pelker RR, Friedlaender GE, Markham TC, et al: Effects of freezing and freeze-drying on the biomechanical properties of rat bone. *J Orthop Res Soc* 11:272, 1986.

39. Hurley LA, Zeier FG, Stinchfield FE: Anorganic bone grafting; clinical experiences with heterografts processed by Ethylenediamine extraction. *Am J Surg* 100:12, 1960.

40. Mulliken JB, Glowacki J: Induced osteogenesis for repair and construction in the craniofacial region. *Plast Reconstr Surg* 65:553, 1980.

41. Mulliken JB, Glowacki J, Kaban LB, et al: Use of demineralized allogeneic bone implants for the correction of maxillocranial deformities. *Ann Surg* 194:366, 1981.

42. Mulliken JB: The use of demineralized bone for reconstruction of a large cranial defect. *Surg Rounds* 5:16, 1982.

43. Urist MR, Dawson E: Intertransverse process fusion with the aid of chemosterilized autolyzed antigen-extracted allogeneic (AAA) bone. *Clin Orthop Rel Res* 154:97, 1981.

44. Chiroff RT, White EW, Weber JN, et al: Tissue ingrowth of replamineform implants. *J Biomed Mater Res Sympos* 6:29, 1975.

45. Holmes RE: Bone regeneration within a coralline hydroxyapatite implant. *Plast Reconstr Surg* 63:626, 1979.

46. Holmes RE, Hagler HK: Porous hydroxyapatite as a bone graft substitute in cranial reconstruction: A histometric study. *Plast Reconstr Surg* 81:662, 1988.

47. Kenney EB, Lekovic V, Ferreira JC, et al: Bone formation within porous hydroxyapatite implants in human periodontal defects. *J Periodontol* 57:76, 1986.

48. Salyer KE, Ubinas EE, Snively SL: Porous hydroxyapatite as an onlay graft in maxillofacial surgery. *Plast Surg Forum* 8:61, 1985.

49. Wolford LM: Interpore 200 porous hydroxyapatite as a bone substitute for orthognathic surgery. Transactions of the 9th International Conference on Oral and Maxillofacial Surgery, Vancouver, B.C., May 21–25, 1986, p 26.

50. Ferraro JW: Experimental evaluation of ceramic calcium phosphate as a substitute for bone grafts. *Plast Reconstr Surg* 63:634, 1979.

51. Ray RD: Bone grafts and bone implants. *Otolaryngol Clin North Am* 5:389, 1972.

52. Tessier P: Autogenous bone grafts taken from the calvarium for facial and cranial applications. *Clin Plastic Surg* 9:531, 1982.

53. Smith JD, Abramson M: Membranous versus endochondral bone autografts. *Arch Otolaryngol* 99:203, 1974.

54. Zins JE, Whitaker LA: Membranous versus endochondral bone: Implications for craniofacial reconstruction. *Plast Reconstr Surg* 72:778, 1983.

55. Longacre JJ, Converse JM, Knize DM: Transplantation of bone. In Converse JM (ed): *Reconstructive Plastic Surgery*. 2nd ed. Philadelphia, WB Saunders, 1977, Vol 1, p 334.

56. Longacre JJ, DeStefano GA: Further observations of the behavior of autogenous split-rib grafts in reconstruction of extensive defects of the cranium and face. *Plast Reconstr Surg* 20:281, 1957.

57. Wolfe SA, Kawamoto HK: Taking the iliac bone graft. *J Bone Joint Surg [Am]* 60:411, 1968.

58. Crockford DA, Converse JM: The ilium as a source of bone grafts in children. *Plast Reconstr Surg* 50:270, 1972.

59. Reid RL: Hernia through an iliac bone graft donor site. *J Bone Joint Surg [Am]* 50:757, 1968.

60. Lotem M, Maor P, Haimoff H, et al: Lumbar hernia at an iliac bone graft donor site. *Clin Orthop* 80:130, 1971.

61. Massey EW: Meralgia paresthetica secondary to trauma of bone graft. *J Trauma* 20:342, 1980.

62. Ghent WR: Further studies on meralgia paresthetica. *Can Med Assoc J* 85:871, 1961.

63. Reale F, Gambacorta D, Mencattini G: Iliac crest fracture after removal of two bone plugs for anterior cervical fusion. *J Neurosurg* 51:560, 1979.

64. Breine U, Johanson B: Tibia as donor area of bone grafts in infants. *Acta Chir Scand* 131:230, 1966.

65. McGrath MH, Watson HK: Late results with local bone graft donor sites in hand surgery. *J Hand Surg* 6:234, 1981.

66. Enneking WF, Eady JL, Burchardt H: Autogenous cortical bone grafts in the reconstruction of segmental skeletal defects. *J Bone Joint Surg [Am]* 62:1039, 1980.

67. Taylor GL, Miller GDH, Ham FJ: The free vascularized bone graft. A clinical extension of microsurgical technique. *Plast Reconstr Surg* 55:533, 1975.

68. Ostrup LT, Fredrickson JM: Distant transfer of a free living bone graft by microvascular anastomoses. *Plast Reconstr Surg* 54:274, 1974.

69. Goldberg VM, Shaffer JW, Field G, Davy DT: Biology of vascularized bone grafts. *Orthop Clin North Am* 18:197, 1987.

70. Brown K, Marie P, Lyszakowski J, et al: Epiphyseal growth after free fibular transfer with and without microvascular anastomosis. *J Bone Joint Surg [Br]* 65:4, 1983.

71. Zaleske DJ, Ehrlich MG, Pilliero C, et al: Growth plate behavior in whole joint replantation in the rabbit. *J Bone Joint Surg [Am]* 65:2, 1982.

72. Adelaar RS, Soucacos P, Urbaniak JR: A study of autologous cortical bone grafts with microsurgical anastomosis of periosteal vessel. Paper read at the Surgical Forum, American College of Surgeons Meeting, Miami, Florida, 1974. Quoted in: Taylor GL: Microvascular free bone graft transfer, a clinical technique. *Orthop Clin North Am* 8:425, 1977.

73. Berggren A, Weiland AJ, Dorfman H: Free vascularized bone grafts: Factors affecting their survival and ability to heal to recipient bone defects. *Plast Reconstr Surg* 69:19, 1982.

74. Moore JB, Mazur JM, Zehr D: A biomechanical comparison of vascularized and conventional autogenous bone grafts. *Plast Reconstr Surg* 73:382, 1984.

75. Taylor GL: Microvascular free bone transfer: A clinical technique. *Orthop Clin North Am* 8:425, 1977.

76. Weiland AJ, Daniel RK: Microvascular anastomoses for bone grafts in the treatment of massive defects in bone. *J Bone Joint Surg [Am]* 61:98, 1979.

77. Weiland AJ, Kleinert HE, Kutz JE, et al: Free vascularized bone grafts in surgery of the upper extremity. *J Hand Surg* 4:129, 1979.

78. McCarthy JG, Zide BM: The spectrum of calvarial bone grafting: Introduction of the vascularized calvarial bone flap. *Plast Reconstr Surg* 74:10, 1984.

79. Antonyshyn O, Colcleugh RG, Hurst LN, Anderson C: The temporalis myoosseous flap: An experimental study. *Plast Reconstr Surg* 77:406, 1986.

80. Cutting CB, McCarthy JG: Comparison of residual osseous mass between vascularized and nonvascularized onlay bone transfers. *Plast Reconstr Surg* 72:672, 1983.

81. LaTrenta GS, McCarthy JG, Cutting CB: The growth of vascularized onlay bone transfers. *Ann Plast Surg* 18:511, 1987.

82. Antonyshyn O, Colcleugh RG, Anderson C: Growth potential in suture bone inlay grafts: A comparison of vascularized and free calvarial bone grafts. *Plast Reconstr Surg* 79:1, 1987.

83. Bos KE: Bone scintigraphy of experimental composite bone grafts revascularized by microvascular anastomoses. *Plast Reconstr Surg* 64:353, 1979.

84. Marx RE, Snyder RM, Kline SN: Cellular survival of human marrow during placement of marrow-cancellous bone grafts. *J Oral Surg* 37:712, 1979.

85. Jacob CH, Berry JT, Pope MH, et al: A study of the bone machining process-drilling. *J Biomechanics* 9:343, 1976.

86. Thompson HC: Effect of drilling into bone. *J Oral Surg* 16:22, 1958.

9

Basic Principles of Tendon Grafting

Paul M. Weeks, M.D., F.A.C.S. and Jeffrey P. Groner, M.D.

Introduction

Tendon function is best restored by direct repair of the severed tendon. The status of the wound, the tendons, and the pulley system determine if primary repair is dictated. The factors precluding primary repair include: (a) infection; (b) loss of the A2 or A4 pulleys; (c) loss of more than 1 cm of tendon length; and (d) inadequate soft tissue coverage. Delayed primary repair is precluded by (a) infection; (b) loss of tendon length; (c) swelling of proximal end of the tendon, which prevents passage through the A2 and A4 pulleys; (d) collapse and obliteration of the tendon sheath by scar; and (e) the presence of stiff joints. Delayed primary repair 5 to 6 weeks after injury is usually precluded by thickening of the proximal tendon end (preventing passage through the digital sheath) and shortening of tendon length. However, delayed primary repair at 48 years after injury has been reported (1).

Flexor tendon grafting is considered only if primary or delayed primary repair is not feasible. If only profundus function has been lost, other methods of management are available, including: (a) fusion of the distal interphalangeal (DIP) joint or (b) tenodesis of the profundus distal stump across the DIP joint. Procedure selection is dependent upon age, occupation, the finger involved, patient awareness of the time commitment, realistic expectations, and complications associated with each procedure. The prime consideration is the functional gain expected from each procedure. If only tendon substance is lost, flexor tendon grafting can be performed immediately. More often, loss of the A2 or A4 pulleys accompanies such an injury, and these pulleys must be reconstructed over a Silastic rod. Flexor tendon grafting is precluded by a scarred tendon bed, stiff joints, or loss of the A2 or A4 pulleys. Fusion of the proximal interphalangeal (PIP) joint in any position has been unsatisfactory in our experience, especially in laborers. A ray amputation is less detrimental to function in these people.

Contraindications to flexor tendon grafting include: (a) stiff joints (with exceptions noted later); (b) adherent extensor tendons; or (c) loss of the A2 and/or A4 pulley (either traumatic loss or collapse and obliteration by scar). If flexor tendon grafting is indicated but cannot be performed acutely, grafting should be delayed until the tissues have softened and the joints are supple. This usually requires 6–8 weeks but can be longer, depending upon the injury. Occasionally, joint stiffness is due to extrinsic factors (e.g., tendon adhesions or skin loss), which prevent obtaining supple joints preoperatively. This can be determined with some confidence based on the type and extent of injury, the surgery performed, the postoperative course, and the examination of the patient (2).

If joint stiffness is due to intrinsic factors (collateral ligament shortening, volar plate adherence, or dorsal pouch fibrosis), a capsulotomy is performed under local anesthesia. Range of motion (ROM) obtained at surgery must be maintained with aggressive therapy. Tendon grafting is delayed until the joints are supple. Joint contractures due to adhesions about injured flexor tendons are released by tenolysis or excision of the scarred tendon and either tendon grafting or rod insertion. The nonsalvageable tendons are removed while preparing the bed for tendon grafting; this allows a single-stage final tendon reconstruction. Salient operative features in flexor tendon grafting are summarized in Table 9.1.

Flexor Tendon Grafts Traversing the Digital Sheath—Operative Procedure

SKIN INCISIONS

All previous incisions and lacerations are marked before planning the incision required for tendon grafting. The incision is planned to utilize, if possible, part or all of the previous laceration sites and to avoid basing flaps on previous lacerations or incisions. We have abandoned the midlateral approach for the volar zig-zag incision. The latter provides excellent exposure, and if a tenolysis is required, the same volar zig-zag incision provides rapid, safe, clear visualization under local anesthesia. A dart is used to prevent formation of an annoying scar contracture across the flexion crease at the web space (Fig. 9.1). A semilunar incision is continued into the palm to the level of the superficial vascular arch.

RETRIEVING THE TENDON ENDS

The skin flaps are reflected to expose the digital sheath throughout the finger. A flap of sheath that includes the C1 and A3 pulleys is reflected between the A2 and A4 pulleys. One must be careful to enter the sheath anterior to its reflection from the volar plate (rather than cutting into the volar plate) and not to enter the joint space by cutting through the accessory collateral ligaments. The

Table 9.1
Flexor Tendon Grafting

Timing
   Edema has subsided
   Scar soft
   Joint supple

Incision
   Bruner incorporating laceration site

Digital Sheath
   Preserve normal sheath
   Preserve all pulleys

Superficialis Tendon
   Minimal gap
      Distal repair of tendon
      Nerve repair
      Proximal repair of tendon
   Large gap
      Distal repair of tendon
      Nerve graft
      Proximal repair of tendon

Tendon Graft
   Palmaris
   Plantaris

Repair
   Distal
      Equal-size tendons (end-to-end)
      Unequal-size tendons
         Drill hole
         Bunnell suture
         Pullout wire
   Proximal
      Equal-size tendons (end-to-end)
      Unequal-size tendons (Brand repair)

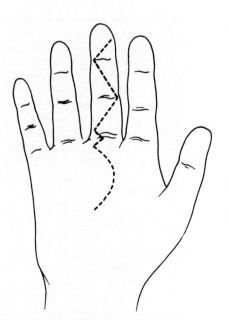

FIGURE 9.1. A dart is incorporated in the volar zig-zag incision to preclude scar contracture across the crease.

plane of dissection is not clear when there is extensive scarring in this area. If the tendons are adherent beneath the A1 or A2 pulley, the interval between the A1 and A2 pulleys is opened. A window of palmar fascia is excised over the flexor tendons of the involved finger. Frequently, there is exuberant synovium within the palm, particularly when the proximal end of the tendon has withdrawn into the palm. This synovium is resected, and the proximal end of the tendon is drawn into the palm. The excursion of the muscle is determined. The sheath is opened over the DIP joint, and the tendon is drawn distally from beneath the A4 pulley. If the profundus tendon is adherent beneath the A4 pulley, the adhesions are divided with a Freer elevator, and the tendon advanced proximally under gentle traction. Every possible millimeter of digital pulley is preserved.

SOURCE OF TENDON GRAFTS

The sources of tendon grafts in descending frequency of preference are the palmaris longus, the plantaris, the long extensors of the middle three toes, and all others (3). Thick tendons are undesirable because they undergo greater central necrosis and form more dense, nonyielding adhesions. The *palmaris longus* is preferred because: (*a*) it is thin; (*b*) its internal structure permits its fibers to be spread laterally to aid in repair; and (*c*) it is readily accessible in the field of surgery. Its presence is determined by active opposition of the thumb to the little finger and flexion of the wrist. Harvey et al. (4) examined 658 cadavers for the presence of the palmaris and/or plantaris tendons. The palmaris was absent in 20.9% of all forearms. One should always remember that the median nerve has been harvested inadvertently, thinking it was the palmaris longus tendon (5). The tendon may be thin or the muscle belly long, reducing its usefulness as a graft. The muscle arises from the medial epicondyle of the humerus and inserts into the palmar aponeurosis and the transverse carpal ligament. Its insertion is exposed through a transverse incision in the distal wrist crease. One must identify all fibers of the palmaris before attempting removal with a stripper. After removal, a clamp is placed on each end of the specimen, and the muscle trimmed from the graft. Usually, it is of sufficient length for one palm or distal wrist-to-fingertip graft.

The *plantaris* tendon is used when a longer graft or several grafts are needed. In Harvey's study, the plantaris tendon was absent in 18.7% of limbs studied. If the plantaris tendon was absent on one side, the chance of finding it on the other side was one in three. There was no difference in males or females. There was no statistical correlation between the presence of palmaris and plantaris tendons; one cannot predict or determine the presence of the plantaris preoperatively. The plantaris may not be suitable for use as a graft due to variability in diameter or muscular attachments, which makes retrieval in one piece difficult. It usually provides sufficient length for two or three palm-to-fingertip grafts or one forearm-to-fingertip graft. The plantaris muscle originates from the linea aspera of the femur (just above the lateral condyle) and the articular capsule of the knee. Its tendon, which is frequently three or four times the length of the muscle belly, traverses the leg, passing medially between the gastrocnemius and soleus muscles. Distally, the tendon emerges from beneath the deep fascia on the medial aspect of the Achilles tendon before inserting into the calcaneus. The tendon is exposed through a transverse incision posterior to the medial malleolus. The deep fascia should be split as far proximally as possible before using the tendon stripper.

The *extensor digitorum longus* arises as a common muscle from the anterior crest of the fibula, the interosseus membrane, and the crural fascia. It inserts into the dorsal aponeurosis of the second through the fourth toes. The common tendon splits into individual tendons after it has passed under the cruciform ligament. The middle three toes have both long and short extensors, permitting removal of the long extensors for grafting. These tendons are always present and are of good quality and diameter as grafts. Occasionally, the tendons fuse proximally, making harvesting difficult. The long toe extensors will provide three and possibly four tendon grafts. Removal of the long extensor of the little toe is usually avoided because there is no short extensor. There is little functional loss from using the toe extensors, although some flexion deformity and lateral deviation occurs when shoes are not worn.

Aulicino et al. (6) reported an independent long extensor of the fifth toe in 39 (50%) of 78 extremities. The length of usable tendon (range of 16–29 cm, mean of 23 cm) was greater than that obtainable from the commonly fused long toe extensors. As a last resort, they suggested harvesting this tendon and preserving fifth toe extension by transfer of the fourth toe long extensor.

We avoid use of the superficialis tendons as grafts. The little finger superficialis tendon can be used but is not sacrificed if intact. The remaining superficialis tendons are not suitable for use as free grafts because of size. The extensor indicis proprius and the extensor digiti minimi provide flat but short tendons that can be used as free grafts. There is no reason to sacrifice function when other tendons are available.

Flexor Tendon Grafts for Isolated Profundus Injury

Many hand surgeons have decried the use of tendon grafts for isolated profundus injury (7). Other authors (8) have recommended a two-stage approach as originally discussed by Gaisford et al. (9).

OPERATIVE PROCEDURE

The tendon ends are exposed and isolated as described earlier. The profundus stumps are withdrawn proximally and distally. A 3-mm Silastic rod is inserted into the digital sheath from the palm to the distal phalanx. If the decussation of the superficialis tendon is obliterated, the rod is placed along the superficialis tendon. If the decus-

sation of the superficialis tendon is open, the surgeon may elect to pass the rod through it. The tendon graft is sutured to the proximal end of the Silastic rod. The rod is advanced distally, pulling the tendon graft through the sheath. The distal end of the graft is temporarily sutured to the pulp skin for support while the proximal repair is being performed. The method of proximal suture is dependent upon the size discrepancy between the graft and the profundus tendon. If there is no discrepancy, an end-to-end repair with a modified Bunnell suture is preferred. If the graft is significantly smaller than the profundus, the suture technique of Pulvertaft (10) is useful. This technique is easy to perform, provides a smooth transition from profundus tendon to graft, and has excellent holding power. The palmar and digital skin wounds are closed to the level of the PIP joint, leaving the distal incision open over the middle and distal phalanges before tension is adjusted in the graft. Determining proper tension is described later, as well as attachment of the tendon to the distal phalanx.

RESULTS AFTER GRAFTING FOR ISOLATED PROFUNDUS INJURY

Stark et al. (11), utilizing the palmaris tendon preferentially, passed the graft through the superficialis in 22 fingers and alongside in three. If the superficialis bifurcation was scarred, the graft would be placed alongside. The distal end of the graft was attached to the terminal phalanx with a pullout suture. Postoperatively, the wrist was immobilized in 30° of palmar flexion with digital extension blocked. The splint was maintained for 4 weeks; the pullout wire removed after 3 weeks. Flexion against resistance was not allowed until 8 weeks postoperatively. Two fingers obtained flexion to the midpalmar crease, eleven to 1.25 cm, nine to 2.5 cm, and one to 3.2 cm. Two fingers had less flexion after operation. In 22 of the 25 patients, useful active flexion of the DIP joint was present, and active independent flexion of the DIP joint was possible. They felt that 20 of 25 patients (80%) had a satisfactory result.

McClinton et al. (12) reported 100 tendon grafts for isolated flexor digitorum profundus injuries in 96 patients, 86% of whom were 40 years of age or younger. Preoperatively, all fingers had full passive range of motion. The palmaris longus tendon was used in 80 cases, and the extensor digitorum communis in 10. The tendon graft was passed around the superficialis decussation in 93 cases and through it in 7 cases. A Bunnell pullout wire was used at the distal juncture, and either a Pulvertaft tendon weave or Bunnell tendon suture was used proximally. Tension was set to maintain a normal digital cascade with the hand in repose. They preferred 30 mm of passive excursion of the muscle tendon unit as a prerequisite to grafting to minimize PIP joint flexion contracture. The hand was immobilized for 1 week postoperatively, after which full passive motion of the PIP joint with the metacarpophalangeal (MP) joint flexed was begun. Rehabilitation was advanced to full flexion and extension at 4 weeks and resisted flexion at 8 weeks. Forty-five patients were able to flex to the distal palmar crease; an additional 24 could flex to within 1.3 cm. More than 90% of the fingers obtained greater than 20° of flexion at the DIP joint. Fifty-five patients lost less than 10% of PIP joint extension, three lost 11–20%, and six lost 21–30%. According to Stark's criteria (a satisfactory result had flexion to at least 3.2 cm of the midpalmar crease, 20° voluntary DIP flexion, and lacked no more than 30° PIP extension; combined PIP/DIP extensor lag was not to exceed 40° for the index or middle finger and 60° for the ring or little finger), greater than 90% of the patients had a satisfactory result.

Jaffe and Wekesser (13) reported 30 patients, ages 1.5 to 61 years when treated. Preoperatively, all fingers had passive ROM to within 0.5 cm of the distal palmar crease. The palmaris tendon was used in 23 patients and the plantaris in seven. Grafts were placed through the superficialis decussation. Graft tension was set at slightly greater flexion than in the normal digital cascade. Three weeks of immobilization were followed by active and passive flexion and then passive extension. Seventeen out of 30 had good or excellent results, while six had poor results. This includes patients who required tenolyses, all of whom achieved a good result.

Bora (14) reported flexor tendon grafting in 20 fingers of children ranging from 4 months to 13 years of age. Full passive ROM was present prior to surgery. The plantaris was used in 19 patients, the profundus in one. The graft was placed through the bifurcation, after which the hand was immobilized with an axilla-to-fingertip cast for 3 weeks. He obtained 17 satisfactory results.

Pulvertaft (15) reported 68 cases, using the plantaris in 46 and the long toe extensor tendon in the remainder. An attempt was made to place the graft through the superficialis decussation; however, if it was too tight, one slip of the superficialis was excised. Tension was set at slightly increased normal flexion in repose. The hand was immobilized for 3 weeks with the digit in response. Sixty-eight percent (33 grafts) were good or excellent, and 83% (57 grafts) were worthwhile. There were 11 poor results, and the digital function was worse in two patients. Poorer results were noted after age 31.

Single-stage profundus grafting in the presence of an intact superficialis provides a reasonable opportunity to improve function. The digit must be supple, and the patient should exhibit the need and possess the commitment to obtain a satisfactory result. Aggressive postoperative therapy is a necessity.

Tendon Graft When Profundus and Superficialis Tendons Are Injured

OPERATIVE PROCEDURE

Exposure is gained through a volar zig-zag incision. A rectangular flap of digital sheath is reflected between the A2 and A4 pulleys. Care is taken to preserve the distal stump(s) of the superficialis tendon. The volar plate is exposed. The level of tendon laceration is determined by inspection of the sheath and knowledge of the digital posture at the time of injury. The distal end of the profundus

tendon is usually between the A2 and A4 pulley or may have retracted beneath the A4 pulley. The synovial lining of the sheath is opened distal to the A4 pulley, and the distal end of the tendon is identified.

The superficialis and profundus tendons and the opening of the A1 pulley are exposed by excising a window of palmar fascia. Scar about the tendons is excised, and the proximal end of the tendons may be retrieved into the palm. If this cannot be easily done, either the vinculum longus or scar is responsible. Adhesions beneath the A1 or A2 pulleys are released with a Freer elevator or tenotomy scissors. If the superficialis tendon has been cut distal to its decussation, excellent flexion at the PIP joint can be obtained if the superficialis is repaired. If the vinculum is intact, direct repair of the superficialis can be performed, and the profundus is grafted, if needed, as described under Profundus Isolated Injury. If the superficialis cannot be repaired, the proximal ends of the distal segment are sutured to the distal edge of the A2 pulley with the PIP joint in 10° flexion. This will prevent hyperextension deformity of the PIP joint. If the distal stump of the superficialis is too short, a slip of superficialis is resected and sutured across the PIP joint to prevent hyperextension.

Adjusting Tension in a Tendon Graft

There are several methods for estimating proper graft length. The following two have proven reliable in our experience. In the first, the finger is fully extended, a clamp is placed on the distal end of the tendon graft, and tension is applied to fully extend the muscle. The repair site is marked on the graft. A modified Bunnell suture is inserted so that the mark is between the criss-crosses. This compensates for the accordion effect that occurs when the suture is tied. The digital cascade of the injured hand serves as a guide to appropriate resting tension. A tendon graft should never be left too long. It is acceptable (and some even consider it desirable) to have the tension slightly greater because the repair site can elongate several millimeters.

In the second method, a clamp is placed on the distal end of the tendon graft, and the excursion of the tendon is marked under maximum and minimum tension with the wrist in neutral position and the fingers at rest. The distal attachment of the graft should be at the midpoint. The wrist and MP joints are flexed, allowing the tendon graft to be advanced distally for easy suture. The methods for distal attachment of a tendon graft are described below. Again, if the tension is too loose (i.e., if the graft is too long), the patient will never get a good result. If the finger is extended relative to its appropriate stance, the distal suture is removed, and the tension is readjusted.

Distal Attachment of the Tendon Graft

The method of distal attachment is determined by the length of profundus stump remaining attached to the distal phalanx.

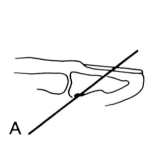 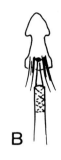 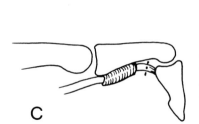

A   B   C

FIGURE 9.2. **A,** A drill hole is made in the distal phalanx from the site of profundus attachment angling dorsally and exiting distal to the lunula. **B,** The profundus stump is split, a hole drilled in the distal phalanx, and the tendon advanced into the hole. The profundus slips can be sutured to the graft for added fixation. **C,** The site of tendon repair must not impinge on the A4 pulley when the DIP joint is fully flexed.

NO PROFUNDUS STUMP AVAILABLE

A drill hole is placed through the base of the distal phalanx at the site of profundus insertion. This hole is angled distally so that the germinal matrix of the nailbed will not be injured (Fig. 9.2A). The suture is attached to the tendon, threaded through the drill hole with a Keith needle, and tied over a padded button.

LESS THAN 1 CM OF PROFUNDUS STUMP

The stump is split longitudinally to the bone. The bone is roughened and slightly grooved with a chisel. A drill hole is made between the split tendon ends to exit dorsally distal to the germinal matrix (Fig. 9.2B). A suture is secured to the tendon graft, passed through the drill hole, and tied over a padded button. The split ends of the profundus are sutured to the tendon graft while being careful not to cut the tendon suture with the needle.

AT LEAST 1 CM OF PROFUNDUS STUMP

After the suture has been attached to the tendon graft, it is criss-crossed through the tendon stump using only 5 mm for suture attachment. Thus, the normal tendon insertion is preserved. The repair site must not impinge on the A4 pulley when the DIP joint is fully flexed (Fig. 9.2C).

With each method, a single throw is placed in the tendon suture and held taut while the wrist is flexed and extended. The graft is not trimmed. The fingers should flex and extend in concert. If the operated finger is extended relative to its normal position in the digital cascade, the distal tendon attachment is taken down. The tendon graft is too long, and the distal suture must be placed more proximally on the graft. The maneuvers outlined above are repeated until proper tension has been obtained. If the tendon graft is too short (a slight discrepancy is tolerated and even preferred by some), the suture is removed, tension determined, and the suture reinserted. If the distal tendon has been trimmed before tension assessment and too little length is left to make the necessary adjustments, a second graft must be harvested. If the DIP joint assumes 30 to 40° of flexion after the tendon graft has been attached distally, the DIP joint is transfixed in extension with a K wire. The wire is left in

place for 6–10 weeks. DIP joint flexion deformity noted at the operating table only becomes more pronounced in the future.

Once the tendon is marked under the desired tension, the suture must be placed to ensure that tension is preserved. A modified Bunnell suture is started 8 mm proximal to the mark and is exited 3 mm distal to the mark. As the suture is tied, the tendon is compressed while maintaining proper tension. The wrist and MP joints are flexed, and the forearm is held midway between pronation and supination to allow excellent exposure for closure of the skin wound over the middle and distal phalanges without placing tension on the graft.

Tendon Grafts Not Traversing the Digital Sheath—"Bridge Grafts"

Infrequently, there is loss of flexor tendon length proximal to the A1 pulley, and the distal tendons are free of adhesions within the digital sheath. Only the proximal portion of the digital sheath is exposed through a semilunar palmar incision. The skin flaps are reflected from the palmar fascia, and the palmar fascia is resected over the involved tendons. The proximal and distal ends of the tendons are identified. The distal stump of the superficialis is cut and allowed to retract into the sheath. If the superficialis is already within the sheath and joint extension is not restricted, the tendon is left undisturbed. If the profundus has been cut distal to the lumbrical and the lumbrical has not been severed, the proximal end of the tendon can be retrieved through the palmar incision. The lumbrical is excised. If the tendon has been cut proximal to the lumbrical or the latter severed, the proximal end usually retracts into the carpal canal or forearm. Under these circumstances, two incisions (palmar and distal forearm) are preferred, rather than opening the carpal canal. The profundus tendon is identified in the forearm, and a Hager dilator is passed through the carpal canal in the proper plane into the palm and directed toward the involved finger. The tendon graft is sutured to the profundus tendon, and its distal end is sutured to the proximal end of the dilator and guided through the carpal canal into the palm. Tension is determined as follows: (*a*) gentle traction is placed on the distal segment of profundus tendon with the finger held in full extension; (*b*) traction is placed on the tendon graft to provide maximal extension of the muscle belly; (*c*) the tendons are marked where they overlap proximal to the edge of the A1 pulley; and (*d*) the tendon ends are repaired with a modified Bunnell suture.

If the tendons are not gliding freely within the digital sheath, the tendon graft should be extended to the distal phalanx. The digital sheath is exposed throughout the finger through a volar zig-zag incision. A rectangular flap of sheath is reflected over the PIP joint, and the sheath is opened over the DIP joint. A tenolysis is performed, and the profundus is extracted distally, maintaining its insertion. The superficialis insertion is left intact. The decussations are sutured to the distal edge of the A2 pulley to prevent PIP joint hyperextension. Tendon grafting is performed as described under Profundus Tendon Injury.

Flexor Tendon Grafts in Children

Some surgeons defer tendon grafting until a child is 3 or 4 years of age or older, when control is possible (16, 17). Our experience has been that the younger child uniformly develops an excellent result if prevented from breaking the tendon repair. Indications and operative procedure for tendon repair or grafting are the same for children and adults.

Dressing

COOPERATIVE ADULTS

The wrist is held in neutral or slight flexion with the MP joints at 70–90° of flexion and the PIP and DIP joints in full extension. Opened 4 × 4 sponges are placed between the fingers. The PIP joint(s) of the operated finger(s) is maintained in slight (15–20 °) flexion. An ABD pad is cut with a thumb hole and wrapped around the wrist. A second pad is required around the wrist and forearm. Cotton or Dacron batting is placed in the palm, and more opened 4 × 4 sponges are placed between the fingers and over the batting. A KLING gauze is wrapped snugly to cover the entire dressing. COBAN is applied to provide gentle, even pressure.

CHILDREN

Immobilization is accomplished with a small, snug, bulky dressing incorporating an aluminum splint. After the tendon graft has been performed, the nonoperated fingers are taped in extension to a padded aluminum splint without intervening dressings. The operated finger is flexed to 70° at the MP joint. Padding is placed in the palm. A strip of tape is applied dorsally, extending over the fingertip into the palm and up the volar forearm. This holds the grafted finger in flexion (45° at the PIP and 30° at the DIP joint). While this is certainly a position to be avoided in adults, it has no deleterious effect in young children. The dressing is reinforced weekly as needed. At 4 weeks, the dressings are discarded, and the parents are instructed in gentle extension exercises and told to en-

courage the child to grasp objects. No formal therapy is given. The child is allowed normal use of the hand. We have not had rupture of a tendon graft when treated as outlined above.

Postoperative Management after Flexor Tendon Grafting (Adults)

Postoperative management is determined by the status of the superficialis tendon. If it is intact, the dressing is discarded after 3–5 days, and a splint is fabricated to hold the wrist in neutral and all fingers in the protective (intrinsic plus) position with the PIP joint of the operated finger held in slight (15–20°) flexion. Active isolated flexion of the grafted finger superficialis tendon is begun. The grafted profundus is not disturbed. The splint is removed frequently, and the nonoperated fingers are exercised. At 3 weeks, profundus motion is begun as described below.

If the superficialis is not intact, a snug, noncompressive dressing that extends from the fingertips to the antecubital fossa is applied. The wrist is in a neutral or slightly flexed position, and the digits are maintained in the intrinsic plus position. No active or passive motion is permitted. After 3 weeks of complete immobilization, the dressing and sutures are removed.

During the first week after dressing removal, the following exercises are begun: (*a*) passive flexion of the MP, PIP, and DIP joints; (*b*) gentle active PIP joint flexion with the MP joint stabilized in flexion; (*c*) gentle active DIP joint flexion with the MP and PIP joints stabilized in flexion; (*d*) massage of the fingers and hand without forcing the fingers into extension; and (*e*) massage of the palmar or wrist scar in a proximal-to-distal direction during active finger flexion.

During the second through the fourth weeks, when the patient is performing exercises (*b*) and (*c*) above, the MP and PIP joints are stabilized in gradually increasing amounts of extension. By the fifth week, resistance is applied to these flexion exercises. During this time, massage as described above is applied with increasing force. These basic exercises are continued until the patient has reached full recovery.

During the second week of rehabilitation, gentle passive extension of the PIP joint is obtained with the MP and DIP joints flexed. Similarly, the DIP joint is extended with the MP and PIP joints flexed. Active flexion of the PIP and DIP joints with the MP joint stabilized in flexion is initiated. During the third week, gentle passive extension of both the PIP and DIP joints is encouraged with the MP joint first in flexion, then in increasing amounts of extension. Active extension of the fingers is encouraged. All patients are encouraged to exercise frequently during the day for periods of 5–20 minutes.

Splints are fabricated as soon as the dressing is removed. A static dorsal protective splint maintains the operated finger in flexion and prevents extension. With the splint in place, the patient can continue to work on active flexion and move his other fingers freely. Two weeks after dressing removal, this splint is discarded.

Within 4 weeks after removal of the dressing, individual patient problems begin to appear. Passive extension of the PIP and DIP joints is often not possible. If indicated, dynamic splinting of these joints is begun during the 4th week after dressing removal. Dynamic force is applied through the use of a rubber band in an outrigger hand splint or with piano wire in a spring-type finger extension splint. Dynamic splinting does not exceed 7–8 oz of pull with a rubber band splint or 9–10 oz with a piano wire splint. Patients are encouraged to use their hands gradually for functional activities and to perform daily activities as soon as they can tolerate them.

Rate of Recovery of Tendon Gliding after Grafting

This has been documented only when the superficialis and profundus are severed and the profundus grafted (18). In a series of 24 tendon grafts, within 6 weeks the average patient regained 50% of preoperative gross grip strength and 115° total active motion, which was 50% of the motion obtained at 1 year. By 12 weeks after grafting, the average patient had regained 66% of preoperative gross grip strength and 176° of total active motion (77% of the motion attained at 1 year). The rate of recovery was greatest during the first 4 months. As expected, motion at the MP joint approached normal within 6–8 weeks after surgery. DIP joint motion recovered more slowly than PIP joint motion.

Results after Flexor Tendon Grafting

Boyes and Stark analyzed the results of graft flexor reconstruction in 607 fingers (19). They found that the most important factor was the preoperative condition (scarring, joint contracture, multiple injuries) of the finger. Patients 40 years of age and older had poorer results. A similar analysis by Kunzle et al. (20) agrees with these findings. In our series of 24 grafts, the average patient obtained a final result at 1 year of 160% of preoperative gross grip strength and 227° of total active motion (18). Nineteen patients could flex to within 3.5 cm of the distal palmar crease, seven of these to 1.2 cm or less.

Results after "Bridge Graft"

Stark et al. reported 41 flexor tendon grafts (37 fingers, 10 thumbs, 6 grafts used to repair two tendons) in 31 patients aged 3 to 69 years (21). There was loss of tendon substance between the musculotendinous junction and the distal palmar crease outside the digital sheath. The assessment criteria were modified so that satisfactory results included finger flexion to within 5 cm or less of the midpalmar crease. Thumb IP active flexion would have to equal 75% of the uninjured thumb with acceptable MP and full IP extension. In the 37 fingers, the superficialis tendon was used 20 times, the palmaris 10 times, and the extensor indicis proprius once. In six patients, a single graft was applied to both the ring and little fingers. Of the 37 fingers, 35 could flex to within 5 cm of the midpalmar crease. Seven of the 35 were unsatisfactory due to limited extension, though five of the seven patients felt that the operation had improved use of the hand. Satisfactory function was obtained in 8 of 10 thumbs.

Management of Unsatisfactory Result after Flexor Tendon Graft

Management decisions are based on the results obtained. To determine progress properly, active and passive range of motion should be recorded at least every 4 weeks. When the rate of recovery reaches a plateau, this should be verified over 1–2 months. If the patient is displeased with the functional result, we recommend use of an algorithm to provide an orderly approach to the problems (Fig. 9.3).

Indications for Tenolysis and/or Capsulotomy

A determination must be made as to whether lack of function is due to adhesions limiting tendon gliding, rupture of the tendon graft, or to stiff joints. This decision is based on the total range of motion and the relationship between passive and active joint motion. Individual motivation is a consideration in adults who must work diligently to maintain the gains accomplished at surgery. Children usually form soft adhesions following tenolysis and capsulotomy, and these procedures are routinely used when indicated without consideration of cooperativeness. If passive joint flexion is limited but exceeds active motion, adhesions are restricting flexor tendon gliding. The cause of limited passive joint flexion must be determined. It may be due to adhesions involving the extensor tendon or scarring of the dorsal joint capsule and/or the dorsal one third of the collateral ligaments. The extent of involvement can only be determined at the time of surgery.

If passive joint flexion is normal and exceeds active joint flexion, a flexor tenolysis is required. If passive and active joint motion are equal but inadequate, both tenolysis and capsulotomy are required. Both flexor and extensor systems may require tenolysis. If passive PIP joint extension is normal and exceeds active PIP joint extension, an extensor tenolysis is required.

Thus, the operative procedure required may be: (*a*) capsulotomy; (*b*) capsulotomy and extensor tenolysis; (*c*) capsulotomy and flexor tenolysis; (*d*) capsulotomy and flexor and extensor tenolysis; (*e*) extensor tenolysis; (*f*) extensor and flexor tenolysis; or (*g*) flexor tenolysis.

CAPSULOTOMY AND LOCAL TENOLYSIS

This operative procedure is routinely performed under local anesthesia as an outpatient. Digital or wrist-block anesthesia is established utilizing 1% xylocaine (*without*

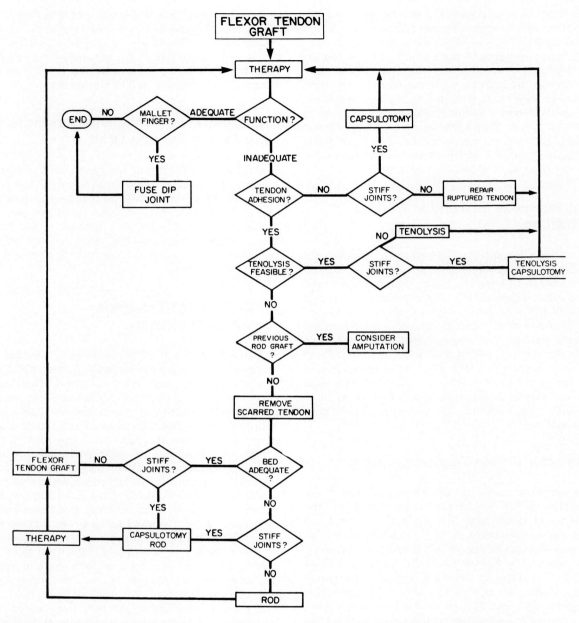

FIGURE 9.3.   An algorithm for management after flexor tendon graft is shown. This approach is used by the authors as an aid to orderly evaluation and restoration of function.

epinephrine). If wrist block anesthesia is used, the intrinsic contribution to digital function will not be present. After blood has been expressed from the upper extremity, an arm tourniquet is inflated to 75–100 mm Hg above the patient's systolic pressure. A dorsal serpentine incision over the PIP joint is used if the joint is stiff in extension. A volar zig-zag incision over the proximal and middle phalanges is used if the PIP joint is stiff in flexion. The volar incision is marked to the level of the distal palmar crease, but initially only the distal portion of the incision is made. If the joint is still in flexion and extension, only a volar approach is used.

The procedure usually takes 20–30 minutes, and the patient is able to actively extend and flex the fingers. If the tourniquet becomes uncomfortable, it is released and reinflated in 10 min. Alternatively, a sterile forearm tourniquet may be used and inflated just prior to arm tourniquet release (22). At the end of the procedure, bleeding is controlled by coagulation of vessels and elevation and compression of the hand for 15 min. The surgical drapes are lowered, and the range of motion under anesthesia is demonstrated to the patient as a realistic goal. The wounds are closed, and a light dressing applied. A plaster splint may be used to maintain digital positioning until a plastic splint is fabricated at the first rehabilitation session, which is usually later that day.

FINGER STIFF IN EXTENSION

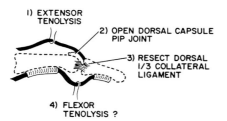

FIGURE 9.4. The order of procedure for releasing the PIP joint stiff in extension is noted.

PROCEDURE IF JOINT IS STIFF IN EXTENSION

A dorsal serpentine incision is made over the proximal interphalangeal joint. The skin flaps are reflected, and the free edges of the extensor hood identified. An incision is made along the free edge of the lateral bands from the midproximal phalanx to the midmiddle phalanx. The lateral bands are freed, and the insertion of the central slip is identified and preserved. The extensor tendon is inspected proximally, and a tenolysis is performed if necessary (Fig. 9.4-*1*). An incision is made into the dorsal capsule of the joint (Fig. 9.4-*2*). After each structure is freed of adhesions, the patient's ability to actively flex the finger is evaluated. If flexion is inadequate, the dorsal one-third of the collateral ligaments are incised (Fig. 9.4-*3*). At this point, full passive flexion is possible. If the patient cannot fully flex the finger actively, a flexor tenolysis is performed as described later (Fig. 9.4-*4*). When 90° of active PIP joint flexion has been obtained, it is demonstrated to the patient. The wounds are sutured, and a light dressing applied. Therapy is begun later that day.

PROCEDURE IF JOINT IS STIFF IN FLEXION

A volar zig-zag incision is made extending from the midproximal phalanx to the midmiddle phalanx. The flexor tendon sheath is identified, and the collateral ligaments of the PIP joint are exposed by transecting Cleland's ligaments. The digital sheath over the PIP joint is opened, and tension is placed on the flexor tendons to see if they are adherent (Fig. 9.5). If the tendons are adherent, a flexor tenolysis is performed. If full extension is not possible after flexor tenolysis is complete, the accessory collateral ligaments, including the volar one-third of the collateral ligaments, are divided. Passive extension is tested again, and if inadequate, the volar plate is inspected. If it is taut with the joint extended, the periosteum of the proximal phalanx is freed, maintaining attachment of the volar plate to the periosteum proximally. Care is taken to prevent hyperextension instability of the PIP joint. This is caused by resecting too much collateral ligament and over-releasing the volar plate. If hyperextension occurs, it is corrected by suturing a distally attached slip of the superficialis to the A2 pulley or the periosteum of the proximal phalanx or by maintaining the

FINGER STIFF IN FLEXION

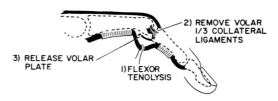

FIGURE 9.5. The order of evaluation of PIP joints stiff in flexion is presented.

PIP joint in slight flexion by dorsal splinting with advancement to full extension over 2–3 weeks (as in treatment of a complete PIP dislocation). If active extension is inadequate after full passive extension has been obtained, the extensor tendon is inspected, and tenolysis is performed through the volar incision.

Postoperative Management: Capsulotomy and Local Tenolysis

Active digital motion is begun during the first 24 hr with a light dressing in place. All patients are instructed in the therapy at this time. If visiting a therapy unit two or three times per week is not feasible, a home therapy program is developed. Such patients are seen as often as possible. Gentle active flexion and extension exercises are outlined for hourly performance. Exercise equipment such as a black roll, dowel stick, and exercise board are utilized. Dynamic and/or static splints are fabricated within the first postoperative day to maintain the gains obtained at surgery. The patient is encouraged to use the hand for light everyday activities. Precautions against sports and heavy lifting are stressed.

During the second week, edema is controlled by a compression stockinette, COBAN wrapping, and massage. Hourly active exercise sessions are continued. Light resistance is added. Additional splints are fabricated if necessary. The patient continues using the hand for light activities. During the third week, scar massage becomes more vigorous. The patient continues hourly active exercises, and more resistance is added. Splinting is advanced as needed, and the patient is encouraged to use his hand for most everyday activities. During the fourth to sixth weeks, scar massage is vigorous. Distal-to-proximal massage is begun. Resistive exercise continues. Appropriate splinting continues, and the patient is encouraged to return to work using his hand without restrictions.

RESULTS AFTER CAPSULOTOMY AND LOCAL TENOLYSIS

In our series of 185 fingers (146 patients), change in active range of motion varied from a loss of 42° to a gain of 100° (23). The average gain in active motion was 23°, 39°, and 12° for the MP, PIP, and DIP joints, respectively. Capsulotomy was limited to the PIP joints. The average pain in passive motion was 20°, 33°, and 13° for the MP, PIP, and DIP joints, respectively.

Extensive Tenolysis After Flexor Tendon Graft

Tenolysis is indicated after flexor tendon graft if (*a*) the passive range of joint motion exceeds the active range of joint motion, and (*b*) the active range of joint motion is insufficient to meet the patient's requirement. Satisfactory skin coverage, skeletal stability, adequate joint function, and at least protective sensation are prerequisite.

It is important to determine as accurately as possible the level of the most significant adhesions that are preventing gliding. The adhesions are almost always more extensive than preoperative examination implies, and one must be prepared to explore the entire length of the tendon at the time of surgery.

The ideal interval between tendon grafting and tenolysis is unknown. Verdan (24) states that, if a satisfactory range of motion is not obtained, tenolysis should be performed 3 months after repair (19, 25, 26). Others have recommended waiting 6 months before performing a tenolysis. The reasons for the delay are twofold: (*a*) tendon function may improve spontaneously up to 6 months after tendon graft, and (*b*) tendon graft rupture may be a greater risk when tenolysis is done only 3 or 4 months postoperatively. Tenolysis in a chicken tendon graft model weakened the tendon at 6 weeks; at 12 weeks, tenolysis did not weaken the tendon and resulted in increased blood supply (27). In our experience, tendon graft rupture does not occur if the tenolysis is delayed for 6 months.

If the joints are supple, evaluation of tendon gliding is much easier. If the joints are stiff, tendon gliding can only be evaluated after the joints have been mobilized. Capsulotomy is performed under local anesthesia. This permits evaluation of active tendon gliding at the operating table. If there are restricting tendon adhesions, a volar zig-zag incision is made from the DIP joint crease to the mid-palmar area. The digital sheath is exposed for the length of the skin incision. A flap of sheath is raised at the PIP joint. Flexor tendons are freed from local adhesions. The interval between the A1 and A2 pulleys is identified, the tendons visualized, and traction applied to the tendons at the PIP level to determine the site of adhesions (Fig. 9.6). Most often, the tendons are adherent under the A2 pulley. If tension on the tendons over the PIP joint fails to produce full DIP joint flexion, the sheath over the DIP joint is opened, and the tendon is elevated with tension applied to it. Frequently, the site of adhesions between the tendon and the middle phalanx becomes obvious and can be divided. A Freer elevator is helpful in dividing adhesions beneath the A2 and A4 pulleys. It is easy to damage or divide the tendon inadvertently beneath the pulleys. Full active tendon gliding must be obtained. The range of active motion is demonstrated to the patient at

FLEXOR TENDON TENOLYSIS

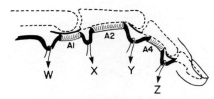

FIGURE 9.6. Tendon gliding is tested at W, X, Y, and Z to determine the level of tendon adhesions.

the operating table to provide added motivation postoperatively. Usually, a capsulotomy and tenolysis can be completed in 20 min. If not, the tourniquet must be deflated to permit voluntary muscle contraction. Alternatively, a second sterile forearm tourniquet may be inflated. Care must be taken to preserve the pulley mechanism. Tenolysis should be continued until the active range of motion is equal to the passive range of motion. Tendon strippers are not helpful and may actually damage the tendon or surrounding structures. Mobilization, rather than devascularization, of the tendon is the goal. The operative procedure is summarized in Table 9.2.

POSTOPERATIVE THERAPY

Active range of motion exercises are begun immediately after surgery. Early active exercises are important in obtaining a satisfactory result. Dynamic splints may aid in the restoration of extension. Active MP, PIP, and DIP joint flexion and extension exercises are performed frequently to prevent recurrent adhesions from restricting motion. Patient education regarding the importance of continuing to exercise throughout the day is essential. The hand is kept elevated over the first 48–72 hr in order to reduce edema. An elastic finger stocking made from an ace wrap is used at night or when the patient is not exercising. An inflatable finger cuff or COBAN wrapping can be used to reduce edema. Cold packs can be applied intermittently to reduce the inflammatory response to exercise. Passive exercises are used to prevent

Table 9.2
Flexor Tendon Tenolysis

1. Local anesthesia
2. Open digital sheath at W, X, Y, and Z (see Fig. 9.6)
3. Traction at W, X, Y, and Z (see Fig. 9.6)
4. Evaluate tendon gliding proximal and distal to traction point
5. Release adhesions
6. Test passive range of joint motion
7. Extensor tenolysis?
8. Capsulotomy?
9. Have patient actively flex and extend finger(s)
10. Show patient result of surgery

joint stiffness. Dynamic splinting is initiated if the patient displays limited motion in flexion or extension of any joint. Scar massage is begun when the incision is healed. As the patient progresses and his tolerance improves, more vigorous and resistive exercises are used to increase hand strength. The goal of therapy is to maintain tendon gliding and joint motion and to promote maximum functional use of the hand.

RESULTS OF TENOLYSIS AFTER TENDON GRAFTING

Kelly (28) reported on the indications for and the effectiveness of tenolysis after tendon grafting. In 71 patients requiring flexor tendon grafts, there were 10 secondary tenolyses. Four had improvement of function following tenolysis, but the degree of improvement was not noted. McCash (29) reported nine tenolyses out of a total of 33 secondary tendon repairs and tendon grafts. Fetrow (30) published the most extensive paper on tenolysis. He reported 220 flexor and extensor tenolyses in 134 patients; 24 patients had tenolysis performed more than once on a given tendon, and 31 patients had simultaneous tenolysis of two or more tendons. Tenolyses were required in 91 of 374 flexor tendon grafts (24%). Almost all of the tendon grafts were performed after repair of tendon lacerations in flexor zone II. Follow-up was obtained on 68 of the 91 tenolyses. A good or excellent result was classified as one in which the fingertip flexed to within 0.5 inch (about 13 mm) of the palm; a fair result was classified as one in which the fingertip flexed to between 0.5 and 1.5 inches (about 38 mm) of the palm; the remainder were classified as poor results. Of the 68 tenolyses, 26% of the patients were improved; 44% were greatly improved; and 30% were unchanged or made worse.

Thompson (31) reported that in five tenolyses required after 100 flexor tendon grafts function was improved in two. He believed that other patients would have been improved by tenolysis, but they either refused surgery or did not return for follow-up. Whitaker (32) reported tenolysis of 26 digits in 26 patients who had previously undergone tendon grafts. Improvement was noted in 81% of the fingers, 66% being good or excellent. Good was rated as 50 to 75% of passive potential being realized as active motion; excellent was greater than 75%.

Determining Tendon Rupture

The patient usually knows when he or she has ruptured the tendon graft. Frequently, a specific event is initially denied, but if pressed, the patient will recall one. When the graft has ruptured, the finger assumes a pronounced extension deformity. DIP joint motion is minimal or nil. There may be discoloration in the subcutaneous tissues due to hemorrhage. Tenderness at the site of disruption often persists for several days.

In a review of 110 tendon grafts, we had nine tendon ruptures in eight patients (33). The events leading to tendon disruption could be grouped as follows: (*a*) exercising—five tendons; (*b*) falling on outstretched hand—

three tendons; and (*c*) loss of button over nail—one tendon. The time of rupture after grafting was: exercise group, 23, 28, 44, 61, and 72 days; fall group, 29, 29, and 45 days; and "button" group, 12 days.

The site of disruption was the distal repair (four tendons), proximal repair (three tendons), and unknown (two tendons—patient refused surgery). In the tendons ruptured at the distal repair site, three were reattached to the distal phalanx and one required a rod-graft. The tendons ruptured at the proximal repair site required a tendon graft in two and a rod-graft in one. The total active ROM in those fingers in which the tendons were reattached was 210°, 221°, and 257°. Those requiring tendon grafts were 158° and 175°. Those requiring a rod-graft obtained 161° and 201°. The two tendon ruptures that were not treated surgically had 151° and 149° motion.

Occasionally, a patient gives a history of loss of motion after exercising accompanied by mild discomfort in the digit. We have found that, if the examination is repeated in 2 days, the patient is often again able to flex the finger actively. This appears to be a fatigue phenomenon with recovery within 2 days. Exploration is recommended if recovery has not occurred by this time. Surgery is recommended immediately when there is obvious rupture. At surgery, the wound over the volar surface of the distal phalanx is opened. If the distal end is not disrupted, an incision is made over the site of proximal repair. Distal disruptions can be resutured, but only if advancement of the tendon graft is minimal and does not significantly alter the balance among the fingers. Proximal disruptions usually require either a tendon graft or a rod-graft.

POSTOPERATIVE MANAGEMENT

There has not been sufficient experience with tendon rupture to develop a best method of postoperative management. If the tendon graft can be directly repaired, we resist immobilizing the hand for an additional 3 weeks. The tendon will have already gained some blood supply from adhesions and its intact anastomosis. Gentle motion may be initiated after reattachment of the tendon. Those receiving a new tendon graft are immobilized for 3 weeks. Those receiving a rod were mobilized within 3 days.

Indications for a Two-Stage Reconstruction of the Flexor Tendon Mechanism

Flexor system grafting in the presence of extensive scarring of the flexor sheath, stiff joints, or an adherent extensor system will not provide an optimal result. Reconstruction of an extensively damaged pulley system is best accomplished over a Silastic rod. Hunter has popularized the staged flexor tendon reconstruction (34). He suggests its main use is in the area of failed flexor tendon surgery or in crushing injuries in which the flexor system has been destroyed. A silicone rubber implant is inserted during the first stage to be replaced by a tendon graft at a second stage.

Table 9.3
Stage 1: Flexor Tendon Reconstruction—Rod-Graft

Pulleys
    Preserve—all
    Reconstruct—A2 and A4
        Tendon weave through sheath remnants

PIP Joint
    Capsulotomy as required

Tendon Management
    Superficialis
        Intact without adhesions
        Intact with adhesions—tenolysis
        Disrupted—suture distal slips to prevent joint hyperten-
            sion
    Profundus
        Resect proximal to lumbricate
        Leave 1.5 cm distal stump

Prosthesis
    Attachment
        Distal—suture beneath profundus stump
        Proximal—none
    Material
        Silastic tube (3 mm)
        Woven Dacron—silicon (5 mm)

Nerve Management
    Direct repair
    Surval nerve graft

A smooth-walled, mesothelium-lined sheath forms about the Silastic rod (35). The fluid produced by this synovial pseudosheath supplies metabolic substrate to the graft while a blood supply develops. Adhesions are vastly reduced. The salient features of the first stage are outlined in Table 9.3.

FIRST-STAGE FLEXOR MECHANISM RECONSTRUCTION

A volar zig-zag skin incision is utilized to expose the tendon sheath. All remaining pulley mechanism is preserved. If the superficialis tendon is intact, it is preserved. If it is adherent, a tenolysis is performed. If disrupted, a distal slip is sutured to the periosteum of the proximal phalanx or to the digital sheath to prevent PIP joint hyperextension. The level of proximal profundus tendon resection is controversial. We resect the profundus proximal to the lumbrical origin because we prefer to do our proximal tendon graft repair in the distal forearm. It is imperative that a distal stump be preserved so that the rod can be sutured between the tendon and the distal phalanx to prevent migration of the rod and erosion through the pulp. If the A2 or A4 pulleys are absent, they must be reconstructed. Synthetic materials have proven to be inadequate. Reconstruction with a tendon graft or extensor retinaculum are current favorites (36, 37). We prefer the former method using a 2 mm-thick slip of the resected profundus tendon. The rod is placed through the carpal tunnel with several centimeters left free in the forearm to make later identification easier. If the digital nerves are injured, direct repair is preferred, but grafts are usually required. Dressings are discarded 2 days after rod placement, and active and passive motion is begun.

DURATION OF ROD IMPLANT

In our series of 29 rod implants followed by tendon grafting, the rod was left in place from 70 to 168 days (median, 110 days). When the percentage recovery in range of motion was plotted against the duration of rod implant, there was no significant difference in the final functional result if the rod had been in place any time between 70 and 168 days (18).

SECOND-STAGE OF FLEXOR MECHANISM RECONSTRUCTION

If the rod cannot be palpated at the distal phalanx preoperatively, a lateral radiograph can be helpful in locating the distal end of the rod. If it has retracted into the palm, the operative procedure will be replacement of the rod. If the rod is in proper position, the operative procedure is outlined in Table 9.4. The skin incision over the DIP joint is reentered, and the distal end of the rod is identified. An L-shaped incision is made over the distal forearm. The forearm fascia is opened, the median nerve and superficialis tendons are retracted, and the appropriate profundus tendon identified. The proximal rod end is identified. The proximal end of the tendon is drawn into the wrist. The end may be trimmed but is left as long as possible. If the proximal end of the profundus tendon has been left long, the palmaris will reach the distal phalanx. If the profundus tendon has been resected in the distal forearm, the plantaris or a toe extensor is required to provide adequate length. After the proximal repair has been accomplished, the graft is sutured to the proximal end of the rod and advanced to the distal phalanx. Tension is determined, and attachment of the graft distally is accomplished as described earlier. Postoperative management is as described under tendon grafting.

Table 9.4
Stage II: Flexor Tendon Reconstruction—Rod-Graft

Incisions
    Distal—over profundus insertion
    Proximal—distal forearm

Tendon Graft (according to level of repair)
    Palm—palmaris
    Forearm—plantaris, toe extensor

Tendon Attachment
    Distal—Drill hole (Bunnell button—pull-out suture)
    Proximal
        Tendon ends equal, end-to-end repair
        Tendon ends unequal, brand repair

RESULTS OF TWO-STAGE FLEXOR TENDON RECONSTRUCTION

Hunter and Salisbury (38) reported significantly better than average results following primary repair in zone 2 injuries. Grafts were placed in 69 fingers (63 patients). Severity of injury varied, although all required two-stage grafting. After recovery, 59 (85.5%) were able to flex to within 3.2 cm of the distal palmar crease, 35 (50%) to 1.9 cm or less.

There is no significant difference between the results of Hunter and Salisbury and those of Boyes and Stark (19) for this entire series of tendon grafts. Nor are there differences between the results of Hunter and Salisbury and Madsen (39) in primary repairs in zone II injuries. If one considers only patients who have had previous tendon surgery, there is no significant difference in the number of poor results reported by Hunter and Salisbury and the number reported by Boyes and Stark. However, the number of excellent and good results of Hunter and Salisbury is significantly higher than that reported by Boyes and Stark.

Wehbe et al. (40) performed two-stage reconstructions in 150 fingers of 136 patients. Of these, 45% were of the most difficult severity level, presenting initially with additional nerve or vascular injury and/or contraction greater than 10° at any joint. The plantaris tendon was used preferentially (49.3%); toe extensors were a second choice (38.7%). The graft was attached to the distal phalanx by a pullout wire tied over a button in 91.8%; a Pulvertaft weave was used for the proximal anastomosis in 93.3%. Preoperatively, the mean palm-to-pulp active distance was 41 mm. At final follow-up, this had improved to 15 mm. The mean grip strength increased from 21% to 70% of normal. Patients less than 21 years of age obtained better results. Results were worse in the more severely damaged fingers and in patients with multiple injured rays. The complication rates were 28.7% and 43.0% for stages I and II, respectively. The most common complication after stage I was synovitis (27% of fingers); after stage II it was bowstringing at the PIP joint (21.5%), followed by tendon rupture and adhesions requiring tenolysis (14.1% and 12.4%).

LaSalle and Strickland (41) reported results on 43 two-stage reconstructions in 39 patients. Preoperative PIP and DIP passive ROM was compared to postoperative active ROM. There were three graft ruptures. The final results were graded as 65% fair or better with 16% excellent. Tenolysis was performed on 20 digits (46.5%). Although there was one graft rupture, no finger was worse after tenolysis, and 12 were upgraded, with final ratings of 36 (83.7%) fair or better and 11 (26.6%) excellent.

In our series (18) of 29 two-stage reconstructions, 62% obtained fair to excellent results, and 38% obtained poor results. All patients were followed for at least 52 weeks. One patient was considered a graft failure because of extensive scar. He regained only 99° of total active ROM. One patient sustained a disruption of the insertion of the tendon graft into the distal phalanx on the 25th day after surgery. This was reattached two days later. At 52 weeks, he had regained 240° of total active ROM in the finger. One rod became exposed and required removal. The rod was reinserted after the skin wound had been healed for three months, and the patient gained 188° of total active ROM at 52 weeks.

TWO-STAGE TENDON GRAFTING FOR ISOLATED PROFUNDUS INJURY

Gaisford et al. (9) first suggested two-stage reconstruction after isolated profundus injury. Versaci (42) reported a series of five patients in which three obtained a near normal DIP active ROM. A fourth patient had nearly as good a result although a pulley reconstruction was required, and a fifth patient obtained approximately 20% of active DIP flexion. It was noted that the patients obtaining the best results had the least damaged fingers preoperatively. Wilson et al. (8) performed 12 profundus grafts in 11 patients. The mean total active motion after operation was 166°; after second-stage grafting, this had increased to 240°. Digital pad-to-palm distance with active flexion was not reported. Eight patients presented with weakened grip compared to the normal hand; postoperatively, all were improved. One patient experienced a tendon graft rupture. All patients were young and highly motivated.

Sullivan (43) performed staged profundus reconstruction on 16 patients ages 19–37 years. Thirteen of the 16 patients obtained a subjectively acceptable result, although only seven of the 16 cases could be judged satisfactory by Stark's criteria (utilizing a 3.2-cm digital pulp-to-midpalmar crease distance). Three additional patients did note some improvement; three had no improvement, and three were made worse. Superficialis function was retained in all patients. There were five complications, including two tendon graft ruptures.

The three patients obtaining the best results in Versaci's series had the best preoperative digital condition. The patients in Wilson's series all had profundus avulsions or lacerations. In Sullivan's series, four sustained profundus avulsions, and 12 sustained zone 1 lacerations. These injuries are basically limited to the injured tendon (44). The best results were obtained in the younger patients. The results are not clearly better than those obtained in a similar patient population utilizing single-stage grafting. The cost of this option is a longer treatment period, a second operation, and the possibility of additional complications associated with the second stage of the procedure.

Inadequate Function After Two-stage Repair

The primary causes of inadequate function after rod-graft repair are mallet deformity (here resulting not from extensor disruption but from mechanical factors contributing to increased flexion moment at the DIP joint), stiff joint, and tendon adhesions. The only treatment we have found adequate for the mallet deformity is fusion of the DIP joint. Prior to fusion, the patient makes a decision regarding the amount of flexion needed in his activities to provide the best function.

DIP JOINT FUSION

Under local anesthesia, the DIP joint is exposed through a dorsal serpentine incision. The extensor tendon is divided 3–4 mm proximal to its insertion. The collateral ligaments are divided. The joint is flexed, and the condyles of the middle phalanx and the base of the distal phalanx are removed with a rongeur. The surfaces are beveled to provide the amount of flexion agreed upon preoperatively. Transverse drill holes are placed across the distal end of the middle phalanx and the distal phalanx in the same plane. A small K wire is drilled out the distal phalanx and retrograde into the middle phalanx. A 24-gauge stainless wire is threaded through the drill holes with the aid of a needle, and the wire twisted on the ulnar side of the joint. The K wire provides alignment in the horizontal plane, and the circumferential wire controls rotation. The K wire is left in place as long as possible, usually 2–3 months. Use of the finger in pinch or grasp is not permitted. Fusion is confirmed by radiography before the patient's return to work.

TENDON ADHESIONS OR STIFF JOINTS

Tendon adhesions and/or stiff joints may develop after a two-stage reconstruction. Hunter and Salisbury (38) reported a 6.7% tenolysis rate; Chamay (45) performed tenolysis in 21% of patients undergoing two-stage reconstruction. Neither study reported results of this procedure. As noted earlier, LaSalle and Strickland's (41) series noted a 46.5% tenolysis rate with one rupture and significant improvement in 60% of these fingers.

We recommend capsulotomy or tenolysis with the recognition that this is the last alternative. If unsuccessful, amputation should be discussed, but the decision should be delayed until the patient requests amputation. Often the need for amputation is only accepted after the patient returns to work. Unfortunately, some patients enter a repetitive cycle of operation and reoperation, undergoing many procedures that do little toward improving function. Use of a second rod, then graft, requires much discussion with the patient because of the time, expense, and generally poorer ultimate outcome. At this point in management, judgment gained by experience, both good and bad, has its greatest impact. The appropriate time to call a halt to operative intervention can only be gained through experience and concern for the patient.

References

1. Jones MW, Matthews JP: Flexor tendon grafting 48 years after injury. *J Hand Surg [Br]* 13:284, 1988.
2. Young VL, Wrap C, Weeks PM: The surgical management of stiff joints in the hand. *Plast Reconstr Surg* 62:835, 1978.
3. White WL: Tendon grafts: A consideration of their source, procurement and suitability. *Surg Clin North Am* 40:403, 1960.
4. Harvey FJ, Chu G, Harvey PM: Surgical availability of the plantaris tendon. *J Hand Surg* 8:243, 1983.
5. Vastamaki M: Median nerve as free tendon graft. *J Hand Surg [Br]* 12:187, 1987.
6. Aulicino PL, Ainsworth SR, Parker M: The independent long extensor tendon of the fifth toe as a source of tendon grafts for the hand. *J Hand Surg [Br]* 14:236, 1989.
7. Holm CL, Embrick RR: Anatomical consideration in the primary treatment of tendon injuries of the hand. *J Bone Joint Surg [Am]* 41:599, 1959.
8. Wilson RL, Carter MS, Holdeman VA, et al: Flexor profundus injuries treated with delayed two-staged tendon grafting. *J Hand Surg* 5:74, 1980.
9. Gaisford JC, Hanna DC, Richardson GS: Tendon grafting: A suggested technique. *Plast Reconstr Surg* 38:302, 1966.
10. Pulvertaft RG: Suture materials and tendon junctures. *Am J Surg* 109:346, 1965.
11. Stark HH, Zemel NP, Boyes JH, et al: Flexor tendon graft through intact superficialis tendons. *J Hand Surg* 2:456, 1977.
12. McClinton MA, Curtis RM, Wilgis EF: One hundred tendon grafts for isolated flexor digitorum profundus injuries. *J Hand Surg* 7:224, 1982.
13. Jaffe S, Weckesser E: Profundus tendon grafting with the sublimis intact. *J Bone Joint Surg [Am]* 49:1298, 1967.
14. Bora FW: Profundus tendon grafting with unimpaired sublimus function in children. *Clin Orthop Rel Res* 71:118, 1970.
15. Pulvertaft GR: Tendon grafting for the isolated injury of flexor digitorum profundus. *Bull Hosp Jt Dis Orthop Inst* 44:424, 1984.
16. Entin MA: Flexor tendon repair and grafting in children. *Am J Surg* 109:387, 1965.
17. Wakefield AR: The treatment of tendon injuries in children. Presented at the annual meeting of the American Society for Surgery of the Hand, Chicago, January 17, 1964.
18. Weeks PM, Wray RC: Rate and extent of functional recovery after flexor tendon grafting with and without silicone rod preparation. *J Hand Surg* 1:174, 1976.
19. Boyes JH, Stark HH: Flexor-tendon grafts in the fingers and thumb. *J Bone Joint Surg [Am]* 53:1332, 1971.
20. Kunzle AL, Brunelli G, Orsi R: Flexor tendon grafts in the fingers. *J Hand Surg [Br]* 9:126, 1984.
21. Stark HH, Anderson DR, Zemel NP, et al: Bridge flexor tendon grafts. *Clin Orthop Rel Res* 242:51, 1989.
22. Strickland JW: Flexor tenolysis. *Hand Clinics* 1:121, 1985.
23. Young VL, Clement R, Weeks PM, et al: Effectiveness of the proximal interphalangeal joint capsulotomy. Proceedings of the American Society for Surgery of the Hand. *J Hand Surg* 9:671, 1984.
24. Verdan CE: Primary and secondary repair of flexor and extensor tendon injuries. In Flynn JE (ed): *Hand Surgery*. Baltimore, Williams & Wilkins, 1966, pp 220–274.
25. Kleinert HE, Kutz JE, Ashbell TS, et al: Primary repair of lacerated flexor tendons in "no-man's land." *J Bone Joint Surg [Am]* 49:577, 1967.
26. Pulvertaft RG: Tendon grafts for flexor tendon injuries in the fingers and thumb. *J Bone Joint Surg [Br]* 38:175, 1956.
27. Wray RC, Moucharafafieh B, Braitberg R, Weeks PM: The optimal time for tenolysis. *Plast Reconstr Surg* 61:184, 1978.
28. Kelly AP Jr: Primary tendon repairs. *J Bone Joint Surg [Am]* 41:581, 1959.
29. McCash CR: The immediate repair of flexor tendons. *Br J Plast Surg* 14:53, 1961.
30. Fetrow KO: Tenolysis in the hand and wrist. *J Bone Joint Surg [Am]* 49:667, 1967.
31. Thompson RV: An evaluation of flexor tendon grafting. *Br J Plast Surg* 20:21, 1967.
32. Whitaker JH, Strickland JW, Ellis RK: The role of the flexor tenolysis in the palm and digits. *J Hand Surg* 2:462, 1977.
33. Kraemer BA, Young VL, Grasse P, et al: Characteristics and management of flexor tendon graft disruption. *Br J Plast Surg* 40:258, 1987.
34. Hunter JM: Staged flexor tendon reconstruction. *J Hand Surg* 8:789, 1983.
35. Rayner CR: The origin and nature of pseudo-synovium appearing around implanted silastic rods: An experimental study. *The Hand* 8:101, 1976.
36. Kleinert HE, Bennett JB: Digital pulley reconstruction employ-

ing the always present rim of the previous pulley. *J Hand Surg* 3:297, 1978.

37. Lister GD: Reconstruction of pulleys employing extensor retinaculum. *J Hand Surg* 4:461, 1979.
38. Hunter JM, Salisbury RE: Flexor-tendon reconstruction in severely damaged hands: A two-staged procedure using a silicone-Dacron reinforced gliding prosthesis prior to tendon grafting. *J Bone Joint Surg* 53:829, 1971.
39. Madsen E: Delayed primary suture of flexor tendons cut in the digital sheath. *J Bone Joint Surg [Br]* 52:264, 1970.
40. Wehbe MA, Hunter JM, Schneider LH, et al: Two-stage flexor-tendon reconstruction. *J Bone Joint Surg [Am]* 68:752, 1986.
41. LaSalle WB, Strickland JW: An evaluation of the two-staged flexor tendon reconstruction technique. *J Hand Surg* 8:263, 1983.
42. Versaci AD: Secondary tendon grafting for isolated flexor digitorum profundus injury. *Plast Reconstr Surg* 46:57, 1970.
43. Sullivan DJ: Disappointing outcomes in staged flexor tendon grafting for isolated profundus loss. *J Hand Surg [Br]* 11:231, 1986.
44. Chang WH, Thoms OJ, White WL: Avulsion injury of the long flexor tendons. *Plast Reconstr Surg* 50:260, 1972.
45. Chamay A, Verdan C, Simonette C: The two-stage graft: A salvage operation for the flexor apparatus (a clinical study of 28 cases). In Verdan C (ed): *Tendon Surgery of the Hand*. London, Churchill Livingstone, 1979, pp 109–112.

10

Principles of Cartilage Grafting

Joel Pessa, M.D. and Ronald Riefkohl, M.D., F.A.C.S.

Autogenous Cartilage

Autogenous cartilage is a versatile, dependable tissue that is readily available from a number of donor sites. These qualities make it an extremely useful tissue for transplantation by the plastic surgeon.

TYPES OF CARTILAGE

There are several types of cartilage categorized according to the characteristics of their intercellular matrix: hyaline, elastic, and fibrocartilage. Each type apparently behaves similarly when transplanted. These autogenous cartilage grafts can be used to achieve three different goals: (*a*) for simple volume replacement, (*b*) for structural support, and (*c*) as architectural support to create new form. Various techniques exist to adapt the cartilage graft to fulfill these usages.

HISTORICAL REVIEW

Although it is presently taken for granted that autogenous cartilage dependably survives transplantation, this is a relatively recent development. Bert (1) is credited with being the first person to transplant cartilage in animals in 1865, and Koenig (2) in 1896 was the first to use autogenous cartilage in humans to repair damaged tracheal cartilage. However, the modern era of cartilage transplantation was ushered in by Lyndon Peer (3) in his classic treatise *Transplantation of Tissues*. Prior to the 1940s, neither otolaryngologists nor plastic surgeons believed that transplanted septal cartilage would survive. In 1941, Peer reported his experiments (4) in which he transplanted autogenous septal cartilage beneath the abdominal skin in patients and found that these grafts survived when examined up to 3 years later. It was further shown that alar, septal, and conchal grafts survived up to 13 years after transplantation (5).

As a result of Peer's work, we now understand that autogenous cartilage, with or without perichondrium, survives transplantation into a well-vascularized bed and does not depend on vascular ingrowth for its survival. Transplanted cartilage will also retain its size and shape, and unlike rib or iliac bone, it does not depend on stress to maintain its volume.

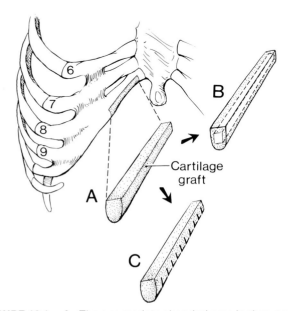

FIGURE 10.1. A, The appropriate chondral area is shown with an excellent source of varied sizes of cartilage. In order to minimize distortion of cartilage, the cone of the cartilage graft is used (**B**) or scoring of the opposite side of the expected distortion is carried out (**C**).

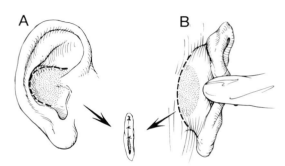

FIGURE 10.2. A, An anterior approach to the chondral cartilage is shown. The curvature of the cartilage in this area is suitable for replacing an orbital defect. **B,** The posterior auricular approach to the ear cartilage is shown. Notice possibility of contouring cartilage for a nasal dorsal graft.

FIGURE 10.3. A, A septal cartilage graft is shown being harvested. Care is taken to use a suitable graft from the lower septum to minimize the possibility of collapse of overlying cartilage. **B,** A chondromucosal graft is satisfactorily obtained from the septum as the donor area.

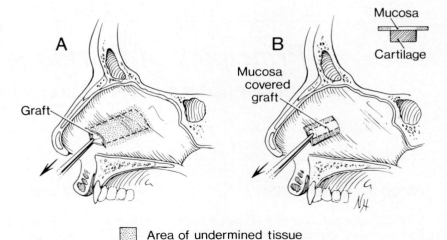

☐ Area of undermined tissue

SOURCE OF CARTILAGE

There are three common sources of autogenous cartilage grafts, and the site is determined by the intended use. Costal cartilage taken from the seventh, eighth, and ninth ribs has been used successfully for ear reconstruction (6–9) (Fig. 10.1). Costal cartilage can be harvested subperichondrially to allow for regeneration in the young patient (10). This cartilage can also be used for nasal alar and dorsal reconstruction (11, 12). A disadvantage of costal cartilage is its tendency to warp unless it is trimmed to balance intrinsic tension forces (13).

Ear cartilage, classified as elastic cartilage, has found widespread use for lower eyelid support (14–16), nipple-

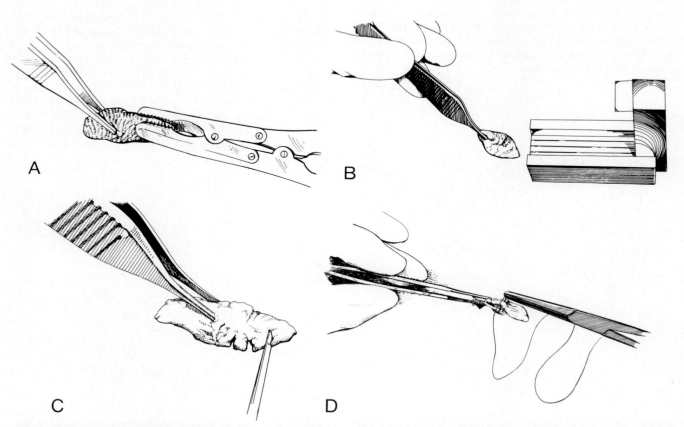

FIGURE 10.4. A, The technique of morselizing and softening the cartilage graft is shown. **B,** The use of the linear morselizer is shown. **C,** The technique of cross-cutting the cartilage is shown. **D,** The morselized cartilage can be shaped and tied with 5.0 nylon sutures.

areola reconstruction (17), and reconstruction of the orbital floor (18, 19). Conchal cartilage is also widely used in nasal reconstruction (20). Conchal cartilage can be harvested by either an anterior or posterior approach (Fig. 10.2). When harvesting conchal cartilage, a firm postoperative dressing is necessary, but drainage is not (14). One must also be careful in harvesting the conchal cartilage graft to avoid a visible step-off deformity (21).

Nasal septal cartilage, an example of hyaline cartilage, is most readily adapted to nasal reconstruction (22). Septal cartilage is harvested by a submucosal dissection; care must be taken to leave a 1-cm strut anterior and caudally to avoid a saddle-nose deformity or retrusive columella postoperatively (Fig. 10.3).

TECHNIQUES

A number of techniques exist to modify the shape of the cartilage graft (Fig. 10.4). Cartilage can be softened by morselizing or crushing the graft (Fig. 10.4A and B). Perichondrium can be scored, and when done on the concave surface, this allows the graft to straighten (Fig. 10.4B). Alternatively, cartilage can be abraded with a similar effect. A more pronounced effect can be obtained by cross-cutting the edges of the cartilage (Fig. 10.4C). Cartilage can also be diced to be used as a volume filler (23) or to reconstruct Montgomery's tubercles (17). Cartilage can be used as single or multi-tiered grafts (Fig. 10.4D). Furthermore, cartilage can be modified by combining it with other tissues as a composite graft (24, 25) or by wrapping it with temporalis fascia to soften the result (26, 27).

The future holds promising new developments in the way of banked cartilage (28), homologous cartilage, and treated xenograft cartilage (29). The perichondrocutaneous graft is an exciting development presently being investigated (30). As for the present, autogenous cartilage grafting is an extremely versatile technique that can be used in myriad ways limited only by the surgeon's experience and creativity.

References

1. Bert P: Sur la greffe animale. *CR Acad Sci* 51:587, 1865.
2. Koenig F: Über reaktive Vorgänge am Knorpel nach verschieden Schädigungen. *Arch Klin Chir* 124:1, 1923.
3. Peer LA: *Transplantation of Tissues.* Baltimore, Williams and Wilkins, 1955.
4. Peer LA: Fate of autogenous septal cartilage after transplantation in human tissues. *Arch Otolaryng* 34:696, 1941.
5. Peer LA: Cartilage grafting. *Surg Clin North Am* 24:404, 1944.
6. Tanzer RC: Total reconstruction of the external ear. *Plast Reconstr Surg* 23:1, 1959.
7. Brent B: The correction of microtia with autogenous cartilage grafts: The classic deformity. *Plast Reconstr Surg* 66:1, 1980.
8. Brent B: The correction of microtia with autogenous cartilage grafts: Atypical and complex deformities. *Plast Reconstr Surg* 66:13, 1980.
9. Fukuda O, Yamada A: Reconstruction of the microtic ear with autogenous cartilage. *Clin Plast Surg* 5:351, 1978.
10. Lester CW: Tissue replacement after subperichondral resection of costal cartilage: Two case reports. *Plast Reconstr Surg* 23:49, 1959.
11. Chait LA, Fayman MS: Treatment of postreconstructive collapsed nasal ala with a costal cartilage graft. *Plast Reconstr Surg* 82:527, 1988.
12. Furlan S: Correction of saddle nose deformities by costal cartilage grafts—a technique. *Ann Plast Surg* 9:32, 1982.
13. Gibson T, Davis WB: The distortion of autogenous cartilage grafts: Its cause and prevention. *Br J Plast Surg* 10:257, 1958.
14. Jackson IT, Dubin B, Harris J: Use of contoured and stabilized conchal cartilage grafts for lower eyelid support: A preliminary report. *Plast Reconstr Surg* 83:636, 1989.
15. Matsuo K, Hirose F, Takahashi N: Lower eyelid reconstruction with a conchal cartilage graft. *Plast Reconstr Surg* 80:547, 1987.
16. Marks MW, Argenta LC, Friedman RJ: Conchal cartilage and composite grafts for correction of lower eyelid retraction. *Plast Reconstr Surg* 83:629, 1989.
17. Brent B, Bostwick J: Nipple-areola reconstruction with auricular tissues. *Plast Reconstr Surg* 60:353, 1977.
18. Stark RB, Frileck SP: Conchal cartilage grafts in augmentation rhinoplasty and orbital floor fracture. *Plast Reconstr Surg* 43:591, 1969.
19. Constantian MB: Use of auricular cartilage in orbital floor reconstruction. *Plast Reconstr Surg* 69:951, 1982.
20. Peck GC: *Techniques in Aesthetic Rhinoplasty.* New York, Thieme-Stratton, Gower Medical Publishing, 1984.
21. Guyuron B: Simplified harvesting of the ear cartilage graft. *Aesthetic Plast Surg* 10:37, 1986.
22. Sheen JH: *Aesthetic Rhinoplasty.* St. Louis, C.V. Mosby Co., 1981.
23. Peer LA: Diced cartilage grafts. *Arch Otolaryng* 38:156, 1943.
24. Lehman JA, Garrett WS, Musgrave RH: Earlobe composite grafts for the correction of nasal defects. *Plast Reconstr Surg* 47:12, 1971.
25. Cosman B: Piggyback composite ear grafts in nasal ala reconstruction. *Ann Plast Surg* 5:293, 1980.
26. Siemian WR, Samiian MR: Malar augmentation using autogenous composite conchal cartilage and temporalis fascia. *Plast Reconstr Surg* 82:395, 1988.
27. Guerrerosantos J: Recontouring of the middle third of the face with onlay cartilage plus free fascia graft. *Ann Plast Surg* 18:409, 1987.
28. Sailer HF: Experiences with the use of lyophilized bank cartilage for facial contour correction. *J Max Fac Surg* 4:149, 1976.
29. Ersek RA, Delerm AG: Processed irradiated bovine cartilage for nasal reconstruction. *Ann Plast Surg* 20:540, 1988.
30. Brent B: The versatile cartilage autograft: Current trends in clinical transplantation. *Clin Plast Surg* 6:163, 1979.

11

Basic Principles of Nerve Grafting

Hano Millesi, M.D.

To achieve function, axons must enter the graft at the proximal site of coaptation, proceed along the graft, cross over to the distal stump, and proceed to the end organ. The nerve graft is not a *substitute* for the lost segment of a nerve; rather, it provides an environment in which axons of the proximal stump can cross the defect. Thus, nerve grafts are akin to a guiding rail. Even though this conceptualization is basically correct, it has been the source of a number of mistakes. Materials other than living nerve tissue might be just as suitable and more efficient if nerve grafts functioned only as a bridging mechanism. Based on this theory, nonvital nerve grafts and alloplastic materials have been used with consistently poor results to date.

Although the nerve graft *is* a guiding rail, this statement must be augmented by specifying those tissues for which it provides a passageway. Axons and axon branches need an environment provided by Schwann cells. A necessary additional function of these cells is the production of myelinated nerve fibers. Only if the Schwann cells have survived the grafting procedure can a viable graft serve as a railway for axons and thereby contain all of the necessary elements identical to a distal nerve stump.

In contrast, a nonviable (preserved) nerve graft provides a rail for a *neuroma* with new growth occurring along the preserved graft. This method of nerve regeneration was studied by Schröder and Seiffert (1) who referred to it as "neuromatous neurotization." For return of function, there is little doubt that this approach offers a less optimal chance of success.

Return of function can only be expected after the axons have crossed both sites of coaptation—the proximal and the distal ends of the graft. Because of this requirement, nerve grafting did not become widely accepted for some time. The basic argument was that if there was difficulty in axons crossing from one stump to another in an end-to-end nerve repair, it would only be compounded by the need to cross two coaptation sites.

In this chapter, some basic principles of nerve grafting are covered, including the anatomy of peripheral nerves, principles of nerve regeneration, and the essentials of nerve repair. A basic understanding of concepts is required because a generally accepted lexicon has not yet evolved and different authors use the same term without a common meaning.

Anatomical Structure of Peripheral Nerves

A *nerve trunk* consists of from one to many *fascicles* embedded in loose connective tissue (interfascicular epineurium) and surrounded by connective tissue (epifascicular epineurium). The *perineurium* consists of layers of mesothelial-like cells and collagen connective tissue. It envelopes the endoneurium and represents the demarcation between nonfascicular and fascicular tissues. It is responsible for the difference between the intrafascicular and extrafascicular environment of the nerve (the barrier function).

The endoneurial tissue within the fascicle contains *nerve fibers* with their endoneurial sheath. The central feature is the *axon,* surrounded by the axolemma. In addition, the nerve fiber consists of Schwann cells with myelin sheath in myelinated nerve fibers, a basal lamina, and a loose collagen framework.

The individual fascicles must be able to move against each other in order to adapt to the deformations during movements of the limb. This possibility is provided by the loose connective tissue of the interfascicular epineurium.

To avoid mechanical irritations, the nerve trunk has to be able to move against the surrounding tissue during joint motions. This possibility is provided by layers of a loose connective tissue, called the paraneurium or adventitia, that surrounds the whole nerve trunk and links the nerve to the surrounding structures. This tissue is regarded as a part of the epifascicular epineurium by some authors, but it can be easily differentiated by its different structure.

The relationship between fascicular and nonfascicular tissue in cross-section is of practical importance. The fascicular pattern changes along the course of a nerve and has great individual variation. Five basic types of *fascicular patterns* can be distinguished:

1. *Monofascicular pattern.* The nerve consists of one large fascicle (Fig. 11.1A).
2. *Oligofascicular pattern with few large fascicles (up to five).* There is only minimal epineurial tissue between the fascicles. The individual fascicles can be handled easily from outside, and exact fascicular coaptation is provided by careful trunk-to-trunk coaptation.

FIGURE 11.1. Basic types of fascicular patterns are shown. **A,** The nerve segment consists of only one large fascicle. There is only marginal epineurial tissue (monofascicular structure). **B,** The nerve segment consists of a few large fascicles. There is only minimal epineurial tissue between the fascicles. Each fascicle can be handled easily from the margin (oligofascicular structure with two to five fascicles). **C,** The nerve segment consists of a certain number of fascicles (six or more). The number is limited, and the size of the fascicles is such that handling is easy. The central fascicle cannot be controlled from the margin. A large quantity of interfascicular epineurium separates the individual fascicles (oligofascicular pattern with six or more fascicles). **D,** The nerve segment consists of many larger and smaller fascicles. Size and number make handling difficult. There is a good quantity of interfascicular epineurium between the fascicles. The fascicles are arranged in groups (polyfascicular pattern *with* group arrangement). **E,** There are many fascicles, varying in size, distributed diffusely over the cross-section, which makes surgical manipulation difficult (polyfascicular pattern *without* group arrangement).

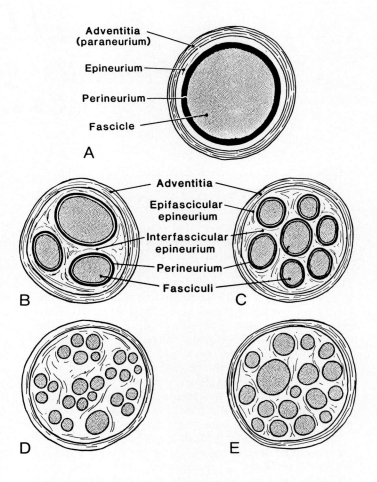

3. *Oligofascicular pattern with more than five fascicles.* If the nerve segment consists of more than five large manageable fascicles, an exact fascicular coaptation is not guaranteed by trunk-to-trunk coaptation. The central fascicles cannot be controlled from the margin. A large quantity of interfascicular epineurium separates the individual fascicles. There is the danger that fascicular tissue may contact nonfascicular tissue. In a nerve trunk the fascicles are large enough to be separated and to be prepared individually for fascicular coaptation. A digital nerve with more than five fascicles does not meet this criterion; rather, it corresponds to a fascicle group (Fig. 11.1*B* and *C*).
4. *Polyfascicular pattern with group arrangement.* The nerve consists of many fascicles of different sizes, arranged in groups with wider spaces of epineurial tissue between the groups (Fig. 11.1*D*).
5. *Polyfascicular pattern without group arrangement.* This pattern is one in which there are many fascicles of different sizes, diffusely arranged over the cross-section without group formation (Fig. 11.1*E*).

For surgical repair, the actual fascicular pattern must be known, and the distribution of motor and sensory fibers over the cross-section of the peripheral nerve is particularly important. Some investigators (2–4) have used electrical stimulation for sensory and motor fiber differentiation. This technique can only be applied during primary repair of the distal stump or with repair of the proximal stump in a conscious patient.

Several investigators (5–7) have used staining techniques in differentiating motor and sensory fibers; a higher content of acetylcholinesterase is indicative of motor fibers. In many cases, a satisfactory image of the fascicular pattern can be obtained by retrograde tracing of the fascicles from the next branching back to the site of transection (8).

Principles of Nerve Regeneration

During nerve regeneration, there are two separate processes that develop simultaneously: (*a*) both stumps must heal to reestablish continuity; and (*b*) axon sprouts must cross from proximal to distal stump to reach the end organs. The gap between the two stumps is filled by fibrin, migrating fibroblasts, and outgrowing capillaries. After a period of 3–4 days, collagen fibers are produced. Fibroblasts originate from epifascicular and interfascicular epineurial tissue, the perineurium, and endoneurial tissue.

There are good reasons to believe that endoneurial and perineurial fibroblasts are more specialized for nerve tissue than epineurial fibroblasts. For example, they produce finer collagen fibrils (diameter of 40–65 nm vs. 60–110 nm) (9). Schwann cells also migrate into the gap. In the normal environment of the axon (the endoneurium), there is a 9 : 1 ratio of Schwann cells to fibroblasts (10). If it can be assumed that this is an optimal relation, then the conclusion may be drawn that it is more favorable to axon sprouts when the tissue between the two nerve stumps contains a considerably higher quantity of Schwann cells than fibroblasts. Among the latter, endoneurial or perineurial fibroblasts are probably more desirable than epineurial fibroblasts. Based on the above analysis, it has been suggested that a strip of epineurial tissue be removed when repairing nerve segments of oligofascicular or grouped polyfascicular patterns (11–15).

Optimal conditions exist for nerve regeneration when axon sprouts can cross the gap between the nerve stumps in the early days after surgery (16). This can only occur when the axon sprouts originate close to the gap. Therefore, all damaged tissue of the proximal stump should be resected; otherwise it becomes fibrotic. Depending on the amount of retrograde degeneration, axon sprouts will then originate far more proximally and must grow along the fibrotic tissue of the stump before a delayed arrival at the gap. In the interim, the gap may be filled with collagen tissue, and the best opportunity for crossing has been lost.

If the axon sprouts do not meet a distal stump, they will form minifascicles with accompanying Schwann cells, fibroblasts, and capillaries, which have the potential to grow over some distance. A regeneration neuroma will be the result. Should the minifascicles meet the distal stump by random chance, there is some possibility of spontaneous healing of a transected nerve. Outgrowth of the minifascicles may be directed toward the distal stump by implanting a segment of an artery, an alloplastic tube, a mesothelial chamber (17), an empty perineurial tube (18), or a vein (19). When minifascicles meet a preserved nerve graft, the possibility of bridging a short defect occurs. Schröder and Seiffert (1) refer to the latter event as "neuromatous nerve regeneration."

Basic Principles of Nerve Repair

In the early days of peripheral nerve surgery, repair was by indirect coaptation ("cum carne"). At that time, surgeons were unwilling to manipulate nerve stumps primarily. Coaptation was achieved by carefully adjusting the edges of other structures to each other. Hueter (20) sutured the tissue around the nerve. It is not clear whether the paraneurium or the epineurium was used for anchoring stitches.

Different techniques have been developed for end-to-end repair of a transected nerve (neurorrhaphy), including:

1. Epineurial suture
2. Perineurial suture
3. Epiperineurial suture
4. Intrafascicular suture
5. Interfascicular guide suture

It becomes evident that the emphasis in labeling these techniques of neurorrhaphy was based on the type of tissue in which the anchoring stitches were placed. Actually, this is of little significance because sutureless techniques have been developed and compare favorably with a suturing approach. Further, to focus on the site of suture anchoring is an oversimplification. The main point is how well the fascicles of the cross-section coapt and not so much where sutures are placed, nor whether sutures or glue are used to secure the coaptation.

Basically, a neurorrhaphy is performed in four steps: (*a*) preparation of the stumps, (*b*) approximation, (*c*) coaptation, and (*d*) maintaining the coaptation.

PREPARATION OF STUMPS

There are essentially two ways in which nerve stumps can be prepared: by resection or by interfascicular dissection.

Resection

Partial excision of the damaged sections of both stumps may be the approach selected in preparing the severed nerve for the next step of the procedure (Fig. 11.2). In secondary nerve repair in which the damage of

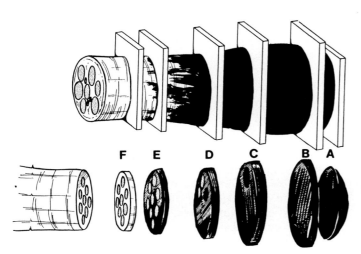

FIGURE 11.2. A nerve stump with eight fascicles and oblique damage is shown. Preparation of the stump is done by *resection*.

the stumps has become apparent by fibrosis, it is important to know whether the initial resection was performed until completely normal tissue was reached or until tissue showing fibrosis but preserved fascicular pattern was apparent in the cross-section (resection into an area of a third-degree damage). In some cases, a very limited resection might reach tissue that does not show a fascicular pattern (damage of fourth degree).

Interfascicular Dissection

In contrast to resection, the two stumps can be prepared by interfascicular dissection, resecting the epifascicular epineurium and separating individual large fascicles in an oligofascicular nerve segment or fascicle groups in a polyfascicular nerve segment with group arrangement.

APPROXIMATION

At this stage of the procedure, the edges of the two stumps are fitted together such that the surfaces of the segments correspond optimally (keeping in mind the topography or fascicular pattern of the severed nerve). Tension at the suture anchoring site(s) is an important consideration when sutures are used. Every effort should be made to keep the tension to a minimum.

COAPTATION

In nerve repair, coaptation can refer to apposition of various anatomical components. For example, the cross-section of two nerve stumps can be coapted; the cross-section of individual fascicles can be coapted; and the cross-section of groups of fascicles can be coapted. The goal of nerve repair is that of coapting the fascicular tissue of one stump as completely as possible with the fascicular tissue of the opposite stump to attain an optimal result. The ideal situation would be that of coapting fascicle to fascicle.

In dealing with a transected *monofascicular* nerve segment, stump-to-stump coaptation is synonymous with fascicle-to-fascicle coaptation. With *oligofascicular nerve segments of up to five fascicles,* stump-to-stump coaptation usually leads to a nearly ideal coaptation of the fascicles. However, in *oligofascicular nerve segments with six to ten fascicles,* the trunk-to-trunk approach does not attain ideal coaptation of the center fascicles of the cross-section. In this situation, interfascicular dissection is executed to separate the fascicles with subsequent coaptation of the larger ones.

Group-to-group coaptation is the most suitable approach for nerve segments with a *polyfascicular grouped pattern,* in the author's experience. In the event of a defect, the ideal coaptation of fascicles within groups would not be feasible because the groups in each stump may be comprised of different numbers of fascicles as a result of a change in pattern over the length of the defect. However, clinical experience has proven that the lack of ideal fascicular coaptation does not influence results (21).

If individual fascicles were isolated and fascicle-to-fascicle coaptation attempted, the surgical trauma would be prohibitive and result in fibrosis and proliferation of connective tissue. Further, it would be very difficult to identify corresponding fascicles.

In a nerve segment with a *nongrouping polyfascicular pattern,* separation of individual fascicles would, again, result in too much surgical trauma. Similarly, identification of individual fascicles would present great difficulty, and with a segmental defect, the number of fascicles is not congruent. Group-to-group coaptation is obviously not realistic in the absence of group formation with this fascicular pattern. Two options remain. A stump-to-stump coaptation may be performed with eventual use of guide stitches. Alternatively, the nerve stumps may be arbitrarily divided into sections, and each coapted with a corresponding section of the opposite stump.

MAINTAINING COAPTATION

Sutures are used to maintain coaptation wherever they are anchored; in the interfascicular epineurium, in the perineurium, or in both the perineurium and the epineurium.

Tissue glues have been used as an alternative to sutures in maintaining coaptation. Concentrated solutions of fibrinogen have been applied to coaptation sites with some success (22, 23). A problem with this technique is fibrinolytic activity, which compromises the intended result. In addition, this technique does not allow for tension; therefore, it has been used most recently only in conjunction with anchoring sutures (24).

Coaptation can also be maintained by placing the two nerve stumps at the ends of a tube (e.g., a vein) some distance from the coaptation site. The tube may be split in a longitudinal direction or remain closed. Application of a tube to the suture site has likewise been suggested as a protective mechanism in preventing adhesions to surrounding tissue. However, no demonstrable advantage has yet been clinically proven.

THE GAP BETWEEN NERVE SEGMENTS (STUMPS)

As applied to nerve repair, *gap* may be defined as the distance between two stumps before restoration of continuity is attempted. When there is a *clean transection* at the time of primary repair, the distance may simply be a function of *elastic retraction.* Only the elasticity of the nerve must be overcome to achieve approximation in this case. When there is *damaged nerve tissue, fibrotic retraction* may result from tissue fibrosis and loss of elasticity. Where there is a *nerve defect,* a segment of nerve tissue has been lost, and the gap will be greater and more difficult to remedy.

Although the terms are often used synonymously, it should be clear that *gap* and *nerve defect* are not the same. When a segment of fibrotic nerve tissue must be resected during the preparation of two stumps, an *additional defect* is created. This, too, increases the gap. A retrospective analysis of factors that have contributed to a final gap may be indeed complex when a secondary repair is being undertaken.

Some methods for remedying gaps between two nerve stumps are:

1. Expand the nerve to its original length to compensate for elastic retraction.
2. Extend nerve tissue beyond its original length to remedy a nerve defect.
3. Mobilize the two stumps to distribute the extension of nerve tissue over a greater distance.
4. Transpose the nerve to provide a shorter route.
5. Change the joint position to approximate two nerve stumps on the flexion side of the joint combined with transposition.
6. Shorten the adjacent bones.
7. Graft the nerve.
8. Interpose a nonvital graft or some type of tube to accomplish neuromatous neurotization.

Basic Concepts of Nerve Grafting

There are a number of aspects of and many ways to perform a nerve grafting procedure. The different conceptual aspects may be classified according to the following criteria: (*a*) mechanical aspects; (*b*) source of nerve grafts; (*c*) blood supply; and (*d*) donor nerves.

MECHANICAL ASPECTS

The distance between two nerve stumps can be bridged in two basically different ways.

1. The length of the graft is selected according to the minimal defect after the two stumps have been approximated to the extent possible by exhausting all other methods for overcoming a gap (mentioned above). The remaining distance is then bridged by nerve grafts. Shorter grafts can be used, but the sites of coaptation offer the same unfavorable conditions for nerve regeneration and end-to-end repairs under tension.
2. The length of the graft is selected according to the maximal gap between the two stumps when the involved limb is in a functional position. Although longer grafts are necessary, optimal conditions are provided at the sites of coaptation. In addition, when mobilization of the limb is resumed, the graft is not exposed to tension, and reengagement of longitudinal movements is not necessary.

SOURCE OF NERVE GRAFTS

Autogenous nerve grafts do not present the immunological problems of the allogenous or xenogenous grafts. The latter types are still in the experimental stage for peripheral nerves. In preserving nerve grafts, the following processes have been used: freezing, irradiation, lyophilization, and cialite solution (1). Allografts are less immunogeneic when preserved by one of the methods listed. Even though they are not vital, they are invaded by nerve fibers (neuromatous neurotization). During the 1960s and early 1970s, experimentation with preserved allografts did not meet with success. Under immunosuppressive therapy with cyclosporine A, allografts survive (25–28). Because even successfully surviving allografts are not completely neurotisized, the results will always be inferior to an autograft transplanted under favorable conditions.

BLOOD SUPPLY

Restored Circulation by Spontaneous Vascularization

After *free grafting,* a nerve segment is initially without blood supply. As with a free skin graft, spontaneous anastomoses take place between vessels on the surfaces of both the graft and the recipient site. Vessels from the recipient site grow into the graft. When the avascular period is short, the graft survives well. During this period, no wallerian degeneration occurs within the graft, and there is no connective tissue proliferation. After circulation has been reestablished, the graft behaves like a distal stump.

When there is a delay in spontaneous revascularization, the fibroblasts survive, but the Schwann cells and other special structures are lost. Such a graft segment becomes fibrotic and can be innervated only by neuromatous neurotization. If spontaneous revascularization fails to occur, the graft becomes necrotic. After free grafting, survival is a function of tissue mass (diameter), surface contact between graft and recipient site, and recipient site vascularity. When the relation is favorable, as with cutaneous nerve grafts, survival is enhanced. If the relation between diameter and surface area is not favorable, such as with a thick trunk graft, fibrosis of the graft occurs.

Preservation of Circulation

Continuity of a nerve can be restored by the two-stage transfer of a *pedicled graft* from a parallel nerve, as in a flap procedure. Circulation within the grafts is preserved during the transfer, and favorable results have been reported to the extent of protective discrimination (29–31).

A nerve segment on its vascular pedicle can be transferred as an *island flap* without interruption of blood supply if the recipient nerve is within range of the pedicle. Many cases that have been discussed as vascularized nerve grafts are, in reality, island flap transfers of peripheral nerves (32, 33).

Restored Circulation by Microvascular Anastomosis (Vascularized Nerve Graft)

The free vascularized nerve graft was introduced by Taylor and Ham (34). If vessels remain patent, the graft behaves like a distal stump at the onset. Important dimensions of the process seem to be that of survival of the paraneurium and the absence of adhesion formation in achieving spontaneous vascularization. The vascularized nerve is independent of vascularity in the recipient site.

Vascularized nerve trunk grafts have been used to bridge large defects. With the reestablishment of circulation, the danger of fibrosis does not occur as is the case when using trunk grafts as free grafts. The disadvantage of such a trunk graft is that the changing fascicular pattern makes it impossible to predict where the nerve fibers at a certain point in the proximal end will leave the graft at the distal end. The superficial branch of the radial nerve has been used successfully alone (34) and in conjunction with free grafts. Microvascular techniques have been developed for use with the sural nerve as a vascularized graft (35, 36). The expectation that vascularized nerve grafts would significantly improve the quality of nerve regeneration over considerable distances has not yet been borne out (Gilbert, personal communications, 1981, 1982; 37). The majority of authors report a somewhat faster regeneration but an equal final result whether either free nerve grafts or vascularized nerve grafts have been used (38–41). Only Terzis et al. (42) reported superior final results. In my personal experience, there was no significant difference as far as the final result is concerned. Undoubtedly, the major advantage of vascularized nerve grafts is the fact that the paraneurium, and consequently the gliding capacity of the nerve graft, is preserved. In contrast, a free graft has to survive by developing adhesions with the surrounding tissue. Also, nerve regeneration is unquestionably better if, along with the nerve graft, the overall circulation (e.g., in an injured finger) is improved by performing a vascularized graft (43).

DONOR NERVES

Nerve Trunk Grafts

The use of nerve trunks as grafts is limited. A major consideration is the functional loss the nerve trunk undergoes when employed as a graft. If two parallel nerves are injured, one may be restored at the expense of the other as with a pedicled nerve graft. Where there is extensive functional loss in selected nerve repairs (e.g., brachial plexus lesions), nerve trunk grafts may be used to advantage.

Nerve trunks cannot be used as free grafts, as noted above, because circulation must be maintained or immediately reestablished. An important disadvantage is the changing fascicular pattern over the length of the graft such that the course of regenerated fibers cannot be predicted from the proximal to the distal end.

Cutaneous Nerve Grafts

Cutaneous nerve grafts have an ideal diameter-to-surface ratio for free grafting and may be regarded as a fascicular group. The ideal donor nerve should have only a few branches. A salient aspect of using cutaneous nerves as donor grafts is the difference in thickness contrasted

with that of the nerve trunk to be repaired. Two possible solutions exist:

1. A *composite nerve graft* may be formed by suturing or gluing together several segments of cutaneous nerve. A cable is designed by uniting several segments of a cutaneous nerve to reach the same size as the nerve to be repaired (44). However, grafts so devised experience a loss in surface dimension available for contact with the recipient site. Further, in the event of a defect, the cross-sections of the two nerve stumps do not correspond, and only a random guiding of axons along the cable graft can occur.
2. *Individual grafts of cutaneous nerve segments* can be used to unite specific sites of the two stumps (11, 45, 46). The entire circumference of the individually placed grafts has good contact with surrounding tissue, and thereby an optimal chance of survival exists. If the topography is known, specific points of the two cross-sections can be connected with individual grafts.

The following nerves have been used as free cutaneous nerve grafts: (*a*) sural, (*b*) saphenous, (*c*) lateral femoral cutaneous, (*d*) medial antebrachial cutaneous, (*e*) medial brachial cutaneous, (*f*) lateral antebrachial cutaneous, (*g*) dorsal antebrachial cutaneous, (*h*) superficial radial, (*i*) cutaneous nerve of the cervical plexus, and (*j*) intercostal nerve.

Techniques of Interfascicular Nerve Grafting

Interfascicular nerve grafting differs significantly from other techniques and is outlined briefly as follows:

1. The length of the graft is selected to bridge the maximal defect in extending position. (See Mechanical Aspects of grafting presented earlier.) No attempt is made to diminish the distance by other methods.
2. If necessary, the nerve stumps are prepared by interfascicular dissection to reduce the amount of nonfascicular tissue.
3. The individual grafts are placed between corresponding fascicles or fascicular groups if the fascicular pattern of the stumps permits.
4. The nerve grafts are individually placed along the entire course to enhance the chance of survival. Since the early days of fascicular nerve grafting, this has been regarded as one of the most important factors for a successful outcome.

Individual steps of the technique are essentially the same as those described for neurorrhaphy (i.e., stump preparation, approximation, coaptation, and securing coaptation).

Cutaneous nerve grafts are provided by excision of one or several of the donor nerves. The two sural nerves are the first choice. Regardless of the anticipated lengths of nerve grafts, the sural nerve is always excised in its total length and transected just below the popliteal area. This locates the transsection site nearest the point of nerve attachment underneath the fascia. Thus, protection is provided for the neuroma that always forms at any site of nerve transsection and prevents exposure to irritation. The donor nerve is segmented according to the distance between the two stumps. The cut ends of the grafts should not be covered with epineurial or perineurial tissue; therefore, these are removed from the cross-sections. Resection of the ends is not necessary because these are free grafts and connective tissue proliferation is delayed. Hence, there is no interference with the coaptation site.

The donor nerve can usually be extended about 10% in length. However, each segmental length is selected in the relaxed state, which allows for additional extension of about 10%.

PREPARATION OF STUMPS

The nerve stumps are prepared in the usual way. Monofascicular and polyfascicular stumps without group arrangements are prepared by resection.

Nerve stumps with an oligofascicular pattern and a few large fascicles that are approximately the same size as the nerve grafts are prepared by resection of the epifascicular epineurium and interfascicular dissection, thus isolating the individual fascicles (Fig. 11.3).

Nerve stumps with a grouped polyfascicular pattern are prepared by resection of the epineurium and separation of the individual fascicle groups by interfascicular dissection.

The technique of interfascicular dissection makes it possible to transect the fascicles or groups of fascicles

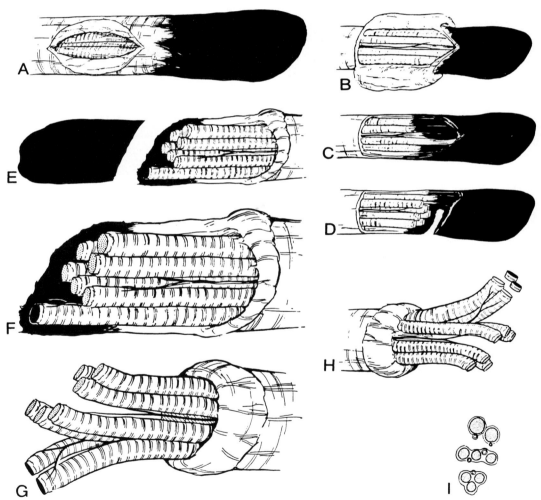

FIGURE 11.3. A nerve stump with eight fascicles and oblique damage is shown. Preparation of the stump is shown by *interfascicular dissection*. **A,** A longitudinal incision of the epifascicular epineurium proximal to the neuroma is illustrated. **B,** The epifascicular epineurium is elevated. A space between the fascicles is seen, indicating the border between groups. **C,** The dissection is extended toward the neuroma. **D,** The fascicles are transected at the point of transition from normal to abnormal appearance. **E,** The neuroma is resected. **F,** Exact inspection reveals the presence of fibrotic tissue around some fascicles and fibrosis of two fascicles. **G,** An epifascicular and interfascicular resection at the back of the stump is performed. The group arrangement becomes clearly apparent. The interfascicular tissue between the fascicles of each group is saved in each vessel. **H,** The two fibrotic fascicles are resected. Finally, a stump is prepared with three fascicular groups. **I,** Only minimal epineurial tissue remains.

exactly at the point of transition from normal to damaged tissue. Donor nerves, such as the sural nerve, have a changing fascicular pattern along their course. It is therefore possible to select segments that closely correspond to the individual fascicle groups of the recipient nerve and thus achieve an optimal match.

APPROXIMATION

The ends of each graft are approximated to corresponding cross-section sites of the two stumps. Site con-

gruency is attained by exploiting all the possibilities previously outlined for defining intraneural topography.

COAPTATION

After approximation has been achieved, maximum care is taken to coapt the fascicular cross-sections as effectively as possible without displacement in either the longitudinal or lateral direction. If the approximation suture is placed ideally and if there is no tension, an optimal contact can be achieved by this single suture without any

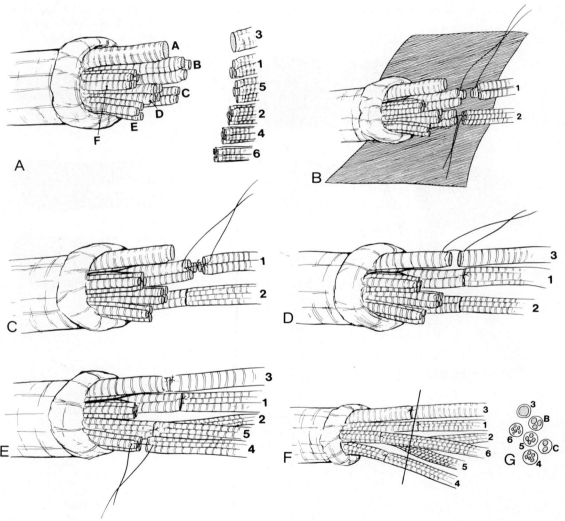

FIGURE 11.4. Interfascicular nerve grafting is illustrated. **A,** The proximal stump is shown after interfascicular preparation. There are 18 fascicles, arranged in six groups, containing one, three, two, four, three, and five fascicles (**A** to **F,** respectively). Six segments of the sural nerve are prepared for grafting (1–6). An attempt is made to select segments that fit best to the stumps, according to their fascicular pattern. **B,** A membrane is placed underneath the stump to provide a smooth surface for the back. Graft segment **1** (three fascicles) is coapted to group **B** (three fascicles). Graft segment **2** (five fascicles) is coapted to group **C** (two fascicles). **C,** Perfect coaptation was achieved with

graft segment **2** with no further activity necessary. For graft segment **1,** a second stitch is necessary to provide optimal coaptation. **D,** Graft segment **3** (one fascicle) is coapted to group **A** (one fascicle). **E,** Graft segment **4** (six fascicles) is coapted to group **E** (three fascicles) by an epiperineurial suture. Graft segment **5** (four fascicles) is coapted to group **D** (four fascicles). No stitch is necessary because coaptation is maintained by side-to-side contact. Graft segment **6** with eight fascicles (not shown) will be coapted to group **F** (five fascicles). **F,** The grafting procedure is completed. **G,** The cross-section upon completion of grafting demonstrates the interdigitation.

deviation in a lateral direction. In this event, approximation and coaptation are performed in a single step. If the graft has a tendency to rotate or deviate laterally and if optimal coverage of the cross-sections cannot be achieved, two or three additional sutures may be necessary to attain and maintain optimal coaptation. The procedure of coaptation between oligofascicular or polyfascicular nerve segments with group arrangement is facilitated if individual fascicles or groups of fascicles have been transected at different levels. In this case, interdigitation between fascicles (or fascicle groups) and grafts occurs and provides side-by-side contact with neighboring fascicles, fascicle groups, and grafts. This is beneficial in preventing dislocation or disruption. Under such ideal conditions, the number of sutures can be reduced to a minimum (Fig. 11.4).

MAINTAINING COAPTATION

If optimal coaptation has been achieved and if tension is eliminated, it is not necessary to use additional sutures or glue to maintain the coaptation. Extreme care must be taken to avoid shearing forces during wound closure and to prevent longitudinal traction. The involved limb is immobilized in the exact position it assumed during the operation.

ALTERNATIVES TO NERVE GRAFTS

As alternatives to nerve grafts, alloplastic nerve conduits (47), venous grafts (Brunelli, personal communication, 1986; 48–52), and degenerated muscle tissue (53) have been used to provide pathways for neuromatous neurotization. According to my personal experience, the results remain under the level of an autogenous free nerve graft under favorable conditions.

Postoperative Care and Follow-up

Immobilization of the affected limb is maintained for 8 days. After this, careful mobilization is initiated without concern for rupture or dislocation. Electrotherapy can be used with exponential current if indicated. Follow-up is extremely important. After 2–3 weeks, advancement of the Tinel and Hoffmann signs along the graft can be observed. It may pause temporarily at the distal end of the graft and then proceed along the distal stump. This is an indication that at least some axon sprouts have crossed the site of coaptation and reached the distal stump. In some instances, a block develops at the distal suture site, and the axon sprouts cannot proceed. The Tinel and Hoffman signs then remain with the maximal point at the distal end of the graft. In some cases after proceeding along the distal stump, the Tinel and Hoffmann signs stop and subsequently retreat to the distal site of coaptation. This phenomenon means that changes within the scar tissue at the distal site of coaptation or along the graft itself have damaged the axon and caused a new axolysis.

In all such cases, surgical exploration is indicated. If a *block at the distal site of coaptation* is found, it is resected, and an end-to-end neurorrhaphy is performed. Sometimes there is only a band of scar tissue or some other cause of compression that interferes with regeneration and requires *neurolysis*. When fibrosis develops along the grafts, it is indicative that they have not survived well and *repeat grafting* will be needed.

The problem of distal site coaptation has attracted the attention of surgeons for some time, and different solutions have been proposed. Some surgeons (54, 55) have emphasized planning the grafting in two stages. At the first stage, only proximal coaptation is performed, and the distal end of the graft is left open. In a second stage the distal end of the graft is coapted to the distal stump. A similar technique has been used in performing a cross-face nerve graft to neurotisize a denervated facial nerve with axons from the contralateral normal nerve (56–58). Coaptation between graft ends and distal stumps of facial nerve branches is carried out 4–5 months later in a second stage. At that time, it can be accurately determined whether the graft has been neurotisized.

In routine cases of nerve repair, this additional precaution (i.e., staging) is not indicated for two reasons:

1. It is relatively easy to direct the nerve grafts from fascicles or fascicle groups of the proximal stump to fascicles of the distal stumps if the procedure is performed simultaneously with both stumps exposed. This is much more difficult to accomplish during a second stage, even if the distal ends of the grafts are carefully marked.

2. In our material, if the grafting procedure is performed carefully and without any tension, a block develops at the distal suture in only 1–2% of cases. It is diagnosed relatively easily, and the problem is solved by resection.

References

1. Schröder JM, Seiffert KE: Die Feinstruktur der neurmatösen Neurotisation von Nerventransplantaten. *Virchows Arch Path Anat (Abt B Zellpath)* 5:219, 1970.
2. Hakstian RW: Funicular orientation by direct stimulation. An aid to peripheral nerve repair. *J Bone Joint Surg [Am]* 50:1178, 1968.
3. Gaul JS Jr: Electrical fascicle identification as an adjunct to nerve repair. *J Hand Surg* 8:289, 1983.
4. Jabaley ME: Presentation at the Meeting of the Sunderland Society at Bishop's Lodge, USA, May 18–22, 1983.
5. Gruber H, Zenker W: Acetycholinesterase: Histochemical differentiation between motor and sensory nerve fibers. *Brain Res* 51:207, 1973.
6. Freilinger G, Gruber H, Holle J, et al: Zur methodik der "sensomotorisch" differenzierten Faszikelnaht peripherer Nerven. *Handchir Mikrochir Plast Chir* 7:133, 1975.
7. Engel J, Ganel J, Melamed R, et al: Choline acetyl transferase for differentiation between human motor and sensory nerve fibers. *Ann Plast Surg* 4:376, 1980.
8. Millesi H, Berger A, Meissl G: Experimentelle Untersuchungen zur Heilung durchtrennter peripherer Nerven. *Chir Plast* 1:1, 174, 1972.
9. Gamble HJ, Eames RA: An electron microscope study of the connective tissues of human peripheral nerve. *J Anat* 98:655, 1964.

10. Ochoa J, Mair WGP: The normal sural nerve in man: Ultrastructure and number of fibres and cells. *Acta Neuropathol* 13:197, 1969.

11. Millesi H: Zum Problem der Überbrükung von defekten peripheren Nerven. *Wien Med Wochenschr* 118:182, 1968.

12. Millesi H, Berger A, Meissl G: Razvoj reparatorno operativnih postupaka kod ozljeda periferinih zivaca. Drugi Simpozij O Bolestima I Ozljedama Sake, Zagreb, 1970, p 161.

13. Millesi H, Meissl G, Berger A: The interfascicular nerve grafting of the median and ulnar nerves. *J Bone Joint Surg [Am]* 54:727, 1972.

14. Millesi H: Clinical aspects of nerve healing. In Gibson T, Van der Meulen JC (eds): *Foundation International Corp in the Medical Science.* Montreux, 1975, p 282.

15. Millesi H: Healing of nerves. *Clin Plast Surg* 4:459, 1977.

16. Cajal SR: *Degeneration and Regeneration of the Nervous System.* London, University Press, 1928, p 168.

17. Lundborg G, Hansson HA: Regeneration of a peripheral nerve through a performed tissue space. *Brain Res* 178:573, 1979.

18. Restrepo Y, Merle M, Michon J, et al: Fascicular nerve graft using an empty perineurial tube: An experimental study in the rabbit. *Microsurgery* 4:105, 1983.

19. Strauch B, Rosenberg B, Brunelli F, et al: Autogenous vein graft substitute in long segment nerve defects. Communication at the Inaugural Meeting of the American Society for Reconstructive Microsurgery. Las Vegas, Nevada, January 17–19, 1985.

20. Hueter K: *Die Allgemeine Chirurgie.* Leipzig, Vogel Verlag, 1873.

21. Millesi H: How exact should coaptation be? In Gorio A, Millesi H, Mingrino S (eds): *Posttraumatic Peripheral Nerve Regeneration. Experimental Basis and Clinical Application.* New York, Raven Press, 1981, pp 301–306.

22. Matras H, Dinges HP, Lassmann H, et al: Zur nahtlosen interfaszikulären Nerventransplantation im Tierexperiment. *Wien Med Woschenschr* 122:517, 1972.

23. Matras H, Kuderna H: Glueing nerve anastomoses with clotting substances. In Marchac D, Hueston JT (eds): *Transactions of the 6th International Congress of Plastic and Reconstructive Surgery* (Paris, August 24–29, 1975). Paris, Masson, Inc, 1976, pp 134–136.

24. Kuderna HP: Communication at the Arbeitstagung fur Handchirurgie. Basel, Switzerland, 1982.

25. MacKinnon SE, Hudson AR, Falk RE, Hunter DA: The nerve allograft response—An experimental model in the rat. *Ann Plast Surg* 14:334, 1985.

26. MacKinnon SE, Hudson AR, Bain JR: The nerve allograft response in the primate, immunosuppressed with cyclosporin A. Presented at the Sunderland Society Meeting, Durham NC, July 1985.

27. Berger A, Schaller E, Mailänder P, Walter A, Wonigeit K, Becker M: The effect of cyclosporine A on free autolog and allogen grafts of the sciatic nerve in the rat. Presented at the 3rd Congress of the International Federation of Societies for Surgery of the Hand, Tokyo, November 3–8, 1986.

28. Schaller E, Mailänder P, Becker M, Walter GF, Berger A: Nervenregenation im autologen und allogenen Transplantat des N. ischiadicus der Ratte mit und ohne Immunsuppression durch Cyclosporin A. *Handchirurgie* 20:7, 1988.

29. Strange FG St C: Case report on pedicled nerve graft. *Br J Surg* 37:331, 1950.

30. Seddon HJ: Nerve grafting. *J Bone Joint Surg [Br]* 45:447, 1963.

31. Brooks D: The place of nerve grafting in orthopaedic surgery. *J Bone Joint Surg [Am]* 37:299, 1955.

32. Birch D: Communication at Symposium on Brachial Plexus, London, January 24–26, 1983.

33. Terzis J: Communication at Symposium on Brachial Plexus Surgery, Lausanne, Switzerland, December, 1984.

34. Taylor GI, Ham FJ: The free vascularized nerve graft. *Plast Reconstr Surg* 57:413, 1976.

35. Fachinelli A, Masquelet A, Restrepo J, et al: The vascularized sural nerve. Anatomy and surgical approach. *Int J Microsurg* 3:57, 1981.

36. Townsend P: Microvascular nerve grafts. Communication at the 4th Congress of the European Section of the International Confederation for Plastic and Reconstructive Surgery, Athens, May 10–14, 1981.

37. Gilbert J: Vascularized nerve grafts. In: Reconstructive Microsurgery. An Indepth Course in Microsurgery, Oklahoma City, May 24–28, 1981.

38. Merle M, Lebreton E, Bour C, et al: Free vascularized nerve transfer in brachial plexus injuries. Communication at the 10th International Meeting of Microsurgery (GAM) and 7th Annual Meeting of the DAM, Strasbourg, May 2–4, 1985.

39. Allieu Y: Joint Meeting of the Groupe pour L'Avancement de la Microchirurgie and the Deutsche Arbeitsgemeinschaft fur Mikrochirurgie, Strasbourg, May 2–5, 1984.

40. Birch D: Communication at Symposium on Brachial Plexus. London, January 24–26, 1983.

41. McCollough CJ, Gagay O, Higginson DW, et al: Axon regeneration and vascularization of nerve grafts. *J Hand Surg [Br]* 9:323, 1984.

42. Terzis JK, Liberson WTH, Maragh HA: Motor cycle brachial plexopathy. In Terzis JK (ed): *Microreconstruction of Nerve Injuries.* Philadelphia, WB Saunders Co, 1987, p 361.

43. Rose E, Kowalski DHA: Restoration of sensibility of unaesthetic scar digits with free vascularized nerve grafts from the dorsum of the foot. *J Hand Surg* 4:514, 1985.

44. Seddon HJ: The use of autogeneous grafts for the repair of large gaps in peripheral nerves. *Br J Surg* 35:151, 1947.

45. Millesi H, Ganglberger J, Berger A: Erfahrungen mit der mikrochirurgie peripherer nerven. *Langenbecks Arch Chir* 316:723, 1966.

46. Millesi H, Galglberger J, Berger A: Erfahrungen mit der Mikrochirurgie peripherer nerven. *Chir Plast Reconstr* 3:47, 1967.

47. Dellon LA, MacKinnon SE: An alternative to the classical nerve graft for the management of the short nerve gap. *Plast Reconstr Surg* 82:5, 849, 1988.

48. Chiu DTW: Autogenous vein graft as a conduit for nerve regeneration. *Surg Forum* 31:550, 1980.

49. Chiu DTW, Janecka I, Krizek TJ, Wolff M, Lovelace RE: Autogenous vein graft as a conduit for nerve regeneration. *Surgery* 91:226, 1982.

50. Rigoni G, Smahel J, Chiu DTW, Meyer VE: Veneninterponat als Leitbahn für die Regeneration peripherer Nerven. *Handchirurgie* 15:227, 1983.

51. Strauch B, Rosenberg B, Brunelli F, Ferder M, de Moura W: Autogenous vein graft substitute in long segment nerve defects. Presented at the Inaugural Meeting of the American Society for Reconstructive Microsurgery, Las Vegas, January 17–19, 1985.

52. Sparmann M: Die Bedeutung des sogenannten Leitschienendefektes für die Regeneration peripherer Nerven über Defektstrecken. Eine tierexperimentelle Untersuchung am N. peronaeus des Kaninchens. Habilitationsschrift aus dem Fachbereich 3—Klinikum Charlottenburg—der Freien Universität Berlin, 1987.

53. Glasby MA, Gschmeissner SE, Hitchcock RJI, Huang CLH, de Souza BA: A comparison of nerve regeneration through nerves and muscle grafts in rats. *Neuro-Orthop* 2:21, 1986.

54. Bsteh FX, Millesi H: Zur kenntnis der zweizeitigen Nerveninterplantation bei ausgedehntem peripherem Nervendefekt. *Klin Med* 15:571, 1960.

55. Bosse JP: Discussional remark. In Gorio A, Millesi H, Mingrino S (eds): *Posttraumatic Peripheral Nerve Regeneration. Experimental Basis and Clinical Implication.* New York, Raven Press, 1981, p 347.

56. Smith JW: A new technique of facial animation. In Hueston JT (ed): *Transactions of the 5th International Congress of Plastic and Reconstructive Surgery* (Melbourne, Australia). London, Butterworths, 1971, p 83.

57. Scaramella L: L'anastomosi tra i due nervi faciali. *Arch Neurol* 82:209, 1972.

58. Anderl H: Reconstruction of the face through cross face nerve transplantation in facial paralysis. *Chir Plast* 2:117, 1973.

12

Biomaterials in Plastic Surgery

Mary H. McGrath, M.D., F.A.C.S.

An alloplastic material is an inert foreign substance implanted within living tissue. Phenomenal expansion in the use of implant materials has occurred since 1945 as industrial improvements in metal alloys and developments in polymer chemistry have been adapted for biomedical application. Over 50 different inorganic materials are in current use in an estimated 2 million patients (1) annually because: (a) they are available when autologous tissue is not (e.g., hydrocephalus shunts or pacemaker units); (b) there is no donor site morbidity or scarring; (c) nonbiodegradable alloplastic materials do not undergo resorption, as do bone or cartilage grafts; (d) biodegradable implant systems are being developed for uses such as controlled-release drug delivery systems.

Fundamental Properties of All Implants

The tissue response to different implants varies with the chemical composition and micro- and macrostructures of the synthetic material, and these differences are used clinically. For example, vigorous tissue ingrowth with Marlex mesh hernia repairs provides a strong and lasting support, while the fibrous encapsulation of a silicone tendon prosthesis ensures free gliding of a tendon graft. However, certain properties and concerns are common to all implants.

NONCARCINOGENIC

Foreign body–induced sarcomas, predominantly fibrosarcomas, can be observed in animals with metal, polymer, and glass implants. This appears to be species-specific, occurring in rats, mice, and hamsters but not in dogs or primates. It is also time-dependent, with a latent period in the rat that corresponds to 10–15 years of human life.

The incidence of rodent tumors is related to the size and the configuration of the implant; there is a higher frequency of tumors with larger implants and with smooth-surfaced implants that evoke a long axis–oriented collagenous shell than with powdered, perforated, or porous forms of the same materials (2–6).

NONTOXIC

Toxicological evaluation of a material includes tissue culture and in vivo testing of cell growth, attachment, and movement parameters as well as histochemical analysis of enzyme activity and solute concentrations in the boundary layer at the implant-tissue interface (7, 8). In general, hydrophilic materials or those with additives such as fillers, plasticizers, antioxidants, and pigments are the most toxic. With the polymeric materials, toxicity can accompany the leaching out of smaller molecular groups when polymerization is not complete (9, 10). Much of the cytotoxicity testing for materials is under regulatory control and includes both cell culture and in vivo studies of mutagenicity and teratogenicity.

NONALLERGENIC

The highest incidence of hypersensitivity reactions to inorganic implants is reported with metallic devices. On skin testing, as many as 6% of patients with metallic prostheses are found to be sensitized to constituent nickel, cobalt, or chromium (11, 12).

NONIMMUNOGENIC

Despite the absence of organic molecules in nonbiological materials, inorganic implants may not be immunologically inert. Theoretically, either a humoral or a cell-mediated immune response could be induced by leaching out of nonproteinous substances stimulating immunoglobulin release and an autoimmune reaction, or by absorption of endogenous proteins into implants, which would alter their conformation in such a way that new antigenic complexes are created. While standard in vitro immunogenicity testing is required for all implants, new interest in implant immunopathology (13) has been stimulated by recent reports of autoimmune connective tissue disease developing after the injection of paraffin or liquid silicone (14). In termed human adjuvant disease, the clinical manifestations are similar to those of scleroderma, rheumatoid arthritis, polymyositis, and others (15). Some clinical discrepancies exist, the association with implants has not been proven, and immunological mechanisms of the disease induction are uncertain.

MECHANICAL RELIABILITY

In addition to mechanical and physical function, biomaterials must demonstrate environmental stability. All of the properties designed into an implant, such as tensile strength, elastic modulus, impact resistance, conductivity, crystallinity, and cross-linking, can be tested during the fabrication process. However, the implant must function in a dynamic biochemical environment where tissue enzymes, free radicals, bacteria, and drugs are present. Screening for hydrolytic resistance, oxidative degradation, extractability, electrical stability, and numerous other factors can make the testing of biomaterials a complex process. Even then, late degradation (as in the mechanical distortion of silicone rubber balls in cardiac valves due to lipid absorption) after years of use cannot always be predicted (16).

BIOCOMPATIBILITY

All implanted materials initially give rise to an inflammatory reaction with migration of macrophages and fibroblasts into the zone around the implant and vascularization to form typical granulation tissue. The course thereafter depends on the chemical composition of the implant, the physical nature of the implant (size, shape, porosity, surface finish), and the tissue in which the prosthesis is implanted.

Absorbable Materials

The degradation of an absorbable material can occur by dissolution, hydrolysis, or enzymatic degradation (17). Macrophage phagocytosis and intracellular digestion clears the residue. As the material is absorbed, granulation tissue replaces it with the eventual formation of a stable scar. The rate of degradation is accelerated by increasing hydrophilic properties, surface charge, or surface energy and/or by adding amino acids (17); all increase material reactivity.

Nonabsorbable Materials

The cellular response around a nonabsorbable substance varies with its chemical composition, reflected in the water content, charge distribution, ion exchange, and protein deposition at its surface (1). Shape affects the in vivo reactivity for unknown reasons (18). Roughness of the surface profoundly affects the adjacent macrophage

behavior and lysosomal enzyme production (19). The absolute size of the implant has less effect than its contiguous distances, or pore size.

These differences in inflammatory cell population and behavior are accompanied by differences in fibroblast activity and collagen deposition. The relatively inert, smooth surface implant becomes encapsulated in a dense collagenous connective tissue sheath. The reactive, rough, woven or knitted implant is incorporated or firmly fixed by the fibrous tissue (Table 12.1) (20).

Theory of Interfacial Behavior

Hench (1) and Ethridge (20) have developed a general theory about interfacial behavior, namely, that the search for inert implants causing the least toxic response in the host will generate smooth surface materials with nonadherent capsules and resultant mechanical instability. For a material that will behave and respond like the tissue it replaces, a stable interfacial bone is needed. Thus, a microporous or controlled surface-reactive biomaterial should be the "ideal"; incorporation of the reparative host tissue within the bioactive layers of the implant surface will parallel the admixing of cellular and acellular components of normal tissues at junctions of the body such as tooth–soft tissue (Table 12.1). The active-surface-chemical viewpoint of a biomaterials goal is in opposition to the historical efforts to develop maximally inert materials, but its application is expanding, particularly in bioactive glass or ceramic coatings or orthopaedic and dental devices.

Classification of Implant Materials

Categorization by chemical composition is the most useful framework for the description and comparison of surgical implants. This materials science approach recognizes that the commonality of different groups of materials arises more from their composition than from the organ systems or clinical disciplines in which they are used. Chemically, there are three major classes of biomaterials: metallic, ceramic, and polymeric. Although they are polymers, biological materials such as collagen must be classified separately because they introduce new considerations of foreign protein antigenicity.

Table 12.1
Interfacial Response to Biomaterials

Surface Chemistry	Surface Structure	Tissue Response
Nonabsorbable Materials		
"Inert"	Smooth surface	Fibrous capsule
"Inert"	Microporous surface	"Controlled" adhesion
Bioactive	Rough, woven, knitted surface	Bonding
Absorbable Materials		
Degradable		Replacement

Metals

Metals are characterized by high thermal and electrical conductivity because of the relative independence of their electrons from parent atoms. Metals are opaque, can be polished to a high luster, and generally are heavy and deformable. Metallic implants serve the *functions* of fixation (as in bone plates, rods, or trays), support (as in suture material and stainless steel meshes), and electrical conduction (as in pacemaker wires and nerve stimulators). Each of these applications makes different demands, but the general *requirements* for a metal device include: mechanical strength for appropriate load-carrying capacity; a suitable elastic modulus for resistance to flexion fatigue in either the rigid or the deformable, flexible implant; density and weight comparable to the surrounding tissue; and resistance to corrosion.

CLINICAL CONSIDERATIONS

The major causes of metallic implant failure are corrosion and implant fracture. Corrosion results from the electrochemical activity of unstable metal ions and electrons in physiological salt solutions. The trace metal ions released into surrounding tissue can elicit fibrosis or fibrous capsule formation at the interface, producing instability of a bone implant. Corrosion products such as iron or chromium can be locally cytotoxic in large concentrations, leading to pain or inflammation. Elements leached out by corrosion, such as nickel, can cause systemic allergic reactions (21).

Corrosion is prevented by an oxide film, termed a passivation film, which forms on the surface of a oxygen-exposed metal. Thus, prepassivation treatment or anodization can be used to stabilize a metal, and factors such as an anerobic environment in the crevices of a scratched implant or fretting from metal-to-metal contact can destroy the oxide film and promote corrosion (21).

Implant fracture is less common than corrosion and may result from: (*a*) improper implant design; (*b*) manufacturing defects such as inclusions, insufficient electropolishing, or mixed metal devices that favor galvanic corrosion; (*c*) improper stress distribution in the bone, causing atrophy and resorption of cortical bone; (*d*) surgical handling that bends (works) the material until brittle spots develop; and (*e*) patient overloading to the point of fatigue fracture at stress risers (20, 22).

METALS IN CURRENT SURGICAL USE

Very few metals have sufficient corrosion resistance or strength to be used in the hostile environment of the living organism (Table 12.2). The noble metals (gold, platinum, iridium) are most stable but lack strength and are limited to use as conductive wires. Most effort has gone into the development of alloys, the mixture of metals or of metal and a crystalline substance, to achieve properties superior to those of any individual constituent. All implant metals are subject to American Society of Test-

Table 12.2
Metals in Clinical Use

Stainless steel—Iron-chromium-nickel
Cobalt-chromium alloys
    Cobalt-chromium-molybdenum (cast Vitallium)
    Cobalt-nickel-chromium-molybdenum (wrought Vitallium)
Titanium
    Unalloyed titanium
    Titanium-aluminum-vanadium (titanium alloy)
Tantalum

ing and Materials standards for metallurgical contents and inclusions.

Stainless Steel

This generic term refers to a large number of iron-chromium alloys. Only austenitic stainless steel is used surgically, and it contains about 60% iron, 20% chromium, and 20% nickel, molybdenum, manganese, and silicon. It is the most widely employed of the metals and is used in the manufacture of artificial joints, bone plates, rods, screws and wires, cranial plates, dental implants, neural electrodes, pacemaker casings, cardiac valves, suture material, hemostatic clips, and meshes for tissue patches (e.g., hernia repair). The advantages of stainless steel are its accessibility and the ease with which it may be worked into complex shapes. Its disadvantages are poorer mechanical strength and fatigue resistance compared with other surgical metals. It is also the most corrosive of the metals in present use (23, 24).

Cobalt-Chromium Alloys

These alloys offer the advantages of superior tensile strength and greater resistance to fatigue fracture (20). Corrosion resistance in body fluids is superior to that of stainless steel (25), but skin tests for metal sensitivity and tests for levels of cobalt (Co) and chromium (Cr) in the hair, blood, and urine indicate that corrosion products are readily dispersed throughout the body (26). The hardness of Vitallium may be a disadvantage because it is extremely difficult to bend or reshape and is most useful in preformed implants. Vitallium is used in the manufacture of artificial joints, bone plates, rods, screws and wires, cranioplasty plates, dental implants, and cardiac valve prostheses.

Titanium and Titanium Alloy

These are superior to stainless steel and Vitallium in several respects: a very low rate of corrosion; lower density, which saves weight and reduces a patient's awareness of the implant; and a low modulus of elasticity, which mean titanium alloy is "springier" and reduces the stresses around the implant by flexing with the bone. Unalloyed titanium has tensile strength comparable to that of stainless steel, but the alloy has superior strength equal to that of cobalt-chromium materials (27). The only disadvantages of titanium are expense and the difficulty in working the metal. It is used in artificial joints, bone plates, screws and wires, dental implants, cardiac valve frames, pacemaker casing, and loops for intraocular lenses.

Tantalum

A unique pure element, tantalum has had limited surgical use because it is a relatively soft metal. It is extremely stable because of a tough oxide surface film, and it compares favorably with ceramics in resisting electrochemical attack. It is used in the manufacture of meshes (e.g., mandibular tray, artificial trachea), cranial plates, dental implants, suture material, staples, and neural electrodes.

Ceramics

The term "ceramic" encompasses materials that contain metallic and nonmetallic elements. They possess high stability and resistance to chemical alteration. Generally, they are harder than metals or polymers, have higher compressive strength, are poor electrical and thermal conductors, and are translucent. Used for some time in dentistry, ceramics are now under vigorous investigation and in limited clinical use as vascular and artificial joint implants (Table 12.3).

GROUPS OF CERAMIC MATERIALS

Carbons

These are dense, inert ceramic materials with properties the same in all directions (isotropic). The strong carbon bonds confer great strength, while the weak bonding between the layers results in an elastic modulus very close to that of bone and significantly lower than that of metals (28). Polished pyrolytic carbons have excellent thromboresistance, although the explanation for this blood compatability is unknown. A number of heart valves have silicon-alloyed pyrolytic carbon discs or coatings, and the remarkable wear resistance of these substances has given rise to the estimate that only 25% of the material will be worn away in 100 years (28). Some artificial hearts have been manufactured from carbon, and the patency of small-diameter carbon-coated Dacron vascular grafts is being evaluated (29). Carbon fibers are woven into a textile that is presently under investigation as a tendon replacement and has been used successfully in composite implants.

Ceramics

Ceramics for bone replacement is one of the most active areas of biomaterials research today. At least 40 to 50 different ceramic materials are under evaluation as implant materials. These are divided into three categories: (*a*) inert, (*b*) reactive or bonding, (*c*) resorbable (20).

Because thin fibrous capsules do form around very *inert* substances, porous forms have been fabricated to allow for bone ingrowth and better stability. Unfortunately, the porosity decreases mechanical strength over time, and this approach has not been put to clinical use. However, hip prostheses partially composed of dense alumina (Al_2O_3) and tooth-root replacements of dense alumina are used clinically (30).

The best known of the *bonding* or *controlled-reactive* biomaterials are the bioglass and bioglass-ceramic compounds whose surfaces interact with and bond to the surrounding tissue. Hench and Ethridge (20) have developed about six different bioglasses that induce a chemical bond at the implant-tissue interface. Bioglasses show similar behavior in soft tissue, with collagenous bonding between the implant and both muscular and subcutaneous tissue. However, the bioglasses' chemical surface features function only under optimal conditions, and any adverse biomechanical factors will shift the tissue response irreversibly from bonding to capsule formation. As a result, clinical applications are awaiting further definition of these factors.

Like an autologous cancellous bone graft or a coral template, the *resorbable* ceramic prosthesis serves as a scaffold for new bone growth and eventually is replaced by living tissue. The advantage of the resorbable material is that there will be no long-term instability or compatibility problems. The disadvantages are strength degradation during the remodeling process, which may cause mechanical implant failure, and the unknown consequences of releasing high concentrations of ions such as aluminum from these reactive substances. Except for dental implants, these resorbable ceramics are in the investigative

Table 12.3
Ceramics

Carbon
    Pyrolytic carbon (pyrolyte)—Dental implants, cardiac valves*
    Vitreous carbon (glassy carbon)—Dental implants*
    Carbon fiber
    Graphite

Inert Ceramics
    Alumina (Al_2O_3)—Dental implant, hip prosthesis*
    Zircon ($ZrSiO_4$)

Surface Reaction Ceramics
    Bioglass (Na_2O-CaF-P_2O_5-SiO_2)
    Durapatite (dense polycrystalline hydroxyapatite)

Resorbable ceramics
    Calcium phosphate [$Ca_3(PO_4)_2$]—Dental implant*
    Calcium aluminate ($CaO \cdot Al_2O_3$)
    Whitlockite ($3CaO \cdot P_2O_5$)
    Plaster of Paris ($CaSO_4$)

* In clinical use.

stage until the metabolic fate of their constituents is known (31, 32).

Polymers

From both the technological and medical standpoint, "plastics" has been the fastest growing area of materials development and application. There are a vast number of these synthetic implants in surgical use. To a large extent, this is due to the ease and low cost of fabrication and because they can be processed easily into tubes, fibers, fabrics, meshes, films, and foams.

CLINICAL CONSIDERATIONS

Some of the polymers are used for bone replacement (e.g., methyl methacrylate, polyacetals, polyethylene), but the majority of these materials are used in soft tissue. Soft tissue applications include (*a*) bulk space fillers for contour restoration, as with nasal, chin, auricular, breast, or chest wall implants; (*b*) devices for transport or encapsulation, such as vascular, tracheal, or ureteral implants or artificial skin; and (*c*) materials that provide structural support (e.g., sutures, tissue glue, meshes).

With the exception of the resorbable polymers, most of the surgical polymers are relatively inert and stimulate fibrous encapsulation. The physical form of the implants, solid versus mesh or smooth versus rough, will determine whether the entire structure is encapsulated as a whole or whether fibrous tissue will penetrate the interstices (18, 19). Tissue reaction to the implant is also influenced by chemical composition and chemical durability of the polymer. Silicone rubber, polytetrafluoroethylene (PTFE), and Dacron are among the most stable of polymers, while nylon, polyurethane, and polyesters undergo substantial degradation (33, 34). Tissue toxicity at the implant interface corresponds particularly well with: (*a*) the concentration of the chemical additives that may be released, although the base polymer itself may be nonreactive; and (*b*) the molecular weight of any polymeric materials available to the tissue. Low-molecular-weight materials are relatively toxic (9).

POLYMERS IN CURRENT SURGICAL USE

Biomedical polymers are classified as either elastomers or plastics (Table 12.4). Although a number of elastomers have been tried as implant materials, silicone rubber and polyether-linked or polyester-linked polyurethanes are the major implant materials in this group.

The nonelastomers are a very large group of materials inclusively termed "plastics" because most are thermolabile with reversible chemical reactions and can be liquified or softened with reheating. Table 12.4 includes the seven major types of plastics but only a handful of the many variants and copolymers now in surgical use.

Table 12.4
Polymers in Clinical Use

Elastomers
  Silicone rubber (Silastic)
  Polyurethane (Estane)
Plastics
  Polyamide (nylon, Supramid)
  Polyester
    Polyethylene terephthalate (Dacron, Mersilene, Mylar)
  Polyethylene (Marlex)
  Polypropylene (Prolene)
  Polyvinyl
    Polyvinyl chloride
    Polyvinyl ether (Ivalon)
  Fluorocarbons
    Polytetrafluoroethylene (PTFE, Teflon, Goretex)
    Polytetrafluoroethylene/carbon (Proplast)
  Adhesives and Cements
    Cyanoacrylate ("tissue glue")
    Polymethyl methacrylate (PMMA, Cranioplast)
  Hydrogels
    Hydroxyethyl methacrylate (HEMA)
    Polyhydroxyethyl methacrylate (Hydron)
  Resorbable polymers and copolymers
    Polyethylene oxide/polyethylene terephthalate (PEO/PET)
    Polyglycolic acid (PGA)/polylactic acid (PLA) (Vicryl)
    Polyglycolic acid (PGA) (Dexon)

Elastomers

Silicone Rubber

Silicone has the advantages of being highly biocompatible (35) and hemocompatible (36), nontoxic and nonirritating, nonallergenic, and almost totally resistant to biodegradation (37). Consequently, the tissue reaction is limited to a mild foreign-body reaction followed by encapsulation of either a bulk elastomer or injectable fluid that distributes itself in small encapsulated droplets (38). Disadvantages of silicone include physiological encapsulation, which may distort soft elastomer implants (39), the absorption of lipids onto elastomers after long-term vascular exposure (cardiac valve poppet wear) (40), and insufficient tensile strength to assure mechanical durability in weight-bearing or heavy stress applications (2.3% fracture rate in finger joint prostheses) (41).

As the most widely used of biomedical materials, silicone is fabricated as: (*a*) elastomer for reconstruction of soft tissue components; (*b*) room temperature vulcanizing (RTV) elastomer for self-curing custom-made implants; (*c*) fluid for lubrication of disposable hypodermic needles and syringes, drug vials, catheters, and other devices; and (*d*) antifoams to defoam blood in extracorporeal bubble oxygenators and as ingredients in oral antacid preparations to reduce flatulence.

Polyurethane

Polyurethane is a generic term applied to a wide variety of materials having in common only that they are formed from the same general classes of starting materials—a diisocyanate and an alcohol. Elastomers and foams result from additional combinations of polyesters, polyethers, and other components (16, 42, 43).

The major breakdown product of the toluene diisocyanate common to all polyurethanes is diaminotoluene. Diaminotoluene is a carcinogen in rodents (44) and a potent respiratory irritant and sensitizer in humans. There is inadequate evidence for the carcinogenicity of the isocyanate to humans (45).

The reactivity of the urethane polymers varies with the component materials and structure. Early cell-culture tests ranked polyurethane with polyvinyl chloride as a less biocompatible material in comparison with silicone, polyethylene, and PTFE (35). The in vivo response to these reactive materials is marked adhesion (34), and the polyester-type materials (Estane) are biodegradable (42). More recent studies of the polyether-type polyurethanes have generated contradictory results. Varying degrees of both enzymatic and oxidative degradation do occur (46), but the magnitude of the biodegradation may be less than thought originally (47).

Clinical applications for polyurethane implants have not been numerous, and the main interest arose because some polyurethanes have shown good thromboresistance. This led to their use in fabricating pumps and balloons to be used in the cardiovascular system (42). In addition, the textured surface afforded by the polyurethane foams has been used on silicone breast implants to promote the attachment of adjacent tissues and to reduce the encapsulation seen with smooth polymeric surfaces. These polyurethane foams do undergo biodegradation in vivo, and the soft tissue exhibits chronic low-grade inflammatory changes (48, 49). Evaluation of new polyurethane textured surfaces continues (50).

Plastics

Polyamide

The nylons are a large group of polymers that show significant degradation in the body. Nylons have been shown to lose 40% of original tensile strength after 17 months in vivo and may be reduced by as much as 80% after 3 years (37). There is a concomitant local inflammatory response (51), and tissues implanted with nylon sheets show marked adhesion and heavy fibroplasia (34). Nylon is used as a suture material and as a velour fabric bonded to less reactive implants, such as silicone or metal electrodes, to achieve soft tissue attachment.

Polyester

The only polyester in common usage is Dacron. It is less reactive than nylon, more reactive than silicone, and there is only mild loss of tensile strength in Dacron sutures after several years in vivo (34, 52). These properties make it suitable for applications that require both tensile strength and tissue ingrowth for stability. Dacron is mar-

keted as Mersilene mesh for abdominal and chest wall reconstruction. It has been used as a sleeve on the stem of silicone small joint prostheses (53) and other silicone implants, and it is the major prosthetic material for arterial vessel replacement (54). Woven or knitted velour grafts are porous to permit fibrous tissue ingrowth and must be preclotted to form thrombus within the interstices. Dacron is relatively thromboresistant, and the graft lumen becomes lined with a thin fibrous capsule.

Polyethylene

Several densities of polyethylene are available, with the chemical resistance, tensile strength, and hardness increasing with the density. Thus, the tissue response to polyethylene depends on the density and the additives present, but in general, it is quite inert, ranking close to silicone in biocompatibility tests (35) and eliciting little adhesion or inflammatory response in vivo (34). It does undergo some degradation, and over time, the ultra-high-molecular-weight polyethylenes used in hip and knee prostheses are subject to wear (55). Polyethylenes of comparatively low molecular weight have been used for facial bone reconstruction. Rubin (56) reports minimal tissue reaction, a thin fibrous capsule, and virtually no loss of the substance of the implant on long-term follow-up. High-density polyethylene mesh (Marlex mesh) is loosely woven and has been reported to show good tensile strength and fibrous tissue infiltration of the spaces in the net for solid anchoring (57).

Polypropylene

This material is extremely nonreactive and undergoes no loss of tensile strength after 2 to 6 years in vivo. It is the strongest, lightest, and most inert suture material available and as a surgical mesh has properties similar to those of polyethylene (57).

Fluorocarbon Polymers

Fluorocarbon materials are resistant to chemical degradation, and only one of these polymers is in common use surgically: PTFE. This material is even less reactive than polyethylene, with no adherence and virtually no inflammatory response in vivo (34). The water repellence of PTFE makes it highly hemocompatible. Because of its thromboresistant properties, PTFE is used in the fabrication of vascular prostheses. It is very effective for venous and small arterial applications but lacks sufficient strength for large arterial implants. Woven meshes of PTFE also have proven inferior to polyethylene mesh in tensile strength (57); Teflon proved to have poor fatigue resistance under loading in hip prostheses (58) and heart valves (58) and has been replaced with high-density polyethylene and pyrolytic carbon, respectively. Where mechanical strength is required, a PTFE coating on a stronger material is effective.

Proplast

A composite material of Teflon and carbon, Proplast I is a black porous scaffold available in sheets or blocks that can be carved to custom shapes for maxillofacial reconstruction. Proplast II was introduced in 1981. It is a PTFE/aluminum oxide analog to Proplast I that is white and, therefore, more suitable for superficial implants. The composite material is nearly inert, but the porous configuration permits collagenous ingrowth for stabilization. There is no induction of osseous tissue (60).

Adhesives and Cements

Cyanoacrylate

Quick-setting, biodegradable tissue adhesives polymerize in contact with tissue to form an adherent polymeric film that "glues" together the margins of a wound or acts as a hemostatic agent in an open wound. The problem with these alkyl cyanoacrylates is toxicity from their degradation products, which can be detected in the urine (20). Other cyanoacrylate types such as isobutyl-2-cyanoacrylate appear to be more biocompatible and are used for repair of cerebrospinal fluid fistulas (61).

Polymethyl Methacrylate

A self-curing acrylin resin, polymethyl methacrylate is used for securing joint components to bone and as a cranial and facial bone substitute (62). It has the advantages of easy surgical manipulation, rapid fixation, density similar to bone, and good long-term soft tissue tolerance. Disadvantages tend to be more pronounced in orthopaedic applications due to larger open wounds and the greater tensile demands placed on the implant material. The in vivo polymerization process is responsible for chemical and thermal injury: it invariably is incomplete and releases unbound monomers that can cause systemic hypotension (63) and local tissue toxicity; it is exothermic, and the heat can induce bone necrosis and possibly lead to eventual loosening of the implant. The major late problem is mechanical failure from implant fracture or deterioration of the polymer-bone interface (20).

Hydrogels

A unique group of hydrophilic acrylic polymers, the hydrogels, incorporate water into their structure, forming soft, pliable, jelly-like structures. Most are based on hydroxyethyl methacrylate (HEMA) and are used in the manufacture of soft contact lenses and semipermeable membranes for graded-release drug implants, wound dressings, and dialysis equipment. Depending on the structure of the hydrogel, 3–90% of its weight can be made up of water (64). Rigid when dry, the hydrogels can be easily machined, but after wetting, the transparent elastic gel form has little mechanical strength. Research may introduce new copolymers for vascular and articular surfaces (65).

Resorbable Copolymers

Biodegradable polymers have several applications: sutures, temporary scaffolds, adhesives, and implantable drug delivery systems (20). The resorbable suture materials based on polyglycolic acid (PGA) and polylactic acid (PLA) are resorbed by hydrolysis of the polymers at a relatively predictable rate. They elicit a milder tissue response and have greater tensile strength than do gut (collagen) sutures of the same diameter (66). These materials are now available as microvascular couplers and are under investigation as resorbable bone plates.

Biological Material

Collagen is the primary biological polymer and is a resorbable material. Its differences from the inorganic polymers are: (a) it is degraded by enzymatic rather than hydrolytic reactions; (b) it is potentially antigenic and requires purification by enzymatic digestion before implantation; and (c) its tensile strength and rate of absorption are related to solubility. It requires tanning to reestablish intermolecular cross-links if it is to exhibit the strength and longevity of insoluble collagen. Monomeric purified collagen is the form of injectable Zyderm collagen implant. For many other applications, the collagen cross-links are replaced by tanning with glutaraldehyde, formaldehyde, dialdehyde starch, or other polymers. The type of agent, its concentration, pH, and temperature will determine the extent of tanning and thus the mechanical and compatibility properties of the collagen. While tanning does not prevent eventual biodegradation, it can delay it for up to 10 years as in the glutaraldehyde stabilized porcine cardiac valves. Immunogenicity of these highly tanned valves has been demonstrated (67).

Collagen preparations include: (a) suspension for dermal injection; (b) microcrystalline collagen (Avitene) topical hemostatic agent; (c) sheets of collagen fibers for wound dressings; (d) collagen sutures from the flexor tendons of cattle; (e) catgut sutures from the fibrous tissue of beef or sheep intestinal wall; (f) collagen gel for periodontal reconstruction; (g) collagen sponges for hemostasis and articular linings; (h) collagen-rich pigskin wound dressings; (i) bovine arteries and cardiac valves (68); and (j) collagen/silicone artificial skin.

Summary

Materials science addresses the systemic and local host-tissue reactions to implant materials; there has been much activity and research in this area in recent years. This review of biomaterials has included only the fundamental principles of implant-host interaction. It does not do justice to the efforts directed at blood-contact surfaces and studies of hemocompatibility and thromboresistance; to transcutaneous device research aimed at developing an implant that will bond with the tissues and resist mechanical manipulation and infection from the outside; or to the ongoing work with external devices such as dialysis membranes or blood oxygenators.

In all of modern materials research, there has been a shift in emphasis from implants for substitution to implants for adaptation (1, 20). The classical goals of mechanical and biochemical stability have broadened to a search for materials with controlled reactive surfaces that will permit active involvement with the host environment rather than mere passive tolerance.

References

1. Hench LL: Special report: The interfacial behavior of biomaterials, 1979. *J Biomed Mater Res* 14:803, 1980.
2. Oppenheimer BS, Oppenheimer ET, Stout AP, Danishefsky I: Malignant tumors resulting from embedding plastics in rodents. *Science* 118:305, 1953.
3. Brand KG, Buoen LC, Johnson KH, et al: Etiological factors, stages and the role of the foreign body in foreign body tumorigenesis: A review. *Cancer Res* 35:279, 1975.
4. Woodward SC: How to relate observations of foreign-body oncogenesis in experimental animals to human health risk. In Rubin LR (ed): *Biomaterials in Reconstructive Surgery*. St. Louis, CV Mosby Co, 1983, pp 17–26.
5. Brand KG: Exploration of implant-associated carcinogenesis in animals. In Rubin LR (ed): *Biomaterials in Reconstructive Surgery*. St Louis, CV Mosby Co, 1983, pp 27–35.
6. Brand KG, Brand I: Risk assessment of carcinogenesis at implantation site. *Plast Reconstr Surg* 66:591, 1980.
7. Autian J: Toxicological evaluation of biomaterials: Primary acute toxicity screening program. *Artif Organs* 1:53, 1977.
8. Rice RM, Hegyeli AF, Gourlay SJ, et al: Biocompatibility testing of polymers. *In vitro* studies with *in vivo* correlation. *J Biomed Mater Res* 12:43, 1978.
9. Blais P: Industrial polymers as implants: Their value and their limitations. In Rubin LR (ed): *Biomaterials in Reconstructive Surgery*. St Louis, CV Mosby Co, 1983, pp 62–72.
10. Park JB: Tissue response to implants. In: *Biomaterials: An Introduction*. New York, Plenum Press, 1979, pp 131–146.
11. Elves MW, Wilson JN, Scales JT, et al: Incidence of metal sensitivity in patients with total joint replacements. *Br Med J* 4:376, 1975.
12. Deutman R, Mulder TJ, Brian T, et al: Metal sensitivity before and after total hip arthroplasty. *J Bone Joint Surg [Am]* 59:862, 1977.
13. Bagnall RD, Arundel PA: A method for the prediction of protein absorption on implant surfaces. *J Biomed Mater Res* 17:459, 1983.
14. Kumagai Y, Shiokawa Y, Medsger TA Jr, et al: Clinical spectrum of connective tissue disease after cosmetic surgery. Observations on eighteen patients and a review of the Japanese literature. *Arthritis Rheum* 27:1, 1984.
15. Van Nunen SA, Gatenby PA, Basten A: Postmammoplasty connective tissue disease. *Arthritis Rheum* 25:694, 1982.
16. Bloch B, Hastings GW: The medical aspects of implantation. In: *Plastic Materials in Surgery*. Springfield, IL, Charles C Thomas, 1972, pp 3–21.
17. Marck KW, Wildevuur CRH, Sederel WL, et al: Biodegradability and tissue reaction of random copolymers of L-leucine, L-aspartic acid and L-aspartic acid esters. *J Biomed Mater Res* 11:405, 1977.
18. Matlaga BF, Yasenchak LP, Salthouse TN: Tissue response to implanted polymers: The significance of sample shape. *J Biomed Mater Res* 10:391, 1976.
19. Salthouse TN, Matlaga PF: Effects of implant surface on cellular activity and evaluation of histocompatibility. In Winter GD, Leray JL, de Groot K (eds): *Evaluation of Biomaterials*. London, John Wiley & Sons, Ltd, 1980.
20. Hench LL, Ethridge EC: *Biomaterials: An Interfacial Approach*. New York, Academic Press, 1982.
21. Williams DF: Electrochemical aspects of corrosion in the physiological environment. In Williams DF (ed): *Fundamental Aspects of Biocompatibility*. Boca Raton, FL, CRC Press, 1981, pp 11–42.
22. Pohler OEM: Degradation of metallic orthopedic implants. In Rubin LR (ed): *Biomaterials in Reconstructive Surgery*. St. Louis, CV Mosby Co, 1983, pp 158–228.
23. Harris B: Corrosion of stainless steel surgical implants. *J Med Eng Technol* 3:117, 1979.
24. Winter GD: Tissue reactions to metallic wear and corrosion products in human patients. *J Biomed Mater Res* 8:11, 1974.
25. Scales JT, Winter GD, Shirley HT: Corrosion of orthopaedic implants: Screws, plates and femoral nail-plates. *J Bone Joint Surg [Br]* 41:810, 1959.
26. Coleman RF, Herrington J, Scales JT: Concentration of wear products in hair, blood, and urine after total hip replacement. *Br Med J* 1:527, 1973.
27. Hille GH: Titanium for surgical implants. *J Mater* 1:373, 1966.
28. Bokros JC: Carbon in prosthetic devices. *Biomed Mater Res Symp Trans* 2:32, 1978.
29. Scott SM, Gaddy LR, Parra S: Pyrolytic carbon-coated vascular prostheses. *J Surg Res* 29:395, 1980.
30. Drummond JL: Histological response to ceramic materials. In Rubin LR (ed): *Biomaterials in Reconstructive Surgery*. St. Louis, CV Mosby Co, 1983, pp 102–108.
31. Ferraro JW: Experimental evaluation of ceramic calcium phosphate as a substitute for bone grafts. *Plast Reconstr Surg* 63:634, 1979.
32. Bajpai PK, Wyatt DF, Gilles NM, et al: Use of calcium aluminate phosphorus pentoxide ceramics as bone substitutes. *Clin Res* 24:524A, 1976.
33. Roggendorf E: The biostability of silicone rubbers, a polyamide, and a polyester. *J Biomed Mater Res* 10:123, 1976.
34. Calnan JS: The use of inert plastic materials in reconstructive surgery. *Br J Plast Surg* 16:1, 1963.
35. Homsy CA: Biocompatibility in selection of materials for implantation. *J Biomed Mater Res* 4:341, 1970.
36. Galletti PM: Application of plastics in membrane oxygenators. *J Biomed Mater Res Symp* 1:129, 1971.
37. Leininger RI: *Plastics in Surgical Implants*. Philadelphia, American Society of Testing and Materials, 1965.
38. Frisch EE: Technology of silicones in biomedical applications. In Rubin LR (ed): *Biomaterials in Reconstructive Surgery*. St. Louis, CV Mosby Co, 1983, pp 73–90.
39. McGrath MH, Burkhardt BR: The safety and efficacy of breast implants for augmentation mammaplasty. *Plast Reconstr Surg* 74:550, 1984.
40. Cuddihy EF, Moacanin J, Roschke EJ, et al: In vivo degradation of silicone rubber poppets in prosthetic heart valves. *J Biomed Mater Res* 10:471, 1976.
41. Swanson AB, Swanson G de G, Frisch EE: Flexible (silicone) implant arthroplasty in the small joints of extremities: concepts, physical and biological considerations, experimental and clinical results. In Rubin LR (ed): *Biomaterials in Reconstructive Surgery*. St. Louis, CV Mosby Co, 1983, pp 595–623.
42. Leininger RI, Bigg DM: Polymers. In vonRecum AF (ed): *Handbook of Biomaterials Evaluation. Scientific, Technical and Clinical Testing of Implant Materials*. New York, Macmillan Publishing Company, 1986, pp 24–37.
43. Lynch W: *Implants. Reconstructing the Human Body*. New York, Van Nostrand Reinhold Company, 1982.
44. Anon: 2-4 Diaminotoluene. *International Agency for Research on Cancer* 16:83, 1978.
45. Anon: Toluene diisocyanate. *International Agency for Research on Cancer* 39:287, 1986.
46. Ratner BD, Gladhill KW, Horbett TA: Analysis of in vitro enzymatic and oxidative degradation of polyurethanes. *J Biomed Mater Res* 22:509, 1988.
47. Bakker D, Van Blitterswijk CA, Daems WTh, Grote JJ: Biocompatibility of six elastomers in vitro. *J Biomed Mater Res* 22:423, 1988.
48. Lilla JA, Vistnes LM: Long-term study of reactions to various silicone breast implants in rabbits. *Plast Reconstr Surg* 57:637, 1976.

49. Smahel J: Tissue reactions to breast implants coated with polyurethane. *Plast Reconstr Surg* 61:80, 1978.
50. Whalen RL: Improved textured surface for implantable prostheses. *Trans Am Soc Artif Intern Organs* 34:887, 1988.
51. Williams DF: The reactions of tissues to materials. *Biomed Eng* 6:152, 1971.
52. Postlethwait RW: Long-term comparative study of nonabsorbable sutures. *Ann Surg* 17:892, 1970.
53. Goldner JL, Urbaniak JR: The clinical experience with silicone-Dacron metacarpophalangeal and interphalangeal joint prostheses. *J Biomed Mater Res Symp* 4:137, 1973.
54. Sawyer PN, Stanczewski B, Hoskin GP, et al: In vitro and in vivo evaluations of Dacron velour and knit prostheses. *J Biomed Mater Res* 13:937, 1979.
55. Ainsworth R, Farling G, Bardos D: An improved bearing material for joint replacement prostheses: Carbon fiber reinforced UHMW polyethylene. *Biomed Mater Res Symp Trans* 1:119, 1977.
56. Rubin LR: Polyethylene as a bone and cartilage substitute: A 32-year retrospective. In Rubin LR (ed): *Biomaterials in Reconstructive Surgery.* St. Louis, CV Mosby Co, 1983, pp 474–493.
57. DeBenedetto A, Fleischer A: Biological properties of surgical mesh. In Rubin LR (ed): *Biomaterials in Reconstructive Surgery.* St. Louis, CV Mosby Co, 1983, pp 819–829.
58. Charnley J: The long-term results of low-friction arthroplasty of the hip performed as a primary intervention. *J Bone Joint Surg [Br]* 54:61, 1972.
59. Silver MD, Wilson GJ: The pathology of wear in the Beall Model 104 heart valve prosthesis. *Circulation* 56:617, 1977.
60. Homsy CA: Biocompatibility of perfluorinated polymers and composites on these polymers. In Williams DF (ed): *Biocompatibility of Clinical Implant Materials.* Boca Raton, FL, CRC Press, Inc, Vol 2, 1981, pp 59–78.
61. Maxwell JA, Goldware SI: Use of tissue adhesive in the surgical treatment of cerebrospinal fluid leaks. *J Neurosurg* 39:332, 1973.
62. Schultz RC: Reconstruction of facial deformities with alloplastic materials. In *Facial Injuries,* 2nd ed. Chicago, Year Book Medical Publishers, Inc, 1977, pp 426–450.
63. Newens AF, Volz RG: Severe hypotension during prosthetic hip surgery with acrylic bone cement. *Anesthesiology* 36:298, 1972.
64. Boretos JW: *Concise Guide to Biomedical Polymers.* Springfield, IL, Charles C Thomas, 1973.
65. Bruck SD: Current activities and future directions in biomaterials research. *Ann NY Acad Sci* 283:332, 1977.
66. Ruderman RJ, Bernstein E, Kairiner NE, et al: Scanning electron microscopic study of surface changes on biodegradable sutures. *J Biomed Mater Res* 7:215, 1973.
67. Bajpai PK, Stull PA, Anderson JM: Immunogenicity of glutaraldehyde cross-linked porcine heart valve xenografts. *Int Res Comm Syst Med Sci* 8:519,1980.
68. Chvapil M, Kronenthal LR, Van Winkle W, Jr: Medical and surgical applications of collagen. *Int Rev Connect Tissue Res* 6:1, 1973.

13

Tissue Expansion

Louis C. Argenta, M.D., F.A.C.S. and Malcolm W. Marks, M.D., F.A.C.S.

Reconstructive surgical procedures are frequently limited by the availability of adequate soft tissue. In the past 10 years, mechanical tissue expansion to provide soft tissue and facilitate reconstructive procedures has become an important modality for overcoming these limitations.

Living skin tissue responds dynamically to mechanical stresses, and the tissue envelope rapidly responds to incorporate an enlarging mass. Selective placement of a silicone prosthesis, which is gradually inflated, allows for the development of new tissue that may be used for reconstructive surgery.

Tissue expansion can be used to provide skin with an almost perfect match of color, texture, sensation, and special adnexal characteristics needed for reconstruction of a specific area. With adequate planning, this procedure results in minimal or no donor scars, a characteristic unique to this technique.

Soft tissue expansion, an important adjunct to the surgeon's armamentarium, allows safe extension of the usual techniques of flap surgery, free flaps, and skin grafts. Tissue expansion has been applied to multiple other tissues of the body, including bladder, intestine, ureter, and blood vessels (1). The ability of the body to create new tissue by responding to mechanical stimulation appears universal and is an area of future investigation for new generations of surgeons.

History

Primitive tribes in Africa and in the Middle East have, for many centuries, stretched lips and ears as a cosmetic ritual. The first published clinical report of tissue expansion was by Neumann in 1957 (2); however, many individuals have come forward with anecdotal claims of having antedated his procedure. Neumann first used a subcutaneous rubber balloon filled through an external transcutaneous tube to achieve expansion of an area of the scalp for ear reconstruction. Despite its success and publication of the case, no further reports ensued until Radovan (3) reported his experience. His technique involved a sophisticated silicone implant that could be placed in a subcutaneous pocket and filled through an attached self-sealing valve by intermittant percutaneous injection. This work went largely unheeded until the first soft tissue expansion seminar was held in Ann Arbor, Michigan in 1982. Over the next 2 years, numerous clini-

cal series (4–9) and experimental studies (10–12) were published, and this led to the widespread acceptance and use of tissue expansion in reconstructive surgery.

Tissue Response to Mechanical Expansion

As the tissue expander is gradually inflated within the body, significant changes take place in the overlying tissues. These have been studied in animals as well as humans (13, 14). There is considerable variation in tissue response, depending on the rate, volume, and duration of the expansion. In general, the changes induced by gradual low-pressure expansion over a longer period of time result in less conspicuous changes than rapid large-volume expansion. Excessive rates of expansion may result in irreversible damage to the overlying tissue, including disruption of skin, fat necrosis, muscle atrophy, stria formation, and neurapraxia.

After the expander has been removed and the reconstructive procedure accomplished, expanded tissue appears to "normalize." Relative thickness and structure of the expanded tissue return to preexpansion levels.

EPIDERMIS

During expansion, epidermis undergoes slight thickening (11) with cellular hyperplasia. Occasional hyperkeratosis and parakeratosis can be found histologically. Electron microscopy reveals a narrowing of intercellular space and an increase in basal lamina undulation that is suggestive of increased mitosis (12). Triitiated thymidine studies in animals have demonstrated a 500% increase in mitotic activity of the basal layer (15).

DERMIS

The most dramatic changes in soft tissue expansion occur in the dermis. Increased fibroplasia, increased collagen deposition, and realignment of collagen fibers are evident. The overall thickness of the dermis decreases 30–50%, resulting in the increased compactness of collagen in both papillary or reticular dermis. Elastic fibers are fragmented, and myofibroblasts increase significantly.

DERMAL APPENDAGES

During normal expansion, there is no significant morphological change in nerve end-receptors, sebaceous glands, hair follicles, or sweat glands. The structures are distracted from one another, but they remain viable and active. With excessively rapid tissue expansion with high pressures, necrosis of these adnexal structures may occur with permanent dysfunction.

MUSCLE

Expansion results in significant changes in overlying muscle. Skeletal muscle becomes thin and compacted, although it remains functional. Sarcomeres become abnormal, and myofibrils become irregular. Mitochondria increase in number and size during muscle expansion, probably as an attempt to compensate for the relative anoxia during expansion.

ADIPOSE

Fat cells atrophy significantly during normal expansion, and there is usually some permanent loss of total fat mass in the area expanded. With aggressive expansion, fat necrosis and fibrosis may occur. Injury incurred by fatty tissue during expansion appears to persist for many years. Later, ingrowth of adjacent fat cells and fibrosis may compensate for contour defects.

VASCULAR RESPONSE

During expansion, there is a significant increase in vasculature. This occurs particularly at the junction of the capsule formed around the prosthesis and the adjacent dermal tissue (Fig. 13.1). Removal of the capsule significantly decreased blood flow in expanded flaps. There is an increase in the number as well as the caliber of capillaries in expanded skin, with a significant increase occur-

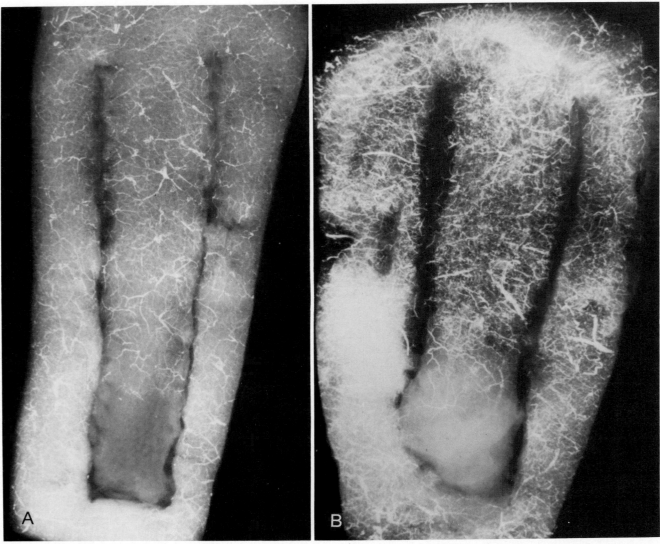

FIGURE 13.1. Barium injections of flaps that have been elevated acutely (**A**) versus flaps that have been expanded (**B**). Note the dramatic increase in vascularity throughout the expanded flap as well as adjacent tissue.

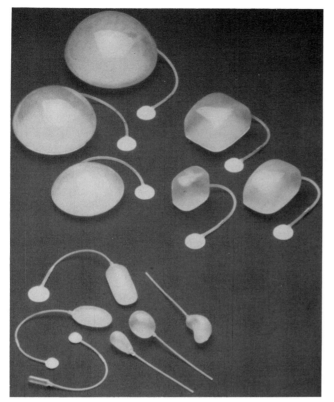

FIGURE 13.2. Tissue expanders are available in a large number of sizes and shapes. Custom implants can be specifically fabricated.

Stock expanders are available in volumes of 20–1000 ml and in round, rectangular, or crescentic shapes. Custom implants of any size and shape can be fabricated by most manufacturers. Most expanders will tolerate two to three times their recommended volumes without rupture.

BASIC TECHNIQUE OF EXPANSION

The object of tissue expansion is to generate a quantity of a particular quality of tissue. Planning so that the proposed area to be expanded can be rotated, advanced, or transposed to the defect with as little risk as possible is critical. As much of the normal adjacent tissue as possible should be used for expansion so that adnexal structures can be more evenly distributed. The expander selection depends more on the surface area to be expanded than on the volume of the device. Several smaller expanders can be inflated more rapidly and more safely than a single larger prosthesis.

Expanders can be placed through any incision that will not interfere with the subsequent reconstruction procedure. Existing scars are preferred. Dissections are carried as homogeneously as possible under the tissue to be expanded to minimize erosion and extrusion. Nerves and

ring in the dermal papillae. An increased survival of expanded random flaps as well as an increase in circulation in the capsule layer has been demonstrated (16). As a consequence of increased vascularity, there is increased resistance to bacterial invasion in expanded versus normal skin (17). Clinical experience has also demonstrated that expanded tissue is highly vascular, in keeping with laboratory observations.

The mechanism of increase of vascularity is poorly understood. Simple mechanical stretch results in new vessel growth proportional to the mechanical force applied to the membrane (18). Ischemia and hypoxia are also strong stimuli for increased blood vessel flow, either by the opening of existing capillaries or by angiogenesis.

Tissue Expanders

Tissue expanders are basically silicone envelopes connected to a self-sealing reservoir through which percutaneous injections of saline are made (Fig. 13.2). The reservoir may be integrated into the envelope itself or at a distance with a tube connecting it to the implant. Recently, textured implants, differential expanders, and polyurethane-covered expanders have been devised. While theoretically interesting, their clinical benefit is still unproven. Attempts at developing self-expanding prostheses (10) are slowly approaching fruition.

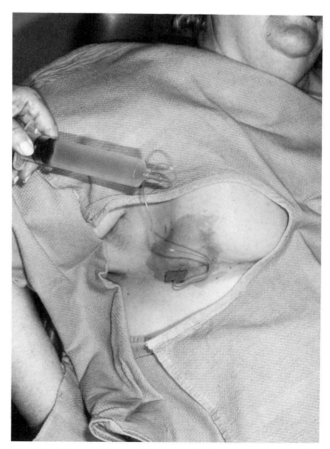

FIGURE 13.3. Inflation of the prosthesis is carried out with a 23-gauge butterfly needle under sterile conditions. Enough isotonic saline is placed to develop tenseness of the skin overlying the prosthesis.

axial vessels are preserved. As large a prosthesis as the wound will comfortably tolerate is placed after hemostasis is achieved. Folds in the prosthesis and abutment of the prosthesis to the wound edges are meticulously avoided because they result in extrusion. The wound is then closed in multiple layers.

Remote valves are situated subcutaneously at distant sites; tissue prominences are avoided. In some cases, reservoirs may be placed externally with the connecting tube exiting the skin (19).

After wound integrity is sufficient, inflation is begun. A 23-gauge or smaller needle is inserted into the reservoir, and sufficient isotonic saline is injected to produce tenseness of the overlying tissue (Fig. 13.3). Excessively aggressive inflation may result in extrusion of the prosthesis or loss of the overlying tissue. Insufficient inflation may result in prolonged expansion. The overlying tissue becomes indurated during expansion; however, this indicates increased vascularity rather than impending infection. After approximately 48 hr, tenseness of the overlying tissue dramatically decreases, and the prosthesis can be felt to move.

Frequent small injections result in a more rapid tissue expansion than infrequent large injections of saline. Continuous infusion with low volumes is safe and generates large areas of tissue at a rapid rate. No precise timetable for inflation should be established. With proper education, selected patients may be able to inflate their own prosthesis, or other family members may learn to help them. If excessive blanching of the overlying tissue occurs, saline may be withdrawn. The use of intraluminal pressures, piezoelectric currents, and laser Doppler have not been particularly useful in assessing the safety of volume inflation.

Breast Reconstruction

The concept of tissue expansion was initially evolved for the reconstruction of postmastectomy breast defects. The acceptance of modified radical mastectomy with preservation of pectoralis muscle and overlying skin allows a large percentage of patients to be successfully reconstructed with a simple expansion technique. It is important that every patient be individualized. Those who can be reconstructed with a simple prosthesis in one stage should be so reconstructed. Patients who have skin grafts, extensive radiation damage to the chest wall, and severely compromised overlying tissues are probably best reconstructed with distant flap procedures such as the rectus abdominis and latissimus dorsi flaps.

In 1990, approximately 70% of postmastectomy breast reconstructions are performed using tissue expansion. The procedure is reliable and minimizes discomfort, hospitalization, and postoperative recovery for the patient. However, multiple visits are required for inflation of the prosthesis. The advent of the "permanent expander" has minimized the need for a secondary procedure for placing a permanent prosthesis. In approximately 60% of patients reconstructed with the Becker implant, a secondary surgical procedure was not necessary after adequate breast development.

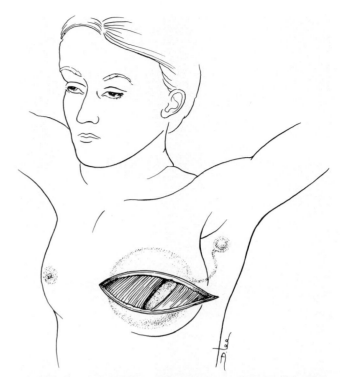

FIGURE 13.4. Reconstruction after mastectomy using tissue expander. The prosthesis is placed submuscularly through the original mastectomy wound. The reservoir is placed in the axilla in the subcutaneous tissue. (From Argenta LC: Reconstruction of the breast by tissue expansion. *Clin Plast Surg* 11:257, 1984.)

Secondary breast reconstruction can be initiated any time after 3 months following the ablative mastectomy. The expander is placed in the prepectoral or, preferably, in the subpectoral space. In patients with thin skin and subcutaneous tissue, it is best to place the prosthesis entirely under muscle, both as a protection for the prosthesis and to minimize the risk of skin compromise. Expansions carried out above the muscle have a higher incidence of capsular contracture than expansion carried out beneath the pectoralis. Textured implants may alter the rate of this contracture.

The expansion prosthesis is usually placed through an incision in the previous scar. This avoids a second incision that will result in a scar placed directly over the apex of the implant. Dissection is then carried down to the pectoralis muscle, which is split in the direction of its fibers laterally. From there, the dissection is carried subpectorally and with sharp dissection is extended under the serratus muscle. In secondary reconstructions with adequate soft tissue coverage, it may not be necessary to dissect beneath the serratus, and the implant is placed only under the pectoral muscle with the inferior lateral 30% of the implant subcutaneous. The inflation reservoir is situated in the axilla or the anterior chest wall beneath the brassiere line (Fig. 13.4).

One to 2 weeks following implant placement, inflation is begun. Sequential inflation is performed until the implant is overexpanded so that the reconstructed breast is approximately 20% larger than the opposite side (20, 21).

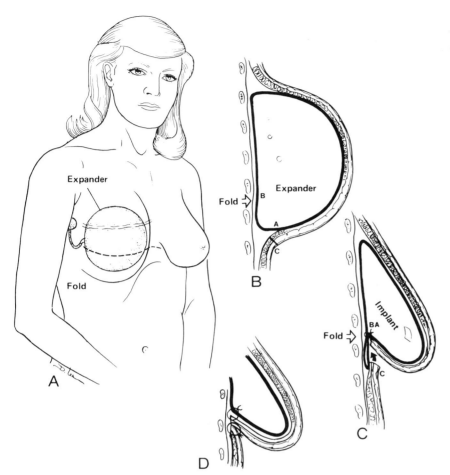

FIGURE 13.5. The procedure for defining the inframammary fold after expansion. **A,** The prosthesis is overinflated and left in place for 3–4 months. **B,** An incision is made at point C, and the expander removed and replaced with a permanent prosthesis whose volume matches the opposite breast. **C,** Point A is moved to an appropriate position along the anterior chest wall to point B to create an appropriate ptotic breast. **D,** The abdominal skin is advanced in a cephalad direction to close the defect.

If more ptosis is needed, the expander is inflated even more. It is important that the overexpanded breast capsule be allowed to mature for approximately 3–4 months. The expander is then deflated until symmetry is reached with the opposite side. If a permanent implant is used, approximately 60% of our patients will have achieved acceptable symmetry without the need of a secondary operative procedure (22).

If the implant has been displaced during expansion or if a more defined inframammary fold is desired, a second procedure is performed. A modification of an abdominal advancement procedure as described in Figure 13.5 is used (23). The expander is replaced with a permanent smaller prosthesis, and vigorous massage is begun as soon as possible after surgery. Nipple reconstruction may be performed 3–4 months following reconstruction of the breast mound.

IMMEDIATE BREAST RECONSTRUCTION

Select patients undergoing modified radical mastectomy in whom the risk of metastatic disease is minimal or patients undergoing subcutaneous mastectomies may have expanders placed beneath the pectoral muscle and fascial extension at the time of their initial surgery (23, 24). Inflation is carried on slowly over the ensuing weeks to minimize the risk of loss of the overlying skin. The procedure is then carried on in a manner similar to that previously described for delayed reconstruction.

Occasionally, patients may develop metastatic disease following the placement of the tissue expander. In these cases, tissue expansion is carried on during the course of chemotherapy at a small-volume, frequent-fill regimen. If radiation treatment for secondary treatment of local recurrence is necessary, this also can be carried on with the expander in situ. Expansion during radiation therapy carries a higher risk of capsular contracture and extrusion, but it is usually successful. Patients who have failed radiotherapy as a primary therapy for breast cancer are poor candidates for expansion. If immediate reconstruction is desirable in these patients, a distant flap is recommended.

Congenital Abnormalities

Expansion is useful in the reconstruction of acquired or congenital breast hypoplasia (25). Unilateral hypoplasia is frequently seen in pubescent females following burns, trauma, Poland's syndrome, and other miscellaneous conditions. Once the asymmetry becomes obvious, a tissue expander may be placed beneath the pectoralis muscle through a transaxillary approach (Fig. 13.6). If the pectoralis is absent as in Poland's syndrome, the prosthesis is placed in the subcutaneous space. The prosthesis is

FIGURE 13.6. Placement of an expander prosthesis through an axillary incision for reconstruction of congenital asymmetry of the breast. Redundancy is left in the connection tubing to avoid tearing the prosthesis during exercise.

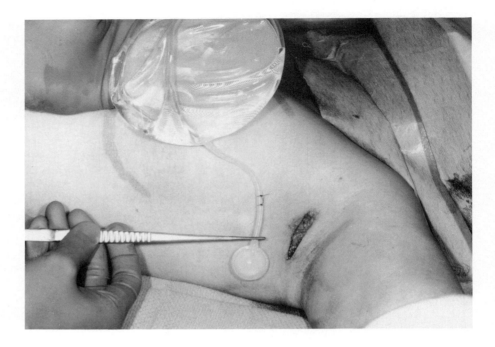

then inflated at appropriate intervals to maintain symmetry until development stabilizes. At 18 or 19 years of age, the expander can be replaced with a permanent implant, and the latissimus dorsi is transposed, if necessary.

This approach has been extremely successful in minimizing psychological trauma in adolescent females. It carries the advantage of recapitulating normal growth of the breast, resulting in enlargement and displacement of the nipple-areola complex to a more caudal position.

Women who have achieved complete breast development and have severe unilateral hypoplasia are also excellent candidates for expansion. The implants are placed subpectorally and gradually inflated until volume symmetry is achieved. The implant is overexpanded to encourage enlargement and migration of the nipple to a more inferior position and the development of ptosis. At a sec-

ond procedure, a latissimus dorsi can be transferred, and the implant is repositioned or replaced, if needed.

Head and Neck Reconstruction

SCALP

The scalp is the only tissue in the human body that has unique hair-bearing qualities. Prior methods of scalp reconstruction resulted in large areas of alopecia, which required multiple sequential excisions over a period of many years if left untreated. Tissue expansion has radically facilitated the reconstruction of large scalp defects associated with congenital abnormalities, tumor, trauma, or male baldness (26; Fig. 13.7).

FIGURE 13.7. Correction of traumatic alopecia using tissue expansion. **A,** A 6 × 8 cm defect in the scalp is covered with a split-thickness skin graft. **B,** The postoperative result after expansion to 600 ml with a single prosthesis and advancement of a hair-bearing flap.

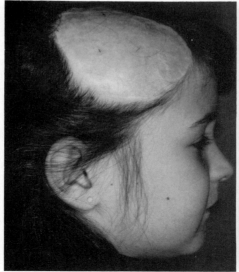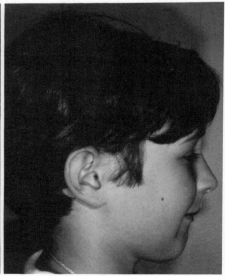

Expansion results in distraction of individual follicles from one another rather than creation of new follicles. Distraction of hair follicles by a factor of two produces no discernible thinness of hair. In blondes, an even greater distraction can be performed without creating obvious scalp thinness. Planning is critical in scalp expansion. The implant should be placed so as to expand as much of the normal hair-bearing scalp as possible. Expanders are placed beneath the galea, through what will be the advancing edge of various flaps (27). Distant incisions may be useful, but they require more meticulous preoperative planning. Expansion of the scalp proceeds quite rapidly after an initial phase of discomfort. At a second procedure, the expanders are removed, and the appropriate rotation, advancement, or specialized flap is created. The surgeon must pay meticulous attention to the direction of hair growth, cowlicks, and temporal and frontal hairlines. Preservation of the major axial blood vessels to the scalp is important to ensure its viability and to minimize ischemic hair loss. Selective incisions of the expanded capsule may be necessary for large defects. Beveling of skin incision and the avoidance of excessive use of cautery minimizes injury to follicles. If defects cannot be completely closed, the expander may be left in place for a second expansion. In adults, serial expansions are very well tolerated. In young children, expansion may be safely performed two or three times sequentially.

Male-Pattern Baldness

Patients with significant male-pattern baldness may be reconstructed using tissue expansion as an adjunct to scalp reduction or the creation of Juri flaps (27). Because there is a period of deformity during expansion, the use of this technique, except in the most motivated patient, is relatively infrequent.

Prostheses are placed beneath the galea in the temporal or posterior occipital areas. If a scalp reduction is contemplated, the expanders are removed at a second procedure, and the flaps are advanced toward the vertex. Occasionally, multiple procedures are necessary. In cases where a frontal hairline requires reconstruction, the use of expanded Juri flaps is most helpful. Wide, anteriorly based expanded flaps are created and transposed to reconstruct the anterior hairline. Expanded temporal scalp is then advanced to fill the donor defect (27; Fig. 13.8).

In all of scalp and forehead reconstruction, it is common to have irregular dog-ears after flap transposition. These should not be excised at the time of reconstruction because their excision may result in compromise of blood flow to flaps. Most dog-ears resolve dramatically over 2–3 months, although some may require a later correction.

FOREHEAD

The forehead interfaces both the soft tissues of the face and scalp and is anatomically similar to the scalp. Pros-

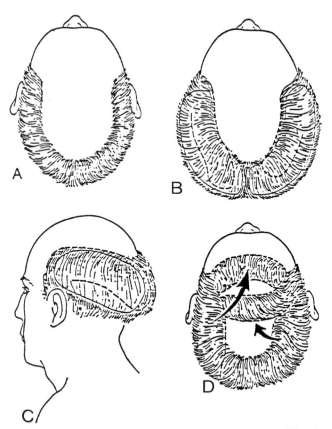

FIGURE 13.8. Correction of male-pattern baldness (**A**) using tissue expanders. **B,** Prostheses are placed under the parietal scalp. **C,** The flaps are then designed over the expanded tissue. **D,** The first flap is transposed to create an anterior hairline. The second is placed behind it, and the expanded tissue is used to close the defect.

theses are placed beneath the frontalis muscle, usually through an incision in the scalp. Expansion of the forehead proceeds quite rapidly, although some patients complain of discomfort during expansion in this area. The frontalis muscle becomes thin; however, it remains animated, and there have been no short- or long-term sequelae. The forehead can be moved laterally, medially, or superiorly to create a symmetrical cosmetic result. Symmetrical positioning of the brows is most important.

EXPANSION OF THE FACE AND NECK

Optimal reconstruction of large facial defects is commonly facilitated by the availability of adequate local tissue. Expansion has become an important modality in the management of these defects. Attention must be directed toward hair-bearing quality of skin or its potential for hair bearing in the case of children. Flaps should be designed so that the suture lines come to rest in areas where they will be minimally visible. Reconstruction should be carried out in anatomical units of the face to minimize patchwork final results.

Prostheses are placed in a subcutaneous tissue over the superficial fascia of the face and neck. Although this skin is quite thin, it is well vascularized and durable, even in children. Despite adjacent facial sensory and motor nerves, neurapraxia is extremely unusual, even in children. With proper low-volume, frequent-interval expansions, children tolerate this procedure extremely well.

The neck is an important source of tissue for reconstruction of the lower face. Implants are best placed above the platysma. If they are placed below, the prosthesis exposes the mandibular branch of the seventh nerve to unnecessary risk and may interfere in the rotation of large flaps. Expanded neck flaps may be moved in a cephalad direction as far as the infraorbital rim. The neck can be expanded to extreme proportions using multiple large expanders without evidence of pressure compromise to underlying vital structures. In designing expansion procedures of the face, all available tissues in the posterior neck below the hairline and behind the ear should be considered. When advanced or rotating expanded flaps are used, they are secured to the underlying fascia or periosteum to minimize subsequent contraction, particularly around the mouth and eyes. Reconstruction should be planned so that the final suture lines rest in the infraorbital area, along the border of the nasal aesthetic unit, and into the nasolabial fold (Fig. 13.9).

NASAL RECONSTRUCTION

Total nasal reconstructions are limited by sufficient skin for both the internal and external lining. Expansion of the forehead flaps greatly facilitates the amount of tissue available for nasal reconstruction and enables the surgeon to obtain primary closure of the donor defect.

A large prosthesis should encompass the entire forehead and is placed beneath the frontalis muscle through the incision in the scalp, which will later be incorporated into the forehead flap. The prosthesis is rapidly inflated until an excess of tissue has been generated. Expansion results in a significant thinning of the forehead flap that allows reconstruction of a more detailed nose over appropriate cantilevered cranial bone graft and conchal cartilage grafts. Thinning of the capsule may be necessary to achieve optimal results on the tip of the nose. If lining is needed, the flap can be doubled upon itself and brought up to about the nasal mucosa. The flap is divided and inset after 3 weeks.

EAR RECONSTRUCTION

Expansion may avoid the need for a temporoparietal flap and skin graft in patients with inadequate nonhair-bearing skin who require ear reconstruction. Custom

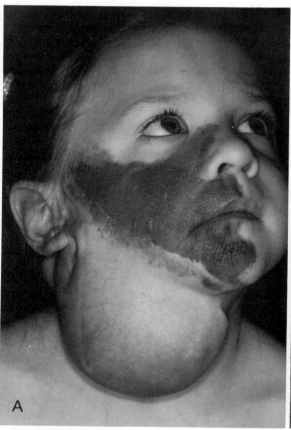
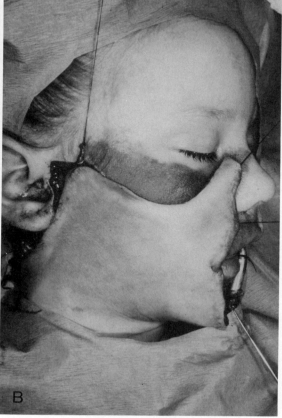

FIGURE 13.9. Reconstruction of the face using a tissue expander. **A,** A large expander is placed in the subcutaneous space in the neck and inflated until adequate tissue is obtained.

B, A large neck/face flap is rotated to cover the entire defect, leaving a final suture line in the infraorbital rim and along the nasolabial crease.

prostheses may be necessary if there are ear remnants that one wishes to preserve. However, if the ear is completely absent, a 100-ml semilunar prosthesis is adequate. Inflation is carried out very carefully because of the thinness of the overlying tissue. Once adequate soft tissue has been generated, the capsule is removed from the flap so that adequate definition of the underlying framework can be obtained over the cartilaginous framework (28).

Expansion of Extremities

Expansion is well tolerated in the upper and lower extremities. Reconstruction by expansion has been effective in facilitating excision of large nevi, tattoos, scars, and skin grafts. The skin over the dorsum of the hand and foot expands readily; however, the palm and plantar surfaces of the foot expand very poorly, and this expansion is very painful. The dorsum of the fingers can be quickly expanded with custom implants for the correction of syndactyly, avoiding all skin grafts (29).

The complication rate in expansion below the knees is significant. Patients who have had extensive degloving or crushing injuries below the knee are particularly poor candidates for expansion, probably secondary to the compromise of lymphatic drainage. Patients who have suffered isolated clean defects of the lower extremity below the knee can be successfully reconstructed.

Expanders are judiciously placed to avoid the thin skin over the pretibial area, the malleoli, the knee, and the peroneal nerve. Reconstruction is particularly facilitated by placing several prostheses radially around a defect and then closing the defect in the vertical direction. Attempts to close defects by moving tissue axially require considerable expansion and much more time.

Trunk

The back and abdomen expand very readily and with a low risk of complication. Standard myocutaneous flaps on the trunk and extremities can be expanded prior to the rotation (30) or prior to their harvesting as free flaps (31). Expansion increases the adjacent random area of such flaps so that extremely large tissue transfers can be accomplished safely. The latissimus dorsi muscle can be expanded bilaterally and then mobilized inferiorly and medially for the closure of large meningocele defects (Fig. 13.10). The latissimus can also be expanded in its anatomical position and then transposed to cover the entire anterior chest wall. Alternatively, it can be transposed to the chest wall and then expanded for breast reconstructions. Expansion has been used to facilitate the closure of abdominal wall defects of both traumatic and congenital origins (32).

Special Uses

EXPANDED FULL-THICKNESS GRAFTS

Preexpansion of a donor site for full-thickness grafts will dramatically increase the potential size of tissue available for such grafts (33). Survival of expanded full-thickness grafts is equal to that of nonexpanded grafts. The prosthesis is placed beneath the prospective donor site and inflated over 4 to 6 weeks. The supraclavicular area is particularly well suited to expansion for full-thickness grafts to the facial area. The groin can be expanded to produce full-thickness skin grafts to cover the foot or hand.

At harvesting, the prosthesis is left in place to facilitate removal of the full-thickness graft. The prosthesis is then removed, and the defect closed primarily after the full-thickness graft has been transferred.

ELONGATION OF PERIPHERAL NERVE

Sensory nerves are routinely successfully lengthened during normal tissue expansion. The Ilizarov technique of bone lengthening has demonstrated that major sensory and motor nerves can be successfully elongated. Laboratory work as well as work in humans has demonstrated that expansion of the proximal or distal segments can be employed to create sufficient nerve to bridge defects (1). Theoretically, elongation of nerves may minimize endoneural fibrosis and facilitate a more uniform distribution of axons within the fascicles.

ELONGATION OF VISCERA BY EXPANSION

The ureter, bladder, and small bowel have all been successfully elongated by expansion. The ureter maintains its patency and may be a viable alternative for future conduit reconstruction. The small bowel and bladder have both demonstrated excessive muscular hypertrophy and compromised function when elongated. The clinical usefulness of these techniques requires further work (1).

SUSTAINED INTRAOPERATIVE EXPANSION

Expanders have been used intraoperatively in an attempt to harness the vasoelastic properties of skin (34). Sequential load cycling of skin by expanding prostheses for several 10-min intervals may be useful in the closure of small defects per primum. Meaningful clinical and experimental work in this area is still wanting.

Complications of Tissue Expansion

Reports of early series have demonstrated a high incidence of complications (9). With development of expertise and appropriate selection of patients, complication rates have decreased dramatically. Of significance is the fact that, even with complications, the vast majority of patients ultimately achieve successful reconstruction using expansion.

PAIN

Transient pain may occur during expansion, but it is usually tolerated with minimal analgesics. The forehead,

FIGURE 13.10.   A, Expansion of bilateral latissimus dorsi myocutaneous flaps to cover a large myelomeningocele. **B,** After transposition of the flaps to cover the defect. Note that there are no donor defects.

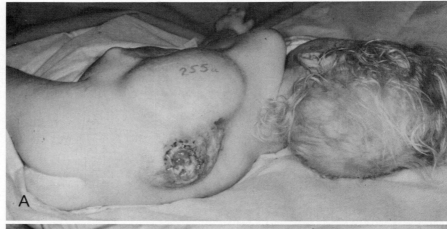

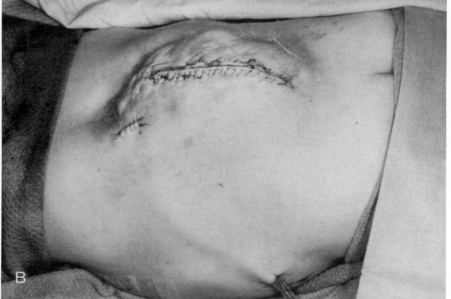

palm, sole of the foot, and genital area are particularly uncomfortable. Frequent small-volume injections are useful in minimizing this discomfort.

NEURAPRAXIAS

Neurapraxias during expansion are unusual, even though nerves may become incorporated in capsule during expansion. The perineal nerve has been reported to develop neurapraxia during expansion. If neurapraxias develop during expansion, the expanders should immediately be deflated.

SEROMAS

Seromas may occur, particularly in the lower extremity and with immediate breast reconstruction. Seromas may be minimized by placing suction drains adjacent to the prosthesis and by the immediate postoperative closure of dead space. Seromas can also be drained by percutaneous aspiration adjacent to the filling reservoir. Placing the reservoir externally allows seromas to drain through the skin, but this also risks colonization.

HEMATOMA

Hematomas are major complications, potentially resulting in flap necrosis. Hematomas are usually the result of inadequate hemostasis at the time of placement of the prosthesis. They may also occur later secondary to vessel erosion by the expander pressure, but this is very rare. Drains should not be depended upon to achieve hemostasis. This complication is an avoidable one.

INFECTION

Foreign bodies within the body are predisposed to infection. Prostheses infected early in the course of expansion should be removed and replaced 4–6 months later. If infection occurs as a result of extrusion late in the course of expansion, it is best to continue filling the prosthesis with low-increment, frequent-volume inflations and proceed. When the expanders are removed, the wound is copiously irrigated, and the flaps turned. Expanded tissues have a remarkable propensity to resist infection.

EXPOSURE

Implants that become exposed early in the course of expansion do so usually through a suture line or a preexisting scar. When this occurs, it is best to abort the attempt, remove the expander, and wait. When exposure occurs late in the course of expansion, the prosthesis can be sequentially filled until adequate tissue can be rotated.

References

1. Manders EK, Saggers GC, Diaz-Alonso P, et al: Elongation of peripheral nerve and viscera containing smooth muscle. *Clin Plast Surg* 14:551, 1987.
2. Neumann CG: The expansion of an area of skin by progressive distention of a subcutaneous balloon. *Plast Reconstr Surg* 19:124, 1957.
3. Radovan C: Adjacent flap development using expandable silastic implants. Presented at the annual meeting of the American Society of Plastic and Reconstructive Surgeons, Boston, September, 1976.
4. Radovan C: Breast reconstruction after mastectomy using the temporary expander. *Plast Reconstr Surg* 69:195, 1982.
5. Radovan C: Tissue expansion in soft-tissue reconstruction. *Plast Reconstr Surg* 74:482, 1984.
6. Argenta LC, Marks MW, Grabb WC: Selective use of serial expansion in breast reconstruction. *Ann Plast Surg* 11:188, 1983.
7. Argenta LC, Watanabe MJ, Grabb WC: The use of tissue expansion in head and neck reconstruction. *Ann Plast Surg* 11:31, 1983.
8. Argenta LC, Marks MW, Pasyk KA: Advances in tissue expansion. *Clin Plast Surg* 12:159, 1985.
9. Manders EK, Schenden MJ, Furrey JA, et al: Soft-tissue expansion: Concepts and complications. *Plast Reconstr Surg* 74:493, 1984.
10. Austad E, Rose GL: A self-inflating tissue expander. *Plast Reconstr Surg* 70:588, 1982.
11. Austad ED, Pasyk KA, McClatchey KD, et al: Histomorphologic evaluation of guinea pig skin and soft tissue after controlled tissue expansion. *Plast Reconstr Surg* 70:704, 1982.
12. Pasyk KA, Austad ED, McClatchey KD, et al: Electron microscopic evaluation of guinea pig skin and soft tissues "expanded" with a self-inflating silicone implant. *Plast Reconstr Surg* 70:37, 1982.
13. Pasyk KA, Argenta LC, Hassett, C: Quantitative analysis of the thickness of human skin and subcutaneous tissue following controlled expansion with a silicone implant. *Plast Reconstr Surg* 81:516, 1988.
14. Pasyk KA, Argenta LC, Austad ED: Histopathology of human expanded tissue. *Clin Plast Surg* 14:435, 1987.
15. Austad ED, Thomas SB, Pasyk K: Tissue expansion: Dividend or loan. *Plast Reconstr Surg* 78:63, 1986.
16. Cherry GW, Austad E, Pasyk K, et al: Increased survival and vascularity of random pattern skin flaps elevated in controlled, expanded skin. *Plast Reconstr Surg* 72:680, 1983.
17. Baker DE, Dedrick DK, Burney RE, Mathes SJ, Mackenzie JR: Resistance of rapidly expanded random skin flaps to bacterial invasion. *J Trauma* 27:1061, 1987.
18. Ryan T, Barnhill R: Physical factors and angiogenesis. In Nigent P: *Development of the Vascular System.* CIBA Foundation Symposium 100, Pitman Books, 1983.
19. Dickson WA, Sharpe DT, Jackson IT: Experience with an external valve in small volume tissue expanders. *Br J Plast Surg* 41:373, 1988.
20. Versaci AD: A method of reconstructing a pendulous breast utilizing the tissue expander. *Plast Reconstr Surg* 80:387, 1987.
21. Versaci AD: Reconstruction of a pendulous breast utilizing a tissue expander. *Clin Plast Surg* 14:499, 1987.
22. Becker H: The permanent tissue expander. *Clin Plast Surg* 14:519, 1987.
23. Argenta L: Reconstruction of the breast by tissue expansion. *Clin Plast Surg* 11:257, 1984.
24. Ward J, Cohen I, Knaysi F, Brown PW: Immediate breast reconstruction with tissue expansion. *Plast Reconstr Surg* 80:559, 1987.
25. Argenta LC, VanderKolk K, Friedman RJ, Marks M: Refinements in reconstruction of congenital breast deformities. *Plast Reconstr Surg* 76:73, 1985.
26. Manders EK, Graham WP, Schenden MJ, et al: Skin expansion to eliminate large scalp defects. *Ann Plast Surg* 12:305, 1984.
27. Adson MH, Anderson RD, Argenta LC: Scalp expansion in the treatment of male pattern baldness. *Plast Reconstr Surg* 79:906, 1987.
28. O'Neal RM, Rohrich RJ, Izenberg PH: Skin expansion as an adjunct to reconstruction of the external ear. *Br J Plast Surg* 37:517, 1984.
29. Van Beek AL, Adson MH: Tissue expansion in the upper extremity. *Clin Plast Surg* 14:535, 1987.
30. Thornton JW, Marks MM, Izenberg PH, Argenta LC: Expanded myocutaneous flaps: Their clinical use. *Clin Plast Surg* 14:529, 1987.
31. Leighton WD, Russell RC, Feller AM, et al: Experimental pretransfer expansion of free flap donor sites. II. Physiology, histology, and clinical correlation. *Plast Reconstr Surg* 82:76, 1988.
32. Byrd HS, Hobar PC: Abdominal wall expansion in congenital defects. *Plast Reconstr Surg* 84:347, 1989.
33. Argenta LC, Marks MW, Iacobucci JJ, et al: Expanded full thickness skin grafts. *Plast Surg Forum* 11:136, 1988.
34. Sasaki GH: Intraoperative sustained limited expansion (ISLE) as an immediate reconstructive technique. *Clin Plast Surg* 14:563, 1987.

14

Lasers in Plastic Surgery

Richard O. Gregory, M.D., F.A.C.S.

General Principles

THE HISTORY OF LASERS

Since the laser was invented in the early 1960s, a variety of applications in medicine have been devised and perfected. Continued evolution of this new modality allows significant advantages over conventional surgery. In fact, it allows the treatment of some lesions that otherwise would probably go untreated. Continued development of new technology will revolutionize the practice of plastic surgery; it is likely that every plastic surgeon will eventually have some use for the laser.

In 1917, Einstein proposed the theory that forms the basis for laser practice. A long lag until the late 1950s occurred until the technology could catch up with the theory. The early lasers were developed in large part for industrial applications. In fact, Bell Laboratories has occupied a central role in the development of lasers. Several laser investigators have earned the Nobel Prize for their developments. Because the earlier lasers were designed primarily for industrial use, they have been adapted to medicine. Thus, they might be less than ideal for medical applications. Unfortunately, the medical laser market, which was estimated to be $60 million in 1989, is probably not sufficient to justify the capital expenditures necessary to create a medical laser, except in a few rare circumstances.

LASERS IN PLASTIC SURGERY

Many medical specialties have been using the laser for a number of years for a variety of applications. Particularly noteworthy in this regard is ophthalmology, which uses the special features available from a laser to accomplish a variety of tasks, including the sealing of retinal vessels, ablation of postcataract membranes, and more recently, radial keratotomies and corneal sculpting. ENT and dermatology, as well as other fields in medicine such as gastroenterology, urology, and pulmonology, have likewise each developed an intrinsic use for the laser.

Although there is much overlap in laser use between plastic surgery and dermatology or otolaryngology, the nature of the average plastic surgery practice, which is largely operating room based, does not lend itself well to the use of an office laser, in contrast to the office-based practice of the dermatologist. Likewise, the plastic surgery establishment seems slow to accept the laser into the

practice. In this regard, however, the climate for lasers in plastic surgery is changing because of increased educational efforts and a growing need to develop new techniques in plastic surgery. Likewise, a change in the technology of lasers has occurred such that the average plastic surgeon could now use the laser frequently in his or her practice. With this change has come a gradual acceptance of the laser by plastic surgery residency program directors and the established plastic surgery community.

The Plastic Surgery Educational Foundation has held nearly annual symposia in order to educate the plastic surgeons in the use of the lasers. These have been well accepted and generally fully enrolled, as have been the educational courses at the annual meeting of the American Society of Plastic and Reconstructive Surgeons (ASPRS), which has for many years had a Laser Committee working to promote the use of lasers in plastic surgery by attempting to convince program directors to incorporate this as part of their training. In many instances, plastic surgery residents can be admitted to the training courses for a reduced fee. In addition, awards have been given at the annual meeting for the best laser-related research paper, and the American Board of Plastic Surgery has been encouraged to include specific questions regarding laser use in plastic surgery in their examinations in order to promote the use of the laser in this discipline.

LASER PHYSICS

Based on Einstein's 1917 theory, the laser emits a very bright light. In fact, the word "Laser" which stands for *L*ight *A*mplification by *S*timulated *E*mission of *R*adiation, is indeed a misnomer. Many medical lasers, for example, the carbon dioxide (CO_2) laser and the neodymium:yttrium-aluminum-garnet (Nd:YAG) laser, emit electromagnetic radiation in the invisible spectrum. There are three primary qualities of laser light that distinguish it from the standard light emanating from an incandescent lamp. One difference is that it is monochromatic; that is, it emits one primary, very pure color.

The laser light is also coherent, both spatially and temporally, implying that laser light beams are "in step." If thought of in terms of a wave form, it would mean that all wave peaks occur simultaneously, as do the troughs. Finally, laser light is collimated or nondivergent. This beam, by virtue of its physical makeup, tends to spread very little as it emanates from the source, unlike the beam from a flashlight or other noncollimated light source. As a result of these three characteristics, laser lights can be used for distinct functions in medicine because of their extremely high power density.

By understanding the principles of lasers as well as the laser light–tissue interaction (physics and physiology), the physician is able to extrapolate this knowledge to other lasers. This makes using the laser of another manufacturer or learning the operation of an additional laser type, such as moving from a CO_2 to a Nd : YAG laser, an easy matter.

As mentioned above, the principles behind the laser were first espoused by Einstein in 1917. This theory of stimulated emission of radiation proposed that light was produced by the shifting of electrons that exist in orbits around the nuclei of atoms or molecules. Electrons usually exist in a baseline or nonexcited state, but they can be excited to change orbits by a variety of electrical, chemical, and physical forces. When elevated to a higher energy position, the electron is termed "excited." Excited electrons will spontaneously decay or fall back into their baseline orbits, thereby producing a photon, which is characteristic of the molecule, atom, or electron within that structure. It is known that electrons in an excited state that is above their baseline energy orbit can be stimulated to fall back into their natural or baseline state. This would thereby trigger the release of the photon. Photons themselves will accomplish this task, but once again, the photons that can trigger release of this energy are characteristic for the particular situation. In essence, one photon entering an excited atom could discharge the energy stored by the excited electron, producing two photons of the same wavelength and other characteristics.

A tungsten incandescent lamp operates in this manner. Electrons flowing through the filament excite the electrons within the filament, and as the electrons collapse, the light is released. This incandescent light could be pictured as undisciplined or random in nature because it is light of a mixture of colors (i.e., frequency) and is not controlled but released randomly into the environment. The atom or molecule can be viewed as a small storage battery. It is charged as an electron becomes excited due to some outside force and discharges when another force releases that energy. When the majority of atoms or molecules have electrons in the excited state within a body, a condition known as population inversion exists. One needs a means of charging the battery and discharging or controlling it at the time of need to take advantage of this population inversion.

All lasers consist of three units. One is a power source, which may be an electrical outlet, a chemical reaction, or indeed, another laser. The second component is the lasing medium. This may be a crystal such as a ruby rod, a gas such as argon or CO_2, or a stream of dye. Solid-state lasers, which create the light within an electronic semiconductor, are now becoming popular. The final main component that every laser has is mirrors at either end of the lasing medium. One is a totally reflecting mirror that is configured to reflect the light striking it from within the cavity back into the cavity of the lasing medium. The other is a partially reflecting mirror that can be used to release light energy from the cavity at will. Of course, depending somewhat on the type of laser, other components may be needed. Certainly a delivery mechanism is important, and in many newer lasers, a fiberoptic bundle provides this delivery mechanism. Unfortunately, carbon dioxide lasers are not presently adaptable to fiberoptic delivery. Instead, they require an articulated arm with a set of gimbaled mirrors within the arm for delivery. Likewise, the laser needs a control mechanism, usually an electronic panel. This, of course, would consist of a means of regulating the power as well as shuttering or turning the beam on or off. Usually, a lens is incorporated into the delivery system to focus the beam to a narrow point. This allows additional control over the laser.

Several characteristics of the laser light require discussion. One of the unique characteristics of laser light is the rather specific wavelength or color of the light emitted. The three commonly used lasers produce light of widely different colors. The carbon dioxide laser emits "invisible light" in the far infrared spectrum at 10,600 nanometers (nm). The Nd : YAG laser emits light at 1,064 nm in the near infrared portion of the electromagnetic spectrum, and the argon laser emits light in the blue-green portion of the spectrum, having two major light spikes or frequencies at 488 nm and 514 nm.

It was mentioned above that these lasers were not conceived initially for use in medicine; therefore, some compromise over what might be an ideal light frequency has been made. This relates in large part to the light-tissue interaction characteristic for that particular wavelength, which will be discussed in further detail below.

The power of the laser is usually measured in watts. It is interesting to contrast the laser to the electric light bulb, which, for instance, may be 60 watts or 100 watts. Because the light from the light bulb is "undisciplined," it does not have any of the laser light characteristics. Furthermore, because it is emitted uniformly throughout the sphere of the environment, this 60 watts creates very little effect on any particular light absorber or surface. However, because the laser is concentrated into a fine beam as a unique color or frequency and is collimated and coherent as mentioned above, the laser light beam can be used with great facility to accomplish certain tasks in medicine.

The watts emitted by the laser are usually controlled by a knob on the control panel and, for a low-power laser such as an argon, may vary from a fraction of a watt to several watts of power (0.1 to 6 or 8 watts). Unfortunately, the argon laser is an inefficient laser and requires a great deal of power input, usually 220 volts at several amperes of current. In addition, because the energy conversion is inefficient, the laser produces a great deal of heat. Therefore, it may require water cooling or certainly air cooling by a fan. In contrast, CO_2 and Nd : YAG lasers tend to be high-power lasers and may emit power to 100 watts or more in medical applications and several hundred watts in industrial applications. These lasers are somewhat more efficient than the argon laser. They convert more power from the power source into light energy. However, they still usually require some form of cooling.

The next feature of the laser light beam that should be mentioned is the duration of the light beam (i.e., the period of time in which the light beam is on). One must be careful, however, to distinguish between a continuously emitting laser such as an argon, which is usually controlled by a switch and a shutter mechanism, and other lasers that emit a series of very high-powered (kilowatts) but very short spikes (nanoseconds), which are emitted so rapidly that the beam appears continuous. This second type of beam, which appears continuous, can be shuttered the same as that of a continuously emitting laser. However, there is a great deal of difference in the laser light–tissue interaction between the two types of beams, even though the two lasers may emit at the same average power over a given period of time.

The power (watts) multiplied by the duration (seconds) gives the resultant energy (joules) delivered to a target. Even though the energy delivered to an object is important, it is even more important that the size of the light beam be taken into consideration. It is easy to understand that a large amount of energy delivered to a large target area may not have nearly as much effect on the target as a relatively smaller amount of energy delivered to a smaller area by a very finely focused beam. The energy delivered to a given target area is termed energy fluence (joules/cm^2), and the power (watts) delivered to a given target area (cm^2) without consideration of the time is termed irradiance (watts/cm^2).

The important characteristics of a laser light beam would then include the frequency of the laser in nanometers, the duration of the delivered light beam in seconds, and the area of the light beam in square centimeters. One must also consider whether the laser beam is delivered in a continuous beam or as tiny spikes of energy that may appear continuous to the casual observer.

To further complicate the physics of the laser, most lasers emit light at more than one frequency, although through various optical and electronic devices, specific frequencies are filtered or accentuated to give the therapist the desired frequency. This is most commonly seen in clinical practice when using the argon laser, which as mentioned above, emits a blue light at about 488 nm as well as a green light at 514 nm. Optical filtering can select out the green light, thereby changing the characteristics of the light-tissue interaction.

LASER LIGHT–TISSUE INTERACTION (PHOTOBIOLOGY)

Knowing the physical characteristics of the laser is only half the story. In order to know the effect that the laser will produce on a given target, one must also know certain characteristics of the target. Unfortunately, animal tissue is heterogeneous and somewhat unpredictable. For example, it is known that there are a number of pigments (chromophores) within the human tissue that will absorb light differently. Blood, for example, absorbs yellow or blue-green light much differently than it absorbs other colors of light. Because tissue is 60% or more water, laser beams that are absorbed heavily by water (e.g.,

from the carbon dioxide laser) will vaporize nearly all types of tissue. Furthermore, the conductivity of the energy in the tissue varies a great deal.

Light striking any object can be refracted, reflected, absorbed, or transmitted. It is actually the laser light that is absorbed that produces an effect on the target; however, for targeted chromophores that are not at the tissue surface, one must be able to transmit the laser light to these greater depths.

Absorption curves have been plotted for a variety of different chromophores. Each absorption curve is known to vary a great deal, depending upon which portion of the electromagnetic spectrum is being studied. For instance, hemoglobin absorbs heavily in the green portion of the spectrum, but it also has some absorption spikes at higher levels. Water tends to absorb heavily in the infrared portion of the spectrum, and melanin, xanthophyll, and other tissue chromophores have their own particular absorption characteristics, which frequently compete with the target for the laser light energy. When a competing chromophore absorbs laser light, there will often be tissue damage that is undesirable and perhaps even detrimental.

Light striking an object can produce a variety of different phenomena. For example, laser light absorbed by most tissue will produce heat within the tissue. Ninety-nine percent of all desirable laser-tissue interactions depend on the thermal effects of the laser light striking the tissue. However, it is possible to use a laser that produces a photobiochemical effect on the tissue or even a photoacoustic or shock-like effect on the tissue, depending on the characteristics of the laser beam, etc. We are only beginning to understand and harness the photobiochemical and photoacoustic effects of laser light striking the tissue, but this is probably where the future of laser medicine lies.

Thermal effects of laser light on tissue may be reversible or may cause irreversible damage to the tissue. A slight warming may produce only "cloudy swelling" in the tissue, which is evidenced by a mild erythema or redness. Likewise, the tissue may increase in heat, producing irreversible thermal damage, including vacuolization. Evidence for this effect can include steam bubbles forming within the tissue, charring, and eventually evaporation of the tissue, which frequently produces a smoke plume.

The effect of the laser light on the tissue depends not only on the amount of heat built up but on how rapidly the tissue can conduct this heat away. A very short pulse of laser light, for example, may have less severe effects than a very long pulse of the same total energy. If the energy is administered over a longer period of time, heat gradually builds up in the tissue and can be dissipated by conduction into the areas adjacent to the lesion being treated. This results in less complete ablation of the lesion and greater damage to the surrounding areas. However, if the energy is administered over a very short period of time, the lesion is totally ablated, and damage to the adjacent tissue is limited because insufficient time has elapsed for appreciable conduction to occur. Thus, even though the same amount of energy may be delivered to a given volume of tissue, the total effects can be quite different if this energy is delivered in a short rather than a long period of time. The term "thermal relaxation time" has been coined to designate the period of time required for a specific tissue to cool to one-half its initial temperature rise after being struck by a laser light beam.

Looking at a cross-section of a tissue volume impacted by a laser light, one will frequently notice a central crater in which the tissue has evaporated, surrounded by a zone of charring, followed by a zone of vacuolization and irreversible damage, and finally, a zone of reversible thermal effect.

Finally, one must factor the human element into the equation of laser medicine. Although a pulsed light of a certain frequency and power striking a given tissue may produce predictable effects, the effect can be influenced by the manner in which the laser operator applies this laser light to the tissue. For example, in a continuous mode, the hand is used to sweep the laser light beam back and forth across a given area of tissue, and the irregular motion of the operator's hand may cause the tissue to absorb the light nonuniformly. Additionally, the diameter of the laser light beam may vary, depending upon the irregular surface of the tissue as well as the unsteadiness of the operator's hand. Much of what we know about laser medicine is empirical and derived from years of experience. Therefore, while one might guess that a laser light–tissue interaction is predictable, there is nevertheless still a certain amount of empiricism and a great deal of experience that is required for a given operator to produce a given effect on the tissue. Unfortunately, a small change in any one of the parameters mentioned above might mean the difference between a beautiful, desired result and a devastating scar as a result of a laser treatment.

SAFETY

A discussion of laser medicine would not be complete without a word about safety. There are many inherent dangers associated with the laser, both to the operator and to the patient. A thorough knowledge of the safety factors is essential and, in fact, comprises a large part of any laser teaching course. The most common safety factor cited in laser usage is the danger to the eyes by the laser beam. This may be corrected by the appropriate use of filtered glasses for the operator or by using an eye shield to protect the patient if the laser therapy is being performed around the eye. There is a fire hazard associated with laser ignition of flammable gases, endotracheal tubes, or even drapes in the operating room. Electrical hazards are also seen with the laser that are more characteristic of laser maintenance. The American National Standards Institute (ANSI) has published a standard ANSI Z-136.3 delineating the safety precautions to be used in laser medicine.

Every laser therapy center, whether within the hospital or an office, should have standard guidelines for use of the laser. Most hospitals with several lasers will have a laser committee that will meet regularly to discuss a variety of factors, including safety, laser organization, laser credentialing, and the purchase, maintenance, and use of lasers within that facility.

Even though laser manufacturers have to satisfy a large number of government regulations in order to sell the laser, the ultimate use of the laser within a clinical setting is the responsibility of the operator. Many laser companies, in their enthusiasm to sell a laser, may not present an objective picture to the unaware potential user, and there are a large number of lasers that go unused for this reason.

Purchasing a laser should be somewhat similar to purchasing computer hardware and software. One should study the applications or needs prior to determining which laser may best fill those needs. Unfortunately, because of the high-tech nature of the equipment as well as the publicity given to lasers in the popular press, the laser frequently is viewed as a gimmick to attract patients and build a practice. Such an approach to laser medicine is detrimental to good patient care.

Specific Laser Types

CARBON DIOXIDE (CO_2) LASER

The carbon dioxide (CO_2) laser has been the most important laser tool in the armamentarium of plastic surgery for a number of years. This attribute derives from its excellent cutting and vaporizing ability as well as from its ability to coagulate smaller vessels in selected cases. In recent years, however, the role of the carbon dioxide laser in some of these functions has been challenged by the neodymium : YAG laser with contact sapphire tips.

The carbon dioxide laser emits laser light in the far infrared band at 10,600 nm. These frequencies are heavily absorbed by water. Because most cells in the body contain a significant proportion of water, nearly every cell will absorb carbon dioxide laser light; therefore, there is very little selectivity in this laser. Consequently, the surface cells absorb the laser light before it has an opportunity to penetrate deeply. Thus, the advantage of the CO_2 laser in cutting and vaporizing is somewhat counterbalanced by its poor penetrability and relatively poor hemostatic or coagulating effect when compared to some of the other lasers.

The carbon dioxide laser is a high-powered laser, and some medical models can emit up to 100 watts of continuous power. In addition, it is capable of delivering power in the milliwatt range, which has been used for tissue welding. Because of the far infrared wavelength of the CO_2 laser, transmission by a fiberoptic bundle is not possible at the present level of technology. This promises to change in the future, but the carbon dioxide lasers presently in clinical service are delivered through a rigid arm that has joints containing mirrors to allow some flexibility. These mirrors create an alignment problem, however, and some of these lasers can be easily knocked out of alignment by vibration or a sudden jolt. Because of this, the CO_2 laser cannot be used in endoscopic procedures.

The laser light delivered through the rigid arm is usually focused through a lens and a handpiece. This allows the laser to be finely focused into a very small spot size (0.1 mm or less) or delivered through a handpiece to allow a focus beam of 1.0 mm or more. The focal distance of the handpiece from the lens to the target likewise can be varied; however, most are set at about 2.5 cm. Other features of note with regard to the carbon dioxide laser are the bottles of carbon dioxide gas required by some lasers. Newer technology, however, has overcome this with the so-called sealed tube. Some carbon dioxide lasers, which are relatively inexpensive, have been packed in a suitcase for portability. Although these may emit only 5–10 watts, they are quite suitable for an office practice. Larger, more expensive CO_2 lasers have added features such as the superpulsed mode.

The superpulsed mode of the carbon dioxide laser permits cooling of the tissue between the very short pulses of laser light. As mentioned earlier, if a large amount of energy can be delivered in a relatively short period of time, there is usually less thermal damage to the tissue surrounding the impact site. When the same amount of energy is delivered over a longer period of time, damage to the surrounding tissue is greater due to heat conduction away from the site of impact. Thus, the operator must overcome the tendency to decrease the power if it appears that too much heat damage is occurring in the tissue at the site of the laser impact. If the power is decreased, a longer duration of application will be necessary to totally ablate the lesion, and conduction of the heat generated during this period of time will result in greater tissue damage in the surrounding areas. In fact, a higher power with a shorter pulse duration might well accomplish the destruction of the lesion while limiting the damage to surrounding tissues. Thus, the superpulsed mode, by producing very short intermittent pulses of laser light, produces clearly delineated areas of injury. This allows the operator to have a greater control over the extent of tissue damage produced.

The carbon dioxide laser has been used for many tasks in the past, and these will be discussed in some greater detail below. Suffice it to say that it has been used for vaporizing many lesions, including benign and malignant skin tumors, vascular tumors, and keloids and for removing tattoos. The incising ability of the carbon dioxide laser allows it to be used for raising flaps and for doing breast surgery as well as other surgery of an incisional nature. In general, pathologists are not accustomed to seeing the thermal damage associated with laser excision of a malignant tumor when they assess the margins of resection. Also, it is difficult to take a very thin section with the CO_2 laser. For these reasons, its use in resecting malignant tumors is not widely accepted.

Finally, the use of the carbon dioxide laser for tissue welding should be mentioned. Certain lasers delivering miniscule amounts of energy in the milliwatt range can be used to coagulate tissue and thus seal two edges together. This technique has many clinical applications, including fertility procedures such as vasectomy reversal, microvascular surgery, and microneurorrhaphies. Other lasers have also been used in tissue welding. However, it is still not widely accepted that this offers a significant advantage over conventional surgical repair techniques.

ARGON LASER

The argon laser, which has been widely used in medicine for a number of years, has found a greater role in dermatology than in plastic surgery. This laser emits in the blue-green portion of the spectrum at 488 as well as 514 nm and has been used for coagulating a variety of different vascular lesions as well as for the treatment of decorative tattoos and some vaporization. Its delivery through a fiberoptic bundle gives it a distinct advantage over the carbon dioxide laser, but there are, in fact, few areas of competition between the two.

The argon laser is a relatively inefficient laser. It emits only a few watts of power but consumes large amounts of energy. The excess energy is then converted to heat energy, which must be accommodated. In the past, this has necessitated bulky cooling hoses running from a water source through the laser to a drain. Newer argon lasers have air-cooled systems to prevent overheating. The traditional role of the argon laser has been in the treatment of superficial vascular lesions such as port wine stains, telangiectasias, and spider angiomas. Because pigments in the skin other than hemoglobin compete for absorption of this argon laser light, there is a considerable buildup of heat in the tissue, and this causes some complications such as depigmentation and scarring. This fact, associated with the somewhat darker lesions in older patients, has led to the exclusion of younger patients with port wine stains from argon laser treatment. Its use in older patients has given an excellent result, and newer techniques may improve the argon laser result. Nevertheless, newer "yellow light lasers," including the flash-pumped tunable dye laser, the argon-pumped dye laser, and the copper vapor laser, are replacing the argon laser in the treatment of many superficial vascular lesions.

Other uses for the argon laser include the treatment of keloids and scars as well as of decorative tattoos. The argon laser has also been used in tissue welding on a limited basis. Many of these roles of the argon laser will be assumed by other newer lasers in the near future.

NEODYMIUM:YAG LASER

The Nd:YAG laser is a laser that emits an invisible light in the near infrared portion of the electromagnetic spectrum. This laser, which emits a major peak at 1,064 nm, combines many of the advantages of both the carbon dioxide and the argon laser. It is absorbed by a variety of pigments within the body and yet is not heavily absorbed by water; thus it has a deeper penetration than the carbon dioxide laser. Because it is absorbed by hemoglobin, it is an excellent coagulating laser. A disadvantage in the past has been that this relatively high-powered laser produced a great deal of scattering and, therefore, heat damage in the tissue. The characteristics of the Nd:YAG laser have been considerably improved for the plastic surgeon by the recent addition of contact tips that can be attached to the end of the fiber through a handpiece or directly to the fiber. These contact tips, which are made of synthetic sapphire and come in a variety of shapes, transfer energy directly from the fiber into the tissue, thus reducing the scattering of the light. Much less energy is required to accomplish a particular task; therefore, the Nd : YAG laser becomes an excellent laser for vaporizing and cutting as well as coagulating. Early models of these contact tips tended to be very fragile. However, more recent models are more durable. The tips were, and still are, quite expensive, and their use was limited by an increased cost per use. Developmental work has continued in this field, and it is likely that the sapphire tips may be improved or replaced by something better in the near future.

Delivery of the Nd : YAG laser light through a fiberoptic bundle enhances its use to the surgeon in the handheld mode or through surgical endoscopes. Uses of the Nd : YAG laser with the sapphire tips would include vaporization of a variety of lesions, including both benign and malignant tumors, decorative tattoos, and vascular lesions, which it readily coagulates.

The Nd : YAG laser has been converted to other wavelengths. In particular, the laser light beam can be passed through a crystal, thereby halving the wavelength to 532 nm or doubling the frequency. This "frequency doubled" laser has found great application in a variety of other surgical fields, but it would seem to offer very little advantage in plastic surgery over other laser types.

YELLOW LIGHT LASERS

As mentioned above, newer lasers arriving on the scene include the so-called yellow light lasers. Three lasers fall into this category; the most widely known is the flash-pumped or tunable dye laser. The argon-pumped dye laser and the copper vapor laser also emit laser light at the frequencies from 577 to 585 nm, which is readily absorbed by hemoglobin but inefficiently absorbed by competing tissue pigments. For this reason, these lasers have been specifically applied to the treatment of port wine stains, particularly in young children, in whom they can selectively coagulate the vessels and do little damage to the surrounding tissue. Much ado has been made about the differences between these three lasers and, in particular, how the laser light temporal characteristics (i.e., pulse duration) affect the tissue. Indeed, there seems to be some minor advantage to rapidly pulsing these lasers. The most rapidly pulsed of these three lasers is the copper vapor laser, which emits pulses of a few nanoseconds in such rapid succession that the laser light beam appears to be continuous.

The flash-pumped dye laser emits laser light of a fixed duration of 450 μsec. This duration is designed to remain below the thermal relaxation time of the tissue, thereby decreasing the heat damage to the surrounding tissue. Finally, the argon-pumped dye laser emits laser light in a continuous beam that can be shutter controlled to tenths of a second or longer periods of time.

Impressive results have been shown using these lasers in port wine stains, particularly in young children. Claims have been made about the relatively painless nature of this laser treatment, but these seem somewhat exaggerated. It should also be appreciated that a considerable number of treatments are frequently needed in order to achieve the optimal results using these lasers. Even the optimal result may not totally erase the vascular lesion, but the treatment will significantly improve it in most instances. Side-by-side comparisons of these various yellow light lasers are currently underway and it is hoped they will resolve some of the disputes relating to the relative effectiveness of the three lasers. One must remember that their benefit compared to that of the argon laser is particularly notable in children but may not be quite so impressive in adults with darker, bumpier lesions.

One has to consider not only the considerable cost of purchasing these lasers but also the operational costs and inconvenience, which, particularly in the dye laser, are significant.

Solid Tumors

WARTS

Verruca vulgaris can occur anywhere on the body. The wart is quite adequately treated by a variety of laser modalities. Most commonly, the CO_2 laser is used to evaporate these warts.

It has been documented that the average recurrence rate for warts treated in the conventional manner with topical medications is approximately 30%. Warts treated with the laser have a documented recurrence rate of approximately 15%. Thus, there is an increased gain over conventional therapy. It should be emphasized that the thoroughness of the laser ablation of the wart controls, to a large extent, the rate of recurrence. Those warts that are incompletely ablated will almost always recur.

The virion of the infectious agent lives in the "cheesy" material at the base of the hyperkeratoses. This should likewise be evaporated with the laser down to the basement membrane. It has been stated that the basement membrane controls the level of pain. If there is ablation of the basement membrane of the skin, there is likely to be a prolonged healing period and excessive pain. This does not occur if the basement membrane is preserved as the wart is being evaporated; however, the laser ablation should not be compromised.

Following ablation of the wart, the wound can be treated with a topical antibiotic ointment and a semiocclusive dressing.

There seems to be less pain with laser ablation of warts, particularly plantar warts, than with conventional therapy. As a result, the patient is usually ambulating and returns to normal activities much sooner.

Condylomata are closely related to warts and also have a viral etiology. They can also be successfully treated with specific laser ablation. As with warts, there will frequently be a tendency for new lesions to appear after treatment, and the patient should be cautioned about this. It would seem most likely that this is persistent infection in areas that were not previously inspected or found to be affected by the virus.

As with treating any viral infection, care should be taken to contain contamination by the wound. An adequate smoke evacuation system is probably the primary means of preventing superinfection or infecting the personnel in the operating room. Newer filtration systems can filter the laser smoke plume to a particle size of less than 1 μm without difficulty. However, these systems require frequent filter changes and may lead to further contamination of the room air unless routine maintenance is carried out. Special laser facemasks as well as gloves, goggles, etc. should be used when treating these lesions.

The treatment plan for the pedunculated type of lesions such as warts or condylomata usually involves the CO_2 laser. This may be used at low to medium power (i.e., 5 to 10 watts or more). Exceptionally large lesions are probably best excised with the laser followed by lasering the base. Smaller lesions can be treated by vaporizing the lesion down to the base with a continuous or intermittent focused beam of 1 mm spot size. Periodically, the area should be cleansed with hydrogen peroxide and perhaps curretted lightly in order to remove charred debris in the base of the wound. When all evidence of the wart has been removed, antibiotic ointment and a light dressing are applied. Postoperative follow-up should occur at frequent intervals in order to ensure that the entire infection has been cleared. Aggressive treatment of recurrent lesions should be undertaken in order to prevent reinfection of those areas that have been adequately treated.

It is inappropriate to treat all warts with the laser. However, it has been found very effective in treating recurrent warts that have failed other treatment methods as well as plantar warts, which tend to be chronic and recurrent.

NEUROFIBROMA

Von Recklinghausen's disease presents as a schwannoma fibroma of the molluscum type and can be readily treated with the laser. The more polypoid the lesion, the easier it is to treat with the laser; those that have a narrow neck can be safely excised with the laser with little discomfort. The wounds are left open to heal secondarily after being dressed with a light coating of antibiotic ointment. More sessile lesions may require more thorough treatment and should be vaporized down deep to beneath the dermis as described above for warts. A substantial number of the deeper, sessile-type lesions will recur unless thoroughly vaporized. These wounds heal rapidly with a relatively minor scar.

The treatment plan for neurofibroma might involve either the carbon dioxide or the Nd : YAG laser with the sapphire contact tips. An effort is made to vaporize the lesion if it is small or can be easily amputated with the laser. Larger lesions can be cured by thoroughly coagulating the lesion by inserting the sapphire tips deep through the lesion into the base near its stalk and administering more energy. Higher power, 10 or more watts, with a relatively high power density (a small beam diame-

ter) is effective in quickly vaporizing these lesions. The sapphire tips may be used at 15 watts to either excise the lesion or to produce necrosis through coagulation. The amount of time of laser application necessary for thermal necrosis of the lesion is quite variable and depends upon the size of the lesion and the depth of the lesion under the skin.

SYRINGOMA, ADENOMA SEBACEUM, ANGIOKERATOMA, PYOGENIC GRANULOMA, AND MISCELLANEOUS BENIGN TUMORS

The list of benign tumors that can be treated with the laser is quite long. In addition to the syringoma, which is characteristic of the lower eyelid, the angiofibroma, which is most commonly found in children with tuberous sclerosis, the random pyogenic granuloma, angiokeratoma, and other lesions can all be well treated with the laser. In essence, these tumors respond to laser treatment similar to the treatment described above for warts. In addition, the more vascular of these lesions (e.g., the pyogenic granuloma, angiokeratoma) can be treated with a coagulating type of laser as well as with the CO_2 and Nd : YAG lasers.

The treatment plan for these types of lesions employs a relatively low power density with the CO_2 laser or the Nd : YAG laser with the contact tips in order to achieve a maximum coagulative effect. The argon laser, however, at a medium to high power density can also be used to coagulate these vascular tumors. Occasionally, a pyogenic granuloma or other small vascular tumor will contain blood under significant pressure that will foil the laser surgeon's attempt to coagulate the tumor. The blood welling up in the field absorbs the laser light and prevents adequate coagulation of the vessels supplying the tumor. Under these circumstances, manual pressure around the base of the vessel can sometimes stem the flow until the laser has had an opportunity to coagulate the vessels. Hemostatic agents such as local anesthetic with epinephrine will also aid in reducing this blood flow sufficiently to allow coagulation of the vessel.

Some lesions may require more than one treatment, and disorders such as tuberous sclerosis will probably require periodic treatment in order to keep the angiofibroma in check.

KELOIDS AND SCARS

Although there have long been claims made for the efficacy of lasers in the treatment of keloids and scars, a controversy persists. The CO_2 laser has been used to treat keloids by excision down to the base followed by treatment of the base with steroids or other adjunctive measures. Likewise, the argon laser has also been used at very high power densities to perforate or "honeycomb" this tissue, thereby perhaps altering the scar chemical makeup or the stresses within the scar. On this basis, the claim has been made that the use of lasers significantly improves the treatment of keloids of various areas on the body. More recently, however, it has been reported that a controlled study of laser treatment of keloid with long-term follow-up has demonstrated no improvement in the treatment with the laser over conventional means. Thus, the controversy continues unabated. It would seem that there may be some slight improvement in the cure rate of keloids treated with the laser in one of these two manners, especially keloids around the ear lobule, which can be readily contoured with the laser. There is insufficient evidence at present, however, to prove that a significant long-term improvement results from the laser treatment of keloids.

Surface contouring of "laserbrasion" of irregular scars of the face and other parts of the body has been demonstrated to be an effective method of leveling these scars. Unfortunately, there is at present also some risk of increasing the scar if the laser is used too aggressively or in a nonuniform manner.

The treatment plan of keloids includes the use of the CO_2 laser at a very small spot size (0.1 mm) and high power density (10–20 watts) with short bursts (0.01–0.1 sec) to effect a honeycomb perforation of the scar. The scar should then be treated with long-acting steroids such as triamcinolone to suppress further scar reaction. Those keloids that are excessively pedunculated or cauliflower-like can be excised with the laser down to and including the bottom of the scar and then injected with steroids and left to heal secondarily.

The treatment of fine scars of the skin by laserbrasion should be effected with the carbon dioxide laser at a relatively high power density (0.1-mm spot size). If available, the superpulsed mode, which effectively shortens the pulse duration to a few nanoseconds, should be used. As mentioned above, care should be taken not to excessively treat any areas of the scar or surrounding skin as this simply would serve to increase the amount of scarring.

NEVI, LENTIGO, ETC.

These lesions can be vaporized with the CO_2 laser, which is essentially nonselective for tissue destruction. Prior to treatment, a histological examination should be made to confirm that the pigmented lesion is not a malignancy.

The treatment plan employs a CO_2 laser in superpulsed mode used at very high power densities with short pulse duration (10–15 watts) for very short periods of time (0.1–0.01 sec). A topical antibiotic ointment is applied after the laser treatment is concluded.

CANCER

Although cancer can be readily excised using the laser, there seems to be very little rationale for doing so. If the laser is used at a low power density, which coagulates the vessels as the cancer is excised, bleeding is decreased. However, this also creates a considerable amount of thermal necrosis in the surrounding bed. It is difficult for the histologist to examine the surrounding bed for persistent cancer cells. When the power density is increased enough to lessen the thermal necrosis, bleeding of the tumor bed is considerable, and the advantages of the laser are lost. Nevertheless, some clinicians advocate the use of the laser to excise malignant skin tumors, and some use it for raising flaps to repair these cancer defects. In most instances, this use of the laser is not justified.

RHINOPHYMA

The excellent results achieved by contouring a rhinophyma with the CO_2 laser merit a description of the technique. While these can certainly be done in a conventional manner, there is usually excessive blood loss, and the appropriate contouring is extremely difficult to achieve. The laser, however, can be used at relatively high power densities to pare down these bulbous formations of acne rosacea to a level of the base of the crypts. Hemostasis is usually easily achieved with this method, and the results tend to be excellent after a short period of healing. Care should be taken not to hone these lesions in an overly aggressive manner because thermal damage to the surrounding tissue with slow healing may occur.

Following excision of the tissue, the nose is dressed with an occlusive antibiotic-impregnated gauze until healing has been effected.

Port-Wine Stains, Telangiectasia, and Other Small Vessel Arteriovenous Malformations

PORT-WINE STAINS

Port-wine stains, also called nevus flammeus, are most frequently located in the trigeminal nerve distribution of the face, although they can occur anywhere on the body. They consist of superficial capillaries in the dermal or subdermal layers. Although they usually will not enlarge as a person ages, the vessels will frequently dilate, thus causing an increasing blue color and bumpiness that result from the presence of arteriovenous shunts within the lesion. Consequently, older patients will have a darker, bumpier lesion than younger patients. For this reason, and because they do not scar as readily, older patients will be somewhat better candidates for laser treatment. However, the new lasers have allowed these lesions to be successfully treated at a much earlier age.

Formerly, the argon laser was commonly used to treat port-wine stains, and it remains an excellent treatment for those older, bumpier lesions. The lasers used most commonly for the treatment of port-wine stains in younger patients are the yellow light lasers, which include the copper vapor laser, the argon pumped-dye laser, and the flash-pumped tunable dye laser. These lasers all emit a yellow light in the 577 nm wavelength range. This yellow light is more selectively absorbed by the hemoglobin and less absorbed by melanin, xanthophyll, and other pigments in the skin.

The laser light entering the vessel heats the blood inside and causes breakdown of the vessel evidenced by clotting and inflammatory response and, finally, by fibrosis of these vessels.

The treatment regimen depends somewhat on which laser is used. As more and more is learned, higher wavelengths, such as 585 nm or above, are favored. Much importance has been attached to the pulsed character of the laser light as contrasted to the continuous nature of the argon pumped-dye laser. Certainly, as indicated earlier in this text, the faster a specific amount of energy can be administered to the tissue (i.e., a higher power density but a shorter pulse duration), the less likely there is to be heat damage to the surrounding tissue. Some of these lasers use a large spot size to treat areas of the port-wine stain; others use a smaller spot size to perform vessel tracing for those lesions that have identifiable vessels in them.

Treatments can be carried out under local or general anesthesia. Topical anesthesia was once advocated, but it seems to be falling into disrepute.

Aftercare is an integral part of the treatment plan and should involve antibiotic ointment in the immediate postoperative period if there is any indication of blistering or crusting. Sunscreen agents should be used during the postoperative period to prevent the hyperpigmentation effects of sun exposure.

By using the yellow light lasers, a good or excellent response should be obtained in 75% or more of patients, depending upon patient selection. In contrast, approximately 50% of patients show good results when treated with the argon laser. Even with these more sophisticated lasers, one should expect that there will be a few patients who do not respond well. Some side effects such as textural change in the skin or alteration in the pigmentation may be noted, and in many patients, a few residual vessels may leave a slight blush after the treatment is finished.

Telangiectasias have been classified into four grades. Generally, grades 3 and 4 can be readily seen at conversational distance. They are most commonly seen around the nose, although other parts of the face and body may be involved. These may be associated with the red nose seen after rhinoplasty as well as with acne rosacea leading to rhinophyma. Although somewhat more resistant to treatment, these telangiectasias nevertheless are very well treated by the yellow light laser, particularly with the vessel tracing type of technique and relatively high power density. Many of these will require more than one treatment in order to achieve satisfactory results. Telangiectasia of the lower extremities are more resistant to treatment and are more likely to recur after treatment; therefore, sclerotherapy remains the treatment of choice for these vessels, although the laser may be a good adjunctive treatment.

Other small arteriovenous malformations, including spider angioma, are also well treated by the laser, but a relatively high power density should be used. In general, these should be treated from the periphery toward the center of the lesion, and extra caution should be taken to assure that the central bump, which represents the arterial shunt, has been thoroughly ablated.

Hemangiomas

Considerable controversy exists over both the need to treat certain hemangioma-type lesions as well as the method of treatment. Much of this results from the confusion about classification of these various lesions. Mulliken and Glowacki (1) generally classify these lesions as either hemangiomas or arteriovenous malformations. The hemangioma is then defined as being that lesion that is likely to shrink. Unfortunately, this classification is primarily retrospective in effect; therefore, lesions may go untreated for many years with the expectation that they will shrink. However, one quarter of them do not, and a large number of them eventually interfere with normal function or develop other complications. Suppression amblyopia in lesions around the eye or interference with the airway or facial disfigurement as tissues are eroded is not uncommon. Perhaps the most common complication is bleeding, which frequently is self-limited but which can be quite severe and may even lead to a coagulopathy. It goes without saying that, if there were an easy way to predict at an early age which of these would develop complications, the decision regarding treatment would be made much easier.

Traditional treatments for these lesions have included selective embolization, ligation, and cryotherapy. A new era in their treatment was introduced when the laser became available. Presently, the treatment of choice is excision with the laser. This can be done with either the carbon dioxide laser or the Nd:YAG laser with the sapphire tips. In general, the laser greatly reduces the blood loss and helps control the hemorrhage.

Many of these lesions spontaneously regress. There is a second method for laser treatment of these hemangiomas that involves the attempt to initiate this coagulation process to produce shrinkage of the lesion. This is sometimes combined with other treatments such as selective embolization. The laser shrinkage treatment usually involves the Nd:YAG laser and can be done via a noncontact method that involves compressing the lesion with a diascope (a clear instrument that compresses the lesion yet transmits the laser light). They can also be treated intralesionally by using the sapphire tips to introduce the laser energy directly into the center of the lesion. In both instances, intralesional steroids are usually added to ensure the best response. Sometimes 10–15 watts of laser energy can be administered with 1–2-sec exposures throughout several areas of these larger lesions. This is then usually followed by injection with a combination of betamethazone and triamcinolone.

Another difficulty with this classification arises from the fact that there are some ''hemangiomas'' that have a cavernous component and are associated with deeper vessels that have no tendency to shrink. Such lesions may also be associated with the Klippel-Trenxaunay syndrome, in which limb or facial hypertrophy occurs secondary to the increased vascularity. These lesions are less likely to respond to the shrinkage therapy and are certainly more difficult to excise with the laser. Nevertheless, the laser still remains the best method of treating these lesions. The shrinkage method may be attempted initially and followed by an excisional treatment if necessary. It is hoped that methods for intravascular laser treatment to close these abnormally large and deep vessels will be developed in the future.

Reconstructive Surgery

FLAPS

Flaps can readily be raised with the laser for a variety of reconstructive procedures. The carbon dioxide laser may be used to incise and elevate these flaps; however, the Nd : YAG laser with the sapphire tips is perhaps a better choice. Several comparative studies have shown that the laser causes less tissue damage than electrocautery. In addition, the electric current generated by the electrocautery can have a deleterious effect on the vascular supply to these flaps, whereas the laser causes no such effect.

Flaps should be raised with the highest power density compatible with the procedure in order to reduce the tissue damage. Larger flaps, such as those normally seen with reduction mammoplasty, abdominoplasty, and other procedures, can be incised with the laser. In general, the skin should initially be incised with a scalpel and the laser then used to incise the deeper tissues. Adequate smoke evacuation as well as traction and countertraction are essential to achieving the best result with flap elevation.

COSMETIC SURGERY

A variety of cosmetic procedures using the laser, including facelift, blepharoplasty, and "laser liposuction," have been described. Well-executed scientific studies of these procedures are lacking; however, publicity surrounding such procedures attracts a great deal of media attention and creates a public demand for these laser cosmetic surgeries. Until well-controlled studies that show the advantages of performing these cosmetics procedures with the laser can be performed, they should not be attempted by the average laser surgeon.

HIDRADENITIS SUPPURATIVA

This infective disease of the apocrine glands is nicely treated using the laser. In most instances, the laser can be used to excise or marsupialize these infected sinus tracts, allowing them to heal from the base of the lesions. Blood loss is usually greatly reduced and healing is rapid following these procedures; however, more than one treatment may be required.

Either the CO_2 or the Nd : YAG laser can be used at 10–15 watts to follow these tracts. After they are opened, they can be either packed or excised.

TATTOOS

Both decorative and traumatic tattoos can be nicely treated with the laser. Although these have been treated primarily with the carbon dioxide laser in the past, a new experimental laser, the ruby-rod laser, seems to be an excellent treatment for them. Argon and Nd : YAG lasers have likewise been effectively used.

The essence of the laser treatment of tattoos is to destroy the pigment within the dermis and subdermal tissues. Unfortunately, this cannot be done with the CO_2 or other available lasers without also destroying the surrounding tissue and thereby causing ghosting type scars and perhaps hypertrophic scars or keloids. Frequently, more than one treatment is required and the patient who desires a tattoo removed may find the procedure cost prohibitive.

The ruby-rod laser has been used experimentally to treat these decorative tattoos. It seems to work best on homemade tattoos of a blue color. It has little effect on some tattoos of other colors, and these may require treatment with the CO_2 or other lasers.

Future of Lasers in Plastic Surgery

A number of laser applications that could be useful in plastic surgery have been described. These include photodynamic therapy and the laser treatment of superficial cancers. Also, tissue welding or tissue fusion to close incisions and lacerations is being investigated to replace suture closure, especially in microsurgical applications such as microvascular anastomosis and microneurorrhaphies. Biostimulation, a low-power laser treatment to induce chronic wounds to heal, has been promoted.

Photodynamic therapy (PDT) has been around for a number of years. This technique involves the administration of a sensitizing dye, frequently a hematoporphyrin derivative (HpD). This dye seems to be selectively retained by malignant tissue. When light of a certain frequency (630 nm when using HpD) then activates the dye, the laser light energy is coupled to create some very active and lethal molecules (singlet oxygen or superperoxides) in the malignant tissue cells. The cell membranes then deteriorate, causing the cells to die. Photodynamic therapy has been used in a variety of primary and metastatic lesions and has been found to be effective. The drawbacks of this technique include photosensitivity in the patient for a prolonged period of time following administration of the dye. In addition, the technique does not penetrate deeply enough to treat very thick tumors; therefore, new methods such as intralesional treatment are being devised. Also, other laser wavelengths and dye combinations are being studied to see if a more effective photodynamic therapy can be developed. The technique promises to revolutionize the treatment of superficial cancers. However, much work remains to be done before it is approved by the Food and Drug Administration for clinical use.

Tissue welding has been accomplished with a variety of different lasers, including the CO_2, the Nd : YAG, and the argon laser. In this technique, the laser energy denatures the protein within the tissue, which then forms a "glue" and fuses the tissue together. The body then gradually reabsorbs the cellular debris or glue and creates a tight tissue bond. Obviously, this is heavily technique-dependent, and while some impressive results have been demonstrated in experimental studies, the expense of the laser and the difficulties in learning the technique provide formidable obstacles to the development of this technique.

The ruby-rod laser, the first laser invented, is being reintroduced to treat decorative tattoos and pigmented lesions. This intense red light at 694 nm has been pulsed very rapidly and used to ablate the pigment-containing cells in the skin. It has been found particularly effective against the dark blue or black pigment of decorative tattoos; however, it apparently has little effect on the other tattoo pigments that might be used. There is some indication that it may be useful in the treatment of melanin-pigmented tumors; however, much work remains to be done to determine its effectiveness in this role.

Biostimulation is a technique for accelerating the healing of damaged or disordered tissues. So-called soft lasers or low-powered lasers have been used for a number of years, particularly outside the United States, for the treatment of chronic or nonhealing wounds. Because there is relatively less governmental regulation in the countries where these techniques have been popularized, exaggerated claims have been made, thus obscuring in part the true effectiveness of these lasers. The helium-neon laser (632 nm), the gallium-arsenide solid-state laser, and other lasers have been used in this role. The present state of knowledge in regard to this laser technique would seem to indicate that there may be a benefit in some instances but it has yet to be defined or characterized.

Reference

1. Mulliken JB, Glowacki J: Hemangiomas and vascular malformations in infants and children: A classification based on endothelial characteristics. *Plast Reconstr Surg* 69:412, 1982.

Suggested Readings

American National Standards Institute, *Safe Use of Lasers in Health Care Facilities* (ANS1 Z136.3), 1988 (Published by Laser Institute of America, 12424 Research Parkway, Suite 130, Orlando, Florida 32826).

Apfelberg DB: *Evaluation and Installation of Surgical Laser Systems.* New York, Springer-Verlag, 1987.

Arndt KA: Treatment techniques in argon laser therapy: Comparison of pulsed and continuous exposure. *J Am Acad Dermatol* 11:90, 1984.

Arndt KA, Noe JM, Rosen S (Eds): *Cutaneous Laser Therapy: Principles and Methods.* New York, Wiley, 1983.

Dover JS, Arndt KA, Geronemus RA, et al: *Illustrated Cutaneous Laser Surgery. A Practitioner's Guide.* East Norwalk, CT: Appleton & Lange, 1990.

Garden JM, O'Banion K, Shelnitz LS, et al: Papillomavirus in the vapor of carbon dioxide laser-treated verrucae. *JAMA* 259:1199, 1988.

Gregory RO, Goldman L: Applications of photodynamic therapy in plastic surgery. *Lasers Surg Med* 6:62, 1986.

Hobby LW: Argon laser treatment of superficial vascular lesions in children. *Lasers Surg Med* 6:16, 1986.

Lanzafame RJ, Hinshaw JR (eds): *Color Atlas of CO₂ Laser Surgical Techniques.* St. Louis, Ishiyoku, 1988.

Noe JM, Barsky SH, Geer DE, Rosen S: Port wine stains and the response to argon laser; successful treatment and the predictive role of color, age and biopsy. *Plast Reconstr Surg* 65:130, 1980.

Tan OT, Sherwood K, Gilchrest BA: Treatment of children with port wine stains using the flash lamp-pulsed tunable dye laser. *N Engl J Med* 320:416, 1989.

Van Gemert MJC, Welch AJ, Amin AP: Is there an optional laser treatment for port wine stains? *Lasers Surg Med* 6:76, 1986.

TWO

Skin and Soft Tissues

15

Repair of Traumatic Cutaneous Injuries Involving the Skin and Soft Tissue

Martin C. Robson, M.D., F.A.C.S. and Lawrence S. Zachary, M.D.

A wound can be defined as a disruption of normal anatomical relationships due to injury. The injury can be an intentional surgical incision or due to accidental trauma. Because man's biological state is not germ-free, there exists a delicate balance that allows him to survive in the presence of a great many species of bacteria, all with the potential of causing infection. The balance is an equilibrium between the factors of host resistance and the bacteria when no infection is present. Once the equilibrium is unbalanced, either by an impairment in host resistance or an increase in the bacterial inoculum, clinical infection results. In any wound, the normal equilibrium between bacteria and host is endangered. The local defense mechanisms are challenged by disruption of the protection provided by the cutaneous barrier. Impediments to local defense mechanisms, such as debris, blood clot, or necrotic tissue, often accompany a large bacterial inoculum in traumatic wounds.

The major advance in the prevention and management of infection in soft tissue has been the understanding that the mere presence of microorganisms in a wound is less important than the level of bacterial growth. A wealth of clinical and experimental data have shown that a level of bacterial growth of greater than 100,000 organisms per gram of tissue is necessary to cause a wound infection and the potential for invasive sepsis for most species of bacteria (1). Only the β-hemolytic streptococcus appears capable of routinely causing infection at levels of less than 100,000 organisms per gram of tissue (2).

The role of the surgeon in managing any soft tissue wound is, first, to evaluate whether the patient's balance is in equilibrium or upset in favor of the bacteria. If in equilibrium, all efforts must be expended to maintain this status and prevent an ensuing infection. If not in equilibrium, infection is present, and the management of the infection is directed at reestablishing the equilibrium.

Infection can be prevented by maintaining the host's defense at peak efficiency. The effect of the interaction between the bacteria and the host, although under systemic influence, is ultimately determined by the local factors in the wound. Among these are necrotic tissue, decreased local wound perfusion, foreign body, hematoma, and dead space. The usual patient presenting with a traumatic wound has little immune defect due to systemic

factors, and the surgeon can do little to influence this defect if it is present. However, the surgeon plays a significant role in eliminating the local deterrents to effective host defense in the wound (3). If local wound factors are not controlled, they upset the equilibrium. Circumstances are then present in which a normally subinfectious inoculum of bacteria may multiply to levels sufficient to produce infection.

All traumatic wounds are contaminated at least to the extent that bacteria can always be identified by cultures performed on tissue biopsies of specimens (4). Normally, the bacterial count of skin is quite high. These bacteria reside both on the surface of the skin and deep in the hair follicles and sweat glands. The amount of bacteria normally present in the recesses is 1000 organisms per gram of tissue (1).

Pulaski et al. (5), in 1941, found on culturing 200 fresh traumatic wounds aerobically and anaerobically that all contained organisms, the dirty wounds more than the clean. Even clean-appearing wounds may harbor organisms with sufficient frequency to suspect their presence in every case. No one can tell which of these wounds is going to develop infection. In a series of 80 wounds, 20% yielded at least 10^5 organisms per gram of tissue (6). However, the mere presence of bacteria is less important than their potential for causing wound sepsis. A great deal of mechanical contamination in the form of debris, necrotic tissue, or sutures can provide the nidus for multiplication of initially small numbers of bacteria to significant levels of growth. Elek (7) has shown that the presence of a single silk will reduce by 10,000 times the number of staphylococci necessary to cause a wound infection. Conversely, the initial inoculum into a wound may be so massive that the local defense mechanisms are overwhelmed from the outset.

It is apparent that a working definition of a truly "contaminated" wound is necessary when dealing with traumatic injuries. A contaminated wound may be defined and identified both by its bacterial flora and by local wound factors. The bacterial level in the tissue is a reflection of the balance between the bacterial invaders and the host defense mechanisms. True contamination leading to wound infection and the potential for invasive sepsis exists when the level of bacterial growth exceeds 100,000 organisms per gram of tissue.

Clinical Evaluation of the Patient and the Wound

Overall care of the individual with a soft tissue injury must begin with a complete evaluation of the patient and history of the accident. The history will give the treating physician a framework to follow as to the severity of injury. Obviously, a patient involved in a high-speed motor vehicle accident with multiple fractures will be at greater risk of associated injuries to other organ systems than will the patient who sustains a laceration from a piece of glass. From a thorough physical examination, a clear picture must be formulated as to the level of the injury (i.e., a superficial laceration with no underlying injury versus a deep laceration with disruption of skin, soft tissue, muscle, and related adnexal structures). Once these parameters have been thoroughly investigated, a plan of management can be initiated.

Radiographic studies, including radiographs, tomography, xeroradiography, and computed tomography (CT) scanning, should be used when appropriate to aid in diagnosis. A patient with a wooden foreign body will benefit from xeroradiography for localization of the fragment, which may be missed on routine radiographs.

The diagnosis of the degree of contamination in a traumatic wound is made on the basis of history and clinical observation and may be confirmed by quantitative bacterial studies. The circumstances of the wounding and character of the wounding agent provide important clues. It is well known that a clean, dry windshield will support little bacterial growth and such a laceration will have a small inoculation. Similarly, a sharp laceration from a clean butcherknife will be unlikely to lead to infection. A crush injury from a machine part that has been well greased presents a different problem, as does a puncture wound from a stake contaminated with soil. The bacterial inoculum from a nonmeat-eating dog bite may be low and allow primary closure, whereas the inoculum from a human bite would be large because human saliva contains as many as 10^8 bacteria/ml.

The location of the wound will reflect the potential of local defense mechanisms to withstand contamination. The excellent blood supply to the face and scalp provides more inherent resistance than is present in the lower extremities. This is why a facial wound with excellent blood supply would be expected to handle an inoculum for a longer period of time than the area at the juncture of the middle and lower thirds of the leg overlying the tibia, where poor blood supply might allow rapid bacterial multiplication.

Time is an important historical factor in diagnosing the potentially contaminated wound. In a series of wounds previously reported, the mean time since injury was 2.2 hr for patients with less than 10^2 bacteria per gram of tissue in their wounds; the mean time was 3 hr for the group with 10^2–10^5 organisms per gram of tissue; and in those with greater than 10^5 organisms per gram of tissue even before being seen, the mean time from wounding was 5.17 hr (6). More importantly, only those in the last group developed infection that prevented primary healing. The "period of grace" or "golden period," of which Pulaski (8) speaks, appears to be that amount of time that is required before an inoculum into a wound reaches the critical level of 10^5 bacteria per gram of tissue. Many local and systemic factors will control the amount of time.

Bacterial Evaluation of the Wound

Because bacteria are present in all traumatic wounds and there appears to be a critical number that results in clinical infection, quantitative as well as qualitative surveillance of the wound seems indicated. This is certainly true for those wounds suspected of having a heavy initial inoculum, those occurring in patients with impaired host defenses, or in those wounds presenting more than 5–6 hr after injury. Surface swabs and cultures of purulent exudates have proven to be unreliable. Surface swabs yield many organisms that have not gained entrance into the tissues. However, if surface organisms are removed, only a single species appears to reach significant tissue levels. Heggers et al. (9), in studying 100 war wounds of the extremities, found 92% yielded single species isolates. The important bacteria are those reaching a significant tissue level.

A tissue culture may be obtained by cleansing the wound surface, removing a specimen, weighing it, flaming it, and homogenizing it after diluting it 10-fold. Serial tube dilutions and pour plates or back plating can then yield an accurate colony count related to a gram of tissue (3). Such detailed analyses are of little value in the Emergency Department situation because they would require 24–36 hr for completion. However, the more important information derived from such a technique can be obtained in 15 min with a rapid slide method (3). Again, a specimen is removed from a wound, weighed, diluted, and homogenized. An aliquot of the suspension is then placed on a glass slide and Gram-stained. The slide is then examined under a microscope. If a single organism is seen on the slide, the bacterial count is greater than 10^5 organisms per gram of tissue in the original biopsy. If no organisms are seen on the slide, the bacterial count is 10^5 or fewer per gram.

Qualitative bacterial cultures are also important. At the time the tissue is homogenized, the homogenate is smeared, Gram-stained, and cultured aerobically and anaerobically. The Gram-stained smear helps to identify streptococci or clostridia, and the culture allows identification of the organisms and performance of antibiotic sensitivities. It is important to identify streptococci and the various clostridia species early. It has been demonstrated that β-hemolytic streptococci prevent satisfactory wound closure primarily, secondarily, or by a graft or flap when they are present in a wound at any level (2). *Clostridium tetani* or *perfringens* must be identified as early as possible to allow for radical débridement and to prevent premature wound closure.

Tetanus Immunoprophylaxis

Guidelines for tetanus immunoprophylaxis have been established by the American College of Surgeons Committee on Trauma and are summarized below. Patients fully immunized who have received their last booster injection within the last 10 years need no booster injection if the wound is not tetanus-prone. Immunized patients with tetanus-prone wounds should receive a 0.5-cc tetanus toxoid booster if their last booster injection was given more than 5 years before injury. Immunized patients who have received no booster injection within the last 10 years need to receive a booster injection for any wound.

Individuals not previously immunized should receive a tetanus booster injection, followed by a full course of immunization, for even the most minor wounds. Patients with tetanus-prone wounds should receive a 0.5-cc booster injection of tetanus toxoid, plus 250 units of tetanus immune globulin, followed by a full course of immunization.

Preparing the Wound for Closure

The sine qua non of any wound is closure, and in all instances, it must be determined if the wound is ready for closure. The bacterial level in the wound is one criterion. Also, one must determine if there is nonviable or potentially nonviable tissue in the wound and any detrimental clot or foreign debris. Sharp débridement remains the most efficient way to prepare a traumatic wound for closure. Débridement removes a large proportion of contaminating bacteria as well as many local deterrents to normal host resistance. If the viability of the tissue remains in question after débridement, intravenous fluorescein can be given, and the wound tissue inspected under ultraviolet light. Tissue fluorescence suggests viability.

Irrigation may be an important adjunct to sharp débridement. Wound irrigation as normally delivered, even with voluminous amounts of solutions, removes little but surface contamination. A pulsating jet lavage is an improved modification. In the experimental animal, when compared to more standard types of irrigation, the pulsating lavage removed significantly more bacteria and resulted in significantly fewer wound infections (10). If a pulsating jet lavage is not available, it has been shown that injection through a high pressure system with a small gauge needle approximates the results obtained with the lavage and is far superior to standard wound irrigation. Irrigation is probably best performed with a balanced salt solution. In 1919, Fleming (11) observed that disinfectants that kill bacteria also kill tissue and, therefore, the solution used to prepare the wound edges should not be used in the wound per se.

Systemic antibiotics have practical and potential value only if a therapeutic blood or, more importantly, tissue level is achieved within the first 4 hr after wounding. Burke (12) has shown that bacterial lodgment is not influenced after that time frame. When antibiotics are begun after the time required for bacterial lodgment, infection

rates are indeed higher. Surgical débridement and freshening the wound would render this restriction less rigid and make antibiotics more effective. However, in traumatic wounds, tissue levels of antibiotics are difficult to achieve rapidly. Adequate tissue levels are further hindered by conditions within the wound such as ischemia or necrotic tissue. Therefore, systemic antibiotics may not be of much use in most cases. Topical antibiotic irrigation affects only surface bacteria and has little influence on tissue lodgment. In controlled studies, it has shown no benefit over the saline irrigation alone (1).

Closure of Acute Traumatic Wounds

Wound closures can be classified as primary, spontaneous, or tertiary. Primary repair represents immediate reapproximation of the wound layers, which can be accomplished by a variety of techniques. After evaluation of the wound, the edges are sharply trimmed to allow for accurate coaptation. The deeper layers such as the fascia are closed with absorbable sutures. No sutures are placed in the subcutaneous tissue as they promote fat necrosis, act as foreign bodies, and may facilitate wound infections. The dermal layer can be closed with simple inverted-interrupted sutures, and a very fine epidermal stitch is used to align the surface. Alternatively, a continuous pull-out suture can be placed, or the edges can be approximated with micropore tape. When the edges of the wound cannot be reapproximated directly without tension, a local flap may be used to close the defect. In certain locations, primary closure can also be obtained by widely undermining the adjacent soft tissue. When this is done, traction on adjacent structures should not result in a subsequent deformity such as an ectropion.

After adequate débridement, wounds that cannot be closed primarily due to contamination or tissue loss can undergo delayed closure or be allowed to close spontaneously. Early reports of delayed closure stressed the necessity of not disturbing the dressing placed on a wound between the time of débridement and the time of delayed closure. Experimentally, the optimal time for a closure has been shown by Edlich et al. (13) to be on or after the fourth postwounding day. We found that, if the bacterial level in the wound is 10^5 or fewer organisms per gram of tissue, successful wound closure can be expected (14). Treatment of the soft tissue should be initiated during the period of delay so as to hasten the decrease in bacterial levels. Occasionally, a wound will be allowed to close spontaneously. This may be preferable in wounds with heavy inocula of streptococci or clostridia. Wound contraction and epithelization will close most defects. Once closure has been accomplished, the need for secondary scar revision can be assessed.

Chronic Wounds

Chronically contaminated wounds, as opposed to the acute potentially contaminated wound, all contain a tissue bacterial flora. Examples are thermal burns and traumatic wounds that were not closed acutely. The characteristic of such wounds is granulation tissue. Granulation tissue does not occur in the absence of bacteria. It is not found beneath the surface of a successfully closed wound. It has been likened to a pyogenic granuloma, and successful closure is predicated on the surgeon's ability to control the level of bacterial flora.

Biopsy cultures have revealed the clinical difficulty in identifying bacteriological healthy granulation tissue (that tissue which contains 10^5 or fewer bacteria per gram). Experimentally and clinically, successful closure of a contaminated wound (by spontaneous epithelialization, wound edge approximation, application of skin grafts, or by pedicle flaps) is directly and consistently related to the surgeon's ability to decrease the bacterial flora in the tissue to 10^5 or fewer bacteria per gram (1, 3). In a series of 50 skin grafts applied to chronically contaminated wounds (regardless of the technique used to prepare the granulations for grafting), a bacterial count of 10^5 or fewer bacteria on the day of grafting resulted in a 94% skin graft take as opposed to 19% when the bacterial counts were above 10^5 per gram of tissue on the day of grafting (15).

Reduction of the bacterial flora is best accomplished by meticulous attention to surgical detail. Frequent débridement and surgical cleansing are critical. Enzymatic débridement may be of some value, but it tends to simultaneously allow rapid bacterial proliferation (16). This is of potential danger, particularly when large areas are involved, such as in thermal burns. Systemic antibiotics do not reach adequate tissue levels in chronic granulation tissue and have been shown experimentally to have no effect on the bacterial level in granulating wounds (17). Conversely, water-based topical antibacterial creams do penetrate the depths of such wounds and have a direct effect on bacterial growth.

Because true bacterial control is only achieved by wound closure, the use of temporary biological dressings for cleansing and temporary closure has been shown to be of value. In a randomized study of 100 delayed wound closures, the authors compared several methods to decrease the bacteria to below the critical level. Temporary biological dressings proved to be the most effective. The biological dressings probably adhered to the wound surface and effected a "biological closure" that allowed the inflammatory tissue to function at peak efficiency and phagocytosis to proceed effectively. Porcine xenografts failed to establish biological union with the underlying tissue and therefore were less effective than allograft skin or amniotic membranes (18). However, the true control of infection in a granulating wound is closure of the wound with autograft tissue.

Techniques of closure in chronically contaminated wounds vary widely, depending on the circumstances. In some wounds, approximation of the wound edges may be accomplished. In others, cutaneous defects may require coverage with skin grafts. Local wound factors other than bacteria, such as exposed bone, marginal blood supply in the recipient site, or previous radiation, may require the use of pedicled flap tissue or free flap coverage.

Dressings

After wound closure, an adequate dressing is applied to the wound. Understanding the function of dressings will help dictate their design and selection. Functions of dressings include: (*a*) protection, (*b*) absorption, (*c*) compression, (*d*) immobilization, and (*e*) provision of an aesthetic wound covering. Protection from mechanical injury of the wound edges and from desiccation is necessary. Also, during the first few hours until the wound is sealed by fibrin, protection from exogenous bacterial contamination is essential. Because all wounds weep during the inflammatory stage of wound healing, absorption of this inflammatory exudate is useful. Likewise, any bleeding from the wound margins needs to be absorbed to prevent maceration. Edema is also part of the inflammatory process. Even compression, but not excessive pressure, is helpful. Attempts to prevent this obligatory edema completely by a pressure dressing or cast should be avoided. Preventing excess motion of the approximated skin edges or of an applied flap or skin graft is a therapeutic imperative. A properly constructed dressing can give the optimal degree of immobilization. This will also decrease the pain associated with the wound. Finally, the dressings should be aesthetically acceptable; this is the portion of wound management that a surgeon first presents to the patient and others. It is the surgeon's signature on his work.

To accomplish the functions addressed above, dressings should be carefully constructed from a variety of materials and thoughtfully applied. The inner layer, in contact with the wound, should be fine-meshed gauze, either plain or impregnated. The purpose of impregnating gauze is not to prevent sticking to the wound because macerating amounts of impregnate are necessary to accomplish this; rather, it provides a coating to the fibers and therefore promotes drainage through to the absorptive layers of the dressing. Plain gauze tends to entrap the drainage and form a coagulum at the innermost layer. Commercially impregnated gauze must be "wrung out" because its heavy impregnation tends to prevent drainage and to macerate tissue. The remainder of the dressing consists of bulky absorptive materials; however, cotton-containing gauze should not be applied next to a weeping wound because later removal is difficult. The dressing can then be completed by the application of firm, even compression using a roller bandage. The use of an Ace or elastic bandage is mentioned only to be condemned. An even, controllable amount of compression is not possible with such a bandage, and dangerously constrictive dressings may result as the wound proceeds through the obligatory edema phase. The dressing is completed by proper positioning and immobilizing in the appropriate position. This may often require the use of plaster splints.

Summary

Basic principles of repair of traumatic cutaneous injuries involving the skin and soft tissue are similar to the principles for repair of an operative incision. The differences are that all traumatic wounds are contaminated and all contain some deterrents to normal wound healing. Therefore, principles must be expanded to include: ascertainment of level of contamination; identification and removal of deterrents to wound healing; and prevention of invasive infections. Once a proper assessment of the level of contamination is made, the bacterial balance of a given wound can be determined. If a wound is in bacterial balance, débridement and irrigation can remove necrotic tissue, clots, and debris, and wound closure can proceed. If a wound is not in bacterial balance, this must be attained while other deterrents to wound healing are being removed. Only then can successful closure of the traumatic soft tissue wound be accomplished and healing proceed.

References

1. Robson MC, Krizek TJ, Heggers JP: Biology of surgical infection. In: *Current Problems in Surgery*. Chicago, Year Book Medical Publishers, 1973.
2. Robson MC, Heggers JP: Surgical infection. II. The β-hemolytic streptococcus. *J Surg Res* 9:289, 1969.
3. Robson MC: Infection in the surgical patient: An imbalance in the normal equilibrium. *Clin Plast Surg* 6:493, 1979.
4. Altemeier WA, Gibbs EW: Bacterial flora of fresh accidental wounds. *Surg Gynecol Obstet* 78:164, 1944.
5. Pulaski EJ, Meleney FL, Spaeth WLC: Bacterial flora of acute traumatic wounds. *Surg Gynecol Obstet* 72:982, 1941.
6. Robson MC, Duke WF, Krizek TJ: Rapid bacterial screening in the treatment of civilian wounds. *J Surg Res* 14:426, 1973.
7. Elek SD: Experimental staphylococcal infections in the skin of man. *Ann NY Acad Sci* 65:85, 1956.
8. Pulaski EJ: *Surgical Infections*. Springfield, IL, Charles C Thomas, 1954.
9. Heggers JP, Barnes ST, Robson MC, et al: Microbial flora of orthopedic war wounds. *Milit Med* 134:602, 1969.
10. Hamer ML, Robson MC, Krizek TJ, et al: Quantitative bacterial analysis of comparative wound irrigations. *Ann Surg* 181:819, 1975.
11. Fleming A: The action of chemical and physiological antiseptics in a septic wound. *Br J Surg* 7:99, 1919.
12. Burke JF: The effective period of preventive antibiotic action in experimental incisions and dermal lesions. *Surgery* 50:161, 1961.
13. Edlich RF, Rogers W, Kasper G, et al: Studies in the management of the contaminated wound. I. Optimal time for closure of contaminated open wounds. II. Comparison of resistance to infection of open and closed wounds during healing. *Am J Surg* 117:323, 1969.
14. Robson MC, Heggers JP: Delayed wound closures based on bacterial counts. *J Surg Oncol* 2:379, 1980.
15. Krizek TJ, Robson MC, Kho E: Bacterial growth and skin graft survival. *Surg Forum* 18:518, 1967.
16. Krizek TJ, Robson MC, Groskin MG: Experimental burn wound sepsis-evaluation of enzymatic débridement. *J Surg Res* 17:219, 1974.
17. Robson MC, Edstrom LE, Krizek TJ, et al: The efficacy of systemic antibiotics in the treatment of granulating wounds. *J Surg Res* 16:299, 1974.
18. Robson MC, Samburg JL, Krizek TJ: Quantitative comparison of biological dressings. *J Surg Res* 14:431, 1973.

16

Scar Revision

Ross Rudolph, M.D., F.A.C.S.

Many patients with unsightly scars have the unrealistic belief that a plastic surgeon can make incisions that will not result in a scar and, in fact, can remove existing scars. Because of this attitude, it is important that the plastic surgeon recognize and clarify for the patients the limitations of scar revision.

The features of a good scar are: (*a*) a fine line (or series of lines) that falls within or is parallel to a skin wrinkle, contour junction, or relaxed skin tension line (RSTL); (*b*) absence of contour irregularities; (*c*) no pigmentation abnormalities; and (*d*) no contractures or distortion of adjacent structures.

The objectives of scar revision are: (*a*) to improve that scar's direction if it is not parallel to an RSTL; (*b*) to decrease the scar's width; (*c*) to divide a long scar into smaller components; (*d*) to correct malalignment or distortion of anatomical units; (*e*) to improve any surface irregularities; and (*f*) to correct any pigmentation abnormalities.

There are several factors to be considered before attempting scar revision.

Time Since Injury. After a skin injury, sufficient time must elapse to allow the third phase of wound healing, that of *maturation* (1), to run its full course. Early scars 2 or 3 weeks old usually are red and raised, as a result of vigorous wound healing. Scar revision at this time almost certainly will lead to recurrence of a red, raised scar. Before revision, 6–12 *months* should elapse to allow maximum spontaneous improvement. In children, maturation may take as long as 12–24 months. Flat, red scars will often fade considerably and need less revision than originally expected, while nodules will soften and flatten. Wide scars, however, will not narrow. The patient and family may insist on early scar revision and should be cautioned about the indications for waiting.

Earlier intervention may be indicated, however, if progressive scar deformity (e.g., traction on an eyelid) is occurring. A foreign body may need early removal to reduce inflammation. Major malalignment (e.g., a badly sutured eyebrow), can also be a legitimate reason for early revision.

The process of scar maturation may be speeded by *judicious* injection of a low-solubility depot glucocorticoid, usually Kenalog (triamcinolone acetonide). Low concentrations, such as 2.5–3.3 mg/ml, should be used to avoid overcorrection, that is, atrophy of a scar as it continues to mature. Care should be taken to keep the injection *within* the scar in order to avoid atrophy or hypopigmentation of the surrounding skin.

Nature of the Injuring Agent and Wound Management. Inquiry about how the scar was caused may help in deciding the outcome of revision. A raised, ragged scar caused by a dog bite that was not sutured may be much improved by careful revision. However, a similar scar resulting from meticulous suture of a clean, sharp glass laceration may recur because it represents the patient's poor reaction to surgical-type wounds. Additional factors to consider are who managed the injury (i.e., if it was managed by a physician skilled in repairing skin), and if wound healing proceeded normally or if complications occurred.

Location. Certain areas of the body are especially prone to scar thickening and spreading after revision. The midsternum (especially in women), deltoid area of the shoulder, and upper large breasts often react to scar revision with less than ideal results. Remember that many descriptions of scar revision are most applicable to the face, and revisions on the trunk or extremities may not heal as well. Scar revision on the extremities and trunk is aided by relieving tension when possible, as with a Z-plasty that changes scar direction.

Age of the Patient. Scar revision in older patients is almost always more successful than in the young, probably because skin healing is less vigorous. No exact demarcation exists, but the mid-20s empirically seem to divide "young" from "old" in doing scar revision. Many of the elegant and complicated scar revision techniques that have historically been described apply mainly to facial scars in older patients, and their use can lead to disastrous results if misapplied to the young.

Ethnic Background of the Patient. When scar revision is done in a person with fair skin and light hair and eyes, the final result may be a relatively thin scar if other criteria of patient selection have been met. In contrast, patients with dark skin, eyes, and hair may develop thicker and more raised scars in response to revision. Scar hyperpigmentation can also be more of a problem in brunettes. In blacks, keloids may develop, but in dark-skinned patients, a mediocre result is more often the result of scar hypertrophy rather than true keloid.

Healing of Prior Scars. If the patient planning scar revision has other scars, how they healed may help guide the surgeon. Thus, the woman who has a fine hairline scar after a cesarean section may heal other scars similarly, whereas one who healed such a wound with a thick ropy scar is less of a candidate for scar revision elsewhere. Of course, no guarantee can be made that one scar will heal like another. A true keloid, though, presages problems in scar revision!

Nature of the Scar. Patients wishing scar revision often complain of "keloids"; however, they may in fact have other types of scars, such as wide spread or hypertrophic scars (2). Wide spread scars are very amenable to the surgical scar revision techniques described below. Hypertrophic scars may be managed with surgery when properly chosen. True keloids must be approached very gingerly with surgery. Large keloids and certain hypertrophic scars may be better managed with pressure, Kenalog injections, or possibly future biochemical approaches rather than with surgery (2).

Whether Any Skin Was Lost. If the surgeon can establish whether skin was not just cut but lost at injury, this can serve as a planning guide. A wound resulting from skin loss such as an avulsion or burn may spring open when released, making revision more difficult and even mandating grafting or flap transfer. Such a situation can be highly uncomfortable for the surgeon if not foreseen. Burns typically heal with scars under tension, and when released, these scars can lead to an unexpectedly large defect. Even if a widely gapping wound can be pulled together, the resulting tension often leads to unacceptable scar spreading. Scar revision should be planned to avoid tension as much as possible.

Perceptions and Expectations of the Patient and Family. As with all surgery, understanding what the patient foresees as a result of surgery is vital. A superb technical result may produce misery if the patient expects miraculous obliteration of scarring. In some ethnic groups, any facial scarring may be viewed as a mark of marital infidelity, leading to unrealistic expectations about surgical outcome (3). Surprisingly, it is usually not hard to learn what the patient expects with gentle and sympathetic questioning. Yet occasionally, mutual misunderstanding and, rarely, outright lying can occur, leading to much unhappiness after surgery.

Surgical Techniques of Scar Revision

When surgical treatment is selected, scars are most often excised, and the wound is then sutured or revised with Z-plasty or W-plasty. Rarely is a large scar excised and the wound resurfaced with a skin graft or a skin flap. Finally, dermabrasion has a role in the management of specific types of scars.

TECHNIQUE OF FUSIFORM SCAR REVISION

Assuming that criteria have been met for scar revision, a number of technical aspects must be considered. *The scar revision should be planned, if possible, so that the final scar will lie in a natural wrinkle, crease, or boundary.* Even if wrinkles are not yet present, scars do best when at right angles to muscle pull (which is where wrinkles form) (Fig. 16.1).

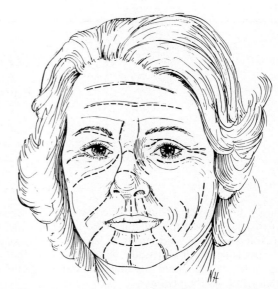

FIGURE 16.1. The locations of the constant facial crease lines are shown. These are important in planning scar revision procedures.

Natural creases such as the nasolabial fold should be paralleled rather than crossed at right angles, while natural boundaries such as the jaw line disguise parallel scars. The notorious semicircular "trapdoor" scar may be best handled by complete excision, if the final scar can be placed in a skin crease. Linear scar excision will be of little help to a poorly oriented scar such as a vertical forehead scar that crosses multiple deep skin wrinkles. In this case, a Z-plasty or W-plasty should be done to change the direction of the scar (4).

In hair-bearing areas, placing incisions to run parallel to the angle of the hair follicles can preserve hair and disguise the final scar. Given a choice, scars should be placed within the hair rather than in visible skin. Avoid shaving hair, if possible, to preserve landmarks. Eyebrows and eyelashes in particular should not be shaved.

Planning should also *avoid tension*. While not always possible, reducing tension to a minimum promotes a final scar that is thin (5).

Anesthesia

Many scar revisions can be done under local anesthesia, a desirable situation because the patient can move muscles to demonstrate skin folds. Lidocaine with epinephrine is preferred, but it should be avoided in the hand because of possible ischemia to the fingertips and in the lip inasmuch as epinephrine may blur the skin-vermilion border of the lip.

Infiltration of local anesthesia distorts the tissues; therefore, skin markings should be done beforehand unless the surgery is so obvious that the plan cannot be lost.

Planning the Revision

No absolute rules can be made, and the surgeon's experience and creativity are vital. In a linear scar revision, the goal should be to remove the old scar with a minimum of normal tissue yet orient the final scar in an ideal direction (Fig. 16.2A).

A valuable basic principle is that obvious landmarks should be preserved (or restored). These include lip vermilion border, hairlines such as eyebrows and eyelashes and scalp, skin creases, and tissue borders such as nasal alar rim or ear helix.

Excision and Undermining

The scar is excised with a scalpel, preferably a no. 15. The cut edges should be perpendicular to the skin surface. Some surgeons complete the excision at the corners with a no. 11 blade (Fig. 16.2B).

In the face and neck, skin undermining is done in the fat close to the skin, whereas on the trunk and extremities more fat is left on the flaps. In either case, the subdermal vascular plexus should be preserved. As a rough guideline, the combined width of the undermining (i.e., on both sides of the wound) should equal the open wound width.

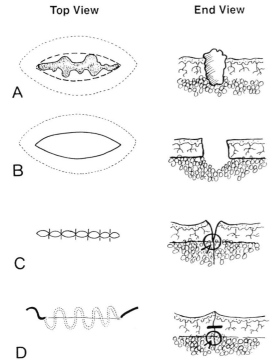

Top View   **End View**

A

B

C

D

FIGURE 16.2. Linear scar revision. **A,** Elliptical (actually lens-shaped) excision outlined around jagged hypertrophic scar is designed to remove all the scar and lie in a natural skin fold. The *outer dotted line* marks the extent of undermining. **B,** The lesion is excised, and undermining is completed. **C,** Deep layer is closed with absorbable suture, the knot is buried, and the dermis is opposed (*left*). The end view (*right*) shows that the wound should be almost fully closed. **D,** Final closure is shown with a buried running subcuticular Prolene suture, superficial in the dermis (*left*). On the *left*, the top view shows suture weaving back and forth across wound in dermis, piercing the epidermis only at each end. The thickness of the suture is exaggerated for clarity.

Undermining frees the normal skin from deep tissues and from remaining scar to allow free movement without tension.

Hemostasis should be obtained with conservative measures. With proper use of epinephrine, allowing 7–15 min to elapse from injection to incision, bleeding is minimal. The small amount of bleeding that occurs can often be controlled by pressure. If not, *selective* electrocautery can help. Random heavy electrocautery should be avoided because it will compromise healing. Rarely, ligation of bleeding vessels may be used, especially if the vessel has retracted into fat or muscle. Hemostatic substances like oxidized cellulose should be avoided.

Closure of the Wound

The wound closure should be with layers of sutures. Staples may cause misalignment and surface scars. Paper strips may be used in place of skin sutures if perfect subcuticular alignment is achieved (which is rarely the case).

The subject of which sutures to use is fraught with legend and strongly held personal opinions. My own preference is to close the deep layers with absorbable sutures, usually 4-0 Vicryl (Ethicon Corp., Somerville, NJ) or Dexon (Davis and Geck, Inc., Danbury, CT). Chromic catgut (but not plain) may be used for the rare patient who is allergic to the synthetic sutures. The most superficial layer of deep sutures (Fig. 16.2C) should be placed into the dermis, with the knot buried, and as close to the dermal-epidermal junction as possible. This will close the wound almost fully so that skin sutures have little or no tension. Drains are rarely used, but *should* be if fluid collection is feared.

Skin sutures ideally should be *running subcuticular* to avoid suture marks yet allow prolonged wound support (Fig. 16.2D). Usually I use 4-0 Prolene (Ethicon Corp., Somerville, NJ). This suture is quite nonreactive. The subcuticular suture can be left as long as 2–3 weeks if not irritated because this prolonged support may reduce scar spreading. Suture tract epithelial ingrowth can occur where the sutures enter and exit the skin; in practice, this is usually not a major problem except around the eyelids. Here sutures should be removed early. Clear Prolene makes the suture less obvious. The ends of the suture can be tied or anchored with sterile paper tape strips, which further support the wound (7). If the incision is long and removal of subcuticular Prolene would be painful, subcuticular running Vicryl may be used instead.

The subcuticular suture is useful only if the wound is relatively straight and if no skin tension exists. Otherwise, interrupted fine, simple, or vertical mattress sutures can be used for closure and edge refinement. Such sutures may be needed around the lips or where facial muscles could cause loosening of a continuous suture. These interrupted surface sutures should be removed as soon as possible to avoid cross-hatching. Usually 4 or 5 days on the face is sufficient, but 7 days on the extremities and longer in areas like palms and soles may be necessary. When sutures are removed early, Steri-strips

(Minnesota Mining & Mfg., St. Paul, MN) can be used for wound support, and the patient should be warned that the wound is not fully healed. Even with a subcuticular suture, such fine surface sutures may also be used and removed at 2 or 3 days, serving to refine the epidermal closure.

At the time of closure, a long-acting steroid like Kenalog (10–20 mg/ml) can be instilled if keloid formation is a major risk because of the patient's history or ethnic group.

"Dog-ear" Excision

With elliptical wound closure, small lumps of folded skin may remain at the ends. While elaborate remedies have been described, the most useful is simple excision following the line of the wound or of major skin creases (Fig. 16.3).

BURIED DERMAL FLAP FOR SUPPORT

Ideally, scar revision should be tension free, yet this is not always possible, especially in the case of a wide scar. As shown in Figure 16.4A–D, a "dermal" flap can be constructed of the deepithelialized scar, which can then be used to anchor and reinforce the scar revision against tension (2). The flap, actually made of scar, has sufficient strength to help prevent scar spreading. This technique is

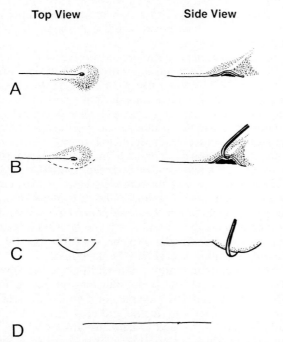

Top View   **Side View**

FIGURE 16.3. Dog-ear excision. **A,** Dog-ear is shown at end of linear scar revision. **B,** The dog-ear is elevated with a hook, and one edge is marked for excision. **C,** One edge is incised, and excess tissue is gently drawn across wound. **D,** Excess tissue is excised, and the wound is closed, extending the scar in the same direction.

End View

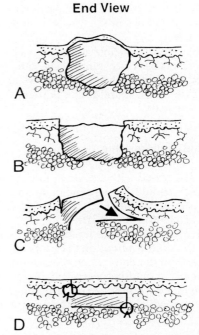

FIGURE 16.4. Buried dermal flap technique. **A,** A wide, hypertrophic scar extends below the skin surface. **B,** The scar is "deepithelialized," with removal of epidermis and a small amount of contiguous scar. **C,** The flap of scar "dermis" is elevated; the opposing skin flap is elevated to accept the dermal flap. Deeper scar has been excised here but may be left if not too bulky. **D,** The flap of dermis (actually scar) is advanced under the skin. It is anchored at both sides with absorbable sutures; a running subcuticular suture can be used for the final skin layer.

especially useful in scars of the trunk and extremities. If the scar is depressed, the entire deepithelialized scar can be left in place and surrounding normal skin advanced over it, to provide more bulk.

THE Z-PLASTY

The double flap rotation known as Z-plasty because of the shape of the design and final scar is an essential component of scar revision (8). It is used primarily for two goals: (*a*) to change the direction of a scar by 90° and, simultaneously, (*b*) to gain length in a scar.

Scars at right angles to skin folds or creases become shortened and thick, and Z-plasty both relieves these deformities and makes recurrence after revision less likely. Innumerable variations have been described, but the most useful is the design in which the limbs of the Z-plasty are equal to the length of the scar (Fig. 16.5A–D) and the limbs make an angle of 60° to the original scar (8).

When designing the Z-plasty, care must be taken to avoid basing it on avascular scar. After the flaps are cut, undermining around the bases helps mobility. The flaps are rotated 90° and sutured (Fig. 16.5).

A major consideration of Z-plasty is that the total amount of scar is lengthened. Obviously, the anticipated improvement must be worth the lengthening of scar. In a

Top View

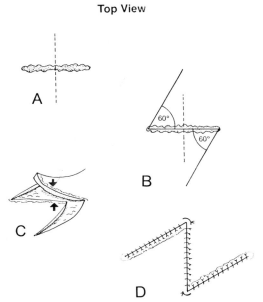

FIGURE 16.5. The classic Z-plasty. **A,** A thick, contracted scar crosses a skin fold. Design is begun by drawing a perpendicular line at the midpoint of the scar; this line helps establish flap incisions, but it is not itself incised. **B,** Completing the design, the limbs of flaps are equal to each other and to the length of the scar. Angles of the flaps are 60°. **C,** Flaps are elevated, preserving the subdermal plexus. Undermining is accomplished around flap bases. The scar is excised unless it is too wide; here a portion of scar is left for clarity in showing flap transposition. **D,** Flaps are transposed and sutured. A three-corner suture (half-buried horizontal mattress) is used to anchor narrow tips without necrosis that could result from simple sutures near tips.

child, where any scar may hypertrophy and be highly visible, the prominent Z scar may be unacceptable. A hypertrophic scar—or worse, a keloid—may not be suitable for Z-plasty because of the risk of the new scar becoming as prominent as the smaller, old scar! Especially on the face, multiple small Z-plasties may be superior to one large one.

THE W-PLASTY

Much the same may be true of the W-plasty, which has been much overused. This technique substitutes a zig-zag scar for a linear one, and it has the potential advantages of disguising a straight scar and of removing wide suture scars (4). Besides discarding normal tissue, the multiple Ws can be highly visible on a young person's face, making the scar revision worse than the original deformity. In the facial area, the W-plasty is most useful in the *older* patient, who may be expected to heal scars well, and appears to have its major value in revision of long, depressed *forehead* scars. The limbs should be about 5 mm, and the angles should be between 60° and 90°, depending on the relationship of the scar to the RSTL (Fig. 16.6A–C). The W-plasty is less likely to produce alternative small ridges and depressions in some areas than multiple Z-plasties.

OTHER TECHNIQUES OF SCAR REVISION

Practically all techniques of plastic surgery may be called into use in scar revision, especially revision of complex scars. Some of the most useful are local flaps, full-thickness skin grafts, and dermabrasion.

Local Flaps

These flaps should be kept in mind, especially if the scar resulted from tissue loss and not just laceration. The surgeon doing scar revision must always have a potential plan for local flap rotation in the unhappy event that, after scar excision, the wound gapes so wide that direct closure is not possible. Often, relatively minor flap rotations are required, yet their execution demands skill and experience. There is no substitute for careful evaluation of local tissue characteristics and preplanning of the scar revision. On the older person's face, local flaps to replace skin grafts or relieve tension can often produce superior results.

Full-Thickness Skin Grafts

Full-thickness grafts are an alternate and often satisfactory way to close a gaping wound if local flaps are not available. Full-thickness skin is preferable to split-thickness skin; it has a more natural feel and appearance (8). Full-thickness skin is harvested from a hairless area and sutured with a bolus tie-over dressing. For the face (the usual location), such skin can be obtained most successfully from behind the ear in all age groups. Older patients may be able to spare upper eyelid or preauricular skin. The latter may avoid the persistent pinkness of grafts from the other donor sites. Upper inner arm full-thickness skin grafts often have a natural facial appearance.

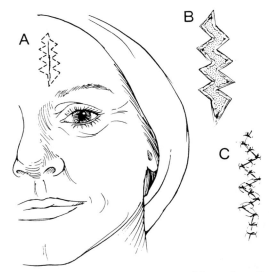

FIGURE 16.6. The W-plasty. **A,** The *dotted lines* show the design for the excision of the scar. **B,** The flaps have now been developed and are ready for interdigitation. **C,** The W-flaps are shown in position.

Dermabrasion

Dermabrasion is a useful adjunct of scar revision. Irregular surface contour defects may be better managed by sanding than by excision, especially if extensive. However, the method is contraindicated if the cutaneous adnexa have been destroyed so that no epithelial resurfacing can occur. Some surgeons lightly dermabrade the wound edges at the time of scar excision in the hope of providing a less visible scar.

Nonsurgical Modalities

In some instances, pressure garments and splints will be useful to prevent recurrent scar hypertrophy or contracture postoperatively (2). Daily massage probably helps soften the subcutaneous nodules and ridges.

An early tendency for hypertrophy after scar revision may be controlled by repeated injections of Kenalog, usually 2.5–3.3 mg/ml. Higher concentrations may be used later if necessary to control recurrence of hypertrophy or keloid. In the case of severe hypertrophy or keloid, concentrations as high as 20 or 40 mg/ml may be used, keeping in mind that tissue atrophy can occur with such doses. Injections should be given 3–6 weeks apart to allow maximum effect of each dose.

For the keloid or hypertrophic scar judged not suitable for scar revision, pressure garments and high-concentration Kenalog injections may be the only current available help (2).

UNDESIRABLE RESULTS FROM SCAR REVISION

The most common problem after scar revision is a recurrence of either hypertrophy or increasing *scar* width. If patient selection is not ideal, this is not a complication but is to be expected. As an extreme example, scar revision of a 3-week-old scar located on the deltoid area in a dark-skinned, 6-year-old patient is doomed to turn out poorly! Yet even with the best of selection and technique, scars may not become thin and inconspicuous. Patients should never be guaranteed results.

Hematoma

Hematoma may result if a dead space is not closed by sutures or dressing compression. Small Penrose drains, rubber band drains, or small suction drains (made from butterfly scalp vein needles and blood-drawing vacuum tubes) may be used to avert this problem.

Infection

Infection is rarely a problem in scar revision of the face, but can be on the trunk or extremities. Antibiotic coverage is rarely used, unless the revision is quite large; even then the value of antibiotics is questionable. Some wounds with retained small foreign bodies appear to be more prone to infection; at scar revision, all such foreign bodies should be removed, if possible.

Hyperpigmentation

Hyperpigmentation may result after scar revision if the scar is exposed to much sunlight. In fact, many scars, especially those with a major component of abrasion, may be visible primarily because of increased pigmentation. We advise patients to apply a good sun-blocking agent (SPF of 15) over the scars for 6 months, after which potential pigmentation problems appear to lessen.

Milia

Milia ("white-heads") are small sebaceous or inclusion cysts. They commonly occur on the face when epithelium grows down suture tracts. Eyelids are especially prone to milia formation; therefore, sutures are removed as early as 4 days postoperatively to prevent milia. After abrasions, milia can form as regenerating epithelium grows over sebaceous duct openings. Treatment consists of unroofing the milia by having the patient scrub the area daily with a rough washcloth. Persistent milia can be unroofed with an 18-gauge needle tip or a no. 11 blade. Once the milia are unroofed and the small sebaceous pellets expressed, they rarely recur.

Dehiscence

Dehiscence, or wound separation, rarely occurs while sutures are in place unless there is excess tension on the wound edges. More commonly, separation is due to mild direct trauma after sutures are removed. When sutures are removed early, patients (or parents of young children) should be informed that the wound is not fully healed and should be protected for another 5–7 days. Often reinforcing Steri-strips are placed on the wound to protect it once sutures have been removed.

References

1. Rudolph R, Fisher JC, Ninnemann JL: *Skin Grafting*. Boston, Little, Brown & Co, 1979, pp 1–2, 19–26, 115–127.
2. Rudolph R: Wide spread scars, hypertrophic scars, and keloids. *Clin Plast Surg* 14:253, 1987.
3. Crikelair GF, Cosman B: Facial scars in Puerto Rican females. *Plast Reconstr Surg* 33:556, 1964.
4. Borges AF: Revision of linear scars. In Goldwyn RM (ed): *The Unfavorable Result in Plastic Surgery*. Boston, Little, Brown & Co, 1972, pp 97–114.
5. Wray RC: Force required for wound closure and scar appearance. *Plast Reconstr Surg* 72:380, 1983.
6. Elliott D, Mahaffey PJ: The stretched scar: The benefit of prolonged dermal support. *Br J Plast Surg* 42:74, 1989.
7. Taube M, Porter RJ, Lord PH: A combination of subcuticular suture and sterile micropore tape compared with conventional interrupted sutures for skin closure. *Ann R Coll Surg Engl* 65:165, 1983.
8. McGregor IA: *Fundamental Techniques of Plastic Surgery*, 3rd ed. London, Churchill Livingstone, 1965, pp 3–52.

17

Cutaneous Carcinomas

Suzanne M. Olbricht, M.D. and Joel M. Noe, M.D., F.A.C.S.

Basal Cell Carcinoma

More than 500,000 new cases of skin carcinomas are identified in the United States per year, an increase of 15–20% over the previous decade. Basal cell carcinomas (BCCs) constitute 65–80% of these cases (1). Local skin cancer detection programs identify presumptive BCC in as many as 28% of participants (2).

The BCC is thought to arise from a pluripotential cell residing in the basal layer of the epidermis or appendageal epithelium (3). Although it has been reported from any cutaneous surface (4), 85% are found on the head or neck areas. The tumor has a variety of biological behaviors. Usually it is a stable, slowly growing lesion present for years. Rapid and destructive growth ("aggressive" tumors) may occur infrequently. Massive silent penetration along deep tissue planes or along nerves is rarely reported (5). Metastasis is quite rare. According to the best figures available (Australia), the risk of metastasis is 0.025% (6).

What induces growth and dictates the behavior of BCC is unknown. That sunlight has a major role is undisputed, but the exact mechanism remains undefined. Chronic cumulative sun exposure, as estimated by the age of the patient and the vocational and recreational exposure history, and complexion (fair, poor tanning ability) are prominent factors (7, 8). Markers for sun-damaged skin, including actinic keratoses, elastosis, localized pigmentary disorders, senile lentigines, freckles, spider nevi, telangiectasia, dry skin, wrinkled skin, and arcus senilis, also define a population at greater risk for BCC than those without evidence of sun damage (11.3% vs. 1.0% in men 65 to 74 years old) (9). Therapeutic, diagnostic, or accidental exposure to radiation has led to the development of BCC. Latent periods as short as 7 years (10) have been reported, but the average is 20–25 years (11, 12). Long-term PUVA therapy (psoralens and ultraviolet-A radiation), used in the treatment of chronic skin diseases such as psoriasis, increases the risk of BCC in a dose-dependent fashion (13). Although rare now, chronic arsenical intoxication from medicaments (14) or well water (15) predisposes to development of tumors. Immunosuppressed patients, including those with acquired immunodeficiency syndrome (16), have both increased incidence and increased metastatic rate of cutaneous tumors (17–19). Miscellaneous predisposing lesions include old burn scars (20), tattoos (21), vaccination scars (22), chronic ulcers and sinuses (23–25), dermatofibromas (26), epider-

mal nevi (27, 28), nevus sebaceous of Jadassohn (29), and areas of trauma (30). The risk of a second cutaneous carcinoma, either BCC or squamous cell carcinoma, is reported to be 20% within 18 months in one study (31), as high as 30% within 2 years in an Anglo-Saxon ethnic group in New York state (32), and 36% within 5 years in a third study (33). BCC may be diagnosed in unexpected patients, such as those less than 29 years old (29) or black individuals (34, 35).

Physical examination readily identifies the BCC in most patients (36). Four primary gross morphologies exist. The most common BCC on the face is a slightly translucent, waxy or pearly papule or nodule with surrounding and overlying telangiectasia and an easily defined border (Fig. 17.1). The superficial (often misnamed "multicentric") BCC, typically present on the back, is an erythematous, telangiectatic, well-demarcated macule with a fine scale (Fig. 17.2). A primary sclerosing BCC (also called a morpheaform or an infiltrating BCC) is relatively rare and appears as an ill-defined flat or hypopigmented or yellowish indurated plaque, sometimes with overlying telangiectasia (Fig. 17.3). On occasion, a BCC may be fibroma-like (fibroepithelioma of Pinkus), presenting as a moderately firm, often slightly pedunculated soft nodule with a smooth, pink surface. Secondary changes may include ulceration, crusting, scaling, pigmentation, erythema, cystic collection, and scarring. A rodent ulcer is a BCC with prominent ulceration and inapparent tumor mass, commonly present around fusion planes of the nose and cheek. Cystic BCC may yield extrusion of mucinous material on puncture. A pigmented BCC mimics a malignant melanoma. A field-fire BCC is a lesion in which the center resolves with scarring and loss of appendages while tumor is found at the edge.

The differential diagnosis of a BCC includes a host of benign tumors (usually nevocellular or appendageal in origin), actinic keratoses, squamous cell carcinomas, malignant melanoma, and rarely an inflammatory condition (e.g., acneiform papule) or traumatic event (e.g., excoriation or shaving cut). Most important to consider is the diagnosis of malignant melanoma; a pigmented BCC (Fig. 17.4) may obviously suggest a malignant melanoma, but an amelanotic melanoma may be difficult to diagnose clinically. Documentation of the presence of a BCC is by pathological examination. The lesion may be sampled by curettage, shave biopsy, punch biopsy (a 2-mm disposable Keyes punch is sufficient), an incisional biopsy, or excision in toto. Curettage yields fragments of disori-

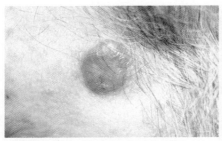

FIGURE 17.1.   Nodular basal cell carcinoma.

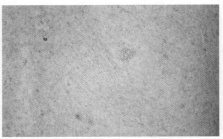

FIGURE 17.2.   Superficial basal cell carcinoma.

FIGURE 17.3.   Morpheaform basal cell carcinoma.

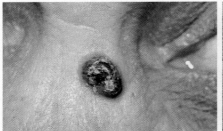

FIGURE 17.4.   Pigmented basal cell carcinoma.

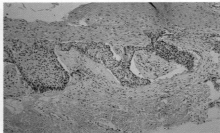

FIGURE 17.5.   Basal cell carcinoma, histology, tumor mass. (Courtesy of Dr. Terence J. Harrist.)

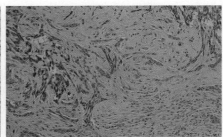

FIGURE 17.6.   Basal cell carcinoma, histology, fibrosis. (Courtesy of Dr. Terence J. Harrist.)

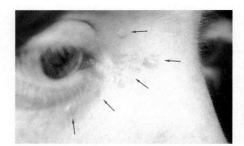

FIGURE 17.7.   Basal cell nevus syndrome.

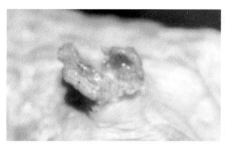

FIGURE 17.9.   Cutaneous horn.

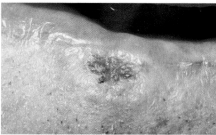

FIGURE 17.10.   Squamous cell carcinoma of lower lip. (Courtesy of Dr. Jessica L. Fewkes.)

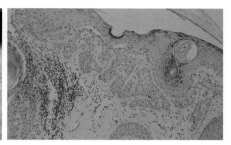

FIGURE 17.12.   Actinic keratosis, histology. (Courtesy of Dr. Terence J. Harrist.)

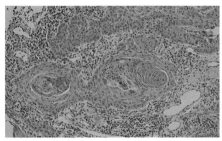

FIGURE 17.13.   Squamous cell carcinoma, histology. (Courtesy of Dr. Terence J. Harrist.)

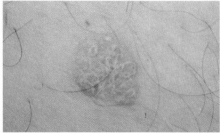

FIGURE 17.14.   Bowen's disease.

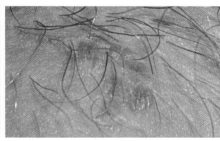

FIGURE 17.15.   Bowenoid papulosis.

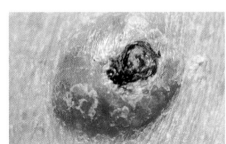

FIGURE 17.16.   Keratoacanthoma.

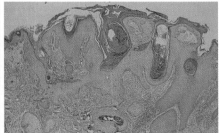

FIGURE 17.17.   Keratoacanthoma, histology. (Courtesy of Dr. Terence J. Harrist.)

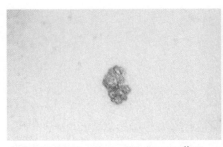

FIGURE 17.18. Superficial spreading melanoma.

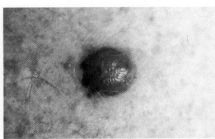

FIGURE 17.19. Nodular melanoma.

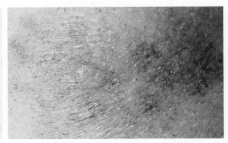

FIGURE 17.20. Lentigo maligna melanoma. (Courtesy of Dr. Jessica L. Fewkes.)

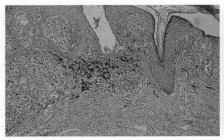

FIGURE 17.21. Superficial spreading melanoma, histology. (Courtesy of Dr. Terence J. Harrist.)

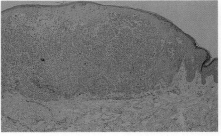

FIGURE 17.22. Nodular melanoma, histology. (Courtesy of Dr. Terence J. Harrist.)

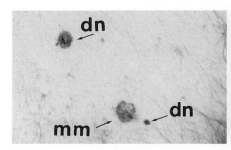

FIGURE 17.23. Small congenital nevus.

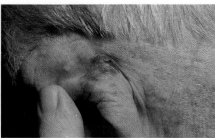

FIGURE 17.24. Dysplastic nevus.

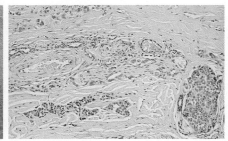

FIGURE 17.25. Lentigo maligna.

FIGURE 17.26. Microscopic satellites. (Courtesy of Dr. Terence J. Harrist.)

ented tissue that are adequate only for documenting a BCC and not for excluding other tumors or disease processes. Shave biopsy is easy to perform, and the site heals well. In addition, the specimen generally contains enough material to enable the pathologist to diagnose an alternative process. If melanoma is being considered in the differential diagnosis, only a punch biopsy of at least 4 mm in diameter or an incisional or excisional biopsy will obtain a specimen appropriate for evaluation.

Microscopic evidence of BCC in an adequately obtained specimen (37) includes cytologically atypical cells with darkly staining, large, oval, elongated nuclei and little cytoplasm collected in masses of various sizes with palisading of the cells at the periphery of the masses and retraction artifact about the masses (Fig. 17.5). Stromal changes include mucin deposition and fibrosis (Fig. 17.6). A cystic BCC will contain large masses of mucin, while fibrosis may be so striking in a morpheaform BCC that the tumor cells are difficult to detect. The tumor may differentiate toward hair structures, sebaceous glands, aprocrine glands, or eccrine glands. Trichoepithelioma, both typical and desmoplastic, may be difficult to differentiate pathologically and should be considered in the histopathological differential diagnosis of a presumed BCC in any young or unusual patient (31).

Three hereditary syndromes of multiple BCC are currently recognized. The basal cell nevus syndrome (38–40) is inherited in an autosomal dominant fashion, although the expression in affected family members may be dissimilar. The cutaneous manifestations include multiple BCC (Fig. 17.7), palmar pits, extreme sensitivity to radiation, and a short latency period of 4–5 years to the onset of numerous tumors (41). Hundreds of BCCs with disastrous consequences can be seen in these patients (42). Jaw cysts, which pathologically are odontogenic keratocysts, are common and usually asymptomatic. Bony abnormalities may include hypertelorism, calcification of the falx cerebri, spina bifida, and bifid ribs. Other hamartomas reported in association are ovarian fibromas with rare malignant degeneration, cardiac fibromas, milia, epidermal cysts, mesenteric cysts, gastric polyps, and tumors such as medulloblastomas, meningiomas, and fatal rhabdomyomas.

The Basex syndrome (43) has rarely been documented in the United States. The inheritance pattern is disputed; both autosomal dominant and *X*-linked dominant genetic transmission have been reported. There is a triad of cutaneous findings: multiple BCC developing between the ages of 15 and 25 years, follicular atrophoderma on the dorsal hands and elbows, and localized areas of anhidrosis. Some patients will also manifest hypotrichosis.

Finally, xeroderma pigmentosum (44) has six known genetic forms, all with autosomal recessive transmission. Biochemical defects in excision repair of ultraviolet (UV) light-induced pyrimidine dimers in DNA or in synthesis of DNA after UV irradiation have been identified. Clinically, the patients manifest acute photosensitivity, photophobia and conjunctivitis, and multiple cutaneous neoplasms, usually before age 10 and often with horrifying results. Some forms also involve microcephaly, progressive mental deterioration, and sensorineural deficits.

Treatment of BCC is primarily surgical and destructive and, in most cases, curative (i.e., no recurrence). Optimal therapy for a primary lesion may depend on multiple factors, including size and location of the tumor, possibility of invasion of vital structures, age and general health of the patient, and the patient's cosmetic concerns. Possible modalities include surgical excision, cryotherapy, electrodesiccation and curettage, radiation, laser surgery, topical application of 5-fluorouracil (5-FU), and Mohs' micrographic surgery.

Of special note is the consideration of adequate margins in planning therapy. In one study of 101 consecutive tumors less than 2 cm in diameter (45), gross margins (marked by electrodesiccation before excision) compared with the histological margins showed concordance within 1 mm in 94% of tumors and within 2 mm in 95%. A later study of 117 cases of untreated, well-demarcated BCC less than 2 cm in diameter determined that a minimum margin of 4 mm was necessary to eradicate the tumor totally in more than 95% of cases (46). Sclerosing BCC present a special problem; a much greater discrepancy was noted in the first study, corroborated by a report (47) in which a staged progressive surgical procedure documented subclinical extension of 7.2 mm ± 3% in 51 biopsy-proven primary morpheaform BCC.

Surgical excision is often the treatment of choice. The recurrence rate after primary excision is 5–6% (48). BCC is most likely to recur if the lesion is greater than 2 cm in diameter, morpheaform (sclerosing), or located in areas of embryonal fusion planes (nasolabial folds, nose-cheek angle, posterior ear sulcus, canal of the ear, periorbital area, and scalp) (49). Only 35% of BCC histologically present at the margin of the surgical specimen recur (50), and recurrence is more common when both lateral and deep margins are involved (51). The decision to reexcise the area of a pathologically diagnosed inadequate excision should be based on the likelihood of recurrence, the location of the original tumor in a cosmetically important area or in an area where recurrence might compromise a vital structure, and either the ability to closely follow a patient or the patient's reliability in examining his or her surgical site.

Standard surgical technique and repair apply to the excision of a BCC. The tumor is outlined with a marking pen prior to the instillation of local anesthesia because resulting vasoconstriction and edema may obscure the edge of the tumor. Finding the tumor edge may also be facilitated by curettage because the mucinous stroma surrounding a BCC allows for easy separation of the diseased tissue from normal skin. A margin appropriate to the type of tumor and anatomical location is then marked around the tumor, and an elliptical excision encompassing the tumor and margin is planned so that the repaired linear wound follows relaxed skin tension lines or hides in a normal wrinkle or anatomical structure. With tension applied to the surgical site, a scalpel is used to incise the planned ellipse perpendicular to the skin surface deep to upper subcutaneous fat. The ellipse is removed with the aid of a curved scissors. Undermining in the upper subcutaneous fat beneath the subepidermal plexus facilitates closure of the wound by standard technique with sutures or staples. The specimen is sent to pathology. Placing a stitch in the most superior position (i.e., 12 o'clock) with a notation on the pathology requisition as well as on the operative report facilitates correlation with the resulting scar should one of the margins be reported as positive. Large defects may require repair with skin grafts or flaps and may be aided by techniques such as tissue expansion. Healing by secondary intention is also acceptable in some wounds. The treatment of difficult or high-risk BCC should be dealt with in two stages: first, removal of the entire tumor with adequate surgical margins, and second, construction of a plan for wound reconstruction (52, 53). Minor modifications in surgical procedures for cosmetic considerations may have devastating consequences for recurrence, requiring secondary procedures or even limiting patient survival.

Alternatives to excision include therapies that deliver a lethal physical insult to tissue within the area to be treated (field destructive techniques). Because these modalities destroy the tumor, biopsy confirmation before treatment is essential. In addition, no specimen will be obtained for histological examination of the surgical margins. Some physicians frequently employ cryotherapy, which is performed with local anesthesia. Liquid nitrogen ($-196°C$) is delivered to the site via spray from a commercially available handheld instrument consisting of a reservoir and an arm with an aperture that can be varied in size (e.g., Kryospray Unit). The field (tumor and margins) is sprayed to complete freezing ($-40°C$ to $-60°C$) of the tissue several millimeters deep, measured either by thermocouple-tipped needles placed in the tumor (54) or by standardized timing of the freeze and thaw cycle (55). The site is usually sprayed and frozen for 30 sec and then allowed to thaw. The best results occur with a thaw time more than 90 sec for each of the two freeze-thaw cycles. The result of cryotherapy is a local frostbite reaction: swelling, pain, and bulla formation for 1–2 days, then an ulcer covered by a crust that separates in 2–6 weeks. Erythema at the site may persist for months. The mature scar, cosmetically acceptable to selected patients in some locations, is hypopigmented, flat or somewhat depressed, and sclerotic. It softens and elevates with time but never regains normal aging lines or skin folds. Complications are few; there may be temporary massive local edema, permanent alopecia, or rare temporary paralysis of the facial nerve if it underlies the treated site (56). The eyelid may be treated if the orbit is protected. The cartilaginous portions of the nose and ear are well preserved unless invaded by the tumor. The recurrence rate is 2–6% in skilled hands (55, 57, 58). Large lesions (greater than 2 cm in diameter) are difficult to treat in this manner and may require division into multiple smaller treatment areas. Difficult tumors such as morpheaform BCC or tumors in sites of developmental fusion planes, as well as any tumors associated with factors likely to lead to recurrence, are usually best treated by excision rather than destruction.

Another common method used for field destruction is curettage and electrodesiccation (59). Under local anesthesia, a curette is used to remove the tumor mass. This procedure is facilitated by the mucinous stroma of BCC,

which easily separates from normal tissue. The material obtained on the first curettage may be sent for pathological evaluation. Heat via electrodesiccation is used to destroy a 1–2-mm rim of tissue in and about the defect. Generally, the eschar is then curetted, and a second 1–2-mm rim of tissue is electrodessicated. Healing is by secondary intention over a 2–6-week period and results in a flat, hypopigmented scar, often with a hypertrophic center. The recurrence rate is 6–10% (60). In a study of BCC in which the lesion was treated first by curettage and electrodesiccation repeated three times in rapid succession and the wound was then excised by shave, residual tumor was found in 8.3% of lesions treated on the trunk and extremities and 46.6% of lesions of the face (61). It may therefore be best to reserve this treatment for tumors of the trunk and extremities.

Curative superficial radiotherapy may be delivered to the field encompassing the tumor and its margins in one to three visits, resulting in acute radiation dermatitis and healing over 4–6 weeks. The result is a hypopigmented, atrophic, telangiectatic scar that tends to worsen cosmetically with time. Because of the high risk of radiation-induced secondary cutaneous carcinoma (average lag time of 15 years) and worsening appearance of the scar, this method of treatment is inadvisable for patients less than 60 years old. Some authors feel that it is an excellent therapy for eyelid lesions (62). In general, the reported recurrence rate is 5–11% (63).

New laser technology provides yet other techniques for field destruction. In one series (64), 42 patients had BCC and its margin vaporized by the carbon dioxide laser with a defocused beam. The surgeons described excellent cosmetic results. Recurrence rate is unknown because only a 6-month follow-up was reported. The neodymium : YAG laser may also prove useful for field destruction (65). Laser light (argon, dye, or heavy metal lasers) has also been used to treat lesions made photosensitive by hematoporphyrin derivative (HPD) administered systematically or by local injection. This technique, called photodynamic therapy (PDT), has been used only for a small number of patients (66, 67) but may hold promise in the future for treatment of multiple, difficult, metastatic, or end-stage invasive lesions.

One useful chemotherapeutic agent is available for the treatment of BCC: 5-FU in a 5% cream is an antimetabolite used systematically in a variety of tumors. The cream may be applied twice a day to a BCC until an endpoint of redness, soreness, and swelling (about 3 weeks for the face, 6 weeks for the legs). The lesion may ulcerate toward the end of the treatment course. Healing time is generally 3–6 weeks and results in a slightly hypopigmented, soft, flat macule, Surrounding normal skin tends to be spared. The recurrence rate is estimated to be 20–50% and is highest for lesions with nodularity or deep foci (68, 69). Better results were obtained in patients in whom curettage of the lesion was performed immediately before chemotherapy was instituted (70). Chemotherapy with 5-FU is therefore primarily indicated for the patient with multiple, superficial lesions, such as superficial spreading BCC of the back, and who may not be a candidate for treatment by another modality. Close follow-up is recommended. In addition to 5-FU, it is possible that, in the future, retinoids may prove useful as primary or adjunctive therapy. Systemic isotretinoin and etretinate and topical tretinoin have been used to treat BCC but have a response rate of 30–40% and a significant incidence of troublesome adverse effects (71–73).

Recurrent BCC may be difficult to treat. Dealing with this problem, Frederick Mohs in 1936 developed a staged procedure (74) in which he removed small amounts of accurately mapped tissue under local anesthesia after fixing the skin in vivo with zinc chloride. He then immediately microscopically examined the inferior margin by horizontal section of tumor and reexcised as necessary. He allowed these wounds to heal by secondary intention.

As practiced today, Mohs' microscopically controlled surgery (75, 76) is a fresh-tissue technique. Under local anesthesia, the tumor is assessed and debulked by curettage. The defect is then excised by saucerization of 1–2 mm of tissue. Hemostasis is accomplished by electrodesiccation or a styptic (usually ferric subsulfate solution). Saucerized tissue is mapped, frozen, and cut in horizontal sections. The entire undersurface of the lateral and inferior margin is systematically reviewed for the presence of tumor. This microscopic review differs from the usual vertical frozen sections of the pathologist and allows for evaluation of all the margins rather than a sampling. Repeat saucerizations are performed the same day until the margins are clear. The wound may be allowed to heal by secondary intention or closed immediately. Large defects may require major reconstructive procedures. The advantages of the Mohs' surgical procedure include maximal preservation of normal tissue and precise delineation of the track of the tumor. Indications for the procedure, therefore, are: (*a*) recurrent tumors (the recurrent rate for the use of other modalities to treat recurrent tumors is 20–50% versus 4–9% for Mohs' surgery) (75–77); (*b*) primary tumors known to have high recurrence rates as above; and (*c*) primary lesions in which maximal preservation of tissue is necessary, such as those involving the eyelid, nose, finger, genitalia, and areas around major facial nerves.

Persistent long-term follow-up care (78) of patients who have had a BCC is important. Visible recurrence at the site of a treated lesion may be delayed; 33% of recurrences are noted at 1 year, 50% at 2 years, but only 66% at 3 years (79). As discussed above, patients are, however, much more likely to develop a second primary than a recurrence of the originally treated lesion; therefore, their entire cutaneous surface should be examined every 6–12 months. Particular attention should be paid to sun-exposed surfaces, sites previously treated with radiotherapy, and areas difficult for the patient to examine. Patients with special risks such as immunosuppression or hereditary disease may need reexamination even more frequently. As noted above, the risk of a second primary is 36% within 5 years. Most importantly, patients need instruction concerning risky behavior *apropos* the sun because cumulative sun exposure is the most common and only preventable inciting factor. The Skin Cancer Foundation (Box 561, Dept. SR, New York, NY 10156) supplies information pamphlets that advise patients to

minimize sun exposure from 10:00 AM to 2:00 PM (11:00 AM to 3:00 PM Daylight Savings Time); to wear a wide-brimmed hat, long-sleeved shirt, and long pants when outside; and to apply a sunscreen with a sun protection factor (SPF) of 15 or more before any exposure to the sun and at least every 2 hr as long as the outdoor activity is continued. It is unclear that sunscreens with SPFs of 20 or 30 are more useful than those with an SPF of 15. Water-repellent or water-resistant sunscreens are especially helpful during sweaty or wet outdoor activities. Significant sun exposure occurs even with brief exposures on overcast days (such as a 30-min outdoor lunch at work). In addition, exposure to artificial sources of ultraviolet radiation, including tanning parlors, should be strictly avoided.

All children, outdoor workers, or fair-skinned individuals who have a tendency to burn should follow these guidelines. It has been calculated that the regular use of a sunscreen with an SPF of 15 for the first 18 years of life would reduce the lifetime incidence of BCC and squamous cell carcinoma by 78% (80). It is generally thought that decreasing sun exposure, even after the first skin cancer has been noted, will decrease the number of new primary cancers diagnosed. Certainly, the use of sunscreen prevents tumor production in animal models (81). Preventative actions will become universally mandatory because the trend toward ozone depletion will give rise to greater intensity of ultraviolet radiation at the earth's surface (82). No adequate or generally useful chemopreventative agent has yet been developed. Oral isotretinoin may prevent carcinomas in some patients with overwhelming risk factors such as arsenic exposure, xeroderma pigmentosum, or the basal cell nevus syndrome, but it also has numerous adverse effects (72, 83). Sparse data exist for etretinate, another oral retinoid (73), and there are no in vivo data in humans substantiating the theoretical chemopreventative properties of tretinoin, a topical retinoid. On the contrary, in one study (84), mice treated with tretinoin and receiving ultraviolet radiation developed more tumors than mice treated with ultraviolet radiation alone. This result is controversial; however, patients using tretinoin to treat photoaging need to be warned so that they can exercise appropriate care in avoiding sun exposure and in making follow-up appointments for examination.

Squamous Cell Carcinoma

Squamous cell carcinoma (SCC) is the second most common type of skin cancer; about 100,000 new cases are diagnosed in the United States each year. It may occur anywhere on the skin or mucuous membranes and arises from atypical epidermal keratinocytes. Rarely occurring in normal skin, it usually appears on sun-damaged skin or in actinic keratoses as a rapidly growing lesion. Up to 14% of older or quickly growing lesions may invade deeply, even extending along nerves (85, 86). The rate of metastasis is debated. Lund (87, 88) estimated that less than 0.1% of SCCs arising in sun-damaged skin metastasize; however, two other studies (89, 90) suggest a metastatic rate of 2–3%. Large lesions of the ear, forehead, temple, and dorsa of the hands have a much greater metastatic rate, calculated to be 10–36% in a group of patients referred for Mohs' micrographic surgery (91). Lip lesions may metastasize at a rate of 11–20% (91–93).

Conditions predisposing to BCC (radiation, arsenic, immunosuppression) also predispose to the development of SCC. In particular, the direct relationship to sun exposure and actinically damaged skin is even more striking. Individuals older than age 50 have a lower BCC:SCC ratio than younger individuals, probably because of greater cumulative sun exposure (94). Using mannequin heads and a chemical system of dosimetry for UV light measurement, Urbach (93) established that the highest incidences of SCC on the head and neck were in the areas of greatest sun exposure. UV-B light has been more strongly implicated, but UV-A probably also plays a role (95). Certainly, patients receiving PUVA therapy develop SCC in a dose-dependent relationship (13, 96) within 5 years. The risk of SCC in immunosuppressed patients is 18 times that of the general population (for BCC, three times) (17). It also correlates with sun exposure and evidence of photodamage (97). Multiple mechanisms have been proposed, including faulty DNA repair after UV light exposure (98), induction of carcinogens from sterols in the skin (99), hyperplasia-inducing factors (100), and immunological alterations (101). Viral infection, particularly with specific subtypes of human papillomavirus, has also been incriminated (102).

Actinic keratoses may be premalignant lesions. One study (103) suggests that 20–25% of patients with actinic keratoses will develop at least one SCC; whether the actinic keratoses mark patients with extensive sun exposure or the actinic keratoses themselves progress is unclear. In a long-term large prospective follow-up study (104), 60% of SCCs arose from lesions previously clinically diagnosed as actinic keratoses, and 40% arose on previously normal skin. The risk of malignant transformation of a solar keratosis to SCC within 1 year was calculated to be less than 1:1,000.

An SCC produced by chronic scarring processes may act more aggressively than an SCC that develops in actinically damaged skin; the metastatic rate for the former is 20–30% (11, 105–108). Such chronic scarring processes include draining sinuses (108), pilonidal sinuses (109), thermally injured skin (106, 110), lichen sclerosus et atrophicus (111), discoid lupus erythematosus (112), porokeratosis of Mibelli (113), and dystrophic epidermolysis bullosa (114). Repeated abrasion gives rise to SCC in an animal model (115), theoretically on the basis of inducing a constantly proliferating epidermal unit. In addition, occupational exposure to tars and polycyclic aromatic hydrocarbons has long been known to predispose to the development of SCC (116).

The primary clinical appearance of SCC is a poorly defined firm nodule, flesh colored to red, with a hyperkeratotic crust (Fig. 17.8). The lesion may ulcerate as it grows. Production of large amounts of compacted parakeratosis may mimic a wart or a so-called cutaneous "horn" (Fig. 17.9). Lesions of the lower lip may be difficult to diagnose both clinically and histologically (117),

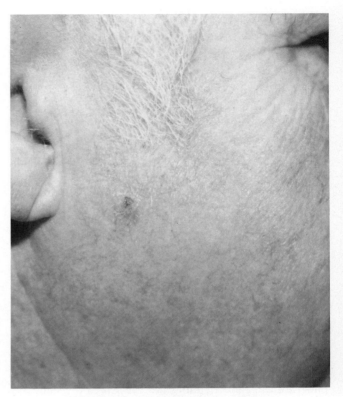

FIGURE 17.8. Squamous cell carcinoma.

appearing as a nonhealing sore, a white plaque (Fig. 17.10), or a rapidly growing inflammatory nodule. The differential diagnosis of SCC includes actinic keratosis, especially the hypertrophic variety, commonly on the dorsum of the hand (Fig. 17.11), and keratoacanthoma. Sometimes it may be difficult to distinguish SCC from BCC, an irritated seborrheic keratosis, or a wart. Pathological examination is again essential for documentation of the exact tumor type. Clinical and histological differences (118) between SCC and actinic keratosis are quantitative rather than qualitative. In an actinic keratosis,

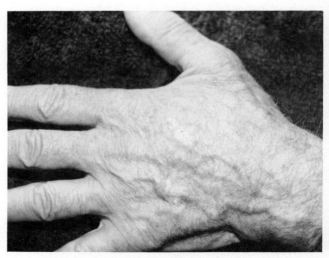

FIGURE 17.11. Hypertrophic actinic keratosis.

atypical keratinocytes proliferate in the lower epidermis in buds that usually grow downward (Fig. 17.12). The upper epidermal cells may be normal, however, indicating the retained ability of the cells to mature. Invasive SCC occurs when the atypical cells invade the dermis in tumor masses, which may contain keratin pearls (Fig. 17.13). It is generally accepted that the changes are progressive with time (119).

Several variants of SCC are recognized. SCC in situ, arising in an actinic keratosis, is a histological variant (120), clinically appearing as a poorly demarcated inflammatory scaling papule or plaque in the midst of marked actinic damage. Bowen's disease (Fig. 17.14), a single lesion of intraepidermal SCC, is clinically manifested as a well-demarcated macule or slightly indurated plaque with a sharp but irregular outline, often with gray-brown hyperpigmentation and fine superficial scaling (121). Although difficult to distinguish from superficial BCC, it generally is more inflammatory (i.e., erythematous) and less telangiectatic. By definition, it does not arise from an obvious preexisting lesion or from skin with actinic damage. With time, the lesion extends peripherally and may tend to clear centrally. It may spread down hair follicles and occasionally develop invasive foci. The older literature states that patients with this lesion have a high incidence of internal malignancy. A recent Danish study (122) reported no relationship; however, a U.S. study (123) found a 29% incidence of internal malignancy in patients with Bowen's disease, an incidence assumed to be higher than that of other patients without Bowen's disease. This latter conclusion may be substantiated by the recent description of 12 patients with perianal Bowen's disease, seven of whom had or developed other malignancy (124). Recently 50 patients with Bowen's disease were compared to 50 patients with BCC and another 50 patients with other dermatoses. No significant increase in internal malignancy was found (125). This was also corroborated by another large retrospective study (126). The controversy continues (127, 128).

Bowenoid papulosis is the name used for single or multiple genital and verrucous papules (Fig. 17.15) that are resistant to therapy and have atypia reminiscent of Bowen's disease on histological examination. The significance of these lesions is unclear (129–131), but it is probable that they are viral induced and have significant malignant potential. Specific subtypes of human papillomavirus (the "wart" virus), usually type 16, are isolated from both invasive cervical cancer and Bowenoid papulosis (132). Erythroplasia of Queyrat (133) signifies an asymptomatic, sharply demarcated, bright red, shiny, slightly indurated plaque on the glans penis with the histological picture of SCC in situ. It develops almost exclusively in uncircumcised men. Progression into invasive SCC has been observed in up to 30% of patients (134) with metastases in up to 20% (135). Carcinoma cuniculatum (136), or verrucous carcinoma, is a warty, slowly growing plaque that develops on the feet. It has no cytological atypia on histological section and may be difficult to diagnose without a deep biopsy to identify the characteristic, broad, invading tumor masses at the base of the lesion (118). Metastases have been reported (137).

The nosology of keratoacanthoma remains controversial. Clinically, it is a well-demarcated nodule with rolled firm borders and a central cup filled with keratinaceous debris (Fig. 17.16). Typically, it grows large quite rapidly, stabilizes over a few months, and then regresses, usually with scarring. The hallmarks of the histological diagnosis (118; Fig. 17.17) include typical architecture (cup-shaped acanthosis), glassy and mildly atypical keratinocytes pushing into the dermis in strands that may even invade perineural space (138), a pronounced inflammatory infiltrate, horn pearls, intraepithelial abscesses, and elimination of elastic tissue in the epithelial tongues. Because architecture and the lack of marked atypia at the base of the lesion are keys to the diagnosis, biopsy should be done either as an excision in toto or as a central wedge incision (139). Available evidence suggests that clinically and histologically, it is difficult to differentiate between a keratoacanthoma and SCC (140), although immunoperoxidase markers may prove useful (141). Some authors advise full excision in each case (142, 143), whereas others (144, 145) will consider careful observation and conservative therapy for selected classic lesions. Data suggest that the daily application of 5-FU topically (146) or the weekly intralesional injection of 5-FU (147) may be effective over a 3-week period and thus avert a surgical or destructive procedure. Multiple keratoacanthomas have been related to internal malignancies (148), photochemotherapy for psoriasis (149), and chronic sun exposure (150).

Hereditary syndromes associated with an increased incidence of SCC are rare. Xeroderma pigmentosum (see above) may develop widely destructive SCC. Epidermodysplasia verruciformis (151) is a rare autosomal recessive disorder in which several subtypes of human papillomavirus induce widespread, polymorphic, and verrucous lesions, beginning in childhood. The warts may develop carcinomatous changes within 2 years of onset. Metastases from SCC and death have been reported. The genetic defect is probably in cell-mediated immunity (152, 153), but the precise delineation has not been made. Interferon may be useful in the treatment of the disorder (154). Muir-Torre syndrome (155, 156) is a recently described, possibly autosomally dominant disorder that is manifested by multiple internal malignancies, cutaneous sebaceous proliferation (adenomas and carcinomas), and keratoacanthomas.

Treatment of SCC follows the same guidelines as discussed for BCC. The primary modalities of therapy are surgical or destructive, and the procedures performed are generally identical to those used in the treatment of BCC. Surgical margins are also chosen similarly. Most data regarding success of therapy for BCC (as detailed above) include small numbers of SCC with similar results, excluding mucous membrane lesions and lesions already metastatic. Factors predisposing to recurrence (157) include size greater than 1 cm in diameter, poorly differentiated cytological features, and histological invasion into deep dermis or fat. Of note is the success of Mohs' surgery in difficult cases (158), with a recurrence rate of 3.3% on the head and neck and 12.5% on the lower extremity in 414 patients. Advanced and multiple SCC have been treated in small numbers with oral isotretinoin, helpful in 11 of 15 reported cases (159, 160).

As with patients who have BCC, much morbidity from actinic damage may be preventable. Patients should be educated about the role of chronic cumulative sun damage in the formation of SCC and be encouraged in the daily use of sunscreen and hats. Individual actinic keratoses can be treated with light cryotherapy (liquid nitrogen applied with a cotton swab for a total freeze and thaw time of 15–30 sec) for cosmetic control of the lesions. Topically applied 5-FU over large areas of exposed skin, dermabrasion, or chemical peeling (161) may eradicate premalignant lesions and maximize time to the development of new lesions. Repeated follow-up examinations of the patient's entire cutaneous surface are also warranted on a long-term basis.

Malignant Melanoma

Malignant melanoma, a neoplasm of neural crest–derived cells that have differentiated toward melanocytes, is a common and sometimes lethal cutaneous tumor. In 1989 (162), an estimated 27,000 melanomas were diagnosed in the United States, resulting in 6,000 deaths. It was the second greatest killer among cancers of males age 15–34 and accounted for 1% of all deaths from cancer. In countries populated by fair-skinned whites, its incidence and mortality rate have risen rapidly (7–15% per year), and more than doubled over the past decade (163–166). Current age-adjusted annual incidence rates per 100,000 population in the United States range from 12 in non-Hispanic whites in New Mexico (167) and 14 in Hawaii (168) to 5.8 in Connecticut (169). One in 250 Americans will have a melanoma diagnosed in his or her lifetime (170). In spite of this grim forecast, the 5-year survival rate has improved from 60% in 1960–1963 to 80% in 1979–1984 (162), probably because of earlier detection and improved diagnostic accuracy. A public education campaign in Scotland was documented to produce a statistically significant rise in the diagnosis of thin melanomas with a good prognosis and a comcomitant fall in the proportion of thick lesions (171). Physicians are also alerted to the need for a complete skin examination, which may detect 6.4 times more melanomas than partial examinations (172).

Like other skin cancers, melanomas have been reported in the setting of immunosuppression (173, 174), xeroderma pigmentosum (175), and chronic scarring lesions (24). It is generally thought that exposure to solar radiation is related to the development of the majority of melanomas based on a series of epidemiological and clinical observations (176). First, the incidence in whites varies inversely with latitude. Second, a large Canadian study (164) that compared patients with melanoma and age-, sex-, and province-matched controls identified blond hair, light color, unexposed skin, and severe freckling to be significant risk factors for melanoma. Another large case control study found a fourfold increase in risk of melanoma of all types when basal cell carcinomas, squamous cell carcinomas, and actinic keratoses were present on the face (177). Furthermore, non-Hispanic whites in New Mexico have six times more melanomas than Hispanics, American Indians, and blacks (167). Melanomas also tend to occur on sites exposed to the sun during recreation (e.g., trunks of men and lower extremities of women). They occur much less frequently on sites covered by bathing suits. Interestingly, the risk of melanoma has been related to annual UV exposure rather than to the cumulative lifetime UV exposure that increases the risk of BCC and SCC. Office workers get more melanomas than outdoor workers. Significantly increased risk has been associated with severe sunburns before age 15, sunbathing, boating, and vacations spent in the sun (178). In Hawaii, where clothing tends to remain the same throughout the year while UV radiation varies with the seasons, 50% more melanomas are diagnosed in July and August than in January and February (179). In addition, the incidence of melanoma has been noted to increase excessively 2 years after peak sunspot activity. Even the incidence of intraocular melanoma has been correlated with sunlight exposure (180). Therefore, UV radiation may act as a short-term promoter of melanoma rather than a dose-dependent initiator as in nonmelanoma skin cancer.

Two major types of melanoma are recognized clinically: superficial spreading melanoma (Fig. 17.18) and nodular melanoma (Fig. 17.19). The former grows radially with or without a vertical growth phase, and the latter only grows vertically. Characteristics (181, 182) that differentiate early lesions from benign pigmented lesions include variegated color (red, white, and blue) or disarray of pigment (reticulated, clumped, and absent all in one lesion), irregular borders (angular indentation or notching), and an irregular surface (verrucous or mixed verrucous and smooth). Patients may complain of change in size or color even in early lesions, but elevation, bleeding, ulceration, tenderness, and itching are symptoms noted with deeply invasive lesions (183). Melanoma may present without pigmentation (amelanotic melanoma), resulting in great diagnostic difficulty. Late lesions, with the highest metastatic rates, have ulceration with or without nodules at the periphery of a plaque or a single nodule without a plaque (the larger the nodule, plaque, or ulcerations the higher the metastatic rate) (184). Loss of skin markings through the lesion also constitutes a late sign associated with deep invasion (185).

Other clinical types of melanoma are relatively less common. Lentigo maligna melanoma (Fig. 17.20) occurs in elderly patients and develops in actinically damaged skin, usually on the head and neck. Clinically, it is manifested by induration or blue-black nodules within a previously slow growing lentigo maligna. Acral lentiginous melanoma (186), the most common melanoma in blacks and other pigmented races, arises principally on the palms and soles. It may be difficult to differentiate from lentiginous nevi, but the same criteria of change in size, shape, color, and surface, and irregular borders apply (187). Desmoplastic melanoma, or its variant neurotropic melanoma, is difficult to diagnose both clinically and histologically. The lesion tends to be located on a sun-exposed site and presents as a poorly defined sclerotic mass only occasionally associated with abnormal pigmentation (188, 189). Of note, there is little evidence to suggest that the Spitz nevus (190), also called benign juvenile melanoma, belongs in this group of malignant lesions, despite its rapid growth over a period of months.

The differential diagnosis of malignant melanoma includes dysplastic nevi, pigmented BCC, seborrheic keratoses, blue nevi, dermatofibromas, pyogenic granulomas, venous lakes, and Kaposi's sarcoma. Excisional biopsies of small lesions or incisional biopsies of large lesions are recommended before definitive wide local excision because as many as 20% of patients diagnosed with melanoma by experienced clinicians may have benign lesions or nonmelanoma skin cancer (191). Biopsy of an even slightly suspicious tumor is highly recommended because these same physicians clinically suspected other types of tumors in 36% of the melanomas diagnosed pathologically. Incisional biopsy and/or use of local anesthesia has not been shown to disseminate tumor or worsen the patient's prognosis (192–194). However, total excision enables the pathologist to study the tumor in a stepwise fashion and improves diagnostic and prognostic accuracy, enabling the surgeon to plan more precisely a definitive therapy. Shave biopsy and curettage are not advised because they may not yield adequate material for diagnosis and will not allow measurement of the depth of penetration of the tumor.

Histologically (Harrist TJ, personal communication), malignant melanoma is composed of dyshesive, polymorphous, and atypical melanocytes of principally epithelioid and spindle-cell types that proliferate along the dermoepidermal junction and spread small nests or single cells (pagetoid array) into the upper epidermis (Fig. 17.21). By definition, nodular melanoma pushes into the dermis as a single tumor mass (Fig. 17.22) with lateral extension only in the epidermis less than three rete pegs from the nodule. In superficial spreading melanoma, the lateral spread is more extensive. Frequent mitoses, both typical and abnormal, may be present with or without lymphocytic infiltrate and fibrovascular response. Malignant melanoma in situ (i.e., lesions in which all atypical cells are confined to the epidermis) is thought to be biologically benign, and some pathologists prefer to use the term "severely atypical melanocytic hyperplasia" or "dysplastic nevus with severe atypia of the intraepithelial component." Borderline melanoma and minimal deviation melanoma are rare pathological diagnoses, and their biological behaviors have not yet been defined. The Spitz nevus may be difficult to distinguish from malignant melanoma histologically because it contains large typical spindle and epithelioid melanocytes and mitotic figures; an astute clinician may need to suggest the diagnosis to the pathologist in the appropriate setting. Spindle cell and desmoplastic melanomas may also be difficult for the pathologist to diagnose because of the relative lack of pigment within the lesion and the abundance of fibroblastic response. They are most commonly confused with spindle cell SCC.

Primary cutaneous malignant melanomas are reported to occur at the sites of preexisting pigmented lesions in 18–85% of cases clinically and 18–72% of cases histologically (195). Because 65% of white adults have at least one nevus, averaging 15 per person (196), much attention has recently been focused on the morphological characteristics of precursor lesions. The number of benign nevi over 2 mm in diameter is directly proportional to the risk of melanoma, although no direct site specificity has been seen (197, 198). Therefore, large numbers of nevi (100 or more) indicate a patient in a high-risk group for melanoma, although that melanoma does not arise directly from any of the nevi (199). In contrast, at least 6% of giant congenital nevi (nevocellular pigmented plaques greater than 10 cm in diameter) degenerate over a lifetime (200), and 50% of the resulting malignancies are said to develop before age three (201). These melanomas may be difficult to diagnose early because even benign areas of congenital nevi tend to have surface lobulation, dark coloration, and hamartomatous nodules. Small congenital nevi (Fig. 17.23) are defined as easily excisable lesions noted by the parents within the first 2 weeks of life. They occur in 1% of newborns (202). Their rate of degeneration is hotly debated but is generally agreed to be increased, perhaps by as much as 5% (203).

Another recognizable precursor of melanoma is the dysplastic nevus, which is generally acquired in adolescence and appears as a pigmented lesion, often greater than 5 mm in diameter. It has irregular or poorly demarcated borders, irregular or very dark coloration (shades of brown and red), and an irregular surface (Fig. 17.24) (204) and often occurs on sun-exposed sites in sun-sensitive individuals (205). The significance of these disorderly appearing nevi was first appreciated in the B-K mole syndrome (206), now called the familial dysplastic nevus syndrome. This is probably an autosomal dominant disorder in which individuals with dysplastic nevi and a family history of melanoma have a relative risk for cutaneous melanoma 148 times that of the general population, approaching 100%, while the risk in the same family of members without dysplastic nevi is not increased (207). Sporadic cases of melanoma are also related to dysplastic nevi (208, 209), and account for as many as 32% of all nonfamilial melanomas (210). The incidence of a single dysplastic nevus in any individual is about 4%, and its significance remains unclear. However, patients with multiple dysplastic nevi may have as much as a 7.7 times relative risk for melanoma (210) and need to be followed carefully, probably by sequential photographs that can document early invasive melanoma by facilitating recognition of subtle morphological changes within a dysplastic nevus (211). The vigilance with which one follows these high-risk patients cannot be relaxed: 10% of all melanoma patients develop second primary malignant melanomas (212), and histological confirmation of dysplasia or melanoma should be frequently employed. Just as dysplastic nevi vary clinically from slightly atypical to severely atypical, a range of atypicality is also appreciated histologically in the characteristics of the nevus cells (cytological atypia) as well as in their arrangement (architectural atypia). Clinicians and pathologists alike are concerned about lesions that are moderately to severely atypical.

Melanomas are not known to develop in other congenital and acquired pigmented lesions such as café au lait macules, mongolian spots, Becker's nevus, lentigines, and epidermal nevi. However, the lengtigo maligna (Hutchinson's freckle) is also considered premalignant. It is an irregularly pigmented and growing macule that occurs on the sun-exposed skin of elderly patients (Fig. 17.25). It is thought to give rise to frank invasive melanoma (lentigo maligna melanoma) in at least one third of cases (213). Progression is very slow, perhaps over 5–10 years.

The biological behavior of malignant melanoma in relation to the risk of recurrence and death is predictable (214, 215). Superficial spreading melanoma has a long period (months to years) of lateral spread (radial growth). Lentigo maligna melanoma may have a decade of radial growth. Acral lentiginous melanoma is thought to have a shorter period of radial growth before vertical growth. The malignancy at first remains localized to the skin (stage 1). It then spreads to regional lymph nodes (stage II) and/or metastasizes to distant sites (stage III), usually skin, brain, lungs, and liver. At the time of diagnosis of the initial primary cutaneous melanoma, staging can be adequately accomplished by a complete physical examination and a baseline chest radiograph; liver function tests, radionuclide liver-spleen and bone scans, whole-lung tomograms, computed tomography (CT) chest scans, and CT brain scans do not add additional information (216). Nearly all patients with stage III disease die within 3 years. Five-year survival in patients with clinical stage II disease is 30%, but 10-year survival is rare.

A combination of histological factors studied by multivariate analysis predicts survival for clinical stage I disease reproducibly. Of these factors, and regardless of tumor type or the presence of microscopic lymph node metastases (217), depth as measured histologically in millimeters from epidermal surface (epidermal granular layer) to deepest tumor margin (Breslow measurement) (218) is by far the most important. The second most important variable is location. Ear and scalp melanomas (219), acral lentiginous melanomas (214), and melanomas on genital or anorectal mucosa (220, 221) have an extremely grave prognosis unexplained by any microstage factors. Lesions on the upper back, posterolateral arms, posterolateral neck, and posterior scalp (BANS locations) may also have a relatively poorer prognosis (222). Other factors associated with unfavorable prognosis include ulceration, deeper level of invasion (Clark levels: II, focal papillary dermis; III, papillary dermis replacement; IV, reticular dermis; and V, subcutaneous fat), high mitotic rate, poor lymphocyte response, presence of microscopic satellites (223), and presence of microscopic metastases in greater than 20% of removed lymph nodes. Most clinicians overvalue the prognostic importance of Clark's levels of invasion; the prognostic information yielded is minimal if measured depth of invasion has already been included in the prognostic model. The presence of microscopic satellites (nests of tumor cells below the principal invasive mass of primary tumor) (Fig. 17.26) is the best predictor of clinically occult metastases in lymph nodes (224). The role of regression as a prognostic factor is debated (225, 226). In summary, the two most important and powerful factors in predicting the outcome in malignant melanoma are the measured depth of inva-

sion of the primary tumor and the location of the primary tumor (Table 17.1).

Surgical excision is the treatment of choice for clinical stage I melanoma; there is no role at present for treating the primary lesion with chemotherapy, radiation, or other destructive techniques. The issue of resection margins has been addressed recently in several studies. Several reports (220, 221, 227–231) have shown that the magnitude of surgical resection margins has no effect on survival, even for high-risk melanomas, although a higher incidence of local recurrences was noted when thicker lesions were excised with less than 3-cm margins. Previous standard surgical practice had dictated excision of most melanomas with a border of normal skin at least 3–5 cm from the edge of the melanoma, but the historical basis for this recommendation is unclear. Some authors (232–234) now suggest much narrower margins based on retrospective data: a 1.5-cm margin is used for all lesions less than 0.85 mm thick and lesions in the non-BANS locations 0.85–1.69 mm thick; all other melanomas are excised with a 3.0-cm radius. The National Institute of Health in Milan, Italy, in conjunction with five other countries, recently accomplished a randomized prospective study (235) of 612 patients with melanomas no thicker than 2.0 mm. These patients were divided into two treatment groups: excision with 1-cm margins and excision with margins of 3 cm or more. Over a mean follow-up period of 55 months, there was no difference in disease-free survival rates, overall survival rates, and subsequent development of metastatic disease. However, duration of follow-up time may have been too brief to be an absolutely definitive study; three patients, all with narrow excisions and a primary melanoma thicker than 1.0 mm, developed local recurrence. A 1.0-cm margin is therefore probably sufficient for all lesions less than 1.0 mm thick and possibly sufficient for lesions less than 2.0 mm thick in the non-BANS locations. All other melanomas should be excised with a 3.0-cm radius. This recommendation should be weighed against cosmetic and functional considerations when dealing with melanomas on the face near vital structures such as the eye, eyelid, nose, ear, or facial nerve. These structures should not be sacrificed unless they are directly invaded. There are no data that show any advantage to removing the deep fascia. Hence, the usual extent of surgery for clinical stage I disease is the epidermis, dermis, and all the fat down to but not including the fascia. Likewise, there are no data

Table 17.1.
Estimated 7.5-Year Survival in Clinical Stage I Melanoma[a]

Thickness (mm)	Non-BANS[b]				BANS[b]
	Extremities	Head and Neck	Trunk	Hands and Feet	
<0.85	99+	99+	99+	99+	98
0.85–1.69	99+	99+	97	99+	78
1.70–3.64	86	64	77	60	58
3.65	83	65	22	0	33

[a] Adapted from Day CL, Mihm C, Lew RE, et al: Cutaneous malignant melanoma: Prognostic guidelines for physicians and patients. *Cancer* 32:113, 1982.
[b] BANS—upper back, posterolateral arms, posterolateral neck, posterior scalp.

showing an advantage to skewing an elliptical excision in the direction of the lymphatic drainage from the site; the orientation of the ellipse, therefore, may be placed for best cosmetic and functional advantage, including lymphatic drainage where feasible.

Surgical excision of the primary tumor is the mainstay of treatment. Lymph node dissection is performed if palpable metastases have developed in regional nodes. Surgical removal of recurrent tumor or easily excisable metastases to lymph nodes or viscera decreases morbidity and prolongs survival (236, 237). In the absence of easily detectable lymph node or distant metastases, there is no consensus about the value of additional surgical or medical therapies such as elective regional lymph node dissection (ERND), isolated regional perfusion, and adjuvant immunotherapy or chemotherapy. No definitive long-term large prospective studies have been done to delineate the effectiveness of ERND. General agreement exists that ERND does not benefit patients with either thin (less than 1.5 mm) or thick (greater than 4.0 mm) lesions (238). Three studies (239–241), all with fewer than 200 patients with lesions of intermediate thickness, did not detect a beneficial effect of ERND. Two other studies (242, 243) appreciated a marked increase in death from melanoma after 5 years for stage I patients with intermediate-thickness lesions treated with wide local excision only as compared to those who also underwent ERND. A more recent report (244) of a prospective randomized study of 171 patients with lesions of all thicknesses treated with local excision with or without ERND revealed no statistical improvement in mortality with ERND in any subset of patients. However, this study included only 28 patients with lesions of intermediate thickness. These studies, the rationale for ERND, and a description of ongoing studies have been reviewed recently (245). If ERND is to be performed, lymphoscintigraphy may be useful in planning the surgical procedure (246).

Unresectable melanomas of the limbs have been treated by isolated regional perfusion with melphalan, and long-term responses of greater than 40% have been achieved. For this reason, it has also been used as an adjuvant therapy for stage I melanomas of the extremity that are thicker than 1.5 mm. The technique (247) requires a surgically created perfusion circuit, anticoagulation, induction of regional hyperthermia, and often a fasciotomy to prevent development of a compartment syndrome. Complications generally result from local or systemic irritation, and the procedure is usually well tolerated even by children. Prior ERND is advisable, particularly in the axillae, where postperfusion scarring may preclude adequate evaluation of lymph nodes by physical examination. Effectiveness is debatable; most reports of a positive response are studies of a small number of patients compared to historical controls (248, 249). A large retrospective study with well-matched controls (250) found no significant difference in patients of any subgroup treated with adjuvant isolated regional perfusion; however, a small prospective study (247) of 37 patients with stage I melanoma found recurrences to be markedly diminished in the perfused group. Because the data do not uniformly document a survival benefit for perfusion as an adjuvant therapy, the procedure is generally reserved for palliative treatment of selected patients with localized advanced disease.

Adjuvant immunotherapy and chemotherapy have been studied in many centers, but their usefulness has never been documented. At best, nonspecific agents are palliative in the setting of metastatic disease (251). It is possible that specific immunostimulatory agents derived by techniques utilizing the patient's own tumor cells may be helpful in the future.

The management of any patient who has had a melanoma includes rigorous repeated examination of the surgical site as well as the entire skin surface, including scalp and genitalia. As noted above, the patient with a thin clinical stage I melanoma has a greater lifetime risk of developing a second melanoma than of developing metastases from the first melanoma. Examinations of the skin should be performed every 6 months for several years, then annually. If the patient has numerous severely atypical nevi and a family history of melanoma, self-examination of the nevi should be performed monthly. In addition, the physician should examine and carefully chart or photograph these nevi every 3 months for the lifetime of the patient. In addition, family members should be examined for precursor lesions and melanomas. Both the patient and family need to refrain from excessive sun exposure; this may entail a change in life-style as well as daily attention to the use of sun-protective topical preparations and clothing. A complete physical examination and annual chest radiograph are sufficient to exclude metastatic disease in a patient who is otherwise well. Specific complaints can be evaluated as indicated by their nature.

Surgical treatment is recommended frequently for precursor lesions. Congenital nevi, especially the large tumors, have a known high rate of malignant degeneration. The surgeon must balance the costs and risks of surgery, general anesthesia, and functional or cosmetic disability against the risk of development of melanoma (252). Because congenital nevi are difficult to follow clinically, excision is frequently performed. Excision in toto with less than 1.0-cm margins is probably sufficient. It should be noted that nevus cells are present in the dermis and subcutaneous fat of these lesions and have been documented to give rise to deep melanomas (253); dermabrasion or superficial laser destruction would not be expected to sufficiently ameliorate the risk of malignancy. Because biologically malignant lesions arise in moderately to severely atypical dysplastic nevi, melanoma in situ, and lentigo maligna, the treatment of choice for these lesions is excision in toto. Not every dysplastic nevus requires excision; particular attention should be paid to new and changing lesions. The exact margin of normal skin to be excised is certainly the same as or less than if the procedure were done for a thin (1.0-mm) melanoma; how much less margin is adequate is unclear.

References

1. Scoto J, Fears TR, Fraument JF: *Incidence of Nonmelanoma Skin Cancer in the United States*. Publication no. 82-2433 (NIH). Washington, DC, U.S. Department of Health and Human Services, 1981.

2. Olsen TG, Feeser TA, Conte ET, et al: Skin cancer screening—a local experience. *J Am Acad Dermatol* 16:637, 1987.
3. Freeman RG: Histopathologic considerations in the management of skin cancer. *J Dermatol Surg Oncol* 2:215, 1976.
4. Robins P, Rabinovitz HS, Rigel D: Basal cell carcinomas on covered or unusual sites of the body. *J Dermatol Surg Oncol* 7:803, 1981.
5. Hanke CW, Wolf RL, Hochman SA, et al: Perineural spread of basal cell carcinoma. *J Dermatol Surg Oncol* 9:742, 1983.
6. Paver K, Doyzen K, Burry N: The incidence of basal cell carcinomas and their metastases in Australia and New Zealand. *Aust J Dermatol* 14:53, 1973.
7. Vitaliano PP, Urbach F: The relative importance of risk factors in nonmelanoma carcinoma. *Arch Dermatol* 116:454, 1980.
8. Giles CG, Marks R, Foley P: Incidence of non-melanocytic skin cancer treated in Australia. *Br J Med [Clin Res]* 296:13, 1988.
9. Engel A, Johnson ML, Haynes SG: Health effects of sunlight exposure in the United States. Results from the first National Health and Nutrition Examination Survey, 1971–74. *Arch Dermatol* 124:72, 1988.
10. Ridley CM: Basal cell carcinoma following x-ray epilation of the head and neck. *Br J Dermatol* 74:222, 1962.
11. Martin H, Strong E, Spiro RH: Radiation-induced skin cancer of the head and neck. *Cancer* 25:61, 1970.
12. Conway H, Huygo NE: Radiation dermatitis and malignancy. *Plast Reconstr Surg* 38:255, 1966.
13. Stern RS, Lange R: Nonmelanoma skin cancer occurring in patients treated with PUVA five to ten years after first treatment. *J Invest Dermatol* 91:120, 1988.
14. Montgomery H, Waisman M: Epithelioma attributable to arsenic. *J Inest Dermatol* 4:365, 1941.
15. Wagner SL, Maliner JS, Morton WE, et al: Skin cancer and arsenical intoxication from well water. *Arch Dermatol* 115:1205, 1979.
16. Sitz KV, Keppen M, Johnson DF: Metastatic basal cell carcinoma in acquired immunodeficiency syndrome-related complex. *JAMA* 257:340, 1987.
17. Gupta AK, Cardella CJ, Haberman HF: Cutaneous malignant neoplasms in patients with renal transplants. *Arch Dermatol* 122:1288, 1986.
18. Marshall V: Premalignant and malignant skin tumors in immunosuppressed patients. *Transplantation* 17:272, 1974.
19. Parnes R, Safai B, Myskowski PL: Basal cell carcinomas and lymphoma: Biologic behavior and associated factors in 63 patients. *J Am Acad Dermatol* 19:1017, 1988.
20. Connolly JG: Basal cell carcinoma occurring in burn scars. *Can Med Assoc J* 83:1433, 1960.
21. Early MJ: Basal cell carcinoma arising in tattoos: A clinical report of 2 cases. *Br J Plast Surg* 36:258, 1983.
22. Marmelzat WL: Malignant tumors in smallpox vaccination scars: A report of 24 cases. *Arch Dermatol* 97:400, 1968.
23. Bowers RF, Young JM: Carcinoma arising in scars, osteomyelitis, fistulae. *Arch Surg* 80:564, 1960.
24. Cruikshank AH, McConnell EM, Miller DG: Malignancy in scars, chronic ulcers, and sinuses. *J Clin Pathol* 16:573, 1963.
25. Lanehart WH, Sanusi ID, Raghunath PM, et al: Metastasizing basal cell carcinoma originating in a stasis ulcer in a black woman. *Arch Dermatol* 119:587, 1983.
26. Bryant J: Basal cell carcinoma overlying long standing dermatofibromas. *Arch Dermatol* 113:1445, 1977.
27. Pack GT, Sunderland DA: Naevus unius lateris. *Arch Surg* 43:341, 1941.
28. Horn MS, Sausker WF, Pierson DL: Basal cell epithelioma arising in a linear epidermal nevus. *Arch Dermatol* 117:247, 1981.
29. Rabbari H, Mehregan AH: Basal cell epithelioma in children and teenagers. *Cancer* 49:350, 1982.
30. Neuman Z, Ben-Hur N, Shulman J: Trauma and skin cancer. *Plast Reconstr Surg* 32:649, 1963.
31. Bergstrasser PR, Halprin KM: Multiple sequential skin cancers: The risk of skin cancers in patients with a previous skin cancer. *Arch Dermatol* 111:995, 1975.
32. Biro L, Price E, MacWilliams P: Basal cell carcinoma in office practice. *NY State J Med* 75:1427, 1975.
33. Robinson JK: Risk of developing another basal cell carcinoma. A 5-year prospective study. *Cancer* 60:118, 1987.
34. Matsuoka LY, Schauer PK, Sordillo PP: Basal cell carcinoma in black patients. *J Am Acad Dermatol* 4:670, 1981.
35. Mora RG, Burris R: Cancer of the skin in blacks: A review of 128 patients with basal cell carcinoma. *Cancer* 47:1436, 1981.
36. Kopf AW, Bart RS, Andrade R: *Atlas of Tumors of the Skin.* Philadelphia, WB Saunders Co, 1978.
37. Lever WF, Schaumberg-Lever G: *Histopathology of the Skin,* 7th ed. Philadelphia, JB Lippincott Co, 1990, pp 622–634.
38. Howell JB, Caro MR: The basal cell nevus syndrome. *Arch Dermatol* 79:67, 1959.
39. Howell JB, Anderson DE: Commentary: The nevoid basal cell carcinoma syndrome. *Arch Dermatol* 118:824, 1982.
40. Gorlin RJ: Nevoid basal-cell carcinoma syndrome. *Medicine* 66:98, 1987.
41. Golitz LE, Norris DA, Leukens CA, et al: Nevoid basal cell carcinoma syndrome: Multiple basal cell carcinomas of the palms after radiation therapy. *Arch Dermatol* 116:1159, 1980.
42. Southwick GJ, Schwartz RA: The basal cell nevus syndrome: Disasters occurring among a series of 36 patients. *Cancer* 44:2294, 1979.
43. Viksnins P, Berlin A: Follicular atrophoderma and basal cell carcinoma. *Arch Dermatol* 113:948, 1977.
44. Robbins JH: Xeroderma pigmentosum: An inherited disease with sun sensitivity, multiple cutaneous neoplasms, and abnormal DNA repair. *Ann Intern Med* 80:221, 1974.
45. Epstein E: How accurate is the visual assessment of basal cell carcinoma margins? *Br J Dermatol* 89:37, 1973.
46. Wolf DJ, Zitelli JA: Surgical margins for basal cell carcinoma. *Arch Dermatol* 123:340, 1987.
47. Salasche SJ, Amonette RA: Morpheaform basal cell epitheliomas: A study of subclinical extension in a series of 51 cases. *J Dermatol Surg Oncol* 7:387, 1981.
48. Bart R, Schrager D, Kopf AW, et al: Scalpel excision of basal cell carcinomas. *Arch Dermatol* 114:739, 1978.
49. Panje WR, Ceilley RI: The influence of embryology of the midface on the spread of epithelial malignancies. *Laryngoscope* 89:1914, 1979.
50. Pascal R, Hobby L, Lattes R, et al: Prognosis of "incompletely excised" versus "completely excised" basal cell carcinoma. *Plast Reconstr Surg* 41:328, 1968.
51. Richmond JD, Davie RM: The significance of incomplete excision in patients with basal cell carcinoma. *Br J Plast Surg* 40:63, 1987.
52. Stanley RB Jr, Burres SA, Jacobs JR, et al: Hazards encountered in management of basal cell carcinomas of the midface. *Laryngoscope* 94:378, 1984.
53. Riefkohl R, Pollack S, Georgiade GS: A rationale for the treatment of difficult basal cell and squamous cell carcinomas of the skin. *Ann Plast Surg* 15:19, 1985.
54. Torre D: Cryosurgery of basal cell carcinoma. *J Am Acad Dermatol* 15:917, 1986.
55. McLean DI, Haynes HA, McCarthy PL, et al: Cryotherapy of basal cell carcinoma by a simple method of standardized freeze-thaw cycles. *J Dermatol Surg Oncol* 4:175, 1978.
56. Elton RF: The course of events following cryosurgery. *J. Dermatol Surg Oncol* 3:448, 1977.
57. Graham FG: Statistical data on malignant tumors in cryosurgery 1982. *J Dermatol Surg Oncol* 9:238, 1983.
58. Holt PJ: Cryotherapy for skin cancer: Results over a 5-year period using liquid nitrogen spray cryosurgery. *Br J Dermatol* 119:231, 1988.
59. Knox JM, Lyles TW, Shapiro EM, et al: Curettage and electrodesiccation in the treatment of skin cancer. *Arch Dermatol* 82:197, 1960.
60. Kopf AW, Bart RS, Shrager D: Curettage-electrodesiccation in the treatment of basal cell carcinoma. *Arch Dermatol* 82:197, 1960.
61. Suhge-dAubermont PC, Bennett RG: Failure of curettage and electrodesiccation for removal of basal cell carcinoma. *Arch Dermatol* 120:1456, 1984.
62. Goldschmidt H, Sherwin WK: Office radiotherapy of cutaneous carcinoma. II. Indication in specific anatomic regions. *J Dermatol Surg Oncol* 9:47, 1983.

63. Bart RS, Kopf AW, Petratos MA: X-ray therapy of skin cancer, evaluation of a "standardized" method for treating basal cell carcinoma. In: *Sixth National Cancer Conference*. Philadelphia, JB Lippincott, 1970, pp 559–570.

64. Walker NP: Carbon dioxide laser treatment of basal cell epitheliomas. *Br J Dermatol* 109:17, 1983.

65. Brunner R, Landthaler M, Haina D, et al: Treatment of benign, semimalignant, and malignant skin tumors with the Nd:YAG laser. *Lasers Surg Med* 5:105, 1985.

66. Tse DT, Kersten RL, Anderson RL: Hematoporphyrin derivative photoirradiation therapy in managing nevoid basal cell carcinoma syndrome. A preliminary report. *Arch Ophthalmol* 102:990, 1984.

67. Keller GS, Doiron DR, Fisher GU: Photodynamic therapy in otolargyngology—head and neck surgery. *Arch Otolaryngol* 111:758, 1985.

68. Reymann F: Treatment of basal cell carcinoma of the skin with 5-Fluorouracil ointment: A ten year followup study. *Dermatologica* 158:368, 1979.

69. Mohs FE, Jones DL, Bloom RF: Tendency of fluorouracil to conceal deep foci of invasive basal cell carcinoma. *Arch Dermatol* 114:1021, 1978.

70. Epstein E: Fluorouracil paste treatment of thin basal cell carcinomas. *Arch Dermatol* 121:207, 1987.

71. Lippman SM, Shimm DS, Meyskens FL: Nonsurgical treatments for skin cancer: Retinoids and alpha-interferon. *J Dermatol Surg Oncol* 14:862, 1988.

72. Peck GL, DiGiovanni JJ, Sarnoff DS, et al: Treatment and prevention of basal cell carcinoma with isotretinoin. *J Am Acad Dermatol* 19:176, 1988.

73. Hughes BR, Marks R, Pearse AD, et al: Clinical response and tissue effects of etretinate treatment of patients with solar keratoses and basal cell carcinoma. *J Am Acad Dermatol* 18:522, 1988.

74. Mohs FE: Chemosurgery. *Microscopically Controlled Surgery for Skin Cancer*. Springfield, IL, Charles C Thomas Co, 1978.

75. Cottel WJ, Proper S: Mohs' surgery, fresh tissue technique. *J Dermatol Surg Oncol* 8:576, 1982.

76. Roenigk RK: Mohs' micrographic surgery. *Mayo Clin Proc* 63:175, 1988.

77. Rigel DS, Robins P, Friedman RJ: Predicting recurrence of basal cell carcinomas treated by microscopically controlled excision. *J Dermatol Surg Oncol* 7:807, 1981.

78. Robinson JK: What are adequate treatment and follow-up care for nonmelanoma cutaneous cancer? *Arch Dermatol* 123:331, 1987.

79. Rowe DE, Carroll RJ, Day CL: Longterm recurrence rates of previously untreated (primary) basal cell carcinoma: Implications for patient follow-up. *J Dermatol Surg Oncol* 15:315, 1989.

80. Stern RS, Weinstein MC, Baker SG: Risk reduction for nonmelanoma skin cancer with childhood sunscreen use. *Arch Dermatol* 122:537, 1986.

81. Kligman LH, Akin FJ, Kligman AM: Sunscreens prevent ultraviolet photocarcinogenesis. *J Am Acad Dermatol* 3:30, 1980.

82. Jones RR: Ozone depletion and cancer risk. *Lancet* 2:443, 1987.

83. Kraemer KH, DiGiovanni JJ, Moshell AN, et al: Prevention of skin cancer in xeroderma pigmentosum with the use of oral isotretinoin. *N Engl J Med* 318:1633, 1988.

84. Forbes PD, Urbach F, Davies RE: Enhancement of experimental photocarcinogenesis by topical retinoic acid. *Cancer Lett* 7:85, 1979.

85. Bourne RG: The spread of squamous cell carcinoma of the skin via the cranial nerves. *Austral Radiol* 24:106, 1980.

86. Goepfert H, Dichtel WJ, Medina JE, et al: Perineural invasion in squamous cell carcinoma of the head and neck. *Am J Surg* 148:542, 1984.

87. Lund HZ: How often does squamous cell carcinoma of the skin metastasize? *Arch Dermatol* 92:635, 1965.

88. Lund HZ: Metastasis from sun-induced squamous cell carcinoma of the skin: An uncommon event. *J Dermatol Surg Oncol* 10:169, 1984.

89. Moller R, Reymann F, Hou-Jensen K: Metastases in dermatologic patients with squamous cell carcinoma. *Arch Dermatol* 115:703, 1979.

90. Katz AD, Urbach F, Lilienfeld AM: The frequency and risk of metastasis in squamous cell carcinoma of the skin. *Cancer* 10:1162, 1957.

91. Dinehart SM, Pollack SV: Metastases from squamous cell carcinoma of the skin and lip. *J Am Acad Dermatol* 21:241, 1989.

92. Mora RG, Perniciaro C: Cancer of the skin in blacks. A review of 36 black patients with squamous cell carcinoma of the lip. *J Am Acad Dermatol* 6:1005, 1982.

93. Urbach F: Ultraviolet radiation and skin cancer. In Montagna W, Dobson RL (eds): *Advances in Biology of the Skin*. New York, Pergamon, 1966, Vol VII, pp 195–214.

94. Yiannias JA, Goldberg LH, Carter-Campbell S, et al: The ratio of basal cell carcinoma to squamous cell carcinoma in Houston, Texas. *J Dermatol Surg Oncol* 14:886, 1988.

95. Epstein JH: Photocarcinogenesis, skin cancer and aging. *J Am Acad Dermatol* 9:487, 1983.

96. Stern RS, Laird N, Melski J: Cutaneous squamous cell carcinoma patients treated with PUVA. *N Engl J Med* 310:1156, 1984.

97. Boyle J, Mackie RM, Briggs JD, et al: Cancer, warts, and sunshine in renal transplant patients. A case control study. *Lancet* 1:702, 1984.

98. Epstein WL, Fukuyama K, Epstein JH: Ultraviolet, DNA repair and skin carcinogenesis in man. *Fed Proc* 30:1766, 1971.

99. Black HS, Douglas DR: Formation of a carcinogen of natural origin in the etiology of ultraviolet light-induced carcinogenesis. *Cancer Res* 33:2094, 1973.

100. Blum HF, McVaugh J, Ward M, et al: Epidermal hyperplasia induced by ultraviolet radiation. *Photochem Photobiol* 21:255, 1975.

101. Kripke ML, Fisher MS: Immunologic parameters of UV carcinogenesis. *J Natl Cancer Inst* 57:211, 1976.

102. Ostrow RS, Shaver MK, Turnquist S, et al: Human papillomavirus 16 DNA in a cutaneous invasive carcinoma. *Arch Dermatol* 125:666, 1989.

103. Montgomery H: Precancerous dermatoses. In *Dermatopathology*. New York, Harper and Row Publishers, Inc, 1967, Vol 2, pp 967–1006.

104. Marks R, Rennie G, Selwood TS: Malignant transformation of solar keratoses to squamous cell carcinoma. *Lancet* 1:795, 1988.

105. Rudolph R, Noe JM: *Chronic Problem Wounds*. Boston, Little, Brown and Co, 1983.

106. Arons MS, Lynch JB, Lewis SR, et al: Scar tissue carcinoma: I. A clinical study with special reference to burn scar carcinoma. *Ann Surg* 161:170, 1965.

107. Sedlin ED, Flemming JL: Epidermal carcinoma arising in chronic ostemyelitic foci. *J. Bone Joint Surg* 45:827, 1963.

108. Johnston WH, Miller TA, Frileck SP: Atypical pseudoepitheliomatous hyperplasia and squamous cell carcinoma in chronic cutaneous sinuses and fistulas. *Plast Reconstr Surg* 66:395, 1980.

109. Sagi A, Rosenberg L, Greiff M, et al: Squamous cell carcinoma arising in a pilonidal sinus. *J Dermatol Surg Oncol* 10:210, 1984.

110. Arrington JH, Lockman DS: Thermal keratoses and squamous cell carcinoma in situ associated with erythema ab igne. *Arch Dermatol* 115:1226, 1979.

111. Eng AM, Jacobs RA: Lichen sclerosus et atrophicus and squamous cell carcinoma. *J Cutan Pathol* 7:123, 1980.

112. Presser SE, Taylor JR: Squamous cell carcinoma in blacks with discoid lupus erythematous. *J Am Acad Dermatol* 4:667, 1981.

113. Oberst-Lehn H, Moll B: Porokeratosis mibelli und Stachelzellencarcinoma. *Hautartz* 19:399, 1968.

114. Carapeto FJ, Pastor JA, Marin J, et al: Recessive dystrophic epidermolysis bullosa and multiple squamous cell carcinomas. *Dermatologica* 165:39, 1982.

115. Argyris TS, Slaga TJ: Promotion of carcinomas by repeated abrasion in initiated skin of mice. *Cancer Res* 41:5193, 1981.

116. Everall JD, Dowd PM: Influence of environmental factors excluding ultraviolet radiation on the incidence of skin cancer. *Bull Cancer (Paris)* 65:241, 1978.

117. LaRiviere W, Pickett AB: Clinical criteria in diagnosis of early squamous cell carcinoma of the lower lip. *J Am Dent Assoc* 99:972, 1979.

118. Lever WF, Schaumberg-Lever G: *Histopathology of the Skin.* Philadelphia, JB Lippincott Co, 1983.

119. Pearse AD, Marks R: Actinic keratoses and the epidermis on which they arise. *Br J Dermatol* 96:45, 1977.

120. Strayer DS, Santa Cruz DJ: Carcinoma in situ of the skin: A review of histopathology. *J Cutan Pathol* 7:244, 1980.

121. Montes LF: Bowen's disease. *J Cutan Pathol* 4:44, 1977.

122. Moller R, Nielsen A, Reymann F, et al: Squamous cell carcinoma of the skin and internal malignant neoplasms. *Arch Dermatol* 115:304, 1979.

123. Callen JP, Headington JT: Bowen's and non Bowen's squamous cell intraepidermal neoplasia of the skin: Relationship to internal malignancy. *Arch Dermatol* 116:422, 1980.

124. Strauss RJ, Fazio VW: Bowen's disease of the anal and perianal area: A report and analysis of twelve cases. *Am J Surg* 137:231, 1979.

125. Chuang T-Y, Reizner GT: Bowen's disease and internal malignancy. *J Am Acad Derm* 19:47, 1988.

126. Reymann F, Ravnborg L, Shou G, et al: Bowen's disease and internal malignant diseases. *Arch Dermatol* 124:677, 1988.

127. Callen JP: Bowen's disease and internal malignant diseases. *Arch Dermatol* 124:675, 1988.

128. Arbesman H, Ransohoff DF: Is Bowen's disease a predictor for the development of internal malignancy? *JAMA* 257:516, 1987.

129. Wade TR, Kopf AW, Ackerman AB: Bowenoid papulosis of the genitalia. *Arch Dermatol* 115:306, 1979.

130. Kimura S: Bowenoid papulosis of the genitalia. *Int J Dermatol* 21:432, 1982.

131. DeVillez RL, Stevens CS: Bowenoid papules of the genitalia. *J Am Acad Dermatol* 3:149, 1980.

132. Kato T, Saijyo S, Hatchome N, et al: Detection of human papillomavirus type 16 in bowenoid papulosis and invasive carcinoma occurring in the same patient with a history of cervical carcinoma. *Arch Dermatol* 124:851, 1988.

133. Goette DK: Erythroplasia of Queyrat. *Arch Dermatol* 110:271, 1974.

134. Mikhail GR: Cancers, precancers, and pseudocancers on the male genitalia. *J Dermatol Surg Oncol* 6:1027, 1980.

135. Graham JH, Helwig EB: Erythroplasia of Queyrat. In Graham JH, Johnson WP, Helwig EB (eds): *Dermal Pathology.* New York, Harper and Row Co, 1972, pp 597–606.

136. Aird I, Johnson HD, Lennox B, et al: Epithelioma cuniculatum—a variety of squamous cell carcinoma peculiar to the foot. *Br J Surg* 42:245, 1954.

137. McKee PH, Wilkinson JD, Corbett MF, et al: Carcinoma cuniculatum: A case metastasizing to skin and lymph nodes. *Clin Exp Derm* 6:613, 1981.

138. Lapins NA, Helwig EB: Perineural invasion by keratoacanthoma. *Arch Dermatol* 116:791, 1980.

139. Bart RS, Kopf AW: Techniques of biopsy of cutaneous neoplasms. *J Dermatol Surg Oncol* 5:979, 1979.

140. Schnur PL, Bozzo P: Metastasizing keratoacanthomas: The difficulties in differentiating keratoacanthomas from squamous cell carcinoma. *Plast Reconstr Surg* 62:258, 1978.

141. Smoller BR, Kwan TH, Said JW, et al: Keratoacanthoma and squamous cell carcinoma of the skin: Immunohistochemical localization of involucrin and keratin proteins. *J Am Acad Dermatol* 14:226, 1986.

142. Sanders GH, Miller TA: Are keratoacanthomas really squamous cell carcinomas? *Ann Plast Surg* 9:306, 1982.

143. Pickrell K, Villarreal-Rios A, Neale H: Giant keratoacanthoma. *Ann Plast Surg* 2:525, 1979.

144. Stranc MF, Robertson GA: Conservative treatment of keratoacanthoma. *Ann Plast Surg* 2:525, 1979.

145. Wolinsky S, Silvers DN, Kohn SR, et al: Spontaneous regression of a giant keratoacanthoma. Photographic documentation and histopathologic correlation. *J Dermatol Surg Oncol* 7:897, 1981.

146. Goette DK: Treatment of keratoacanthoma with topical fluorouracil. *Arch Dermatol* 119:951, 1983.

147. Goette DK, Odom RB: Successful treatment of keratoacanthoma with intralesional fluorouracil. *J Am Acad Dermatol* 2:212, 1980.

148. Snider BL, Benjamin DR: Eruptive keratoacathoma with an internal malignant neoplasm. *Arch Dermatol* 117:788, 1981.

149. Sina B, Adrian RM: Multiple keratoacanthomas possibly induced by psoralens and ultraviolet A photochemotherapy. *J Am Acad Dermatol* 9:686, 1983.

150. Reid BJ, Cheesebrough MJ: Multiple keratoacanthoma. A unique case and review of the present classification. *Acta Derm Venereo* 58:169, 1978.

151. Lutzner MA: Epidermodysplasia verruciformis. An autosomal recessive disease characterized by viral warts and skin cancer. A model for viral oncogenesis. *Bull Cancer (Paris)* 656:169, 1978.

152. Prawer SE, Pass F, Vance JC, et al: Depressive immune function epidermodysplasia verruciformis. *Arch Dermatol* 113:495, 1977.

153. Ostrow RS, Manias D, Mitchell AJ, et al: Epidermodysplasia verruciformis. A case associated with primary lymphatic dysplasia, depressed cell-mediated immunity, and Bowen's disease containing human papillomavirus 16 DNA. *Arch Dermatol* 123:1511, 1987.

154. Androphy EJ, Dvoretsky I, Maluish AE, et al: Response of warts in epidermodysplasia verruciformis to treatment with systemic and intralesional alpha interferon. *J Am Acad Dermatol* 11:197, 1984.

155. Fahmy A, Burgdorf WH, Schosser RH, et al: Muir-Torre syndrome: Report of a case and reevaluation of the dermatopathologoic features. *Cancer* 49:1898, 1983.

156. Finan MC, Connolly SM: Sebaceous gland tumors and systemic disease: A clinicopathologic analysis. *Medicine* 63:232, 1984.

157. Immerman SC, Scanlon EF, Christ M, et al: Recurrent squamous cell carcinoma of the skin. *Cancer* 51:1537, 1983.

158. Robins P, Dzubow LM, Rigel DS: Squamous cell carcinoma treated by Moh's surgery. An experience with 414 cases in a period of 15 years. *J Dermatol Surg Oncol* 7:800, 1981.

159. Levine N, Miller RC, Meyskens FL Jr: Oral isotretinoin therapy. Use in a patient with multiple cutaneous squamous cell carcinomas and keratoacanthomas. *Arch Dermatol* 120:1215, 1984.

160. Lippman SM, Meyskens FL Jr: Treatment of advanced squamous cell carcinoma of the skin with isotretinoin. *Ann Intern Med* 107:499, 1987.

161. Spira M, Freeman RF, Arfai P, et al: A comparison of chemical peeling, dermabrasion, and 5-fluorouracil in cancer prophylaxis. *J Surg Oncol* 3:367, 1971.

162. Silverberg E, Lubera JA: Cancer statistics, 1989, *CA* 39:3, 1989.

163. Roush GC, Schymura MJ, Holford TR: Patterns of invasive melanoma in the Connecticut Tumor Registry. Is the long-term increase real? *Cancer* 61:2586, 1988.

164. Elwood JM, Gallagher RP, Hill GB, et al: Pigmentation and skin reaction to sun as risk factors for cutaneous melanoma: Western Canada melanoma study. *Br Med J* 288:99, 1984.

165. Malec E, Eklund G: The changing incidence of malignant melanoma of the skin in Sweden 1959–1968. *Scand J Plast Reconstr Surg* 12:19, 1978.

166. Freeman NR, Fairbrother GE, Rose RJ: Survey of skin cancer incidence in the Hamilton area. *NZ Med J* 95:529, 1982.

167. Pathak DR, Samet JM, Howard CA, et al: Malignant melanoma of the skin in New Mexico 1969–1977. *Cancer* 50:1440, 1982.

168. Hinds MW, Kolonel LN: Malignant melanoma of the skin in Hawaii, 1960–1977. *Cancer* 45:811, 1980.

169. Houghton A, Flannery J, Viola MV: Malignant melanoma in Connecticut and Denmark. *Int J Cancer* 25:95, 1980.

170. Sober AJ: Diagnosis and management of skin cancer. *Cancer* 51:2448, 1983.

171. Doherty VR, MacKie RM: Experience of a public education program on early detection of cutaneous malignant melanoma. *Br Med J* 297:388, 1988.

172. Rigel DS, Friedman RJ, Kopf AW, et al: Importance of com-

plete cutaneous examination for the detection of malignant melanoma. *J Am Acad Dermatol* 14:857, 1986.

173. Hardie IR, Strong RW, Hartley LC, et al: Skin cancer in Caucasian renal allograft recipients living in a subtropical climate. *Surgery* 87:177, 1980.

174. Tindall B, Finlayson R, Mutimer K, et al: Malignant melanoma associated with human immunodeficiency virus infection in three homosexual men. *J Am Acad Dermatol* 20:587, 1989.

175. Takebe H, Nishigori C, Tatsumi K: Melanoma and other skin cancers in xeroderma pigmentosum patients and mutations in their cells. *J Invest Dermatol* 92 (suppl):236, 1989.

176. Ross PM, Carter DM: Actinic DNA damage and the pathogenesis of cutaneous malignant melanoma. *J Invest Dermatol* 92 (suppl):293, 1989.

177. Green AC, O'Rourke MG: Cutaneous malignant melanoma in association with other skin cancers. *JNCI* 74:977, 1985.

178. Osterlind A, Tucker MA, Stone BJ, et al: The Danish case-control study of cutaneous malignant melanoma. II. Importance of UV light exposure. *Int J Cancer* 42:319, 1988.

179. Hinds MW, Lee J, Kolonel LN: Seasonal patterns of skin melanoma incidence in Hawaii. *Am J Public Health* 71:496, 1981.

180. Tucker MA, Shields JA, Hartge P, et al: Sunlight exposure as risk factor for intraocular malignant melanoma. *N Engl J Med* 313:789, 1985.

181. Mihm MC, Fitzpatrick TB, Lane-Brown MM, et al: Early detection of primary cutaneous malignant melanoma: A color atlas. *N Engl J Med* 289:989, 1973.

182. Sober AJ, Fitzpatrick TB, Mihm MC: Primary melanoma of the skin: Recognition and management. *J Am Acad Dermatol* 2:179, 1980.

183. Sober AJ, Day CL, Kopf AW, et al: Detection of "thin" primary melanomas. *CA* 33:160, 1983.

184. Day CL, Mihm MC, Sober AJ, et al: Skin lesions suspected to be melanoma should be photographed. Gross morphological features of primary melanoma associated with metastases. *JAMA* 248:1077, 1982.

185. Bondi EE, Elder DE, Guerry D, et al: Skin markings in malignant melanoma. *JAMA* 250:503, 1983.

186. Schiffman N, Arndt KA, Noe JM: Acral lentiginous melanoma. *Ann Plast Surg* 5:232, 1980.

187. Coleman WP, Gately LE, Krementz AB, et al: Nevi, lentigines and melanomas in blacks. *Arch Dermatol* 116:548, 1980.

188. Egbert B, Kempson R, Sagebiel R: Desmoplastic malignant melanoma. A clinicohistopathologic study of 25 cases. *Cancer* 62:2033, 1988.

189. Jain S, Allen PW: Desmoplastic malignant melanoma and its variants. A study of 45 cases. *Am J Surg Pathol* 13:358, 1989.

190. Mihm MC, Fitzpatrick TB, Clark WH: Malignant melanoma of the skin, and benign neoplasms and hyperplasias of melanocytes in the skin. In Fitzpatrick TB, Eisen AZ, Wolff K, et al. (eds): *Dermatology in General Medicine*. New York, McGraw-Hill Book Co, 1979, pp 629–654.

191. Kopf AW, Mintzis M, Bart RS: Diagnostic accuracy in malignant melanoma. *Arch Dermatol* 111:1291, 1975.

192. Epstein E, Bragg K, Linden G: Biopsy and prognosis of malignant melanoma. *JAMA* 208:1369, 1969.

193. Jones WM, Williams WJ, Roberts MM, et al: Malignant melanoma of the skin: Prognostic value of clinical features and the role of treatment in 111 cases. *Br J Cancer* 22:437, 1968.

194. Lederman JS, Sober AJ: Does biopsy type influence survival in clinical stage I cutaneous melanoma? *J Am Acad Dermatol* 13:983, 1985.

195. Elder DE, Greene MH, Bondi EE, et al: Acquired melanocytic nevi and melanoma. The dysplastic nevus syndrome. In Ackerman AB (ed): *Pathology of Malignant Melanoma*. New York, Masson Publ Inc, 1981, pp 185–215.

196. Rhodes AR: Pigmented birthmarks and precursor melanocytic lesions of cutaneous melanoma identifiable in childhood. *Pediatr Clin North Am* 30:435, 1983.

197. Weinstock MA, Colditz GA, Willett WC, et al: Moles and site-specific risk of nonfamilial cutaneous malignant melanoma in women. *JNCI* 81:948, 1989.

198. Osterlind A, Tucker MA, Hou-Jensen K, et al: The Danish

199. Holly EA, Kelly JW, Shpall SN, et al: Number of melanocytic nevi as a major risk factor for malignant melanoma. *J Am Acad Dermatol* 17:459, 1987.

200. Lorentzen M, Pers M, Bretteville-Jensen G: The incidence of malignant transformation in giant pigmented nevi. *Scand J Plast Surg* 11:163, 1977.

201. Trozak DJ, Rowland WD, HU F: Metastatic malignant melanoma in prepubertal children. *Pediatrics* 55:191, 1975.

202. Castilla EE, DaGraca-Dutra M, Orioli-Parreiras JM: Epidemiology of congenital pigmented nevi: Incidence rate and relative frequencies. *Br J Dermatol* 104:307, 1981.

203. Rhodes AR, Sober AJ, Day CL, et al: The malignant potential of small congenital nevocellular nevi. *J Am Acad Dermatol* 6:230, 1982.

204. Greene MH, Clark WH, Tucker MA, et al: Acquired precursors of cutaneous malignant melanoma. The familial dysplastic nevus syndrome. *N Engl J Med* 312:91, 1985.

205. Kopf AW, Goldman RJ, Rivers JK, et al: Skin types in dysplastic nevus syndrome. *J Dermatol Surg Oncol* 14:827, 1988.

206. Clark WH, Reimer RR, Greene M, et al: Origin of familial malignant melanomas from heritable melanocytic lesions: The B-K mole syndrome. *Arch Dermatol* 114:732, 1978.

207. Greene MH, Clark WH, Tucker MA, et al: Melanoma risk in familial dysplastic nevus syndrome. *J Invest Dermatol* 82:424, 1984.

208. Elder DE, Goldman LI, Goldman SC, et al: Dysplastic nevus syndrome: A phenotypic association of sporadic cutaneous melanoma. *Cancer* 46:1787, 1980.

209. Mackie RM: Multiple melanoma and atypical melanocytic nevi—evidence of an activated and expanded melanocytic system. *Br J Dermatol* 107:621, 1982.

210. Roush GC, Nordlund JJ, Forget B, et al: Independence of dysplastic nevi from total nevi in determining risk for nonfamilial melanoma. *Prev Med* 17:273, 1988.

211. Rigel DS, Rivers DK, Kopf AW, et al: Dysplastic nevi. Markers for increased risk for melanoma. *Cancer* 63:389, 1989.

212. Mackie RM: Which moles matter. The association between melanocytic nevi and malignant melanomata. *Br J Dermatol* 105:607, 1981.

213. Davis J, Pack GT, Higgins GK: Melanotic freckle of Hutchinson. *Am J Surg* 113:457, 1967.

214. Day CL, Mihm MC, Lew RE, et al: Cutaneous malignant melanoma: Prognostic guidelines for physicians and patients. *CA* 32:113, 1982.

215. Maize JC: Primary cutaneous malignant melanoma: An analysis of the prognostic value of histologic characteristics. *J Am Acad Dermatol* 8:857, 1983.

216. Iscoe N, Kersey P, Gapski J, et al: Predictive value of staging investigations in patients with clinical stage I malignant melanoma. *Plast Reconstr Surg* 80:233, 1987.

217. Day CL, Sober AJ, Lew RA: Malignant melanoma patients with positive nodes and relatively good prognoses. *Cancer* 47:955, 1981.

218. Breslow A: Thickness, cross-sectioned areas and depth of invasion in the prognosis of cutaneous melanoma. *Ann Surg* 172:902, 1970.

219. Wanebo HJ, Cooper PH, Young DV, et al: Prognostic factors in head and neck melanoma. Effect of lesion location. *Cancer* 62:831, 1988.

220. Davidson T, Kissin M, Westburg G: Vulvo-vaginal melanoma—should radical surgery be abandoned? *Br J Obstet Gynaecol* 94:473, 1987.

221. Ward MW, Romano G, Nicholls RJ: The surgical treatment of anorectal malignant melanoma. *Br J Surg* 73:68, 1986.

222. Weinstock MA, Morris BT, Lederman JS, et al: Effect of BANS location on the prognosis of clinical stage I melanoma: New data and meta-analysis. *Br J Dermatol* 119:559, 1988.

223. Day CL, Harrist TJ, Gorstein F, et al: Malignant melanoma. Prognostic significance of "microscopic satellites" in the reticular dermis and subcutaneous fat. *Ann Surg* 194:108, 1981.

224. Harrist TJ, Rigel DS, Day CL, et al: "Microscopic satellites" are more highly associated with regional lymph node metas-

tases than is primary melanoma thickness. *Cancer* 53:2183, 1984.

225. Kelly JN, Sagebiel RW, Blois MS: Regression in malignant melanoma. A histologic feature without independent prognostic significance. *Cancer* 56:2287, 1985.

226. Slingluff CL, Vollmor RT, Reintgen DS, et al: Lethal "thin" melanoma. Identifying patients at risk. *Ann Surg* 208:150, 1988.

227. Cascinelli N, van der Esch EP, Breslow A, et al: Stage I melanoma of the skin: The problems of resection margins. *Eur J Cancer* 16:1079, 1980.

228. Bagley FH, Cady B, Lee A, et al: Changes in clinical presentation and management of malignant melanoma. *Cancer* 47:2126, 1981.

229. Zeitels J, LaRossa D, Hamilton R, et al: A comparison of local recurrence and resection margins for stage I primary cutaneous malignant melanomas. *Plast Reconstr Surg* 81:688, 1988.

230. Schmoeckel C, Bockelbrink A, Bockelbrink H, et al: Is wide excision necessary in malignant melanoma? *J Invest Dermatol* 76:424, 1981.

231. Day CL, Lew RA: Malignant melanoma prognostic factors III: Surgical margins. *J Dermatol Surg Oncol* 9:797, 1983.

232. Day CL, Mihm MC, Sober AJ, et al: Narrower margins for clinical stage I malignant melanoma. *N Engl J Med* 306:479, 1982.

233. Breslow A: The surgical treatment of stage I cutaneous melanoma. *Cancer Treat Rev* 5:195, 1979.

234. Balch CM, Munrad TM, Soong S, et al: Tumor thickness as a guide to surgical management of clinical stage I melanoma patients. *Cancer* 43:883, 1979.

235. Veronesi U, Cascinelli N, Adamus J, et al: Thin stage I primary cutaneous malignant melanoma. Comparison of excision with margins of 1 or 3 cm. *N Engl J Med* 318:1159, 1988.

236. Karakousis C, More R, Holyoke E: Surgery in recurrent malignant melanoma. *Cancer* 52:1343, 1983.

237. Overett TK, Shiu MH: Surgical treatment of distant metastatic melanoma. Indications and results. *Cancer* 56:1222, 1985.

238. Day CL, Lew RA, Mihm MC, et al: A multivariate analysis of prognostic factors for melanoma patients with lesions 3.65 millimeters in thickness. *Ann Surg* 195:44, 1982.

239. Day CL, Mihm MC, Lew RA, et al: Prognostic factors for patients with clinical stage I melanoma of intermediate thickness (1.51–3.99 millimeters). *Ann Surg* 195:35, 1982.

240. Veronesi U, Adamus J, Bandiera DC, et al: Inefficacy of immediate node dissection in stage I melanoma of the limbs. *N Engl J Med* 297:627, 1977.

241. Elder DE, Guerry D, Van Horn M, et al: The role of lymph node dissection for clinical stage I malignant melanoma of intermediate thickness (1.51–3.99 mm). *Cancer* 56:413, 1985.

242. Balch CM, Soong S, Murad T, et al: A multifactorial analysis of melanoma. II. Prognostic factors in patients with stage I (localized) melanoma. *Surgery* 86:343, 1979.

243. Sim FH, Taylor WF, Pritchard DJ, et al: Lymphadenectomy in the management of stage I malignant melanoma: A prospective randomized study. *Surg Gynecol Obstet* 161:575, 1985.

244. Sim FH, Taylor WF, Pritchard DJ, et al: Lymphadenopathy in management of stage I malignant melanoma: A prospective randomized study. *Mayo Clin Proc* 61:697, 1986.

245. Balch CM: The role of elective lymph node dissection in melanoma: Rationale, results and controversies. *J Clin Oncol* 6:163, 1988.

246. Eberback MA, Wahl RL, Argenta LC, et al: Utility of lymphoscintigraphy in directing surgical therapy for melanomas of the head, neck, and upper thorax. *Surgery* 102:433, 1987.

247. Ghussen F, Krüger I, Groth W, et al: The role of regional hyperthermic cytostatic perfusion in the treatment of extremity melanoma. *Cancer* 61:654, 1988.

248. Cumberlin R, DeMoss E, Lassus M, et al: Isolation perfusion for malignant melanoma of the extremity. *J Clin Oncol* 3:1022, 1985.

249. Baas PC, Hoekstra HJ, Koops HS, et al: Hyperthermic isolated regional perfusion in the treatment of extremity melanoma in children and adolescents. *Cancer* 63:199, 1989.

250. Franklin HR, Koops HS, Oldhoff J, et al: To perfuse or not to perfuse? A retrospective comparative study to evaluate the effect of adjuvant isolated regional perfusion in patients with clinical stage I extremity melanoma with a thickness of 1.5 mm or greater. *J Clin Oncol* 6:701, 1988.

251. Legha SS: Current therapy for malignant melanoma. *Semin Oncol* 16(S1):34, 1989.

252. Sweren RJ: Management of congenital nevocytic nevi: A survey of current practices. *J Am Acad Dermatol* 11:629, 1984.

253. Rhodes AR, Wood WC, Sober AJ, et al: Nonepidermal origin of malignant melanoma associated with a giant congenital nevocellular nevus. *Plast Reconstr Surg* 67:782, 1981.

18

Benign Skin Tumors— Clinical Aspects

Vincent Voci, M.D., and Nicholas G. Georgiade, M.D., F.A.C.S.

Benign skin lesions have many varied characteristics as to size, shape, and color differentiation. This chapter describes the variance of these benign tumors and deals primarily with clinical characteristics. The following chapter describes the histopathology of these skin tumors.

Epidermal Appendage Tumors

Lever and Schaumburg-Lever (1) have classified epidermal appendage tumors into four groups according to their type of differentiation: hair, sebaceous, apocrine, and eccrine. These four groups are subdivided into degrees of differentiation: hyperplasia, adenoma, benign epithelioma, and basal cell epithelioma. The most mature are well-differentiated tumors, the hyperplasia and nevi, and the least differentiated are basal cell epitheliomas, often considered malignant.

HYPERPLASIA

Organoid Nevus (Nevus Sebaceous)

The term "organoid nevus" has been applied to this true nevus because it involves the entire skin organ and more than one skin adnexa. The most common site is the scalp, but the face and neck, and rarely the trunk or extremities, may be involved. Mehregan and Pinkus (2) have outlined the natural history of an organoid nevus into three stages.

The first-stage lesion is usually present at birth as a hairless area composed of papillomatous hyperplasia of the epidermis with loss of hair follicles. A second stage develops at puberty with tremendous hyperplasia of sebaceous glands and, occasionally, apocrine sweat glands. It is this character that gave the lesion its name: nevus sebaceous of Jadassohn. The lesion usually has a yellowish cobblestone appearance (Fig. 18.1). A third stage, much later in life, occurs in perhaps 10–20% of cases in which the nevus sebaceous evolves into a benign skin

appendage tumor or a basal cell epithelioma (3). Complete excision before puberty is recommended.

Sebaceous Hyperplasia

The lesion of sebaceous hyperplasia is a small, yellowish, slightly raised nodule that appears on the face, chiefly the forehead, in older individuals. It is composed of enlarged, tightly grouped sebaceous gland lobes. Similar lesions representing ectopic sebaceous glands commonly appear at the vermilion edge in the same group of individuals (4). Treatment consists of excisional biopsy.

ADENOMAS

Sebaceous Adenoma

True sebaceous adenomas are rare. They appear as solitary or multiple lesions. Solitary sebaceous adenomas usually present as small, smooth, slightly pedunculated nodules on the face or scalp in older individuals. Histologically, they consist of lobules of mature sebaceous glands with basaloid cells and germinative cells. Multiple sebaceous adenomas have been associated with multiple visceral carcinomas (5). Excisional biopsy is recommended.

Trichofolliculoma

The trichofolliculoma usually appears as a solitary skin-colored, well-demarcated, dome-shaped nodule on the face of an adult. Many of these lesions have a central pore with woolly white hairs emerging. Histologically, there is a larger, immature central follicle with many surrounding aborted follicles. Treatment consists of simple excision.

SYRINGOMA

Syringomas ordinarily occur in women during puberty or adolescence. They are usually multiple and occur most

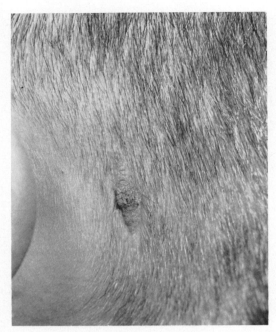

FIGURE 18.1.   An organoid nevus (nevus sebaceous) is shown in the second stage.

often on the lower eyelids but may occur anywhere on the face, neck, or anterior chest. Syringomas appear as small (usually less than 3 mm), firm nodules that are either skin-colored or slightly yellow (Fig. 18.2). Histologically, they consist of multiple small cystic ducts that histochemically resemble eccrine ducts (6). They often increase in size and number during pregnancy and with administration of estrogen. Treatment is necessary only for appearance and may consist of excision or electrical or laser destruction.

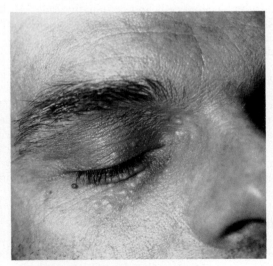

FIGURE 18.2.   Syringomas of face are shown.

BENIGN EPITHELIOMAS

Trichoepitheliomas

Multiple trichoepitheliomas are inherited as an autosomal dominant trait (7). Generally, they are first noticed in adolescence and increase in size and numbers during adult life. These lesions are firm, skin-colored nodules measuring 2–6 mm in diameter, and they sometimes coalesce. Larger lesions may have overlying telangiectasia. The most common location is centrally around the nose, along the nasolabial folds, and over the upper lip. Clinically, they may resemble syringomas, the lesions of the basal cell nevoid syndrome (8), and neurofibromas (Fig. 18.3). Solitary trichoepitheliomas are similar in appearance and location, occur in adulthood, and are not inherited.

Histologically, solitary and multiple trichoepitheliomas resemble basal cell epitheliomas with solid epithelial nests. These nests characteristically have keratinizing centers with multiple immature aborted hair follicles and cysts. Histological differentiation from basal cell epitheliomas may be difficult, and the diagnosis may have to be made on clinical grounds. The trichoepithelioma rarely ulcerates, and when multiple they have a characteristic distribution centrally on the face, unlike the lesions in basal cell nevus syndrome, which may occur anywhere. Treatment of solitary trichoepitheliomas consists of complete excision and pathological examination. Treatment of multiple trichoepitheliomas for cosmetic reasons is very difficult because of their extent and propensity for recurrence.

Calcifying Epithelioma of Malherbe

The calcifying epithelioma of Malherbe was originally described by Malherbe and Chenantais (9) as a tumor of sebaceous gland origin. Forbis and Helwig (10), however, suggested that the term "pilomatrixoma" was more appropriate because these epitheliomas differentiate in the direction of the germinating matrix of hair follicles rather than sebaceous glands. The lesion occurs as a solitary, firm nodule in the deep dermis of the face, neck, or upper extremity. Onset is usually in the first or second decade. They may be less than 1 cm in diameter or grow as large as 4–5 cm. The overlying epidermis appears normal, as with an epidermal cyst. The nodule is often surrounded by a capsule that may extend into the subcutaneous fat (Fig. 18.4).

Histologically, there are three types of cells in this entity. Compact basaloid cells surround a layer of more mature transitional cells that eventually lose their nuclei and appear as "shadow cells" in the central portion of the nodule. Shadow cells are so called because only an unstained area or "shadow" of the cell's original nucleus remains. As the tumor ages, there are more shadow cells and fewer basaloid cells. Foci of calcification sometimes occur in the cytoplasm of the shadow cells. Ossification surrounding these lesions may occur but is uncommon. Treatment consists of surgical excision.

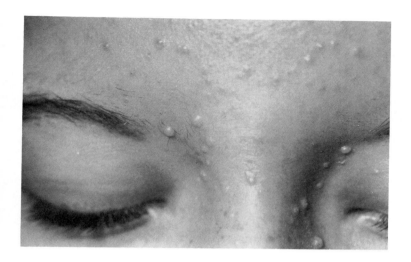

FIGURE 18.3. Multiple trichoepitheliomas, an autosomal dominant inheritance, are shown involving skin of forehead, eyelid, and nasal areas.

Cylindroma

These tumors occur in solitary and multiple forms (11). Most evidence now suggests that their differentiation is toward eccrine glands. Multiple lesions occur as an autosomal dominant inherited trait, usually in females at a young age. Most common in the scalp, they often cover the entire scalp, and in such cases have been given the name "turban tumors" (Fig. 18.5). The nodules are round or lobulated, firm, and pink. When they occur as solitary lesions, they are not inherited, and they may occur on the face or scalp, usually later in adulthood. Histologically, numerous epithelial islands are seen in the dermis, outlined by hyaline sheaths fitting together in a pattern like a jigsaw puzzle. Occasionally, hyaline droplets are also seen. Complete excision is the only treatment recommended.

ECCRINE POROMA

First described by Pinkus et al. in 1956 (12), eccrine poromas are usually solitary lesions but can be multiple. They are fairly common and often appear on the plantar surface of the foot, but they may also appear on the palmar surface of the hand and fingers and, less commonly, in other areas of the body. Adulthood is the typical time of appearance. Clinically, they may have a vascular presentation similar to pyogenic granuloma, but they usually are skin-colored and easily confused with nevi, dermatofibromas, and neurofibromas. They may be sessile or slightly pedunculated.

Typically, on histological section, the tumor lies in both the epidermis and dermis. Occasionally, it may be completely intraepidermal or intradermal. Large amounts of glycogen are usually present within the epithelial cells, and narrow ductal lumina are very common. The cell of origin is probably the intraepidermal eccrine sweat gland. Malignant eccrine poromas have been reported but are rare (13). Treatment consists of complete surgical excision.

Clear Cell Hydradenoma

These benign epitheliomas have been known by many different names, including clear cell myoepithelioma, solid cystic myoepithelioma, nodular hydradenoma, eccrine sweat gland adenoma, and eccrine acrospiroma. They most commonly occur in adults anywhere in the skin as an intradermal skin-colored or bluish nodule and are frequently 1–2 cm in diameter. Histologically, there are multiple lumina and cystic spaces interspersed in

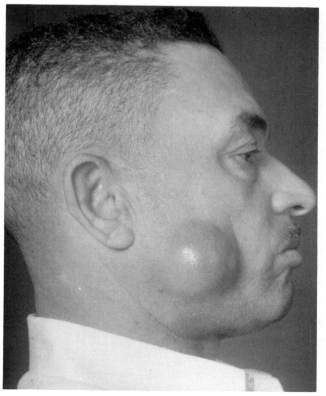

FIGURE 18.4. A calcifying epithelioma of Malherbe of the cheek.

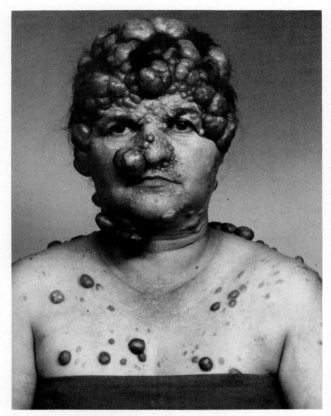

FIGURE 18.5. "Turban" tumors of face and scalp.

ceous duct, or entrapment embryologically along fusion lines. In the latter instance, they are called dermoid cysts and are noted at birth or in early childhood. Traumatic displacement of epidermal cells is uncommon; most epidermal cysts are the result of occluded pilosebaceous units. These cysts occur most commonly on the face, neck, and trunk as a round, dermal or subcutaneous, firm or fluctuant mass, often with a visible umbilicated punctum that represents the occluded follicle. If the cyst ruptures into the dermis, the cheesy contents stimulate an intense foreign body inflammatory reaction. The cysts may also become secondarily infected. In either case, the wall may be partially or completely destroyed. Malignant degeneration is rare (Figs. 18.6 and 18.7).

Histologically, the cyst wall is composed of true epidermal cells with intercellular bridges. The cyst contains laminated keratinous (horny) material. Electron microscopy reveals that differentiation of the epidermal cells in the cyst wall is identical to surface epidermis and the infundibulum of hair follicles (1). Treatment consists of excision with care to remove the entire cyst wall to prevent recurrence. Destruction of a cyst wall by curettage or electrodesiccation is less reliable. When infected, the cyst must be incised and drained. At that time, an attempt may be made to destroy the cyst wall that the infection has not already obliterated. A cyst that is merely inflamed secondary to rupture into the dermis may be observed until cessation of the inflammatory response or treated prophylactically with antibiotics.

lobules with sheets or epithelial cells, many of which are clear cells. Differentiation is toward the eccrine sweat gland. Malignant clear cell hydradenomas are rare but do occur (1). Treatment is complete excision with pathological examination.

ECCRINE SPIRADENOMA

Eccrine spiradenoma usually occurs in young adults as a solitary tumor anywhere on the body (14). It presents as a tender, sometimes painful, firm, small nodule that is skin-colored or slightly bluish. Microscopically, it appears in the deep dermis. There are two cell types: large compact pale cells form cords in line tubules, while smaller basophilic cells are situated in the periphery. Differentiation is toward ductal and secretory elements of eccrine sweat glands. Rare malignant eccrine spiradenomas have been reported (15). Recommended treatment is complete surgical excision and pathological examination.

Cysts of the Epidermis

EPIDERMAL CYST

This is the most common of the epidermal cysts. These cysts may occur at any time in adolescence or adulthood. They are the result of epidermal cells being trapped in the dermis secondary to trauma, occlusion of a piloseba-

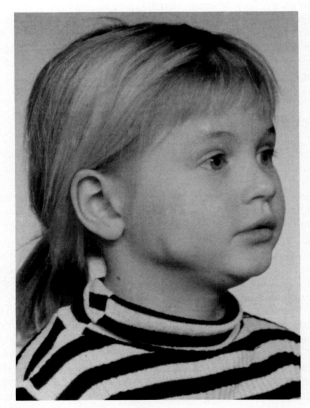

FIGURE 18.6. A single epidermal cyst of the right cheek in a 5-year-old girl.

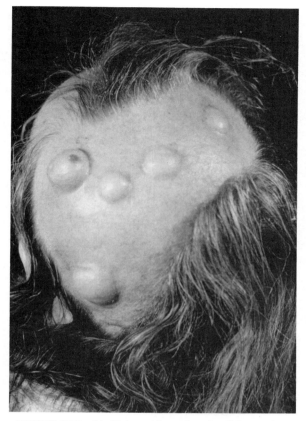

FIGURE 18.7.   Multiple epidermal cysts of the scalp.

PILAR CYST

Occurring most commonly on the scalp (90%), pilar cysts may also present on the face, neck, and trunk (1). Grossly, they are almost identical to epidermal cysts but occur only one tenth as frequently (16). The cyst contents are less solid than epidermal cysts, but they behave in a similar fashion. Malignant degeneration is again very rare. Histologically, pilar cysts are different from epidermal cysts in that the epithelial lining shows no intercellular bridges, and there is no flattening of the innermost cells. In fact, the cells become bulkier and paler as they approach the lumen. They eventually lose their nuclei and fall into the central amorphous nonlaminated keratinous material. A dense basement membrane allows the cell to be easily shelled out.

Initially, pilar cysts were called sebaceous cysts. Then, in 1969, Pinkus (17) showed that these cysts originate from the outer root sheath (trichilemma) of the hair follicle. Thus, "pilar cyst" or "trichilemmal cyst" are more appropriate names. The same treatment is recommended for these lesions as for epidermal cysts.

MILIA

These are very common epidermal cysts that occur de novo, most commonly on the face. Milia may also occur as retention cysts secondary to insults such as burns or bullous eruptions anywhere on the body. They occur as

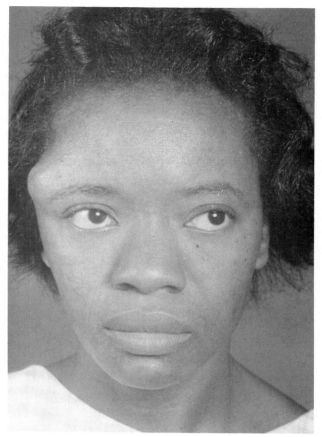

FIGURE 18.8.   A large dermoid cyst at the right frontotemporal suture line.

1–2-mm, very superficial, white, smooth papules. Histologically, they are similar to epidermal cysts. Treatment consists of simply unroofing the cyst.

DERMOID CYST

Dermoid cysts of the skin occur secondary to sequestration of epidermis along lines of embryological fusion. They resemble epidermal cysts and occur most frequently on the head and neck along the lateral brow (Fig. 18.8) and in the midline at the nasal radix. They are situated in the subcutaneous tissue and may adhere to the periosteum. In the nasofrontal region, they may occasionally extend through the bone to the meninges. The cysts usually contain keratin debris and skin appendages. On occasion, bone, teeth, cartilage, and nerve tissue may be present (18, 19). Excision is indicated to prevent secondary infection. Care must be taken to evaluate the depth of the cyst preoperatively.

Mesodermal Skin Tumors

DERMATOFIBROMA

There are very common skin nodules appearing frequently on the extremities, especially the legs, in young and middle-aged women. Approximately 20% of patients

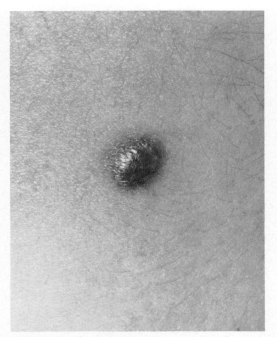

FIGURE 18.9. A dermatofibroma, well circumscribed and slightly raised, is shown.

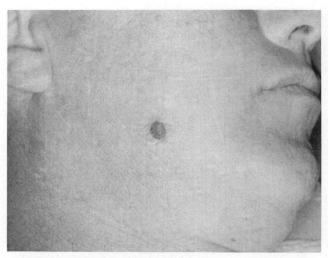

FIGURE 18.10. A squamous papilloma of the right cheek.

can give a history of minor trauma such as an insect bite or small puncture wound (20). Although dermatofibromas are usually solitary, multiple lesions are not uncommon. Typically, a dermatofibroma is a firm, slightly raised, dome-shaped nodule, 1 cm or less in diameter, and brownish-red in color: it may also be yellowish or black. It remains unchanged for many years (Fig. 18.9). Microscopically, there is a cellular type with fibroblasts and histiocytes in varying degrees and a fibrous type with large amounts of collagen. Excision is recommended for biopsy or for cosmetic reasons.

ACROCHORDON (SKIN TAG)

These very common skin lesions occur in two forms. The more common form presents as multiple delicate filiform or pedunculated papular lesions about the face and neck, axilla, and upper chest in middle-aged women (Fig. 18.10). They are usually skin-colored or more darkly pigmented and are usually asymptomatic unless irritated. Less commonly, they occur as large, solitary, soft, plump, pedunculated growths on the extremities or trunk. The filiform lesions histologically are composed of hyperplastic epidermis with loose dermal connective tissue in a stalk. The larger solitary soft fibromas will often have adipose tissue in the central portion. Treatment of the smaller lesion may consist of electrodesiccation or snip excision. Larger lesions can be removed sharply at the surface of normal skin, treating the base with cautery or silver nitrate for hemostasis.

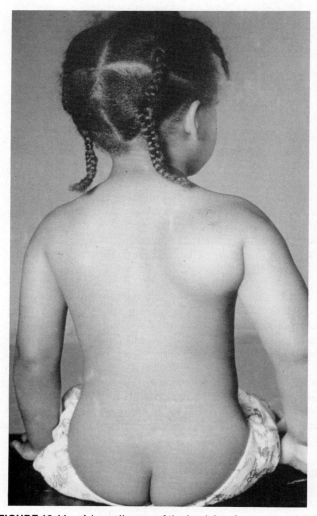

FIGURE 18.11. A large lipoma of the back in a four-year-old girl is shown.

LIPOMA

Lipomas are very common benign adipose tissue tumors of the subcutaneous tissue and may also occur in intramuscular septae and in the thoracic and abdominal cavities. Most are solitary and occur in women. They are usually asymptomatic and are most commonly seen over the posterior neck, trunk, forearms, and buttocks (Fig. 18.11). By contrast, multiple lipomatosis is an inherited condition usually seen in men. It is inherited as an autosomal dominant trait. Multiple lipomas are symmetrically located on the trunk and extremities in most cases. Angiolipomas are a less common variant. They are more vascular, firmer, and usually painful. Otherwise, they are similar to the more common lipoma. Solitary and multiple lipomas have the same histological appearance. They are encapsulated, probably by condensed surrounding connective tissue, and consist of mature adipose tissue. Liposarcomas are very rare in the subcutaneous tissue and do not arise in lipomas. However, liposarcoma may invade subcutaneous tissue from intramuscular locations. Excision is performed for cosmetic or functional reasons.

XANTHOMATOUS TUMORS—XANTHOMA, TUBEROUS XANTHOMA, XANTHELASMA

These terms describe the formation of foam cells in skin lesions caused by an accumulation of an excess of lipids in the body owing to the disturbance of lipid metabolism (Figs. 18.12 and 18.13).

ATYPICAL FIBROXANTHOMA

This interesting common cutaneous lesion (21) is benign, but on histological examination it appears malignant. It most commonly occurs on the face or sun-exposed areas of individuals with light complexions, usually

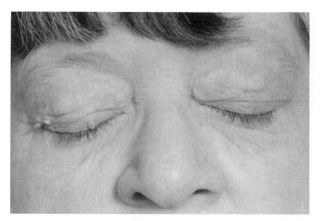

FIGURE 18.13. Extensive xanthomatous plaques of the eyelids.

older men. Irradiated skin has a higher incidence of this lesion as well. It usually consists of a 1–2-cm, soft or firm nodule in the skin, resembling a pyogenic granuloma or basal cell epithelioma. Histologically, there are a number of pleomorphic and atypical bizarre histiocytes, often with mitotic figures. The histological appearance resembles a fibrosarcoma, except that it is present in the dermis and fibrosarcomas more commonly occur in the deep subcutaneous tissues or fascia. Rarely, an atypical fibroxanthoma may metastasize. Complete surgical excision is recommended.

Vascular Tissue Tumors

HEMANGIOMAS

These mesodermal vascular lesions are usually divided into three main groups: *Nevus flammeus* (*port-wine stain*) (Fig. 18.14) is a flat, irregular, pink to dark reddish-blue pigmented lesion and may cover large areas of the body. This lesion can be associated with the Sturge-Weber syndrome. *Capillary hemangioma,* usually bright red in appearance and slightly raised, may be diffusely distributed or isolated to a distinct lesion (Fig. 18.15). It is the most common of the hemangiomata. *Cavernous hemangioma* has the longest subcutaneous collection of vascular spaces. It may attain a large size over a period of months, followed by gradual regression (Fig. 18.16). In unusual instances, a coagulopathy with thrombocytopenia may occur (Kasabach-Merritt syndrome).

PYOGENIC GRANULOMA

This lesion simulates a vascular tumor; however, it is probably a response to an inflammatory process with many vessels and usually one larger "feeder" vessel. It can be treated with extensive cautery or excision (Fig. 18.17).

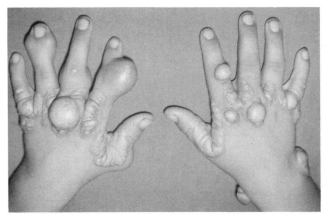

FIGURE 18.12. Extensive xanthomatous nodules of the hands.

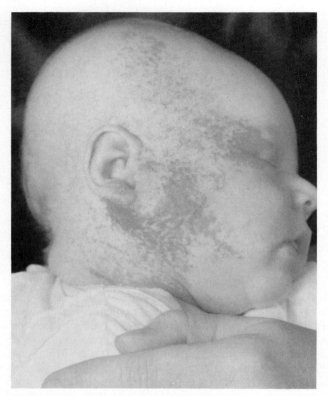

FIGURE 18.14. A extensive nevus flammeus (port-wine stain)

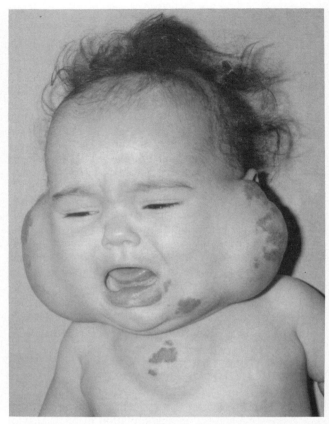

FIGURE 18.16. An extensive bilateral cavernous hemangioma in a 3-month-old infant.

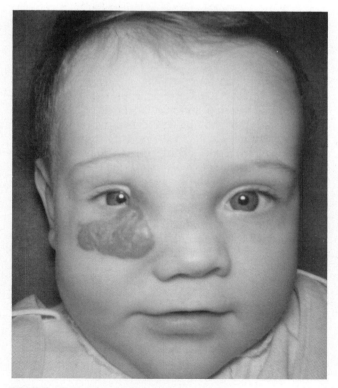

FIGURE 18.15. A capillary (strawberry) hemangioma involving a large area of the cheek.

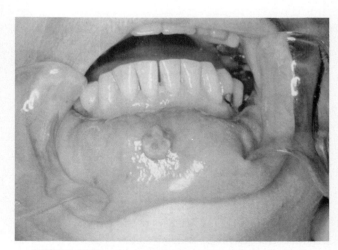

FIGURE 18.17. A pyogenic granuloma of the lower lip.

Tumors of Neural Tissue

NEUROFIBROMA

These may occur as solitary benign lesions or as multiple lesions in neurofibromatosis or von Recklinghausen's disease (22; Fig. 18.18). The latter is an autosomal dominant inherited syndrome of multiple cutaneous neurofibromas arising late in childhood. Of significance in the syndrome are extracutaneous neurofibromas in bone and in cranial, spinal root, and peripheral nerves. In addition, there is a 10% incidence of pheochromocytoma. Café au lait spots may herald von Recklinghausen's disease in early childhood before the appearance of the neurofibromas. There must be at least six or more café au lait spots greater than 1.5 cm in diameter in order to make the diagnosis of von Recklinghausen's disease on this basis.

The cutaneous neurofibroma is usually a globular or pedunculated growth that can vary in size (Fig. 18.19). It is usually skin colored or slightly bluish. Solitary and multiple neurofibromas have a similar appearance clinically and histologically. Microscopically, the tumors are sharply demarcated but not encapsulated in the dermis; they sometimes extend into the subcutaneous fat. There is a delicate network of loose, wavy fibers that consist of nerve and collagen. Electron microscopy has determined that the Schwann cell is the chief constituent of the neurofibroma. Malignant degeneration can occur but is uncommon (23). Excision for diagnostic, cosmetic, or functional reasons may be indicated.

NEUROLEMMOMA

A benign neural sheath tumor arising from cranial sympathetic, or peripheral nerves, the neurolemmoma is most often seen on the head and neck (Fig. 18.20), especially involving the vestibular branch of the acoustic nerve (24). Peripheral nerves in the extremities are also commonly involved, but neurolemmomas of the skin are not very common. Histologically, elongated nuclei and spindle-shaped cells are arranged in a streaming pattern with gaps called Verocay bodies between palisading rows of spindle cells. Enucleation of the neurolemmoma from the nerve with preservation of the nerve is the treatment of choice.

GRANULAR CELL MYOBLASTOMA

Although granular cell myoblastoma was originally thought to be derived from muscle, most authors now agree that the tumor consists of Schwann cells. It most commonly occurs in the tongue (40% of cases), skin, and subcutaneous tissue as a solitary tumor. Lesions arising in the dermis are usually discrete, firm nodules less than 2 cm in diameter, slightly raised, and nontender but sometimes painful. Approximately 8% are multiple, and 3% are malignant (25). Microscopically, they are composed of large pale cells with numerous characteristic granules. They appear to infiltrate muscle or collagen fibers. Complete surgical excision is indicated.

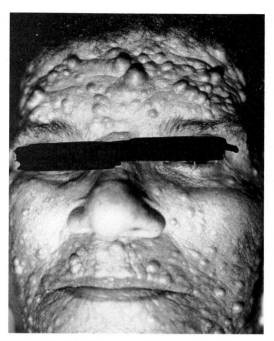

FIGURE 18.18. Multiple neurofibromas involving extensive areas of the scalp and face in von Recklinghausen's disease.

Tumors of the Epidermis

KERATOACANTHOMA

This is a benign but invasive squamous cell tumor that is self-limited and results in an atrophic scar. It resembles a squamous cell carcinoma (SCC) in both its clinical and its microscopic appearance. Clinically, the keratoacanthoma is a well-circumscribed, round, firm, pink or skin-colored bulging nodule with a constricted base and an umbilicated center. The center is usually filled with a keratinous plug covered with crust (Fig. 18.21). The clinical history differs from SCC in that it appears abruptly in previously normal skin. Growth is rapid over 4–8 weeks. This rapid period of growth is usually followed by an 8-week latency period, finally resulting in an 8-week period of regression. The typical keratoacanthoma is only 1.0–1.5 cm in diameter, but it will occasionally attain a much larger size.

The histopathological differentiation of keratoacanthoma and squamous cell carcinoma can be very difficult. The architecture of the entire lesion is very important in making the diagnosis. Biopsy, if it cannot be excisional, must contain at least the edge on both sides, the base, and the central portion of the nodule. In the early lesion, there is a horn-filled invagination of epidermis centrally. In the base, there are usually many atypical cells with mitoses resembling SCC, but there is often a high degree of keratinization that is more typical of the keratoacanthoma. The clinical history of abrupt onset and rapid growth may help the pathologist make the final differentiation between SCC and keratoacanthoma. The more mature keratoacanthomas are sometimes more easily distinguished from SCCs than the early lesions. The central portion of a mature keratoacanthoma is a center filled

FIGURE 18.19. An extensive pedunculated neurofibroma involving the face and neck.

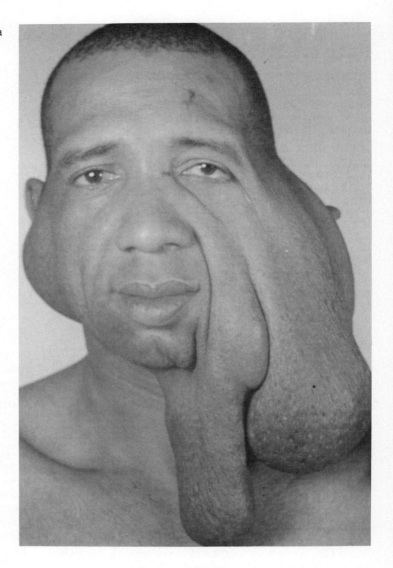

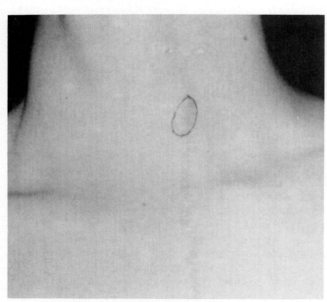

FIGURE 18.20. A small neurolemmoma in the neck skin.

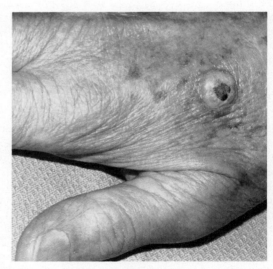

FIGURE 18.21. A keratoacanthoma of the hand is shown. Note the resemblance to a squamous cell carcinoma.

with a keratin plug, and there are few atypical cells at the base and more advanced keratinization. The rolled epidermal edge around the crater is also very characteristic.

Solitary, multiple, and eruptive keratoacanthomas exist as three related but different entities. The solitary are common; the multiple very uncommon; and the eruptive keratoacanthomas are rare. The average ratio of solitary keratoacanthomas to SCCs is approximately 1:4, although estimates of this ratio vary widely.

Solitary keratoacanthomas arise in older Caucasians. They are three times more common in males than in females, and they occur most frequently on exposed skin, namely, the central face and dorsal surface of the hands and forearms. Multiple and eruptive keratoacanthomas are more widely distributed over the body and occur in younger individuals. The eruptive lesions are usually much smaller than the solitary and multiple ones. The multiple form (Ferguson Smith syndrome) may be inherited (22).

The treatment of keratoacanthoma is tempered somewhat by the self-limiting history, but there are several excellent reasons to excise these lesions early. It is often difficult to differentiate keratoacanthomas from SCC without an excisional biopsy. In addition, one cannot predict how much larger the lesions will become before involution if it is, in fact, a keratoacanthoma. Also, the linear scar after excision is almost always preferable to the round, atrophic scar that results from spontaneous resolution.

SEBORRHEIC KERATOSIS

As the most common skin tumors in older individuals, these benign, keratotic lesions do not evolve into malignant lesions. Seborrheic keratoses are usually multiple and may be present in large numbers in some individuals. Sun exposure, chronic irritation, and heredity may be etiological and developmental factors. The trunk, face, scalp, and proximal extremities are the most common locations. Early lesions are flat, discrete, and light brown with a velvety texture. They often grow to several centimeters in diameter and become darker and thicker, with a waxy scale. Classically, the lesions appear as though they could be picked off the skin easily. Crusting and induration may occur if they become irritated (Fig. 18.22).

Histologically, the seborrheic keratosis is characterized by hyperkeratosis, acanthosis, and papillomatosis to varying degrees in different lesions. Horn cysts are characteristic, as is the appearance of the tumor lying on top of normal skin. Treatment of seborrheic keratoses consists of removal either with a curette and cauterization of the base, or with the application of liquid nitrogen. The cosmetic result is usually excellent because they are very superficial lesions. Excisional biopsy is indicated if the diagnosis is uncertain.

Dermatosis papulosa nigra is very similar to seborrheic keratosis histopathologically, but the two differ clinically. Dermatosis papulosa nigra is much smaller, more hyperpigmented, and papular. It occurs in 35% of black people, beginning in adolescence (26). It usually is multi-

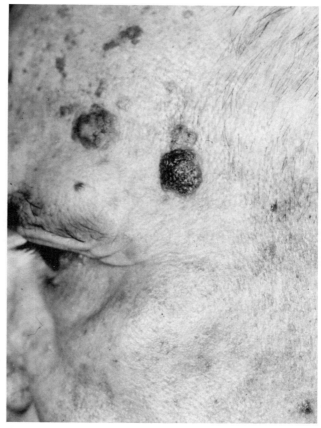

FIGURE 18.22. Multiple raised, brown lesions of the skin typical of seborrheic keratoses.

ple and occurs predominantly on the face, especially over the cheek in zygomatic areas.

ACTINIC KERATOSIS (SOLAR)

Actinic keratoses are the most common premalignant skin tumors, and 20–25% eventually develop into SCCs (16). They are usually multiple and occur in sun-exposed skin such as the bald scalp, face, ears, and dorsum of the hands in older individuals with fair complexions. Actinic cheilitis is the counterpart on the lower lip. Actinic keratoses are usually 1 cm or less in diameter. They are usually erythematous and rough, and sometimes scaly and crusted (Fig. 18.23). Indications of malignancy include thickening, ulceration, and rapid growth alone or in combination.

Histologically, actinic keratosis is characterized by hyperkeratosis and parakeratosis. There are often atypical epidermal cells proliferating into the superficial dermis. Transformation into SCC is characterized by deeper penetration and breaking away of these cells with increased growth. Electrodesiccation and curettage and cryotherapy with liquid nitrogen are satisfactory methods of treatment. For wide areas of involvement, 5-fluorouracil cream is more appropriate. If there is doubt concerning the possibility of an invasive SCC, then incisional or excisional biopsy should be pursued.

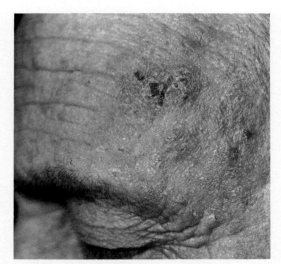

FIGURE 18.23. Actinic keratosis characterized by scaly, encrusted lesions and skin pigmentary changes.

Pigmented Skin Lesions

Pigmented skin lesions represent one of the most common skin disorders seen by the plastic surgeon. The term "nevus" is often misunderstood and misused. Before the actual nevus cell was identified, the term "nevus" was used to describe any pigmented "mole" or tumor. In 1980, Masson (27) defined nevi as "cutaneous malformations in which all the constituents of the integumentum may take part." Nevus sebaceous consists of a localized excess of sebaceous glands and thus satisfies such a definition. Unlike the melanocyte, the nevus cell is an abnormal component of skin; therefore, the common nevus-cell nevus, or "mole," is actually a benign neoplasm, not a malformation or nevus. Although this paradox of terms is confusing, we shall continue to refer to the nevus-cell nevus by that name because of its widespread use.

Another common misunderstanding is the difference between the nevus cell and the melanocyte. Both epidermal and dermal melanocytes are derivatives of the prenatal neuroectodermal melanoblast and are normal constituents of skin. Epidermal melanocytes are responsible for freckles (ephelides) and pigmented macular lesions of the lip. These are true malformations or nevi. Epidermal melanocytes also give rise to lentigo senilis and lentigo maligna, which are true neoplasms. Dermal melanocytes are responsible for the blue nevus, nevus of Ota, and the mongolian spot. These can be considered malformations or nevi (28).

NEVUS-CELL NEVUS

The average American has 15 nevus-cell nevi (29). This very common benign pigmented skin tumor is composed of nevus cells derived from the neuroectoderm. One theory (30) suggests that they are derived from nevoblast stem cells, in contrast to an earlier theory by Masson (27), who postulated that the nevus cell in the epidermis was derived from epidermal melanocytes and those in the

dermis from Schwann cells. Nevus cells differ from melanocytes in that they are round, usually nondendritic, and form nests. Melanocytes are fusiform and dendritic and are usually solitary. Nevus-cell nevi can be divided into junctional nevi, compound nevi, and intradermal nevi. Variants include: (*a*) the halo nevus; (*b*) spindle and epithelioid cell nevus (benign juvenile melanoma); and (*c*) the congenital giant pigmented nevus.

The natural history of a nevus cell is very interesting. Few are present at birth; they appear during the first decade of life and reach their peak numbers in early adulthood. The *junctional* nevus appears first and, therefore, is most common in children. As the nevus cells drop deeper into the skin from the lower epidermis to the deep epidermis and superficial dermis, the junctional nevus evolves into the *compound* nevus, characteristically during young adulthood. This stage is followed by an almost completely dermal location of nevus cells in the *intradermal* nevus of more mature adulthood. Subsequently, regression occurs, and few, if any, nevus-cell nevi are present in the elderly individual (FIg. 18.24).

JUNCTIONAL NEVUS

The nevus cells of the junctional nevus form nests in the lower epidermis. These nests often lie slightly below the epidermis, but still in contact with the epidermis. The

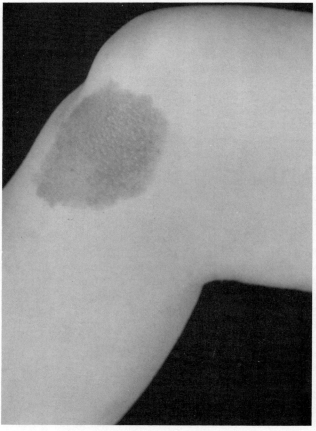

FIGURE 18.24. A typical nevus-cell nevus is shown.

junctional nevus is usually flat, smooth, and irregularly pigmented. These benign neoplasms are seen in the lip vermilion, palms, soles, and the glans penis or the vulva in all age groups because in these locations they do not appear to evolve.

COMPOUND NEVUS

The combined histological character of the junctional and intradermal nevus are possessed by the compound nevus. Nevus-cell nests are found in the epidermis and free in the dermis. Compound nevi are usually well circumscribed and slightly elevated.

INTRADERMAL NEVUS

Few if any junctional nevus cells will be found in the intradermal nevus. The upper dermis will have nests and cords of nevus cells, and the deeper dermis will often have spindle-shaped nevus cells that contain no melanin. Papillomatous, polypoid, and dome-shaped nevi will almost always be intradermal. These are most common in adults as the last stage in the evolution of the nevus-cell nevus before regression.

Unlike other pigmented lesions (discussed later), nevus-cell nevi only rarely deteriorate into malignant lesions. Even the junctional nevi on palms and soles, which at one time were thought to be premalignant, need not be excised prophylactically (31). If there are suspicious changes in any nevus, such as darker color, pigmentation spreading to normal surrounding skin, or unprovoked bleeding or ulceration, then biopsy is indicated. The small suspicious lesions should be treated with a complete excisional biopsy, the larger lesions with a full-thickness incisional or punch biopsy.

Most nevi are removed for cosmetic reasons or because of frequent irritation. Shaving or electrodesiccation of nevi for cosmetic reasons is inadequate because of occasional recurrence. There is no evidence to suggest that incomplete removal will result in malignant transformation (32). Recurrent pigmentation in the wound is of concern to both the patient and the physician, and complete excision is recommended.

GIANT CONGENITAL PIGMENTED NEVUS

This is an uncommon nevus-cell nevus that is present at birth and can be quite extensive. It is often called the "bathing trunk nevus" because it may involve the skin over the entire pelvis. It may also involve an entire extremity, the trunk, or a smaller area anywhere on the body (Fig. 18.25). The lesions may be flat, elevated, or verrucoid; most often they contain coarse hair. Three unique features include association with neurofibromatosis; leptomeningeal melanocytosis and seizures, and melanoma. The latter association makes treatment of the giant congenital pigmented nevus controversial. The actual

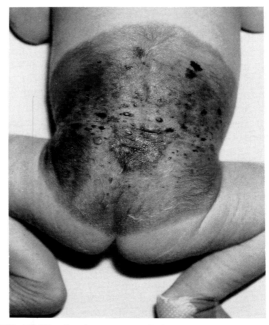

FIGURE 18.25. A giant congenital pigmented nevus in a 2-month-old infant.

incidence of malignant transformation is not known. The largest series is from Denmark, where the incidence in a countrywide survey over a 60-year period was calculated to be 4.6% (33). The incidence in other series varies from 2 to 31% (34), and most authors agree that the actual incidence is probably 2–4%. Melanoma may occur anywhere this nevus is involved, including the central nervous system. Approximately 60% of malignant transformations occur before the age of 10 years, and most of these before 5 years of age (35).

The histological picture is usually similar to the intradermal nevus or the compound nevus. In addition, it may have nevus cells, neuroid nevus cells, and melanocytes deep in the dermis and often extending into the subcutaneous fat. The lesion often extends microscopically beyond the gross margin in the skin peripherally and deep into the fat.

Even though the actual incidence is low, mortality from melanomas arising from the giant congenital pigmented nevus is very high, virtually 100% (33–35). Most of these melanomas occur before the age of 5. Complete prophylactic excision, therefore, is warranted before school age. This can be done in stages with or without skin grafts. In addition to the preventive justification, excision of these oftentimes conspicuous and unattractive lesions may provide significant psychological benefits.

SPINDLE AND EPITHELIOID CELL NEVUS (BENIGN JUVENILE MELANOMA)

Most commonly seen in young children (occasionally at birth), this type of nevus may also be seen for the first time in adolescents or adults. It presents as a pigmented red papule or nodule, typically on the face, and is usually smooth but sometimes scaly. It initially grows rapidly but rarely exceeds 1–2 cm in diameter (36) and usually remains stable.

The spindle and epithelioid cell nevus is histologically similar to the compound nevus. The nevus cells, however, are often large. Mitoses are sometimes seen, and an inflammatory infiltrate is common. These features are similar to those seen in malignant melanoma and, for this reason, these lesions were formerly called "benign juvenile melanoma." Spitz (37) was the first to elucidate the benign nature of this lesion. Other common names include Spitz nevus, spindle-cell nevus, and epithelioid nevus. Treatment consists of complete excision and pathological examination.

HALO NEVUS

A halo nevus is a nevus-cell nevus surrounded by an area of depigmented skin (Fig. 18.26). The depigmentation represents a reduction in melanin and a heavy inflammatory infiltrate consisting of lymphoid cells, histiocytes, and macrophages. The central nevus usually undergoes regression and ultimately disappears along with the halo. The halo nevus is most common in younger people and is frequently seen on the back (38). This process probably represents an immunological phenomenon (39). Approximately 20–30% of nevi regress during the lifetime either by atrophy, fibrosis, fatty replacement, or the halo phenomenon (28). The most common lesion to develop a halo is a compound nevus; however, malignant melanoma, neurofibroma, and blue nevi may also develop similar halos. Treatment is not necessary unless the diagnosis of the central lesion is in doubt, in which event the entire lesion should be excised. Excision should include the halo for aesthetic reasons because it can persist in some cases.

Melanocytic Nevi and Benign Tumors

BLUE NEVUS

The blue nevus, also called the blue nevus of Jadassohn-Tieche (40), is a slate blue or black, often well-circumscribed, smooth papular nodule, usually 1 cm or less in diameter. It occurs most frequently over the head and neck area, upper extremity, feet, and buttocks. It consists of a localized collection of melanocytes deep in the dermis. The blue nevus occurs most often in the female. It can be present at birth or develop later (Fig. 18.27).

A less common variant, called the cellular blue nevus, is usually larger and presents more commonly over the presacral and buttock areas. The cellular blue nevus is important to recognize because it has a low incidence of malignant transformation (41).

Histologically, the blue nevus is composed of spindle-shaped melanocytes in the mid and deep dermis, often with little pigment. Most of the pigment is usually within macrophages. The cellular blue nevus also has densely

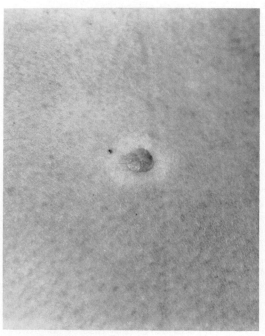

FIGURE 18.26. A characteristic halo nevus is shown.

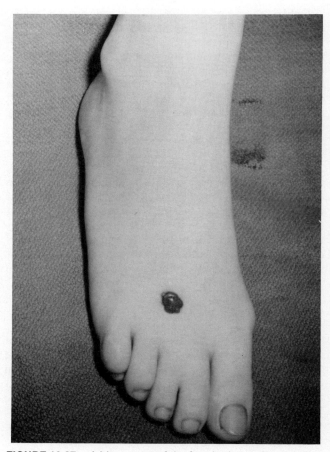

FIGURE 18.27. A blue nevus of the foot is shown. Note similarity to melanoma.

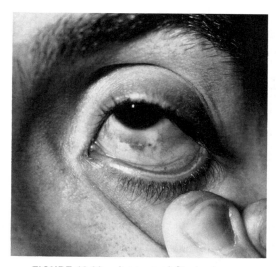

FIGURE 18.28.   A nevus of Ota is shown.

packed larger rounded cells. Treatment is complete excision and pathological evaluation.

NEVUS OF OTA

This is an area of brown or bluish discoloration that is usually unilateral and occurs in the distribution of the first and second branch of the trigeminal nerve. It therefore involves the periorbital area, and occasionally the sclera and conjunctiva (Fig. 18.28). The cornea, retina, oropharynx, and nasal mucosa are rarely involved. Approximately 80% of cases are female, and 5% are bilateral (42). It can be present at birth or appear later in childhood. The nevus of Ito is a similar lesion that occurs on the shoulder. Only a rare malignant transformation has been reported. In a thin, lightly pigmented nevus of Ota, the melanocytes are spindle shaped and widely dispersed in the reticular dermis. In thicker darker lesions, the histological pattern is similar to a blue nevus. No treatment is indicated except for cosmetic improvement.

MONGOLIAN SPOT

Typically an area of bluish discoloration in the lumbosacral skin, a mongolian spot is present at birth and is most often found in orientals and blacks. It affects about 95% of black American infants (43). Occasionally, multiple mongolian spots may occur anywhere over the back. Microscopically, the mongolian spot resembles a light nevus of Ota. Because these lesions are self-limited, treatment is not indicated. Melanocytes become inactive, and the spots disappear after 3 or 4 years. Only a rare spot will persist.

FRECKLES

Freckles (ephelides) are small brown macules consisting of overreactive epidermal melanocytes in skin

exposed to sun. The number of melanocytes and the histological picture of the skin is otherwise normal. Pigmentation deepens with sun exposure.

NEVUS SPILUS

This is a light brown macule (lentigo) present from birth and histologically identical to a freckle. However, it does not darken in response to sunlight. A café au lait spot (the term usually given to the light brown macule associated with neurofibromatosis) is considered a nevus spilus. The brown macules or lentigines of Albright's syndrome are also in this category.

LENTIGO SIMPLEX AND LENTIGO SENILIS

Lentigo simplex and lentigo senilis are similar to the freckle and nevus spilus, but they differ in that they have an increased concentration of melanocytes and elongated rete ridges. Lentigo simplex macules usually appear in childhood in varying degrees and are probably universal (28). The multiple dark brown macules of Peutz-Jeghers syndrome (44) and the leopard syndrome (45) belong in the category of lentigo simplex, as well.

Lentigo senilis is histologically very similar to lentigo simplex, but the lentigines associated with lentigo senilis usually occur later in life and mostly in areas exposed to

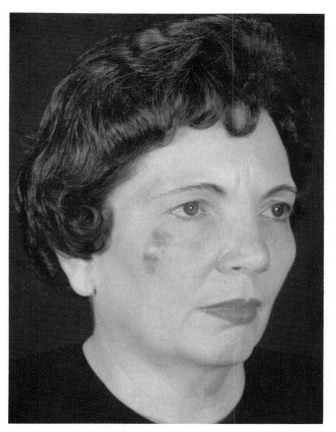

FIGURE 18.29.   A Hutchinson's freckle of the face.

sun. They may be very small or may coalesce into larger lesions and are commonly called age spots or liver spots. These macules may thicken somewhat and resemble seborrheic keratoses. Differential diagnosis must also include lentigo maligna. Lentigo senilis may be treated with a lightening agent such as 3% hydroquinone topical solution or with liquid nitrogen, and this is indicated only for aesthetic appearance.

LENTIGO MALIGNA

Lentigo maligna, or Hutchinson's melanotic freckle, is a brown macular lesion that usually arises in sun-exposed skin, typically on the face of older individuals. It begins as a small macule but progressively enlarges radially to a diameter of several centimeters. Its borders are very irregular, and pigmentation varies within each lesion from light brown to black (Fig. 18.29).

Histologically, the epidermis appears thinned, without ridges, and there are atypical melanocytes in the basal layer. These lesions remain flat, growing radially for many years. Approximately one third will eventually become malignant (46). The transformation is often noticed as a thickening or a more rapid period of radial growth. Increase in pigmentation may also indicate malignant transformation. The melanoma arising in a lentigo maligna has a more favorable prognosis than a de novo or nevus-cell nevus melanoma (46). Obviously, a lentigo maligna should be excised before malignant degeneration occurs. Complete excision without extensive margins is all that is necessary.

Acknowledgments. Appreciation is extended to dermatologist Allan Kayne, M.D., who kindly contributed many of the photographs used in this chapter.

References

References 1, 20, and 28 are recommended as general references.

1. Lever WF, Schaumburg-Lever G: *Histopathology of the Skin,* 5th ed. Philadelphia, JB Lippincott Co, 1975.
2. Mehregan AH, Pinkus H: Life history of organoid nevi. *Arch Dermatol* 91:574, 1965.
3. Jones EW, Heyl T: Naevus sebaceus: A report of 140 cases with special regard to the development of secondary malignant tumors. *Br J Dermatol* 82:99, 1970.
4. Miles AEW: Sebaceous glands in the lip and cheek mucosa of man. *Br Dent J* 105:235, 1958.
5. Leonard DD, Deaton WR: Multiple sebaceous gland tumors and visceral carcinomas. *Arch Dermatol* 110:917, 1974.
6. Hashimoto K, Gross BG, Lever WF: Syringoma: Histochemical and electron microscopic studies. *J Invest Dermatol* 46:150, 1956.
7. Anderson DE, Howell JB: Epithelioma adenoides cysticum: Genetic uptake. *Br J Dermatol* 95:225, 1976.
8. McNamara R: Nevoid basal cell carcinoma syndrome. *Cutis* 18:205, 1976.
9. Malherbe A, Chenantais J: Note sur l'épithéliome calcifié des glandes sebacées. *Bull Soc Anat (Paris)* 5:169, 1880.
10. Forbis R Jr, Helwig EB: Pilomatrixoma (calcifying epithelioma). *Arch Dermatol* 83:606, 1961.
11. Crain RC, Helwig EB: Dermal cylindroma (dermal eccrine cylindroma). *Am J Clin Pathol* 35:504, 1961.
12. Pinkus H, Rogin JR, Goldman P: Eccrine poroma: Tumors exhibiting features of the epidermal sweat duct unit. *Arch Dermatol* 74:511, 1956.
13. Bottles K, Sagebiel RW, McNutt NS, et al: Malignant eccrine poroma: Case report and review of the literature. *Cancer* 53:1579, 1984.
14. Kersting DW, Helwig EB: Eccrine spiradenoma. *Arch Dermatol* 73:199, 1956.
15. Evans HL, Su WPD, Smith JL, et al: Carcinoma arising in eccrine spiradenoma. *Cancer* 43:1881, 1979.
16. McGavran MH, Binnington B: Keratinous cysts of the skin. *Arch Dermatol* 94:499, 1966.
17. Pinkus H: "Sebaceous cysts" are trichilemmal cysts. *Arch Dermatol* 99:544, 1969.
18. Brownstein MH, Helwig EB: Subcutaneous dermoid cysts. *Arch Dermatol* 107:237, 1973.
19. New GB, Erich JB: Dermoid cysts of the head and neck. *Surg Gynecol Obstet* 65:48, 1937.
20. Moschella SL, Pillsbury DM, Hurley HJ: *Dermatology.* Philadelphia, WB Saunders Co, Vol 2, 1975.
21. Fretzin DF, Helwig EB: Atypical fibroxanthoma of skin: A clinicopathologic study of 140 cases. *Cancer* 31:1541, 1973.
22. Jelinek JE: Aspects of heredity, syndromic associations, and course of conditions in which cutaneous lesions occur solitarily or in multiplicity. *J Am Acad Dermatol* 7:526, 1982.
23. Knight WA III, Murphy WK, Gottlieb JA: Neurofibromatosis associated with malignant neurofibromas. *Arch Dermatol* 107:747, 1973.
24. Das Gupta TK, Brasfield RD, Strong EW, et al: Benign solitary schwannomas (neurilemomas). *Cancer* 24:255, 1969.
25. Strong EW, McDivitt RW, Brasfield RD: Granular cell myoblastoma. *Cancer* 25:415, 1970.
26. Hairston MA Jr, Reed RJ, Derbes VJ: Dermatosis papulosa nigra. *Arch Dermatol* 89:655, 1964.
27. Masson P: My conception of cellular nevi. *Cancer* 4:9, 1951.
28. Pinkus H, Mehregan AH: *A Guide to Dermatohistopathology,* 3rd ed. New York, Appleton-Century-Crofts, 1981.
29. Pack GT, Lenson N, Gerber DM: Regional distribution of moles and melanomas. *Arch Surg* 65:862, 1952.
30. Mishima Y: Macromolecular changes in pigmentary disorders. *Arch Dermatol* 91:519, 1965.
31. Allyn B, Kopf AW, Kuhn M, et al: Incidence of pigmented nevi. *JAMA* 186:890, 1963.
32. Schoenfeld RJ, Pinkus H: The recurrence of nevi after incomplete removal. *Arch Dermatol* 78:30, 1958.
33. Lorentzen M, Pers M, Bretteville-Jensen G: The incidence of malignant transformation in giant pigmented nevi. *Scand J Plast Reconstr Surg* 11:163, 1977.
34. Kopf AW, Bart RS, Hennessey P: Congenital nevocytic nevi and malignant melanomas. *J Am Acad Dermatol* 1:123, 1979.
35. Kaplan EN: The risk of malignancy in large congenital nevi. *Plast Reconstr Surg* 53:421, 1974.
36. Kopf AW, Andrade R: Benign juvenile melanoma. In: *Yearbook of Dermatology 1965–1966.* Chicago, Year Book Medical Publishers, 1966, pp 7–52.
37. Spitz S: Melanomas of childhood. *Am J Pathol* 24:591, 1948.
38. Frank SB, Cohen HJ: The halo nevus. *Arch Dermatol* 89:367, 1964.
39. Copeman PWM, Lewis MG, Phillips TM, et al: Immunological associations of the halo naevus with cutaneous malignant melanoma. *Br J Dermatol* 88:127, 1973.
40. Dorsey CS, Montgomery H: Blue nevus and its distinction from mongolian spot and the nevus of Ota. *J Invest Dermatol* 22:225, 1954.
41. Rodriguez HA, Ackerman LV: Cellular blue nevus: Clinicopathologic study of 45 cases. *Cancer* 21:393, 1968.
42. Kopf AW, Weidman AT: Nevus of Ota. *Arch Dermatol* 85:195, 1962.

43. Jacobs AH, Walton RG: The incidence of birthmarks in the neonate. *Pediatrics* 58:218, 1976.
44. Jeghers H, McKusick VA, Katz KH: Generalized intestinal polyposis and melanin spots of the oral mucosa, lips and digits: A syndrome of diagnostic significance. *N Engl J Med* 241:993, 1949.
45. Gorlin RG, Anderson RC, Blaw M: Multiple lentigines syndrome. *Am J Dis Child* 117:652, 1969.
46. Wayte DM, Helwig EB: Melanotic freckle of Hutchinson. *Cancer* 21:893, 1968.

Suggested Readings

Ackerman AB, Troy JL, Rosen LB, Jerasutus S, White CR Jr, King DF: *Differential Diagnosis in Dermatopathology*. Philadelphia, Lea & Febiger, 1988.
Mehregan A: *Pinkus Guide to Dermatopathology*. 4th ed. Norwalk, CT, Appleton-Century-Crofts, 1986.
Lever F, Lever GS: *Histopathology of the Skin,* 7th ed. Philadelphia, J. B. Lippincott Co., 1990.

19

Benign Skin Tumors: Histopathology

Robin T. Vollmer, M.D.

Benign tumors of the skin fall naturally into five categories, depending on their tissue origin or character: tumors of skin appendages, cysts, tumors of soft tissue elements, keratoses of epidermis, and pigmented tumors (Table 19.1). In this chapter, I present lesions in each of these categories, and I describe their clinical appearance, their histology, important clinical associations, their differential diagnosis, and in some instances their treatment, which for the most part is simple excision.

Skin Appendage Tumors

FOLLICULAR DIFFERENTIATION

Trichoepithelioma (Fig. 19.1)

Trichoepitheliomas are either solitary or multiple and inherited. They occur as 2–20-mm, translucent, white to pink papules most commonly on the face about the nose and mouth, but they can occur anywhere.

Histologically, they resemble basal cell carcinoma; their epithelial component is basaloid (small to medium-sized with dark, uniform nuclei and small amounts of cytoplasm). It is not uncommon for them to be misdiagnosed by the pathologist as basal cell carcinoma; therefore, beware the pathologist's diagnosis of basal cell carcinoma on a biopsy of a small pink papule in a child or of

Table 19.1.
Benign Tumors of Skin

Skin appendage tumors
Follicular differentiation
Sebaceous differentiation
Eccrine differentiation
Apocrine differentiation
Cysts
Soft tissue tumors
Fibrous tissue tumors
Fatty tissue tumors
Smooth muscle tumor
Neural tissue tumors
Vascular tissue tumors
Uncertain origin
Keratoses
Pigmented skin tumors

a single papule on the face of a young black person! What discriminates trichoepitheliomas is their formation of usually multiple, small, uniform, keratin-containing microcysts with lining epithelium that often mimics the base of new hair follicles and a surrounding thin layer of cellular stroma. Furthermore, they lack the superficial patterns, solid patterns, and mucinous materials often seen in basal cell carcinoma. Sometimes the keratin in their microcysts is calcified. A variant is the desmoplastic trichoepithelioma, in which the epithelium is reduced to thin strands embedded in a sclerotic stroma, so that the discrimination of this variant from morphea basal cell carcinoma is difficult if the microcysts are sparse. Other variations include tumors with few microcysts and ones with sebaceous, apocrine, or eccrine-like epithelium. At the extreme of the spectrum in number of keratin-filled microcysts lies the trichoadenoma, which has many microcysts and little or no follicular differentiation.

Solitary trichoepitheliomas tend to occur in older persons, so that their confusion with basal cell carcinoma is both greater and probably of lesser consequence because simple excision cures either. Multiple trichoepitheliomas are clinically distinctive, and one half to two thirds of patients will remember that some family members have had the same (autosomal dominant) lesions. Thus, even when the pathologist misdiagnoses the biopsy as basal cell carcinoma, clinical information should place the diagnosis back on track.

Solitary trichoepitheliomas are easily treated by excisional biopsy, but unless all the tumor is removed, it may regrow. Multiple trichoepitheliomas are more difficult. The patient may be reassured after one excisional biopsy that he or she does not have skin cancer; however, the patient may not be happy with all the remaining tumors intact or with the scars that complete removal might imply. Treatments recommended include multiple shave excisions, dermabrasion, and carbon dioxide laser vaporization, but any technique that leaves some residual tumor at the base risks regrowth of the tumor.

Trichofolliculoma (Fig. 19.2)

Trichofolliculoma is an uncommon tumor that occurs only on the head or neck. It presents as a solitary 3–5-mm nodule with a central pore that sometimes extrudes white hairs.

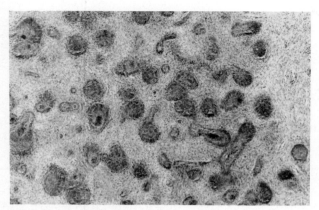

FIGURE 19.1. Trichoepithelioma is composed of epithelial strands mimicking rudimentary follicles. The cellular connective tissue surrounding these is key for the diagnosis.

Histologically, the trichofolliculoma is also composed of basaloid epithelium; therefore, like trichoepithelioma, it too may be misdiagnosed as a basal cell carcinoma. However, it is distinguished by its appearance as a cystically dilated hair follicle with more basaloid epithelium than usual and with peripherally arranged rudimentary follicle-like epithelial protrusions. Excision is curative.

Tricholemmoma

Tricholemmoma appears as a small, warty papule or papules around the mouth, nose, ears, or other parts of the head and neck. Although the clinical appearance may be that of a wart, the histological appearance differs. Rather than showing a papillomatous proliferation of epidermis, the tricholemmoma shows an endophytic lobulated proliferation in the high dermis, attached to the epidermis but comprised of cells with clearer-appearing cytoplasm that mimics the outer root sheath of the follicle. Furthermore, there is a thickening of the basement membrane region, and this also resembles the outer root sheath. In 1980, Ackerman generated some controversy about this lesion by suggesting that it was nothing other than an aged wart affecting follicular epithelium (1). Others were quick to disagree with him, and most texts

still describe it as a tumor. The importance to this issue is the occurrence of this lesion in Cowden's syndrome.

Cowden's syndrome is a rare inherited condition characterized by numerous papules on the face (mostly tricholemmomas), fibroepithelial polyps of the oral mucosa, keratoses of the palms and soles, and an increased tendency to breast cancer in women. Some suggest that the incidence of breast cancer in the syndrome exceeds 50%. Other reported associations include goiter, thyroid adenomas, ovarian cysts, uterine leiomyomas, and colonic adenomas. Brownstein (2) goes so far as to suggest that it is malpractice not to recognize and act on the association between tricholemmoma and breast cancer. Thus, the distinction and diagnosis of this lesion could be quite important.

Other "Tumors" of Follicular Differentiation

Dilated pore of Winer and pilar sheath acanthoma appear to differ little from comedoes with unusual pseudocarcinomatous hyperplasia of lining follicular epithelium. Tumor of follicular infundibulum appears both clinically and histologically as a variant of seborrheic keratosis. Perifollicular fibroma appears similar to the fibrous papule that is most common on the nose.

ECCRINE AND APOCRINE DIFFERENTIATION

Eccrine Poroma

Eccrine poroma is an uncommon tumor occurring most commonly on the palms or soles. It presents at variable sizes (up to 3 cm) and variable thickness and height above the skin. Sometimes it is ulcerated. Histologically, it is comprised of relatively uniform and mildly atypical basaloid cells that thicken the epidermis into broad interconnecting strands. In this regard, the pattern is not unlike Bowen's disease, except that the cytological atypica is less than usual for Bowen's disease. Like Bowen's disease, the tumor tends to follow and engulf adnexal epithelium, including sweat ducts, into the dermis. It seldom involves the deeper layers of the dermis, but when it does, it is sometimes designated "dermal duct tumor."

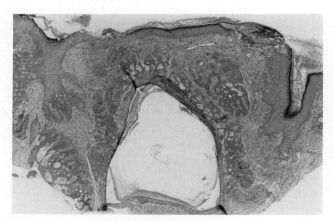

FIGURE 19.2. Trichofolliculoma is a cystically dilated, follicle-like structure with peripheral protuberances of smaller, rudimentary follicle-like structures.

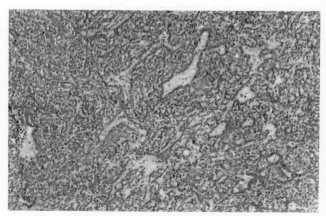

FIGURE 19.3. Eccrine spiradenoma is a solid dermal nodule of basaloid cells arranged in trabeculae and hinting at acinar structures.

Of greatest concern is its occurrence as "porocarcinoma." Here, it shows a pagetoid pattern in the epidermis, invades the deeper layers of the dermis, and often involves lymphatics at the original site. In this form, the tumor metastasizes.

Eccrine Spiradenoma and Cylindroma (Fig. 19.3)

Although most authors consider eccrine spiradenoma to be of sweat duct origin and cylindroma to be of apocrine origin, both the histologies and clinical circumstances of these two tumors merge; therefore, it is reasonable to consider them as two ends of a spectrum. Both present as dermal nodules that can be painful (this is especially true for the eccrine spiradenoma.) The spiradenoma occurs anywhere. The cylindroma occurs mainly on the scalp, and it often is multiple and part of an inherited trait that can include multiple trichoepitheliomas. In older patients, the scalp cylindromas sometimes coalesce into the "turban" tumor appearance. Nevertheless, both tumors occur most commonly as single tumors, and both can coexist on the same patient.

Histologically, both tumors are comprised of two cell types: a basaloid cell and a clearer, more squamoid cell. In narrower epithelial trabeculae, the basaloid cell will be peripherally located, and the squamoid cell will be centrally located. These trabeculae or wider lobules of similar epithelium are bordered by a distinctive, dense, pink-staining band of altered collagen. Thus, especially in the cylindroma, the pattern resembles a mosaic tile or stained glass picture. If anything distinguishes the histology of the spiradenoma, it is the predominance of more solid-appearing lobules of epithelium in this lesion.

As solitary tumors, these are easily cured by complete excision. There probably is no adequate cure for the multiple turban-type tumors, but in some cases the entire scalp is excised.

Nodular Hidradenoma (Figs. 19.4 and 19.5)

The designation "nodular hidradenoma" may include several entities, but all present as a single solid or cystic dermal mass that histologically is comprised of at least

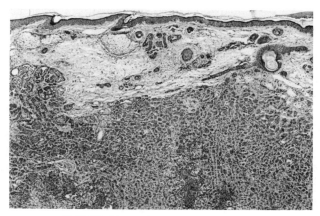

FIGURE 19.5. Nodular hidradenoma.

two cell types: one round with pink cytoplasm and large nuclei, the other with clear cytoplasm and smaller, darker nuclei. Sometimes ductular structures lined by columnar cells are present, and there may be mucinous differentiation. There is a variable amount of accompanying hyalinized stroma. Malignant variants have been reported and may represent diagnostic confusion with either poorly differentiated squamous carcinoma or true adenosquamous carcinomas presenting in the skin. Nodular hidradenomas showing two distinct cell populations, both without cytological atypia, should be curable by simple excision.

Syringoma (Fig. 19.6)

Syringomas possess both clinical and histological features that are distinctive. Clinically, they most often present as multiple 0.1–0.5-cm pink papules on the lower eyelids of young women, but they may appear as either single or multiple papules in broader sites, including the face, neck, anterior trunk, fingers, and genitals. They can occur in either sex. Sometimes, they are familial, and they are also associated with Down's syndrome. They may occur as part of a larger organoid cutaneous nevus that involves several types of tissues.

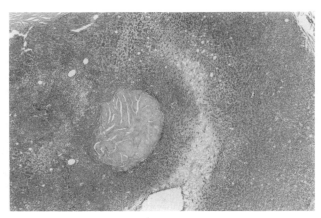

FIGURE 19.4. Nodular hidradenoma.

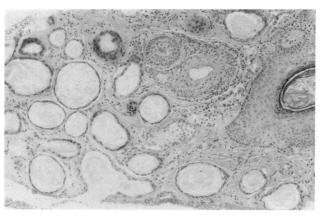

FIGURE 19.6. Syringoma. Note the multiple microcysts with thin epithelial lining of cells, some of which have clear cytoplasm.

Histologically, syringomas are comprised of strands and ducts of epithelium intercalated in the dermis. Most often, two cell types are present: an inner clear cell surrounding a lumen empty or filled with amorphous material, and an outer cell with darker cytoplasm. These strands are curved into comma shapes and "Y" shapes, and some form microcysts. Occasional keratin microcysts similar to those in trichoepithelioma suggest an organoid nevus.

Suggested treatments of multiple syringomas include carbon dioxide laser and ophthalmic scissor excisions, but simple excision works well for the single syringoma.

Mixed Tumor (Chrondroid Syringoma) (Fig. 19.7)

Mixed tumor presents most commonly as a single nodule in the dermis of the head or neck, and it shows the same histology as the mixed tumor of the salivary glands: strands and ducts of epithelium embedded in a mucoid and sometimes cartilaginous stroma. Simple excision is curative.

Papillary Syringadenoma (Syringocystadenoma Papilliferum)

Papillary syringadenoma occurs most commonly on the scalp and appears as a moist verrucal growth. It also occurs on the face and neck and is often part of an organoid nevus first noticed in childhood. Histologically, it is a large cystic break in the epidermis with extension into the underlying dermis. The cystic space is partly filled by blunt papillae composed of vascular stroma rich in plasma cells and lined by epithelium that is often two-cell layered and apocrine-like. Although simple excision is curative, neither surgeon nor pathologist should ignore the broader abnormality of an organoid nevus that may surround this tumor.

Papillary Hidradenoma (Hidradenoma Papilliferum)

Although both papillary syringadenoma and hidradenoma are lined by apocrine-type epithelium, the hidradenoma's name emphasizes its more apocrine distribution on the body. It occurs most commonly in the female perineum, especially the labia majora. It can also occur on the nipple, the anus, the eyelid, and the external auditory canal. Histologically, it is a large cystic space in the dermis with numerous inward papillary thin projections of vascular stroma (without many plasma cells) lined by apocrine-like cells. Surgical excision is curative.

Papillary Eccrine Adenoma and Tubular Apocrine Adenoma

Some authors consider these rare tumors to be the same entity even though papillary eccrine adenoma occurs on the arms and legs of blacks, whereas tubular apocrine adenoma is said to occur most commonly on the scalp. Histologically, they are composed of ducts and

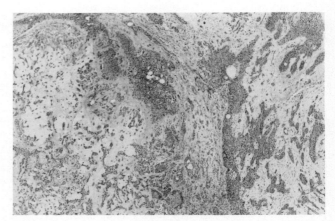

FIGURE 19.7. Mixed tumor reveals strands of epithelium embedded in a stroma rich in mucin and cells, which mimics early cartilage.

lobules of epithelium intercalated through the dermis and with lining epithelium of two cell layers, each of which fails to show cytological atypia.

Aggressive Digital Papillary Adenoma

Aggressive digital papillary adenoma overlaps benign and malignant categories. In its most benign form, it is composed of cystic areas with a minimal epithelial lining. In its more malignant, and often recurrent, form, it shows more solid masses of epithelium in the walls of the cystic areas.

Malignant Variants of Sweat Gland Tumors

Many of the tumors listed above have malignant counterparts that may merge in clinical and histological appearances with these benign tumors. Thus, there is the malignant eccrine poroma (porocarcinoma), the malignant eccrine spiradenoma, the malignant clear cell hidradenoma, several versions of eccrine adenocarcinoma, malignant mixed tumor, hidradenocarcinoma, and adenoid cystic carcinoma, to mention just a few.

SEBACEOUS DIFFERENTIATION

Sebaceous Adenoma, Sebaceous Epithelioma, and Sebaceous Carcinoma

Histologically, at least, these tumors appear as a spectrum. The sebaceous adenoma (Fig. 19.8) shows a circumscribed collection of immature-appearing sebaceous glands, but cells showing fatty, vacuolated, sebaceous-like cytoplasm predominate. The sebaceous epithelioma shows fewer of such cells and more basaloid cells, and the sebaceous carcinoma shows marked cytologic atypia but some evidence of sebaceous cytoplasmic morphology. Because the carcinoma is largely confined to the eyelids, whereas the adenoma and epithelioma occur on the rest of the face, these can be separated somewhat on

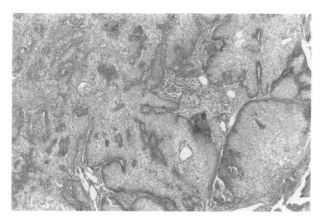

FIGURE 19.8. Sebaceous adenoma. Like sebaceous epithelium, the cells of this tumor are large and vacuolated. Unlike normal sebaceous epithelium, its cells have larger nuclei and more basophilic cytoplasm, and it is arranged in more massive lobules.

the basis of their site alone. Nevertheless, the separation of adenoma from epithelioma, which is more aggressive and likely to recur, is tricky, and I have misplaced at least one tumor in this binary discrimination.

Cysts of Skin

Epidermoid Cyst and Comedone (Fig. 19.9)

The epidermoid cyst is the most common cyst of the skin. It is thought to arise from the upper, or infundibular, portion of hair follicles and in fact merges clinically and histologically with simple comedones. It occurs most commonly on the head, neck, and upper trunk but can occur anywhere. Sometimes it maintains a drainage tract to the skin surface, and the patient reports periodic exudate of cheesy material (keratin debris). It sometimes becomes ruptured and inflamed.

Multiple epidermoid cysts occur in Gardner's syndrome with polyposis coli, osteomas of the jaw, and intestinal desmoid tumors. Some epidermoid cysts result from prior trauma that leaves invaginated fronds of epi-

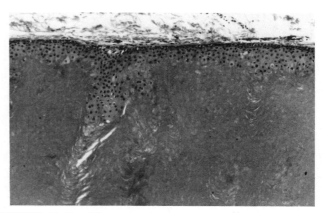

FIGURE 19.10. Pilar cyst. The inner cells of this cyst are plumper than those of an epidermoid cyst, and the luminal material appears less flaky.

dermis unnaturally within the dermis. For example, these cysts sometimes occur at sites of prior suturing and burns.

Histologically, an epidermoid cyst is lined by mature squamous epithelium that forms a thin granular (bluestaining) layer and abundant keratin debris. If ruptured, it may be enveloped in heavy, and often granulomatous, inflammation. In fact, probably the most common cause of granulomatous inflammation in the skin is the rupture of either a hair follicle or an epidermoid cyst.

Pilar Cyst (Fig. 19.10)

Ninety percent of pilar cysts occur on the scalp, but the pilar cyst is still less common on the scalp than the epidermoid cyst. In 75% of patients, there will be a familial history of (dominantly) inherited pilar cysts. Histologically, the pilar cyst is lined by squamous epithelium that, unlike the epidermoid cyst, matures to a plump cell with light-staining cytoplasm. The center of the cyst contains more homogeneous debris than the flaky material typical for keratin in an epidermoid cyst. The pilar cyst is often miscalled a ''sebaceous'' cyst.

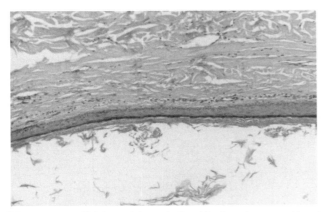

FIGURE 19.9. Epidermoid cyst is lined by keratinocytes identical to those of the epidermis, and it is filled with keratin debris.

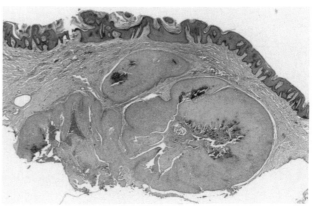

FIGURE 19.11. Proliferating pilar cyst that was removed from the scalp. Note the massive lobules of keratinocytes having mild, but definite, cytologic atypia.

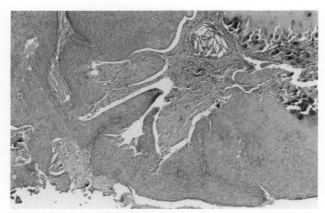

FIGURE 19.12. Proliferating pilar cyst (high magnification). The keratinocytes have atypia similar to that of a well-differentiated squamous carcinoma or keratoacanthoma.

Proliferating Pilar Cyst (or Tumor) (Figs. 19.11 and 19.12)

This is a cystic tumor rather than a simple cyst. Like the pilar cyst, it occurs on the scalp. Unlike the pilar cyst, the proliferating pilar cyst histologically has a complex, thick, and atypical squamous lining that merges with well-differentiated squamous carcinoma. In fact, some proliferating cysts have been reported to metastasize. Whether this tumor-like behavior truly belongs to this entity or merely emphasizes its morphological confusion with squamous carcinoma is unclear. What is clear is that it requires careful and complete excision.

Hydrocystoma (Fig. 19.13)

Clinically, hydrocystoma usually is a single, translucent fluid-filled cyst on the face. Its lining epithelium may appear either eccrine or apocrine, and the innermost cells often have a columnar morphology with clear cytoplasm.

Dermoid Cyst

Dermoid cyst often occurs near the upper eyelid and may be present from birth. Its lining is squamous epithelium that includes hair follicles and sebaceous glands, and its lumen is filled with both keratin debris and hairs.

Steatocystoma Multiplex

Steatocystoma multiplex cysts are usually multiple and part of an autosomal-dominant inherited condition. In males, the cysts of steatocystoma multiplex occur most commonly on the anterior chest and scrotum. In females, they occur most commonly in the axilla and groin. Histologically, their lining is a thin squamous epithelium containing frequent flattened sebaceous glands and small hair follicles, and their lumina are filled with light-staining low-density debris with small hairs.

Branchial Cyst (Fig. 19.14)

Branchial cyst occurs exclusively in the anterolateral neck. It is lined by squamous epithelium with often prominent lymphoid tissue similar to adenoid tissue of the pharynx. It is thought to result from residual embryonic branchial cleft tissue.

Bronchial Cyst

Bronchial cyst occurs most often in the skin above the sternal notch in a child. It is lined by pseudostratified ciliated columnar epithelium.

Thyroglossal Duct Cyst

Thyroglossal duct cyst occurs in the anterior midline of the neck near the hyoid bone. It is lined by columnar epithelium, and there may be thyroid tissue in the surrounding tissue.

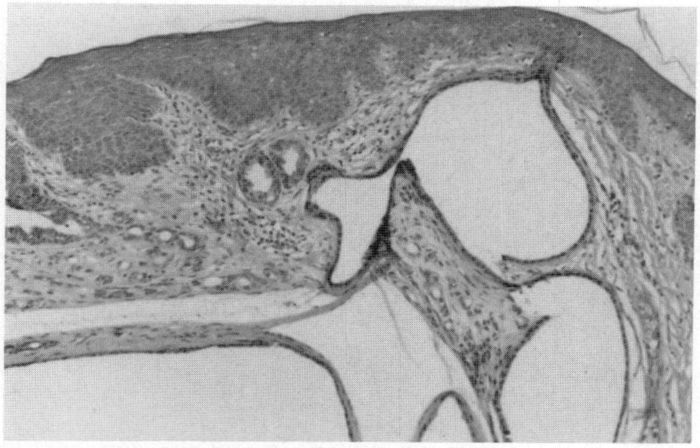

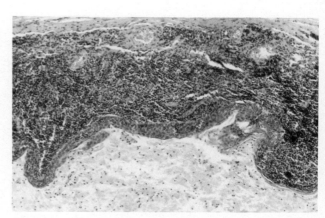

FIGURE 19.13. Hydrocystoma is lined by a thin cell layer and filled with loose proteinaceous fluid.

FIGURE 19.14. Branchial cyst. The lining to this cyst is composed of a complex of keratinocytes and lymphoid tissue.

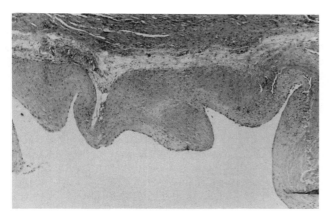

FIGURE 19.15. Ganglion cyst. The lining has no epithelium, just dense connective tissue.

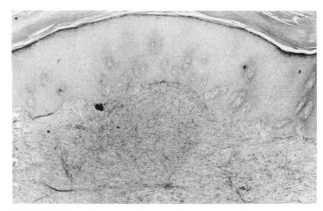

FIGURE 19.16. Dermatofibroma. Note the epidermal hyperplasia and the nodule of stromal cells in the dermis.

Cutaneous Ciliated Cyst

Cutaneous ciliated cyst is a rare cyst occurring on the legs of women. It is lined by ciliated columnar to low columnar epithelium and is thought to be related to misplaced müllerian duct tissue.

Penile Cyst

Penile cyst, also called median raphe cyst, occurs on the ventral midline of the glans as a nodule or translucent cyst present from birth. It is lined by pseudostratified columnar epithelium.

Digital Mucinous Cyst and Ganglion (Fig. 19.15)

These are soft tissue accumulations of mucopolysaccharide rather than true cysts; they are lined by a mucin-rich stroma rather than epithelium. They may originate from synovial or other joint tissues because the digital cyst overlays the distal interphalangeal joint and the ganglion cyst overlays the wrist.

Tumors of Connective Tissue Differentiation

FIBROUS TISSUE TUMORS

Dermatofibroma (Fig. 19.16)

Dermatofibroma is a common lesion that may be little more than exaggerated repair of the skin after simple trauma, rather than a true tumor. However, because it appears clinically as a small (typically 3–5-mm), firm nodule on the legs or arms of adults, it is often discussed with tumors. Although it is usually single and isolated, it sometimes appears as multiple nodules. It most often has a stable size and appearance, but sometimes it may grow slowly.

Histologically, dermatofibroma combines epidermal hyperplasia with a complex of cells and altered collagen in the dermis. In the epidermis, increased basalar cells mimic basal cell carcinoma or the changes of an organoid nevus. In the dermis, increased fibroblasts, endothelial

cells, and macrophages concentrate in the center of the lesion. Toward the periphery, they intermix with distinctive collagen that is shorter, narrower, and more tortuous than usual so that it appears as small, tight curls among fibroblasts. Sometimes, vessels are so numerous that the lesion is called sclerosing hemangioma.

Dermatofibrosarcoma Protruberans (Fig. 19.17)

Dermatofibrosarcoma protruberans is a low-grade (I out of III) soft tissue sarcoma whose histology can be confused with dermatofibroma. In contrast to dermatofibroma, dermatofibrosarcoma is a larger, deeper tumor composed of more homogeneous cells. It often involves the subcutaneous fat, and its moderately sized spindle cells are concentrated into whorled fasicles. Dermatofibrosarcoma requires complete excision and often skin grafting. If the surgical margins are not free of tumor, it will recur. In some cases it metastasizes.

Acrochordon (Skin Tag)

Acrochordons are such common and trivial lesions that to call them tumors inflates their importance. Their bulk consists of normal connective tissue, including collagen,

FIGURE 19.17. Dermatofibrosarcoma protruberans shows dense swirls of spindle cells with mildly atypical nuclei and an overall homogeneity not apparent in dermatofibromas.

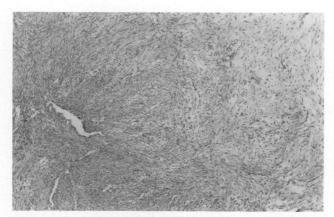

FIGURE 19.18. Nodular fasciitis. In some foci, this tumor looks sarcomatous. Recognizing it as benign requires examination of its entirety.

blood vessels, and a few leukocytes. Their covering is a corrugated hyperplastic and hyperkeratotic epidermis that can merge with that of squamous papillomas and seborrheic keratoses. Acrochordons occur most commonly on the neck and in the axillae, and probably because of this, they sometimes are traumatized by the edges of clothing and jewelry.

One may excise acrochordons with scissors or shave them off with a scapel blade. Excising smaller ones may not even require anesthesia. Freezing them with liquid nitrogen or electrodesiccating them makes them drop off after several days.

Nodular Fasciitis (Fig. 19.18)

Like dermatofibroma, nodular fasciitis is probably an exaggerated repair rather than a true tumor. Unlike dermatofibroma, its histology looks sarcomatous. Nodular fasciitis begins in the subcutaneous tissues and grows rapidly, but also regresses spontaneously. Histologically, it is a vascular, myxomatous connective tissue with such infiltrative edges and foci of such cytologic atypia that it mimics grade I fibrosarcoma. Nevertheless, the arrange-

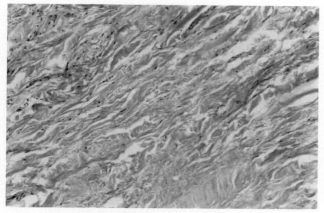

FIGURE 19.19. Elastofibroma. Note the faintly stained elastin within the collagen of this tumor.

ment of these tissues and their maturation suggest a benign process. To resolve an uncertain diagnosis, additional biopsy tissue and/or follow-up may be needed to decide if the lesion is enlarging like a tumor, or regressing like an injury.

Infantile Digital Fibroma

Infantile digital fibroma is a nodular growth on the dorsa or lateral aspects of the fingers or toes of infants less than 3 years old. It may be either a single nodule or multiple nodules. It is composed of fascicles of spindle cells and dense collagen, and the cytoplasm of these cells contains bright pink inclusions that are thought to be bundles of myofilaments. This tumor can attach to periosteum and recurs when incompletely excised, but it does not metastasize.

Elastofibroma (Fig. 19.19)

Elastofibroma occurs in the deep connective tissue beneath the scapula of elderly patients. It consists of pink, loose fibriller connective tissue with modest numbers of spindle cells, and high-magnification microscopy or special stains show numerous elastin fibers. Although it attaches to ribs, it behaves benignly and does not require aggressive excision.

FATTY TISSUE TUMORS

Lipoma and Angiolipoma

Lipomas sit in the subcutaneous fat and present as soft nodules. They are composed of mature fat cells and, if numerous capillaries are present, are called angiolipoma. Lipomas can be easily excised, and smaller ones may be gently expressed through a small excision over the nodule. They have also been treated by liposuction.

Spindle Cell Lipoma (Fig. 19.20)

Spindle cell lipoma is important because, like nodular fasciitis, it is sometimes misdiagnosed as a sarcoma. It presents as a subcutaneous mass on the neck, shoulder, or upper back. Histologically, it combines fatty tissue and myxoid spindle cell tissue that infiltrates among collagen fibers, and the spindle cells cytologically mimic those of grade I fibrosarcoma. The tissue arrangement and composition are distinctive, if taken together.

SMOOTH MUSCLE TUMORS

Leiomyoma and Angioleiomyoma (Fig. 19.21)

Leiomyomas may occur either singly or, more commonly, as groups. They occur on the arms, anterior trunk, nipples, and genitals, and often they are painful and tender. Histologically, they are composed of interlacing fascicles of spindle cells with pink cytoplasm but with-

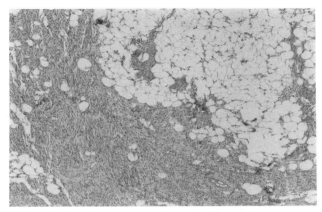

FIGURE 19.20. Sclerosing or fibrosing lipoma. Note the intimate combination of lipocytes and spindle cells.

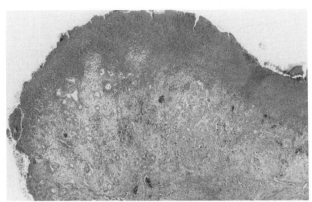

FIGURE 19.22. Pyogenic granuloma is an exophytic mass of capillaries forming granulation tissue with an ulcerated epidermis.

out atypia. These cells fill the dermis and sometimes involve the subcutis. If thick-walled vessels are integral to the tumor, it is probably an angioleiomyoma. Leiomyoma is distinguished from leiomyosarcoma by lower cell density, less nuclear atypia, and the absence of mitotic figures.

XANTHOMATOUS TUMORS

Juvenile Xanthogranuloma

Juvenile xanthogranuloma presents most often as multiple papules or nodules about the head, neck, and upper trunk of infants less than 1 year old, and they usually regress within a year. Histologically, they are composed of many foamy-appearing macrophages filling the dermis and accompanied by multinucleated giant cells. This tumor has also been described in adults, and here it must be discriminated from granulomatous inflammations and infections.

Xanthoma, Tuberous Xanthoma, Xanthelasmata

Xanthomas often reflect hyperlipidemia because they wax and wane with the lipid levels in the blood. They

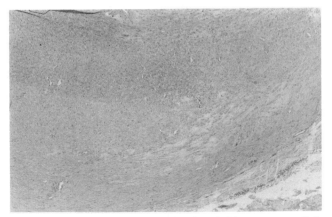

FIGURE 19.21. Leiomyoma. The cells of this tumor are light staining and spindle shaped. They form a circumscribed nodule in the dermis.

present in crops on the buttocks, shoulders, arms, or legs, but the common xanthelasmata occur on or about the eyelids and are less often tied to hyperlipidemia. Unless inflamed, xanthomas are yellow nodules or plaques. If inflamed, they appear red. Histologically, they contain large macrophages with foamy-appearing cytoplasm, and there may also be many leukocytes. Older lesions of tuberous xanthoma show fibrosis. Although xanthelasmata are thin and superficial, tuberous xanthoma is thick and deep enough to involve the subcutis.

Small xanthomas due to hyperlipidemia are best treated by reducing the blood lipids. Larger xanthomas, those not associated with hyperlipidemia, and those disfiguring the face can be excised, electrodesiccated and curetted, frozen with liquid nitrogen, or reduced with topical trichloroacetic acid.

VASCULAR TUMORS

Pyogenic Granuloma (Fig. 19.22)

Pyogenic granuloma is not a tumor, but another exaggerated tissue repair. It presents as a large bleeding nodule that has broken through the surface of the skin on the fingers, face, or other sites. It is composed of granulation tissue, not granuloma; therefore, it has numerous capillaries, a loose connective tissue framework, and often numerous leukocytes. Shave excision to include the visible edges of the lesion is adequate for treatment and diagnosis, but complete excision to include a border of normal skin, electrocautery, and liquid nitrogen have also been used. Because pyogenic granuloma can histologically overlap with Kaposi's sarcoma, it is desirable to remove enough tissue to allow complete histological exam.

Hemangiomas (Fig. 19.23)

Hemangiomas are divided in at least three different ways: by their clinical syndrome, by their clinical or gross appearance, and by their histology. For example, their gross appearance varies from a small red papule, to a

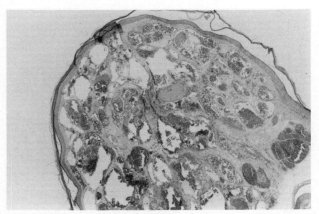

FIGURE 19.23. Cavernous hemangioma. Beneath the epidermis are numerous dilated capillaries.

large, flat, dark-red lesion, to a large, pedunculated, disfiguring tumor. Their histology varies from a simple hyperplasia of normal capillaries (telangiectasia), to a tumor of cellular capillaries lined by plump endothelial cells (capillary hemangioma), to a complex of widely dilated capillaries (cavernous hemangioma), to a complex of thick-walled, muscular vessels (arteriovenous malformation or venous hemangioma). In this discussion, they are divided by their clinical syndrome.

Small Hemangiomas in Infancy

Small hemangiomas are common in infancy. Usually, they are small red macules or papules on the head or neck. Some have a central prominent vessel that feeds smaller and radially arranged vessels (spider hemangioma). Histologically, most are capillary hemangiomas, and because more than 90% involute by age 7, most require no treatment.

Large, Disfiguring Hemangiomas in Infancy

Fortunately, large, disfiguring hemangiomas are uncommon in infants. Unfortunately, they sometimes require treatment before they have involuted because they threaten to disrupt or destroy vital tissues such as the eye, ear, or mouth. Nevertheless, the consensus opinion is that their removal should be postponed until puberty. Histologically, they are mostly cavernous hemangiomas.

Port-Wine Stains

Port-wine stains are variably sized, flat, and purple to red in color. They are present from birth and usually located on the face and head. Histologically, they are telangiectasias, which do not involute. Smaller ones can be excised; larger ones have recently been successfully treated with a tunable laser.

Some patients with port-wine hemangiomas on the head have Sturge-Weber syndrome, with vascular proliferations in the meninges, calcifications in the brain, and epilepsy. Patients with port-wine hemangiomas on the extremities may have Klippel-Trenaunay syndrome, with hypertrophy of bone and soft tissue of the affected limb.

Adult Cherry-Red Hemangiomas

Cherry-red hemangiomas are common, often multiple, 1–3-mm red papules on the trunk, neck, or face of middle-aged patients. Histologically, they are mostly capillary hemangiomas. They require no treatment except to improve appearance, and such treatment can be shave excision, electrodesiccation, or topical liquid nitrogen.

Maffucci's Syndrome

Maffucci's syndrome combines multiple subcutaneous cavernous hemangiomas with severe defects in ossification of bones. There are marked bony deformities, osteochondromas, and even chondrosarcomas.

Blue Rubber Bleb Syndrome

Blue rubber bleb syndrome combines multiple soft superficial cavernous hemangiomas with hemangiomas of the mouth and intestines, and the patient may be anemic as a result of chronic loss of blood from the gastrointestinal tract.

Glomus Tumor (Fig. 19.24)

Glomus tumor may occur at any age and on any site; however, it is most common on the fingers of adults. It appears as a painful, sometimes exquisitely painful, dark red nodule. The subungual site is commonly involved. Histologically, it is a collection of uniform small cuboidal cells arranged closely about a complex of capillaries. Although it occurs most often as a single lesion in an adult, less commonly it occurs as multiple tumors in children as part of an inherited trait.

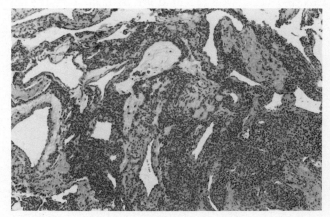

FIGURE 19.24. Glomus tumor. The distinguishing feature for this tumor is the nests of uniform small cells located next to vessels.

Angiokeratoma

Angiokeratoma presents as either single or multiple red, scaly papules. Histologically, the epidermis is hyperplastic with hyperkeratosis, and closely abutting the epidermis are dilated, blood-filled capillaries.

Depending on clinical distribution, age of onset, inheritance, and associated biochemical abnormalities, this tumor sorts itself into several subtypes. Angiokeratoma corporis diffusum is sex-linked, is due to a deficiency of ceramide trihexosidase, and is located on the thighs, buttocks, back, and penis of children. Angiokeratoma Mibelli is located on the fingers and toes of children or adolescents. Angiokeratoma of the scrotum is located on the scrotum of adults. Papular angiokeratoma is located most often on the legs of young adults.

Cavernous Lymphangioma

Cavernous lymphangioma presents as a subcutaneous soft mass or cyst-like structure, most often in the neck (cystic hygroma). It consists of cystically dilated lymph vessels lined by endothelium and situated in the connective tissues, including within muscles. Other sites for this tumor include the tongue and lips.

NEURAL TUMOR

Neurofibroma (Fig. 19.25)

Cutaneous neurofibromas present as single, or less often as multiple, soft, fleshy protuberances. Histologically, the dermis is replaced by a loose fibrillar-myxomatous tissue with numerous small spindle cells having delicate curved nuclei. Capillaries are also numerous.

Any patient with a cutaneous neurofibroma, especially those with multiple neurofibromas, could have von Recklinghausen's disease (spontaneously occurring or autosomally dominant inherited traits of multiple neurofibromas, café-au-lait spots, sometimes mental retardation,

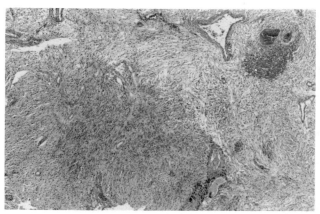

FIGURE 19.26. Schwannoma. The low magnification shows both densely cellular and less cellular areas typical for this tumor.

sometimes central nervous system tumors, bone tumors, and soft tissue sarcomas).

Schwannoma (Figs. 19.26 and 19.27)

Schwannoma is also called neurilemmoma, and it is a tumor of peripheral nerves. It begins in the subcutaneous tissues of the head, neck, or limbs as a solitary, sometimes painful, mass. Histologically, its distinctive feature is a dense spindle cell tissue (Antoni A), in which cell nuclei line up in intermittent parallel rows (Verocay bodies), like battle lines in a 19th century infantry assault. This Antoni A tissue is often joined by a loose myxomatous tissue (Antoni B), but nowhere is there atypia. Like neurofibroma, schwannoma can occur in von Recklinghausen's disease.

TUMORS OF UNCERTAIN ORIGIN

Granular Cell Tumor

Granular cell tumor occurs more frequently in the tongue than in the skin; however, it can occur in the skin

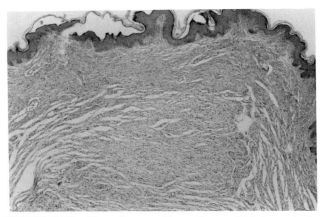

FIGURE 19.25. Neurofibroma. The softness of this tumor is due to its delicate, mucin-rich stroma with thin fibers and small spindle cells.

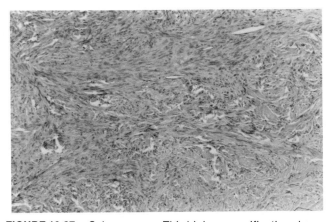

FIGURE 19.27. Schwannoma. This higher magnification shows how the cell nuclei concentrate like waves of fish in a school.

and especially on the arms of women. What distinguishes the granular cell is its abundant granular pink cytoplasm that stains positively for S100 antigen. In granular cell tumor, these cells fill the dermis, and the epidermis is hyperplastic to the point of imitating a carcinoma (pseudocarcinomatous hyperplasia). Nevertheless, there is no cytologic atypica.

Keratoses

Seborrheic Keratosis (Fig. 19.28)

Seborrheic keratoses are common in older adults. They present as multiple, pigmented, elevated verrucal lesions seemingly stuck to the skin. Histologically, seborrheic keratosis is a complex epidermal hyperplasia of keratinocytes with basaloid morphology, and the epidermal pattern often seems a broad band with entrapped dermal papillae and keratin debris (pseudocysts). Often, there is inflammation similar to that of lichen planus (lichen planus–like keratosis), and seborrheic keratosis can undergo such hyperplasia and squamous metaplasia that it imitates squamous carcinoma (irritated seborrheic keratosis). It is easily removed by shave excision, but whenever there is clinical doubt about the presence of melanoma, it is best to do an excisional biopsy because this provides deeper tissue for histological examination.

Solar Keratosis (Fig. 19.29)

Solar (or actinic) keratosis is a dysplasia or carcinoma in situ of the epidermis, but because it can be treated by shave biopsy or topical liquid nitrogen like a benign lesion, it is included here. Histologically, it is an atypical maturation of the keratinocytes in the epidermis, and the atypia ranges from mild, involving just the basal cells of the epidermis, to moderate, involving most of the epidermis, to severe (or hyperplastic solar keratosis), with papillary extensions of atypical rete processes into the level of the papillary dermis. The involved keratinocytes have larger, darker nuclei whose orientation deviates from the

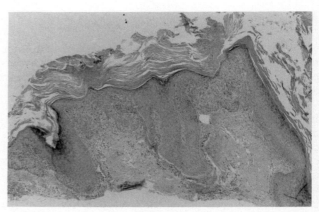

FIGURE 19.29. Solar keratosis is an altered maturation of the keratinocytes in the epidermis in sun-damaged skin. The changed cells have enlarged and atypical nuclei, especially in the lower layers of the epidermis, but there is no invasion of the dermis.

usual, and these cells are less cohesive to neighboring cells (acantholytic solar keratosis).

Pigmented Tumors

Melanocytic Nevi (Figs. 19.30 and 19.31)

Melanocytic nevi are common on white persons, begin to appear in childhood, reach a maximum number (average: 25) by middle age, and then disappear. Histologically, they are classed as junctional, compound, or intradermal. The junctional nevi are usually flat and have collections of melanocytes at the tips of rete ridges. Both compound and intradermal nevi are dome-shaped elevations, and both have melanocytes in the dermis. Although the compound nevus has junctional melanocytes, the intradermal nevus appears to lack these.

The major problem with melanocytic nevi is their discrimination from malignant melanoma, and this difficulty

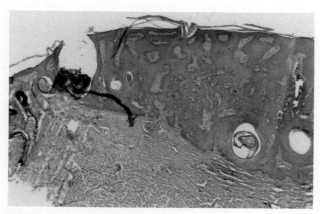

FIGURE 19.28. Seborrheic keratosis has a broad hyperplasia of basaloid keratinocytes in the epidermis with intermittent islands of dermis or keratin. There is no atypia.

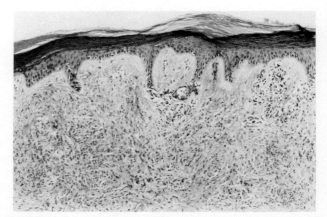

FIGURE 19.30. Compound melanocytic nevus. At the bottom of the epidermis are collections of melanocytes with clear-appearing cytoplasm. The dermis contains many smaller melanocytes.

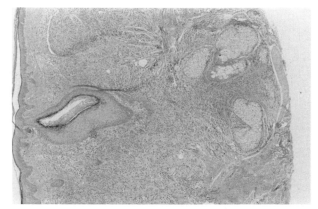

FIGURE 19.31. Congenital melanocytic nevus. The melanocytes follow a hair unit deep into the dermis.

has worsened with the rising incidence of melanoma and with the recognition of clinically and histologically atypical, or dysplastic, nevi that overlap the definitions of nevus and melanoma. Clinically, the smaller the nevus (e.g., 4 mm or less), the more uniform its color, the rounder and sharper its border, and the more stable its growth, the more likely it is to be benign. Histologically, the lower its cell mass, the less cytological atypia it has, the more vertical maturation pattern it has, and the sharper its border with the normal skin is, the more likely it is to be benign (Table 19.2). Fortunately, most common lesions occur at either end of the benign-malignant spectrum (i.e., they are either clearly benign nevi or clearly malignant melanoma), but there are a small number of atypical nevi and thin early melanomas that merge both clinical appearances and histologies to the point that pathologists will disagree about the diagnosis. Often, patients with these difficultly diagnosed lesions will have large numbers of nevi (greater than 50); they will have nevi that are clinically atypical because of large diameter (7 mm or greater), varying color, and irregular contour; and they will have a family or personal history for melanoma. In short, they will have the dysplastic nevus syndrome. Because of all these issues, no nevus should be excised or treated without histological examination.

Congenital Nevus (Fig. 19.31)

The congenital nevus is a compound or intradermal melanocytic nevus present at birth (or appearing shortly after birth). Its diameter often exceeds 1 cm, and its melanocytes are spread through more of the dermis and more intimately surround deep dermal structures such as hairs. Sometimes, congenital nevi become speckled with many dark spots sprinkled across a tan or slightly discolored large area of skin (nevus spilus).

Because approximately 6% of congenital nevi are said to evolve into melanoma, there is greater concern about their management. Particularly difficult to treat are the large "bathing-trunk" nevi, for which the risk of melanoma is said to be 15%, but for which complete removal results in disfigurement. The exact incidence of melanoma and the best treatment for these lesions is unclear and controversial. If a large congenital nevus is disfiguring and can be removed so that the scar site is cosmetically superior to the nevus, there seems little doubt that excision, even if in stages, is the best course. If complete excision implies even more disfigurement, it may be more prudent to follow the lesion. If the congenital nevus is small, the decision whether or not to excise it can be left to the judgment of the patient and the clinician. However, as a national policy, it is probably unwise to excise all small, congenital nevi because they probably number 15,000 per year.

Blue Nevus (Mongolian Spot) (Figs. 19.32 and 19.33)

The common blue nevus is a 5-mm, round, elevated, blue-black nodule most often located on the dorsa of hands or feet of darker skinned women—for example, on Oriental females. They may also occur on the buttocks, face, and other sites on the arms and legs. Histologically, they are heavily pigmented spindle cells (dentritic melanocytes and macrophages) intercalated throughout the collagen of the reticular dermis and sometimes into the subcutaneous fat.

A variant is the cellular blue nevus. This is a larger, more atypical, lesion that can clinically and histologically overlap with, or even evolve into, malignant melanoma. It is large—1–2 cm—and is comprised in part of large, pale spindle cells replacing much of the reticular dermis.

Table 19.2.
Clinical Features Helpful in Discriminating Nevi from Melanoma

	Nevi	Melanoma
Size	1–4 mm	>6 mm
Color	Uniform brown	Variable (white, black, brown, red, blue)
Border	Smooth & round	Irregular & nonrounded
Thickness	Even or smooth dome	Irregular (flat with nodules)

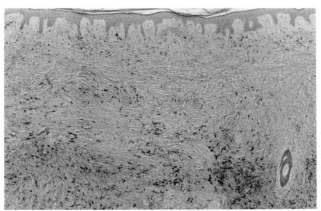

FIGURE 19.32. Blue nevus. The dermis contains numerous heavily pigmented spindle cells without atypia.

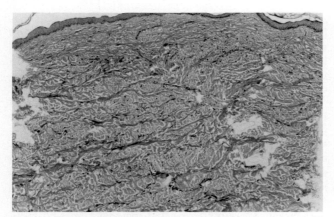

FIGURE 19.33. Mongolian spot. Embedded throughout the collagen are sparse numbers of pigmented spindle cells.

Spitz Nevus (Juvenile Melanoma) (Figs. 19.34 and 19.35)

Nowhere within skin tumors is there a greater difficulty in histological differential diagnosis than with the Spitz nevus. Its histology looks malignant, but its behavior is benign. The biggest clue to its identity is probably its clinical appearance as a red, round, dome-shaped nodule that is often mistaken for a pyogenic granuloma. In fact, the clinician's preoperative diagnosis of pyogenic granuloma coupled with the pathologist's diagnosis of melanoma is a scenario so common that it by itself suggests the diagnosis of Spitz nevus.

Spitz nevi occur more commonly in infancy and childhood than during adult life. They are most often round, sharply and smoothly bordered, pink to red nodules less than 6 mm in diameter. They occur most commonly on the face and legs and are most often a single lesion.

Histologically, Spitz nevi are sharply circumscribed, have large, often spindle-shaped, cells with large nuclei and abundant pink cytoplasm, have moderate maturation

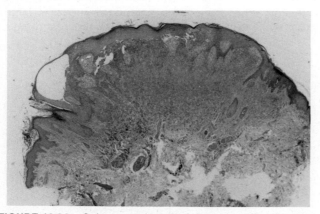

FIGURE 19.34. Spitz nevus is one of the most difficult lesions to diagnose. It is a circumscribed lesion with symmetry to its growth, with clefts at the epidermal junction and evidence of maturation of the cells toward the base. At the junctional clefts are pink, amorphous globules. This histology suggests a Spitz nevus; however, accurate diagnosis requires clinical information and probably follow-up.

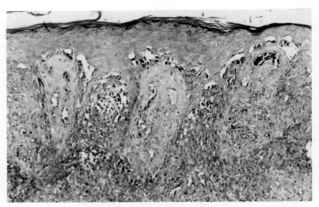

FIGURE 19.35. Spitz nevus.

to smaller cells in the deeper dermis, have epidermal hyperplasia with large cleft spaces at the epidermal-dermal junction, and have round, pink globules also located at the junction (Kamino bodies). They lack a lateral junctional component, pagetoid spread of melanocytes within the epidermis, and significant numbers of mitotic figures. Yet there is probably no set of histological features that safely discriminates all Spitz nevi from melanoma.

Freckle (or Ephelis)

The freckle is the most common pigmented lesion of the skin, but it is not a tumor of anything, let alone a melanocyte. Freckles are often multiple. They occur on sun-exposed skin, increase with age, increase with summer exposure, are probably an inherited trait, and certainly occur more commonly on fair-skinned persons (blondes and redheads). Freckles are 1–2 mm, flat, tan spots, and histologically they are a mild increase in pigmentation of keratinocytes. They may result from a different type of melanosome (the cytoplasmic organelle responsible for melanin synthesis), rather than from any increase in melanocytes.

Lentigo and Solar Lentigo

Like freckles, lentigos are flat, small, pigmented lesions occurring with sun damage. Unlike freckles, lentigos appear darker and histologically show elongated rete ridges and melanocytic hyperplasia. They merge morphologically with junctional nevi and, in some instances, with dysplastic nevi and lentigo maligna (a form of melanoma in situ).

Café-au-Lait Spot

The café-au-lait spot varies from millimeters to over 20 cm. It is uniformly light tan, flat, and has sharp, but often irregular, borders. Neither its distribution nor its behavior relates to sun exposure. Whereas 90% of patients with von Recklinghausen's disease have café-au-lait spots, less than 0.5% of patients with a café-au-lait spot have von Recklinghausen's disease; therefore, the single spot is a sensitive, but nonspecific, marker for the disease. On the other hand, multiple café-au-lait spots are both sensitive and specific because it is seldom that an individual has over six café-au-lait spots over 1.5 cm unless he or she also has von Recklinghausen's disease. The histology of the café-au-lait spot is similar to a freckle, and like the freckle, the café-au-lait spot may be due to an altered melanosome (sometimes giant melanosomes) rather than to any change in the number of melanocytes.

Becker's Nevus

Becker's nevus is a large, hairy, pigmented abnormality most often located on the shoulder and chest. It is a malformation rather than a tumor and may represent an organoid nevus. Its histology comprises subtle abnormalities of epidermis (mild hyperplasia and corrugation), hairs (increased number), smooth muscle (increased in some), and possibly melanocytes (subtly increased in some).

References

1. Ackerman AB, Wade TR: Tricholemmoma. *Am J Dermatopathol* 2:207, 1980.
2. Brownstein MH: Tricholemmoma. Benign follicular tumor or viral wart? *Am J Dermatopathol* 2:229, 1980.

Suggested Readings

Hashimoto K, Mehregan AH, Kumakiri M: *Tumors of Skin Appendages.* Boston, Butterworths, 1987.
Lever WF, Schaumburg-Lever G: *Histopathology of the Skin.* Philadelphia, JB Lippincott, 1983.
McKee PH: *Pathology of the Skin with Clinical Correlations.* Philadelphia, JB Lippincott, 1989.
Roenigk RK, Roenigk HH: *Dermatologic Survey, Principles and Practice.* New York, Marcel Dekker, Inc, 1989.
Maize JC, Ackerman AB: *Pigmented Lesions of the Skin, Clinicopathologic Correlations.* Philadelphia, Lea & Febiger, 1987.

20

Surgical Management of Cutaneous Melanoma

Hilliard F. Seigler, M.D., F.A.C.S.

Cutaneous melanoma represents a disease entity that is experiencing a true increase in incidence. Historically, this malignancy comprised approximately 3% of all neoplastic diseases. Over the past decade, melanoma has increased in our population by more than 90%. At the turn of the century, approximately 1 in 1,500 Americans developed melanoma, and at the present, approximately 1 in 128 will develop the disease. The reconstructive surgeon is involved both with the management of the primary disease and reconstructive procedures and with the surgical therapy of metastatic disease. Questions concerning biopsy procedures, operative management of the primary lesion, the role of regional lymphadenectomy, and the type of reconstruction depend on both clinical presentation and histopathological features. The prognostic factors and indicators for cutaneous melanoma have been investigated thoroughly and are of utmost importance to the surgeon in devising a comprehensive treatment plan for the patient.

Clinical and Pathological Features

There are four histopathological types of cutaneous melanoma: (*a*) lentigo maligna melanoma (Fig. 20.1); (*b*) superficial spreading melanoma (Fig. 20.2); (*c*) acral lentiginous melanoma (Fig. 20.3); and (*d*) nodular melanoma (Fig. 20.4). With the exception of nodular melanoma, all others demonstrate an intraepidermal component. In a clinical sense, the early growth phase is in a radial direction, and only nodular melanoma exhibits vertical growth from its inception. If early diagnosis could be established for the first three types before vertical growth and involvement of the vascular structures takes place, most could be cured by simple excision alone. Unfortunately, diagnosis is often delayed and, thus, the prognosis is less favorable. The histological features of the different types of cutaneous melanoma are well characterized. Lentigo maligna melanoma demonstrates junctional activity and prominent solar elastosis. Pagetoid cells are uncommon (Fig. 20.5). Superficial spreading melanoma is characterized by the presence of pagetoid cells. Solar elastosis is not prominent, and again, junctional activity is usually present (Fig. 20.6). Acral lentiginous melanomas have only recently been described. These lesions have junctional activity and abundant atypical melanocytes. Solar elastosis is absent (Fig. 20.7). Nodular melanomas do not

have a junctional component and are characterized by vertical growth patterns (Fig. 20.8).

Adequate tissue representation obtained by a biopsy is the responsibility of the surgeon. The pathologist can be helpful only if the tissue he or she receives is representative of the most severe involvement of the primary tumor process. Whenever possible, excisional biopsy is preferred. However, should the lesion be in a difficult location or quite large, an incisional biopsy should be done in the area of the primary tumor that exhibits the most severe clinical involvement. The indications for biopsy are dictated by changes that have taken place in the pigmented lesions. These changes are characterized by irregular surfaces, irregular borders, and change in pigmentation. Scaling and ulceration are also important clinical characteristics.

The pathologist should make careful notations concerning the depth of invasion, tumor thickness, tumor ulceration, type of primary, and the presence or absence of satellitosis. Each of these histopathological features represents an important prognostic factor. The contribution of Clark et al. (1) on the importance of level of invasion is well recognized (Table 20.1). In terms of reproducibility and clinical correlation, tumor thickness as described by Breslow (2) carries with it a greater statistical significance (Fig. 20.9).

Balch et al. (3) have reported the importance of tumor ulceration. If the tumor is confined to the epidermis and measures less than 0.7 mm in thickness, simple excision alone will cure more than 90% of the patients. If microsatellitosis is absent in this group, as is usual, then a margin of 1 cm is adequate. If the tumor is of intermediate thickness, margins of 2 cm are generally recommended. Only large primaries with either microscopic or macroscopic satellitosis will require broader tissue margins. Regional

Table 20.1.
Description of Tumor Invasion by Clark's Levels

Clark Level	Description
1	All tumor cells above basement membrane
2	Invasion into loose connective tissue of papillary dermis
3	Tumor cells at junction of papillary and reticular dermis
4	Invasion into reticular dermis
5	Invasion into subcutaneous fat

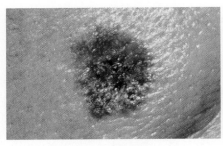

FIGURE 20.1.   Lentigo maligna melanoma of the right cheek.

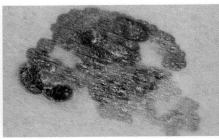

FIGURE 20.2.   Superficial spreading melanoma.

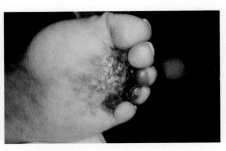

FIGURE 20.3.   Acral lentiginous melanoma.

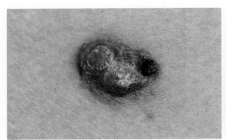

FIGURE 20.4.   Nodular melanoma.

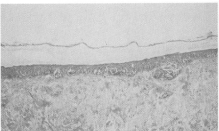

FIGURE 20.5.   Lentigo maligna melanoma demonstrating junctional activity and solar elastosis.

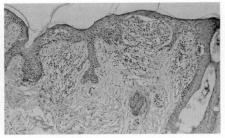

FIGURE 20.6.   Superficial spreading melanoma demonstrating presence of pagetoid cells and junctional activity.

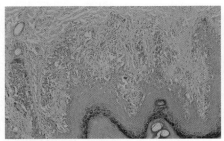

FIGURE 20.7.   Acral lentiginous melanomas demonstrating junctional activity with abundant atypical melanocytes.

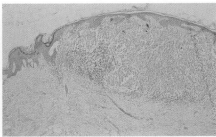

FIGURE 20.8.   Nodular melanomas characterized by vertical growth patterns.

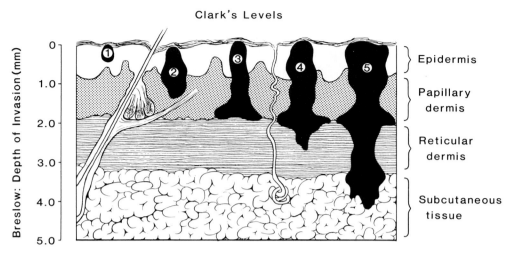

FIGURE 20.9. Prognostic factors showing Clark's level of invasion and Breslow's depth of invasion.

lymph node dissection is discussed in a subsequent section.

Association of Pathological Types with Clinical Presentation

Lentigo maligna has a tendency to occur in older individuals and is commonly seen on sun-exposed areas of the body. The most common location is the head and neck; however, this type of melanoma can occur on the dorsa of the hands and feet. The biological behavior demonstrates a prolonged radial growth phase. The lesion has a tendency to exist for a number of years before undergoing rapid changes that direct the patient to seek medical attention. Not all of the typically large pigmented area is, in fact, malignant or invasive. If the lesion involves the dorsa of the hands and feet, excision and skin grafting is usually the treatment of choice. If the lesion involves the skin of the face, excision and either cosmetic grafting or flap coverage is recommended. If the lesion covers a broad area of the face, the biopsy should be done in the area of vertical growth, and the resection can be limited to the malignant portion of the pigmented primary process. If the lesion is quite thin, lymph nodes do not need to be addressed. Overall, the prognosis of lentigo maligna is excellent.

Superficial spreading melanoma and *nodular melanoma* have a tendency to occur in similar areas of the body. Nodular melanomas can usually be excised and the wound closed primarily because of the absence of radial growth, whereas large superficial spreading melanomas may require skin grafts or skin flaps if adequate tissue margins are to be attained. Areas of the body requiring specialized therapy with these two pathological types are generally confined to the head and neck. Most other areas can be excised with 1–2-cm margins, and primary closure is technically feasible. If the scalp is involved and the tumor is small, excision of the primary lesion with flap coverage is preferable. If the lesion has a wide diameter, an excision extending to the galea and skin grafting are

FIGURE 20.10. Composite graft showing reconstruction of nasal melanoma.

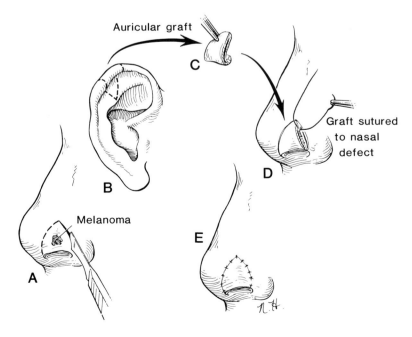

FIGURE 20.11. **A,** Wide local excision of primary melanoma. Two-centimeter margins represent adequate measurement for excision. **B,** Split-thickness skin grafting providing wound closure.

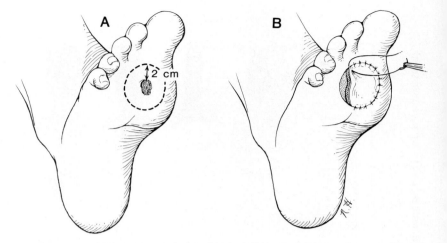

usually necessary. Because of the rich lymphatic and vascular supply, scalp lesions have a tendency to recur locally if adequate borders are not accomplished by the surgeon. Lesions involving the ala of the nose or the pinna of the ear are associated with a guarded prognosis and a high incidence of local recurrence and regional metastasis. It is recommended that amputation in these areas be completed.

Reconstruction can be accomplished for nasal primaries using composite grafts (Fig. 20.10), but standard reconstructive procedures should be done if the large portion of the ear has been deleted in an effort to gain control of the primary. Fortunately, eyelid primaries are extremely rare. If the lid is involved, excision with standard lid reconstruction is the recommended procedure for lesions greater than 1 mm in thickness. If lesion thickness is less than 1 mm, excision and thin split-thickness skin grafting can be accomplished.

Acral lentiginous melanomas occur in the subungual area, the palms, plantar surfaces, mucous membranes, and anorectal junction. Palmar and plantar acral lentiginous primaries require wide local excision and thick split-thickness skin grafting (Fig. 20.11). Coverage using skin

flaps is discouraged. If the area of involvement is near a digit, wide local excision with partial amputation and filleting of the dorsal skin of the digit for local flap coverage is associated with excellent control and functional wound coverage.

Lesions involving mucous membranes are associated with a poor prognosis. Not only is local control difficult to achieve, but the likelihood of systemic spread of the disease is quite high. If the lesion is confined to the mucous membranes of the genital tract, excision with 2-cm margins should be planned. The type of closure will be dictated by the area of the primary lesion. If the glans penis or clitoris is involved, amputation is necessary.

Melanoma occurring in the mucous membranes of the nose and sinuses should be approached more conservatively because the prognosis is ultimately poor. Usually, local excision followed by adjuvant therapy is the most justifiable treatment regimen. If the primary is located at the anorectal junction, local excision and closure for small and thin lesions is adequate; however, abdominoperineal resection might well be required for large primary lesions.

Pigmented lesions in the subungual position should be biopsied if they persist beyond 3–4 weeks. If the diagnosis of subungual melanoma is established, amputation at the distal interphalangeal joint should be accomplished. No attempt at local control by excision and cross-digit flap should be entertained. If the lesion is quite large and advanced to the area of the distal joint, total deletion of the digit might well be necessary. If the thumb is involved, attempts should be made to preserve opposition (Fig. 20.12). A reasonable functional result can be realized if the amputation is done at the level of the interphalangeal joint.

Elective Versus Therapeutic Lymph Node Dissection

The question concerning the efficacy of elective lymph node dissection in patients with melanoma has been refuted and defended over the years. Only recently have randomized trials, statistical techniques, and sufficient

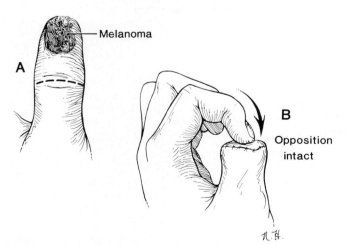

FIGURE 20.12. **A,** Partial thumb amputation for subungual melanoma. **B,** Thumb amputation permits functional digital opposition.

data bases permitted the accurate assessment of this difficult topic. If those patients who stand to benefit from this procedure can be identified, a therapeutic benefit is possible. Univariant and multivariant statistical analyses indicate that patients with thin melanomas (less than 1.5 mm) have little to gain from elective node dissection. The likelihood that micrometastases are present in this group of patients is so small that lymph node dissection on an elective basis is usually not justified.

Those patients who have a thick melanoma, whether ulcerated or nonulcerated, also have little to gain. A Breslow tumor thickness of 4.0 mm or greater suggests the probability of systemic disease that exceeds the potential therapeutic benefit of performing elective node dissection. Patients with tumor thicknesses ranging from 1.5 to 4 mm appear to have the most to gain from elective node dissection (4). Lymph node groups typically involved include cervical, axillary, and ilioinguinal nodes. Patients with intermediate-thickness melanoma primaries who undergo elective node dissection realize an approximate 15% increase in remaining disease free.

There is little argument of the prognostic value derived from a lymphadenectomy. Patients with a single positive lymph node have a 60% risk of recurrent disease. Those with two to four positive nodes have approximately a 75% risk factor, and those with greater than four positive lymph nodes are at greater than 90% risk of recurrent disease. If the lesion occurs on the lower extremity, a superficial inguinal node dissection is probably adequate. Removal of deep iliac nodes adds to limb morbidity and resection and probably does not add significantly to the disease-free interval. If the deep iliac nodes are involved, the probability of systemic disease usually dictates the eventual outcome, and more than 90% of patients die secondary to their disease. If the lesion occurs on the upper extremity, standard axillary dissection preserving the pectoralis major and minor muscles is recommended.

If the primary tumor occurs on the head, neck, or trunk and exhibits an ambiguous area of lymph node drainage, diagnostic lymphoscintigraphy can assist in identifying the site of lymph node drainage (5). Technetium-99m–labeled antimony trisulfide scan is a simple, standardized technique that can assist in accurate identification of axillary versus inguinal or supraclavicular lymph node drainage in ambiguous truncal lesions, as well as anterior versus posterior lymph node drainage from scalp lesions. In most instances, the lymph nodes can be identified and the dissection done at the time of definitive management of the primary tumor.

Chemotherapy

Chemotherapeutic drugs can be administered either systemically or by regional infusion. They can be given for an adjuvant effect in patients at high risk with no evidence of disease or to those patients with obvious tumor burdens in a treatment modality. Adjuvant systemic chemotherapy, either with a single drug or multiple drugs in different combinations, has proven to be of little significant clinical benefit in patients at high risk of developing recurrent disease. A number of studies have been reported from a variety of institutions, and all demonstrate little benefit from adjuvant chemotherapy.

Patients with documented tumor burden have demonstrated therapeutic benefit from systemic chemotherapy. The two most beneficial combinations include DTIC, CCNU, vincristine, and bleomycin administered over a 5-day period each 6 weeks (6) or cisplatin, DTIC, BCNU, and tamoxifen administered monthly (7). The complete response rate of either regimen is approximately 10%; an additional 30% of patients will realize a partial response. Chemotherapy has been most efficacious for those patients with metastatic disease involving skin, subcutaneous tissue, lymph nodes, and lungs. Anatomical areas of involvement associated with a poor response include brain, bone, liver, and the gastrointestinal tract. More recently, high-dose chemotherapy with autologous bone marrow reconstitution has been attempted with some clinical success. The response in patients with systemic disease undergoing this more aggressive treatment has approached 60–70%. Unfortunately, the long-term outlook continues to be guarded.

Regional drug infusion, either at normothermic or hyperthermic temperatures, has undergone numerous clinical trials. Limb perfusion for high-risk patients in an adjuvant setting has clear benefit in this patient population. Additionally, limb perfusion has been reported to show a significant therapeutic benefit in patients with local recurrent disease, in-transit lesions, or numerous metastatic lesions involving only the affected extremity (8, 9). The major shortcoming of this technique is that patients are at high risk for the development of systemic disease. Failures in the regional form of therapy usually lead to the development of distant disease. For this reason, many oncologists recommend systemic combination chemotherapy for patients receiving regional perfusion. The morbidity of limb perfusion can also be significant. Problems including muscle compartment syndromes, major skin loss, and decrease in range of motion have all been reported. These are serious side effects and must be weighed carefully when recommending regional therapy for patients treated in the adjuvant mode.

Immunotherapy

In a classical sense, immunotherapy can be administered either passively or actively. Passive immunotherapy includes passive serotherapy and passive cellular therapy. Active immunotherapy includes nonspecific immunogens as well as a specific immunogen. Until recently, the passive administration of specific antibody could be practically managed only in a limited sense. However, with the advent of monoclonal antibody technology, this has become an area of intense research and may lead to clinical application. A phase I clinical trial has been reported with some clinical benefit (10). The passive administration of host lymphocytes modified in vitro has been under intense investigation over the past 5 years. For the most part, this has included lymphokine-activated lymphocytes, expanded tumor-infiltrating lymphocytes, and specific cytotoxic T cells. Patients receiving lymphokine-activated lymphocytes in conjunction with interleukin-2 have realized approximately 20% therapeutic benefit (11). More recently, utilization of tumor-infiltrating lymphocytes has been associated with approximately 35% clinical response. This area of tumor immunobiology is certain to undergo additional scrutiny in the near future. Most of the lymphokines have been successfully produced by recombination into bacteria. Thus, reasonable amounts of very pure reagents are now available for expanded clinical trials. At the present time, interleukins 1 through 6 are available for study.

Traditionally, the most efficient means of producing clinically relevant immunity has been in the area of specific active immunization. Melanoma patients have been immunized with either intact autologous or allogeneic melanoma cells or with a viral oncolystate prepared from such cells (12, 13). The data suggest that statistically significant therapeutic benefit is produced in high-risk stage I and stage II patients treated in the adjuvant mode. Specific active immunization administered directly into the lymphatic systemic has also been reported to be of some benefit in patients with macroscopic stage II disease (14).

References

1. Clark WH Jr, From L, Bernardino EA, et al: The histogenesis and biologic behavior of primary human malignant melanomas of the skin. *Cancer Res* 29:705, 1969.
2. Breslow A: Thickness cross-sectional areas of depth of invasion in the prognosis of cutaneous melanoma. *Ann Surg* 172:902, 1970.
3. Balch CM, Soong S, Murad TM, et al: A multifactorial analysis of melanoma. III. Prognostic factors in melanoma patients with lymph node metastases (stage II). *Ann Surg* 193:377, 1981.
4. Reintgen DS, Cox EB, McCarty KS Jr, et al: Efficacy of elective lymph node dissection in patients with intermediate thickness primary melanomas. *Ann Surg* 198:379, 1983.
5. Reintgen DS, Sullivan D, Coleman E, et al: Lymphoscintigraphy for malignant melanoma: Surgical considerations. *Ann Surg* 198:379, 1983.
6. Seigler HF, Lucas VS, Pickett NJ, et al: DTIC, CCNU, bleomycin and vincristine (BOLD) in metastatic melanoma. *Cancer* 46:2346, 1980.
7. McClay EF, Mastrangelo MJ, Sprandio JD, Bellet RE, Berd D: The importance of tamoxifen to a cisplatin-containing regimen in the treatment of metastatic melanoma. *Cancer* 63:1292, 1989.
8. McBride CM, Sugarbaker EV, Hickey RC: Prophylactic isolation-perfusion as the primary therapy for invasive malignant melanoma of the limbs. *Ann Surg* 182:316, 1975.
9. Stehlin JS, Smith JL, Jing B, et al: Melanomas of the extremities complicated by in-transit metastases. *Surg Gynecol Obstet* 122:3, 1966.
10. Houghton AN, Mintzer D, et al: Mouse monoclonal 1g G3 antibody detecting GD3 ganglioside: A phase 1 trial in patients with malignant melanoma. *Proc Natl Acad Sci USA* 82:1242, 1985.
11. Rosenberg SA, Lotze MT, Muul LM, et al: A progress report of the treatment of 157 patients with advanced cancer using lymphokine-activated killer cells and interleukin-2 or high-dose interleukin-2 alone. *N Engl J Med* 316:889, 1987.
12. Seigler HF, Cos E, Mutzner F, et al: Specific active immunotherapy for melanoma. *Ann Surg* 190:366, 1979.
13. Cassel WA, Murray DR, Phillips HS: A phase II study on the postsurgical management of stage II malignant melanoma with a Newcastle disease virus oncolysate. *Cancer* 52:856, 1983.
14. Giuliano AE, Moseley HS, Morton DL: Clinical aspects of unknown primary melanoma. *Ann Surg* 191:98, 1980.

21

Management of Benign and Malignant Primary Salivary Gland Tumors

Mark S. Granick, M.D., F.A.C.S., Dwight C. Hanna, M.D., F.A.C.S., and E. Douglas Newton, M.D., F.A.C.S.

Primary neoplasms of the salivary glands are uncommon, comprising less than 3% of all head and neck tumors (1). Their diverse range of pathology, the complex interrelationships between the tumors, their location adjacent to various critical anatomical structures, and the variable biological behavior of the different histopathological tumor types all complicate their management.

Proper treatment begins with an accurate histopathological diagnosis. Foote and Frazell (2) were the first authors to attempt a comprehensive pathological classification of parotid tumors. Batsakis and coworkers (3) have redefined and clarified this categorization into the currently accepted standard (Table 21.1).

A number of large series have been published during the past 30 years, and in general, the distribution and percentage of histopathological types are similar. The larger glands have the most tumors and the highest percentage of benign tumors (Table 21.2). The most common benign tumor in all of the salivary glands is by far the pleomorphic adenoma (benign mixed tumor). Mucoepidermoid carcinoma is the most common parotid malignancy, and adenoid cystic carcinoma is the most common malignancy in the submandibular and minor salivary glands.

Preoperative Evaluation

The most common presentation is that of a painless mass (Fig. 21.1). A fluctuant or soft mass is most commonly associated with the benign Warthin's tumor. A mass bulging behind the lateral oropharyngeal wall frequently represents a parotid deep lobe tumor. Associated symptoms may include pain or facial weakness, which are both suggestive of underlying malignancies, but even the most experienced examiners cannot reliably determine whether a mass is benign or malignant. Duration of symptoms is more than a year in 50% of the patients (4, 5).

Gallia and Johnson (6) demonstrated that as many as 85% of submandibular and 27% of parotid lesions treated by excision were inflammatory disorders. At least two thirds of the patients with submandibular gland disease gave a history of recurrent postprandial pain, erythema, swelling, and purulent discharge. Examination of each patient should include careful examination of the oral cavity and oropharynx. Warthin's and Stensen's ducts and orifices must be viewed and palpated for signs of inflammation, tumor, scarring, sialolithiasis, and saliva flow. Lack of resolution with appropriate medical treatment of a mass suspected of being inflammatory demands histopathological analysis.

The tonsillar fossa and soft palate must be examined for the presence of deep lobe parotid involvement. Direct palpation of the individual glands must be done bimanually to appreciate intraglandular masses. Bilateral comparison of the glands is important to detect subtle abnormalities. The neck needs to be thoroughly examined for nodal involvement. In addition, potential primary sites that can metastasize to the salivary glands, such as the scalp, face, and distant sites (7–9), must be examined.

Preoperative radiographic studies may delineate a mass lesion but are useless in deciding whether or not it is malignant (10). Ultrasonic analysis is not clinically valuable at this time (11). Radionuclide imaging is only able to detect mass lesions greater than 1.5 cm in diameter (12). Warthin's tumor and oncocytoma specifically concentrate technetium-99m, but this is not presently of clinical use.

All salivary gland tumors should be excised as a rule. The value of preliminary biopsy is controversial. Eneroth (13) and others (14) have advocated fine-needle aspiration, reporting a 74–92% accuracy. Almost all of the lesions should be excised, regardless of the result of fine-needle biopsy, because only positive diagnoses are significant (15).

Indications for large-core needle or incisional biopsy include differentiation of inflammatory from neoplastic masses and diagnosis of inflammatory masses. Frozen section diagnosis of malignant salivary neoplasms is unreliable in some hands (16, 17). In our experience, frozen section analysis has been accurate and useful, particularly in those instances in which we are debating the necessity of facial nerve resection. The accuracy rate of frozen section at our institution, based on 462 salivary tumors, is 95.7% (18).

Table 21.1.
Classification of Epithelial Salivary Gland Tumors[a]

Type of Lesion	Variations
Benign	Mixed tumor (pleomorphic adenoma)
	Papillary cystadenoma lymphomatosum (Warthin's tumor)
	Oncocystoma oncocytosis
	Monomorphic tumors
	Basal cell adenoma
	Glycogen-rich adenoma (?)
	Clear-cell adenoma (?)
	Membranous adenoma
	Myoepithelioma
	Sebaceous tumors
	Adenoma
	Lymphadenoma
	Papillary ductal adenoma (papilloma)
	Benign lymphoepithelial lesion
	Unclassified
Malignant	Carcinoma ex pleomorphic adenoma (carcinoma arising in a mixed tumor)
	Malignant mixed tumor (biphasic malignancy)
	Mucoepidermoid carcinoma
	Low grade
	Intermediate grade
	High grade
	Adenoid cystic carcinoma
	Adenocarcinoma
	Mucus-producing adenopapillary and nonpapillary carcinoma
	Salivary duct carcinoma (ductal carcinoma)
	Other adenocarcinomas
	Oncocytic cell carcinoma (malignant oncocytoma)
	Clear-cell carcinoma (nonmucinous and glycogen containing or non-glycogen containing)
	Primary squamous cell carcinoma
	Hybrid basal cell adenoma/adenoid cystic carcinoma
	Undifferentiated carcinoma
	Epithelial myoepithelial carcinoma of intercalated ducts
	Miscellaneous (includes sebaceous lesions, Stenson's duct lesions, melanoma, and carcinoma exlymphoepithelial lesions)
	Metastatic
	Unclassified

[a] From Batsakis JG, Regezi JA: The pathology of head and neck tumors: Salivary glands part 1. *Head Neck Surg* 1:59, 1978–1979.

Staging

The current American Joint Committee on Cancer (19) clinical staging system for cancer of the salivary gland is based on five clinical variables that influence survival rates over a 10-year period. These variables include tumor size, local extension, presence of distant metastases, palpability of regional nodes, and "suspicion of metastatic carcinoma" in regional nodes (Table 21.3). The 5-year survival probabilities range from 85–90% for stage II and III tumors to 9% for stage IV tumors (Table 21.4).

Table 21.2.
Distribution of Salivary Gland Tumors

Gland	% Salivary Gland Tumors	% Malignant Tumors
Parotid	80	25
Submandibular	15	35
Minor salivary glands	5	50

Clinical Management

PAROTID BENIGN TUMORS

Pleomorphic Adenoma (Mixed Tumor)

Pleomorphic adenomas are the most common salivary gland tumors. Rauch's (20) review of 4,245 pleomorphic adenomas revealed that 84% of them occur in the parotid gland. In Spiro's evaluation of 2,807 salivary gland tumors, 70% of the parotid and 45% of all of the tumors were benign mixed (15). Clinically, they appear as firm, discrete, gradually enlarging parotid masses. Rarely, pain or facial paralysis may occur. Grossly, the tumors appear to be solid and encapsulated. Histologically, however, the capsule is actually composed of compressed tumor cells. There are, in addition, multiple projections and sometimes multicentric foci of tumor in the gland (21). The cell types composing this tumor consist of a spectrum ranging from epithelial to myoepithelial cells (3).

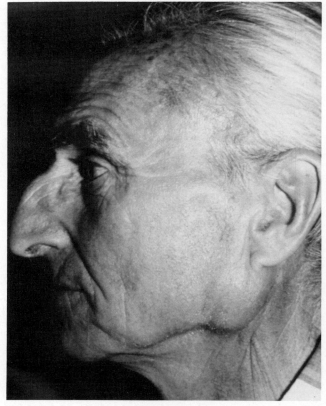

FIGURE 21.1. Most salivary gland tumors present as a painless mass.

Table 21.3.
Proposed Staging System for Major Salivary Gland Cancer (Parotid and Submandibular)[a]

Code	Criterion
T0	No clinical evidence of primary tumor
T1	Tumor less than 2.0 cm in diameter without significant local extension
T2	Tumor 2.1–4.0 cm in diameter without significant local extension
T3	Tumor 4.1–6.0 cm in diameter without significant local extension
T4a	Tumor more than 6 cm in diameter without significant local extension
T4b	Tumor of any size with significant local extension
N0	No evidence of regional lymph node involvement (including palpable but not suspicious regional lymph nodes)
N1	Evidence of regional lymph node involvement (including palpable and suspicious regional lymph nodes)
NX	Regional lymph nodes not assessed
M0	No distant metastases
M1	Distant metastases such as to bone, lung, etc.

Stage I	T1N0M0
	T2N0M0
Stage II	T3N0M0
Stage III	T1N1M0
	T2N1M0
	T4aN0M0
	T4bN0M0
Stage IV	T3N1M0
	T4aN1M0
	T4bN1M0
	Any T, Any N, and M1

[a] From Levitt SH, McHugh RB, Gomez-Martin O, et al: Clinical staging system for cancer of the salivary gland. A retrospective study. *Cancer* 47:2712, 1981.

When a pleomorphic adenoma recurs, the morbidity of the tumor and additional therapy increases dramatically. Recurrent benign mixed tumors are generally locally aggressive and infiltrative. O'Dwyer et al. (22) cited a 26% incidence of facial nerve sacrifice in recurrent tumor excisions and claimed that the major morbidity associated with benign mixed tumors is in managing recurrence. Because of the high risk to the facial nerve as well as the aggressive nature of recurrent benign tumors, Piorkowski and Guillamondegui have advocated radiation treatment for these lesions (23).

Pleomorphic adenomas tend to recur if inadequately excised, and there is a potential for malignancy in long-standing tumors (24–27), predicating their management by generous excision. Lanier et al. (24) demonstrated that there was a 70% recurrence rate in enucleated tumors, whereas after superficial parotidectomy, there was a 3.6% recurrence rate. Adequate surgical removal of pleomorphic adenoma consists of superficial or total parotidectomy. Dawson and Orr (27) demonstrated that irradiation was useful to prevent recurrences in difficult surgical situations such as in deep lobe tumor, poor margins of resection, or tumor adjacent to the facial nerve (27).

Warthin's Tumor (Papillary Cystadenoma Lymphomatosum)

Warthin's tumor is the second most common benign parotid neoplasm, accounting for 15% of all parotid tumors. It is a tumor of the salivary oncocyte, a cell that is thought to be an epithelial cell mutant, rarely present in parotid tissues before 40–50 years of age (3). In addition, there is a lymphoid stroma in these lesions. The tumors are multicentric and/or bilateral in 10–15% of patients (28). Patients are generally middle-aged men with a soft, cystic-feeling mass in the tail of the parotid. Adequate therapy consists of superficial parotidectomy. In spite of the apparent localization of the tumor in the tail of the parotid in many patients, the high incidence of multicentricity dictates against limited parotid resections.

PAROTID MALIGNANT TUMORS

The best staging parameters, the appropriate extent of surgery, the management of the facial nerve, the treatment of the clinically negative neck, and the use of adjuvant therapy are all issues of current concern in parotid cancer. Tumor histology is an important predictor of survival; mucoepidermoid carcinoma and acinic cell carcinoma have the best survival statistics (29). Histological grading is also a critical predictor; low-grade tumors have a 90% 10-year survival, and high-grade tumors have a

Table 21.4.
Stage Grouping in Salivary Gland Cancer (Using Five Clinical Variables)[a,b]

TNM Set	No. of Patients	5-year Survival Probability (%)	SE (%)
Stage I			
T1N0M0	136	90.1	2.6
T2N0M0	151	85.9	2.9
Overall	287	87.9	2.0
Stage II			
T3N0M0	51	56.9	6.9
Overall	51	56.9	6.9
Stage III			
T1N1M0	4		
T2N1M0	16	0.0	0.0
T4aN0M0	30	40.2	9.3
T4bN0M0	106	45.2	4.9
Overall	156	39.4	4.0
Stage IV			
T3N1M0	8		
T4aN1M0	12	17.7	10.8
T4bN1M0	38	7.9	4.4
Any T, Any N, and M1	8		
Overall	66	9.1	3.5

[a] From Levitt SH, McHugh RB, Gomez-Martin O, et al: Clinical staging system for cancer of the salivary gland. A retrospective study. *Cancer* 47:2712, 1981.
[b] Combination of five variables: *primary tumor:* size, local extension; *regional lymph nodes:* palpability, suspicion; *metastasis:* distant metastasis.

25% 10-year survival (15). Interestingly, TNM staging also correlates with prognosis; the 10-year survivals are 90%, 65%, and 22% for stages I, II, and III tumors, respectively (15).

The best result in terms of local tumor control still consists of wide local excision. Superficial parotidectomy with facial nerve preservation is the minimum treatment. The extent of surgery depends on the extent of disease rather than histology (15, 29, 30). The facial nerve should be excised if it is involved with malignant tumor. All additional tumor-involved tissue, including adjacent skin, bone, and muscle, should be similarly ablated. Some authors suggest elective neck dissection as a staging aid (31). The use of adjuvant irradiation to the primary site and ipsilateral neck for advanced, high-grade, or marginally resected tumors has provided significant improvement in locoregional control, but it has not improved long-term survival (29, 32–35).

Mucoepidermoid Carcinoma

This malignant tumor accounts for 50% of the parotid malignancies (29). It arises from interlobular and intralobular ductal epithelium and is mucin producing. There is a spectrum of biological activity, with low-grade or well-differentiated types acting in an almost benign fashion. The intermediate-grade tumors are less differentiated and tend to be locally invasive. The high-grade or poorly-differentiated tumors are very cellular and may be confused with squamous cell tumors. These lesions are very aggressive locally, have a high recurrence rate, and tend to metastasize.

Patients usually present with a painless solitary parotid mass present for a year or less. As many as 20% of patients with high-grade tumors have facial nerve dysfunction (36).

The factors most influencing survival of these patients are the histological grade of the tumor, the presence of clinically positive cervical nodes, and the clinical stage of the tumor.

Appropriate therapy consists of parotidectomy with excision and immediate nerve grafting of the facial nerve only if the tumor involves the nerve. Cervical lymphadenectomy is reserved for patients with palpable nodes. Radiation therapy to the primary site and lateral neck is advisable at 3–5 weeks postoperatively for moderate- or high-grade tumors.

Malignant Tumor in Pleomorphic Adenoma

Malignant tumors in pleomorphic adenomas comprise 10–20% of salivary malignancies. This neoplasm is highly malignant with a tendency to metastasize. In the series by Spiro et al. (37), 25% of the patients had cervical node metastases, and 32% had distant metastases to brain, bone, and lung. The presence of metastatic disease was usually associated with death within 1 year. Tortoledo et al. (38) demonstrated that survival was related to the degree of extension of malignant disease beyond the benign aspect of the tumor. Tumor extension greater than 8 mm was uniformly fatal, whereas those patients with extension less than 6 mm all survived.

A malignant tumor in a pleomorphic adenoma is of controversial histopathological origin (3). Six histological subtypes with differing prognoses have been identified (38). The common type occurs in long-standing or recurrent benign mixed tumor (Fig. 21.2). Treatment includes total parotidectomy, resection and immediate grafting of the facial nerve if it is involved with tumor, and neck dissection if there are nodal metastases.

Adenoid Cystic Carcinoma

This lesion is relatively uncommon in the parotid (7–15% of malignancies) but is the most common malignant tumor of the submandibular and minor salivary glands (35%). Adenoid cystic carcinoma has a variable histological pattern, ranging from cellular to cystic even within the same tumor.

Early perineural invasion with local spread is common, and later distant metastases, especially to the lung, contribute to long-term failure. Recurrences or metastases may occur after 20 or more disease-free years following initial treatment.

The accepted form of treatment for this tumor is similar to that for other parotid malignant tumors. Particular attention must be paid to the facial nerve because of this tumor's tendency for perineural spread. Postoperative radiation therapy has improved locogregional control, but it has not improved long-term survival because of poor control of distant metastases (39, 40). Our current philosophy of management is wide local excision and radiation therapy in all cases.

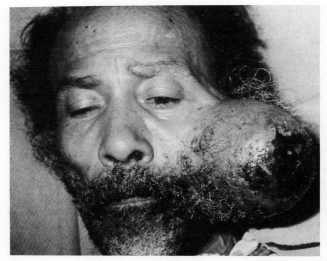

FIGURE 21.2. This 67-year-old patient had a long-standing stable parotid mass that suddenly began to rapidly enlarge. The pathology revealed malignant tumor in pleomorphic adenoma.

Other Malignant Tumors

There are a variety of additional but less common cancers that occur in the parotid (3, 5, 41–44; Table 21.1). Acinic cell carcinoma is locally aggressive but rarely involves the facial nerve or metastasizes to the neck. Adenocarcinoma (45) and epidermoid carcinoma often require facial nerve resection and cervical lymphadenectomy. Lymphoma may present in the partoid and is the only nonsurgically treated parotid cancer (46). Tumors that can metastasize to the parotid include squamous cell carcinoma in the watershed area draining through the gland (47). Additional distant sources of metastases include lung, breast, kidney, colon, stomach, pancreas, prostate, and distant melanoma (9, 47). A recently recognized source of parotid tumors is the lymphadenopathies related to the acquired immunodeficiency syndrome (48, 49).

Strategy for Management of Parotid Tumors

Our philosophy includes a number of basic concepts, little changed from those proposed in 1975 (4), from which decisions can be formulated for the management of specific cases.

1. Excisional biopsy is accomplished by superficial or total parotidectomy.
   A. Preliminary biopsy is rarely indicated.
   B. Superficial parotidectomy is performed for all tumors.
   C. Deep lobe tumors require superficial parotidectomy for exposure of the facial nerve, followed by resection of the deep lobe.
   D. Frozen section analysis of the tumor is routinely performed as an aid in determining the extent of surgery.
2. Management of the facial nerve:
   A. Possible facial nerve dysfunction following surgery is explained to all patients.
   B. Sacrifice of the facial nerve trunk or branches is necessary only when malignant tumor invades or is directly adherent to the nerve.
   C. Immediate nerve graft reconstruction is performed in all cases following nerve resection.
3. Management of malignant tumors:
   A. Total parotidectomy with facial nerve preservation is appropriate for most malignant tumors.
   B. See 2B.
   C. Cervical lymphadenectomy is performed when there is palpable cervical adenopathy associated with a malignant neoplasm.
   D. Radical resection of all tumor-involved tissue is required if extraglandular spread has occurred.
   E. Postoperative radiation therapy is advisable for all moderate to high-grade malignancies.

SUBMANDIBULAR GLAND TUMORS

Submandibular gland tumors are less common than parotid tumors, but they are more likely to be malignant (Table 21.3). The histopathological types are the same as those of the parotid, but adenoid cystic carcinoma is the more common malignancy (4, 50, 51). Benign pleomorphic adenoma is by far the most common benign neoplasm. Total gland excision is the biopsy technique. In small tumors, this may be adequate treatment. If frozen section diagnosis discloses malignancy, an upper neck dissection should be performed to assure adequate resection and to sample the upper neck nodes and nerves. Indicators of poor prognosis include extraglandular spread, cervical metastases, and high-grade mucoepidermoid or adenoid cystic carcinoma (52).

STRATEGY FOR MANAGEMENT OF SUBMANDIBULAR GLAND TUMORS

1. Excisional biopsy is accomplished by total glandular excision.
   A. Preliminary biopsy is not indicated.
   B. Frozen section analysis of the tumor is routinely performed as an aid in determining the extent of surgery.
2. Management of adjacent nerves:
   A. Possible postoperative dysfunction of the marginal mandibular branch of the facial nerve, the hypoglossal nerve, and the lingual nerve is explained to all patients.
   B. Sacrifice of any of the adjacent nerves is performed only when malignant tumor invades or is directly adherent to a nerve.
   C. Immediate nerve graft reconstruction should be performed, if possible.
3. Management of malignant tumors:
   A. Excision of the submandibular gland with submental and submandibular lymphadenectomy is appropriate for most malignant tumors.
   B. See 2B.
   C. Cervical lymphadenectomy is performed when there is palpable cervical adenopathy associated with a malignant neoplasm and for high-grade, T3 or T4 malignant tumors.
   D. Radical resection of all tumor-involved tissue is performed if extracapsular spread has occurred.
   E. Postoperative radiation therapy is advisable for all moderate- to high-grade malignancies.

MINOR SALIVARY GLAND NEOPLASMS

Benign pleomorphic adenoma is the most common benign neoplasm of the minor salivary glands. However, more than half of the neoplasms are malignant, and most of these are adenoid cystic carcinoma (53). The palate is the most commonly involved site (54, 55). These lesions generally present as firm, smooth, asymptomatic submucosal masses. Neither the history nor the gross physical appearance of these tumors is predictive of their histopathology.

Necrotizing sialometaplasia, which commonly occurs as an ulcerated palatal mass, is a benign lesion but can be mistaken for mucoepidermoid or undifferentiated carcinoma on histological examination. The histopathological features that characterize this entity are squamous metaplasia of necrotic seromucinous glands with maintenance of lobular architecture, nonanaplastic nuclear morphology, and prominent acute and chronic inflammation (56). This lesion is a reactive metaplasia apparently related to local ischemia. Necrotizing sialometaplasia heals spontaneously and does not require excision (56–59).

STRATEGY FOR MANAGEMENT OF MINOR SALIVARY GLAND TUMORS

1. Biopsy:
   A. Excisional biopsy with a small margin of normal tissue is performed for most lesions less than 4 cm in diameter.
   B. Preliminary incisional biopsy is advisable prior to definitive resection for lesions larger than 4 cm in diameter or for masses that are suspected of being necrotizing sialometaplasia.
   C. Frozen section analysis is routinely obtained as an aid in determining the extent of surgery and for control of the margins of resection.
2. Management of malignant tumors:
   A. Local excision of the tumor with a small margin of adjacent normal tissue is appropriate for most malignancies.
   B. Cervical metastases are rare, and cervical lymphadenectomy should be performed only for palpable cervical adenopathy.
   C. Immediate reconstruction of the excisional defect with local or distant tissue should be performed.
   D. Postoperative radiation therapy is advisable for all moderate- to high-grade malignancies, all malignant tumors larger than 4 cm, all cases of neural invasion, all cases associated with cervical metastases, and all instances of positive surgical margins.

PEDIATRIC SALIVARY TUMORS

Salivary gland tumors in infants and children are rare, and the topic is not widely covered in the literature. The Mayo Clinic experience showed a proportion of benign parotid lesions similar to that for adults (60), while the Iowa series had a 70% malignancy rate (61), and the Johns Hopkins experience demonstrated a 50% malignancy rate (62).

Benign pleomorphic adenoma was the most common benign tumor, followed by hemangioma, lymphangioma, and cystic hygroma (60). Mucoepidermoid carcinoma was the principle malignancy. A large survey of salivary gland lesions in children revealed that 61% of 430 lesions

were inflammatory (63). The evaluation of a child with a salivary gland mass should be directed toward establishing whether the mass is inflammatory. If there is any doubt or if the lesion is apparently a tumor, the treatment of choice is surgical excision.

Treatment

PAROTIDECTOMY—OPERATIVE TECHNIQUE

The key to parotidectomy is accurate, safe localization of the facial nerve. This has traditionally been performed by locating the main trunk of the nerve proximal to the parotid gland. We have found a distal nerve localization technique to be more expeditious in most cases. The consistent location of the distal facial nerve branches allows them to be identified easily, and the majority of tumors overlie the main trunk, which makes nerve identification under that area more difficult. Additionally, the trunk is more difficult to identify proximally within its surrounding connective tissue than are the peripheral branches, which are surrounded by loose areolar-type tissue.

Preoperative planning should anticipate the possibility of total parotidectomy, facial nerve grafting, temporal bone resection, mandibulectomy, or cervical lymphadenectomy. Usually, however, superficial parotidectomy is the operation that is performed.

The patient is placed in a supine position with the head of the table elevated. The head is turned away from the side of the lesion so that the entire side of the face can be prepped into the operative field.

General endotracheal anesthesia is the preferred method of anesthesia, but local anesthesia may sometimes be used. Any interference with facial nerve function makes its preservation more difficult. Facial nerve activity is closely monitored during surgery by observing the movement of facial muscles. Therefore, muscle relaxants commonly used in anesthesia should be avoided except for short-acting agents during induction.

The incision begins at the helical insertion of the ear, continues inferiorly to below the earlobe, and curves anteriorly, paralleling the angle of the jaw and approximately 2 cm below it. Sharp dissection is carried out anteriorly at the level of the superficial parotid fascia, with electrocautery of bleeding vessels. When this flap has been raised to the anterior border of the gland, it is sutured to the cheek, retracting it anteriorly (Fig. 21.3). Dissection continues posteriorly and inferiorly, exposing the remaining gland and the anterior border of the sternocleidomastoid muscle. At this point, the great auricular nerve is identified and as much of it as possible is preserved. This nerve not only supplies sensation to the ear lobule, but it is also the best source for nerve graft should it be needed. When operating on recurrent tumors, the scar of the previous surgery should be excised in continuity with the deeper specimen. On rare occasions, a deep lobe tumor may displace the facial nerve to a superficial position just below the lobule of the ear, where it can be easily injured by the unwary surgeon. Normally, however, the nerve is deep within the gland and becomes superficial only along the anterior border of the gland.

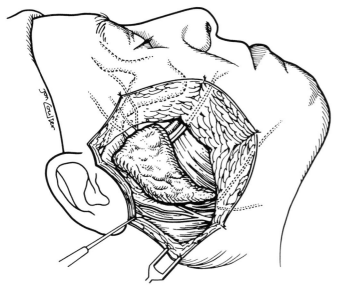

FIGURE 21.3. This schematic illustration demonstrates complete exposure of the parotid gland and the peripheral branches of the facial nerve.

Actual dissection of the facial nerve begins peripherally. A straight hemostat is used to bluntly separate the overlying tissue from the nerve branches by inserting the jaws of the instrument along the path of the nerve and spreading (Fig. 21.4). The operator should extrapolate the direction and approximate location of the radiating nerve branches and proceed along each branch in this fashion. This method of blunt dissection, when properly executed, should not injure normal nerve tissue. Stensen's duct is dissected free, clamped, divided, and ligated. Early identification and division of the duct facilitates quick mobilization of the anterior portion of the gland. The peripheral branches of the nerve are easily located lying on the temporalis muscle fascia superiorly and the masseter muscle fascia anteriorly. The marginal branch is found within the fibrofatty tissue of the upper neck overlying the facial vessels and submandibular gland (Fig. 21.3). The temporal branch of the facial nerve

crosses the superficial temporal vein and artery just below the level of the mandibular condyle (Fig. 21.5).

During dissection, care must be taken to manipulate the specimen as little as possible in order to prevent rupture of the tumor as well as stretching of the facial nerve. If dissection should become slow in one area, or if landmarks are unclear, it is always wise to progress to another location in which dissection is found to be easier and then to return to the area that had been more difficult.

When the tumor is located in the superficial portion of the gland, generally very little parotid tissue is found in the deep lobe. However, when the tumor is located in the deep portion of the gland, the facial nerve will be found stretched over the top of the tumor after the superficial portion has been removed. At this point, the nerve should be carefully teased off the tumor and the tumor removed from the fossa. On rare occasions, it has been necessary for us to divide the jaw just distal to the mental foramen in order to obtain enough exposure to remove the tumor.

Following the removal of the tumor, frozen section diagnosis is obtained in order to confirm the adequacy of the procedure that has been done or to indicate the need for further operative procedure. The facial nerve is sacrificed only when malignant or recurrent tumor directly involves the nerve. If the nerve is divided during the procedure, microneurorrhaphy under no tension should yield a 60–90% return of function. Our experience has been that microsurgical nerve grafting using the greater auricular nerve should yield similar results.

When the bleeding has been controlled, the wound is carefully flushed with saline and closed with a suction drain brought out through a stab wound inferior to the incision. The external auditory canal is carefully flushed in order to remove any blood that may have entered the canal during the procedure. The use of a suction drain eliminates the need for a pressure-type dressing.

SUBMANDIBULECTOMY: OPERATIVE TECHNIQUE

The patient is placed supine on the operating table, and general endotracheal anesthesia is administered. As for

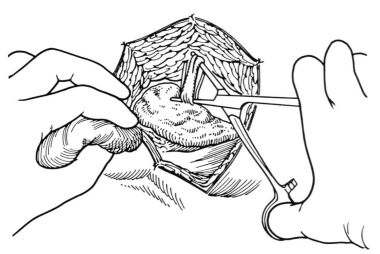

FIGURE 21.4. The technique of dissection consists of bluntly separating the overlying parotid tissue from the branches of the facial nerve.

FIGURE 21.5. This diagram demonstrates the vascular and neural anatomy in the operative field after removal of the superficial parotid lobe.

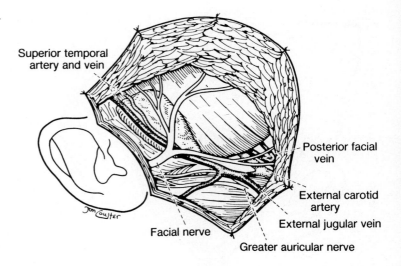

Superior temporal artery and vein

Posterior facial vein

External carotid artery

External jugular vein

Facial nerve

Greater auricular nerve

parotidectomy, precautions about the use of paralytic agents should be observed. The patient's head is turned, and the entire neck and lower face is prepped and draped into the operative field.

The submandibular gland is approached through an incision along a line that begins at the level of the mastoid process and is carried anteriorly 2 cm below the lower border of the mandible to the midline at the point of the chin. The actual incision is usually only 6 cm long overlying the gland, but it can be extended as necessary along this line, which also serves as the upper limb of a MacFee incision if a neck dissection is performed.

The incision is carried down through the platysma muscle, leaving the platysma attached to the skin flap unless there is adherence of the tumor to this tissue. As the flap is elevated, the marginal branch of the facial nerve will be found just deep to the platysma muscle and superficial to the facial vessels. The position of the nerve is variable in relation to the gland. The safest way to avoid nerve injury is to divide the posterior facial vein inferiorly and to raise the flap in the plane just deep to this vessel. In this way, it is possible to elevate the nerve while leaving it attached to the platysma muscle and thus preserving its function.

Dissection of the submandibular gland is then begun at the level of the hyoid bone where the lower border of the gland can be visualized. Deep to the gland and just superior to the digastric muscle, the hypoglossal nerve and accompanying ranine veins will be found. Dissection is continued superiorly until the facial artery is encountered exiting the gland anteriorly. The artery is clamped and divided at this point and ligated. Retraction of the myelohyoid muscle anteriorly will reveal the lingual nerve pulled inferiorly by the submandibular ganglion and accompanying vessels attached to the gland. This pedicle must be divided and ligated carefully, in order to preserve the main trunk of the lingual nerve. Warthin's duct will also be seen in this field and should be clamped, divided, and ligated. This allows for complete removal of the gland with any adjacent lymph nodes that might be attached to the gland.

Following removal of the submandibular gland, the wound is flushed out with saline and a layered closure is

performed along with placement of a suction drain. Again, this eliminates the necessity for a compression dressing.

COMPLICATIONS OF SURGERY

The primary complication that all surgeons should try to avoid is tumor recurrence. This is, unfortunately, not always preventable, even with excision that is considered adequate at the time of surgery. In our experience, locally recurrent tumor has been related almost exclusively to an inadequate initial extirpation.

Several reports detail the surgical precautions necessary to prevent common intraoperative complications such as bleeding, injury to the ear canal, and poor exposure. Injury to the facial nerve is an avoidable complication if proper surgical technique is used. However, if the nerve is inadvertently divided, it should be repaired immediately under magnification (4, 64, 65).

Frey syndrome is a common complication following parotidectomy. This is manifested by a spectrum of symptoms from erythema related to eating to copious gustatory sweating. Its etiology is thought to be aberrant connection of the regenerating salivary parasympathetic fibers to the sweat glands of the overlying skin flap. Numerous treatment plans have been proposed: irradiation, division of the glossopharyngeal or auriculotemporal

Table 21.5.
Salivary Gland Cancer Indications for Postoperative Radiation[a]

1. Highly malignant tumors
2. Extraglandular extension of tumor: neural, perineural, lymphatic invasion
3. Regional nodal metastases
4. After resection of recurrent tumor
5. Parotid deep lobe tumor
6. Tumor adjacent to facial nerve
7. Gross residual tumor after resection

[a] From Guillamondegui OM, Byers RM, Luna MA, et al: Aggressive surgery in treatment for parotid cancer: The role of adjunctive post-operative radiotherapy. *AJR* 123:49, 1975.

nerves, topical applications of atropine-like creams, and insertion of synthetic materials, fascial grafts, or vascularized tissue under the skin flap. None of these techniques have been useful in our hands. Most patients, fortunately, adapt well to this condition.

Postoperative complications such as seroma, hema-

toma, salivary fistula, and wound healing problems are uncommon. Temporary paralysis of all or a portion of the facial nerve is common and probably results from partial devascularization of the nerve, direct trauma to the nerve, or postoperative inflammation. Temporary paresis generally recovers within a few weeks but may take as

Table 21.6.
Comprehensive Treatment Plan for Salivary Gland Tumors

A. Parotid Gland

Tumor Characteristics	Parotidectomy	Facial Nerve	Neck Dissection	Radiation	Chemotherapy
			Management		
Low-grade mucoepidermoid carcinomas Benign tumors; T1 + T2 low grade; acinic cell carcinoma	Superficial or total	Preservation	No	No	No
T1 and T2 moderate to high grade; malignant mixed; adenocarcinoma; undifferentiated; epidermoid carcinoma	Total	Resection and immediate nerve graft only if nerve is involved by tumor	Yes, when there is palpable lymphadenopathy	Yes	No
T3; recurrent malignancy	Total	Resection and immediate nerve graft only if nerve is involved by tumor	Yes, when there is palpable lymphadenopathy	Yes	Possible
Any size tumor with extraglandular spread or T4	Radical (with involved adjacent tissues)	Resection and immediate nerve graft if nerve is involved by tumor	Yes, when there is palpable lymphadenopathy	Yes	Possible

B. Submandibular Gland

Tumor Status	Surgery	Radiation	Chemotherapy
		Management	
Benign tumors, T1 and T2	Total gland excision; limited upper cervical lymphadenectomy for malignant tumors without palpable adenopathy and full cervical lymphadenectomy if palpable nodes	Yes, if moderate- to high-grade malignancy or adenoid cystic carcinoma	No
Any size with extraglandular spread, T3, T4	Radical gland excision; excision of involved adjacent tissue; cervical lymphadenectomy	Yes	Possible

C. Minor Salivary Gland

Tumor Status	Surgery	Radiation	Chemotherapy
		Management	
T1 and T2	Local excision with clear margin	Yes, if moderate- to high-grade malignancy or adenoid cystic carcinoma	No
T3 and T4	Radical resection of all tumor-involved tissues, immediate reconstruction after surgical margins are confirmed	Yes	Possible

long as 6 months. Patients reconstructed with nerve grafts may develop inappropriate twitching or pain several years postoperatively.

Surgery of the submandibular gland exposes the hypoglossal nerve and the lingual nerve to potential injury. In addition, the mandibular branch of the facial nerve can be injured during the approach to the gland. The technique of submandibular gland excision is specifically designed to avoid unintentional injuries to these important structures.

RADIATION THERAPY

Surgical excision is the primary treatment of salivary neoplasms. Radiation therapy is a very useful adjunctive treatment modality following surgery (31–35, 40, 66). The improved locoregional control in patients receiving postoperative radiation shows that small foci of residual tumor cells are radiosensitive. Indications for postoperative radiation depend on the tumor type and stage (Table 21.5).

CHEMOTHERAPY

Chemotherapy should be reserved for advanced tumors that are not likely to benefit from surgery. Chemotherapy of recurrent, locally advanced, or metastatic tumor has not enjoyed a high response rate. Partial responses in 35–50% of patients were noted, but there has not been any survival advantage (67–70). Adenocarcinoma, mixed tumors, and acinic cell carcinomas responded better to adriamycin, cisplatinum, and 5-fluorouracil; mucoepidermoid and squamous carcinoma responded better to methotrexate and cisplatinum (68, 70).

SUMMARY OF TREATMENT PLAN

Our treatment plan is presented as a guideline. It cannot account for the many individual social and physical patient factors that will influence the course of therapy.

Johns (71) summarized the data of several large series and developed a management plan for parotid malignancies. Our comprehensive plan for treatment of salivary gland neoplasia (Table 21.6) differs from that of Johns in that it includes nonparotid salivary malignancies and specifically lists the appropriate use of surgery, radiation, and chemotherapy. In addition, our management scheme does not include prophylactic neck dissection.

References

1. Leegaard T, Lindeman H: Salivary gland tumors: Clinical picture and treatment. *Acta Otolaryngol* 263:155, 1970.
2. Foote FW Jr, Frazell EL: Tumors of the major salivary glands. *Cancer* 6:1065, 1953.
3. Batsakis JG, Regezi JA, et al: The pathology of head and neck tumors: Salivary glands parts 1–4. *Head Neck Surg* 1:59, 167, 260, 340, 1978–1979.
4. Richardson GS, Dickason WL, Gaisford JC, et al: Tumors of

salivary glands: An analysis of 752 cases. *Plast Reconstr Surg* 55:131, 1975.
5. Spiro RH, Huvos AA, Strong EW: Cancer of the parotid gland: A clinicopathologic study of 288 primary cases. *Am J Surg* 130:452, 1975.
6. Gallia LJ, Johnson JT: The incidence of neoplastic versus inflammatory disease in major salivary gland masses diagnosed by surgery. *Laryngoscope* 91:512, 1981.
7. Storm FK, Eilber FR, Sparks FC, et al: A prospective study of parotid metastases from head and neck cancer. *Am J Surg* 34:115, 1977.
8. Rees R, Maples M, Lynch JB: Malignant secondary parotid tumors. *South Med J* 74:1050, 1981.
9. Yarington CT: Metastatic malignant disease to the parotid gland. *Laryngoscope* 91:517, 1981.
10. Kushner DC, Weber AL: Sialography of salivary gland tumors with fluoroscopy and tomography. *AJR* 130:941, 1978.
11. Baker SR, Krause CJ: Ultrasonic analysis of head and neck neoplasms correlation with surgical findings. *Ann Otol* 90:126, 1981.
12. Bladh WH, Rose JG: Nuclear medicine in diagnosis and treatment of diseases of the head and neck. I. Salivary and parathyroid gland disease and one identification and staging of head and neck tumors. *Head Neck Surg* 4:129, 1981.
13. Eneroth CM, Franzen S, Zajicek J: Aspiration biopsy of salivary gland tumors. A critical review of 910 biopsies. *Acta Cytol* 11:470, 1967.
14. Sismanis A, Merriam JM, Kline TS, et al: Diagnosis of salivary gland tumors by fine-needle biopsy. *Head Neck Surg* 3:482, 1981.
15. Spiro RH: Salivary neoplasms: Overview of 35 year experience with 2807 patients. *Head and Neck Surg* 8:177, 1986.
16. Hillel AD, Fee WE Jr: Evaluation of frozen section in parotid gland surgery. *Arch Otolaryngol* 109:230, 1983.
17. Miller RH, Calcaterra TC, Paglia DE: Accuracy of frozen section diagnosis of parotid lesions. *Ann Otol* 88:573, 1979.
18. Granick MS, Erickson ER, Hanna DC: Accuracy of frozen section diagnosis in salivary gland lesions. *Head and Neck Surg* 8:177, 1986.
19. Levitt SH, McHugh RB, Gomez-Marin O, et al: Clinical staging system for cancer of the salivary gland. A retrospective study. *Cancer* 47:2712, 1981.
20. Rauch S: *Die Speicheldrusen des Meuschen.* Stuttgart, Thieme, 1959.
21. Conley J, Clairmont AA: Facial nerve in recurrent benign pleomorphic adenoma. *Arch Otolaryngol* 105:247, 1979.
22. O'Dwyer PJ, Farrar WB, Finkelmeier WR, et al: Facial nerve sacrifice and tumor recurrence in primary and recurrent benign parotid tumor. *Am J Surg* 152:442, 1986.
23. Piorkowski RJ, Guillamondegui OM: Is aggressive surgical treatment indicated for recurrent benign mixed tumors of the parotid gland. *Am J Surg* 142:434, 1981.
24. Lanier VC, McSwain B, Rosenfeld L: Mixed tumors of salivary glands: A 44-year study. *South Med J* 65:1485, 1972.
25. Judd ES: Development of cancer in mixed tumors of salivary glands. *Postgrad Med* 21:112, 1952.
26. Beahrs OH, Woolner LB, Kirklin JW, et al: Carcinomatous transformation of mixed tumors of the parotid gland. *Arch Surg* 75:605, 1957.
27. Dawson AK, Orr JA: Long-term results of local excision and radiation therapy in pleomorphic adenoma of the parotid. *Int J Radiat Oncol Biol Phys* 11:451, 1985.
28. Lamelas J, Terry JH, Alfonso AE: Warthin's tumor: Multicentricity and increasing incidence in women. *Am J Surg* 154:347, 1987.
29. Tran L, Sadeghi A, Hanson D, et al: Major salivary gland tumors: Treatment results and prognostic factors. *Laryngoscope* 96:1139, 1986.
30. Friedman M, Levin B, Grybauskas V, et al: Malignant tumors of the major salivary glands. *Otol Clin North Am* 19:625, 1986.
31. Jackson GL, Luna MA, Byers RM: Results of surgery alone and surgery combined with postoperative radiotherapy in the treatment of cancer of the parotid gland. *Am J Surg* 146:497, 1983.
32. Sullivan ZMR, Breslin K, McClatchey KD, et al: Malignant

parotid gland tumors: A retrospective. *Otolaryngol Head Neck Surg* 97:529, 1987.

33. Reddy SP, Marks JE: Treatment of locally advanced high grade malignant tumors of major salivary glands. *Laryngoscope* 98:450, 1988.
34. McNaney D, McNeese MD, Guillamondeguie OM, et al: Post-operative irradiation in malignant epithelial tumors of the parotid. *Int J Radiat Oncol Biol Phys* 9:1289, 1983.
35. Eapen LJ, Gerig LH, Catton GE: Impact of local radiation in the management of salivary gland carcinomas. *Head Neck Surg* 10:239, 1988.
36. Spiro RH, Huvos AG, Berk R, et al: Mucoepidermoid carcinoma of salivary gland origin: A clinicopathologic study of 367 cases. *Am J Surg* 136:461, 1978.
37. Spiro RH, Huvos AF, Strong EW: Malignant mixed tumor of salivary origin. A clinicopathologic study of 146 cases. *Cancer* 39:388, 1977.
38. Tortoledo ME, Luna MA, Batsakis JG: Carcinomas ex pleomorphic adenoma and malignant mixed tumors. *Arch Otolaryngol* 110:172, 1984.
39. Matsuba HM, Spector GJ, Thawley SE, et al: Adenoid cystic salivary gland carcinoma. *Cancer* 57:519, 1986.
40. Nascimento AG, Amaral ALP, Prado LAF, et al: Adenoid cystic carcinoma of the salivary glands. *Cancer* 57:317, 1986.
41. Bardwil JM: Tumors of the parotid gland. *Am J Surg* 114:498, 1967.
42. Eneroth CM: Histopathological and clinical aspects of parotid tumors. *Acta Otolaryngol (Suppl)* 191:1, 1964.
43. Lambert JA: Parotid gland tumors. *Milit Med* 136:484, 1971.
44. Skolnick EM, Friedman M, Becker S, et al: Tumors of the major salivary glands. *Laryngoscope* 87:843, 1977.
45. Matsuba HM, Mauney M, Simpson Jr, et al: Adenocarcinoma of the major and minor salivary gland origin: A histopathologic review of treatment failure patterns. *Laryngoscope* 98:784, 1988.
46. Schusterman MA, Granick MS, Erickson ER, et al: Lymphoma presenting as a salivary gland mass. *Head Neck Surg* 10:411, 1988.
47. Kucan JO, Frank DH, Robson MC: Tumors metastatic to the parotid gland. *Br J Plast Surg* 34:299, 1981.
48. Ryan JR, Ioachim HL, Marmer J, et al: Acquired immune deficiency syndrome-related lymphadenopathies presenting in the salivary gland nodes. *Arch Otolaryngol* 111:554, 1985.
49. deVries EJ, Kapadia SB, Johnson JT, et al: Salivary gland lymphoproliferative disease in acquired immune disease. *Otolaryngol—Head and Neck Surg* 99:59, 1988.
50. Eneroth CM: Salivary gland tumors in the parotid gland, submandibular gland, and the palate region. *Cancer* 27:1415, 1971.

51. Spiro RH, Hajdu SI, Strong EW: Tumors of the submaxillary gland. *Am J Surg* 132:463, 1976.
52. Byers RM, Jesse RH, Guillamondegui OM, et al: Malignant tumors of the submaxillary gland. *Am J Surg* 126:458:1973.
53. Spiro RH, Koss LG, Hajdu SI, et al: Tumors of minor salivary gland origin. *Cancer* 31:117, 1973.
54. Weisberger E, Luna MA, Guillamondegui OM: Salivary gland cancers of the palate. *Am J Surg* 138:485, 1979.
55. Tran L, Sadeghi A, Hanson D, et al: Salivary gland tumors of the palate: The UCLA experience. *Laryngoscope* 97:1343, 1987.
56. Abrams AM, Melrose RJ, Howell FV: Necrotizing sialometaplasia. *Cancer* 32:130, 1973.
57. Granick MS, Pilch BZ: Necrotizing sialometaplasia in the setting of acute and chronic sinusitis. *Laryngoscope* 91:1532, 1981.
58. Gahhos F, Enriquez RE, Bahn SL, et al: Necrotizing sialometaplasia: Report of five cases. *Plast Reconstr Surg* 71:650, 1983.
59. Granick MS, Solomon MP, Benadetto AV, et al: Necrotizing sialometaplasia masquerading as residual lip cancer. *Ann Plast Surg* 71:650, 1988.
60. Chong GC, Beahrs OH, Chen MLC, Hayles AB: Management of parotid gland tumors in infants and children. *Mayo Clin Proc* 50:279, 1975.
61. Schuller DC, McCabe BF: The firm salivary mass in children. *Laryngoscope* 87:1891, 1977.
62. Shikhani AH, Johns ME: Tumors of the major salivary glands in children. *Head and Neck Surg* 10:257, 1988.
63. Krolls SO, Trodahl JN, Boyers RC: Salivary gland lesions in children: A study of 430 cases. *Cancer* 30:459, 1972.
64. Gaisford JC, Hanna DC: Parotid tumor surgery. In Goldwyn RM (ed): *The Unfavorable Result in Plastic Surgery*. Boston, Little, Brown & Co, 1984, p 419.
65. Rankow RM, Polayes IM: Complications of surgery of the salivary glands. In Conley JJ (ed): *Complications of Head and Neck Surgery*. Philadelphia, WB Saunders Co, 1979, p 196.
66. Guillamondegui OM, Byers RM, Luna MA, et al: Aggressive surgery in treatment for parotid cancer: The role of adjunctive post-operative radiotherapy. *AJR* 123:49, 1975.
67. Rentschler R, Burgess MA, Byers R: Chemotherapy of malignant major salivary gland neoplasms. *Cancer* 40:619, 1976.
68. Suen JY, Johns ME: Chemotherapy for salivary gland cancer. *Laryngoscopy* 92:235, 1982.
69. Creagan ET, Woods JE, Rubin J, et al: Cisplatin-based chemotherapy for neoplasms arising from salivary glands and contiguous structures in the head and neck. *Cancer* 62:2313, 1988.
70. Kaplan MJ, Johns ME, Cantrell RW: Chemotherapy for salivary gland cancer. *Otolaryngol Head Neck Surg* 95:165, 1986.
71. Johns ME: Parotid cancer: A rational basis for treatment. *Head Neck Surg* 3:132, 1980.

22

Surgical Management of Soft Tissue Sarcomas

John M. Harrelson, M.D. and William J. Barwick, M.D.

Soft tissue sarcomas are rare, comprising approximately 1% of all malignant disease. Of all soft tissue sarcomas, 50% occur in the lower extremities with the majority of this group occurring in the thigh. The upper extremity accounts for 10%, with the remaining 40% occurring in the head, neck, trunk, and retroperitoneum. Although these lesions are categorized histologically by their connective tissue cell of origin (fat, muscle, fibrous tissue, vascular, neural, synovial), the specific cell type is usually not important from a therapeutic standpoint because the biological behavior of these lesions and their response to treatment is similar. The peak incidence of soft tissue sarcoma is in the fifth and sixth decade of life, with males predominating (1, 2).

Biological Behavior

Local patterns of growth and the mechanism of metastatic spread govern the treatment of soft tissue sarcomas. In addition to invading the structure of origin, these lesions expand centripetally, compressing normal tissues at their periphery. This expansile growth produces a "pseudocapsule" at the margins of the lesion consisting of compressed muscle and fascial structures. Neural, vascular, and osseous elements in the path of an expanding lesion may become embedded in this pseudocapsule. In addition to expansile behavior, these lesions demonstrate invasive properties. Both the pseudocapsule of the lesion and local vascular structures may be penetrated by tumor. Satellite lesions may develop external to the pseudocapsule and physically separate from the primary lesion either by capsular penetration or by seeding within the venous drainage of the primary tumor. Lymphatic invasion and nodal metastasis is rare because muscle contains only sparse lymphatics (3).

The site of origin governs to some extent the potential distribution of satellite lesions. Primary soft tissue sarcomas may arise (*a*) within major anatomical compartments (intracompartmental), (*b*) within fascial planes separating major anatomical compartments (extracompartmental), or (*c*) within the subcutaneous tissue. Intracompartmental primary lesions place at risk all tissue within the anatomical compartment, with the likelihood of satellite lesions increasing with proximity to the primary lesion. Extracompartmental lesions expose the fascial plane of origin and all bordering structures to potential tumor spreading. Subcutaneous primary lesions expose the subcutaneous tissues surrounding the lesion and also have a greater likelihood of lymphatic spread. Usually, major fascial planes serve as a barrier to local invasion of sarcoma, and penetration into an adjacent major compartment is rare (4). Similarly, subcutaneous primaries rarely involve the underlying muscle.

Clinical Presentation

Most patients with soft tissue sarcoma present with complaints of a painless, slowly enlarging mass. Aching discomfort with local tenderness, overlying venous distention, and local erythema may be present in long-standing lesions. Occasionally, patients may present with a history of the sudden appearance of a painful mass when hemorrhage occurs in a previously unrecognized lesion. Symptoms of neural and vascular compression are rare unless the primary is of neural origin or is situated in an area such as the popliteal fossa, femoral triangle, or antecubital fossa, where neurovascular structures cannot be easily displaced as the lesion expands. Weight loss and other systemic symptoms are similarly rare because metastasis at the time of diagnosis is infrequently encountered. Fever and chills occasionally may be observed in patients with large lesions in which central hemorrhage and necrosis have occurred.

Staging of Soft Tissue Sarcomas
PREBIOPSY IMAGING

In the patient presenting with an extremity mass, certain anatomical information must be gathered before biopsy of the lesion is undertaken. In addition to local physical examination, radiographic imaging studies aid in determining the site (intracompartmental, extracompartmental, subcutaneous), the proximity to major neural, vascular, and osseous structures, and the vascularity of the lesion. All of these factors are of extreme importance in planning the subsequent biopsy and surgical treatment.

Routine radiographs of the tumor should be obtained but are of limited benefit. Only when the lesion contains calcium, has eroded adjacent bone, or is of fat density will these studies be informative.

Computed tomography (CT) scanning has proved invaluable in the assessment of tumor location (5). Scans should be performed at 1-cm intervals with and without intravenous vascular enhancement in order to assess the density of the lesion relative to adjacent normal tissues

FIGURE 22.1. An enhanced CT scan shows a hypervascular mass in the deep posterior compartment.

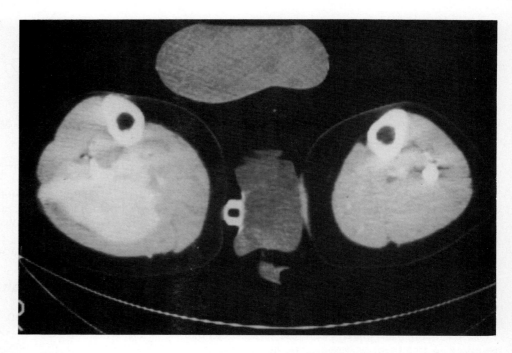

and to obtain some measure of its vascularity (Fig. 22.1). In tumors arising in muscle that are themselves of muscle density, the enhancement study may outline the pseudocapsule, which frequently contains hypervascular granulation tissue (Fig. 22.2). The scan should encompass the entire anatomical compartment in which the tumor arises in order to appreciate the full extent of the lesion and the presence or absence of edema within the muscle. Large satellite lesions occasionally may be demonstrated, although they are most frequently too small for detection. The enhanced phase of the study demonstrates the proximity of major vascular structures to the pseudocapsule of the tumor. Neural structures (other than the sciatic nerve) are often difficult to identify on CT scan. Mixed density of the lesion on the unenhanced study with irregular areas of low and high density suggest that necrosis has occurred and sarcoma should be strongly suspected. However, when such lesions cross major fascial planes and involve muscles in separate anatomical compartments, infection becomes a more likely etiology.

Radionuclide imaging with technetium-99 polyphosphate is also a useful adjunct in the evaluation of soft tissue sarcoma (6, 7). The study should be performed in three phases with immediate scan after injection, a delayed blood pool image at 15 min, and a delayed bone scan at 3 hr. In this manner, the arterial supply to the

FIGURE 22.2. An enhanced CT scan shows a hypervascular reactive pseudocapsule about the periphery of the lesion with a low-density area, which indicates central necrosis.

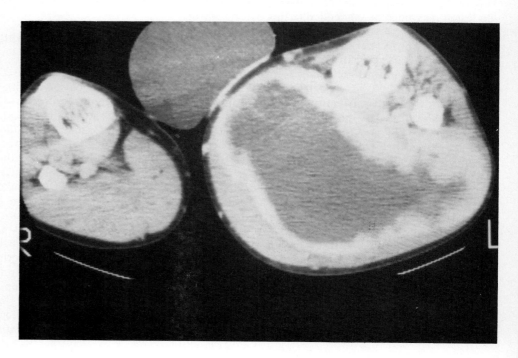

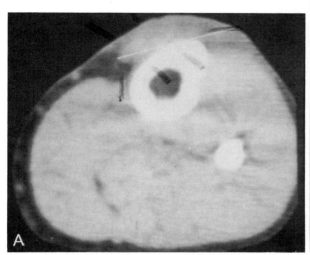

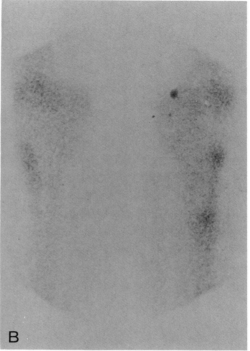

FIGURE 22.3.   A, A CT scan shows a subcutaneous high-grade sarcoma immediately adjacent to the anterior tibia. **B,** An ante- rior radionuclide scan shows increased uptake in the right mid- tibia. This indicates that the reactive capsule is involving bone.

lesion, the venous pooling within the lesion, and the ef- fect of the lesion on adjacent osseous structures can be appreciated. Increased uptake in bone on the delayed scan indicates involvement of that bone with the pseudo- capsule of the tumor (Fig. 22.3). In fat-density lesions, retention of radionuclide on the delayed scan is a strong indication of liposarcoma because lipomas have not been observed to retain the isotope.

When the CT scan and bone scan do not provide con- clusive information regarding the blood supply of the le- sion or the proximity of the lesion to major vessels, angi- ography is beneficial and should be performed in two planes in order to assess vessel displacement fully (8).

Lymphangiography is rarely indicated as a staging study. Although synovial sarcoma and subcutaneous pri- maries have a predisposition for lymphatic spread, CT evaluation will usually encompass the lymphatic drainage of the primary lesion. If enlarged, suspicious nodes are observed on CT scan, then lymphangiography may be considered (9). Although magnetic resonance (MR) imag- ing of soft tissue sarcomas has not been fully evaluated, this technique may also be of benefit in anatomical staging.

BIOPSY

Biopsy for diagnosis and histological grading is under- taken only after anatomical localization of the lesion has been accomplished. Biopsy is of equal importance to the definitive surgical procedure and must be planned care- fully (10). Although direct local invasion and vascular penetration are the natural modes of tumor spread, it has

been our experience that tumor dissemination by injudi- cious biopsy is a far more common occurrence. There- fore, one must consider what type of definitive surgical resection will be performed and place the biopsy incision in a location that will allow its complete extirpation at the time of definitive surgery. Because virtually all tumor excision in the extremities is accomplished through longi- tudinal exposure, transverse incisions are to be avoided because their excision is difficult and requires the sacri- fice of more skin and soft tissue. In the same way that natural vascular dissemination may produce satellite le- sions, hemorrhage from the biopsy incision is contami- nated with tumor cells and can produce recurrent tumor within the field of biopsy hematoma. Thus, both the placement of the biopsy incision and contamination re- sulting from the biopsy procedure may adversely affect the prognosis by increasing the extent of definitive sur- gery required and by increasing the chances of local re- currence. A potentially salvageable limb may require am- putation if these factors are not considered (Fig. 22.4).

Using the imaging data to select an exposure for defini- tive resection, the biopsy incision is placed in line with the chosen resection incision and sharp dissection is used to expose the tumor. Care is taken not to undermine the adjacent skin or to dissect within the tumor pseudocap- sule, which makes an inviting plane through which to "shell out" the lesion. Only in lesions of 3 cm or less is excisional biopsy recommended. An adequate sample of tumor is removed and frozen section utilized to assure that viable, diagnostic tissue has been obtained. Meticu- lous hemostasis is then achieved with electrocautery and, if necessary, with local thrombotic agents. If definitive

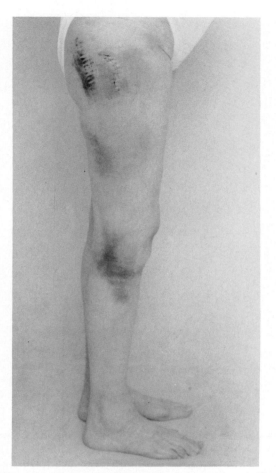

FIGURE 22.4. This patient had a biopsy of a high-grade liposarcoma over the right greater trochanter 1 week earlier. Contaminated hematoma extends from the midcalf to above the iliac crest.

surgery is immediately to follow the biopsy based on the frozen section diagnosis, the wound is closed and dressed, the limb reprepped and draped, and new instruments, gowns, and gloves used for the definitive resection (Fig. 22.5). If delayed resection is planned, a small suction drain inserted in line with the biopsy incision and exiting the skin 1–2 cm from the end of the incision is utilized to avoid the accumulation of hematoma.

Needle biopsy has been used with increasing frequency in the assessment of pulmonary, hepatic, and renal lesions. Particularly, fine-needle aspiration of breast lesions has been successful in establishing a diagnosis. However, for a variety of reasons, needle biopsy (by either core or aspiration technique) is not advised for intramuscular masses suspected of being sarcoma. First, sarcomas are intrinsically cohesive neoplasms and do not shed cells as freely as a carcinoma. Only occasionally is a diagnosis of malignancy established by fine-needle aspiration, and histological determination of tissue type (carcinoma versus sarcoma) may not be possible. Second, the vascularity of most sarcomas makes hemorrhage inevitable after core needle biopsy. This hemorrhage is not

controllable and, for reasons described previously, may contaminate areas of uninvolved tissue both in the subcutaneous regions surrounding the biopsy and along fascial planes crossed by the procedure. Finally, sarcomas are not homogeneous. Broad zones of fibrosis and necrosis may constitute a significant percentage of lesion. The limited amount of specimen obtained by core biopsy technique is often insufficient for diagnosis.

HISTOLOGICAL GRADING

Numerous schemes for histological grading have been described (11). Most of these divide malignant lesions into at least four categories based on progressive pleomorphism and atypia. From a practical point of view, surgical decisions regarding soft tissue sarcomas can be based on a knowledge of whether the lesion is low grade (Broders I and II) or high grade (Broders III and IV). The majority of soft tissue sarcomas are classified as high-grade lesions. When frozen section is utilized for immediate definitive surgery, it is important that a specific histological diagnosis be achieved. Soft tissue deposits of both carcinoma and lymphoma, for which surgical extirpation would be inappropriate, have been encountered. Therefore, a frozen section diagnosis of ''undifferentiated malignancy'' should await permanent sections and further definition before proceeding with surgical treatment.

STAGING SYSTEM

As with histological grading, numerous systems for staging sarcomas have been described (12). Most of these have been patterned after staging systems for carcinomas. Thus, they usually include categories for tumor size and nodal metastasis, factors that are not significant in the treatment of soft tissue sarcomas. Enneking et al. (13, 14) have described a staging system (adopted by the Musculoskeletal Tumor Society) that takes into account those factors necessary to make a surgical decision. Thus, staging is based on (*a*) anatomical location (intracompartmental, extracompartmental), (*b*) histological grade (low grade, high grade), and (*c*) the presence or absence of metastasis. Low-grade lesions are designated I; high-grade lesions II; intracompartmental lesions A and extracompartmental lesions B; any lesion with metastases is designated stage III (Table 22.1).

Table 22.1.
Surgical Staging System[a]

Stage	Grade	Site	Metastases
IA	Low	Intracompartmental	None
IB	Low	Extracompartmental	None
IIA	High	Intracompartmental	None
IIB	High	Extracompartmental	None
III	Any	Any	Regional or distant

[a] Adapted from Enneking et al. (14).

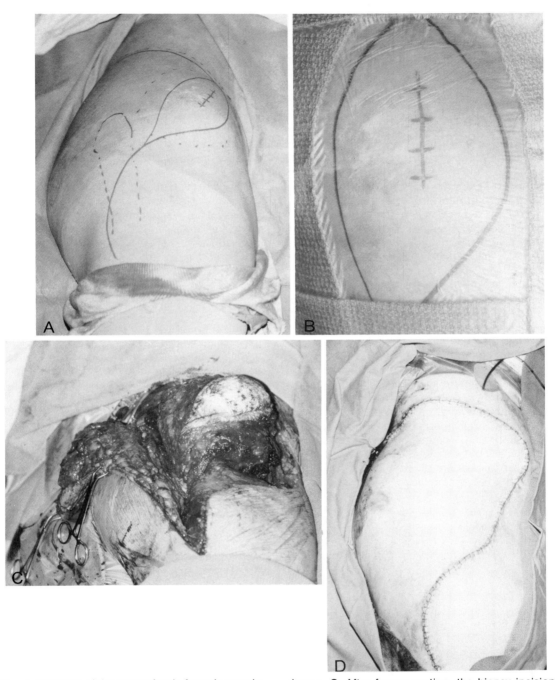

FIGURE 22.5. **A,** Sarcoma of the tensor fascia femoris muscle. The femur is outlined with a *dotted line;* the biopsy incision is shown as a *cross-hatched line* with a major resection ellipsing the biopsy planned from the iliac crest above to the lateral femur below. **B,** The biopsy incision has been isolated with adhesive drapes. **C,** After frozen section, the biopsy incision has been closed and isolated with a sterile plastic drape. The major resection includes the biopsy site. **D,** Wound closure from iliac crest to femur. Loss of muscle bulk allows tension-free skin closure despite biopsy ellipse.

Surgical Alternatives

Historically, surgery has been considered the definitive treatment for soft tissue sarcomas (15, 16). Within the past decade, the role of surgery and the role of adjunctive radiotherapy and chemotherapy have undergone extensive reevaluation (17–19). It is important that the surgeon understand the definition of each surgical procedure and the potential for local recurrence with each of these procedures for both high-grade and low-grade lesions.

Marginal excision is defined as tumor removal through or adjacent to the reactive capsule at the pushing margin of the tumor. This ''shelling out'' of the lesion leaves microscopic tumor and, for high-grade lesions, results in predictable local recurrence. Marginal excision would, therefore, not be considered therapeutic in the treatment of soft tissue sarcomas.

Wide local excision is defined as removal of the lesion with a cuff of normal tissue, including any biopsy incision. The tumor is not visualized during the surgical procedure. For low-grade lesions and subcutaneous sarcomas of low or high grade, this excision results in less than 10% local recurrence. For high-grade lesions, in the absence of any other form of adjunctive treatment, wide local excision results in approximately 40% local recurrence, which is most likely the result of satellite lesions within the compartment of origin or contamination by venous efflux from the tumor during surgery.

Radical excision is defined as complete removal of the major anatomical compartment in which the tumor arises without violation of the major fascial boundaries of that compartment. For high-grade sarcomas, radical (compartmental) excision results in less than 10% local recurrence.

The importance of these definitions must be emphasized. Note that the question of amputation is not addressed by the definition of these surgical procedures. While above-knee amputation for a lesion of the quadriceps is a "radical" operation, it achieves only a wide local margin because a portion of the quadriceps muscle remains. A radical margin for such a lesion would involve removal of the entire anterior compartment of the thigh whether or not amputation was a part of that procedure.

The selection of a surgical procedure requires analysis of the factors outlined. Localization of the lesion to a major anatomical compartment, extracompartmental site, or subcutaneous location; the proximity of the tumor pseudocapsule to bone; major blood vessels and neural structures; and the histological grade of the lesion are all considered. When the tumor pseudocapsule is in contact with major neural or vascular structures or produces increased uptake on bone scan, any surgical procedure that spares these structures will result in a marginal excision and guaranteed local recurrence. In certain situations, it may be possible to include the involved bone as a part of the resection (Fig. 22.6) or to resect a major vessel en bloc with the tumor and perform vascular bypass. In general, procedures that require sacrifice of a major nerve (sciatic, median, ulnar) produce a degree of disability equal to amputation, and limb salvage in such situations is not advised. This situation arises most frequently with extracompartmental tumors of the popliteal fossa, femoral triangle, and antecubital fossa and large tumors of the posterior compartment of the thigh where the sciatic nerve is involved.

Recent studies utilizing preoperative irradiation and wide local excision as a means of local tumor control have produced local recurrence figures equivalent to those achieved with radical compartmental excision (less than 10%) (20). This combination may be particularly useful in tumors of the posterior thigh where the sciatic nerve is separated from the tumor pseudocapsule by uninvolved muscle, because it may allow preservation of the sciatic nerve and salvage of the limb. In the anterior compartment of the thigh (quadriceps) ultimate function of the limb is the same for either procedure because minimal if any quadriceps function would be preserved by wide local excision after irradiation.

Major anatomical compartments in the upper extremity are the deltoid muscle, the anterior compartment (biceps, brachialis, coracobrachialis), posterior compartment (triceps), volar forearm (profundus, sublimis, flexor

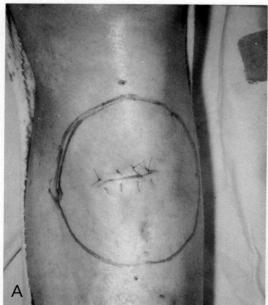
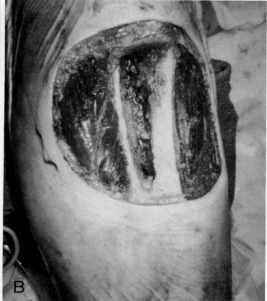

FIGURE 22.6. A, Planned resection of biopsy site and lesion shown in Figure 22.3. The anterior tibia is involved according to the bone scan. **B,** Resection includes the anterior tibial cortex. Closure accomplished by gastrocnemius rotational flap and split-skin coverage.

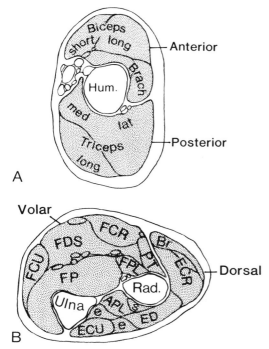

FIGURE 22.7. **A,** Major anatomical compartments in the upper arm. Brach, brachialis. **B,** Major anatomical compartments in the forearm. Volar compartment: FCR, flexor carpi radialis; FCU, flexor carpi ulnaris; FDS, flexor digitorum superficialis; FP, flexor profundus; FPL, flexor pollicis longus; PT, pronator teres. Dorsal compartment: APL, abductor pollicis longus; Br, brachioradialis; ECR, extensor carpi radialis; ECU, extensor carpi ulnaris; ED, extensor digitorum.

carpi ulnaris, flexor carpi radialis), and dorsal forearm (brachioradialis, extensor digitorum communis, extensor carpi radialis longus and brevis, extensor carpi ulnaris) (Fig. 22.7).

In the lower extremity, the major anatomical compartments are the gluteus maximus; the abductors (gluteus medius, gluteus minimus, tensor fascia femoris); the anterior (quadriceps), posterior (biceps femoris, semitendinosus, semimembranosus), and medial (adductor longus, adductor brevis, adductor magnus, gracilis, sartorius) compartments of the thigh; and the posterior (gastrocnemius, soleus, flexor digitorum communis, flexor hallucis longus, posterior tibialis), anterior (tibialis anterior, extensor digitorum communis, extensor hallucis longus, peroneus tertius), and peroneal (peroneus longus, peroneus brevis) compartments of the leg (Fig. 22.8).

Sarcomas of the hand and foot are uncommon, and the proximity of these lesions to neural, osseous, and vascular structures make partial salvage difficult to accomplish. Sarcomas of these structures most frequently result in amputation.

Subcutaneous sarcomas demonstrate a different biological behavior than those located in deep muscular structures and are less likely to exhibit metastatic behavior. Subcutaneous lesions do not arise in a true anatomical compartment and rarely penetrate the underlying fascia. Wide local excision for these lesions, with a 5-cm margin around the biopsy incision and fascia and an underlying layer of muscle, is considered adequate treatment.

The goal of surgery in the treatment of soft tissue sarcomas is the eradication of the primary lesion. While, in a direct sense, surgical treatment does not affect the development of metastatic lesions, it should be understood that those patients who develop local recurrence after a definitive surgical procedure experience a twofold increase in the incidence of subsequent pulmonary metastases. This consequence is not surprising because local recurrence means that the patient has harbored the tumor for a longer period of time with greater exposure to vascular invasion and dissemination.

In general, low-grade lesions of either intracompartmental or extracompartmental origin (IA, IB) are adequately treated by wide local excision. Adjunctive radiotherapy and chemotherapy are usually unnecessary. High-grade lesions of intracompartment or extracompartmental origin (IIA, IIB) may be treated either by achieving a radical margin or by wide local excision after preoperative radiotherapy. The recurrence rate for these two procedures is similar and the choice between them is dependent on the anatomical location of the tumor, its proximity to neural, vascular, and osseous structures, and the predicted function of the limb. Wide local excision does

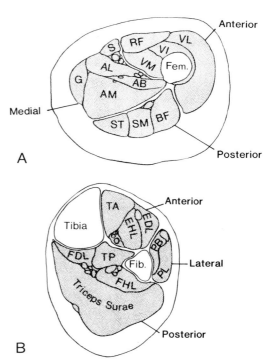

FIGURE 22.8. **A,** Major anatomical compartments of the thigh. Anterior: RF, rectus femoris; VI, vastus intermedius; VL, vastus lateralis; VM, vastus medialis. Medial: AB, adductor brevis; AL, adductor longus; AM, adductor magnus; G, gracilis; S, sartorius. Posterior: BF, biceps femoris; SM, semimembranosus; ST, semitendinosus. **B,** Major anatomical compartments of the lower leg. Anterior: EDL, extensor digitorum longus; EHL, extensor hallucis longus; TA, tibialis anterior. Lateral: PB, peroneus brevis; PL, peroneus longus. Posterior: FDL, flexor digitorum longus; FHL, flexor hallucis longus; TP, tibialis posterior.

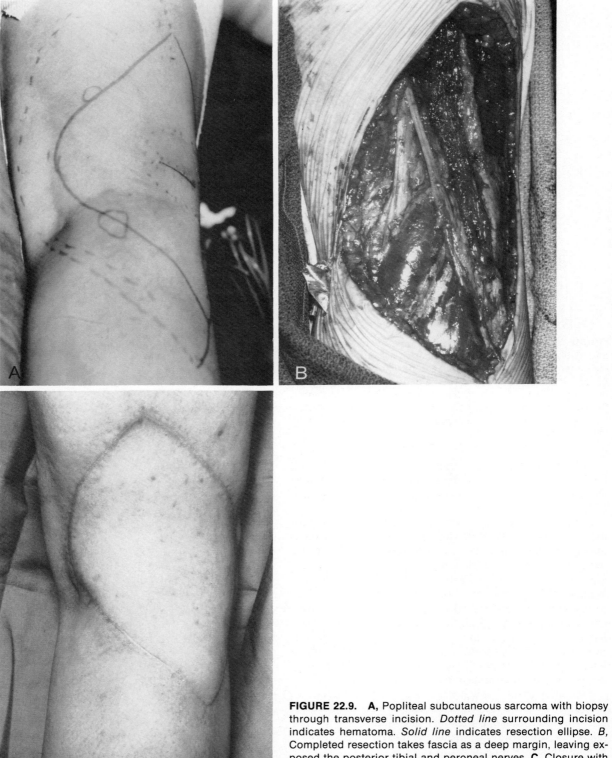

FIGURE 22.9. **A,** Popliteal subcutaneous sarcoma with biopsy through transverse incision. *Dotted line* surrounding incision indicates hematoma. *Solid line* indicates resection ellipse. *B,* Completed resection takes fascia as a deep margin, leaving exposed the posterior tibial and peroneal nerves. **C,** Closure with free scapular flap provides excellent coverage.

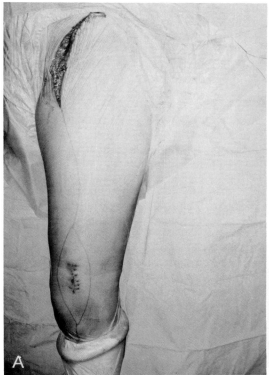

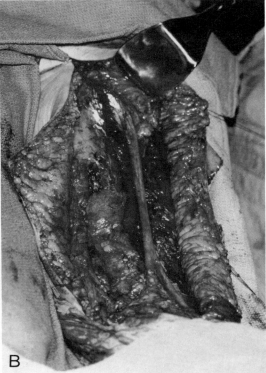

FIGURE 22.10. A, Planned resection of high-grade quadriceps sarcoma. The resection begins at the anterior superior iliac spine and ends at the patellar tendon, ellipsing the biopsy. **B,** The completed resection leaves the femur exposed from the femoral condyles to the lesser trochanter. The medial and lateral intermuscular septae have been excised. The bed of the wound consists of the femur, portions of the adductors, and hamstring muscles.

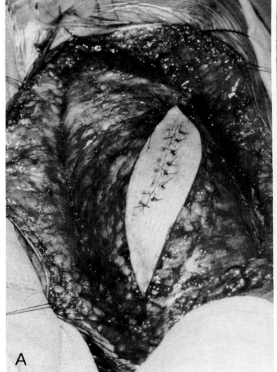

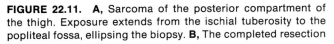

FIGURE 22.11. A, Sarcoma of the posterior compartment of the thigh. Exposure extends from the ischial tuberosity to the popliteal fossa, ellipsing the biopsy. **B,** The completed resection shows the sciatic nerve from the sciatic notch to the popliteal fossa.

not necessarily guarantee better function than radical (compartmental) excision.

The patient should be apprised of the factors that govern the choice of a surgical procedure as well as the expected limb function after surgery (21). Contingency plans should be established preoperatively to deal with unexpected findings. Transgression of the tumor or the presence of hematoma from the previous biopsy extending along the fascial planes results in a contaminated wound and the equivalent of a marginal or intralesional excision. It may be necessary to abandon the attempted resection and resort to more radical resection or amputation at a higher level.

Reconstruction

The goal of surgical treatment of soft tissue sarcomas is eradication of local disease. When this can best be accomplished by amputation, closure and prosthetic rehabilitation are routine. When limb salvage by either compartmental excision or wide local excision are undertaken, the tumor surgeon must not let concerns for wound closure and limb function compromise the quality of surgical excision. We have found it advantageous to use a team approach with one surgeon performing the excision and another the reconstruction. Preoperative planning by both teams is mandatory. In recent years, technological advances in free vascularized tissue transfer have offered a broad range of options for reconstruction.

When wide local excision is performed or when compartmental excision is performed for large lesions and split-skin grafting or free tissue transfer is required, it is important to establish clean surgical margins before potential contamination of the donor site if the margins are involved. This examination is best performed by multiple inked sections about the periphery of the resection specimen and examination of permanent slides. It is difficult to perform this examination on frozen section. Thus, when margins are in question, delayed reconstruction after thorough specimen examination is advised.

Subcutaneous sarcomas treated by wide local excision with underlying fascia and muscle as a deep margin can usually be treated by split-thickness skin grafting. However, when these lesions occur around joints (popliteal fossa, patella, antecubital fossa), joint function may be compromised by simple skin grafting.

Because most compartmental and wide local excisions are performed through longitudinal incisions ellipsing the biopsy, a significant amount of muscle bulk is removed, and if subcutaneous dissection allows medial and lateral flap preservation, most of these wounds can be closed primarily. However, transverse or oblique biopsy incisions that require a wide ellipse, radiation skin changes that produce problems with wound healing, or loss of circulation to the medial or lateral flap may require the use of tissue transfer for wound reconstruction (Fig. 22.9).

The most common site of soft tissue sarcomas is the anterior compartment of the thigh. When primary closure in this area is not possible, one is usually faced with a wound that cannot be grafted either, because the femur forms the base of the wound (Fig. 22.10). An option here is the use of the rectus abdominis, either as an island muscle or musculocutaneous flap. The inferior epigastric artery, which supplies the flap, enters from the inferior end. Its origin from the region of the inguinal ligament permits rotation of the muscle downward almost to the knee. If the rectus cannot be used because of previous groin or abdominal surgery, the best alternative is free tissue transfer.

FIGURE 22.12. Excision of the dorsal forearm compartment with skin loss requires free tissue transfer of a latissimus myocutaneous flap. The radial nerve is preserved proximally in the wound for anastomosis to the motor nerve of the latissimus.

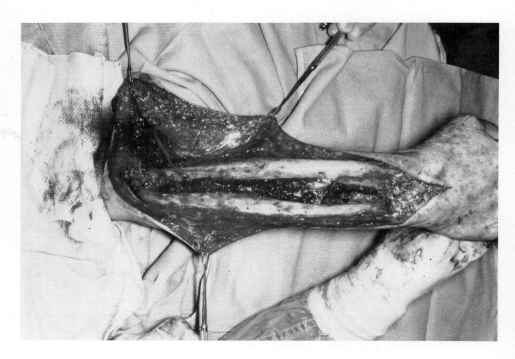

A similar situation arises in the posterior thigh, where a skin graft will not suffice after compartmental resection and inability to close wounds primarily. Flap options for closure depend on the size, shape, and location of the defect, but there are not many readily available local flaps to use (Fig. 22.11).

In the upper extremity and pectoral girdle, an island lattissimus flap has an arc of rotation that allows coverage to almost all the arm and the scapular and deltoid areas. The latissimus muscle provides good coverage of the shoulder, especially when radiation therapy has been part of the treatment. In the forearm, even with loss of muscle bulk, primary closure is difficult and free tissue transfer is usually preferable (Fig. 22.12).

In addition, skin grafts in these areas have a tendency to break down frequently. Therefore, some type of flap will usually be necessary (Fig. 22.9). There are a variety of muscle, musculocutaneous, and fasciocutaneous flaps available for regional coverage of joint areas. For example, it may be possible to resurface a wide local excision of the antecubital fossa with a latissimus dorsi musculocutaneous pedicle flap. However, in the extremities local muscle flaps usually can bring only a limited amount of tissue. Moreover, there may have been preoperative radiation, making the flap more risky. Strong consideration should be given to the use of free vascularized tissue transfer in these areas, either as immediate or delayed reconstuction.

References

1. Enneking WF: *Musculoskeletal Tumor Surgery.* New York, Churchill Livingstone, 1983.
2. Eilber FR: Soft tissue sarcomas of the extremity. *Curr Prob Cancer* 8:3, 1984.
3. Simon MA, Enneking WF: The management of soft tissue sarcomas of the extremities. *J Bone Joint Surg [Am]* 58:317, 1976.
4. Enneking WF, Spanier, SS, Malawer MM: The effect of the anatomic setting on the results of surgical procedures for soft parts sarcoma of the thigh. *Cancer* 47:1005, 1981.
5. Schumaker TM, Genant HK, Korobkin M, et al: Computed tomography—its use in space-occupying lesions of the musculoskeletal system. *J Bone Joint Surg [Am]* 60:600, 1978.
6. Galasko BSB: The pathologic basis for skeletal scintigraphy. *J Bone Joint Surg [Br]* 57:148, 1975.
7. Kirchner PT, Simon MA: The clinical value of bone and gallium scintigraphy for soft-tissue sarcomas of the extremities. *J Bone Joint Surg [Am]* 66:319, 1984.
8. Hudson TM, Haas G, Enneking WF, et al: Angiography in the management of musculoskeletal tumors. *Surgery* 141:11, 1975.
9. DeSantos LA, Wallace S, Finklestine JB: Angiography and lymphangiography in peripheral soft tissue sarcomas. In: *Management of Primary Bone and Soft Tissue Tumors.* Chicago, Year Book Medical Publishers, 1977, p 235.
10. Makin HJ, Lange TA, Spanier SS: The hazards of biopsy in patients with malignant primary bone and soft tissue tumors. *J Bone Joint Surg [Am]* 64:1121, 1982.
11. Broders AC: The microscopic grading of cancer. In Pack GT, Arrel IM (eds): *Treatment of Cancer and Allied Diseases.* New York, PB Hoeber, 1964.
12. American Joint Committee: *Manual for Staging of Cancer.* Chicago, American Joint Committee, 1977.
13. Enneking WF, Spanier SS, Goodman MA: Current concepts review. The surgical staging of musculoskeletal sarcoma. *J Bone Joint Surg [Am]* 62:1027, 1980.
14. Enneking WF, Spanier SS, Goodman MA: A system for the surgical staging of musculoskeletal sarcoma. *Clin Orthop* 153:106, 1980.
15. Pack GT, Arrel IM: Principles of treatment of tumors of the soft somatic tissues. In Pack GT, Arrel IM (eds): *Treatment of Cancer and Allied Diseases.* New York, PB Hoeber, 1964.
16. Bowden L, Booher RJ: The principles and techniques of resection of soft parts for sarcoma. *Surgery* 44:963, 1958.
17. Eilber FR, Morton DL, Eckardt J, et al: Limb salvage for skeletal soft tissue sarcomas. Multidisciplinary preoperative therapy. *Cancer* 53:2579, 1984.
18. Eilber FR, Mirra JJ, Grant TT, et al: Is amputation necessary for sarcomas? A seven year experience with limb salvage. *Ann Surg* 192:431, 1980.
19. Mantravadi RV, Trippon MJ, Patel MK, et al: Limb salvage in extremity soft tissue sarcoma: Combined modality therapy. *Radiology* 152:523, 1984.
20. Rosenberg SA, Tepper J, Glatstein E, et al: The treatment of soft tissue sarcomas of the extremities: Prospective randomized evaluations of limb sparing surgery plus radiation therapy compared with amputation in the role of adjuvant chemotherapy. *Ann Surg* 196:305, 1982.
21. Sugarbaker PH, Barofsky I, Rosenberg SA, et al: Quality of life assessment of patients in extremity sarcoma clinical trials. *Surgery* 91:17, 1982.

23

Treatment of Hemangioma

David P. Apfelberg, M.D., F.A.C.S.

Vascular neoplasms constitute the largest group of hamartomas of childhood. Their pathogenesis is not entirely clear, and the biological mechanism of spontaneous involution that some of these lesions exhibit has yet to be well defined. Numerous superficial vascular lesions develop in adulthood as well. A familiarity with vascular cutaneous lesions and a knowledge of their natural history can direct the surgeon toward appropriate treatment.

The laser is becoming an invaluable tool for the treatment of various vascular lesions. The unique hemostatic properties of the carbon dioxide laser and the neodymium : yttrium-aluminum-garnet (YAG) laser transmitted and focused with synthetic sapphire scalpels allows virtually bloodless excision of hemangiomas and vascular malformations. YAG laser photocoagulation is effective for thick hypertrophic lesions, and argon laser light, selectively absorbed by hemoglobin pigment, results in photocoagulation of many cutaneous vascular lesions. Tunable dye lasers allow safe and effective treatment of hemangiomas in infants and young children.

Classification and Description of Hemangiomas (Table 23.1)

Hemangiomas may vary from inconspicuous, harmless blemishes to large lesions that threaten the life of the patient (1). The incidence of vascular abnormalities in infants is estimated to be 1 : 1,500 (2). Innes (3) considers these lesions to be hamartomas arising from a mass of vasoformative tissue. The great majority are present at birth or appear shortly thereafter. Their enlargement during the first year after birth is due to the establishment of a new blood flow and canalization in adjacent tissue (4–7). There is a positive family history in 3–10% of the cases but little correlation to complications of pregnancy or delivery. Hemangiomas occur more than twice as often in girls than in boys, and one half of the lesions develop in the head and neck (8).

Hemangiomas may be classified as histological types and clinical entities (3, 9). Capillary hemangiomas account for 75% of the hemangiomas seen in children and adults. *Strawberry marks (hemangioma simplex)* are bright red or purple capillary hemangiomas with well-defined margins consisting of many tiny capillaries. Generally present at or shortly after birth, the lesions clinically are soft, slightly raised, and usually bright red. Histologically, they are composed of masses of endothelial cells exhibiting a modest amount of differentiation, frequently without discrete capillary formation. They tend to increase in size rapidly during the first 6 months of life and then to stabilize for a period. At about 1 year of age, they often show evidence of spontaneous involution with a change to a more mottled appearance. Fleshy gray areas of "herald spots" augur eventual complete or near-complete involution. In cases of larger lesions, atrophic skin may be the only remaining evidence of their former presence. Capillary hemangiomas may persist into adulthood without involution or may arise de novo as primary vascular tumors.

Among other capillary hemangiomas are senile (cherry) hemangiomas (Campbell-DeMorgan's spots), which present as small, raised, discrete, red or purple lesions about 1–2 mm in diameter. They are commonly seen on the trunk and extremities in middle-aged and older patients. These lesions are composed of dilated capillaries in the dermis that are surrounded by fibrous stroma.

Pyogenic granulomas are superficial polypoid lesions composed of inflammatory capillaries in an edematous matrix much like granulation tissue. They may occur at any age in either sex and are said to have an infectious origin, although this is unproven. They are found most commonly on the face and extremities and appear as bright red or red-brown vascular tumors that are often covered by crusts. They are firm with variable pain and tenderness and bleed easily with trauma. Often, a considerable number of them are deep in the dermis. Histological studies reveal the presence of distinct lobules of capil-

Table 23.1.
Classifications of Hemangioma

Capillary vessels
  Strawberry mark of infancy
  Campbell-DeMorgan cherry spots
  Pyogenic granuloma
  Telangiectasia (nevus araneus)
  Livido reticularis
  Salmon patch (erythema nuchae)
  Port-wine hemangioma (nevus flammeus)
  Acne rosacea
Cavernous vessels
  Cavernous hemangioma
  Blue rubber bleb nevus
Vascular hamartoma (mixed hemangioma)
Arteriovenous fistula
Cirsoid-racemose aneurysm

laries separated by a fibromyxomatous stroma, as opposed to the radially arranged capillaries in granulation tissue. This characteristic appearance has been recently described as "lobular capillary hemangioma." Traditionally, they are treated by excision or electrocautery, but recurrences are common.

Telangiectasia (*nevus araneus*) are red lesions that consist of a central vascular punctum from which capillary vessels radiate. They may be associated with systemic conditions (cirrhosis, vitamin deficiency, or imbalance of sex hormones).

Livido reticularis (*cutis marmorata congenital*) is a transient, bluish, mottled discoloration of the skin in a characteristic reticulated pattern associated with cold exposure. The mottling is asymptomatic, improves with elevation of the extremity, and may persist for years.

The *salmon patch* (*erythema nuchae*) and *port-wine stain* (*nevus flammeus*) are histologically similar lesions composed of mature capillaries and venules within the dermis and usually covered by normal-appearing epithelium. The major difference between them is the much greater concentration of vessels per area of skin with the port-wine stain. The salmon patch, a pink or salmon-colored macular lesion, is visible at birth. The color deepens with crying and other maneuvers that increase venous pressure. These lesions are present in 20–40% of newborns and are generally situated on the face (forehead and eyelids) and the posterior aspect of the neck. As the children grow, the lesions become less noticeable and often seem to resolve completely.

Port-wine stains are flat initially, but over years they may take on a more pebbly appearance as capillaries dilate or hemodynamics change. They vary from deep red to purple, and the color depends somewhat on the depth of the capillaries and venules within the dermis. The face is the most common site, and lesions frequently are situated over the distribution of two or more branches of the trigeminal nerve. Any of several well-known systemic syndromes may be associated.

Lesions composed of larger vascular channels are often referred to as *cavernous hemangiomas*. Frequently, they lie deep to the dermis and may involve muscle or other underlying tissue. The rarity with which these lesions exhibit regression suggests that they are composed of vessels lined with mature endothelial cells. These large lesions are differentiated from arteriovenous malformations primarily on the basis of the vessels involved. In an arteriovenous malformation, mature arterial and venous structures can be identified with aberrant interconnections and fistulas; however, the cavernous malformation is composed primarily of mature venous structures. The lesions are often associated with systemic syndromes and may cause gigantism of an involved extremity or underlying body structure secondary to the increased blood supply to the area.

Cavernous hemangiomas are less common than capillary lesions and are commonly deeper in the dermis, with larger vascular channels and less distinct clinical margins. They are easily compressed and show little tendency toward spontaneous involution. The thick, spongy, compressible tissue with blue-tinged subcutaneous appearance appears at birth or shortly thereafter and may go through the same phases as the capillary hemangioma, although spontaneous involution is much less certain and more variable. Cavernous hemangiomas of the face and scalp have been observed to involute very infrequently. Wisnicki (10), in an encyclopedic summary of the subject, suggested that cavernous hemangiomas have the same potential for spontaneous involution as do capillary hemangiomas. However, he noted that the residual deformity "may be significant" and that "in many instances, cavernous involution may be incomplete." Matthews (11) observed that cavernous hemangioma is capable of more rapid growth than any other hemangioma and that it can fade spontaneously on occasion but more rarely than capillary lesions. He believed that the extreme variability in behavior, as well as the grossly disfiguring continued extension of its growth, which causes secondary deformity, may argue in favor of its treatment. Williams (12) reported 7 patients with facial bony changes secondary to hemangioma and believed spontaneous resolution was unlikely in such cases of hemangioma (mainly cavernous). Pasyk (13) found minimal levels of estrogen receptors in cavernous hemangiomas that were classified as more resistant to hormonal treatment. Pasyk also observed that cavernous hemangiomas do not show mitotic activity typical of capillary hemangioma histology: "They are indolent and more persistent in growth and rarely undergo spontaneous involution" (14). The experience of the authors in evaluating and following the course of over 100 patients with capillary/cavernous hemangiomas has not demonstrated any significant fading or spontaneous resolution of the purely cavernous component. Many hemangiomas are mixed capillary-cavernous hemangiomas (vascular hamartoma).

Acne rosacea is a chronic skin disease of the face characterized by vascular (erythema and telangiectasia) and acneiform (nodules and pustules) components. There may be an accompanying hyperplasia of the soft tissue of the nose (rhinophyma). Onset is insidious, and the skin of the nose and cheeks is primarily involved. Pathological studies reveal vascular dilation and a nonspecific dermal lymphocyte infiltrate in the erythematous areas, with a typical picture of acne vulgaris in the acneiform areas.

Arteriovenous (AV) *fistulas* and *cirsoid/racemose aneurysms* are vascular deformities characterized by abnormal vascular connections and grossly dilated pulsatile masses of vessels.

A recent classification based on endothelial characteristics provided predictive information, which can, in turn, define appropriate therapy (9; Table 23.2). It divided the lesions into two groups: hemangiomas, characterized by immature endothelial cells that exhibit an increased rate of proliferation and mitotic activity; and vascular malformations, characterized by mature endothelial cells that demonstrate a normal, more stable cell cycle. The vascular malformations, whether composed primarily of arterial, venous, or capillary components, exhibit histologically mature and identifiable vessels. This simplification in classification helps to eliminate the question of which hemangiomas can be expected to involute; that is, by definition, all would be predicted to invo-

Table 23.2.
Classifications of Cutaneous Vascular Lesions

Hemangiomas
    Strawberry mark
Vascular malformations
    Salmon patch (erythema nuchae)
    Port-wine stain (nevus flammeus)
    Senile (cherry) hemangioma (DeMorgan's spots)
    Pyogenic granulomas
    Spider angioma (nevus araneus)
    Telangiectasia
    Cavernous malformations
    Arteriovenous malformations

Table 23.3.
Complications of Hemangiomas

Infection
Bleeding
Necrosis and ulceration
Gigantism
Disfigurement
Congestive heart failure (arteriovenous fistula)
Malignancy

lute to some extent. Vascular malformations would be expected to change minimally.

Natural History of Hemangiomas and Complications

Payne et al. (6) have described the stages in development of hemangiomas. In the first stage, the lesion is a pale, well-demarcated, nonelevated area that reddens during crying. In the next stage, a small telangiectasia progresses to a vascular stain or to the typical irregular, pebbly hemangioma. Full development requires 2 weeks to 1 year and is quite rapid during the first year of life. Spontaneous regression of hemangiomas has long been recognized. Lampe and Latourette (2) described the initial signs of regression as a change in color from a brilliant red to a dull red-gray. The fading begins in the center of the lesion and then spreads to the periphery (herald spots). Later, the lesion decreases in bulk and tenseness, and the overlying skin appears slightly wrinkled. The lesion then gradually decreases in thickness but not in size. It has been estimated that 60–90% of hemangiomas involute spontaneously within 5 years. Bowers et al. (5) concluded that hemangiomas that do not show signs of regression by 6–8 years of age are not likely to regress further spontaneously.

Although no one knows for certain, approximately 80–90% of involution is said to occur by the age of 6, and it is unusual for further spontaneous involution to occur after the age of 6–8. Recently, however, this fact has been reevaluated. Grabb and associates (15) studied 69 children with hemangiomas at the University of Michigan Medical Center from 1964 to 1978. Twenty patients with strawberry hemangiomas were studied. Complete involution occurred in only five patients, the earliest being at age 3 and the latest at age 18. Partial involution occurred in six additional patients (mainly nasal tip and dorsum of the nose). Nine others had operative excision; therefore, the natural history of the lesion was not known. All authors agree that capillary hemangiomas of the strawberry type will undergo a natural involution and leave a minimal residual deformity of a shiny, crinkled, atrophic skin texture. The most elegant study of these lesions has been provided by Pasyk et al. (13, 14). These authors have documented by biopsy studies that cellularly dynamic vascular malformations such as capillary hemangiomas

contain several specific elements that may explain their subsequent disappearance. There is an abnormally high number of mast cells, precursors to fibrous replacement. Secondary estradiol-17β receptors are found in increased numbers in these lesions, possibly explaining their unusually high response to hormone (13, 14). Kaplan (16), in detailed pathological studies of these lesions, has found that involuting hemangiomas have an embryonal form of endothelium, while the more permanent hemangiomas have an "adult" type of endothelium. Complications of hemangioma are listed in Table 23.3.

Associated Hemangioma Syndromes

Associated hemangioma syndromes are listed in Table 23.4. Sturge-Weber syndrome consists of port-wine hemangiomas in the trigeminal distribution and vascular malformation of the leptomininges, often associated with focoepileptic seizures and variable mental retardation. Kasabach-Merritt syndrome represents a diffuse intravascular coagulopathy (DIC) with platelet and fibrinogen consumption in a rapidly expanding cavernous hemangioma of the trunk or extremities. The resultant bleeding disorder can be treated with steroids, x-rays, compression, and occasionally heparin. Kippel-Trenauney syndrome is a triad of superficial port-wine hemangiomas and varicose veins, hypertrophic soft tissue, and overgrowth of bone, most often in an extremity. Abdominal viscera may have associated tumors. Maffucci syndrome consists of multiple cavernous hemangiomas plus dyschondroplasia of bones and joints and multiple enchondroma. Hemangiomas of the skin along with retinal and cerebellar hemangiomas that result in central nervous system (CNS) and visual problems are features of the Von Hippel-Lindau syndrome. Weber-Osler-Rondu he-

Table 23.4.
Associated Hemangioma Syndromes

Sturge-Weber
Kasabach-Merritt
Klippel-Trenauney
Maffucci
Von Hippel-Lindau
Weber-Osler-Rondu hereditary hemorrhagic telangiectasia
Ollier's
Beckwith-Wiedeman
Blue rubber bleb nevus
Multiple neonatal hemangiomatosis

reditary hemorrhagic telangiectasia patients may have alarming bleeding from the oral mucous membrane and gastrointestinal (GI) mucosa multiple telangiectasia along with similar skin lesions. Patients with Ollier's syndrome exhibit enchondromas often associated with malignant changes into osteosarcomas along with cutaneous hemangiomas. The Beckwith-Wiederman syndrome consists of port-wine hemangiomas of the face, macroglossia, and defects of the pancreas, liver, and kidney. Also associated with lesions of the GI tract, liver, spleen, and CNS in the form of bleeding cavernous hemangiomas and painful skin cavernous hemangiomas is the blue rubber bleb nevus syndrome. Children both with multiple superficial strawberry hemangiomas and similar bleeding lesions of the brain and viscera, occasionally leading to lethal bleeding, exhibit multiple neonatal hemangiomatosis syndrome.

Indications for Intervention

Aside from cosmetic concern to the patient and family, many hemangiomas require no special treatment other than family counseling. Certainly, asymptomatic, spontaneously involuting lesions fall into this category. Indications for intervention are shown in Table 23.5 and may be divided into absolute and relative indications. Any complications of the associated hemangioma syndromes, such as DIC in the Kasabach-Merritt syndrome, obviously require rapid treatment because of life-threatening problems. Uncontrolled growth far beyond the natural history of hemangioma growth may necessitate intervention, as may local wound-healing problems such as ulceration with subsequent sepsis and frequent bleeding. Pain is an infrequent complication of hemangiomas and should be investigated by a biopsy in adults as a possible indication of malignant change. Cardiac enlargement or congestive heart failure as a result of an AV fistula can be reversible with adequate control of the peripheral lesion. Any interference or obstruction of a vital orifice with

Table 23.5.
Absolute and Relative Indications for Intervention in Cutaneous Vascular Lesions

Absolute
  Life-threatening complications
    Disseminated intravascular coagulation (DIC)
    High-output cardiac failure
    Obstruction of body orifice
    Actual or suspected malignant change
    Sepsis secondary to disseminated infection
  Local complications
    Recurrent bleeding
    Ulceration
    Infection
  Functional deformity
    Gigantism of involved area
    Visual obstruction (periorbital lesion)
Relative
  Family concern
  Cosmesis

subsequent functional loss (e.g., eyelid hemangioma blocking vision and resulting in amblyopia, oral cavity hemangioma interfering with feeding or respiration, genital hemangioma obstructing bladder or bowel function) necessitates intervention. Special consideration should be given to any periorbital hemangioma that may cause visual disturbances in infants, even if sight is not blocked totally. The mass itself may result in compression of the globe and astigmatism. Treatment consists of selective patching of the good eye and consideration of the use of steroids.

Relative indications for intervention in hemangioma include family concern and correction or prevention of present or future deformity. It seems desirable to alleviate or prevent up to 6 years of ridicule and embarrassment for a child with a visual facial birthmark. Certainly, it is hard for a child to grow up with constant questions and comments from family and strangers about their "bruise" or "mark." Similarly, it is difficult for a child with a visual facial deformity to start school without some regard for peer ridicule or curiosity and resulting embarrassment or loss of self-esteem about being different. This is especially the case if the birthmark can be easily and safely treated and if final results are not significantly different than those that occur after spontaneous involution. Occasionally, when hemangioma removal is simple and easy and secondary deformity is minimal, surgical removal may be considered.

Nonlaser Methods for Hemangioma Treatment

Many interventive and noninterventive methods of hemangioma treatment have been utilized in the past and are being recommended today. They are summarized in Table 23.6. X-ray therapy (17) should be reserved for life-threatening conditions such as DIC with subsequent hemorrhage in the Kasabach-Merritt syndrome or rapidly growing laryngeal lesions that threaten total airway obstruction. X-ray radiation of a superficial lesion may be associated with undesirable side-effects, including additional damage to the skin, epiphysis, breast, gonad, lens, or thyroid (18). Surgical methods of treatment include partial or complete excision, often accompanied by flaps or grafts. Steroid control of hemangiomas has been promulgated by Zarem and Edgerton (19) and gives better than excellent response in 90% of younger patients (infants less than 18 months). Dosages of 40 mg of prednisone every second day are tapered rapidly, although rebound growth under the critical dose of 20 mg every other day is not uncommon. Mazzola (20) has demonstrated a similar dramatic reduction of hemangioma growth by injection of intralesional methylprednisone in selected lesions. Kushner (21) was able to produce marked to moderate involution in periorbital infantile hemangiomas with intralesional corticosteroids.

Selective ligation of peripheral vessels and AV fistulas located directly in the hemangioma has been used effectively by Bingham and associates (22, 23) in conjunction with Doppler localization by the percutaneous route.

Table 23.6.
Methods of Hemangioma Treatment

X-ray
Surgery
Steroids
Selective ligation
Compression
Injection sclerosants
Cryotherapy
Embolization
Tattooing
Laser—argon, CO_2, neodymium : YAG, tunable dye

Other authors caution against selective proximal ligation of feeder vessels because they believe it is largely ineffective and may cause steals or shunts from new vessels as well as prevent future embolization. Miller and associates (24) have demonstrated the beneficial effect of continuous pressure as a primary treatment or in conjunction with other treatments such as steroids for control of large or complicated hemangiomas. Embolization with gel foam, dura, silicone beads, and the like along with selective arteriography has been advocated by Iricheff and Berenstein (25) and Schrudde and Petrivici (26), usually as an adjunct to surgery in control of rapidly growing, markedly deforming hemangiomas. A variety of sclerosing agents, including hot water, hypertonic saline, sodium morrhuate, and others, have been injected into hemangiomas but are not used frequently now. Ethibloc, a compound composed of natural amino acids plus alcohol, has been reported to change the vessels of hemangiomas into a putty-like fibrous mass (27). It must be directly injected into the hemangioma under arteriographic control and is usually followed by excisional surgery after 2 weeks. Port-wine hemangiomas have been camouflaged with surgical tattoo, but the results have not been permanent.

Laser Treatment

At present, a variety of lasers offer great promise for a wide variety of hemangioma treatment (Table 23.7). The most effective and applicable lasers for use in hemangioma include the argon, carbon dioxide, YAG, and tunable dye lasers. Each has a special mechanism of action.

Table 23.7.
Laser Treatment of Hemangiomas

Hemangiomas amenable to argon laser
Port-wine hemangioma
Strawberry mark
Acne rosacea
Telangiectasia
Hemangiomas amenable to CO_2 laser
Cavernous hemangioma
Hemangiomas amenable to argon/CO_2 lasers
Pyogenic granuloma
Campbell-DeMorgan spots

The argon laser produces intense blue-green light between 488 and 514 nm. This laser light is selectively absorbed by hemoglobin, which has a relatively high coefficient of light absorption at about 500 nm. The argon laser light is able to penetrate intact the overlying skin and is absorbed by the hemoglobin-laden abnormal hemangioma vessels. Light absorption is then converted to heat, which coagulates the abnormal vessels, sparing skin appendages such as sweat glands and pilosebaceous glands. Thus, photocoagulation is the mechanism of the argon laser's action. It has been used successfully to treat adult hemangioma, including port-wine hemangioma, in thousands of patients for more than 8 years (28–33).

Studies have also shown that argon lasers are able to produce involution in hemangiomas in children, merely at an accelerated pace. The characteristic texture of the skin in the laser-treated hemangioma versus that of one that has spontaneously involuted 3–4 years later is identical, as demonstrated by Apfelberg et al. (30) for the argon laser. Precedents for treatment of the capillary component of hemangiomas in infants have been previously established for the argon laser by Apfelberg et al. in 1981 (30). This work was validated and expanded by the work of Hobby (34) and Achauer (35) in 1985. These authors demonstrated the laser's ability to induce thrombogenesis in hemangiomas in infants, later followed by accelerated spontaneous involution. There were no significant residual scars reported in any series.

The carbon dioxide laser produces intense light in the invisible infrared spectrum (10.6 nm), which is capable of being absorbed by water. Because the water content of biological tissue, especially hemangioma, is 75–90%, the laser acts by vaporizing tissue at its focal point, leaving adjacent tissue practically unaffected. The primary advantage of the carbon dioxide laser in hemangioma surgery is the ability to cut as a knife and seal small vessels at the same time. Larger vessels do require clamping, but defocusing the laser beam accomplishes cautery, thus reducing blood loss during surgery—a critically important factor for pediatric patients. Postoperative scarring is similar to that with conventional techniques, and postoperative pain and edema are reduced appreciably (36–39).

The neodymium : YAG laser may be used in either contact or noncontact modes. This laser produces continuous-wave power output of 1,064 nm in the near-infrared light spectrum. This laser can produce tissue reactions to depths of 5–7 mm into the dermis in the noncontact mode. The scattering (forward and backward) effect within the tissue heats up a large volume and causes tissue coagulation and necrosis over a large area. Hypertrophic capillary-cavernous hemangiomas, particularly in the oral cavity, may be successfully photocoagulated with this laser (40, 41). The YAG laser energy may also be finely focused for precise excision and outstanding hemostasis through synthetic sapphire scalpel peripheral devices. This allows relatively bloodless excision of massive cavernous hemangiomas and vascular tumors. This adaptation to the YAG laser fiberoptic cable is the only laser modality that uses direct tissue contact; all others depend on light from a distance to accomplish either photocoagulation or incision. Apfelberg and colleagues have recently demonstrated the beneficial effect of YAG laser photocoagulation plus direct intralesional instillation of steroids for the treatment of capillary-cavernous hemangiomas of infancy. Thirteen patients were treated between one and three times. Treatments were done under general anesthesia as an outpatient. Five of the 13 patients experienced dramatic blanching and shrinking of the hemangioma with one treatment. Six patients experienced mild to moderate shrinkage. Complications of mild scarring occurred in two patients (42).

The tunable dye laser shows great promise in the treatment of port-wine hemangiomas and telangiectases of infants and young children and those on the trunk and extremities of children and adults. Traditional argon laser therapy results in a greater incidence of scarring and minimal fading in these situations. The tunable dye laser produces yellow light at 577–585 nm. This light is selectively absorbed by dermal vascular structures but does not affect the overlying epidermis. Very low power densities (3–20 joules/cm^2) and rapid pulses (300 μsec to 200 msec) serve to decrease thermal injury, thus markedly diminishing the tendency toward scarring. Several series (43, 44) have now demonstrated near-total blanching of port-wine stains in infants and children with a negligible incidence of scarring using the tunable dye laser. Between one and eight separate treatments of the same area may be necessary to achieve the final results.

Lasers have been used safely in surgery for more than 20 years in many fields. Laser light is nonionizing. Apfelberg (45) has demonstrated in fibroblasts grown in tissue culture and exposed to argon and carbon dioxide lasers that no significant malignant transformation of the cells resulted from the exposure.

References

1. Levy DM, Apfelberg DB: Hemangiomas in children. *Am Fam Physician* 5:89, 1972.
2. Lampe I, Latourette HB: Management of cavernous hemangiomas in infants. *Pediatr Clin North Am* 6:511, 1959.
3. Innes FLF: Classification of haemangiomata. *Br J Plast Surg* 6:76, 1953.
4. Bivings L: Spontaneous regression of angiomas in children. Twenty-two years' observation covering 236 cases. *J Pediatr* 45:643, 1954.
5. Bowers RE, Graham EA, Tomlinson KM: The natural history of strawberry nevus. *Arch Dermatol* 82:667, 1960.
6. Payne NM, Moyer F, Marcks KM, et al: The precursor to hemangioma. *Plast Reconstr Surg* 38:64, 1966.
7. Phelan JT, Grace JT Jr: Conservative management of cutaneous capillary hemangioma. *JAMA* 185:246, 1963.
8. Margileth AM: Developmental vascular abnormalities. *Pediatr Clin North Am* 18:773, 1971.
9. Mulliken JB, Glowaki J: Hemangiomas and vascular malformations in infants and children. A classification based on endothelial characteristics. *Plast Reconstr Surg* 69:412, 1982.
10. Wisnicki JL: Hemangiomas and vascular malformations. *Ann Plast Surg* 12:41, 1984.
11. Matthews DN: Hemangiomata. *Plast Reconstr Surg* 41:528, 1968.
12. Williams HB: Facial bone changes with vascular tumors in children. *Plast Reconstr Surg* 63:309, 1979.
13. Pasyk KA, Cherry GW, Grabb WC, et al: Quantitative evalua-tion of mast cells in cellularly dynamic and adynamic vascular malformations. *Plast Reconstr Surg* 73:69, 1984.
14. Pasyk KA: Classification of clinical and histopathological features of hemangiomas and other vascular malformations. In Ryan TJ, Cherry GW (eds): *Vascular Birthmarks*. London, Oxford University Press, 1987, p 23.
15. Grabb WC, Dingman RO, Oneal RM, et al: Facial hamartomas in children: Neurofibroma, lymphangioma, and hemangioma. *Plast Reconstr Surg* 65:509, 1980.
16. Kaplan EN: Hamartomas. In Kernahan DA, Vistnes LM (eds): *Biological Aspects of Reconstructive Surgery*. Boston, Little, Brown & Co. 1977, p 213.
17. Pyesmany A, Ekert H, Williams K, et al: Intravascular coagulation secondary to cavernous hemangioma in infancy: Response to radiotherapy. *Can Med Assoc J* 100:1053, 1969.
18. Li FP, Cassady JR, Barnett E: Cancer mortality following irradiation in infancy for hemangioma. *Radiology* 113:117, 1974.
19. Zarem HA, Edgerton MT: Induced resolution of cavernous hemangiomas following prednisolone therapy. *Plast Reconstr Surg* 39:76, 1967.
20. Mazzola RF: Treatment of haemangiomas in children by intralesional injections of steroids. A long term follow-up. *Chir Plast (Berl)* 4:161, 1978.
21. Kushner BJ: The treatment of periorbital infantile hemangioma with intralesional corticosteroid. *Plast Reconstr Surg* 76:517, 1985.
22. Bingham HG, Lichti EL: The Doppler as an aid in predicting the behavior of congenital cutaneous hemangioma. *Plast Reconstr Surg* 47:580, 1971.
23. Bingham HG; Predicting the course of a congenital hemangioma. *Plast Reconstr Surg* 63:161, 1979.
24. Miller SH, Smith RL, Shochat SJ: Compression treatment of hemangiomas. *Plast Reconstr Surg* 5:573, 1976.
25. Berenstein A, Iricheff II: Therapeutic vascular occlusion. *J Dermatol Surg Oncol* 4:11, 1978.
26. Schrudde J, Petrovici V: Surgical treatment of giant hemangioma of the facial region after arterial embolization. *Plast Reconstr Surg* 68:878, 1981.
27. Riche MC, Hadjean E, Tran-Ba-Huy P, et al: The treatment of capillary-venous malformations using a new fibrosing agent. *Plast Reconstr Surg* 71:607, 1983.
28. Apfelberg DB, Kosek J, Maser MR, et al: Histology of port wine stains following argon laser treatment. *Br J Plast Surg* 32:232, 1979.
29. Apfelberg DB, Maser MR, Lash H, et al: The argon laser for cutaneous lesions. *JAMA* 245:2074, 1981.
30. Apfelberg DB, Greene RA, Maser MR, et al: Results of argon laser exposure of capillary hemangiomas of infancy, preliminary report. *Plast Reconstr Surg* 67:188, 1981.
31. Cosman B: Experience in the argon laser therapy of port wine stains. *Plast Reconstr Surg* 65:119, 1980.
32. Goldman L, Dreffer R: Laser treatment of extensive mixed cavernous and port wine stains. *Arch Dermatol* 113:504, 1977.
33. Noe JM, Barsky SH, Gerr DE, et al: Port wine stains and the response to argon laser therapy: Successful treatment and the predictive role of color, age, and biopsy. *Plast Reconstr Surg* 65:130, 1980.
34. Hobby LW: Further evaluation of the potential of the argon laser in the treatment of capillary hemangiomas of infancy. *Plast Reconstr Surg* 71:481, 1983.
35. Achauer BM, Vander Kam VM: Argon laser treatment of strawberry hemangioma in infancy. *West J Med* 143:628, 1985.
36. Aronoff BL: The use of lasers in hemangiomas. *Lasers Surg Med* 1:323, 1981.
37. Kaplan I, Sharon U: Current laser surgery. *Ann NY Acad Sci* 267:247, 1976.
38. Oshiro T: The CO$_2$ laser in the treatment of cavernous hemangioma of the lower lip. *Lasers Surg Med* 1:337, 1981.
39. Slutzki S, Shafir R, Borenstein L: Use of the carbon dioxide laser for large excisions with minimal blood loss. *Plast Reconstr Surg* 60:250, 1977.
40. Apfelberg DB, Smith T, Lash H, et al: Preliminary report on use of the neodymium : YAG laser in plastic surgery. *Lasers Surg Med* 7:189, 1987.

41. Apfelberg DB, Smith T: Study of the benefits of the Nd:YAG laser in plastic surgery. In Ogura Y, Joffee S (eds): *Advances in Nd:YAG Laser Surgery*. New York, Springer-Verlag, 1987.

42. Apfelberg DB, Maser MR, White DN, et al: A preliminary study on the combined effect of neodymium:YAG laser photocoagulation and direct steroid instillation in the treatment of capillary/cavernous hemangiomas of infancy. *Ann Plast Surg* 22:94, 1989.

43. Garden JM, Tan OT, Parrish JA: The pulsed dye laser: Its use at 577 nm wavelength. *J Dermatol Surg Oncol* 13:134, 1987.

44. Tan OT, Sherwood K, Gilchrest BA: Treatment of children with port-wine stains using the flashlamp-pulsed tunable dye laser. *N Engl J Med* 320:416, 1989.

45. Apfelberg DB, Chadl B, Maser MR, Lash H: Study of carcinogenic effects of in vitro argon laser exposure of fibroblasts. *Plast Reconstr Surg* 71:93, 1982.

24

Lymphatic Malformations

A. Jay Burns, M.D.

Lymphatic malformations are a varied group of ill-defined vascular anomalies often confusing to the student reader and the clinician. The foundation for a better understanding of these interesting lesions is proper terminology. While a number of different names are used to describe them (e.g., lymphangioma, cystic hygroma, hemangiolymphangioma, lymphangioma circumscriptum, lymphangioma diffusum), they all share a common histology and embryology. They are congenital defects of the lymphatic system.

The histories of the many terms used to describe lymphatic malformations give us clues to their positions in modern classification schemes. The first report of a cervicofacial lymphatic malformation dates to Redenbacker in 1828, who called it "ranula congenita" (1). In the head and neck, lymphatic malformations are usually referred to as "cystic hygromas." This was the term initially used by Wernher in 1843 when he distinguished cystic hygromas from brachial cleft cysts and thyroglossal duct anomalies on histological grounds (2). Twenty years later, Virchow perpetuated the misnomer by assuming that they were tumors capable of rapid cell proliferation and independent growth (the Greek suffix "*-oma*" implies a potential for growth by cellular mitosis and proliferation) (3). A student of Virchow, Wegner, in 1877 detailed a histomorphological classification for lymphatic anomalies that is often referred to today as types of *lymphangioma:* "simplex," "cavernous," and "cystoides" (4). In 1889, Morris introduced the term "lymphangioma circumscriptum" to describe a localized lymphatic anomaly presenting with vesicular skin lesions (5).

The terms "lymphangioma" and "cystic hygroma" suggest that these lesions have a propensity for cellular proliferation and recurrence after excision. Unfortunately, this belief permeates the literature, although the evidence is strongly against it. Thymidine labeling studies of excised lymphatic anomalies do not show increased cellular turnover (6). It is also extremely difficult to grow endothelium from tissue specimens of lymphatic anomalies, and this reinforces the classification system that places these lesions under true malformations rather than neoplasms (7).

In 1982, Mulliken and Glowacki published an innovative classification scheme that greatly simplifies the nomenclature of vascular anomalies. Their scheme is clinically useful and is solidly based on both the cellular biology and the natural history of these lesions (6). The authors restrict the use of the term "hemangi*oma*" to vascular tumors that enlarge through rapid cellular proliferation (as predicted by its suffix); all other vascular birthmarks are classified as malformations. Vascular malformations are further categorized as capillary, venous, arterial, and lymphatic anomalies; a combination of two or more of these subgroups is common.

Lymphatic malformations exhibit a normal rate of endothelial cell turnover and are true structural anomalies that betray their origins as errors of vascular morphogenesis. Because they are congenital, they are usually detected at birth or shortly thereafter and grow commensurately with the developing child. (Occasionally, lymphatic anomalies will show a rapid increase in size but not as a result of cellular hyperplasias, as is discussed later.) The logic and practicality of the Mulliken and Glowacki classification scheme is easily seen when one applies it in the clinical setting. The terms "lymphangiohemangioma" and "hemangiolymphangioma" have been incorrectly given to lesions that on pathological examination show a mixture of lymphatic and blood-filled spaces. These lesions exhibit a slow growth rate commensurate with the growth of the child and no abnormal cellular proliferation; therefore, "lymphaticovenous" or "venolymphatic malformation" is a more appropriate descriptor.

In discussing lymphatic malformations in this chapter, we follow the classification system of Mulliken and Glowacki. For the reasons mentioned above, "lymphangioma" is a misnomer, and the term should be discarded in favor of "lymphatic malformation." For descriptive purposes, and because they are entrenched in the literature, we occasionally use the names "lymphangioma circumscriptum" and "cystic hygroma" to ease the transition to the more accurate nomenclature (Fig. 24.1).

Anatomy

The human body is supplied with a rich lymphatic network. Lymphatic vessels are found in the skin and subcutaneous layer as well as deep to the fascia. Three layers of lymphatics have been described in the dermis: (*a*) the superficial plexus in the upper third of the dermis, composed of small vessels of uniform caliber and devoid of valves: (*b*) an intermediate plexus in the middle third of the dermis with vessels of varying caliber, also devoid of valves: and (*c*) a deep dermal plexus of vessels of varying and sometimes quite large caliber, containing valves at

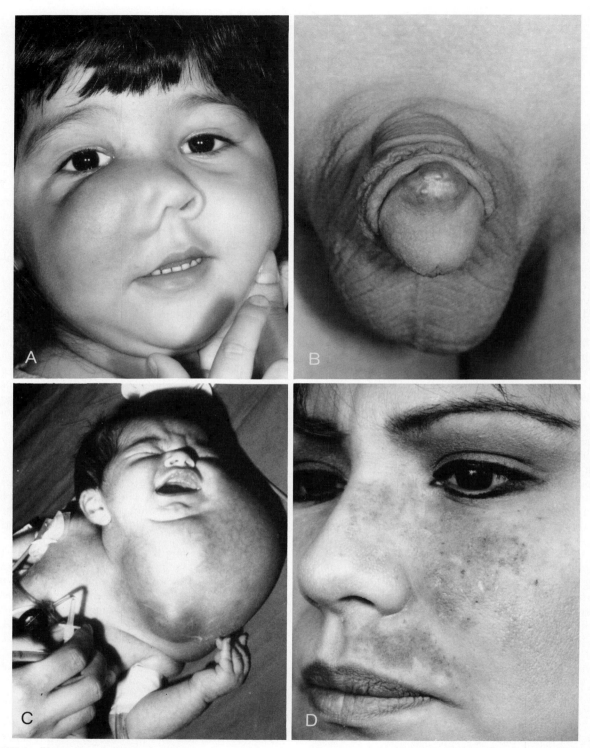

FIGURE 24.1. Examples of past and present nomenclature of common vascular malformations. **A,** Six-year-old girl with swelling of right cheek deforming right nasal rim. Past: "lymphangioma"; present: lymphatic malformation. **B,** Four-year-old boy with mass on distal penis that was present at birth and has grown commensurately since birth. Past: "cavernous hemangioma"; present: venous malformation. **C,** Newborn infant with large cystic swelling of left cheek and neck. Past: "cystic hygroma"; present: lymphatic malformation. (Courtesy of Dale, Coln, M.D.) **D,** Forty-year-old woman with vascular stain of left cheek present since birth. Past: "port-wine stain"; present: capillary malformation.

the junction of the dermis with the subcutaneous tissue (8). The subcutaneous tissues are linked by horizontal arcades that empty into the main lymphatic trunks close to the deep fascia. Deep to the fascia, lymphatic trunks run in the intermuscular planes in association with the main blood vessels of the limb.

The superficial and subfascial lymphatic trunks connect at only two points: a supratrochlear lymph node in the arm and a popliteal lymph node in the leg. Open communication between the superficial and deep systems is otherwise nonexistent by virtue of the segregating deep fascia.

Embryology

Lymphatics are thought to arise from the venous system as epithelial buds off the anterior cardinal vein, the mesonephric vein, and the veins from the deep edge of the wolffian body (9). Sabin observed that lymphatic vessels in fresh pig embryos grow out of lymph sacs that were derived from veins (10). Working separately, Lewis confirmed this finding in rabbit embryos (11). Their anatomical studies at the turn of the century formed the basis for the *centrifugal theory* of lymphatic development.

Shortly thereafter, Huntington and McClure challenged the validity of this deep-to-superficial sequence of lymphatic development when they concluded from their work with cat embryos that lymphatic channels arise from clefts in the primitive mesenchyme and only secondarily communicate with the venous system (12). This process they called the *centripetal theory* (superficial to deep). Subsequent studies in human embryos by van der Putte (13), however, reestablished Sabin's centrifugal theory as the true mechanism of embryogenesis of the

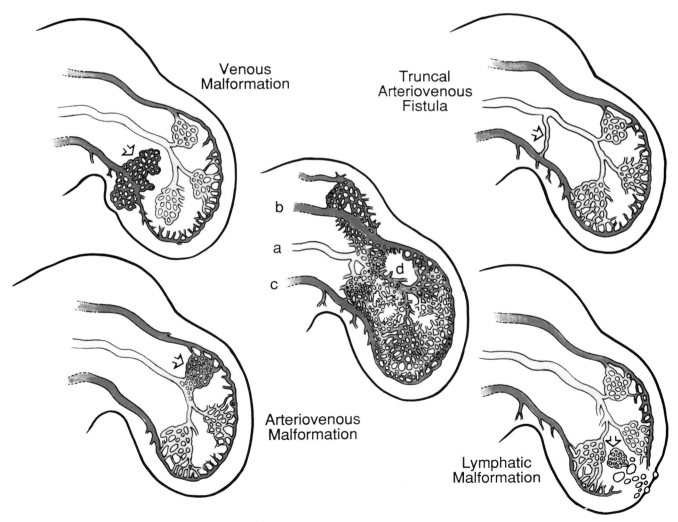

FIGURE 24.2. Drawing of injected 12-mm pig embryo showing early development of blood vessels in anterior appendage bud (equivalent to 6-week human embryo). (After Woollard HH: The development of the principal arterial stems in the forelimb of the pig. *Contr Embryol Carnegie Instit* 14:139, 1922.) Drawing is modified to show possible vascular malformations. **a,** Retiform central (axial) artery (persists as volar interosseous artery); **b,** cephalic vein; **c,** basilic vein; **d,** primitive capillary plexus undergoing resorption. (From Mulliken JB, Young AE: *Vascular Birthmarks: Hemangiomas and Malformations.* Philadelphia, WB Saunders Co, 1988, p 111.)

lymphatic system, and it is still widely held as such today (Fig. 24.2).

The lymphatic system begins as two sets of paired lymph sacs, the jugular and iliac, as well as two sets of unpaired sacs, the retroperitoneal and the cisterna chyli. Eventually, these four sacs join and form the three major lymphatic ducts (thoracic, right lymphatic, and cisterna chyli). The paired jugular lymph sacs appear in the sixth week, sprouting from the primitive venous plexus between the anterior cardinal (internal jugular) veins and the subclavian veins. For a short period of time these lymph sacs become isolated and lose their connections with the vascular system of their origin, but shortly afterward they become reconnected between the sixth and seventh week of fetal life (14). Once the connection is reestablished, the jugular sacs and their tributaries continue to spread and eventually join the subclavian or axillary lymph sacs.

The cisterna chyli begins at the junction of the two major lumbar lymph trunks that drain the lower extremities. The cisterna chyli drains the lateral aortic lymph nodes and intestines and continues upward to the level of L2, where it enlarges through the aortic hiatus and becomes the thoracic duct. The thoracic duct is a continuous channel by the ninth week; cranially, it joins the left jugular bud and hence drains into the junction of the internal jugular and subclavian veins. Except for the right lymphatic duct, the thoracic duct serves as the common trunk for all lymph vessels. The right lymphatic duct drains the right upper extremity, right side of the head and neck, thorax, lungs, heart, and diaphragm.

Other connections are known to exist between the lymphatic system and the central venous system at the level of the inferior vena cava, renal, portal, azygos, and hemiazygos veins (8, 9, 15, 16).

Pathogenesis

Based on what we know of normal lymphatic embryogenesis, one can envision that cystic cervicofacial and axillary lymphatic anomalies ("cystic hygroma") stem from errors of morphoigenesis of the primitive lymph sacs in the jugular, subclavian, and axillary regions. Failure of these lymph sacs to reestablish venous connections in the sixth and seventh weeks of fetal life is a possible cause of these anomalies.

There is mounting evidence to suggest that lymphatic anomalies present as a wide spectrum of deformities, from lymphedema on one end to large cystic malformations on the other. We will not attempt here to give a detailed overview of lymphedema, which is the subject of another chapter. We limit our discussion to a recounting of Crockett's observations regarding the pathological anatomy seen in lymphedema (8). Crockett studied normal and edematous limbs using two techniques: injection of contrast media in amputated limbs and x-ray lymphangiography in living subjects. All patients with clinically "pure"—noninfectious, nontraumatic—lymphedema were found to have gross anatomical abnormalities of the lymphatic vessels, such as absence, hypoplasia, discontinuity, varicosity with valvular incompetence, or obstruction. Extremities with edema from causes other than lymphedema do not show these changes.

Between the two extremes of lymphedema and large cystic lymphatic malformations range from a number of anomalies such as lymphangiomas, lymphangiectasia, and lymphangioma circumscriptum. One could theorize that these lesions are perhaps the result of an interruption in the peripheral lymphatic embryological development. Bill and Sumner (17) suggested that the various morphological types of lymphatic malformation can be explained by their anatomical locations. For example, lesions occurring in areas with distinct tissue planes and loose areolar tissue (e.g., the neck, axilla, and mediastinum) are able to expand and form cystic structures. Conversely, lymphatic malformations in the lips, cheek, and tongue are bound by a more restrictive organization of tissues and will present as compact lesions. Although this theory is widely accepted, it has yet to be proven experimentally.

Thompson and Keiller in 1923 thought that the rapid growth of lymphatic anomalies in utero and after birth

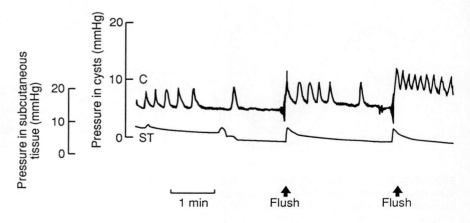

FIGURE 24.3. Pressure tracing from a cannula inserted into the cistern of a cutaneous lymphatic malformation. It demonstrates regular pulsations at the rate of about 4/min. The small fluctuations in the trace are those of respiration. The lower tracing is from a control cannula inserted into the subcutaneous fat adjacent to the lymphatic malformation. The minimal pressure difference between the malformation and the surrounding tissues suggests that the malformation maintains a small but constant tone, as well as contracting intermittently. (From Browse NL, Whimster IW, Stewart G, et al: The surgical management of lymphangioma circumscriptum. *Br J Surg* 73:585, 1986, with permission of Butterworth Publishing Co.)

was due to excessive secretion from the endothelial lining and not to cellular proliferation (18). Goetsch in 1938 accepted that lymphatic anomalies were true developmental malformations, but he believed that the cystic walls of the lymphatic vessels retained their ''embryonic power'' for neoplastic growth based on histological studies of excised specimens (19). Willis disagreed with the cellular proliferation theory and stated that lymphatic malformations expanded as a result of fluid accumulation, cellulitis, or inadequate drainage of anomalous lymphatic channels (20). This correlates well with the empirical conclusion that the vast majority of lymphatic malformations grow commensurately with the child; rapid growth of the lesions is usually found in association with a viral upper respiratory infection or other infectious processes.

In 1980, McHale et al. discovered spontaneous contractions in the mesenteric lymphatics of cattle (21). Whimster and Browse recorded spontaneous pressure waves of 5–15 mm Hg at a frequency of 3–5/min in lymphatic malformations (22). Indwelling catheters were placed in human foot lymphatics, and regular pressure waves of 20 mm Hg, which sometimes rose to 50 mm Hg, were recorded (23; Fig. 24.3). These studies strongly suggest that human lymphatics have an intrinsic contractility themselves and that this capability is seen in lymphatic malformations as well.

Histopathology

Lymphatic malformations present histologically in diverse forms, and Mulliken and Young detailed these in a succinct review (24).

Microscopically, cystic spaces of lymphatic malformations may be unilocular, multilocular, or diffuse. Regardless of the specific pattern of loculation, all the cysts are lined with a single layer of endothelium. The cyst fluid stains acidophilic and is protein rich. Blood cells are often present in the cystic fluid and may indicate recent hemorrhage into the lymphatic cavity or a combined lymphaticovenous malformation (6). Mural thrombi and lymphoid reaction are frequently seen in lymphatic malformation specimens.

The vessel walls of lymphatic malformations vary in thickness; although some are quite thin, more frequently the walls are thickened with the fibromuscular layering of both striated and smooth muscle.

Abnormal lymphatic tissue can be seen *within* large nerves and *within* the walls of local blood vessels.

Epidemiology

In a series of 112 patients with lymphatic malformations, Gross found that 65 (58%) of the malformations were present at birth, 80% were diagnosed by 1 year of age, and 90% had become evident by 2 years of age. Males and females were equally affected (25).

Lymphatic malformations can affect all areas of the body, but most are concentrated in the head, neck, and axilla. Seventy-five to 90% of cystic lymphatic malformations (cystic hygromas) occur in the cervical region, and the majority of these are in the posterior triangle. If found in the anterior triangle, these lesions carry a poor prognosis because they are often intertwined with complex vascular and neural structures. Approximately 0.5% of all neck masses are eventually diagnosed as cystic hygroma; 10% of these have a mediastinal component.

Lymphatic malformations are the most common cause of congenital tongue enlargement (macroglossia), lip enlargement (macrocheilia), and ear enlargement (macrotia).

NATURAL HISTORY

The frequency with which lymphatic malformations undergo spontaneous involution has been variously reported from <1% (26) to 16% (27); Grabb et al. (28) reported 41% total and 29% partial involution by 5 years of age in 17 patients. The latter authors also quoted a published incidence of involution ranging from 15% to 70% in the first 20 years of life.

Large cystic lymphatic malformations are brought to the physician's attention primarily because of their size and appearance. Although they generally grow proportionately with the child, sudden and rapid increases in the size of the lesions are common, usually following an upper respiratory or soft tissue infection.

Diagnosis

CYSTIC CERVICOFACIAL LYMPHATIC MALFORMATION (CYSTIC HYGROMA)

With improved prenatal care and refinements in ultrasonographic technique, many lymphatic malformations can be diagnosed at an earlier age. Large cystic cervicofacial masses can be detected and their characteristic features clearly identified as early as the 12th week of embryonic life (29). Of 17 cases of fetal cystic hygroma diagnosed by ultrasound examination, Pijpers et al. found nine instances of associated abnormalities. Subsequent karyotyping revealed normal findings in six, Turner's syndrome in eight, and Edward's syndrome in one.

In another article, Rodis et al. (30) described a case of cystic hygroma diagnosed by ultrasound between 14 and 16 weeks of gestation (Fig. 24.4). Upon karyotyping, the fetus was found to have trisomy 21, and the pregnancy was terminated shortly afterward. Gross and pathological examination of the specimen revealed only mild webbing of the neck, supporting the hypothesis that redundant skin of the fetal neck represents early cystic hygromas. Besides the previously mentioned chromosomal aberrations, cystic hygromas may be associated with Klippel-Feil syndrome. It should be noted that, although there are case reports of spontaneous resolution of prenatally detected cystic neck masses in fetuses with normal karyotypes and normal outcomes (31), cystic hygroma, especially when associated with fetal hydrops, carries a grim prognosis. Nonseptated cystic lymphatic malformations tend to follow a more benign course than septated masses.

There are multiple differential diagnoses for neck

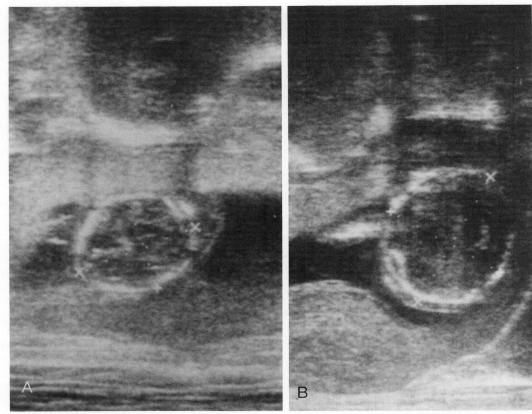

FIGURE 24.4. Spontaneous resolution of cystic hygroma between 14 weeks **(A)** and 16 weeks of **(B)** gestation. Arrows indicate occiput. (From Rodis JF, Vintzileos AM, Campbell WA, Nochimson DJ: Spontaneous resolution of fetal cystic hygroma in Down's syndrome. *Obstet Gynecol* 71:977, 1988, with permission of the American College of Obstetricians and Gynecologists.)

masses in children. Inflammatory masses are most common, but one must keep in mind the possibility of a thyroglossal duct cyst, sternocleidomastoid masses, hemangioma, and other vascular malformations of nonlymphatic origin. Neuroblastoma is the third most common tumor of childhood; therefore, it should be considered, as should teratoma and lymphoma. Thyroid masses are typically in the midline, which is an unusual presentation for cystic lymphatic malformations.

The larger cystic lymphatic malformations are usually translucent on radiographic examination, but a combination of hemorrhage, fibrosis, and chronic inflammation may change their typical appearance and mask their true lymphatic nature (32). Deep, localized lymphatic malformations may be extremely difficult to diagnose. If a lymphatic malformation is suspected, magnetic resonance (MR) imaging and/or contrast-enhanced computed tomography may be performed to rule out other etiologies: lymphatic malformations usually have a characteristic tissue density on MR imaging but they can sometimes be confused with lipomatous tissue. However, the finding of septae is evidence for their loculated cystic nature. In the parotid region, all masses must be considered neoplasms until proven otherwise. It is not uncommon for lymphatic malformations in the cervical area, particularly those occupying the floor of the mouth region, to become contaminated with oral flora. Because growth commensurate with the child's is the rule in lymphatic malformations,

several office visits may be required to ascertain this growth pattern. Abrupt enlargement of the mass may follow an upper respiratory infection or intralesional hemorrhage.

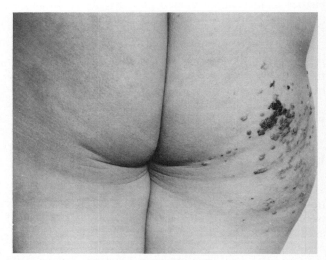

FIGURE 24.5. Localized lymphatic malformation of the buttock (lymphangioma circumscriptum). (From Mulliken JB, Young AE: *Vascular Birthmarks: Hemangiomas and Malformations.* Philadelphia, WB Saunders Co, 1988, p 223.)

LYMPHANGIOMA CIRCUMSCRIPTUM

In 1889, Morris first used the term "lymphangioma circumscriptum" to describe a disorder of subcutaneous lymphatic cisterns communicating through dilated lymphatic channels with superficial and cutaneous vesicles (5). In classic lymphangioma circumscriptum, the characteristic vesicles are noted at birth or soon thereafter. In some cases, the appearance of vesicles may be preceded by the palpation of a subcutaneous mass or swelling consistent with a deep-seated lymphatic malformation.

The classic lesion can occur anywhere, but it is prone to localize over the proximal parts of the limbs and the corresponding adjacent parts of the limb girdle. The size of the lesion is extremely variable (Fig. 24.5). In contrast, localized lymphangioma circumscriptum is well defined and may become apparent for the first time at any age. Furthermore, the area of involvement is usually 1 cm² or less. These circumscribed lesions are the exception rather than the rule.

In Bauer et al.'s (33) words,

[T]he (classic) lesion consists of scattered or grouped vesicles ranging in size from minute to 5 mm in diameter. Clear vesicles may be present on apparently normal skin or may top small papules. On occasion, there may be a plaque appearance or a super-imposed warty hyperkeratosis. Blood-filled capillary tufts may be seen through the clear vesicular contents, and some vesicles may contain varying amounts of blood mixed with lymph, giving them a pink or red color. Coagulation of blood within the vesicles may produce a purple or black appearance. (Fig. 24.6)

Whimster has shown histologically that lymphangioma circumscriptum has a deep component of large cystic spaces that give rise to the superficial vesicles through thin-walled channels (22). The large spaces are called cisterns and are usually surrounded by a thick, muscular coat. Spontaneous pressure waves of 5–15 mm Hg at a frequency of 3–5/min have been recorded in lymphatic

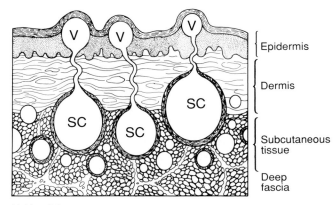

V Vescicles
SC Subcutaneous cisterns

FIGURE 24.7.   Diagram to illustrate the histological findings of circumscribed lymphatic malformations (lymphangioma circumscriptum). The dermis in the subcutaneous area is packed with thick, muscular-walled, deep cisterns that feed the superficial vesicles through short channels lined by lymphatic endothelium. The deep cisterns may extend well beyond the area of the superficial vesicles, and the channels feeding the vesicles are usually more complex than portrayed here. (From Browse NL, Whimster IW, Stewart G, et al: The surgical management of lymphangioma circumscriptum. *Br J Surg* 73:585, 1986, with permission of Butterworth Publishing Co.)

malformations (22, 23). The superficial manifestations of dermal lymphatic malformations (a.k.a. lymphangioma circumscriptum) are misleading, and the cutaneous vesicles are usually but the tip of the iceberg obscuring extensive intradermal and subcutaneous pathology (Fig. 24.7). Interestingly, the pathology seems to be demarcated by the surrounding muscle, and the dermal cystic spaces do not communicate with adjacent subcutaneous lymphatics, which appear to be normal in every respect. This gives further evidence to the finding that these lymphatic malformations may be a result of a failure to involute or establish normal connections in utero (34). Flanagan and Helwig's data revealed that there was a 25% recurrence rate after initial excision of lymphangioma circumscriptum (35). In most cases, recurrences occurred in less than 14 months and over half were in fact found within 3 months. For these reasons, Bauer et al. (33) recommended excising all dermal lymphatic malformations (lymphangioma circumscriptum) with frozen section control.

Electrocautery is usually recommended for the cutaneous vesicles of lymphangioma circumscriptum; however, the technique is plagued by high recurrence rates and moderate to severe scarring.

Special Considerations

COMBINED MALFORMATIONS

Lymphatic malformations are sometimes seen in combination with other vascular anomalies. The *Klippel-Trenaunay syndrome* consists of a dermal capillary malformation (port-wine stain) of the lower extremity with an underlying venolymphatic malformation, usually asso-

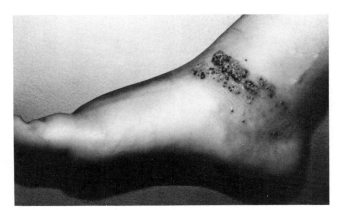

FIGURE 24.6.   Young child born with "constriction rings" at the ankles. One can see the Z-plasty release scars above the medial malleolus. The skin changes are typical of *dermal lymphatic malformations* (e.g., note the dark red vesicles secondary to bleeding in the abnormal dermal lymph channels). These lesions were previously termed lymphangioma circumscriptum. (Courtesy of John B. Mulliken, M.D.)

ciated with bony overgrowth and limb hypertrophy (Fig. 24.8). The syndrome is usually restricted to one lower extremity, but it may extend into the lower abdomen and trunk. A similar symptom complex may be seen occasionally in the upper limbs, either unilaterally or bilaterally.

If a lower extremity presents with all the findings of Klippel-Trenaunay syndrome, but in addition has arteriovenous fistula(s), the condition is known as *Parkes-Weber syndrome* applies. One should rule out the presence of arteriovenous fistulas in any patient with Klippel-Trenaunay syndrome because this finding drastically increases the expected morbidity.

SECONDARY DEFORMITIES

A vascular anomaly affecting some part of the skeleton is most likely a lymphatic malformation. Boyd et al. report skeletal hypertrophy and distortion in 80% of cystic hygromas by the age of 10 years (36). Typically, there is anterior distortion of the mandible or maxillary enlargement that results in prognathism, open bite, or other complex malocclusion (Fig. 24.9). The mechanism for bone overgrowth is not known, but it is theorized that direct pressure on the bone by the expanding mass redirects the bony growth. Increased blood flow is not believed to cause the osseous changes, although the lymphatic malformation may also be found within the bone itself (36). Osborne et al. reported their experience with orthognathic correction of mandibular deformities associated with large cystic hygromas. They recommended postponing surgery if at all possible until mandibular growth has completed because there is a high recurrence rate in these patients. They also recommended attempting surgery after the tumor has been adequately debulked and is no longer growing. Obviously, this status is difficult to predict because a slow but steady commensurate growth rate is the rule (37).

ACQUIRED PROGRESSIVE LYMPHANGIOMA

The so-called acquired progressive lymphangioma is thought to be a lymphatic malformation that slowly develops over a course of several years. The cutaneous manifestation is that of a flat, erythematous patch that may resemble lymphangioma circumscriptum, and it is usually first diagnosed in young children (38). The condition may be the same entity as a low-grade angiosarcoma, and the prognosis is favorable. An incision with 1-cm margins has shown to be effective and to prevent recurrence in these lesions.

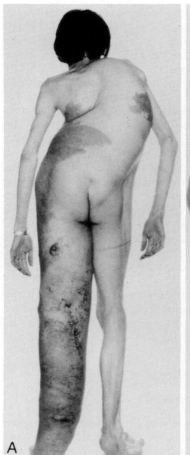
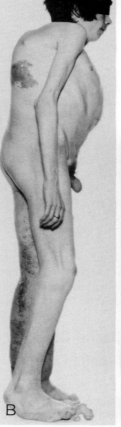
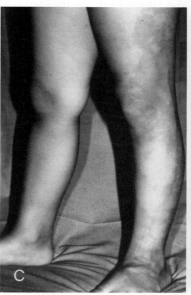
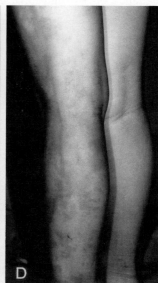

FIGURE 24.8. **A and B,** Klippel-Trenaunay syndrome of the left leg with gross associated lymphatic and skeletal abnormalities; in particular, the commonly associated feature of giant toes in this patient is found on the opposite side, suggesting that the vascular anomaly was not itself the cause. (From Mulliken JB, Young AE: *Vascular Birthmarks: Hemangiomas and Malformations.* Philadelphia, WB Saunders Co, 1988, p 255.) **C and D,** Klippel-Trenaunay syndrome in a 4-year-old boy. Venolymphatic component is subtle, but diagnosis can be made by large portwine stain and prominent lateral vein in this mildly hypertrophied limb.

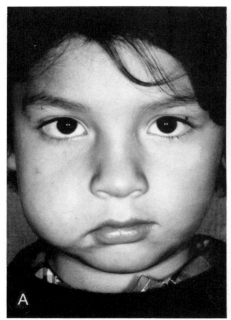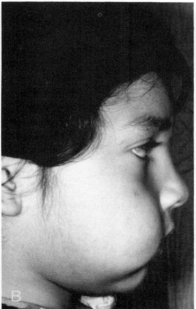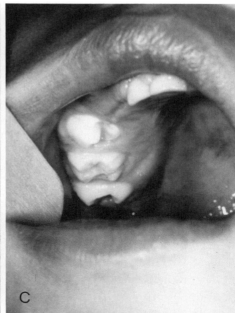

FIGURE 24.9. **A and B,** Five-year-old boy with mild lymphatic malformation. MR imaging diagnosis was lipomatous tissue; however, diagnosis of lymphatic malformation can be made by noticing secondary bony changes as depicted in **C. C,** Enlarged maxillary alveolar ridge as well as tooth deformity.

Treatment

SURGERY

Complete extirpation of the lesion by surgical means is the objective but, unfortunately, this goal is rarely achieved. In well-demarcated, unilocular, posterior triangle cysts, total excision can be carried out with relative ease, minimal morbidity, and a low recurrence rate. However, for larger or multiloculated masses, particularly those in the anterior triangle, a meticulous dissection is imperative, and care should be taken to avoid injury to the marginal mandibular branch of the facial nerve and to the greater auricular, spinal accessory, and phrenic nerves. In these lesions, it is often best to confine surgery to one anatomical area and to stage serial debulkings (Fig. 24.10).

The timing of surgery directly affects the outcome and must be tailored to the type of lesion and patient factors. Higher recurrence rates are reported when surgery is postponed to await natural involution of the lesion; however, the older the patient the safer the operation and the better the aesthetic result (27, 28). Grabb et al. emphasized that one must be reluctant to operate and recommended absolutely no surgery before the age of 3 years (28). If any evidence of involution is noted by this time, the child should be followed and photographed at yearly intervals. Transient enlargement of the mass secondary to infection should not force one to operate unless the infant's airway is compromised. In this case, a tracheostomy is recommended, and the infectious process is managed conservatively with warm packs and antibiotics. Finally, if no involution of the lymphatic malformation is noted by 3 years of age, partial excision can be carried out, although Grabb et al. still prefer to wait until the patient is 5 years old, if at all possible.

In contrast to the slow and cautious approach of Grabb and coworkers, Ravitch and Rush (39) and Vistnes (40) suggested early complete excision, believing that cure rates of 80% can be achieved. Obviously, an individualized treatment plan must be devised for each patient because no two malformations are identical.

RADIOTHERAPY

At the present time, irradiation is not indicated for the treatment of lymphatic malformations because it has been clearly shown that cellular proliferation is not a component of the pathological process. The morbidity associated with radiotherapy only adds to the argument against it.

SCLEROSING AGENTS

Sclerosing injections of boiling water, sodium morrhuate, sugar solutions, hypertonic saline, and oil have been ineffective. In general, sclerosing injections are not met with enthusiasm in the literature, although the recent Japanese experience with sclerotherapy for large cervicofacial lymphatic malformations in children has been extensive and largely favorable. Tanigawa et al. (41) reported on their experience with bleomycin fat emulsion. The bleomycin fat emulsion was injected in 0.3–0.5-ml increments once every 4–6 weeks. Clinical responses were defined as "excellent" if the tumor diminished to

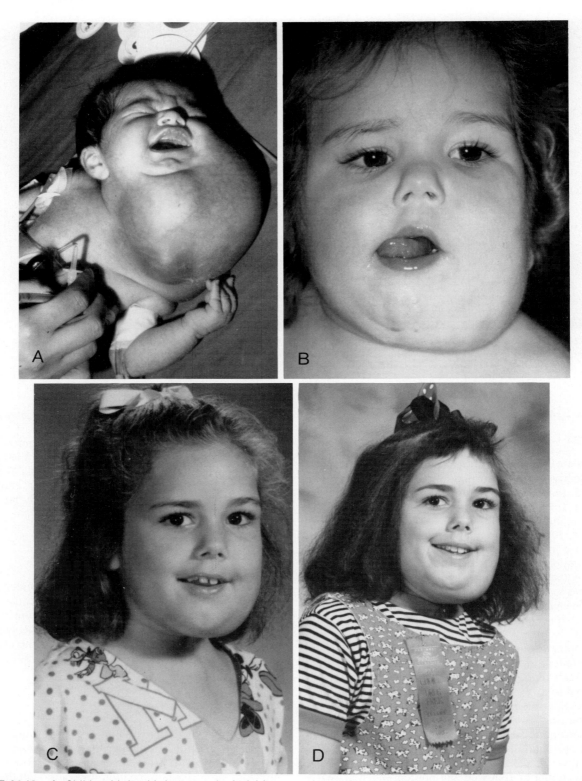

FIGURE 24.10. **A,** Child at birth with large cervicofacial lymphatic malformation (cystic hygroma). Patient underwent subtotal excision and bleomycin injection of residual. **B,** Same patient at 22 months of age prior to receiving second injection of bleomycin. **C and D,** Same patient at 6 and 8 years of age, respectively. No further treatment has been carried out.

symmetry with the contralateral side and "good" if the tumor shrank more than 50% of its original volume. If the tumor regressed less than 50%, it was considered a "no response." Satisfactory (good to excellent) results were noted in 27 of 33 patients (41). Cervicofacial lymphatic malformations have the highest response rates compared to lesions on the chest wall and leg. Fifty-five percent of these patients experienced fever as a result of treatment; diarrhea, local infection, and vomiting were additionally noted in a small number of patients. One patient suffered marked swelling and subsequent airway compromise in what was presumed to be an anaphylactic reaction to the sclerosing agent and required an emergency operation. This patient had a mediastinal component to the cervical lymphatic mass.

Ogita et al. report intracystic injection of OK-432, which they describe as a new sclerosing agent for cystic hygroma in children (42). OK-432 is a familiar sclerosant used in Japan, usually for the treatment of pleural effusion by intracavitary injection. Derived from specially treated group A *Streptococcus pyogenes* of human origin, OK-432 is thought to be safe and has fewer side effects than bleomycin. Its mechanism of action is reported to involve activation of the complement system, resulting in the release of anaphylotoxins and causing an intense inflammatory response. OK-432 does produce transient fever lasting 2–3 days, which may be controlled with antipyretics. Complete regression of the cystic hygroma was observed in eight patients within 2–3 months; three of eight patients required a second injection of OK-432 to bring about the desired response. The remaining patient showed marked but incomplete regression of the lesion. Although these reports are promising, sclerotherapy should still be approached with caution.

LASER

Laser therapy is rapidly becoming an important option in the management of all vascular anomalies; therefore, it is no surprise that it is being applied to lymphatic malformations as well.

CO_2 Laser

White and Adkins (43) reported three patients with cystic hygroma who were treated with the CO_2 laser by an intraoral approach. The water-like character of the fluid in these cystic lesions apparently makes them particularly susceptible to the CO_2 laser. The CO_2 laser has also proven to be effective in the treatment of the cutaneous vesicles of dermal lymphatic malformations (lymphangioma circumscriptum), but it is not curative in these cases because of the deep pathology in the cistern mechanism, which is inaccessible to the laser. Patients who are poor surgical risks or who refuse operation, however, may benefit from laser therapy of their lymphatic malformations. Use of the CO_2 laser in the treatment of lymphatic malformations is purported to cause less edema, less trauma, less bleeding, and less postoperative pain than conventional surgery.

Neodymium: YAG Laser

Apfelberg et al. (44) stated that the neodymium: yttrium-aluminum-garnet (Nd: YAG) laser, with its new sapphire tip technology, "allows resection of very difficult and massive hemangiomas previously considered unresectable by standard techniques." According to the authors, a major advantage of laser surgery in the management of congenital vascular lesions is decreased blood loss; however, they support this conclusion by their experience with only four patients, one with involuted hemangioma and three with lymphatic malformations, neither of which entities is especially prone to excessive bleeding. Although the Nd: YAG laser has proven effective in obliterating certain intradermal vascular anomalies, one should be careful to champion its use in deeper lesions consisting of large vascular channels. These channels may be beyond the reach of the laser, and excessive scar may result from the extensive thermocoagulation necessary to eradicate the anomalous vessels. At the present time, good evidence supporting the superiority of the Nd: YAG laser over standard surgical extirpation in the treatment of large, subdermal vascular lesions is lacking.

References

1. Redenbacker EAH: *De ranula sub lingua, speciali, cum casu congenito.* Monachii: Lindhauer, 1828.
2. Wernher A: *Die angebornen Kysten-Hygrome und die ihnen verwandten Geschwulste in anatomischer, diagnosticher und therapeutischer Beziehung.* Gissen, GF Heyer, Vater, 1843.
3. Virchow R: *Die Krankhaften Geschwulste,* vol III. Berlin: A Hirschwald, 1863, p 170.
4. Wegner G: Ueber Lymphangiome. *Arch Klin Chir* 20:641, 1877.
5. Morris M: Lymphangioma circumscriptum. In Unna PG, Morris M, Duhring LA, et al (Eds): *International Atlas of Rare Skin Diseases.* London: HK Lewis, 1889, p. 2.
6. Mulliken JB, Glowacki J: Hemangiomas and vascular malformations in infants and children: A classification based on endothelial characteristics. *Plast Reconstr Surg* 69:412, 1982.
7. Mulliken JB, Zetter BR, Folkman J: In vitro characteristics of endothelium from hemangiomas and vascular malformations. *Surgery* 92:348, 1982.
8. Crockett DJ: Lymphatic anatomy and lymphedema. *Br J Plast Surg* 18:12, 1965.
9. Kobayashi MR, Miller TA: Lymphedema. *Clin Plast Surg* 14:303, 1987.
10. Sabin FR: On the origin of the lymphatic system from the veins and the development of the lymph hearts and thoracic duct in the pig. *Am J Anat* 1:367, 1902.
11. Lewis FJ: The development of the lymphatic system in rabbits. *Am J Anat* 5:95, 1905.
12. Huntington GS, McClure CFW: The development of the main lymph channels of the cat in their relation to the venous system. *Anat Rec* 1:36, 1907.
13. van der Putte SCJ: The development of the lymphatic system in man. *Adv Anat Embryol Cell Biol* 51:3, 1975.
14. Patten BM: *Human Embryology,* ed 3. New York: McGraw-Hill Book Co, 1968, p 532.
15. Pick JW, Anson BJ, Burnett HW: Communications between lymphatic and venous systems at renal level in man. *Q Bull Northwestern Univ Med School* 18:307, 1944.
16. Szabo G, Magyar Z: The relationship between tissue fluids and lymph: Enzymes in tissue fluid and lymph. *Lymphology* 11:101, 1978.
17. Bill AH Jr, Sumner DS: A unified concept of lymphangioma and cystic hygroma. *Surg Gynecol Obstet* 120:79, 1965.

18. Thompson JE, Keiller VH: Lymphangioma of the neck. *Ann Surg* 77:385, 1923.
19. Goetsch E: Hygroma colli cysticum and hygroma axillare. Pathologic and clinical study and report of twelve cases. *Arch Surg* 36:394, 1938.
20. Willis RA: *Pathology of Tumors,* ed 3. London: Butterworth and Co, Ltd, 1960, p 716.
21. McHale NG, Roddie IC, Thornbury KD: Nervous modulation of spontaneous contractions in bovine mesenteric lymphatics. *J. Physiol.* 309:461, 1980.
22. Whimster IW: The pathology of lymphangioma circumscriptum. *Br J Dermatol* 94:473, 1976.
23. Olszewski WL, Engeset A: Intrinsic contractility of leg lymphatics in man. *Lymphology* 12:81, 1979.
24. Mulliken JB, Young AE: *Vascular Birthmarks: Hemangiomas and Malformations.* Philadelphia, WB Saunders Co, 1988.
25. Gross RE: *The Surgery of Infancy and Childhood.* Philadelphia: WB Saunders Co, 1964.
26. Ninh TN, Ninh TX: Cystic hygroma in children: Report of 126 cases. *J Pediatr Surg* 9:191, 1974.
27. Broomhead IW: Cystic hygroma of the neck. *Br J Plast Surg* 17:225, 1964.
28. Grabb WC, Dingman RO, O'Neal RM, Dempsey PD: Facial hamartomas in children: Neurofibroma, lymphangioma and hemangioma. *Plast Reconst Surg* 66(4):509, 1980.
29. Pijpers L, Reuss A, Stewart PA, Wladimiroff JW, Sachs ES: Fetal cystic hygroma: Prenatal diagnosis and management. *Obstet Gynecol* 72(2):223, 1988.
30. Rodis JF, Vintzileos AM, Campbell WA, Nochimson DJ: Spontaneous resolution of fetal cystic hygroma in Down's syndrome. *Obstet Gynecol* 71(6 Pt 2):976, 1988.
31. Distell BM, Hertzberg BS, Bowie JD: Spontaneous resolution of a cystic neck mass in a fetus with normal karyotype. *Am J Roentgenol* 153(2):380, 1989.
32. Sumner TE, Volberg FM, Kiser PE, Schaffner L de S: Mediastinal cystic hygroma in children. *Pediatr Radiol* 11:160, 1981.
33. Bauer BS, Kernahan DA, Hugo NE: Lymphangioma circumscriptum—a clinicopathological review. *Ann Plast Surg* 7:318, 1981.
34. Edwards JM, Peachey RDG, Kinmonth JB: Lymphangiography and surgery in lymphangioma of the skin. *Br J Surg* 59:36, 1972.
35. Flanagan BP, Helwig EB: Cutaneous lymphangioma. *Arch Dermatol* 113:24, 1977.
36. Boyd JB, Mulliken JB, Kaban LB, et al: Skeletal changes associated with vascular malformations. *Plastic Reconstr Surg* 74:789, 1984.
37. Osborne TE, Levin LS, Tilghman DM, Haller JA: Surgical correction of mandibulofacial deformities secondary to large cervical cystic hygromas. *J Oral Maxillofac Surg* 45(12):1015, 1987.
38. Tadaki T, Aiba S, Masu S, Tagami H: Acquired progressive lymphangioma as a flat, erythematous patch on the abdominal wall of a child. *Arch Dermatol* 124(5):699, 1988.
39. Ravitch MM, Rush BF Jr: Cystic hygroma. In Ravitch MM, Welch KJ, Benson CD, et al (Eds): *Pediatric Surgery.* Chicago, Year Book Medical Publishers, 1979, p 368.
40. Vistnes LM: Treatment of lymphangiomas and cystic hygromas. In Williams HB (Ed): *Symposium on Vascular Malformations and Melanotic Lesions.* St. Louis, CV Mosby, 1983, p 186.
41. Tanigawa N, Shimomatsuya T, Takahashi K, et al: Treatment of cystic hygroma and lymphangioma with the use of bleomycin fat emulsion. *Cancer* 60:741, 1987.
42. Ogita S, Tsuto T, Tokiwa K, Takahashi T: Intracystic injection of OK-432: A new sclerosing therapy for cystic hygroma in children. *Br J Surg* 74:690, 1987.
43. White B, Adkins WY: The use of the carbon dioxide laser in head and neck lymphangioma. *Lasers Surg Med* 6:293, 1986.
44. Apfelberg DB, Maser MR, Lash H, White DN: Sapphire tip technology for YAG laser excisions in plastic surgery. *Plast Reconstr Surg* 84:273, 1989.

25

Burn Injury

Joseph A. Moylan, M.D., F.A.C.S.

The management of an individual with a burn injury presents a challenge to the physician because this injury runs the gamut of clinical presentation from simple small, superficial injuries to those major burns that result in significant metabolic, cardiovascular, and organ dysfunction. A large percentage of burn injuries can be treated by a physician on an outpatient basis (1). Those patients involved in burn accidents that produce major surface damage require a team approach and coordination to minimize complications and optimize survival. The emphasis of this chapter is to provide the treating physician with an overall approach to the triage, initial management, and disposition of all burn patients.

The most common kind of burn injury results from thermal damage to the skin from a heat source such as flame, hot liquids, or heated objects. Of patients with these types of burns, 20–30% require hospitalization, but the larger portion can be treated as outpatients. Surface injuries could be categorized as minor, intermediate, and major (Table 25.1). *Minor burns* involve less than 15% of total body surface (TBS) and are primarily second degree. The third-degree component is less than 2–3% of total body surface and does not involve the eyes, hands, feet, or perineum. *Intermediate-size burns* are defined as second-degree burns up to 25% of the TBS with a slightly larger percentage of the total area being third degree (i.e., up to 10%). It has been suggested that moderate-size burns can be treated in the community hospital, particularly where there are physicians with burn care experience. *Major burns* include burns over 25% of the TBS, any burns of which 10% or more are third degree, burns involving vital structures such as the hands, face, feet, ears, and perineum, and those patients with inhalation injuries or other trauma. These patients should be initially stabilized and then transferred to a definitive burn care facility.

Table 25.1.
Burn Classification and Triage

Minor	Total burn—15% TBS or less	Ambulatory clinic
	Third degree less than 3%	
Moderate	Total burn—25% TBS or less	Community hospital
	Third degree less than 10%	
Major	Total burn—greater than 25% TBS	Burn center
	Third degree more than 10%	
	Complex injuries	

Mechanism of Injury

The extent and depth of thermal injuries depend upon the distribution of the heat source, the temperature, and the duration of exposure. Exposure to a heat source of greater than 160°F for 1–2 sec will produce a full-thickness injury. The distance of the agent from the skin, the configuration of the heat source, and any insulating agents such as clothes may modify the depth of the injury. The larger the burn size the more associated systemic complications occur. However, a team approach that involves nutritional support and the effective treatment of shock and infection has drastically minimized the mortality rate in recent years.

Systemic effects of burn injury can be divided into early, intermediate, and late effects. Early effects occur primarily in the first 24–48 hr and focus on the cardiovascular and the pulmonary systems (2). There is increased capillary permeability, resulting in the loss of protein-rich fluid into the extravascular space. The mechanism of this increased permeability appears to be cellular disruption from thermal injury as well as the release of vasoactive substances. Edema occurs throughout the whole body, even in uninjured areas. The volume of fluid changes are proportional to the size of the burn injury. Cardiac output may fall because of the loss of protein-rich fluid from the intravascular space as well as changes in the systemic resistance (3). Burn shock resulting in decreased cardiac output and associated with decreased urine output, confusion, and hypoxia is evident. Deficits in plasma volume may last from 24 to 48 hr because of arteriovenous shunting, even though cardiac output has been returned to normal levels.

While 8–10% of red cells may be destroyed by the thermal surface contact, the hematocrit falls over the intermediate phase of burn injury primarily as a result of volume replacement and shortened red cell life. Changes in the immune response as well as clotting parameters are also intermediate-phase complications occurring between the 3rd and 14th days after injury. Burns have a much higher incidence of infection than other types of trauma, not only because of the skin barrier disruption but also because of alterations in cellular and humoral immune responses (4).

Pulmonary abnormalities occur in both the early and intermediate phases. Initially, most early complications are due to either inhalation injury, which is discussed in more detail later; carbon monoxide poisoning; or those mechanical effects due to increasing edema under circumferential third-degree burns on the chest wall. This produces mechanical restriction, resulting in the requirement for increased pressure for ventilation. The use of chest escharotomies is therapeutic in this group of patients and should be performed when respiratory excursion of the chest wall is limited because of a tight eschar. A shield-like chest escharotomy should be performed through the full-thickness circumferential burned areas of the thorax. During the intermediate phase of burn case, most pulmonary complications are due to either sepsis, such as localized pneumonia, or systemic infection, which produces secondary postseptic acute respiratory distress syndrome.

Hypermetabolism secondary to hormonal and chemical alterations begins in the early phase but reaches its peak during the intermediate phase (5). Patients remain hypermetabolic until the wound is totally healed. Other late metabolic and endocrine disruptions are influenced by sepsis as well as by the burn wound itself.

Emergency Department Care

The goal of the Emergency Department care is to treat life-threatening complications of burn injury, to determine the disposition of the patient based on size and depth of injury, and to begin treatment of the burn injury and any systemic complications (Fig. 25.1). Implementation of the ABCs of the standard trauma protocol is appropriate for the patient with a major burn injury (6). The presence of severe inhalation injury, apnea, or significant carbon monoxide poisoning requires immediate endotracheal intubation with mechanical ventilation. Assessment of the patency of the airway, removal of any foreign material from the upper airway, and assessment of the adequacy of ventilation and gas exchange are primary goals in this as well as other types of trauma care. Once the

primary survey has been completed, depending upon the size of the injury (i.e., moderate or major burn), one or more intravenous lines will be required and should be placed in a nonburned area. All patients should be weighed prior to beginning intravenous resuscitation because most burn shock therapy is based on the size of the burn injury as well as the weight of the patient. The magnitude of the burn injury can be assessed by the "rule of nines" (Fig. 25.2), and the proportions of partial-thickness and full-thickness burns can be assessed by using criteria that include the etiology of the acident, the appearance and color of the wounds, and the presence of moisture and sensation. Other important diagnostic and therapeutic maneuvers in the early phase of burn care include placing a urinary Foley catheter in patients with larger burns and obtaining an electrocardiogram, particularly in patients over 45 years of age and those with pre-existing cardiovascular disease or other associated trauma injuries.

Initial treatment of the burn itself includes gently washing damaged skin with a mild soap that does not contain alcohol. Frequently, this will require use of analgesia, preferentially intravenous, because of the painful nature of the treatment. There is controversy over whether bullae should be débrided, especially in minor burns. In large burns, this can be accomplished with minimal difficulty. For those patients with minor burns who are treated as outpatients, many physicians favor the closed treatment using a dressing of a nonadherent fine mesh gauze and then a bulking dressing. A closed technique appears to provide the patient with more comfort and lessens the requirement for oral analgesia. Serial inspection of the wound over the first week is necessary in this group of patients, and careful written instructions should be provided to the outpatient. Topical antibacterial agents and systemic antibiotics are usually not required for minor burns because of the minimal risk of infection. However, all patients with burn injuries should receive appropriate

FIGURE 25.1. Patient with 30% chest, back, and head burns with associated intrathoracic and closed head injury from flaming automobile accident.

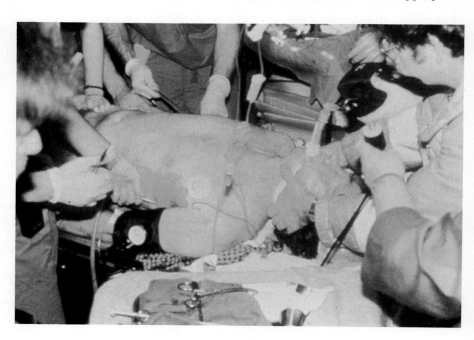

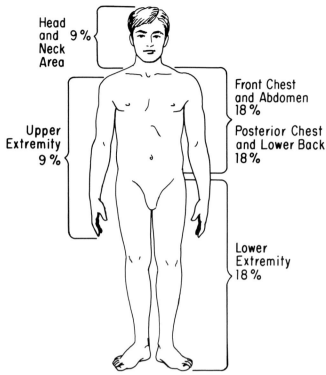

Head and Neck Area 9%

Upper Extremity 9%

Front Chest and Abdomen 18%

Posterior Chest and Lower Back 18%

Lower Extremity 18%

FIGURE 25.2. "Rule of nines" used to assess areas of burn involvement.

tetanus prophylaxis. Burn injuries should be considered a moderate risk for tetanus development.

Therapy

SHOCK RESUSCITATION

Treatment of burn shock has evolved over the past 30 years. Modern therapy focuses on the use of electrolyte solutions in either hypo-, iso-, or hypertonic sodium concentrations (Table 25.2). Intravenous resuscitation is required for patients with burns greater than 15% of TBS because this group frequently has ileus, vomiting, and complications of low cardiac output. While many different formulas have been suggested over the past 30 years, all are based on the size of the burn injury and the initial weight of the patient. Accurate patient weights are a priority to instituting resuscitation. Clinical experience and supporting animal studies have demonstrated that various concentrations of sodium and water are effective in replenishing cardiac output (CO) and can be expressed in the following formula:

$$CO = K[Na^+] + [volume]$$

The most commonly used formula is the Parkland formula, which administers hypotonic Ringer's lactate solution at 4 ml/kg of body weight/percent TBS burned (7). This hypotonic resuscitative program results in approximately 20% body weight gain by the end of 48 hr. However, extensive experience with this formula demonstrates that it is safe and has a low incidence of renal failure.

Isotonic resuscitation administers sodium chloride at between 150 and 160 mEq Na/liter. The experience at Duke University with this formula is extensive and has provided a wide margin of safety (8). This solution is prepared by adding half an ampule of sodium bicarbonate to Ringer's lactate, giving a sodium concentration of 150 mEq Na/liter. The solution is administered at 3 ml/kg/% TBS burned and has very low incidence of pulmonary edema, ileus, and cerebral edema because patients only gain approximately 10% of their preburn weight by 48 hr.

Hypertonic resuscitation using a sodium solution of 225–250 mEq Na/liter has been suggested and is utilized in some centers (9). The solution is administered at 2.0–2.5 ml/kg/% TBS burned and has a low minimal weight gain, approximately 7–9% of the preburn weight by 48 hr. However, because this formula depends upon recruiting extravascular fluid to fill the intervascular space, its margin of safety is less, and it is not recommended for routine use unless the individual burn doctor has extensive experience with this technique.

Colloid is not routinely employed in any of these formulas in the first 24 hr because capillary permeability is increased during this time and the colloid particles fail to remain within the intervascular space. After 24 hr colloid may be helpful, and its use has been suggested by those employing the Parkland formula. They administer 20–60% of the fluid in the second 24 hr as colloid in the form

Table 25.2.
Burn Shock Resuscitation

Agent	Rate	Colloid	Advantage	Morbidity
Hypotonic solution of lactated Ringer's 130 mEq Na (liter)	4 ml/kg/% TBS	After 24 hr	Safe with large experience	Large weight gain
Isotonic lactated Ringer's and 1/2 ampule NaHCO₃ (150 mEq Na/liter)	3 ml/kg/% TBS	If serum albumin >2 mg/dl after 24 hr	Safe	Low weight gain
Hypertonic sodium solution (225–250 mg Na/liter)	2 ml/kg/% TBS	No	Limits fluids	Under resuscitation renal failure

of plasma, plasmanate, or diluted salt-poor albumin. However, the value of colloid in early resuscitation has been seriously questioned unless the serum albumin falls below 2 g/dl.

The purpose of all formulas is to provide a guide for initiating resuscitation. Careful monitoring of the general condition, vital signs, and specifically hourly urinary output dictates the rate of volume resuscitation in burn shock. Urinary output between 30 and 50 ml/hr in the adult and 1 ml/kg in children less than 30 kg is advised. If urinary output is less than these parameters, the volume of solution should be increased. Low urinary output is indicative of inadequate volume replacement; therefore, diuretics are rarely indicated unless the patient has a documented history of use of these agents or has congestive heart failure. Initial therapeutic response to low urinary output is to increase the volume of electrolyte solution until adequate urinary output is achieved. If urinary output exceeds 75 ml/hr in the adult or 2 ml/kg/hr in the child, the volume resuscitation should be decreased unless this diuresis is due to glucosuria. Excessive resuscitation results in increasing risk of tissue swelling, particularly pulmonary, cerebral, and gastrointestinal.

After 24 hr, if the patient is stable, the solution should be reduced in a stepwise manner in order to maintain urinary output between the parameters described above. Careful monitoring of the urine for sugar is important because glucosuria may give a false sense of adequate resuscitation (10). Steps should be taken to correct glucosuria, primarily by administering sugar-free solutions. Insulin is rarely required. Glucose-containing solutions should be reinstituted, particularly in children, after evidence of glucosuria disappears.

PHYSIOLOGICAL MONITORING

Monitoring during the initial phase of resuscitation focuses on cardiopulmonary dynamics, extremity circulation, and adequacy of ventilation. Standard cardiopulmonary monitoring of a burn patient includes frequent checking of vital signs, hourly urinary output determinations, and assessment of generalized stability, especially mental function. Initial laboratory tests include serum electrolytes, blood gases, creatinine, blood urea nitrogen, and blood sugar. Serial hematocrits may not be as helpful as previously suggested, and it is not uncommon for an initial hematocrit to be in excess of 55 ml/dl. This parameter tends not to return to normal levels in the first 24 hr, even in adequately resuscitated patients. However, a sharp fall in hematocrit may indicate hemolysis or gastrointestinal bleeding and should be investigated. Daily chest radiographs are employed to monitor any early infectious pulmonary complications as well as pulmonary edema.

Central venous monitoring is rarely indicated in major burns because of the risk of infection as well as the possibility of creating a nidus for seeding of the endocardium or valves on the right side of the heart. Indications for invasive vascular monitoring should be limited to those patients who, in spite of large volumes of resuscitation,

fail to achieve adequate urinary output; those on a ventilator requiring high ventilating pressures; and individuals with a history of congestive heart failure who are on major cardiac medications.

Monitoring of extremity circulation is extremely important in those patients who have circumferential burns to the extremity (11). As edema increases, interstitial pressure also rises, compromising venous return as well as arterial inflow. Prevention or minimization of edema formation is extremely important in these patients. All circumferentially burned limbs should be elevated to provide adequate venous drainage. In addition, active limb exercise every 4 hr over the first 24 hr augments venous return and minimizes edema. Monitoring of the extremity blood flow can be accomplished using a Doppler ultrasonic flowmeter; this is more accurate than the usually employed clinical signs of cyanosis, prolonged capillary refill, paresthesia, or deep tissue pain. Audible flow sounds with placement of this instrument over the distal palmar arch of the hand or the posterior tibial artery of the lower extremity indicate adequacy of perfusion. Loss of Doppler sounds in these areas is an indication for escharotomy.

Escharotomies can be performed at the bedside and should only be performed through full-thickness injuries (Fig. 25.3). The incision is carried down through the full-

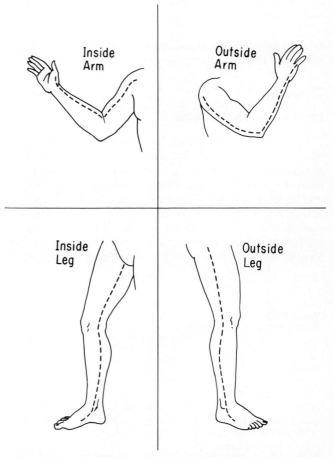

FIGURE 25.3. Upper and lower extremity escharotomies of medial and lateral aspects of limb.

thickness injury into the subcutaneous tissue and need not go through the fascia in thermal burns. Fasciotomies are required only for electrical injuries, not thermal injuries. Extension of this escharotomy on the medial and lateral aspects of the upper extremity down to the thenar eminence is frequently beneficial. On the lower extremities, such extension is done on the medial and lateral aspect of the leg to below the malleolus.

PULMONARY ASSESSMENT

The focus of pulmonary monitoring is on detecting two potential early complications related to the restrictive effects of circumferential full-thickness burns on the chest wall and to the presence of an inhalation injury. Full-thickness circumferential burns to the chest wall, like those of the extremity, can result in a tight eschar and restriction of respiratory excursion, resulting in decreased tidal volumes, hypercapnia, and hypoxia. If the chest wall reveals significant tightness, then escharotomy should be carried out. It is usually carried out on the anterior thorax in a shield-like manner with the vertical limb extending along the anterior axillary line and the horizontal limbs across the costochondral margin inferiorly. As with limb escharotomies, this should be performed only through full-thickness injury and needs only to go to the subcutaneous tissue. Bleeding can be controlled with direct pressure, suture, or electrocautery and is usually minimal. Escharotomy wounds are treated with topical antibacterial agents and skin grafting, in the same manner that other segments of the burn injury are treated.

Inhalation injury, depending upon the level of involvement in the respiratory tree, can result in either upper airway occlusion, tracheobronchitis, pneumonia, or abnormalities in oxygen and carbon dioxide exchange (12). Inhalation injuries have been reported in as many as 30% of people with major burn injuries and occur not from direct thermal insult, but from the chemical burn of the airway caused by the inhaled products of incomplete combustion.

Inhalation injury can be divided into three areas anatomically: (*a*) injuries to the upper airway, involving the pharynx and larynx down to the level of vocal cords; (*b*) injuries to the major airways that involve the tracheobronchial tree; and (*c*) parenchymal inhalation injuries involving the capillary alveolar membrane. The pathophysiology of this injury includes mucosal damage, edema, upper airway occlusion, tracheobronchitis, mucosal plugs, and pneumonia. Rarely, initial hypoxia may be a manifestation of damage to the capillary membrane. Presently, all patients with a major burn should be suspected of having an inhalation injury. Clinical signs include head and neck burns, production of sooty sputum, hoarseness, wheezing, or bronchorrhea. These may not be present at the time of initial presentation of the patient in the Emergency Department.

Common techniques used to diagnose inhalation injury include fiberoptic bronchoscopy, xenon or lung scan, and pulmonary function testing. The most commonly used approach is fiberoptic bronchoscopy (13). This procedure can be accomplished transnasally with topical anesthesia in the Emergency Department. If there is evidence of upper airway edema in the 48 hr following injury, a nasotracheal tube can be inserted using the bronchoscope as a guide (Fig. 25.4). Bronchoscopic evaluation below the level of the vocal cords in patients with inhalation injury will show edema, soot, and mucosal damage. At the initial bronchoscopy, mucosal plugs and other debris may be aspirated from the airway to minimize the risk of early atelectasis and superimposed infection.

Lung scans and pulmonary function tests have been suggested by some, but at the present time, they have limited use because of the unavailability of xenon gas and the nonspecificity of pulmonary function tests in diagnosing inhalation injury (14).

Careful monitoring of patients with a diagnosis of an inhalation injury over the first 24–48 hr includes observation for upper airway occlusion and the development of hypoxia. Initial treatment of airway occlusion is to maintain the patency of the airway, and this can be accomplished with a nasotracheal tube.

Treatment of inhalation injury is based on the severity and intensity of the inhalation injury itself. This can be determined at the time of initial bronchoscopy. The use of humidified air or oxygen will promote mobilization of secretions. Vigorous pulmonary toilet, including endotracheal suction, is frequently necessary. Repeat bronchoscopy is indicated if atelectasis develops over the first few days. Progressive hypoxemia will necessitate endotracheal intubation and positive end-expiratory pressure ventilation. Prophylactic antibiotics are usually not helpful and may predispose to bacterial superinfection. Specific antibiotics are indicated based on serial sputum cultures (15).

Daily chest radiographs are important to follow potential complications, including pneumonia, atelectasis, and acute respiratory distress syndrome. Careful regulation of fluid resuscitation is particularly important in patients with inhalation injuries because overhydration may produce significant pulmonary edema. Careful attention to

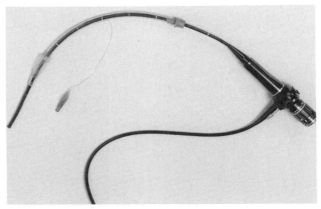

FIGURE 25.4. Fiberoptic bronchoscope with nasotracheal tube in place prior to bronchoscopic examination. Tube can be inserted at time of bronchoscopy if intubation is necessary.

many small details is important to minimize this major determinant of morbidity and mortality following burn injury.

BURN WOUND MANAGEMENT

The burn wound and its management still remains the major focus after initial resuscitation. This colonized wound is the chief source of infectious complications, including bacteremia, septicemia, pneumonia, and embolic focal abscess formation throughout the body. The goal of treatment is to convert this surface wound from an open, contaminated wound to a closed, healed wound as rapidly as possible.

It must be remembered that both topical and systemic antibacterial agents do not sterilize the wound but maintain colonization at an acceptable level so that burn wound sepsis does not occur. As the granulation tissues develop and the eschar separates, protection of the burn wound with either early skin grafting or the use of biological dressings will prevent secondary desiccation and pseudoeschar formation.

The goal of burn wound management is a controlled or planned separation of the eschar from the underlying viable tissue. This is accomplished by either of two methods. The first is the use of topical systemic agents to control the density and type of bacteria and allow separation of the burned eschar when granulation tissue develops. This is followed by biological dressings such as homografts or heterografts as the granulation bed evolves. The other approach is early excision before colonization takes place and the use of either biological or autologous grafting at that time. Both approaches have a role in minimizing the morbidity and mortality of burn injury.

Topical agents used in the present era include Silvadene, which is a 1% silver sulfadiazine compound; sulfamylon cream, which is a 10% methylated sulfonamide cream; and silver nitrate solution, which is a 0.5% inorganic silver salt solution. Each agent has some specific advantages and disadvantages.

The most commonly used agent is Silvadene, which is a cream employed with or without dressings to the surface of the wound and is mechanically removed by washing each day (16; Figs. 25.5 and 25.6). It is an effective broad-spectrum agent against the usual bacteria found colonizing the burn wound. It is pain-free and causes no respiratory depression. The major disadvantage is its topical allergenic sensitivity, which is low, however. Initially, it was thought that Silvadene caused leukopenia; however, continued clinical experience with this agent shows that the initial fall in white count following burns is the result of the burn and not the Silvadene.

Sulfamylon remains the most effective topical antibacterial agent. It has a broad spectrum of activity against Gram-negative and Gram-positive organisms (17). However, because of its carbonic anhydrase inhibition and significant pain associated with topical application, its use is limited. It has been employed in those patients with progressively increasing bacterial counts as well as in those with demonstrated burn wound invasion. It is applied as a cream to the wound twice a day and can be washed off in a bath or shower. Topical sensitivity to sulfur is experienced in approximately 5% of patients.

The other commonly used agent is 0.5% silver nitrate solution (18). It is employed using a dressing technique. It is pain-free but requires intensive nursing care. The silver nitrate solution may leak sodium, potassium, chloride, and calcium from the wound, and this may result in alkalosis, mineral deficits, and water loading. A discoloration

FIGURE 25.5. Silvadene application to lower extremity following third-degree wound.

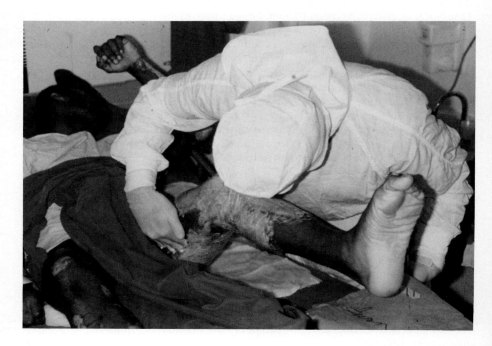

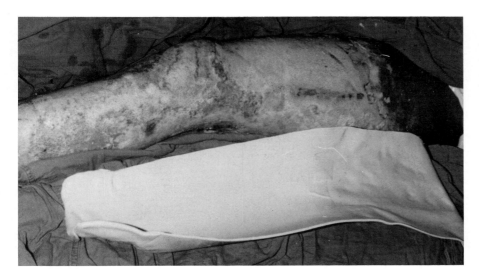

FIGURE 25.6. Same wound after removal of Silvadene by gentle washing. The wound is carefully examined prior to each new application of topical cream to detect any evidence of burn wound sepsis.

of the burn wound and the environment occurs with this agent.

Most burn units today use rotation of the agents to prevent the development of resistant organisms. Silvadene and sulfamylon are the two primary agents; the use of 0.5% silver nitrate solution is reserved for those patients with sulfa allergies.

INFECTIOUS COMPLICATIONS

The burn wound itself is the primary source of local or systemic infectious complications; therefore, careful daily attention focusing on changes in bacterial density and activity is mandatory. The approach to management of the burn wound itself is multiple, including different topical agents, use of biological dressings, timing of removal of the eschar, and appropriate surface coverage following escharectomy, either with autograft or biological dressings. Optimal results are best obtained with repeated use of a single organized technique. However, every physician treating multiple burn patients should have the capability of understanding both the advantages and limitations of each technique.

Over the initial 3–4 weeks following burn injuries, the surface burn undergoes many changes. The most serious adverse change is conversion of a partial-thickness to a full-thickness burn as a result of bacterial invasion of the underlying viable tissue. The presence of black or dark hemorrhagic discoloration in a previously normal-appearing burn wound is indicative of burn wound sepsis. Other signs include eschar separation that is more rapid than usual, bleeding into the subcutaneous tissue, systemic signs of sepsis, fever, leukocytosis, and increasing edema in unburned areas.

The presence of burn wound sepsis can be confirmed by an elliptical biopsy of the eschar and underlying unburned tissue (19). The specimen should be of sufficient size so that half can be sent for quantitative culturing and the other half for frozen sectioning, looking for invasion

of bacteria into unburned viable tissue. This technique, compared to serial quantitative surface cultures, is more accurate in diagnosing burn wound sepsis.

Treatment of burn wound sepsis depends upon location, extent, and depth of the invasive process. Changing the topical agent is the usual first step. The addition of specific parenteral antibacterial therapy should be instituted based on available microbiological information. It is suggested that new cultures of the burn wound as well as blood cultures be obtained at the time of institution of parenteral therapy. In addition, subeschar infusion of an antibiotic solution such as carbenicillin solution as a broad-spectrum antibiotic should be instituted. One-half the total doses should be given initially; the remaining half is given after 12 hr.

If there is evidence that the burn wound sepsis extends into the underlying subcutaneous tissue, excision is advised. The excision should be limited to the burn eschar area itself, although, in a totally burned extremity, amputation may be required. Systemic antibiotics should be instituted preoperatively and continued to limit the progression of hematogenous spread in these situations. Mortality and morbidity in burn wound sepsis is significant, and every effort should be carried out on a daily basis to prevent this serious complication.

REMOVAL OF ESCHAR

Débridement of the wound is accomplished each day using either scissor or scalpel as the eschar begins to separate. Aggressive débridement should be avoided because exposing underlying tissue that does not have adequate granulation tissue will lead to desiccation. Using Using topical antibacterial agents, separation usually begins at 2–3 weeks following the burn accident. As the eschar begins to separate and the burn wound appears ragged, dressings can be applied to achieve mechanical débridement of the small amount of residual necrotic debris.

FIGURE 25.7. Freshly excised wound with mesh skin graft in place.

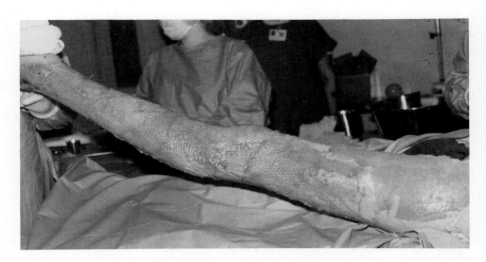

WOUND EXCISION

Surgical excision of the burn eschar and immediate closure can be implemented to achieve rapid closure of the burn wound, minimize the risk of burn wound invasion, and shorten hospital stay. A variety of techniques have been suggested, including scalpel incision and the use of dermatomes or other types of excision apparatus, including lasers. The goal of excisional therapy is to remove the burn eschar and graft the wound as early as possible before significant colonization occurs (Fig. 25.7). All excision techniques have been associated with significant blood loss, the inability to define the depth of the burn wound itself (which may be variable), and the expense of the operating room and the anesthesia time used (20). Currently, excisions have been used primarily for full-thickness burns of less than 20% of the TBS for which an adequate donor site is available. Experience with excision in larger burns has been limited to centers in which homograft, skin culture lines, or other types of major support is available. Excisional therapy and immediate therapy in full-thickness burns of less than 15% TBS has achieved shorter hospitalization than standard therapy of similar injuries (21). Experience with larger burn injuries has shown less convincing benefit from excisional treatment.

BIOLOGICAL DRESSING

A variety of biological dressings are available, including homograft, heterograft, and synthetic membranes. Homograft tissue remains the biological dressing of choice because its effectiveness in preventing desiccation and water loss is optimal (22). This biological dressing also has an inherent ability to minimize bacterial proliferation due to adherence of underlying granulation tissue. Additional benefits of homografts include control of wound pain and increased motion. Homograft skin from cadavers should be harvested in the operating room using a sterile technique. Contraindications to cadaveric harvest include systemic infection or viral disease, cutaneous malignancies, or jaundice. The skin can be stored in a refrigerator for up to 2 weeks. The biological dressing is left in place for 3–5 days and should be removed before dense adherence occurs because significant bleeding can occur with removal after that point.

Cutaneous xenograft is sold commercially, and is frequently used because it is more available than homograft tissue. It is less effective than homografts in controlling bacterial proliferation. However, it has advantages similar to those of homografts in terms of water evaporation, pain control, and wound desiccation.

Synthetic membranes are now available. Their use is primarily limited to healing a second-degree burn and donor sites. Many are impregnated with an antibacterial agent, which adds to their effectiveness. Commercial availability of these products has made their use more widespread; however, major advantages of synthetic membranes over homografts or heterografts have not been defined at the present time.

Cell culture techniques to grow epithelium are being developed (23). This area is promising; however, the membrane is not available for general use at the present time.

Whenever biological dressings are employed, regardless of type, careful observation of the wound is necessary, especially following the initial application. Bacterial overgrowth may be extensive, and the risk of burn wound sepsis occurs at this time. At any time, if sepsis occurs, the biological membrane should be removed and either topical antibacterial agents reinstituted or a new biological dressing applied.

Systemic Complications of Burn Injury

METABOLIC HYPERMETABOLISM

Following a major burn injury, there is a significant hypermetabolism producing elevated cardiac output, hyperthermia, and significant catabolism. A supermetabolic state secondary to higher catecholamine production and excretion extends through the intermediate and late phases until the burn wound is either closed or healed. Catabolism, primarily of muscle protein, may result in weight loss unless adequate attention is paid to nutritional support (24). Energy requirements are high and are met primarily by muscle breakdown using the gluconeogenic pathway to produce energy.

Attempts have been made to control this hypermetabolic state using pharmacological agents (25). Such drug manipulation has not resulted in fewer complications or lower morbidity. Rather than drug manipulation, the primary approach should be to supply adequate carbohydrates and protein (26). Estimation of nutritional needs in the form of calories and protein can be calculated based on weight and size of burn injury. Early implementation of a nutritional support program using primarily the enteral route has been shown to improve survival and decrease complication rate. Loss of 10% or more of preburn weight has been associated with serious infectious complications and death.

Although intravenous parenteral nutrition offers another route to nutritional support, it should be avoided because of the high incidence of sepsis (27). The use of oral or tube feedings is preferred. Diarrhea is not an unusual complication of early feeding and usually can be controlled with oral antidiarrheal agents such as Paregoric.

GASTROINTESTINAL COMPLICATIONS

Gastrointestinal complications in burn patients are similar to those that occur in other patients with major metabolic stresses. These include duodenal ulceration, bleeding, and acalculous cholecystitis. Early implementation of feeding as well as the use of antacids has been shown to be effective in preventing gastric and duodenal ulceration (28). Type 2 histamine receptor antagonists are not more effective than the above program and may actually be associated with a higher incidence of nosocomial infections, particularly pneumonia. No effective preventive program for acute acalculous cholecystitis has been documented; however, early feeding may be beneficial because biliary stasis appears to be a prominent factor in the development of this poststress complication (29).

INFECTIOUS COMPLICATIONS

Pneumonia remains the most common infectious complication other than those involving the burn wound. Because of the high incidence of inhalation injury as well as a depressed immune response, this group of patients is at risk of developing bronchial pneumonia (30). Gram-negative organisms are most common in this group of patients. Careful use of aseptic technique, particularly in pulmonary toilet, is mandatory. Daily physical examination and the use of frequent chest radiographs are important in the early diagnosis of an infiltrative process. Prophylactic antibiotics are not only of no benefit, but they have also been shown to result in the development of superimposed infection. Serial endotracheal cultures of those individuals at high risk following inhalation injury are indicated in defining specific antimicrobial therapy when an infiltrate appears.

The incidence of hematogenous pneumonia is decreasing as a result of better attention to the burn wound itself and to other potential sources of hematogenous spread of bacteria. This type of pneumonia is extremely lethal and requires treatment not only of the pneumonia itself but also of the source of sepsis to prevent recurrent bouts.

SUPPURATIVE THROMBOPHLEBITIS

The requirement for continuous intravenous (IV) support during the early phases of care, particularly in large burns where the IV access is limited, places the burn patient at risk of suppurative thrombophlebitis. This occurs because of direct introduction of organisms at the IV site into an immunocompromised patient. The presence of induration at the IV site and along its course as well as purulent drainage at the time of catheter removal are signs of suppurative thrombophlebitis. This type of complication is usually not responsive to systemic antibiotics alone and requires total surgical excision of the vein segment to the first open tributary. Gram-negative organisms are the primary pathogens in this complication.

BLOOD-BORNE INFECTIONS

Septicemias are a common phenomenon in burn patients. This primarily occurs from the burn wound itself as the eschar separates and the burn wound undergoes daily care. Signs of infection in this group of patients include hyperthermia or hypothermia, tachycardia, and confusion. Serial blood cultures should be obtained if any of these signs appear. Septic shock has had a higher mortality in burn patients; therefore, immediate institution of antibiotics covering both Gram-positive and Gram-negative organisms is suggested (31). As specific culture data become available, appropriate therapy can be directed. Prolonged use of broad systemic antibiotics should be avoided because the development of resistant organisms may lead to a lethal outcome.

Summary

Improvement in survival as well as optimal functional and cosmetic results following major burn injury require a carefully organized and implemented team plan for burn care that begins with understanding the pathophysiology of burn injury and implements effective and systematic initial care. Careful attention to fluid resuscitation, topical wound and physiological monitoring, and awareness of the early complications during early burn care allows an increased survival in severely burned patients during the phase of highest risk. Implementation of either a program of controlled separation of the burn eschar using topical agents or excision and early grafting both have distinct advantages and disadvantages. Awareness of the complications of these techniques and individualization of the technique for each patient assures optimal care. Continued support during the intermediate and late phase and anticipation of infectious, gastrointestinal, and metabolic complications based on current therapy are also important aspects of care. Overall, the mortality and morbidity rates in recent years have been significantly improved and will continue to decrease with attention to these factors.

References

1. Moylan JA: Outpatient treatment of burns. *Postgrad Med* 73:235, 1983.
2. Asch MJ, Feldman RJ, Walker HL, et al: Systemic and pulmonary hemodynamic changes accompanying thermal injury. *Ann Surg* 178:218, 1973.
3. Pruitt BA Jr, Moylan JA: Current management of thermal burns. *Adv Surg* 6:237, 1972.
4. Winkelstein AU: What are the immunological alterations induced by burn injury? *J Trauma* 24:S72, 1984.
5. Wilmore DW, Long JM, Mason AD Jr, et al: Catecholamines: Mediator of the hypermetabolic response to thermal injury. *Ann Surg* 180:653, 1974.
6. Baxter CT, Waecker JF: Emergency treatment of burn injury. *Ann Emerg Med* 17:1305, 1988.
7. Baxter CR: Crystalloid resuscitation of burn shock. In Stone H, Polk HA (eds): *Contemporary Burn Management*. Boston, Little, Brown and Co., 1971.
8. Moylan JA: Resuscitation and early management of the acutely burned child. In Serafin D, Georgiade N (eds): *Pediatric Surgery*. Philadelphia, WB Saunders Co, 1984, p 112.
9. Gunn ML, Hansbrough JF, Davis JW, Furst SR, Field TO: Prospective, randomized trial of hypertonic sodium lactate versus lactated Ringer's solution for burn shock resuscitation. *J Trauma* 29:1261, 1989.
10. Yu CC, Hua HA, Tong C: Hyperglycemia after burn injury. *Burns* 15:145, 1989.
11. Moylan JA, Inge WW Jr, Pruitt BA Jr: Circulatory changes following circumferential extremity burns evaluated by the ultrasonic flometer: An analysis of 60 thermally injured limbs. *J Trauma* 11:763, 1971.
12. Moylan JA, Chan CK: Inhalation injury—an increasing problem. *Ann Surg* 188:34, 1978.
13. Moylan JA, Birnbaum M, Abid K: Fiberoptic bronchoscopy following thermal injury. *Surg Gynecol Obstet* 140:541, 1975.
14. Moylan JA, Wilmore DW, Mounton DE, Pruitt BA Jr: Early diagnosis of inhalation injury using Xenon 133 lung scan. *Ann Surg* 176:477, 1972.
15. Pruitt Ba Jr, Erickson DR, Morris A: Progressive pulmonary insufficiency and other pulmonary complications of thermal injury. *J Trauma*, 15:369, 1975.
16. Baxter CT: Topical use of 1.0% silver sulfadiazine. In Polk HC, Stone HH (eds): *Contemporary Burn Management*. Boston, Little, Brown and Co, 1971.
17. Moncried JA: Topical antibacterial therapy of the burn wound. *Clin Plast Surg* 1:563, 1974.
18. Monafo WW: The management of burns: The silver nitrate method. *Curr Probl Surg.* Feb:53, 1969.
19. Pruitt BA Jr: The burn wound. In Cameron JL (ed): *Current Surgical Therapy*. Philadelphia, BC Decker, 1984, p 513.
20. Herndon DN, Barrow RE, Rutan RL, Rutal TC, Desai MH, Abston S: A comparison of conservative versus early excision. Therapies in severely burned patients. Ann Surg 209:547, 1989.
21. McManus WF, Mason AD Jr, Pruitt BA Jr: Excision of the burn wound in patients with large burns. Arch Surg 124:718, 1989.
22. Shuck JM: Biologic dressings. In Artz CP, Moncrief JA, Pruitt BA Jr (eds): *Burns—A Team Approach*. Philadelphia, WB Saunders Co, 1979, p 211.
23. Cuono C, Langdon R, McGuire J: Use of cultured epidermal autografts and dermal allografts as skin replacement after burn injury. *Lancet* 1 (pt 2):1123, 1986.
24. Jahoor F, Desai M, Herndon DN, Wolfe RR: Dynamics of the protein metabolic response to burn injury. *Metabolism* 37:330, 1988.
25. Herndon DN, Barrow RE, Rutan TC, Minifee P, Jahoor F, Wolfe RR: Effect of propranolol administration on hemodynamic and metabolic responses of burned pediatric patients. *Ann Surg* 208:484, 1988.
26. Wolfe RR: Glucose metabolism in burn injury: A review. *J Burn Care Rehab* 6:408, 1985.
27. Herndon DN, Stein MD, Rutan TC, Abston S, Linares H: Failure of TPN supplementation to improve liver function, immunity, and mortality in thermally injury patients. *J Trauma* 27:195, 1987.
28. Rath T, Walzer LR, Meissl G: Preventive measures for stress ulcers in burn patients. *Burn Incl Therm Inj* 14:504, 1988.
29. McDermott: MW, Scudamore CH, Boileau LO, Snelling CF, Kramer TA: Acalculous cholecystitis: Its role as a complication of major burn injury. *Can J Surg* 28:527, 1985.
30. Zoch G, Hamilton G, Rath T, et al: Impaired cell mediated immunity in the first week after burn injury: Investigation of spontaneous blastogenic transformation, PHA IL-2 response and plasma suppressive activity. *Burns Incl Therm Inj* 14:7, 1988.
31. Hansbrough JF, Field TO Jr, Gadd Ma, Soderberg C: Immune response modulation after burn injury: T cells and antibodies. *J Burn Care Rehab* 8:509, 1987.

26

Principles and Management of Injuries from Chemical and Physical Agents

Anthony J. DeFranzo, M.D., F.A.C.S.

Chemical Injuries

In any industrialized society, injuries from chemical agents pose an ever-present hazard. Chemical products are commonly used in the home, in agriculture, in scientific laboratories, in industry, and in the military. More than 25,000 products capable of producing chemical injury are marketed today. Annually in the United States, accidental contact and/or criminal assault with chemicals produce more than 60,000 cases that require medical attention. More than 3000 deaths occur each year from internal or external chemical injuries (1). Yet, comprehensive reports on the treatment of common chemical injuries are few, and many physicians are not aware of important and specific treatments for common chemical injuries.

ACID INJURIES

In most acid burns, the moiety responsible for injury is the hydrogen ion. Common strong acids, such as sulfuric acid, nitric acid, hydrochloric acid, and trichloroacetic acid, produce similar injuries and require similar methods of treatment. The hydrogen ion produces an exothermic reaction, cellular dehydration, and precipitation of proteins. Coagulation necrosis is the result. Fortunately, in acid burns, the hydrogen ion appears to be neutralized at the point of initial tissue reaction (2). The injuries are proportional to the concentration of the acid and the length of time the acid is in contact with the tissue.

Acid burns are extremely painful, and the pain lasts a long time. It does not disappear until the neutralization of hydrogen ions has been completed (3). As in thermal burns, the appearance of the acid burn varies with the severity of the injury. Minor acid burns appear erythematous and soft in texture; major burns are gray, yellow-brown, or black and are leather-like in texture.

Common acid injuries should be treated with copious water irrigation. Dilute solutions of sodium bicarbonate may follow as a neutralizing agent (2). Water irrigation should begin at once, and the area of the acid injury should not be underestimated. Spills or splatters are the most frequent acid injuries and may involve several remote patches of skin. The immediate removal of all clothing that may contain acid and the use of a shower stall is most effective. Bromberg et al. (4) recommended hydrotherapy for several hours. Blisters and nonviable tissue are débrided, and topical antibiotics are applied, as in thermal burns. Primary excision and grafting of severe but small localized burns is a time- and cost-effective treatment. Acid burns of the upper extremities, such as the dorsum of the hands, are common and lend themselves to the above management.

Systemic complications of common acid burns are not usually significant. However, hydrofluoric acid and phenol (carbolic acid) burns may result in severe systemic complications. Burns from these chemicals are not uncommon. Thus, the complicated pathophysiology and treatment of each are dealt with separately.

Hydrofluoric Acid Burns

Hydrofluoric acid is one of the strongest of all inorganic acids (5). Its expanded uses have led to increased numbers of related injuries. Hydrofluoric acid has been used since the 17th century for the frosting and etching of glass. Currently, it is used in the manufacturing of tanning agents, dyes, germicides, fire-proofing materials, solvents, plastics, and semiconductors. Other uses include rust removal, the removal of sand from castings in foundries, and the removal of glazing defects from pottery. Hydrofluoric acid is also used in photography, chemical milling, ore digestion, graphite processing, metal electropolishing, pipe cleaning, and beer brewing, and as a laboratory reagent.

The pathophysiology of the hydrofluoric acid burn distinguishes it from all other acid burns. The hydrogen ion plays only a small part in the chemical burn (i.e., cellular dehydration, protein precipitation, and coagulation necrosis). The freely dissociable fluoride ion quickly penetrates skin to reach the deep tissues, producing liquefaction necrosis and decalcification and erosion of bone. The pain associated with tissue damage is excruciating, although with dilute concentrations, the onset of pain may be delayed for many hours. Without proper treatment, the pain persists for several days. Klauder et al. (6) suggested that the excruciating pain is due to the mobilization of calcium ions in the tissues, which leads to a shift of potassium ions and intense nerve stimulation.

The clinical appearance of hydrofluoric acid burns begins with simple erythematous, swollen, and painful areas similar to those of other acid burns. With concentrated solutions or with neglected burns from more dilute solutions, progressive tissue destruction occurs. The affected area becomes firm, edematous, and pasty white to yellow-white. Blisters form, containing a white, caseous, necrotic material. Erythema surrounds this area of severe tissue destruction (Fig. 26.1). Full-thickness tissue loss may occur with severe, permanent scarring.

The hands and upper extremities are the most common sites of hydrofluoric acid burns (5, 7). Untreated or improperly treated hand injuries may result in erosion of the distal phalanx and destruction of the nail bed. Gangrenous loss of a finger is not uncommon (8, 9). Shewmake and Anderson (9) pointed out that hydrofluoric acid will easily pass through pinholes in protective rubber gloves and penetrate subungual tissues. This exposure may go unrecognized by the patient for 6–24 hr, until severe pain begins. Leather gloves offer no protection and cannot be decontaminated. They must be destroyed, or further burns may occur when they are worn again. Subungual burns are of particular concern because the tissue has no stratum corneum. The remainder of the hand, especially the palm, is much more resistant to acid penetration. Hydrofluoric acid rapidly penetrates the nail matrix and, if

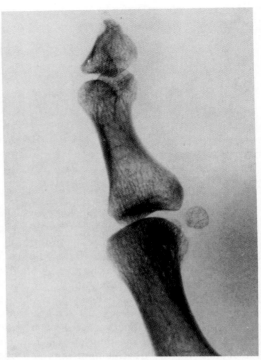

FIGURE 26.2. Roentgenogram shows destruction of 60% of the distal phalanx of the right thumb from subungual involvement with 30% solution of hydrofluoric acid. (From Blunt CP: Treatment of hydrofluoric acid skin burns by injection with calcium gluconate. *Indust Med Surg* 33:869, 1964.)

allowed to progress, will rapidly destroy the soft tissue and distal phalanx (Fig. 26.2). Subungual tissue destruction causes intolerable pain, which may seem out of proportion to the clinical impression of the inexperienced physician.

The effective treatment of a hydrofluoric acid burn differs from that of other acid burns. Treatment must deactivate both the hydrogen ion and the powerful fluoride ion. In addition to initial dilution and neutralization of the acid with copious amounts of water or dilute solutions of sodium bicarbonate or alkaline soap, treatment must also be directed specifically toward the fluoride ion. Many salts are formed by hydrofluoric acid, but only calcium fluoride and magnesium fluoride are insoluble in tissue and therefore neutralizing (2). All other fluoride salts dissociate freely, allowing the destructive effects of the fluoride ion to continue.

Opinions differ somewhat as to the best method of neutralizing the fluoride ion. Cold itself is thought to decrease blood and lymph flow, hinder the development of edema, and slow the penetration of fluoride ion through the tissue. Topical agents include: (*a*) magnesium oxide ointment; (*b*) cold 25% magnesium sulfate soaks; (*c*) cold Hyamine chloride soaks (a quaternary ammonium compound that exchanges chloride for fluoride, producing a nonionized fluoride complex); (*d*) cold Zephiran soaks (benzalkonium chloride, which has an action similar to that of Hyamine); and (*e*) calcium gluconate gel (2, 5, 10). Another topical agent, calcium carbonate gel, is made from calcium carbonate tablets and K-Y jelly. This gel is

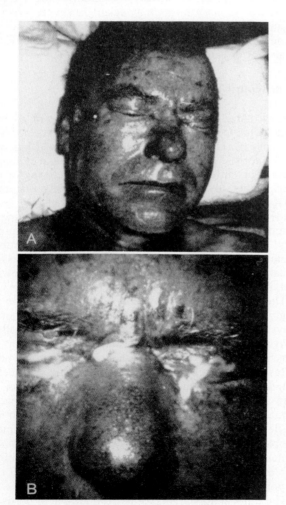

FIGURE 26.1. A, Burn of face with 70% hydrofluoric acid, is shown 45 min after the exposure. There is swelling, erythema, and severe pain. **B,** The face, except for the nose, was treated with calcium gluconate injections some 2 hr later. The erythema and swelling are much worse in the untreated nose. (From Iverson RE, Laub DR, Madison MS: Hydrofluoric acid burns. *Plast Reconstr Surg* 35:85, 1971.)

easy to prepare and may be poured into a surgeon's glove, which is put on the hand and changed every 4 hr (11).

In severe hydrofluoric acid burns injectable agents are required. Calcium gluconate, in a 5–10% solution, has been shown to be the most effective injectable agent, although 25% magnesium sulfate may be used instead (12). Trevino et al. (13) believed calcium gluconate in concentrations stronger than 5% causes severe pain and tissue damage and may itself cause severe scarring and keloids. Injections should be done within, under, and around the injured area using a 30-gauge needle (9). The injections should extend 0.5 cm beyond the area of obvious injury into uninjured tissue (14). Severe pain may be eliminated within 15 min, and the tissue destruction is abruptly halted. However, precautions must be taken because overinjection in burned tissue will cause distention and subsequent necrosis. The minimum amount of calcium gluconate injected that effectively stops pain is adequate even if less than 0.5 ml/cm² of surface area is in-

jected. Injections must be carefully controlled in the fingers and nail beds, which have little soft tissue (Fig. 26.3). A local or regional block given before injection may prevent the pain experienced with calcium gluconate injection (5, 9). However, pain is a valuable symptom to follow; if it recurs, reinjection is indicated immediately (5).

The severity of burns from hydrofluoric acid injury depends, as with any acid, on the concentration of the acid and the duration of the exposure. The decision simply to use topical therapy or to inject calcium gluconate is made with knowledge of the concentration of the hydrofluoric acid causing the injury. The National Institutes of Health has classified hydrofluoric acid burns on the basis of acid concentration. This can be useful in management and in the prediction of the clinical course of the burn (15; Table 26.1). Determining the concentration may avoid undertreating the injury.

There is general agreement that burns caused by hydrofluoric acid concentrations of less than 20% can be

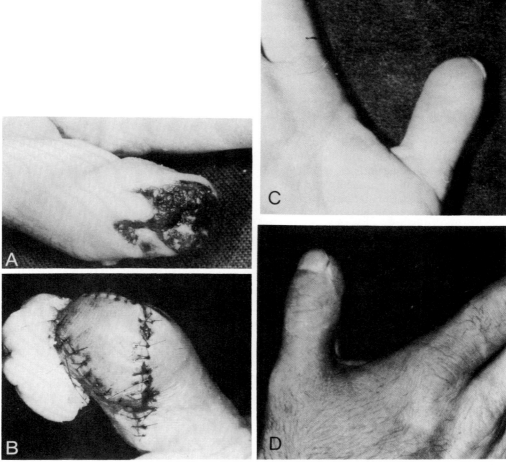

FIGURE 26.3. Hydrofluoric acid burns of thumb requiring reconstruction. **A,** Débridement of necrotic portion 6 days after injury. **B,** Repair with V-Y advancement flap. **C** and **D,** Appearance 9 months after repair. (From Kleinert HE, Bronson JL: Hydrofluoric acid burns of the hand. *Med Times* 104:75, 1971.)

Table 26.1.
Classification of Hydrofluoric Acid Burns Proposed by Division of Industrial Hygiene, National Institutes of Health[a]

Concentration	Human Burn
0–20%	This burn manifests itself by pain and erythema as late as 24 hr after burn.
20–50%	This burn becomes apparent 1–8 hr after exposure to the acid.
Greater than 50%	This burn is felt immediately, and tissue destruction is rapidly apparent.

[a] From Dibbell DG, Iverson RE, Jones W, Laub DR, Madison MS: Hydrofluoric acid burns of the hand. *J Bone Joint Surg [Am]* 52:931, 1970.

treated safely with iced Zephiran or Hyamine chloride soaks for 1–4 hr (14). Calcium gluconate in a 2.5% gel may also be used, and the patient, if treated as an outpatient, should be instructed to reapply the gel whenever pain returns to the burned area (13). Burns known to result from concentrations greater than 20% should be treated with calcium gluconate injections. If pain or skin changes become apparent with hydrofluoric acid exposures of concentrations less than 20%, calcium gluconate should be used. Calcium gluconate injections that could not be initiated until 36 hr after exposure have still provided prompt pain relief and arrest of tissue destruction (14). Following calcium gluconate injections, severely burned areas that are demarcated may be débrided under appropriate anesthesia. Routine topical antibiotic treatment should be initiated, and the burned area should be placed in a bulky dressing and elevated. Fingernails should be removed if subungual burns are present in order to facilitate the rapid neutralization of hydrofluoric acid in the nail bed.

If the total burn area is greater than 50–100 cm², hospitalization for optimal care is suggested. Burn areas greater than 100–150 cm² can cause systemic complications and require close monitoring in a burn unit or an intensive care unit (13). Systemic treatments must be directed specifically at pulmonary (inhalation) injuries and electrolyte imbalance that may result in cardiac dysfunction. Pulmonary injuries should be treated immediately with 100% oxygen by face mask. A 2.5–3.0% calcium gluconate solution should be given by inhalation using a nebulizer or intermittent positive pressure breathing machine (13).

The patient should be watched expectantly for 24–48 hr for the development of severe upper airway edema and/or pulmonary edema. Intubation may become mandatory if pulmonary edema develops. Calcium gluconate should continue by inhalation in the intubated patient, and positive end-expiratory pressure (PEEP) ventilation should be initiated (13). Systemic antibiotics and steroids may be helpful. The acute pulmonary injury from hydrofluoric acid continues for several weeks, and dyspnea with moderate physical activity may last for 9 months. Steroid therapy every third day has been advocated for 3 months after inhalation injury (13). Pulmonary function tests may reveal permanent damage in severe injuries.

Electrolyte imbalance must be carefully monitored with frequent serum calcium and magnesium level determinations. The fluoride ion rapidly penetrates tissue after severe hydrofluoric acid injuries to the skin or respiratory tree. Intravenous (IV) calcium gluconate therapy should maintain the calcium level at or above the upper limit of normal. Continuous electrocardiogram, liver function, blood urea nitrogen (BUN), and creatinine monitoring must also be instituted. Hepatic and renal toxicity may develop rapidly in severe hydrofluoric acid exposures to the skin and respiratory tree. Hemodialysis may become essential.

Vapor or liquid hydrofluoric acid injuries to the face may severely damage the eye. Hydrofluoric acid vapor alone may cause extensive injury to the cornea and conjunctiva. A 1% calcium gluconate solution should be used to wash the eye as soon as possible (13). As in the management of all other significant injuries to the eye, an ophthalmologist should be consulted as soon as possible.

Phenol (Carbolic Acid of Hydroxybenzene) Burns

The toxic effects of phenol have greatly restricted its use in modern medicine. It is now used for chemical face peels, for nerve injections, and as a topical anesthetic and antipruritic (6). However, phenol is used extensively today in the plastics industry, in cosmetics, in cleaning agents, and in the production of fertilizers, dyes, and explosives (16). Treatment of severe phenol exposure from industrial accidents requires the physician to be well attuned to the local systemic effects of phenol.

Phenol is quickly absorbed through intact skin and mucous membranes, and phenol vapor is readily absorbed through the lungs. The rate of absorption is directly proportional to the concentration of phenol vapor in the lungs, the surface area of skin in contact with phenol, and the time of exposure. Concentrated phenol solutions produce rapid necrosis in the epidermis and upper dermis. The necrotic avascular tissue produces a barrier to further phenol absorption. Dilute solutions damage the skin more slowly, allowing a longer period of time for phenol to be absorbed systemically. The toxic actions of phenol include alterations in cell membranes and coagulation of cell proteins (16). The effect of phenol on the skin has been described as "keratocoagulation" (17; Fig. 26.4).

The body rids itself of toxic phenol in three ways: conjugation, oxidation, and excretion. Phenols are conjugated in the intestine, liver, kidneys, and red blood cells. Dietary phenols are conjugated in the intestine to phenol sulfates and glucuronide before reaching the portal blood stream. Oxidation into CO_2 and H_2O disposes of 25–50% of sublethal doses of phenol in experimental animals. A small amount of catechol and quinol are also formed in the oxidative process. These moieties, in turn, are conjugated and excreted in the urine (16, 18).

Phenol has a toxic effect on the hypothalamus, causing hypothermia within a few hours after exposure. Hypothermia may last 24 hr. The effect on the cardiovascular system may also be dramatic. Blood pressure may rise initially and then fall precipitously as a result of central vasomotor collapse. Phenol also causes a decrease in cardiac output via a direct toxic effect on the myocardium.

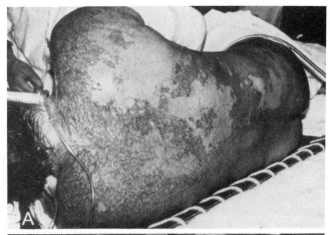

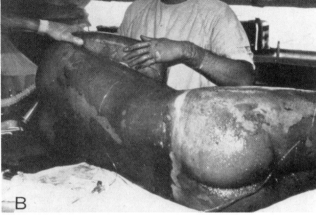

FIGURE 26.4. **A,** Partial-thickness burns of the back due to phenol exposure. (From Pardoe R, Minami RT, Sato RM, et al: Phenol burns. *Burns* 3:29, 1976.) **B,** Partial-thickness burns due to phenol exposure.

Circulating phenol may cause hemolysis of red blood cells because of its damaging effect on cell membranes. Methemoglobin, Heinz bodies, and a decrease in red cell glutathione are noted (16). The lungs exhibit a picture of edematous chemical pneumonitis, and ulceration of the trachea may be noted on bronchoscopy. Renal damage is caused by cardiovascular collapse, leading to renal ischemia; by hemolysis of red blood cells with the precipitation of hemoglobin in the glomeruli and tubules, forming obstructive casts; and by the direct excretion of free unconjugated phenol, which is toxic to glomeruli and tubules. Pardoe et al. (16) noted gross hematuria, hemoglobinuria, and oliguria within 1 hr after injury. Phenol toxicity in the liver results in central lobular necrosis, which impairs the liver's ability to detoxify phenol by conjugation. Serum bilirubin levels are increased.

The treatment of phenol burns is first directed at minimizing exposure. The patient should be immediately removed from the site of the accident, where there may still be contact with phenol in liquid or vapor form. All clothing should be removed, and a high-flow shower initiated. (The phenol should not be diluted with water unless a high-flow shower is used.) The skin should then be cleansed with a solvent to remove phenol. Solvents in

order of preference are polyethylene glycol, propylene glycol, glycerol, vegetable oil, and soap and water. The hair of the scalp or face may trap diluted phenol and allow further absorption. Contaminated hair should be removed (16).

Intubation and ventilation with a volume-controlled respirator using PEEP may be required early. Steroids and antibiotics are given for the chemical respiratory burn. A large volume of intravenous fluids is required early to counter vasomotor collapse and to maintain urine output. Diuretics such as mannitol may be essential to prevent renal failure. A high urine output is ideal to remove hemoglobin and also to promote the excretion of free unconjugated phenol as rapidly as possible. The hematocrit may fall steadily over the first 10 days because of continued hemolysis, and blood is transfused as needed. Alkalinization of the urine with sodium bicarbonate may decrease hemoglobin precipitation in the renal tubules. Phenol also has the direct effect of producing metabolic acidosis, which may require sodium bicarbonate. Dopamine may be beneficial by increasing cardiac output and renal blood flow. If stimulation rather than depression of the central nervous system is a continuing problem, intravenous diazepam (Valium) and barbiturates may be required to prevent convulsions.

The surface burn caused by phenol is usually partial thickness, but full-thickness injury may occur (Fig. 26.5). Hydrotherapy, débridement, topical antibiotics, and, when necessary, split-thickness skin grafting are performed as per the usual routine treatment for burns of the skin. Phenol may cause depigmentation of the skin as seen in chemical face peeling. Depigmentation is due to competitive inhibition of the enzyme tyrosinase in the oxidation of tyrosine and dopa to melanin, and a selective injury to melanocytes (19; Fig. 26.6).

ALKALI INJURIES

The vast majority of alkali injuries occur during personal quarrels. In a study of 416 patients with alkali inju-

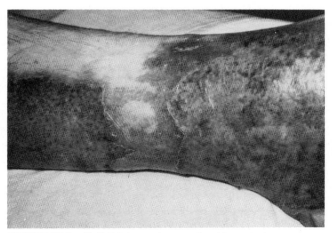

FIGURE 26.5. Full-thickness burns of ankle region due to phenol exposure. (From Pardoe R, Minami RT, Sato RM, et al: Phenol burns. *Burns* 3:29, 1976.)

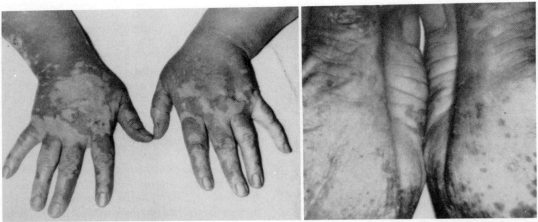

FIGURE 26.6. Hands of hospital employee after using phenolic germicide. (From Kahn G: Depigmentation caused by phenolic detergent germicides. *Arch Dermatol* 102:177, 1970. Copyright 1970, American Medical Association.)

ries, only 9 had been injured in industrial accidents (20). Strong alkalis such as caustic potash (KOH) and caustic soda (NaOH) are available in any supermarket. Alkalis can be fabricated into cheap, disfiguring weapons referred to as "12-cent pistols" (21).

The moiety responsible for alkali burns is the hydroxyl ion (OH⁻). Erythema and epidermal bullae appear early in the wound, and an eschar may form later (Fig. 26.7). The wound is painful to palpation and is soapy and slippery to the touch. Burns produced by common strong alkalis are more penetrating than burns produced by acids other than hydrofluoric acid and phenol. In common acid burns, the hydrogen ion is inactivated immediately by its chemical reaction with tissue; however, in alkali burns, the hydroxyl ion is not. Alkali proteinates, which are formed in alkali-tissue reactions, are soluble (2). Thus, the hydroxyl ion may continue to pass more

deeply into tissue, denaturing one protein molecule after another. This penetrating injury has been called a liquefaction necrosis.

The total picture of alkali injury includes saponification of fats and cellular dehydration, resulting in cell death. Saponification is an exothermic reaction that produces a significant amount of heat, which is the cause of the tissue damage. Destruction of fat allows increased water penetration through the alkali burn eschar, negating the natural water barrier that lipid provides (20). Untreated alkali injuries will often penetrate the full thickness of the skin, destroying all ectodermal elements such as hair follicles and sweat glands (Fig. 26.8). Regeneration of skin, therefore, can occur only from the edge of the wound because skin islands usually do not develop in the center of the wound. An eschar may form and, if untreated, may continue to harbor alkali, which may penetrate into the

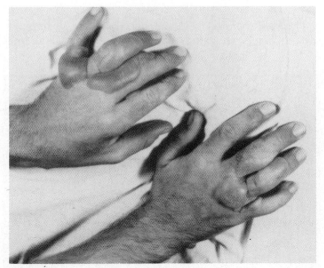

FIGURE 26.7. Bullae on dorsa of hands secondary to alkali injury. These blebs should be unroofed and topical chemotherapy applied following irrigation. (From Orcutt TJ, Pruitt BA: Chemical injuries of the upper extremity. *Major Prob Clin Surg* 19:84, 1976.)

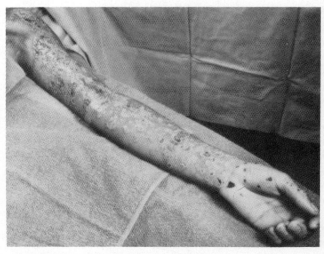

FIGURE 26.8. Extensive lye burns of the left arm. After initial copious irrigation and débridement of grossly necrotic tissue, a topical antimicrobial agent is applied. (From Orcutt TJ, Pruitt BA: Chemical injuries of the upper extremity. *Major Prob Clin Surg* 19:84, 1976.)

deeper tissues and cause further damage (4). In alkali injuries, there seems to be a significant latent period during which proper therapy can be administered advantageously (22). Progressive and immediate hydrotherapy is the best treatment, and it serves the following purposes: (*a*) washing away or diluting the offending agent; (*b*) decreasing the rate of chemical reaction; (*c*) decreasing tissue metabolism and thus decreasing the inflammatory reaction; (*d*) minimizing dehydration; and (*e*) restoring normal skin pH (4). Some heat is given off with dilution, making high water flow important. The length of time for hydrotherapy is another important consideration. Because the hydroxyl ion is soluble in tissue over long periods and may be quantitatively significant in the eschar, Bromberg et al. (4) have advocated prolonged water irrigation in a shower stall. In their study, patients underwent hydrotherapy for periods ranging from 6 hr to 6 days. The elapsed time between injury and initiation of hydrotherapy ranged from immediate to 12 hr.

During and after hydrotherapy, nonviable tissue that may contain alkali should be débrided immediately to prevent further penetration of alkali and to increase the effectiveness of hydrotherapy. Early excision of small full-thickness injuries with delayed closure or split-thickness skin grafting is advantageous. Open wounds should be treated with topical antibacterial agents. Sulfamylon is the agent of choice because it is bacteriostatic; it also combines with active alkali to form sodium acetate and sulfamylon radicals. These reactions give off no heat, and the products are innocuous to the wound (20).

The penetrating nature of lye injuries has been associated with special complications, including tympanic membrane perforations, parotid fistulas, severe keloid formation, and the early development of Marjolin's ulcers. Although the average time to development of a Marjolin's ulcer in a thermal injury scar is 34 years, these ulcers occurred at 3, 7, and 9 years after injury in a series of lye burns reported by Wolfort et al. (20).

Phosphorus Burns

Burns caused by white phosphorus, also called yellow phosphorus, deserve special attention. White phosphorus is used in the military as an incendiary device or an igniter for munitions. It is found in various weapons such as artillery shells, mines, hand grenades, and mortar rounds (12). In the military, human or mechanical errors as well as battlefield action account for a significant number of phosphorus burns (1). In civilian life, white phosphorus is used to manufacture munitions, insecticides, fertilizers, and rodent poisons (23). Industrial accidents as well as military accidents may lead to explosions that embed phosphorus particles in the skin.

White phosphorus burns are caused by both liquids and solids. When a weapon containing phosphorus explodes, it spreads flaming droplets of inorganic phosphorus, which become embedded in the skin (24). Phosphorus is highly lipid soluble and may spread quickly beneath the dermis. There, it will continue to oxidize until removed by débridement or consumed by oxidation (23). The pain

associated with burning white phosphorus is extreme. Tissue damage is mainly due to the heat of combustion. However, phosphorus pentoxide, which is formed by the oxidation of phosphorus, is also damaging because it is intensely hygroscopic. Furthermore, phosphoric acid, the end product of phosphorus combustion, is corrosive (24). In military injuries, tissue is frequently damaged by shell fragments and sustains significant areas of third-degree burns. Clinically, the burn wounds become necrotic and yellowish and may fluoresce. The wound may give off a white vapor and has a characteristic garlic-like smell (12; Fig. 26.9).

A patient burned with phosphorus requires immediate treatment. All contaminated clothing should be removed to prevent further contact of phosphorus with the skin. The wound should be irrigated copiously with water, and all identifiable particles of phosphorus should be removed. These particles should be placed under water to avoid their spontaneous ignition upon drying. A thick layer of wet gauze should be placed over the wound, and the patient should be transported directly to an operating room, where definitive removal of all phosphorus must proceed meticulously. Smoke may aid in the localization of embedded phosphorus; however, phosphorus can burrow deeply, and its detection may be difficult.

Copper sulfate solutions ranging in concentration from 0.5% to 5.0% have been advocated to aid in the identification of phosphorus particles (12, 21, 23, 24). The chemicals react to form cupric phosphide, which is black. The formation of cupric phosphide may also slow the oxidation reaction of phosphorus. It must be pointed out, however, that copper is toxic and may cause massive hemolysis, gastrointestinal disturbances, hepatic necrosis, and cardiorespiratory collapse. A 1% copper sulfate solution is sufficient to tag the phosphorus particles (2). Copper

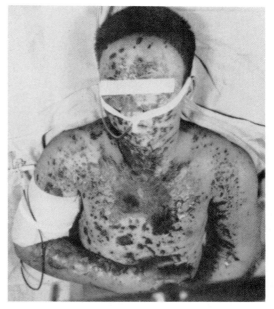

FIGURE 26.9. White phosphorus burn injury. (From Summerlin WT, Walder AI, Moncrief JA: White phosphorus burns and massive hemolysis. *J Trauma* 7:476, 1967.)

sulfate soaks or baths should not be employed. A brief irrigation of phosphorus burns with 1% copper sulfate should be followed by copious amounts of water to remove excess copper sulfate solution. More than one session of débridement may be required to remove all phosphorus particles. Small areas of full-thickness burns are treated effectively by primary excision with delayed closure or split-thickness skin grafting. The subsequent management of the burn wound is similar to that of any other burn wound.

Systemic toxicity from phosphorus burns has been somewhat unpredictable and mysterious. In Vietnam, there were reports of sudden, unexpected deaths with phosphorus burns of only 10–15% of total body surface area (25). The literature does not report consistent systemic toxicity resulting from absorption of elemental phosphorus from the burn wound. However, toxicity resulting from ingestion or inhalation of this substance has been well documented. Ingestion has been known to induce generalized petechiae, seizures, electrocardiographic changes, hematuria, oliguria, icterus, and acute yellow atrophy of the liver (24).

Massive hemolysis has been reported by Summerlin et al. (24) in patients with phosphorus burns of 29%, 12.5%, and 7.5% of body surface. Whether hemolysis was due to systemic toxicity from phosphorus or from copper is not clear. All patients with phosphorus burns, therefore, should be monitored closely, even if the burn surface area is small. The patient should be placed in an intensive care unit or well-equipped burn unit, and particular attention should be directed to electrocardiographic changes, calcium-phosphorus shifts, and precipitous falls in hematocrit as a result of hemolysis.

Physical Injuries

SUNLIGHT

Since ancient times, man has worshipped the sun. Sunlight is the very basis of life, but as we now know, it can cause reactions in the skin that adversely affect health.

The relationship between sunlight and cutaneous malignancy has long been recognized (26–28). The incidence of nonmelanoma skin cancers in the United States is approximately 400,000–450,000 new cases per year (29). A majority of skin cancers develop on sun-exposed areas such as the head and neck area and the arms and hands. Most nonmelanoma skin cancers have had a better than 95% cure rate and rarely, if ever, are metastatic. Numerous theories linking excessive sun exposure to skin cancer have been proposed.

One such theory has to do with wavelengths and energy. The energy of the sun's rays is inversely proportional to their wavelengths. The shorter wavelengths, which have more energy, are potentially more damaging than the longer wavelengths. Approximately one third of the radiation emitted from the sun is reflected, scattered, and absorbed by the atmosphere before it reaches the earth's surface. However, the remaining two thirds are transmitted to the earth. Forty percent of sunlight is dissipated in the infrared spectrum and is known as heat from the sun. Fifty percent is visible light, which allows differentiation of colors by the reflective patterns therein. The remaining 10% is ultraviolet light, and it is this light that concerns the plastic surgeon.

Wavelength Ranges of Ultraviolet Light

Ultraviolet light has three wavelength ranges:

1. UVA: ultraviolet light with a wavelength spectrum of 320–400 nm
2. UVB: ultraviolet light with a wavelength spectrum of 280–320 nm
3. UVC: Ultraviolet light with a wavelength spectrum of less than 280 nm

The *decreasing* order of these wavelengths represents an *increasing* order of energy.

Approximately 99% of ultraviolet light is UVA. This spectrum stimulates immediate pigment darkening and melanogenesis, which lead to tanning. Approximately 1% of ultraviolet light is UVB, which causes burning, and it is believed that UVB acts synergistically with UVA in stimulating melanogenesis. It is this fraction of ultraviolet light that is the primary factor in premature skin aging and skin carcinogenesis. A small fraction of 1% of ultraviolet light consists of UVC. This is fortunate because UVC is carcinogenic and causes severe erythematous reactions in the skin. Most of the UVC from the sun is absorbed in the atmosphere, where it interacts with oxygen and is held in the ozone layer. UVC has a germicidal effect and is emitted from cold quartz lamps, which have been used to help maintain sterile conditions in operating rooms. These lamps have been used in several university hospitals (30). Although the correlation between ultraviolet light and melanoma is not clear, it may be that the UVC component of ultraviolet light plays a very important role in the etiology of melanoma.

Important observations of human skin type have been made. The incidence of human skin cancers, especially basal cell and squamous cell carcinomas, is related to the physical characteristics of pigmentation (31, 32). Light eye color (i.e., hazel, gray, green, or blue), light hair color, and fair complexion are coupled with poor tanning ability and a higher incidence of nonmelanoma skin cancers. Having parents of British ancestry with light-colored eyes also predisposes a person to skin cancer. On the other hand, skin cancer is rare in the black race, probably because of the photoprotection provided by the large amount of melanin in the skin (33). Skin has been classed as follows:

Type 1: Always burns and never tans
Type 2: Always burns and slightly tans
Type 3: Sometimes burns and always tans
Type 4: Never burns and always tans

The potential for developing skin cancer decreases from type 1 to type 4 (34).

The development of all types of skin cancers, including melanomas, is related to exposure. The exposure of skin to solar ultraviolet light is a growing problem in the United States because of the increasing population of the sunbelt, the increasing number of vacations being taken in warmer areas, and the popularity of sunbathing, tanning salons, and outdoor sports. The greater life expectancies in most industrialized countries will also raise the lifelong exposure of many persons to the sun.

Acute skin-damage sunburn is primarily caused by exposure to UVB, and the most erythemogenic wavelength is 297 nm. Compared to a control population, skin cancer patients exposed to erythemogenic doses of UVB radiation usually have a prolonged duration of erythema, lasting for 2–3 weeks. UVA is also capable of causing erythema, but not as efficiently as UVB. Between 10:00 AM and 12:00 noon during July, the amount of UVA is 100 times that of UVB, but the UVB is 1000 times more erythemogenic than the UVA. The physiological mechanisms of producing erythema by ultraviolet light are not known, but they may be mediated by prostaglandin, which in turn causes dermal blood vessels to dilate.

With a life-style of increased sun exposure, the incidence of malignant melanoma is rising at an alarming rate in the United States and in other countries as well. In Norway, for example, it has been projected that, within 15 years, malignant melanoma could account for as much as 10% of all cancers. Currently, the incidence of melanoma and its mortality rate are doubling every 10–17 years. Before the 1960s, it was rare for a physician to see one case of melanoma during his or her whole medical practice.

The ability to modify sunlight and therefore to decrease the chances of carcinoma in patients prone to sunburn should be understood by all physicians. One of the many factors responsible for modifying the intensity of sunlight is the ozone layer, which shields the earth from solar ultraviolet radiation. Much concern has been raised recently about the fact that the stratospheric ozone layer appears to be decreasing. The role played by high-altitude aircraft, above-ground nuclear explosions, and chlorofluoromethanes from refrigerants and aerosol sprays is a major concern. Because UVC has the most severe cutaneous effect and most of the UVC from the sun is screened by the ozone layer, concern is justifiable about any loss of ozone. One anticipated effect would be an increase in some types of skin cancer in humans (35).

The most important factor in modifying the amount of solar ultraviolet light exposure is the distance of the sun from the earth, a distance that is directly related to the seasons of the year and the geographical latitude, longitude, and altitude of the person receiving the radiation. Obviously, the intensity of the ultraviolet light increases as one approaches the equator. For every 1000 feet above sea level, the exposure to ultraviolet light increases approximately 5% because the sunlight is filtered through a thinner atmospheric layer. The time of day, or the height of the sun above the horizon, is also important. The intensity of the ultraviolet rays is believed to be strongest between 10:00 AM and 3:00 PM. Atmospheric clouds and smog will decrease the intensity of solar ultraviolet light but to what extent is unclear. Water vapor may allow transmission of about 80% of UVB. Therefore, it is possible to sunburn on a cloudy day.

Glass transmits UVA with wavelengths greater than 320 nm (i.e., visible light, infrared, and beyond), but it filters the shorter wavelength UVB. Snow reflects 85 to 90% of sunlight, almost doubling the exposure. Therefore, people who enjoy winter sports can get sunburn in frigid temperatures. Sand at the beach, however, is a poor reflector, being only 15–20% efficient. Water will transmit 50% of UVB and most of UVA. Therefore, one can get sunburned under water. Water will also reflect sunlight, but as a reflector, it is only about 5% efficient. However, as the angle of the sun to the water decreases (i.e., at sunrise and sunset), the amount of reflection approaches 100%.

The amount of clothing worn during exposure to ultraviolet light is also important. There are new bathing suit materials that transmit light while looking opaque. Wet cotton shirts transmit both UVA and visible light; therefore, they do not protect against sunburn. The burns through these fabrics may be particularly severe because the underlying skin has had little sun exposure and, therefore, has little protective melanin.

The ability to suntan ranges widely. UVA and UVB are both capable of inducing melanogenesis, but neither is as effective alone as they are together. A few hours after exposure to ultraviolet light, immediate pigment darkening occurs as a result of oxidation of the existing preformed melanin (leukomelanin) into melanin. This reaction contributes little to the development of a lasting suntan because it fades within a few hours, but the reaction does lead to the most important aspect of suntanning—melanogenesis. New melanin production begins 48 hr after exposure to ultraviolet light and will not become maximal for approximately 2–3 weeks. This tanning reaction is believed to be one physiological way in which the body protects itself from the ultraviolet light. Exposure to UVB causes the stratum corneum, or the outer layer of the cells, to thicken threefold. This is another protective mechanism; the thickened stratum corneum is an effective UVB absorber.

UVB exposure and the physiological response to it give rise to the thick, leathery skin noticed in those chronically exposed to the sun. The constant solar radiation is damaging to the elastic tissue in the dermis and causes an overall loss of its resiliency, subsequent wrinkling, and the weather-beaten appearance that is so noticeable in aging persons who have spent a lot of time outdoors. These changes are most noticeable around the corners of the mouth and the eyes and along the posterior and lateral aspects of the neck. The older sun worshipper frequently presents this aging phenomenon to the plastic surgeon, and it is a direct result of chronic solar radiation.

Multiple skin lesions, malignant and benign, have been associated with skin exposure. The most common of the cutaneous neoplasms is the basal cell carcinoma (BCC), which has been covered in Chapter 17. BCCs are usually 98% curable with local surgical procedures, but they can become a problem for the plastic surgeon because they occur so frequently near vital structures such as eyes, ears, nose, and mouth. Squamous cell carcinomas (SCC) of the skin are also common, and they may metastasize if they are not secondary to actinic keratosis. The most common precancerous skin lesion among Caucasians is actinic keratosis (senile or solar keratosis). It is found in nearly all elderly Caucasians and in many fair-skinned young whites in the sunbelt. It is a reddish or yellow-brown macule or papule with a smooth, scaly, or verrucous surface. Actinic keratoses may hypertrophy with hyperkeratosis to form a cutaneous horn. Those squamous cell carcinomas that arise secondary to actinic keratosis rarely ever metastasize. SCCs have likewise been covered in Chapter 17. They are treated with local excision, and the cure rate is above 90%. It has been estimated that 25–30% of actinic keratoses (precursors of SCC) will degenerate into SCC if left untreated. Malignant melanoma is well covered in Chapter 17.

Benign skin lesions are also linked to sun exposure. Freckles are accumulations of melanin, and they are believed by some to protect the skin from actinic damage (36). Most freckles are benign, except for the Hutchinson's melanotic freckle, which is irregular in shape and variegated in color. These should be treated as malignancies. The so-called liver spots (lentigo) are essentially large freckles that appear in areas of sun-exposed skin. Seborrheic keratoses are also believed to be the result of sun-damaged skin. These are usually crusted, verrucous, tan to brown papules that have a "stuck-on" appearance and are frequently greasy. These are common on the face and trunk and are benign, with little, if any, potential for malignant degeneration.

Many skin diseases are photosensitive. These diseases may occur as a result of chemicals or medicinal drugs. They are always in a sun-exposed area of the skin and are most prominent on the cheeks, nose, sides of the neck, chest, and extensor surfaces of the forearms. The treatment of these diseases is the providence of the dermatologist rather than the plastic surgeon.

Sunburn should be treated with cool water compresses, topical creams, and analgesics. However, the biggest factor in treating sunburn and skin cancer is prevention. For those persons who insist on getting a suntan, gradual exposure over long periods of time is a must. Probably the most effective physical reflector of sunlight is clothing that shades the body continuously. It must be emphasized again that meshed clothing or light clothing, especially if wet, will transmit ultraviolet light. *Para*-aminobenzoic acid (PABA), esters of PABA, and benzophenones (all found in suntan lotions) absorb UVB and will prevent burning but allow tanning. Benzophenones have a wider spectrum than PABA and absorb both UVA and UVB; however, their efficiency in the UVB range is less than that of PABA. Zinc oxide ointment is a reliable chemical reflector, especially useful in small, prominent sites such as the nose.

All sunscreens are now rated by a sun protection factor (SPF). These factors vary from 2 (with least protection) up to 30 and higher (providing the greatest protection). If a product has an SPF of 15, one can stay 15 times longer in the sun before burning than one could stay in the sun without a sunscreen. Products with a higher SPF, such as 30, will frequently prevent tanning as well as erythema. Agents containing PABA work best when applied 1 hr before exposure and again after getting wet. Contrary to popular belief, tanning agents such as mineral oil and baby oil with iodine offer no protection against sunburn.

OTHER IRRADIATION

Sources of radiating damage other than the sun include nuclear explosions, radioisotopes, particle accelerators, and x-ray machines. Plastic surgeons must be aware of the frequency and types of radiation accidents. More than 100 radiation accidents involving more than 500 persons have occurred since 1940 (37). With the increasing use of radioisotopes and radiation devices in industry as well as their transportation by rail and highway, it is probable that an increasing number of accidents will occur in the coming years. The major cause of radiation accidents in the United States has been exposure to radioisotope sources, x-ray generators, radar generators, and accelerators. Approximately 7% of all accidents with radiation devices have occurred with radioisotope sources such as the radium-192, cobalt-60, and cesium-137 devices that are used by radiographers to check the integrity of welds and of oil, gas, and steam pipelines. Other exposures have occurred when sources have been picked up by unsuspecting children (38–42). Such radiation sources should always be labeled clearly but sometimes are not. Injuries incurred by these "accidental pickup" exposures obviously vary with the amount of radiation received. Unfortunately, while the total body radiation exposure remains quite low, thousands of rads with an extremely destructive effect may be delivered to the hands.

X-rays, alpha particles, and beta particles are forms of radiation other than sunlight. X-rays were initially labeled as such because their exact nature was not understood. It is now known that x-rays are actually gamma rays, which are uncharged photons of energy that travel at the speed of light. These rays have the ability to penetrate deeply; therefore, they are the core of radiation therapy. Alpha particles are another form of radiation and are positively charged helium nuclei; they do not penetrate deeply because of their relatively large size. However, tissue penetrated by alpha rays may be more severely damaged than that penetrated by gamma rays because of the size of the alpha particles and the damage done to DNA, RNA, and enzymatic proteins in the cell (43). The third known type of radiation particle is the beta particle. It is negatively charged and is actually an electron traveling at high speed. It generally penetrates to a depth of 1 cm. Biological damage to the cell from radiation is believed to be due to enzymes and to DNA. When damage occurs, it is difficult for the cell to repair itself, and cell breakdown occurs.

The rad (the most common unit of measurement in radiation) is the amount of energy absorbed per unit of mass of an irradiated tissue by the individual ionizing particles, whether alpha, beta, or gamma. All of these particles may cause systemic or local damage or both.

Patients with a history of exposure to radiation, whether it be from an industrial accident or a nuclear explosion, must be treated for the direct radiation problem and possible radiation sickness. In 1897, Walsh (44) first described radiation sickness after total body irradiation. Additional information was derived from study of the victims of the atomic bomb explosions at Hiroshima and Nagasaki. The systemic results of such irradiation have been called the "acute radiation syndrome." Manifestations of the syndrome depend upon dosage, body distribution, and duration of exposure. Acute radiation syndrome is normally divided into four phases: the prodromal phase, the latent phase, the manifest illness, and the recovery phase.

The transitory prodromal phase usually begins within minutes to hours after exposure, and the interval depends on the dosage. The effects during this stage are probably due to acute radionecrosis, which releases vasoactive substances such as bradykinins and histamines. Other neurohumoral agents may cause systemic manifestations. Signs and symptoms of the prodromal phase include anorexia, nausea, vomiting, diarrhea, intestinal cramps, excessive salivation, and dehydration. Fatigue, apathy, and sweating may follow with hypotension, resulting in cardiovascular shock from neurovascular dysfunction. It is usually estimated that a minimal dosage of 50–100 rads will produce the prodromal symptoms, and this phase almost always occurs when the dosage is greater than 400 rads. Thus, after excessive exposure to irradiation, the amount of exposure in rads should be determined as nearly as possible.

After the prodromal phase, a latent phase of relative well-being occurs. It essentially reflects the time necessary for the development of sustained disturbances in organ function through depletion of cells. This depletion is species dependent and is generally slower in humans than in laboratory animals.

Manifest illness follows the latent phase. Initial management of patients in this phase should include hospital admission. Isolation is essential because lymphocytes often disappear within 24 hr, granulocytes within a few days, and platelets within approximately 10 days, rendering the patient highly vulnerable to infection.

The epithelium of the small intestine is almost as radiosensitive as the bone marrow and plays a role in determining whether the patient will survive (45). A dosage of 100 rads of total body radiation, for example, results in gastrointestinal injury with decreased cell production in the small intestinal crypts and loss of intestinal integrity. Bacteria are thereby permitted to penetrate the denuded villa and enter the portal circulation. Death from sepsis may result secondary to infection coupled with the diminished defenses from white blood cell depletion. Epithelial injury also leads to significant fluid loss and to vomiting, diarrhea, and electrolyte disturbances.

In addition to the hematopoietic failure and the loss of the gastrointestinal mucosa, injury to the central nervous system (CNS) may occur. The peripheral nerves and CNS are moderately resistant to radiation therapy, and deaths typically are not attributed to direct CNS damage. Fanger and Lushbaugh (38) described two deaths in which injury to the CNS may have influenced the outcome. Death was attributed to increased intracranial pressure, cerebral anoxia, and cardiovascular shock, causing massive peripheral edema and collapse. It is believed by most neuroradiologists that greater than 5500–6000 rads to the brain or CNS can result in acute death.

In addition to the hematological, gastrointestinal, and CNS problems, damage to the reproductive organs also must be considered in radiation accidents. Chromosomal analysis of the patient must be done, and the possibility of sterility in male patients must be evaluated. Radiation dosimetry should be carried out as soon as possible.

The treatment of total body radiation injury is basically one of support and management of electrolytes and fluid volumes as well as the infection. Treatment can result in survival only in instances in which the total body radiation is less than 300–400 rads (LD_{50} = 300–400 rads) and when there is some shielding of the bone marrow so that some stem cells can regenerate themselves. If the treatment of the manifest illness is successful (i.e., if infection is controlled, bone marrow replenished, and normal gastrointestinal function restored), the patient usually survives.

Radiation injury to the skin and adnexa is certainly the best studied and best known response to radiation in humans. It has been noted that about 50% of the people who are exposed to radiation will experience epilation after 300 rads, erythema after 600 rads, dry desquamation after 1000 rads, and wet desquamation after 2000 rads (46, 47). The erythema is secondary and is very similar to a second-degree burn. However, the wet desquamation is transepidermal and is very similar to a third-degree burn. The extent of medical intervention depends on the severity, size, and location of the lesion. Skin necrosis, which always occurs, is similar to a severe chemical burn when exposure is greater than 2000 rads. Usually, it is accompanied by a much more excruciating pain, which must always be treated. In all radiation skin and adnexa injuries, the common histological denominator is obliterative endarteritis, which results in ischemia, necrosis, and secondary infection.

As for the care of radiation burns, it should be realized that such injuries are usually deeper than first assumed, and that débridement will remove more than just skin and subcutaneous tissue. Thus, the defect will be larger than initially believed. The hands frequently are involved in such accidents. Because it is often difficult to obtain total dosimeter readings, lesions on the hands must be watched. Frequently, they appear similar to contact thermal burns but tend to evolve more slowly. Radiation lesions become apparent over the first several days, then may break down after 4–5 days. After adequate débridement, the lesions may slowly heal, and granulation-type tissue may develop over the next month. An outstanding symptom of this whole process is constant pain. Repeated débridements, flap coverage, or amputation may be necessary.

The most common radionecroses seen by the plastic surgeon are those in patients who have had radiotherapy for carcinoma of the uterus, cervix, or vulva, or those in patients who have had radiation to the abdomen or the chest wall for breast cancer delivered by orthovoltage radiation equipment used prior to the mid 1960s. This older equipment frequently caused severe skin damage. In the treatment of head and neck cancers, this radionecrosis often involves the mandible. In such cases, most surgeons will remove the involved necrotic tissue and bring in a new blood supply with a local pedicle flap, a myocutaneous flap, or, when necessary, a free flap to provide the best coverage and prevent further breakdown of this tissue (48). These new methods of bringing in a new blood supply have allowed better healing in patients who might otherwise continue to have the chronic cycle of breakdown, infection, and drainage. As noted by several investigators (42, 44), the possibility of late carcinoma developing in irradiated tissues is always present.

LIGHTNING

Lightning kills approximately 200 people per year in the United States, causing more deaths directly than any other phenomenon associated with the weather (49). The mortality is approximately 30%; death is usually related to paralysis of the cardiorespiratory system (50–54). Most people who are struck by lightning survive, but two thirds of survivors have permanent sequelae. Lightning causes injury in four ways: direct strike, flash discharge, ground current, and shock wave. Direct strikes are frequently fatal. A flash injury suffered when lightning strikes a nearby object may cause severe burns similar to electrical burns. Electrical current may move along the ground and enter a patient's legs, causing electrical burns. A shock wave damages tissue in a manner similar to an explosion.

Lightning may injure almost any organ in the body. Of interest to the plastic surgeon are lightning burns. Body injuries from lightning differ from high-tension electrical injuries. Lightning is instantaneous and brief, and the voltage may be from several hundred million volts to a billion volts. Amperage generally ranges from 12,000 to 200,000 (52). These energies are seldom obtained in the high-tension electrical injury. On the other hand, lightning is a direct current, which is much less dangerous than the alternating current that is most frequently associated with electrical accidents. Alternating current may also link the victim to the source, causing catatonic contraction of the muscles, severe internal burns, and charring of tissue (55). Contact during a lightning injury is brief. The management of lightning burns involving the skin and underlying muscle compartments is similar to that for electrical burns, which is discussed in the next section. An interesting injury to the skin specific to lightning burns is known as ''feathering'' or ''lightning prints.'' These marks are fernlike and erythematous; they do not blanch and will fade away over several days (56). These marks are caused by the ''flash-over'' phenomenon, which occurs when lightning passes over the outside of the victim, vaporizing skin moisture and damaging clothing but sparing underlying tissue. The recognition of lightning prints in a comatose patient may make the diagnosis of a lightning injury.

Lightning damages numerous organ systems. Cardiovascular effects include myocardial depolarization and arrest (56). Marked vasoconstriction causing tissue ischemia also occurs from the passage of current. Respiratory arrest with hypoxia follows, making resuscitation difficult. Severe myocardial necrosis has been reported (50, 57–60). The central nervous system is damaged directly by electric current or by associated trauma. Three fourths of lightning-injured patients lose consciousness, and two thirds have a paralysis of the arms or legs, which usually is temporary.

As for other effects of being struck by lightning, tympanic membrane rupture, often accompanied by hearing loss, is seen in over half of patients. Cataracts may be produced either by the light itself or by the direct effect of the heat. Therefore, it is vital that all patients who have been struck by lightning be evaluated carefully for these injuries. Myoglobinuria and hemoglobinuria with acute tubular necrosis and renal failure also have been reported (61); however, these are much less frequent than with lower voltage electrical injuries. In Cooper's recent review of 66 victims of lightning strikes (62), the prognosis was poor for those who had suffered leg injuries (mortality 30%), cranial burns (mortality 38%), or cardiopulmonary arrest (mortality 77%). Permanent sequelae were found in 74% of the surviving patients.

ELECTRICAL INJURIES

Electricity causes two basic types of burns of interest to the plastic surgeon: those caused by electrical arc, or flash, and those caused by the passage of current through the patient's body. Electrical injuries account for approximately 1000 deaths per year in the United States. Male workers in the third and fourth decades of life are most frequently injured. Electrical injuries are very complex, and despite the typical health and youth of the patient, the mortality rate from electrical injuries reaches 15% (56).

Basic terms and equations necessary to understand electrical injuries are:

Voltage: electrical energy potential produced by a power source
Amperage: current flow per unit of time
Resistance: impedance to current flow, measured in ohms

$$\text{Resistance} = \frac{\text{Voltage}}{\text{Amperage}}$$

$$Amperage = \frac{Voltage}{Resistance}$$

Most electrical injuries seen today are the direct result of alternating current (63, 64). This type of current essentially has replaced direct current because it is inexpensive to produce and can be transformed into any required voltage. Use of direct current is limited to streetcars, subways, ships, metallurgy, and the chemical industries. Alternating current is produced with a cyclic change in the direction of electron pressure (voltage). The pressure pushes, then pulls, electrons, resulting in alternating current (65). The current frequency in Hertz (Hz) is the number of complete forward and reverse electron cycles in 1 sec. For example, the typical 120-volt wall outlet is 60-cycle current, 60 forward flows and 60 reverse flows per second.

Alternating current is more dangerous than direct current at low voltage for two reasons. First, the skin offers lower resistance to alternating current than to direct current, and second, alternating current has a tetanizing effect on muscles, which increases the duration of contact. At high voltage, direct current is as dangerous as alternating current.

As the amperage progressively increases, the sensation of contact with alternating current increases from a tingling to a shock to a feeling of muscle contraction to an actual tetany of voluntary muscle contraction. These muscle contractions can be strong enough to cause fractures and dislocations. The point at which the muscle contractions are so severe that an individual grasping the electrical conductor cannot let go is called the "let go" threshold. Muscle contractions are most pronounced between the frequencies of 15 and 150 Hz. Household current, at 60 Hz, can therefore be dangerous. The "let go" threshold at 60 Hz for men and women is 15.9 and 10.5 mA, respectively (64). The inability to let go of the conductor is the main cause of prolonged heat buildup and tissue damage in low-tension accidents. If the alternating current increases above 20 mA, there usually is a fairly sustained contraction of the muscles of respiration, leading, in time, to respiratory asphyxiation and death. When the flow increases above 40 mA, ventricular fibrillation may be induced. It has been found that the threshold of ventricular fibrillation is inversely proportional to the square root of the duration of the shock and directly proportional to the victim's body weight.

The most common electrical injury seen today is due to high-voltage alternating current. High-voltage injuries are classified as those injuries arising from a source of greater than 1000 volts; low-voltage injuries arise from a source of less than 1000 volts (66). High-tension electrical injuries are frequently associated with an arc, or flash of light, formed between the high-voltage power source and the body, which is usually grounded (67). The temperature of this arc may be as high as 4000°C, and the flash may ignite the victim's clothing. This temperature is even high enough to melt bone. In high-tension accidents, the victim does not hold the conductor but is thrown away from it and may sustain traumatic injuries to the arms, head, or legs. Most injuries from high-tension contact are not caused by sustained contact because the circuit is completed by arcing before the victim even touches the voltage power sources. For every 10,000 volts, electrical current can arc 1 inch (56).

The second type of electrical burn injury is caused by the passage of an electrical current between the power source and the patient's exit wound—that is, within the patient's body (67). Direct injury to cells from the current itself occurs in nerves, blood vessels, and muscle. In addition, tissue resistance to the passage of current causes the buildup of intense heat. Skin represents an initial barrier to current and serves as a relatively good insulator, or resistor, against a low-voltage, but not a high-voltage, source. Skin resistance is related directly to skin moisture. A moist hand is 10–100 times less resistant than a dry hand. The production of heat as current enters the body through the skin results in necrosis of skin and underlying tissues. Once the resistance of the skin is overcome, the current enters the underlying tissues and flows through the body with negligible resistance to flow except when it encounters bone. In decreasing order, tissue resistance is as follows: bone, fat, tendon, skin, muscle, vessels, and nerve. A high-voltage current can produce temperatures greater than 1000°C along bone, causing bone destruction and deep tissue necrosis (56). Because almost all current is concentrated at the entrance to the body and again before exiting, more severe tissue damage occurs at the sites of entrance into and exit from the body. Baxter (67) pointed out that high-tension electrical entrance wounds are usually charred and centrally depressed with severe eschar; exit wounds are more likely to be exploded. Entrance wounds may show a central charred area surrounded by a grey-white zone, which in turn is surrounded by a red zone of coagulation. All three zones are full-thickness injuries.

The amount and type of injury between the entrance and the exit wounds must be determined by the plastic surgeon called to treat the surface burns. Almost every organ in the body can be injured by an electrical current. Most common low-voltage burns are exclusively of the contact type and are localized basically to the hands and the mouth. Local voltage burns of the hand are small and deep and usually involve blood vessels, tendons, and nerves. Involvement may be severe and may necessitate amputation or débridement of skin and muscle in this area.

Burns of the lips and mouth lead to scar contracture. Such burns are common in children from 3 months to 3 years of age and occur most often in boys and in the 1–2-year-old group. Most are the result of a child's biting an electrical cord or an infant's sucking an electrical cord socket. The electrical injury thus sustained is believed to be a combination of flash burn, contact burn, and the electrical arc. The commissures are the most frequently damaged sites of entrance involved (in about 50% of children with electrical injuries). The injury is local and usually not accompanied by systemic side effects. Significant perioral edema occurs during the first week. During the second and third weeks after an oral electrical burn, tissue slough occurs. During this period, 20% of such patients bleed from the labial artery and parents must be warned of that possibility and instructed to apply firm digital pressure to control any hemorrhage that occurs. Most physicians now believe that a conservative surgical approach is indicated and that reconstructive surgical procedures should be delayed until the eschar has separated and the scar has softened and remodeled over 6 months. Some advocate the use of intraoral prostheses that may later reduce the possibility of microstomia or labial alveolar adhesions (68). Splinting should be maintained for as long as 6 months. Treatment for tetanus is necessary, but prophylactic antibiotics usually are not required.

In higher tension injuries and acute electrical injuries with greater damage, the patient must be hospitalized, have a Foley catheter inserted, and be watched carefully. The condition of the entrance and exit wounds is a clue to the extent of local destruction of deeper tissues. Muscle necrosis within a compartment has a severe systemic sequela. Myoglobin pigment from the damaged muscle cells and hemoglobin released from injured red cells enter the circulation. Thus, the kidney is exposed to significant pigment loads, and the absorption of this pigment may lead to acute renal shutdown. Attempted prevention of this sequela by early fasciotomy and débridement, even in a limb that may later require amputation (67), is most important. The presence of dark, tea-colored urine is almost diagnostic of the presence of myoglobinuria. Mannitol has been used to enhance pigment excretion after adequate urine output has been established through volume replacement. Usually, the mannitol treatment consists of a 25-g loading dose followed by 12.5 g/hr for several hours. Baxter (67) reported that the duration of myoglobinuria can be used to predict morbidity. In his series of 19 patients with electrical injury who had myoglobinuria for longer than 6 hr, high amputation of one extremity or more or wide excision of trunk musculature was necessary.

The presence of rhabdomyolysis gives a clue to the extent of muscle damage. Technetium-99m stannous pyrophosphate scintigraphy appears to be a sensitive and reliable diagnostic tool. This test can be performed in almost any hospital with a nuclear scanner. Increased uptake of this radioactive material identifies the muscle damage, but it does not necessarily predict death. Areas with no uptake are devoid of blood supply and are obviously necrotic.

In patients with severe muscle damage and deteriorating renal function, there can be a disproportionate rise in the serum creatinine concentration in relation to the serum urea concentration. Baxter (67) also noted that these patients may have a severe acidosis that will complicate resuscitation. A specific alkalizing agent, such as sodium bicarbonate, may be needed in addition to mannitol during the first 24 hr. Serial monitoring of arterial blood gas values is also necessary for maintaining good respiratory physiology. Unless corrected, marked hyperphosphatemia can occur along with severe hyperkalemia, acidosis, and subsequent death. Severe hypocalcemia also is seen in many patients and is probably related to the hyperphosphatemia, although it may occur during the di-

uretic phase of the acute renal failure. Management of the acute renal failure is accomplished either by hemodialysis or by peritoneal dialysis.

Other problems associated with electrical burns are neurological, abdominal, cardiovascular, and pulmonary, and there may be extensive damage to the extremities. The neurological complications are probably the most common in electrical burns. Both acute and delayed central nervous system problems have been described. Unconsciousness is very common; according to Skoog (63), 70% of the patients in his series were rendered unconscious by high electrical voltage. Intracerebral injury, hemiplegia, epilepsy, and headaches have occurred after such injuries; however, most victims recover and do well. Peripheral nerve injuries may also be involved in electrical injuries. Most are transient and recover completely if the nerve is not involved in local tissue injury. However, permanent injury to the nerve can occur when the tissue around it has been injured by a severe electrical burn. In this situation, the prognosis for recovery is certainly unfavorable.

Spinal cord damage due to electrical injuries has also been described (65). Neurological deficits may occur immediately, and total quadriplegia or hemiplegia may develop within 2–3 days after the injury. Signs suggestive of amyotrophic lateral sclerosis and transverse myelitis have also been seen. Motor deficits are more common than sensory losses. Most experimental animal studies (69–71) demonstrate that the electrical injury may cause perivascular hemorrhage around the myelin sheath and reactive gliosis and subsequent death in the neuronal sheath.

Nausea and vomiting are probably the most common gastrointestinal symptoms and are usually seen in about 25% of patients. Necrosis of the gallbladder as well as injury to the small bowel have been reported. Gallstones have been reported several years after electrical injuries; most likely, they are the result of large amounts of pigment mobilized from necrotic muscle. High-voltage destruction of the abdominal wall musculature may involve the underlying bowel directly. The urinary bladder may be injured, as may the liver and the spleen. Although pancreatic injury is rare in abdominal electrical injuries, Baxter (67) reported that 4 of 45 patients with electrical burns had prolonged ileus and hyperamylasemia. Both can be treated medically. The complication rate after abdominal surgery is somewhat higher than that of routine abdominal surgery, for the most part because of leakage of bowel anastomoses. Wound dehiscence is also higher in electrical burn injuries.

The two other major systems that are often injured in electrical burns are the cardiovascular system and the pulmonary system. The most common electrocardiographic abnormalities associated with electrical burns are sinus tachycardia and nonspecific ST segment–T wave alterations; these may persist for several weeks. Myocardial infarction is an uncommon complication of electrical injury, but it has been known to develop as late as 36 hr after the patient's contact with a high-tension wire. Thus, every patient with a high-tension electrical injury should have electrocardiographic monitoring for the first 3–4 days after injury. Electrical injuries of the anterior chest wall can also directly involve the myocardium as well as the lung if an actual burn is present. Acute pulmonary complications are due to pleural damage, which results in effusions and pneumonitis.

A major problem of interest to the plastic surgeon is the treatment of severe electrical burns of the extremities. Large blood vessels within the extremity may remain patent, but damage to the intima and media may have occurred, leading to the formation of surface thrombi. Delayed hemorrhage and/or thrombosis may result. Segmental portions of the large vessels may remain patent. Microsurgical replacement of damaged vessel segments in the extremities has been described (72). Small blood vessels show severe vessel wall injury with complete thrombosis and necrosis. Muscle necrosis occurs as a result of decreased inflow and direct heat damage from adjacent bone. After a few hours, this causes the interstitial pressure of the compartment so involved to rise, and that, in turn, exceeds the capillary perfusion pressure. Ischemia develops in the muscles involved, and after 6 hr, muscle damage is irreversible (67). Compartment pressure should be measured, and frequently immediate fasciotomy is indicated.

The sequence of increased interstitial pressure, suppressed capillary perfusion pressure, and ischemia can be interrupted by early fasciotomy. This increases blood supply and limits ischemic injury. Most patients with a severe electrical injury to the arm should have fascial decompression of the forearm, hand, and carpal tunnel within the first 4 hr, and no later than the first 6 hr. Dead tissue should be débrided in the area as far as it can be seen. The use of magnification during débridement may help determine muscle viability. All visible devitalized tissue should be excised, and the débridements should be repeated at 3-day intervals until only viable tissue remains. Whether an electrical injury is progressive is still controversial. Robson et al. (73) suggested that increased production of arachidonic acid metabolism in distal sites near an entrance wound of an electrical burn causes vasoactive substances such as thromboxane to be elevated. This, in turn, causes progressive necrosis and explains why the wound may need to be débrided every 2–3 days.

Complications of the eye and of the bone are rare after electrical injury, but they can occur. Even with the high resistance of bone, certain areas can be damaged, and disruption of the calcium-phosphate matrix and devitalization of the periosteum can occur. This type of injury may subsequently lead to devascularization. Injury to the outer table of the skull has been seen with high-tension injuries to the scalp. Cataracts can result from voltage higher than 220 volts near the area of the eye. The time of onset of the symptoms has been from 3 weeks to 2 years after the electrical shock. Thus, the ocular lens system needs to be watched for some time.

References

1. Curreri PW, Asch MJ, Pruitt BA: The treatment of chemical burns: Specialized diagnostic, therapeutic, and prognostic considerations. *J Trauma* 10:634, 1970.
2. Orcutt TJ, Pruitt BA: Chemical injuries of the upper extremity. *Major Probl Clin Surg* 19:84, 1976.
3. Artz CP, Moncrief JA: Chemical burns. In Artz CP, Moncrief JA (eds): *The Treatment of Burns*, ed 2. Philadelphia, WB Saunders Co, 1969, p 224.
4. Bromberg BE, Song IC, Walden RH: Hydrotherapy of chemical burns. *Plast Reconstr Surg* 35:85, 1965.
5. Iverson RE, Laub DR, Madison MS: Hydrofluoric acid burns. *Plast Reconstr Surg* 48:107, 1971.
6. Klauder JV, Shelanski L, Gabriel K: Industrial uses of compounds of fluorine and oxalic acid. Cutaneous reaction and calcium therapy. *Arch Indust Health* 12:412, 1955.
7. Blunt CP: Treatment of hydrofluoric acid skin burns by injection with calcium gluconate. *Indust Med Surg* 33:869, 1964.
8. Kleinert HE, Bronson JL: Hydrofluoric acid burns of the hand. *Med Times* 104:75, 1976.
9. Shewmake SW, Anderson BG: Hydrofluoric acid burns. A report of case and review of the literature. *Arch Dermatol* 115:593, 1979.
10. Reinhardt CF, Hume WG, Linch AL, et al: Hydrofluoric acid burn treatment. *J Chem Educ* 46:A171, 1969.
11. Chick L, Borah G: Topical calcium carbonate gel for treatment of hydrofluoric acid burns to the hand. *Proc Am Burn Assoc* 21:159, 1989.
12. Ben-Hur N, Giladi A, Neuman Z, et al: Phosphorus burns—a pathophysiologic study. *Br J Plast Surg* 25:238, 1972.
13. Trevino MA, Herrmann GH, Sprout WL: Treatment of severe hydrofluoric acid exposures. *J Occup Med* 25:861, 1983.
14. Dibbell DG, Iverson RE, Jones W, et al: Hydrofluoric acid burns of the hand. *J Bone Joint Surg [Am]* 52:931, 1970.
15. Division of Industrial Hygiene, National Institute of Health: Hydrofluoric acid burns. *Indust Med* 23:634, 1943.
16. Pardoe R, Minami RT, Sato RM, et al: Phenol burns. *Burns* 3:29, 1976.
17. Campbell RM: Surgical and chemical planing of the skin. In Converse JM (ed): *Reconstructive Plastic Surgery, General Principles*, ed 2. Philadelphia, WB Saunders Co, 1977, vol I, p 442.
18. Deichmann WB: Local and systemic effects following skin contact with phenol. A review of the literature. *J Indust Hygiene* 31:146, 1949.
19. Kahn G: Depigmentation caused by phenolic detergent germicides. *Arch Dermatol* 102:177, 1970.
20. Wolfort FG, DeMeester T, Knorr N, et al: Surgical management of cutaneous lye burns. *Surg Gynecol Obstet* 131:873, 1970.
21. Ben-Hur N, Giladi A, Applebaum J, et al: Phosphorus burns. The antidote: A new approach. *Br J Plast Surg* 25:245, 1972.
22. Davidson EC: The treatment of acid and alkali burns. An experimental study. *Ann Surg* 85:481, 1927.
23. Konjoyan TR: White phosphorus burns: Case report and literature review. *Milit Med* 148:881, 1983.
24. Summerlin WT, Walder AI, Moncrief JA: White phosphorus burns and massive hemolysis. *J Trauma* 7:476, 1967.
25. Bowen TE, Whelan TJ Jr, Nelson TG: Sudden death after phosphorus burns: Experimental observations of hypocalcemia, hyperphosphatemia and electrocardiographic abnormalities following production of a standard white phosphorus burn. *Ann Surg* 174:779, 1971.
26. Unna PG: *The Histopathology of the Diseases of the Skin*. Edinburgh, WF Clay Company, 1896, p 719.
27. Shield AM, Cantab MB: A remarkable case of multiple growths of the skin caused by exposure to the sun. *Lancet* 1:22, 1899.
28. Hyde JN: Special article on the influence of light in the production of cancer of the skin. *Am J Med Sci* 131:1, 1906.
29. Silverberg E: Cancer statistics, 1981. *CA* 31:13, 1981.
30. Glazer SF: Adverse reactions to sunlight. *Compr Ther* 7:44, 1981.
31. Hall AF: Relationships of sunlight, complexion and heredity to skin carcinogenesis. *Arch Dermatol Syphilol* 61:589, 1950.
32. Urbach F, Rose DB, Bonnem M: Genetic and environmental interactions in skin carcinogenesis. In *Environment and Cancer. A Collection of Papers Presented at the Twenty-fourth Annual Symposium on Fundamental Cancer Research, 1971.* Baltimore, Williams & Wilkins Company, 1972, p 355.

33. Fleming ID, Barnawell JR, Burlison PE, Rankin JS: Skin cancer in black patients. *Cancer* 35:600, 1975.
34. Fitzpatrick TB: Soleil et peau. *J Med Esthétique* 2(7):33, 1975.
35. Kripke ML: Speculations on the role of ultraviolet radiation in the development of malignant melanoma. *J Natl Cancer Inst* 63:541, 1979.
36. Wilson PD, Kligman AM: Do freckles protect the skin from actinic damage? *Br J Dermatol* 106:27, 1982.
37. Sagan LA, Fry SA: Radiation accidents: A conference review. *Nuclear Safety* 21:562, 1980.
38. Fanger H, Lushbaugh CC: Radiation death from cardiovascular shock following a critical accident. Report of a second death from a newly defined human radiation death syndrome. *Arch Pathol* 83:446, 1967.
39. Andrews G: Mexican Co-60 radiation accident. *Isotopes Radiat Technol* 1:200, 1963.
40. Ye GY, Liu Y, Tien N, et al: The People's Republic of China Accident in 1963. In Hubner KF, Fry SA (eds): *The Medical Basis of Radiation Accident Preparedness.* New York, Elsevier/North-Holland, Inc, 1980, p 81.
41. Conklin JJ, Walker RI, Hirsch EF: Current concepts in the management of radiation injuries and associated trauma. *Surg Gynecol Obstet* 156:809, 1983.
42. Jammet H, Gongora R, Poullilard P, et al: The 1978 Algerian accident: Four cases of protracted whole-body irradiation. In Hubner KF, Fry SA (eds): *The Medical Basis of Radiation Accident Preparedness.* New York, Elsevier/North-Holland, Inc, 1980, p 113.
43. Warren S: *The Pathology of Ionizing Radiation.* Springfield, IL, Charles C Thomas, 1961, p 3.
44. Walsh D: Deep tissue traumatism from roentgen ray exposure. *Br Med J* 2:272, 1897.
45. Prasad KN: *Human Radiation Biology.* New York, Harper & Row, 1974.
46. Hubner KF, Fry SA (eds): *The Medical Basis for Radiation Accident Preparedness.* New York, Elsevier/North-Holland, Inc, 1980.
47. Langarn WH: Radiobiological factors in manned space flights. Report of the Space Radiation Study Panel of the Life Sciences Committee, Space Science Board, National Academy of Science, National Research Council Publication no. 1487, Washington, DC, National Academy of Science, 1967.
48. Ariyan S, Krizek TJ: Radiation effects, biological and surgical considerations. In Converse JM (ed): *Reconstructive Plastic Surgery.* Philadelphia, WB Saunders Co, 1977, p 531.
49. McCrady-Kahn VL, Kahn AM: Lightning burns. *West J Med* 134:215, 1981.
50. Myers GJ, Colgan MT, VanDyke DH: Lightning-strike disaster among children. *JAMA* 238:1045, 1977.
51. Apfelberg DB, Masters FW, Robinson DW: Pathophysiology and treatment of lightning injuries. *J Trauma* 14:453, 1974.
52. Bennett IL Jr: Electrical injuries. In Wintrobe MM, Thorn GW, Bennett IL, et al (eds): *Harrison's Principles of Internal Medicine,* ed 6. New York, McGraw-Hill Co, 1970, p 720.
53. Strasser EJ, Davis RM, Menchey MJ: Case reports. Lightning injuries. *J Trauma* 17, 315, 1977.
54. Kleiner JP, Wilkin JH: Cardiac effects of lightning stroke. *JAMA* 240:2757, 1978.
55. Masters FW, Robinson DW, Ketchum LD: Management of electrical burns. In Lynch JB, Lewis SR (eds): *Symposium on the Treatment of Burns.* St. Louis, CV Mosby Co, 1973, vol 5, p 82.
56. Demling RH, LaLonde C: *Burn Trauma (Trauma Management, vol IV).* New York, Thieme Medical Publishers, Inc, 1989, p 221.
57. Hanson GC, McIlwraith GR: Lightning injury: Two case histories and a review of management. *Br Med J* 3:271, 1973.
58. Kravitz H, Wasserman MJ, Valaitis J, et al: Lightning injury: Management of a case with ten-day survival. *Am J Dis Child* 131:413, 1977.
59. Jackson SHD, Parry DJ: Lightning and the heart. *Br Heart J* 43:454, 1980.
60. Shaw GP Jr, Atkinson LS: Hearing loss secondary to lightning strike. *J & SC Med Assoc* 77:233, 1981.
61. Yost JW, Holmes FF: Myoglobinuria following lightning strike. *JAMA* 228:1147, 1974.
62. Cooper MA: Lightning injuries: Prognostic signs for death. *Ann Emerg Med* 9:134, 1980.
63. Skoog T: Electrical injuries. *J Trauma* 10:816, 1970.
64. Nichter LS, Bryant CA, Kenney JG, et al: Injuries due to commercial electric current. *J Burn Care Rehab* 5:124, 1984.
65. Langworthy OR: Necrosis of the spinal cord produced by electrical injuries. *Bull Johns Hopkins Hosp* 51:210, 1932.
66. Peterson RA, Gibney J: Electrical burns. In Grabb WC, Smith JW (eds): *Plastic Surgery,* ed 3. Boston, Little, Brown and Company, 1979, p 489.
67. Baxter CR: Present concepts in the management of major electrical injury. *Surg Clin North Am* 50:1401, 1970.
68. Colcleugh RG, Ryan JE: Splinting electrical burns of the mouth in children. *Plast Reconstr Surg* 58:239, 1976.
69. Harman JW: The significance of local vascular phenomena in the production of ischemic necrosis in skeletal muscle. *Am J Pathol* 24:625, 1984.
70. Seddon HJ: Volkmann's ischaemia in the lower limb. *J Bone Joint Surg [Br]* 48:627, 1966.
71. Langworthy OR: Abnormalities produced in the central nervous system by electrical injuries. *J Exp Med* 51:943, 1930.
72. Xue-wei W, Yong-hua S, Nai-ze W: Early reconstructing blood circulation of wrist to prevent upper extremity necrosis after electrical injuries with the wrist as the injury center: A new surgical consideration. *Proc Am Burn Assoc* 16:47, 1984.
73. Robson MC, Murphy RC, Heggers JP: A new explanation for the progressive tissue loss in electrical injuries. *Plast Reconstr Surg* 73:431, 1984.

THREE

Head and Neck

27

Embryology of the Head and Neck

Ellen Beatty, M.D.

In the span of the fourth to eighth weeks of development, the normalcy of the embryo's face and pharynx is determined by the timing and completeness of cell growth and migration. During the fourth week of embryonic development, the human face and pharynx begin forming with closure of the anterior neuropore. This is the time that the ectodermal cells, known as the neural crest cells, located adjacent to the neural plate will migrate peripherally. These neural crest cells are responsible for facial, muscular, and skeletal elements, in contrast to their lesser role in other areas (1, 2). This chapter is a summary of the development of the head and neck.

The branchial arches are the basic structures from which the face and pharynx develop. They can be recognized in an embryo at the 10-somite stage. They form in pairs flanking the stomodeum and pharynx (Fig. 27.1). The first and largest arch is known as the mandibular arch. This arch has a small superior portion that contributes to the maxilla and a larger inferior portion that will contribute to the mandible, malleus, and incus. The second and only other named arch is the hyoid arch. Its contribution is to the body of the hyoid, the stapes, and adjacent neck structures. The remaining arches are smaller, and the fifth and sixth arches are rudimentary. The hyoid arch will actually grow caudally over the third and fourth arches. This process creates a temporary cervical sinus. Rarely, a persistence of this sinus communi-

cates with the second pharyngeal pouch, providing a fistula that will track between the internal and external carotid to drain in the skin at the anterior border of the sternocleidomastoid (3; Fig. 27.2).

These arches have a common structure (Fig. 27.3). Each arch is composed of internal and external walls of endoderm and ectoderm, respectively. The center of each arch is filled with mesoderm. At the time of migration, neural crest cells go from a compact collection to dispersed isolated cells when they arrive in the branchial arches. They travel between ectoderm and mesoderm initially and then proceed throughout the mesoderm, with the exception of the central mesodermal core, which they go around (2). The other components of the mesoderm of each arch include an artery, nerve, cartilaginous bar, somitic mesoderm for muscle formation, and cranial nerve. The arches appear as definite ridges along the future neck early in the fourth week of embryonic development. By the end of the fourth week, there are four distinct arches and two rudimentary arches with little future contribution.

Externally, each arch is bounded by a groove, which eventually smoothes out to yield a normal neck contour. The internal surface of each arch is bounded by a pharyngeal pouch (Fig. 27.4). Each pouch follows an arch, making four pouches and a last rudimentary pouch after the small final arch. The pouches provide recesses for vital

FIGURE 27.1. Branchial arch differentiation in the early embryo. *CR,* crown-rump length. (Redrawn from embryo 6502 in the Carnegie Collection.)

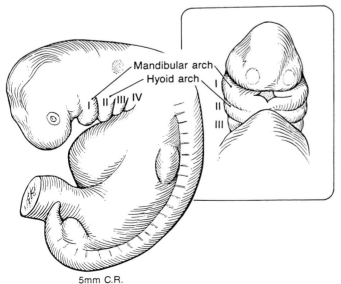

Mandibular arch
Hyoid arch
I
II III IV
I
II
III

5mm C.R.

FIGURE 27.2.   The cervical sinus. **A,** a side view of a 4-week embryo depicts location of cervical sinus. **B,** Cross section of an embryo demonstrates overgrowth of the third and fourth arches by hyoid arch. **C,** A longitudinal section of neck shows persistent cervical sinus tracking between the internal and external carotid.

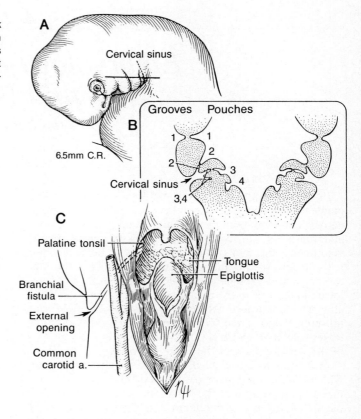

pharyngeal structures (Fig. 27.5). The first pouch lengthens and includes the middle ear ossicles. The long channel will be known as the Eustachian tube. The distal end of the pouch will contribute to the tympanic membrane as it grows to meet the first branchial groove, which is concurrently forming the external auditory canal. The second pharyngeal pouch becomes the tonsillar fossa. Its endoderm will proliferate to cover the lymphoid tissue of the tonsil, which forms in the fifth month of development (4). The third pouch has elongated and lost its opening

into the pharynx. The dorsal portion of this pouch will proliferate into the inferior parathyroid as the ventral pouch is obliterated by expanding thymic tissue forming there. The tissue of this pouch migrates caudally, and the inferior parathyroids will join the posterior thyroid while the thymus continues into the mediastinum. The fourth pharyngeal pouch allows the formation of the superior parathyroids. These glands also migrate caudally to a position on the posterior thyroid surface at a level above the third pouch derivatives. The ventral portion of this fourth

FIGURE 27.3.   Branchial arch structure in cross section.

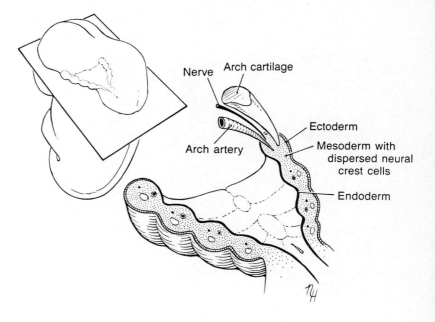

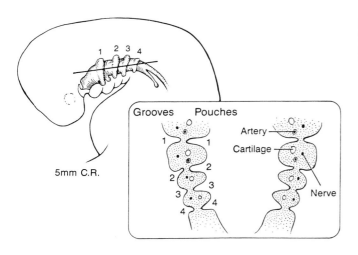

FIGURE 27.4. Branchial pouches in 4-week embryo. (Modified from Patten BM: Ductless glands and pharyngeal derivatives. In *Human Embryology,* ed 3. McGraw-Hill Book Company, New York, 1968, p 432.)

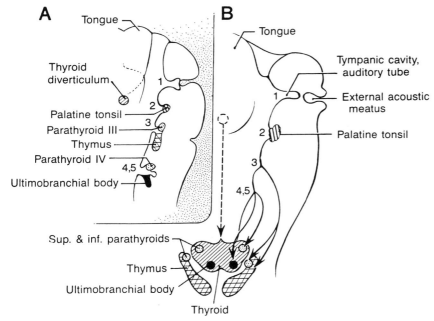

FIGURE 27.5. Derivatives of the pharyngeal pouches. **A,** Cross section. **B,** Frontal view. (Modified from Moore KL: *The Developing Human.* Philadelphia, WB Saunders Co, 1977, p 163.)

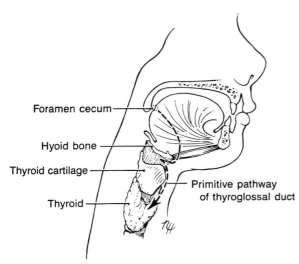

FIGURE 27.6. The development of the thyroid involves migration of these endodermal cells from their origin in the foramen cecum to their destination in the neck.

pouch will develop into the ultimobranchial bodies, which will join to the forming thyroid to provide the parafollicular cells of this gland (3). The fifth pouch coalesces with the fourth or disappears. Although the thyroid is not derived from a pharyngeal pouch, it does form in the third week of development as a diverticulum in the pharyngeal floor (Fig. 27.6). These endodermal cells proliferate and migrate as the neck and pharynx mature and straighten to their usual position anterior to the trachea. The site of the early thyroid diverticulum will become the foramen cecum. Incomplete migration of any of these glandular cells formed in pharyngeal pouches or diverticula will result in ectopic tissue located in the usual path of migration. In the case of the thyroid, the thyroglossal duct may remain patent with a trail of thyroid leading to the isthmus.

The cartilaginous bars in the branchial arches differentiate into the initial cartilages of the head and neck (Fig. 27.7). The dorsal portion of the first bar will ossify and become the malleus and incus. The ventral portion of the first bar is known as Meckel's cartilage and will form

FIGURE 27.7. Derivation of the cartilaginous component of the branchial arches.

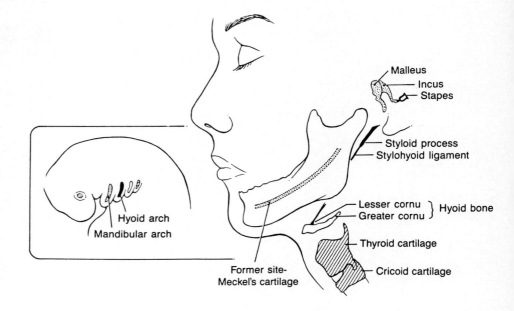

FIGURE 27.8. Formation of facial features. (Modified from Patten BM: In Schaeffer JP (ed): *Morris' Human Anatomy,* ed 10. Philadelphia, McGraw-Hill Book Co, Blakiston Division, 1942, p 27.)

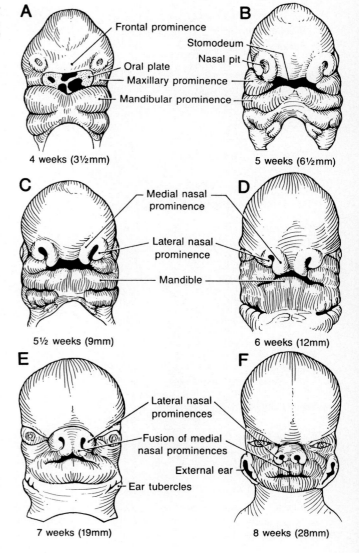

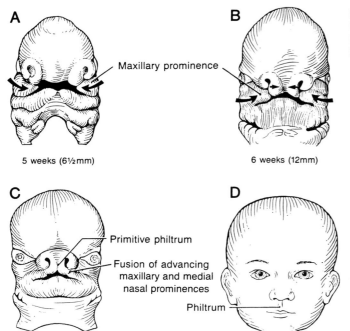

A

Maxillary prominence

5 weeks (6½mm)

B

6 weeks (12mm)

FIGURE 27.9. Fusion of the facial prominences. (Modified from Patten BM: In Schaeffer JP (ed): *Morris' Human Anatomy*, ed 10. Philadelphia, McGraw-Hill Book Co, Blakiston Division, 1942, p 27.)

C

Primitive philtrum

Fusion of advancing maxillary and medial nasal prominences

7 weeks (19mm)

D

Philtrum

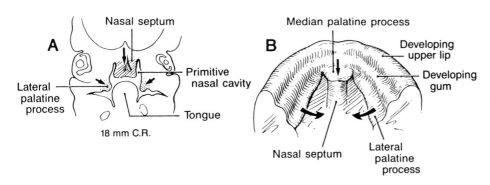

A

Nasal septum

Lateral palatine process

Primitive nasal cavity

Tongue

18 mm C.R.

B

Median palatine process

Developing upper lip

Developing gum

Nasal septum

Lateral palatine process

FIGURE 27.10. The primary and secondary palate form by fusion of lateral palatine shelves with the median palatine process. (Modified from Moore KL: The branchial apparatus. In *The Developing Human*, ed 2. Philadelphia, WB Saunders Co, 1977, p 173.)

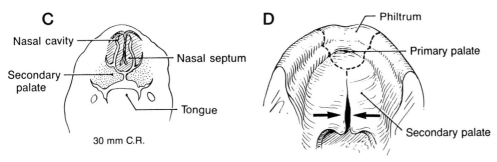

C

Nasal cavity

Secondary palate

Nasal septum

Tongue

30 mm C.R.

D

Philtrum

Primary palate

Secondary palate

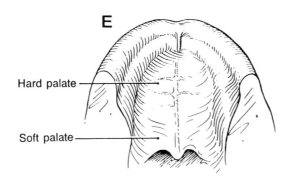

E

Hard palate

Soft palate

Table 27.1.
Derivatives of the Branchial Arches

Arch	Nerve	Muscles	Skeleton
First	Trigeminal (V)	Muscles of mastication Mylohyoid and anterior belly of digastric Tensor tympani Tensor veli palatine	Malleus Incus
Second	Facial (VII)	Muscles of facial expression Stapedius Stylohyoid Posterior belly of digastric	Stapes Styloid process Lesser cornu of hyoid Upper part of body of the hyoid bone
Third	Glossopharyngeal (IX)	Stylopharyngeus	Greater cornu of hyoid Lower part of body of the hyoid bone
Fourth and sixth	Superior laryngeal branch of vagus and recurrent laryngeal branch of vagus, respectively (X)	Pharyngeal and laryngeal	Laryngeal cartilages

the mandible by intramembranous ossification. The dorsal portion of the second bar will become known as Reichart's cartilage and will osiffy to form the stapes and styloid process. The lesser cornu and upper part of the body of the hyoid are formed from the ventral portion of the second bar. The third cartilaginous bar contributes its ventral portion, which ossifies to the greater cornu and lower body of the hyoid. A fusion of the ventral portions of the fourth and sixth bars forms the laryngeal cartilages, except for the epiglottis. The epiglottis forms from mesenchyme derived from the third and fourth branchial arches (3).

The branchial arches are each supplied by a cranial nerve (Table 27.1). The nerve to the first arch is the trigeminal, whose branches innervate the facial skin. The maxillary and mandibular branches supply the teeth, the mucous membranes of the oral and nasal cavities, and the tongue. The second arch is supplied by the facial nerve, which supplies the facial expression muscles. The glossopharyngeal nerve supplies the third branchial arch. The fourth arch is supplied by the superior laryngeal branch

of the vagus, and the recurrent laryngeal branch supplies the rudimentary fifth and sixth arches.

The musculature of the face and neck are derived from the somitic cells of the branchial arches' mesodermal core (Table 27.1). The first arch will contribute the muscles of mastication, which include the temporalis, masseter, and medial and lateral pterygoids, along with the mylohyoid, anterior belly of the digastric, and the tensors veli palatini and tympani. The second arch supplies the muscle cells for the facial expression muscles (orbicularis oris and oculi, frontalis, platysma, auricularis, and buccinator), the posterior belly of the digastric, stapedius, and the stylohyoid. The sole muscle originating from the third arch is the stylopharyngeus. The pharyngeal and laryngeal muscles are derivatives of the fourth and sixth arches.

Formation of the face begins in the third week of development with the genesis of the branchial arches and growth of the frontonasal prominence (Fig. 27.8). Kissel et al. (1) described a streaming of neural crest cells into the mesoderm of the early facial and frontonasal promi-

FIGURE 27.11.   The differentiation of the first and second branchial arches for the formation of the ear. (After Streeter GL: Development of the auricle in the human embryo, *Carnegie Contrib Embryol* 14:111, 1922.)

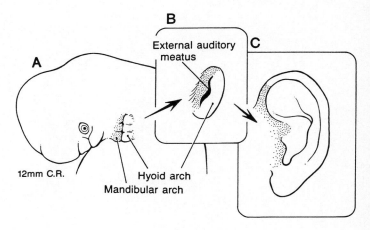

nences and laterally into the first and second branchial arches, which will become the maxilla and mandible. These neural crest cells are believed to be responsible for the fusion of the facial prominences. The frontonasal prominence will contribute the philtrum and primary palate (Fig. 27.9) when it fuses with the maxillary prominences in the sixth to seventh weeks of development. The maxillary prominences are responsible for the lateral upper lip and maxilla and the secondary palate. The palate forms from two lateral palatine shelves that initially lie in a vertical plane adjacent to the tongue (Fig. 27.10). With differential growth of the face, the shelves are normally able to grow to a horizontal plane, allowing fusion of the shelves in the midline to form the secondary palate and fusion with the triangular primary palate anteriorly. The nasal septum will form from the fusing of the medial nasal prominences and grow downward to join the fused palatal shelves. This growth and fusion process should be complete by the 12th week of development.

While the facial prominences are developing, the remainder of the sense organs also form. The external auditory canal forms from the first branchial groove. The first and second arches provide the mesoderm to form the auricle (Fig. 27.11). The second arch contributes the major portion of the auricle, and the innervation will come from branches of the cervical plexus (3). The ear forms in the area of the branchial arches and grooves, but differential growth of the head will allow the auricle to move gradually from the neck to the level of the eye.

The eyes begin development in the third week as grooves over optic vesicles from the forebrain. The retina, neurovascular bundle, and lens develop prior to the formation of eyelids in the late embryonic period. The lids form from ectodermal folds that grow and will fuse until the sixth month of fetal development (3).

This summary of normal head and neck development provides a basis for understanding the consequences of failed or incomplete formation. The clefts, pits, tags, sinus, cysts, and asymmetries should be thought of in these terms before we attempt correction in order to avoid oversight of a more serious related anomaly.

References

1. Kissel P, André JM, Jacquier A: *The Neurocristopathies*. New York, Masson Publishing, 1981.
2. Moore KL: *The Developing Human*. Philadelphia, WB Saunders Co, 1977.
3. Slavkin HD: *Developmental Craniofacial Biology*. Philadelphia, Lea & Febiger, 1979.
4. Johnson MG, Sulik KK: Embryology of the head and neck. In Serafin D, Georgiade NG (eds): *Pediatric Plastic Surgery*. St. Louis, CV Mosby Co, 1984, p 184.

28

Unilateral Cleft Lip

Don La Rossa, M.D., F.A.C.S. and Peter Randall, M.D., F.A.C.S.

Cleft lip and/or palate has been the second most frequently occurring of the major congenital anomalies (1 : 750 to 1 : 1,000 live births), with club foot being the most common (1, 2). Clefts of the lip result from a failure of mesenchymal penetration and fusion of the nasofrontal and lateral facial processes of the developing face at 4–7 weeks of gestation (3). This condition is expressed in those structures anterior to the incisive foramen: the prepalate alveolus, maxilla, lip, and nasal structures, sometimes up to and including the lacrimal ducts. The degree of expression varies considerably from the typical wide, gaping cleft of the alveolus and lip structures straddled by a stretched and flattened ala, to a mere "scar" of the minimal incomplete cleft with the lip almost fused to normalcy. An absolute deficiency is seen in all tissues involved in the cleft: skin, muscle, mucous membranes, maxillary and nasal bones, and nasal cartilages. The quantitative differences vary with the severity of the cleft. It is up to the surgeon to evaluate how much tissue remains and to rearrange and augment the remnants to create a "near normal"–appearing lip.

"Cleft lip" is a diminutive term and often does not properly describe or emphasize the extent of the deformity. A more appropriate term might be "prepalatal cleft" because the nose and alveolus are integral parts of the anomaly (4). Indeed, the maxilla should be included in the definition because the bony infrastructure of the cleft has a great impact on the external soft-tissue appearance. Maxillary orthopaedics and orthodontics, with or without bone grafting, play an integral part in successful management of the cleft lip patient. Thus, these areas are covered in a later section.

Fortunately, many normal anatomical landmarks and "clues" remain to aid in the repair. Each lip is different and each retains some anatomical features that can be incorporated into the repair. The surgeon must search diligently for them and analyze the unrepaired lip to identify them. Cardosa (5) emphasized the need to recognize and save the "Cupid's bow" remnants, which were often disregarded and discarded in earlier repairs. The outcome was lips that had symmetry but lacked adequate horizontal dimension, were "too tight," and lacked a normal Cupid's bow (6, 7).

Fara (8) delineated the abnormal architecture of the orbicularis oris muscle in the cleft, leading to the incorporation of muscle repairs in cleft lip surgery by Randall et al. (9) and others (10–13).

Pool (14) noted that it is not the width of the cleft but the vertical height discrepancy between the cleft and noncleft sides that determines the difficulty of repair. The surgeon must bring into balance the peak or Cupid's bow on the cleft and noncleft sides. The surgical principle involved in correcting the cleft lip defect is to lengthen the cleft side, so that it equals the vertical dimensions of the noncleft side. A tissue rearrangement is designed to borrow tissue from the lateral element of the cleft, where there is usually available tissue, and introduce it into the medial element, which is deficient. Modern techniques lengthen the medial side of the cleft by opening incisions into which flaps from the lateral side of the cleft are introduced. The most commonly used flap designs can be categorized as triangular, quadrangular, or rotation advancement types. The success of the repair depends largely on the skill of the surgeon in assessing the abnormal anatomy, identifying remaining anatomical details and landmarks, and using these "key points" to recreate the missing lip structures (15–20).

A cleft lip can be repaired at any time after birth in an otherwise healthy infant. Most surgeons adhere to the pediatric surgical dictums of 10 weeks of age, 10 lb in weight, and 10 g of hemoglobin. General anesthesia is preferred because it allows the surgeon to work in a precise fashion. However, in selected patients, repairs can be accomplished under local anesthesia supplemented by sedation and intermittent feeding with a bottle to soothe the infant during surgery. In the anesthetized patient, an uncuffed oral Rae tube (Rae preformed tracheal tube; NCC division—Mallinckrodt Inc., Argyle, NY) is used. Care must be taken to tape it precisely in the midline to minimize distortion of the lips. The tape is kept inferior to the commissures.

The head and face remain accessible to the surgeon. Marking is conveniently done with methylene blue dye and a straight pen. Key points are tattooed into the skin with the pen point or a hypodermic needle to finalize the operative plan *before* injection with vasoconstrictive agents. Epinephrine 1 : 100,000 or 1 : 200,000 should be injected locally to reduce bleeding and to facilitate the accuracy of the repair. Commercial preparations of epinephrine mixed with 1% or 0.5% lidocaine are the most convenient way to use these agents. Care must be exercised because of the toxic effects of both drugs. The maximum dose of lidocaine is 7 mg/kg. Seven minutes, by the clock, are required for the full vasoconstrictive effect.

Anatomy of Repair

The markings begin with a careful and accurate identification of the normal and abnormal landmarks in the cleft lip (Fig. 28.1). The key points to identify are:

Point 1: the midline point of the arch of Cupid's bow
Point 2: the peak of Cupid's bow on the noncleft side
Point 3: the proposed peak of Cupid's bow on the cleft side (distance from *1* to *2*)
Point 4: the midline of the columella
Points 5 and 6: the base of the columella on the cleft and noncleft sides
Points 7 and 8: the points at which the alar bases insert into the nostril sill
Point 9: the point at which the white roll and vermilion begin to thin out or disappear on the lateral lip element. This point should be at the same level as the peak of Cupid's bow on the normal side (2) and should be where the roll is still well developed.

The difference in distance from the base of the columella to the peak of Cupid's bow on the cleft (3) and

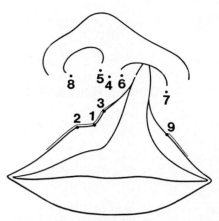

FIGURE 28.1.   Anatomy of the normal and unrepaired unilateral cleft lip indicate "key points" used for planning repair: **(1)** lowest point in arch Cupid's bow, midline of the lip; **(2)** peak of Cupid's bow on the noncleft side; **(3)** proposed peak of Cupid's bow; **(4)** midpoint of the columella; **(5)** and **(6)** base of columella; **(7)** and **(8)** inset of alar base into nostril sill; **(9)** point of disappearance of white roll of the vermilion cutaneous junction (at the same level as point **2** and where the roll is well developed).

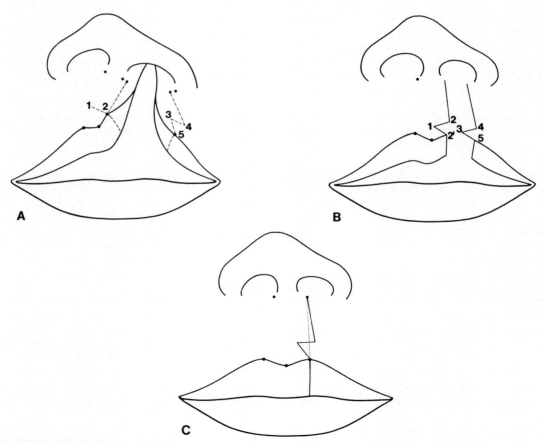

FIGURE 28.2.   Triangular flap technique. The medial lip element is lengthened by a back-cut **(1–2)** and a triangular flap **(3–5)** on the lateral lip element is introduced into it. The lengthening achieved is equal to the base of the triangular flap **(4–5)** for practical purposes.

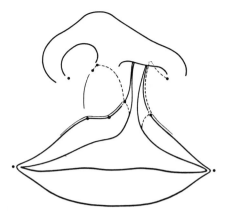

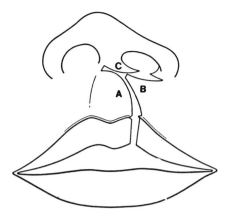

FIGURE 28.3. Techniques of rotation advancement. The flap (**A**) on the medial lip element rotates downward to achieve the necessary lengthening and the flap (**B**) from the lateral lip ele- ment advances into the defect. A small pennant-shaped medial flap (**C**) can be used as needed to restore the nostril sill or to lengthen the columella.

noncleft (2) side—measured in millimeters—is the lengthening that must be achieved to produce symmetry. Triangular, quadrangular, or rotation advancement flaps are modern techniques of repair used to achieve this effect in all cases with the exception of minimal cleft lips. The Rose-Thompson (21, 22) slightly curved line repair may be used for the latter.

Techniques of Repair

TRIANGULAR FLAP TECHNIQUE (TENNISON-RANDALL)

Originally described by Tennison (16), the geometry of this technique was explained by Randall (18). It permits the relatively inexperienced cleft lip surgeon to obtain reproducible results. Lips repaired by this method are sometimes slightly long on the cleft side. If this occurs, secondary revisions can be achieved by selective excisions in the horizontal limb of the triangular flap (Fig. 28.2).

ROTATION ADVANCEMENT TECHNIQUE (MILLARD)

Described as a "cut as you go" technique by Millard (19, 20), this method places most of the scar in a more anatomically correct position along the philtral column (Fig. 28.3). It is not as easy as the triangular flap method for the beginner to master. Insufficient lengthening is sometimes a problem in the cleft lip, with a marked discrepancy in height between the cleft and noncleft sides. A small Z-plasty just above the white roll can be added at the time of primary repair or as a secondary procedure.

Helpful Details

1. To gain extra length in a rotation advancement repair of the cleft with marked discrepancy of vertical height, the medial side of the cleft (*point 3* in Fig. 28.1) should be moved 1 mm medially and the lateral side of the cleft (*point 9* in Fig. 28.1) should be moved 1 mm laterally when marking the proposed Cupid's bow (Fig. 28.4*A*).

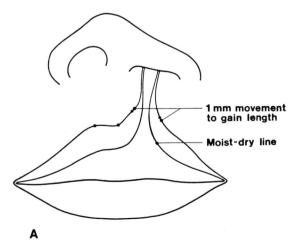

1 mm movement to gain length

Moist-dry line

A

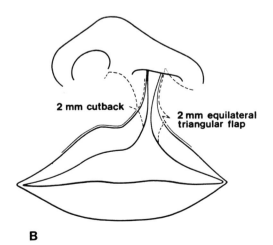

2 mm cutback

2 mm equilateral triangular flap

B

FIGURE 28.4. **A,** Double marks where the incisions cross the vermilion cutaneous junction aid in realignment during lip clo- sure. **B,** A 2-mm equilateral triangular flap just above the vermilion cutaneous junction aids in achieving proper lengthening.

FIGURE 28.5. **A,** Original technique is shown for reorientation of displaced or orbicularis oris muscle bundles at the time of primary lip repair. **B,** Division of the muscle bundle into three tails, which are interdigitated. The uppermost bundles are attached to dermis along the philtrum. The inferior two are sutured to each other to minimize tightness at the free border. **C,** Division of the muscle into an upper triangular portion and lower rectangular portion is shown. The triangular portions are interdigitated like a Z-plasty, lengthening the lip. The rectangular portions are sutured end-to-end. We have abandoned technique **A** and are using **B** and **C.**

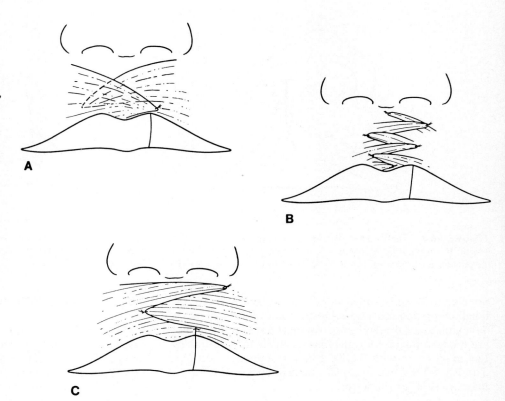

2. *Point 9* should be level with the Cupid's bow point on the noncleft side (*point 2*) and where the roll is well developed. This will help restore a full roll across the entire repaired lip. It will also help to set the proper vertical height on the repaired side.
3. The distance from the commissure to the peak of Cupid's bow on each side need not be equal.
4. Double marks should be made at these two sites, leaving a tattoo mark adjacent to the incision to serve as a guide for accurate alignment of the vermilion cutaneous junction at the time of lip closure.
5. In a rotation advancement repair, a 2-mm triangular flap from the lateral lip element can be introduced into a 2-mm backcut of the medial lip at the junction of skin and vermilion. This will add length and emphasis to the white roll as well as improve the lip profile. The angle of the backcut is designed to place the endpoint in the depression above the vermilion-cutaneous roll. (Fig. 28.4*B*).
6. The point on the lip where moist and dry vermilion (red-line) meet should be lined up (23; Fig. 28.4*A*).
7. The nose and the lip should always be repaired from the inside out. The temptation to close the lip skin to assure that the repair will work should be suppressed.

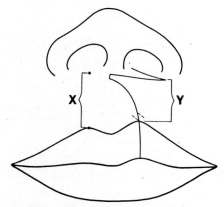

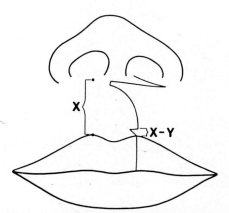

FIGURE 28.6. Most commonly seen after rotation advancement repairs, a Z-plasty can be used to lengthen the short scar. The Z should be introduced just above the vermilion cutaneous junction where it will help improve the profile of the lip in the region of the white roll.

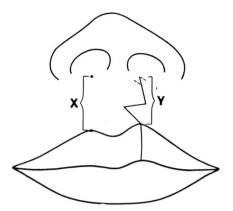

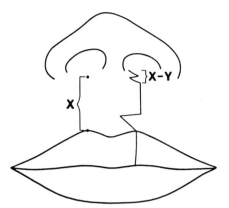

FIGURE 28.7. When this deformity follows a triangular flap or quadrangular flap repair, a Z-plasty can be introduced at the upper end of the lip scar, or the triangular flap can be advanced further toward the midline.

Reorientation of the Orbicularis Muscle

In describing the anatomy of the orbicularis oris musculature in cleft lips, Fara (8) pointed out that the muscle fibers parallel the margin of the cleft in the vast majority of instances. Delaire, Lathum, Nicolau, and others have further elucidated the complex anatomy of the orbicularis oris (10–13). If the margins of the cleft are "pared" and closed side to side, as was done in the early repairs of cleft lips, the abnormal attachments of the muscle persist. The result is the "orbicularis bulge" seen in the lateral lip element, typical of many repaired cleft lips. Additionally, such lips show distorted muscle pull and distortion during speaking, grimacing, smiling, and whistling. Detaching the muscle from its dermal and mucosal attachments and reorienting it has been advocated by many authors. Results have not been fully evaluated, and the proper method of muscle reorientation is not yet clear. Current techniques are shown in Figure 28.5.

Revisional Surgery of the Unilateral Cleft Lip

The timing of revisional procedures should be guided by the conspicuousness of the deformity. Once scar maturation has occurred, an accurate assessment of the deformity can be made, and a plan for correction and its timing developed. Some of the more common defects after primary cleft lip surgery are presented in Figures 28.6 through 28.11).

1. Lips that are "too short" (Figs. 28.6 and 28.7).
2. Lips that are "too long" (Fig. 28.8).

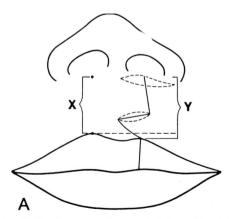

A

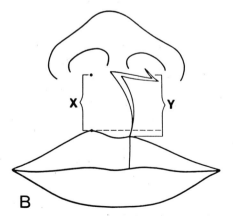

B

FIGURE 28.8. **A,** Most commonly seen in triangular and quadrangular flap repairs, all or most of the repair may have to be redone, or an elliptical segment equal to about twice the amount of shortening desired can be excised from the transverse incision along the superior edge. **B,** In the rotation advancement technique, the flaps are recut and the amount of rotation reduced by trimming the lateral flap an appropriate amount.

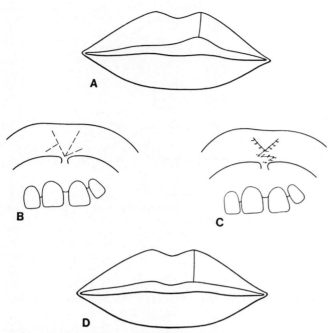

FIGURE 28.9. The off-center, elevated vermilion-free border at the site of cleft repair is referred to as the whistling deformity because it simulates the configuration of the upper lip when whistling. In most instances, a V-Y advancement of mucosa can correct the deficiency of tissue. Incorporation of a Z-plasty in the verticle limb of the Y aids in preventing relapse. Care should be taken to include the mucous glands of the lip in the mucosal flaps to prevent the complications of a chronically dry, scaling lip. If a muscle dehiscence is present, it should be closed as well. For more severe defects, composite musculo-mucosal "pendulum flaps" bordering the area of depression can be brought together to restore an even, vermilion-free border (24).

3. The "whistling deformity" (Figs. 28.9 and 28.10).
4. The "orbicularis bulge" (Fig. 28.11).

Cleft Effects on Nasal Cartilages and Bone

The cleft lip nasal distortion is a reflection of nasal cartilage and bone deformity and displacement. The reconstruction, therefore, depends on remodeling this underlying infrastructure (Fig. 28.12). The timing of intervention remains controversial. Some repositioning of the distorted tip cartilages can be done at the time of primary lip closure, although it is frequently postponed and treated secondarily. Proponents of early correction suggest that early realignment of malpositioned cartilages will facilitate more normal growth (25–31). Opponents express concern about injury to the fragile infant cartilages and subsequent interference with normal growth by surgical scar, making the eventual rhinoplasty more difficult (32–34).

The deformity, as described by Huffman and Lierle (27) and others (28), consists of a flattened and splayed-out alar cartilage, loss of the normal overlapping relation-

ship of the upper lateral and alar cartilages, lateral displacement of alar base, nasal septal deviation to the noncleft side, and retrodisplacement of the pyriform aperture. After lip repair, a characteristically flattened and depressed nasal tip persists. Further, the alar rim hangs below the normal position, a ridge or fold projects into the nasal vestibule, and the deficient bony platform at the pyriform aperture causes an inward displacement of the alar base.

Principles involved in correction of the cleft lip nasal deformity (Fig. 28.12) include:

1. Elevation of the medial crus and dome of the alar cartilage to even parity or to a slightly overcorrected position relative to the noncleft side; on-lay grafts of auricular, septal, or contralateral alar cartilage on the depressed dome.
2. Reestablishment of the overlap of the upper and lower lateral cartilages.
3. Medial repositioning of the laterally displaced alar base.
4. Forward advancement of the alar base by augmentation of the bony platform at the pyriform aperture with bone or cartilage grafts or artificial implants (silicone, proplast, or hydroxyapatite).
5. Straightening of the deflected caudal portion of the nasal septum.

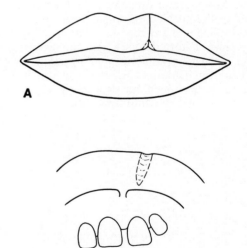

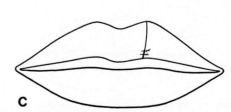

FIGURE 28.10. Often an attempt to preserve too much tissue is made at the original operation, utilizing vermilion that does not have full thickness. The segment of excess vermilion may need to be excised to achieve an even, full vermilion.

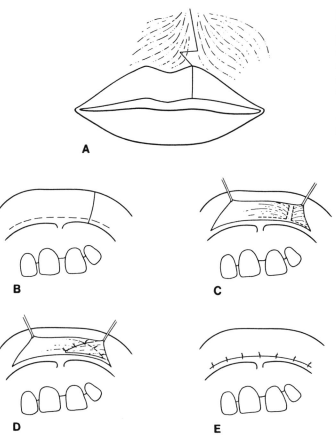

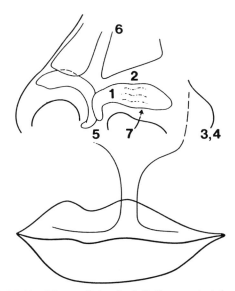

FIGURE 28.11. The orbicularis bulge is often a major clue to the presence of a cleft, even in the most elegantly repaired lips. It is caused by the abnormal position and "bunching up" of the orbicularis oris muscle on the cleft side. The muscle can be detached and reoriented in a secondary procedure via a labial sulcus approach. **A,** Abnormal muscle position is shown in a cleft lip repaired without muscle reorientation. **B,** Buccal sulcus incision gives access to the orbicularis oris muscle. **C,** The muscle is detached from mucosa and skin is divided at the repair site. **D,** The muscle is reoriented from a vertical to a horizontal position. **E,** Mucosa is closed.

FIGURE 28.12. The unilateral cleft lip nasal deformity: **(1)** hypoplastic alar cartilage with depressed dome; **(2)** loss of normal overlap of upper and lower lateral cartilages; **(3)** laterally displaced ala; **(4)** hypoplasia and retrusion of the bony platform at the pyriform aperture; **(5)** deviation of the nasal spine and caudal septum to the noncleft side; **(6)** flattening and displacement of the nasal bones and upper lateral cartilage; **(7)** buckling of the lateral crus of the lower lateral cartilage creating a web in the vestibule.

6. Osteotomy of the bony pyramid when the dorsum is broad (rhinoplasty).
7. Reduction of the internal vestibular ridge or web, often with a Z-plasty in the vestibule.

Cleft Lip Nasal Deformity

The management of the cleft lip nasal deformity remains the most difficult, involved, and challenging aspect of cleft lip surgery. The conservative approach of delaying nasal tip surgery until more growth has occurred has withstood the test of time, but it is often not accepted by the growing child. No primary or secondary repair method has fully solved the problem.

TECHNIQUES FOR PRIMARY CORRECTION

1. The medial and lateral crura of both alar cartilages are widely undermined through the medial lip incision at the base of the columella and the incision used to release the attachment of the lateral lip element to the maxilla to free their skin attachments. An intercartilaginous incision should be avoided because of the risk of nostril stenosis in the growing child. The lateral crus dome and medial crus are pulled superiorly over the upper lateral cartilage to restore the normal overlap. Internal through-and-

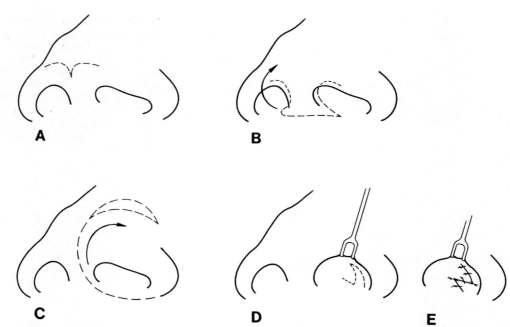

FIGURE 28.13. Approaches for correction of nasal tip deformity. **A,** Gull-winged incision gives good exposure but often leaves conspicuous scars. **B,** Rim plus transcolumellar incision gives excellent exposure, hides incisions well, especially if columellar incision is at the nasolabial angle. Incorporation of the sill flap in a rotation advancement technique permits columellar lengthening. This is our preferred approach. **C,** Tip incision permits a rotation of the entire alar complex. Although this often heals well, it can leave an unacceptable scar. **D and E,** Z-plasty of the vestibular skin and alar cartilage is performed to correct the vestibular web. It is often incorporated in the above repairs of the nasal tip.

through absorbable mattress sutures along the ridge of overlap of the upper and lower alar cartilages (internal valve) or external sutures on bolsters as described by McComb may be used to maintain the new anatomy during healing (31).

A "pennant"-shaped mucosal flap of lateral lip vermilion, based on the lateral maxillary segment, can be introduced into any gap that results from release of the floor of the nose from the maxilla. This leaves a permanent fistula that requires secondary closure.

2. The lateral crus and nasal floor are advanced medially.

3. A Z-plasty of the vestibular web is performed, if needed (Fig. 28.13).

TECHNIQUES FOR SECONDARY CORRECTION

1. A Berkeley-type tip incision can be performed; however, the external tip scar is a detractor (Fig. 25.13).

2. A number of other surgical exposures and techniques have been proposed to accomplish this goal (29, 35–37). The most useful of these is the open tip technique, which permits direct visualization and manipulation of the affected cartilage. Septal correction can be done through this approach as well. The transcolumellar incision can be placed at the columellar-lip angle, incorporating the sill flap from a Millard rotation advancement repair for columellar lengthening. Many surgeons prefer an incision at the columellar waist (Fig. 25.13).

Maxillary Orthopaedics and Orthodontics in the Management of Cleft Lip

CLEFT EFFECTS ON MAXILLA

The extent of maxillary clefting is proportional to the severity of the cleft lip deformity. Clefts of the prepalatal structures can extend to the incisive foramen posteriorly and into the nasal bones superiorly. Incomplete cleft lips may have minimal bone deficiency. When alveolar bone is involved, the lateral incisor tooth in the area of the cleft is usually malpositioned, malformed, or absent. The process of surgical repair reestablishes the soft tissue and muscular forces on the displaced maxillary segments, forcing them together. Scar from dissection of the hard and soft palate mucoperiosteum during palate repair may exacerbate the collapse. The result is displacement of the alveolus into cross-bite, and depression in the region of the pyriform aperture, maxilla, and zygoma on the cleft side. The overall management plan seeks to remedy these deficiencies.

Early management may include presurgical orthopaedics or lip adhesion procedures. The principle involves the use of external pressure on the displaced alveolus, substituting for the discontinuity of the lip. This can be accomplished by use of a head cap and elastic traction and is most often applied in bilateral clefts, although it can be used in unilateral clefts as well.

Lip adhesion procedures are a physiological means to this end. Done early in infancy (0–3 months) under general or local anesthesia, this procedure restores tension across the cleft, helping to mold the maxillary segments, and seeks to convert a complete cleft to an incomplete one, thereby facilitating the final repair (38).

The use of traction devices or lip adhesion is often combined with the use of intraoral appliances to guide the movement of the maxillary segments into an ideal position as advocated by McNeil (39), Burston (40), and Georgiade and Latham (41). This approach can facilitate eventual lip and palate closure or can be used to prepare for early bone grafting. Although still controversial, proponents of early bone grafting have demonstrated minimal harmful effects from rib grafts inserted into the alveolar cleft after minimal undermining of the alveolar mucoperiosteum (42). If not stabilized by bone grafts, the alveolar segments must be held in retention throughout childhood. Otherwise, alveolar collapse and crossbite will reappear. This treatment program is only feasible with motivated parents and available skilled orthodontic and prosthodontic support.

More commonly, alveolodental abnormalities are bone grafted during mixed or secondary dentition, ages 8–10 years, after standard orthodontic techniques, modified for the peculiarities of clefts, are used to realign the teeth and alveolar segments. Rib, iliac cortical, cancellous, and most recently cranial bone have been successfully used (43; Kawamoto, personal communication). The grafts fill the bony defect, stabilize the maxillary segments, and provide bone for the eruption, stabilization, and growth of teeth. At the same time, on-lay bone grafts can be used to augment the hypoplastic bone of the pyriform aperture and malar regions to help restore facial symmetry and to reposition the alar base on the cleft side.

An alternative method involves orthodontic realignment followed by orthognathic surgical movement of displaced, hypoplastic, or hyperplastic dentoalveolar elements. In some patients, these techniques provide the only solution to disordered dentoalveolar relationships. In particular, older patients with severe class III malocclusion, open-bite deformity, or prognathism (true or pseudo) will need orthognathic surgery to bring the facial profile into harmony. Such procedures are deferred until facial growth and tooth eruption is complete. Radiographs for bone age and dental age are helpful in determining when this has occurred.

Nonosteoplastic methods involve orthodontic repositioning of malpositioned segments. The repositioned structures are then held in position by fixed or removable bridgework. These appliances, fashioned by a prosthodontist, maintain and complete the functional and cosmetic dental restoration in the cleft patient. It is clear from the foregoing that expertise from orthodontic and prosthodontic cleft palate team members is essential throughout the entire treatment period in patients with clefts involving the maxilla.

References

1. Ivy RH: Modern concept of cleft lip and cleft palate management. *Plast Reconstr Surg* 9:121, 1952.
2. Fogh-Anderson P: *Inheritance of Harelip and Cleft Palate.* Copenhagen, Ejuar Munksgaard Forlag, 1943.
3. Stark RB: The pathogenesis of harelip and cleft palate. *Plast Reconstr Surg* 13:20, 1954.
4. Stark RB: Embryology, pathogenesis, and classification of cleft lip and cleft palate. In Pruzansky S (ed): *Congenital Anomalies of the Face and Associated Structures.* Springfield, IL, Charles C Thomas, 1961.
5. Cardoso AD: A new technique for harelip. *Plast Reconstr Surg* 10:92, 1952.
6. Blair VP, Brown JB: Mirault operation for single harelip. *Surg Gynecol Obstet* 51:81, 1930.
7. Brown JB, McDowell F: Surgical repair of cleft lips. *Arch Surg* 56:750, 1948.
8. Fara M: The importance of folding down muscle stumps in the operation of unilateral clefts of the lip. *Acta Chir Plast (Praha)* 13:162, 1971.
9. Randall P, Whitaker LA, LaRossa D: The importance of muscle reconstruction in primary and secondary cleft lip repair. *Plast Reconstr Surg* 54:316, 1974.
10. Latham RA, Deaton TG: The structural basis of the philtrum and the contour of the vermillion border: A study of the musculature of the upper lip. *J Anat* 121:151, 1976.
11. Delaire J, Fève JR, Chateau JP, Courtay D, Tulasne JF: Anatomie et physiologie des muscles et du frein médian de la lèure supérieure. *Rev Stomatol Chir Maxillofac* 78:821, 1977.
12. Kernahan DA, Bauer BS: Functional cleft lip repair: A sequential layered closure with orbicularis muscle realignment. *Plast Reconstr Surg* 72:459, 1983.
13. Nicolau JP: The orbicularis oris muscle: A functional approach to its repair in the cleft lip, *Br J Plast Surg* 36:141, 1983.
14. Pool R Jr: Analysis of the anatomy and geometry of the unilateral cleft lip. *Plast Reconstr Surg* 24:311, 1959.
15. LeMesurier AB: A method of cutting and suturing the lip in the treatment of complete unilateral clefts. *Plast Reconstr Surg* 4:1, 1949.
16. Tennison CW: The repair of the unilateral cleft lip by the Stencil Method. *Plast Reconstr Surg* 9:115, 1952.
17. Marcks KM, Travaskis AE, daCosta A: Further observations in cleft lip repair. *Plast Reconstr Surg* 12:392, 1953.
18. Randall P: A triangular flap operation for the primary repair of unilateral clefts of the lip. *Plast Reconstr Surg* 23:331, 1951.
19. Millard DR: A primary camouflage of the unilateral harelip. In: *Transactions of the International Society of Plastic Surgeons,* First Congress, 1955. Baltimore, The Williams & Wilkins Co, 1957, p 160.
20. Millard DR Jr: Cleft craft: The evolution of its surgery. In *The Unilateral Deformity.* Boston, Little, Brown & Co, Vol 1, 1976.
21. Rose W: *Harelip and Cleft Palate.* London, HK Lewis and Co, 1976.
22. Thompson JE: An artistic and mathematically accurate method of repairing the defect in cases of harelip. *Surg Gynecol Obstet* 14:498, 1912.
23. Noordhoff MS: Reconstruction of vermilion in unilateral and bilateral cleft lips. *Plast Reconstr Surg* 73:52, 1984.
24. Kapatansky KI: Double pendulum flaps for whistling deformities in bilateral cleft lips. *Plast Reconstr Surg* 47:321, 1971.
25. McIndoe AH: Correction of the alar deformity in cleft lip. *Lancet* 1:607, 1938.
26. Brown JB, McDowell F: Secondary repair of cleft lips and their nasal deformities. *Ann Surg* 114:101, 1941.
27. Huffman WC, Leirle DM: Studies on the pathologic anatomy of the unilateral harelip nose. *Plast Reconstr Surg* 4:225, 1949.
28. Berkeley WT: The cleft lip nose. *Plast Reconstr Surg* 23:576, 1959.
29. Berkeley WT: Correction of secondary cleft-lip nasal deformities. *Plast Reconstr Surg* 44:234, 1969.
30. Millard DR: The unilateral cleft lip nose. *Plast Reconstr Surg* 34:169, 1964.

31. McComb H: Primary correction of unilateral cleft lip nasal deformity. A 10-year review. *Plast Reconstr Surg* 75:791, 1985.
32. Peet EW, Patterson TJS: *Essentials of Plastic Surgery.* Oxford, Blackwell Scientific Publications, 1963.
33. Marcks KM, Travaskis AE, Berg EM, et al: Nasal defects associated with cleft lip nasal deformity. *Plast Reconstr Surg* 34:176, 1964.
34. Matthews D: The nose tip. *Br J Plast Surg* 21:153, 1968.
35. Brauer RO, Foerster DW: Another method to lengthen the columella in the double cleft patient. *Plast Reconstr Surg* 38:27, 1966.
36. Rethi A: Raccourissement dir nez trop long. *Rev Chir Plast* 2:85, 1934.
37. O'Connor GB, McGregor MW, Tolleth H: The nasal problems in cleft lips. *Surg Gynecol Obstet* 116:503, 1968.
38. Randall P: A lip adhesion operation in cleft lip surgery. *Plast Reconstr Surg* 35:371, 1965.
39. McNeil CK: *Oral and Facial Deformity.* London, Pitman, 1954.
40. Burston WR: The early orthodontic treatment of cleft palate conditions. *Dental Pract* (*Bristol*) 9:41, 1958.
41. Georgiade NG, Latham RA: Maxillary arch alignment in the bilateral cleft lip and palate infant, using the pinned coaxial screw appliance. *Plast Reconst Surg* 56:52, 1975.
42. Rosenstein SW, Monroe CW, Kernahan DA, et al: The case of early bone grafting in cleft lip and cleft palate. *Plast Reconstr Surg* 70:927, 1982.
43. Abyholm FE, Bergland O, Semb G: Secondary bone grafting of alveolar clefts. A surgical/orthodontic treatment enabling a nonprosthodontic rehabilitation in cleft lip and palate patients. *Scand J Plast Reconstr Surg* 15:127, 1981.

29

Repair of the Bilateral Cleft Lip

William S. Garrett, Jr., M.D., F.A.C.S.

The bilateral cleft lip, with its often severe tissue deficits and anatomical distortions, offers one of the greatest challenges in the field of cleft surgery. Ideal repairs are difficult to design and even harder to execute. At this time, there are no techniques permitting full repair in one operation of a complete bilateral cleft lip and the associated short columella. Constructing a Cupid's bow and vermilion tubercle, completing the continuity of the interrupted orbicularis oris muscle, and lengthening the columella require incising the periphery of the prolabium and undermining it. The only way to avoid amputation of the prolabium is to divide the repair into at least two stages. Even more sittings may be required.

However, the biggest obstacle to satisfactory repair of the complete double cleft lip is not the prolabium or the columella; it is the protruding premaxilla.

Protruding Premaxilla

In the complete bilateral cleft lip, the premaxilla, if protruding as it usually is, can distort skeletal support for the upper lip, making repair without tension difficult and compromising the surgeon's ability to make the aesthetic value judgments necessary for a satisfying result.

GENESIS

Atherton (1) has made some interesting observations helpful for understanding and managing the protruding premaxilla. He noted that the protruding premaxilla is unique to humans, even though bilateral clefting of the lip and palate is not. In lower mammals with complete double clefts, the normal relationships of the premaxilla to the lateral palatal shelves remain virtually undisturbed.

The normal human, in contrast to lower mammals, does not have a premaxillary-maxillary growth suture. The result is that forward growth of the premaxilla ordinarily is restricted, even though forward growth of the nasal septum does occur and causes development of the anterior nasal spine and columella, which are also unique characteristics of humans. In the human with a complete bilateral cleft, the cleft acts as a premaxillary-maxillary suture and allows forward growth of the premaxilla. This results in a long upper jaw, an absent anterior nasal spine, a short or absent columella, and a flat, nonprojecting nasal tip. The configuration closely resembles that seen in lower mammals, in which a premaxillary-maxillary su-

ture allows the premaxilla to grow forward to produce a muzzle or snout. It is curious that, with regard to premaxillary position, the normal human is the mammalian variant and the infant with complete double cleft is the norm. This general concept involves considerable oversimplification of the complexities of growth and development, but it does give a useful working theory to bear in mind.

The details of development of the protruding premaxilla are complicated and involve both anterior positioning of the premaxilla and rotation of this structure on its transverse axis. Many specialists, particularly orthodontists interested in facial growth and development, have contributed to our understanding of the problem. Several reports have provided an overview of thought development in this area (1–6). These authors cite other valuable material in their own references.

PLAN OF MANAGEMENT

A general rule for dealing with the protruding premaxilla is to control it orthopaedically, if possible. Otherwise, the surgeon should try to work around it, leaving it in place. If it is not possible to work around a protruding premaxilla, it should be set back surgically but only as a last resort.

Orthopaedic Control

The advantages of repairing a double cleft lip under conditions that permit the closure to be free of tension and the lip to be normally supported by a well-aligned upper jaw scarcely need to be explained. Attempts to control the protruding premaxilla by infant maxillary orthopaedic techniques are worth the effort. Unfortunately, perfect results are difficult to achieve, but here even limited successes can be very useful.

The goal of orthopaedic control of the protruding premaxilla probably is best conceived as the restraint of further anterior growth of the premaxilla during a period when there is rapid anterior growth of the lateral palatal segments. In other words, an attempt should be made to rein in the premaxilla so that the lateral segments can be allowed to catch up. Treatment should be gentle. Force should not be applied so vigorously to the premaxilla that the septum buckles. Maxillary collapse behind the protruding premaxilla will sabotage the project and must be prevented if any degree of success is to be achieved.

The earlier treatment is started, the better. Sometime during the first week or two of life seems ideal. The failure rate probably rises sharply past this time. One commonly used management technique utilizes gentle restraining pressure applied to the premaxilla with an elastic ribbon attached at earlobe level to a baby bonnet that is held in place with a chin strap (Fig. 29.1). Both ribbon and bonnet can be obtained at an ordinary department store. The elastic strap crossing the premaxilla should be relatively wide and nonirritating. An ordinary rubber band is likely to cut into the prolabium.

An alternative approach uses three segments of adhesive tape, one on the premaxilla and one on each cheek. The segments are connected across the clefts by elastic bands to provide a simple traction device. Care must be taken to avoid irritation of the skin by the adhesive tape. There is no question that these appliances and their many variations have their shortcomings and require patience and perseverance for successful use. Cooperative and intelligent parents are essential.

An intraoral maxillary expansion device can be used concurrently with extraoral strapping to guide catch-up growth of the lateral segments and to prevent their medial collapse behind the protruding premaxilla. There is debate about which is more important, the extraoral strapping or the intraoral appliance. Hotz and Perko (7) report good results using the intraoral appliance alone. Vargervik (6) reported using extraoral strapping alone. Experiences with combined maxillary expansion and premaxillary traction are reported by several authors (8–12). Georgiade et al. (13, 14) have reported on the use of an ingenious pin-fixed intraoral coaxial screw appliance that controls movement of both the premaxilla and the lateral segments.

At this time, data that clearly demonstrate the superiority of any one technique of management over another do not exist. Ross (15) has made a plea for the use of simple and gentle approaches, which he suspects work as well as any and avoid the risks inherent in aggressive treatment.

Lip Repair over a Protruding Premaxilla

There comes a time when maximum benefit from orthopaedic control is reached and the surgeon may be faced with the problem of lip repair over a better positioned but still protruding premaxilla. In our clinic, we seem to reach this point at 10–16 weeks, a time consistent with the observations of Robertson et al. (10). However, Peat (8), Manchester (16), and Hotz and Perko (7) have continued preoperative orthopaedic management longer and have deferred initial lip surgery until 5–6 months of age. At this point, Manchester closed the hard palate and lip in one stage, Hotz and Perko closed only the alveolar process and nostril floor, putting off definitive lip repair still longer.

There are no hard and fast rules to guide the surgeon, who ultimately must face the responsibility of making decisions based on personal experience and assessment of tissues. Aside from possible surgical setback of the premaxilla, the surgeon for the initial operation has three choices: (*a*) lip adhesion; (*b*) unilateral closure to be followed by closure of the remaining side at a later date; and (*c*) bilateral lip closure.

When protrusion of the premaxilla is severe, tissues are scant, and tension on any kind of repair promises to be critical, surgery that establishes continuity of the lip but does not accomplish definitive aesthetic or anatomical correction merits consideration. Surgery of this type commonly is called lip adhesion. It can be carried out in a variety of ways and serves to establish physiological restraining forces on anterior growth of the premaxilla. In essence, it is the ideal extraoral strapping device, although it may accelerate maxillary collapse, a complication that usually can be controlled with an intraoral appliance. So that important tissue is not wasted, it is necessary to plan the adhesion with the definitive repair in mind. Bilateral lip adhesions carried out under tension are inclined to disrupt. Staged adhesion, first on the worse side and subsequently on the other, may be advisable in severe cases. The definitive repair then is put off for a few months or even a few years. Walker et al. (17) and Hamilton et al. (18) were early advocates of this approach, and several others (7, 19, 20) have supported it in principle.

Two-stage closure of first one side and then the other, usually the worse side first, is an alternative to lip adhesion, especially when the repair to be used is of the simplest straight line type. Repair in this way closely resembles staged lip adhesion, but it usually gives a better early or aesthetic result. This is an advantage if one is going to defer definitive correction for a few years. With staged

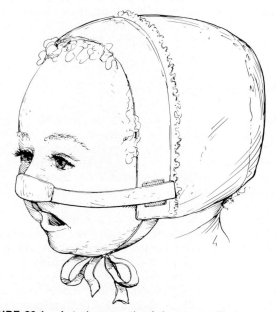

FIGURE 29.1. Anterior growth of the premaxilla is restrained with an elastic strap and baby bonnet. The attachment of the strap to the bonnet should be adjustable to permit change in tension. Molded plastic pillows and soft pads can be added to the strap to distribute pressure evenly on the premaxilla and prolabium.

closure, corrections of the wide prolabium, the short columella, the shallow labial sulcus, and the muscle deficit in the central lip generally are left until later, just as in bilateral lip adhesion. Aside from the fact that the lip must be reentered later for definitive prolabial and columellar revisions, the chief disadvantage of this approach is the problem of maintaining symmetry. Tensions exerted on the lip by the first stage cause distortions that must be compensated for at the second. Although this is a nuisance, it usually can be accomplished satisfactorily. Trusler et al. (21) and Horton et al. (22) have described variations of this technique.

If premaxillary protrusion is moderate, bilateral lip closure usually is possible. The decision depends on the clinical judgment of the surgeon.

Surgical Setback of the Protruding Premaxilla

Surgical setback of the premaxilla as a preliminary step to lip repair is a salvage operation. Occasionally, it may be performed as a primary procedure if the surgeon judges that there is no alternative. Perhaps it is performed better secondarily when conservative maxillary orthopaedics and attempted staged bilateral lip adhesion have failed to establish lip continuity.

Setback of the premaxilla is accomplished by septal resection posterior to the bulbous portion containing the premaxillary-vomerine suture (Fig. 29.2). The resection in profile can be designed as a rectangle (shown) or as a truncated triangle, according to the amount of rotational deformity to be corrected. The goal is to provide just enough correction to make simultaneous lip repair without tension possible. Cronin (23) suggested that the recession be 3–4 mm less than the measured protrusion. Precise immobilization of the retropositioned premaxilla is difficult and probably is not necessary. Wire loops are hard to insert and tighten accurately. Fixation with a Kirschner (K) wire passed in an anterior-to-posterior direction can be treacherous. Our clinic has followed one case, and has heard of others, in which the posterior tip of a K wire migrated intracranially. Fortunately, in the case we saw, the patient never had symptoms; the migration of the wire was discovered on a routine follow-up radiograph, and extraction was accomplished uneventfully with a neurosurgeon standing by. Investigation of old radiographs showed the wire was not improperly positioned by the original surgeon. Presumably, it was forced posteriorly by a forgotten minor accident or by repeated minor movements of incompletely immobilized fragments.

The results of carefully planned and performed setbacks are not as bad as one might expect. Certainly, crude surgery can produce gross retardation of midface growth, but with good work calamity usually can be avoided. Several articles (24–26) and numerous plastic surgeons have reported favorable clinical results. Most orthodontists, however, have tended to be critical. Some clinicians (6, 27, 28), in examining cases available to them, concluded that surgical setback of the premaxilla very clearly retarded midface growth and development and resulted in identifiable midface retrusion. This position is widely supported by knowledgeable dentists.

In fairness to both points of view, it should be stated that the number of patients in any series is small. Furthermore, the variables in the patients, their surgeons, and their orthodontists are enormous, and meaningful controls are not possible. Also, plastic surgeons and orthodontists sometimes base their compromises on different value systems. It is reasonable to conclude that surgical setback should be performed only as a last resort and,

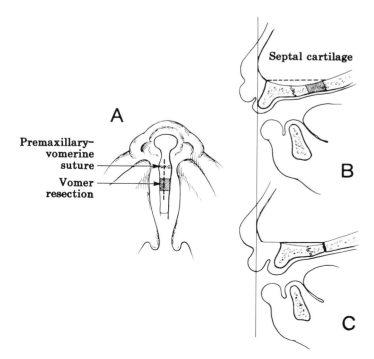

Premaxillary-vomerine suture

Vomer resection

Septal cartilage

FIGURE 29.2. The protruding premaxilla is set back surgically. **A and B,** An appropriately shaped block of vomer is removed posterior to the premaxillary-vomerine suture, and the septal cartilage is incised. **C,** Retrodisplacement of the premaxilla and correction of any malrotation are carried out.

when inevitable, should be carried out as conservatively as possible.

Soft Tissue Repair

COMPLETE CLEFTS

The evolution of bilateral lip repair has been reviewed in detail by Millard in *Cleft Craft* (29), a unique encyclopedia of cleft lip and palate surgery that is likely to stand for a long time as the most comprehensive reference work available. Despite the complexity of the subject, there are certain relatively simple basic principles that can be applied to guide surgeons in performing operations best suited to their own skills, the needs of their patients, and the resources of their cleft palate teams.

Timing

At some time during the first few months of life, most surgeons will repair the lip—perhaps at 10–16 weeks, perhaps later if preliminary adhesions have been carried out or if progress is still being made in conservative management of the protruding premaxilla. Most lips are probably repaired during the first year; however, some surgeons delay longer (19).

Straight Line Repair

Cronin (23), in an important review of the literature and his own experience, summarized the guiding principles of straight line closure. He emphasized that the prolabium should form the full vertical dimension (height) of the central portion of the repaired lip. Although he allowed the introduction of lateral vermilion, he advised against introduction of lateral skin into the prolabium. The prolabium of the unrepaired cleft can appear minute, but it has a surprising ability to stretch. Adding skin to it tends to produce a long lip that is difficult to shorten and gives intrusive scars marring the hoped-for illusion of a philtrum.

In 1957, Cronin and many of his colleagues were confident that the vermilion–cutaneous ridge (white roll) of the prolabium should be preserved to form the central portion of the constructed Cupid's bow. Furthermore, they believed that only vermilion should be introduced from the lateral segments to provide a tubercle inferior to the tiny strip of vermilion usually found on the prolabium. Today, attitudes are more flexible, and it is recognized that, in many cases, more pleasing results can be obtained by bringing lateral vermilion *and white roll* into the prolabium to construct a Cupid's bow. This saves the prolabial vermilion to augment the tubercle inferior to the lateral vermilion flaps. Because the white roll of the prolabium often is faint as compared to that of the lateral segments, this latter method can give a cleaner sweep of white roll by eliminating a central hypoplastic segment. The method also substitutes one fairly easy central white roll approximation for two often difficult paramedian

ones, thereby reducing the incidence of annoying malapproximations of the vermilion–cutaneous ridge. The price for these gains is a fairly obvious skin scar that sometimes results just above the white roll of the central lip. Each surgeon must make his or her own compromises.

The bilateral straight line repair really is little more than an elegant lip adhesion (Fig. 29.3). There are good things to be said for it: it is safe and can be carried out with precision by the experienced plastic surgeon who treats only occasional cases of bilateral cleft; it is forgiving and can be carried out under moderate tension when control of the protruding premaxilla has been disappointing; and it lends itself readily to staging. The bad features are ones of omission: it does not introduce orbicularis oris muscle into the prolabium, where muscle characteristically is absent in complete bilateral clefts; it does not deepen the labial sulcus; it does not shape the prolabium to mimic a philtrum; and it makes no special provision for subsequent lengthening of the columella. The net result is that the lip almost certainly will have to be revised, possibly in stages, by the time the patient reaches school age.

Myoplastic Repair with Provision for Columellar Lengthening

Millard (29, 30) described an operation derived from straight line closure, as advocated by Cronin (23), but designed to correct problems the older operation ignores. The Millard operation is complicated and can be difficult to execute well. It is applied best by experienced cleft surgeons to ideal cases, particularly to cases in which excellent control of the protruding premaxilla has been achieved. Although the operation does not lengthen the columella, it provides for subsequent columellar lengthening without reentry into the lip. This operation is the current touchstone of bilateral complete cleft lip repair (Fig. 29.4).

Technical Modifications

Manchester (16) described a straight line repair that Broadbent and Woolf (31) and others have found useful. In the Manchester operation, a transverse incision in the sulcus allows the prolabium to be lifted off the premaxilla as a superiorly based flap. The prolabial mucosa is released and allowed to drift inferiorly. A tubercle effect is created by augmentation of the prolabium with deepithelialized "tag" flaps without the introduction of additional vermilion. This method is compatible with sulcus deepening and advancement of orbicularis oris into the prolabium as well as with prolabial narrowing and banking of tissues for columellar lengthening. Good contours of the free border of the lip can be obtained. The significant defect is that mucosa can be advanced into a visible position on the prolabium. The resulting appearance can be discordant because vermilion and mucosa have different textures and shades of color. Because mucosa does not tolerate exposure well, chapping also can be an annoying problem in dry or cold climates.

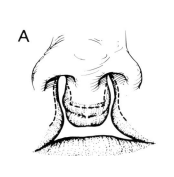

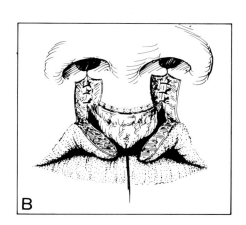

FIGURE 29.3. The simplest type of bilateral straight line lip repair. **A,** Sight judgments guide incision placement. Measurements may be helpful, but the flabbiness of the prolabium tends to make them unreliable. Incisions on the prolabium are gently curved medially to give a little extra length and to reduce the tendency of this repair to give a circular prolabium with trap-door puffiness. **B,** The lip is sutured in three layers; mucosa to mucosa, lateral muscle to prolabial subcutaneous tissue, and skin to skin. **C and D,** The extremely thin vermilion of the prolabium is augmented by lateral vermilion flaps. The lateral flaps may be butted end on or interdigitated to create a vermilion tubercle. Vermilion must be distinguished precisely from mucosa in this difficult step of the repair or an ugly patchwork of mismatched colors and textures will result. **E,** An alternative is the sacrifice of the prolabial white roll and the creation of a Cupid's bow effect by interpolation of both lateral vermilion *and white roll* (see text).

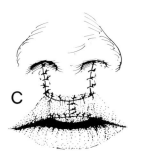

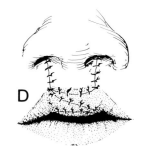

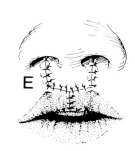

All of these described repairs are interrelated, and features may be adapted from each by the surgeon to fit the needs of an individual patient. The guiding principles are that the tissues be treated gently and that every scrap of tissue be preserved and used to advantage.

Complications

An adhesion or one side of a straight line repair may rarely disrupt, perhaps shortly after the skin sutures are removed. The cause usually is tension produced by a protruding premaxilla that has not responded well to conservative management. When this complication occurs, it is important for the surgeon to keep a cool head. The temptation to perform immediate resuture should be resisted. Suturing of the inflamed and friable tissue is not likely to hold and is likely to cause conspicuous stitch marks that are impossible to revise. There is little point in repeating a failed operation; therefore, a change in plan is indicated. Surgical setback of the premaxilla may be a necessity. If the setback and repeat lip surgery are carried out after tissues have softened, scars of good quality can be expected, and a year or two later one probably will not be able to distinguish the disrupted side from the other.

Scar Quality

Much has been said about the quality of surgical scars. Many surgeons believe that the infant possesses unique healing characteristics that give the scars of primary lip repair a superior quality that can never again be equaled. Other surgeons are skeptical of this theory, and at this time it is neither proved nor disproved. The important point is that if, through foresight and advance planning, a surgeon can perform an initial repair that avoids reentry into the lip, he or she would be foolish not to do so. However, there may be times when the surgeon, after thinking problems through, will find reentry into the lip necessary. In such cases, the surgeon should proceed without guilt and anticipate a pleasing long-term result, although months of annoying scar maturation must be expected.

INCOMPLETE AND ASYMMETRICAL CLEFTS

Incomplete bilateral lip clefts occur in infinite variety from forms that closely resemble complete clefts to *formes frustes,* which closely resemble normal lips. Asymmetries range from minor degrees to the extreme of a complete cleft on one side and a *forme fruste* on the other. Fortunately, in incomplete and asymmetrical clefts, there is at least some tissue continuity on one side, and this partially restrains forward growth of the premaxilla. As a result, the protruding premaxilla usually is not the problem that it is in complete bilateral clefts. In incomplete clefts, the surgeon must adapt techniques of unilateral and bilateral cleft lip repair to suit the particular requirements of the individual patient.

If a philtral dimple is present with a true Cupid's bow, which may be a bit offset in alignment, then bilateral

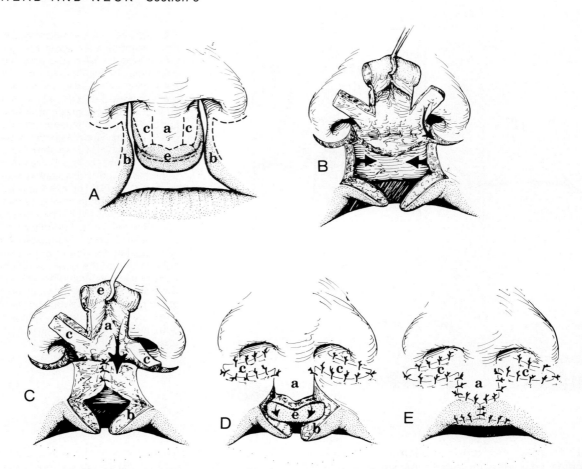

FIGURE 29.4. Basic myoplastic repair with provision for later columellar lengthening. **A,** Incisions are made that narrow the prolabium to mimic a philtrum (*flap a*) and preserve the lateral excesses (*flaps c*) as "whisker" flaps to be banked and used subsequently for columellar lengthening. The prolabial white roll is discarded by an incision that shapes the inferior margin of flap a into the central portion of a Cupid's bow. This incision must be shallow because the subcutaneous attachments of *flap e* to *flap a* must be preserved. The lateral vermilion *flaps b* carry lateral white roll with them. **B,** The prolabial flaps *a, c,* and *e* are released *en bloc* from the underlying premaxilla by an incision placed in the rudimentary labial sulcus and shown as a dotted line along the inferior margin of flap e in A. This step allows the sulcus to be deepened at the time of lip repair but converts flap e to a subcutaneously based island pedicle. Less courageous surgeons may prefer to omit this step and deepen the sulcus at a later time, perhaps at the time of palate repair or columellar lengthening. **C and D,** The lip then is repaired in three separately dissected layers. Lateral mucosa is closed to lateral mucosa in the midline if the sulcus is to be deepened, or to prolabial mucosa if it is not. Lateral muscle is closed to lateral muscle in the midline. Skin then is draped for surface repair. **E,** The completed repair shows the c flaps banked as "whiskers" in incisions made along the nostril sills; the Cupid's bow effect created by the lateral b flaps, which include vermilion and white roll; and a tubercle effect created by flap e. The c flaps will be used subsequently for columellar lengthening by a modified forked flap technique.

adaptation of unilateral lip repair techniques may be helpful. In these cases, it may be convenient to begin with the less severe side and then move on to try to make the more severe side match. An annoying problem here can be a shortage of lateral vermilion to interpolate across a vermilion notch for plumping up a thin tubercle. A good vermilion contour may be difficult to achieve in minimal clefts.

If there is no philtral dimple, if the prolabium is flabby and devoid of muscle, or if the vermilion-cutaneous ridge is hypoplastic with no trace of a defined Cupid's bow, then adaptation of a bilateral lip repair technique may become the procedure of choice. A decision must be made as to whether or not eventual columellar lengthening will be required. If it will be, tissue should be reserved for the purpose. If it will not be, planning can be simpli-

fied (Fig. 29.5). In asymmetrical clefts of this more severe type, there will be a disconcerting tendency for repair to result in the less severely cleft side being too long. The treatment for this problem is shortening the less severely cleft side by transverse wedge excision of the lateral segment along the nostril sill. In these cases, it usually is convenient to work with the worse side first and then repair the less severe side to match. Here too, shortage of lateral vermilion for prolabial augmentation may be a problem.

Columellar Lengthening

The short columella is an integral part of the bilateral cleft lip anomaly. In complete and many incomplete

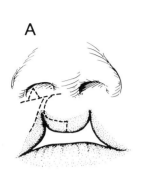

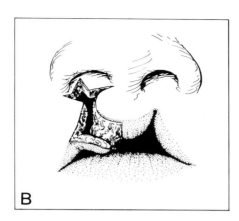

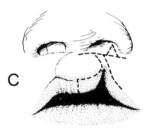

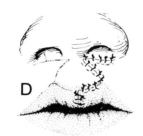

FIGURE 29.5. Repair of a bilateral incomplete cleft lip in which columellar length already is adequate, as described by Millard (29). Note wedge excisions to narrow the nostril floors. In some cases, it might be useful to leave the nostril floors broad in order to allow for the subsequent use of the excess tissue in a Cronin columellar lengthening operation. Discrepancies in lip length can be equalized by transverse excision of lateral flap tissue along the nostril floor and by appropriate rotations of the prolabium as in unilateral rotation-advancement repair. To avoid an undesirably long lip, it is wise to leave at least a sliver of connection between the columella and prolabium. When the configuration of the cleft allows preservation of only a minimal connection between prolabium and columella, the repair should be carried out in two operations a month apart, first on one side and then on the other. Otherwise, necrosis of the prolabium secondary to compromise of blood supply may result.

cases, columellar lengthening eventually will be necessary. Primary lip repairs should be carried out with this problem in mind. Columellar lengthening can be performed by the interpolation of local flaps, the transfer of distant flaps, and the introduction of free composite grafts. However, the best results are achieved by the advancement of local tissue, either from the nostril sill as described by Cronin (32) or from the lip as described by Millard (33). Any advancement from the lip must preserve the prolabium and work through existing lip scars. Operations advancing the entire prolabium into the columella are obsolete. The Cronin and Millard operations have won wide acceptance because they provide good results with smooth contours and unobtrusive scars.

TECHNIQUES

The Cronin operation for the bilateral cleft lip nasal deformity is akin to the widely used nostril rotations for the unilateral deformity described by Gillies and Kilner (34) and subsequently much modified by many surgeons. Overcorrection with disagreeable nostril exposure is difficult to achieve. Alar base corrections can be carried out simultaneously. Usually reentry into the lip along old scar lines is required to tailor out fullness produced by medial advancement of the alar bases (Fig. 29.6).

The Millard operation often permits greater correction, even overcorrection. Its principal disadvantages are that healing problems and contour irregularities can occur at the base of the lengthened columella where the tips of five flaps meet (Fig. 29.7). These difficulties are lessened when the forked flaps are banked adjacent to the nostril sills at the time of primary lip repair.

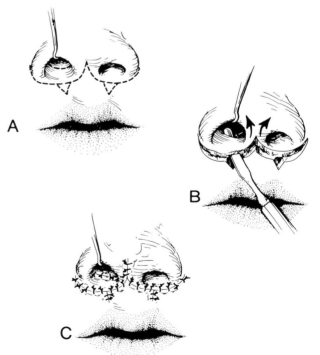

FIGURE 29.6. The Cronin columellar lengthening operation. **A and B,** Through appropriate incisions, the nasal floor and alar bases are mobilized on each side as bipedicled flaps. It is desirable to carry the incision in the floor of the vestibule deep laterally so that the lateral base of each flap is thicker than the medial. This incision also is carried along the caudal margin of the quadrilateral cartilage to permit generous mobilization of the columella and nasal tip from the septum. **C,** Rotation of the nostrils lengthens the columella and narrows the distance between the alar bases. Darts must be taken from the upper lip to compensate for this latter correction.

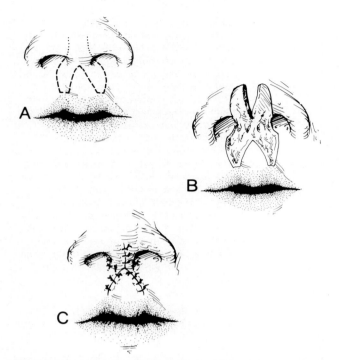

FIGURE 29.7. The Millard forked flap columellar lengthening operation. **A,** The forked flap is elevated from the prolabium along existing scar lines or from the banked "whisker" position (see Fig. 29.4). **B,** The dissection is continued to release the short columella from the caudal margin of the septum. **C,** The forked flaps are advanced into the columella, and the donor defects are closed.

The columella also can be lengthened from the dorsum. The "gull wing" operation described by Brauer and Foerster (35) is one of the best known corrections of this type.

Mulliken (36) has proposed an interesting columellar lengthening in which banked forked flaps are transposed intranasally and the alar cartilages are repositioned to give projection to the tip. He has not yet published long-term follow-up information.

TIMING

Lengthening of the columella by tissue advancement from the nostril sills or lip necessarily requires that the connection between columella and lip be divided. Changes in lip posture can result, often with apparent lip lengthening as pointed out by Millard (29). It probably is helpful to deal with this potential problem by deferring columellar lengthening until facial features, especially the jaws, are fairly mature and problems with the underlying dental arch have stabilized.

Another timing consideration is psychological. Children during the "terrible twos, threes, and fours" seem to have few concerns about appearance and are not interested in aesthetic refinements. In addition, they find hospitalization threatening and respond by being difficult and uncooperative patients. Elective facial revisions are inappropriate at this time. However, as children enter kinder-

garten and first grade, they become aware of differences and become concerned about appearance and peer pressure. Treated sympathetically and stressed cautiously, they can become willing and cooperative patients. For reasons both anatomical and emotional, these latter years are good ones for carrying out revisions in preparation for the competitive school life ahead.

Occasionally, a child who is a candidate for columellar lengthening or some other facial revision also is a candidate for a pharyngeal flap. The operation to improve speech should take precedence over the one to improve appearance.

Miscellaneous Revisionary Operations

After primary lip repair and columellar lengthening have been completed, residual irregularities may persist. These irregularities usually can be corrected in modest touch-up revisions that are individualized to suit the patient.

VERMILION

The most common vermilion problem encountered is residual thinness or notching of the central portion—the "whistle" deformity. Various V-Y advancements and Z interpolations have been designed to improve the contour, often at the expense of exposing mucosa. The bilateral pendulum flap operation described by Kapetansky (37, 38) avoids exposure of mucosa by augmenting thin central vermilion with the often redundant lateral vermilion.

CUPID'S BOW

Because it has no philtral dimple and no sign of philtral columns, the complete bilateral cleft lip has not even a vestige of a true Cupid's bow. Cupid's bow effects must be created by surgical draping of the vermilion–cutaneous ridge. The effects are not always successful; the most common defect is that of the white roll extending as an unbroken arc from commissure to commissure. Operations such as the one described by Gillies and Kilner (34), which create bow effects by advancing vermilion superiorly to an artistically drawn line after sacrifice of intervening white roll and skin, tend to produce unnatural, painted-on effects. Usually, better results can be obtained by the composite advancement superiorly of both vermilion and white roll after low excisions of skin just above the roll. Vecchione (39) described a modification in which the white roll is transposed as a bipedicled flap and skin and vermilion are repositioned as free grafts. Operations that change the position of the white roll may be especially useful if they can be limited to short segments with avoidance of long and possibly conspicuous skin scars.

If vermilion–cutaneous ridge flaps are intolerable and cannot be solved by minor adjustments, as in those cases in which the prolabium has been sacrificed and the white roll consists of just the two lateral segments meeting at a single peak in the midline, an Abbé cross-lip flap merits serious consideration. This operation is remarkably safe but can be difficult to execute artistically. Fortunately, current high standards of primary repair have made Abbé flap revisions rarely indicated today. The experience of the University of Pittsburgh Cleft Palate Center with this operation has been reviewed by Garrett and Musgrave (40).

PHILTRUM

The philtral dimple and its defining columns are subtle structures that to date have defied precise construction by plastic surgical techniques. In the normal lip, superficial fibers of the orbicularis oris muscle enter laterally and meet fibers from the opposite side near the midline to form a compact intermingling revealed as the dimple. They then proceed to insert in the skin of the opposite side to produce a column. Detailed descriptions of this anatomy have been published (41–43). The surgeon can thin deep tissues to create a dimple and can augment with dermal and other deepithelialized flaps to produce columns, and such efforts are worthy. However, the caution must be made that delicate, meticulously executed operations may make no discernible difference. In addition, aggressive surgery may produce gross lumps and depressions more disturbing to the beholder than a flat prolabium. Arriving at the appropriate compromise is difficult.

Even if a detailed dimple with delicate columns cannot be achieved, the prolabium at least should be tailored to mimic a philtrum. The scars of repair should suggest columns, and although they may curve medially, they should never bow laterally to give a circular prolabium predisposed to trap-door effect.

Revision to achieve the ideal may not be easy, largely because of the tendency of revisions to add undesirably to lip length. Tailoring lip length by shortening excisions along the nostril sill may be necessary and gives incisions similar to bilateral rotation-advancement repair; however, rotational lengthening of the prolabium usually should be avoided. If one is going to perform extensive revisions of the skin repair in a lip in which muscle repair has never been carried out, serious thought should be given to simultaneous muscle repair in an attempt to avoid recurrent prolabial distortion from tension caused by unopposed action of the lateral muscle segments.

MUSCLE

In recent years, there has been considerable interest in the role of muscle in lip repair. It has long been recognized that the prolabium in complete clefts contains no muscle; however, the prolabium in incomplete clefts contains muscle inversely proportional in amount to the severity of the cleft. This finding is consistent with the observation that muscle in embryonic development enters the prolabium from the lateral lip segments and is impeded from doing so by a cleft. Failure to introduce mus-

cle into the prolabium at the time of bilateral cleft lip repair can produce several problems: noticeable lack of animation in the central portion of the lip; bulging of the lateral segment masses, which lack normal drape and opposing forces; excessive stretching of the prolabium; and spreading of the scars of repair, which bear the strain of unopposed activity of the lateral muscle segments. Several authors (44–46) have described the use of the Millard primary myoplastic lip repair as a secondary or revisionary operation when failure to carry out early repair of the muscle has produced identifiable problems. If failure to perform a primary muscle repair has not led to identifiable problems, there is no need to intervene.

SUPERIOR LABIAL SULCUS

Although establishment of a good superior labial sulcus at the time of primary lip repair may be difficult, at the time revisions are considered, there usually is enough mucosa available to permit sulcus deepening by mucosal flap advancements and interpolations. Only rarely is free grafting necessary.

NOSE

Even after the short columella has been lengthened, the patient with a bilateral cleft lip is likely to have serious problems with nasal appearance, particularly in the tip, which may be large, thick skinned, poorly projecting, and lacking in details. Treatment of these problems utilizes rhinoplasty techniques that are not exclusive to the cleft field and hence are beyond the range of this discussion. It is worth noting, however, that the open rhinoplasty now enjoying widespread revival is proving indispensable in secondary cleft surgery because it permits meticulous shaping of the existing cartilages and precise placement and fixation of cartilage grafts. Puckett and Wells (47) and Daniel (48) have published recent reviews and innovations.

Conclusion

In the long-range management of the bilateral cleft lip, the many variables and uncertainties present make treatment as much an art as it is a science. Wilson (49) emphasized that each patient has a unique combination of deformities and management requires the individualized modification and combination of various surgical operations. Just as the patients are diverse, the results are variable. This fact was emphasized by Pruzansky (50), who in a general reference to all aspects of cleft management pointed out that "even within a single cleft type there is sufficient variation between patients to affect prognosis."

References

1. Atherton JD: The natural history of the bilateral cleft. *Angle Orthod* 44:269, 1974.

2. Scott J: The cartilage of the nasal septum. *Br Dent J* 95:37, 1953.
3. Friede H, Pruzansky S: Longitudinal study of growth in bilateral cleft lip and palate from infancy to adolescence. *Plast Reconstr Surg* 49:392, 1972.
4. Ross RB, Johnston M: *Cleft Lip and Palate.* Baltimore, Williams & Wilkins, 1972, p 84.
5. Latham R: Development and structure of the premaxillary deformity in bilateral cleft lip and palate. *Br J Plast Surg* 26:1, 1973.
6. Vargervik K: Growth characteristics of the premaxilla and orthodontic principles in bilateral cleft lip and palate. *Cleft Palate J* 20:289, 1983.
7. Hotz M, Perko M: Early management of bilateral total cleft lip and palate. *Scand J Plast Reconstr Surg* 8:104, 1974.
8. Peat J: Early orthodontic treatment for complete clefts. *Am J Orthod* 65:28, 1974.
9. Peat J: Effects of presurgical oral orthopedics on bilateral complete clefts of the lip and palate. *Cleft Palate J* 19:100, 1982.
10. Robertson N, Shaw W, Valp C: The changes produced by presurgical orthopedic treatment of bilateral cleft lip and palate. *Plast Reconstr Surg* 59:86, 1977.
11. Reisberg D, Figueroa A, Gold H: An intraoral appliance for management of the protrusive premaxilla in bilateral cleft lip. *Cleft Palate J* 25:53, 1988.
12. Rutrick R, Black P, Jurkiewicz M: Bilateral cleft lip and palate: Presurgical treatment. *Ann Plast Surg* 12:105, 1984.
13. Georgiade N, Latham R: Maxillary arch alignment in the bilateral cleft lip and palate infant, using the pinned coaxial screw appliance. *Plast Reconstr Surg* 56:52, 1975.
14. Georgiade N, Mason R, Riefkhol R, Georgiade G, Barwick W: Preoperative positioning of the protruding premaxilla in the bilateral cleft lip patient. *Plast Reconstr Surg* 83:32, 1989.
15. Ross RB: Discussion of preoperative positioning of the protruding premaxilla in the bilateral cleft lip patient. *Plast Reconstr Surg* 83:39, 1989.
16. Manchester W: The repair of double cleft lip as part of an integrated program. *Plast Reconstr Surg* 45:207, 1970.
17. Walker J, Collito M, Mancusi-Ungaro A, Meijer R: Physiologic considerations in cleft lip closure: The C-W technique. *Plast Reconstr Surg* 37:552, 1966.
18. Hamilton R, Graham W, Randall P: The role of the lip adhesion procedure in cleft lip repair. *Cleft Palate J* 8:1, 1971.
19. Spina V, Kamakura L, Lapa F: Surgical management of bilateral cleft lip. *Ann Plast Surg* 1:497, 1978.
20. Rintala A, Haataja J: The effect of the lip adhesion procedure on the alveolar arch. *Scand J Plast Reconstr Surg* 13:301, 1979.
21. Trusler H, Bauer T, Tondra J: The cleft lip–cleft palate problem. *Plast Reconstr Surg* 16:174, 1955.
22. Horton C, Adamson J, Mladick R, Taddeo R: The upper lip sulcus in cleft lip. *Plast Reconstr Surg* 45:31, 1970.
23. Cronin T: Surgery of the double lip and protruding premaxilla. *Plast Reconstr Surg* 19:389, 1957.
24. McDowell F: Late results after long term growth in cleft lip repairs. *Plast Reconstr Surg* 38:444, 1966.
25. Monroe C, Griffith B, McKinney P, Rosenstein S, Jacobson B: Surgical recession of the premaxilla and its effect on maxillary growth in patients with bilateral clefts. *Cleft Palate J* 7:784, 1970.
26. Cronin T, Penoff J: Bilateral clefts of the primary palate. *Cleft Palate J* 8:349, 1971.
27. Bishara S, Olin W: Surgical repositioning of the premaxilla in complete bilateral cleft lip and palate. *Angle Orthod* 42:139, 1972.
28. Friede H, Pruzansky S: Long-term effects of premaxillary setback on facial skeletal profile in complete bilateral cleft lip and palate. *Cleft Palate J* 22:97, 1985.
29. Millard DR: *Cleft Craft: Bilateral and Rare Deformities, Vol II.* Boston, Little, Brown and Co, 1977.
30. Millard DR: Closure of bilateral cleft lip and elongation of columella by two operations in infancy. *Plast Reconstr Surg* 47:324, 1971.
31. Broadbent TR, Woolf R: Bilateral cleft lip repairs. *Plast Reconstr Surg* 50:36, 1972.
32. Cronin T: Lengthening columella by use of skin from nasal floor and alae. *Plast Reconstr Surg* 21:417, 1958.
33. Millard DR: Columella lengthening by a forked flap. *Plast Reconstr Surg* 22:454, 1958.
34. Gillies H, Kilner TP: Hare-lip: Operations for correction of secondary deformities. *Lancet* 223:1369, 1932.
35. Brauer R, Foerster D: Another method to lengthen the columella in the double cleft patient. *Plast Reconstr Surg* 38:27, 1966.
36. Mulliken J: Principles and techniques of bilateral complete cleft lip repair. *Plast Reconstr Surg* 75:477, 1985.
37. Kapetansky D: Double pendulum flaps for whistling deformities in bilateral cleft lips. *Plast Reconstr Surg* 47:321, 1971.
38. Kapetansky D: Animation and cosmetic balance in repair of congenital bilateral cleft lip: A modified technique. *Cleft Palate J* 11:219, 1974.
39. Vecchione T: Construction of the Cupid's bow. *Plast Reconstr Surg* 65:830, 1980.
40. Garrett W, Musgrave R: The Abbé flap: A twenty year cumulative experience. In Georgiade NG, Hagerty RF (eds): *Symposium on Management of Cleft Lip and Palate and Associated Deformities.* St. Louis, CV Mosby, 1974, p 295.
41. Monie I, Cacciatore A. The development of the philtrum. *Plast Reconstr Surg* 30:313, 1962.
42. Latham R, Deaton T: The structural basis of the philtrum and the contour of the vermilion border: A study of the musculature of the upper lip. *J Anat* 121:151, 1976.
43. Briedis J, Jackson I. The anatomy of the philtrum: Observations made on dissections in the normal lip. *Br J Plast Surg* 34:128, 1981.
44. Oneal R, Greer D, Nobel G: Secondary correction of bilateral cleft lip deformities with Millard's midline muscular closure. *Plast Reconstr Surg* 54:45, 1974.
45. Lehman J: Secondary repair of bilateral cleft lip deformities: A two-stage approach. *Br J Plast Surg* 29:116, 1976.
46. Meijer R: Secondary repair of the bilateral cleft lip deformity. *Cleft Palate J* 21:86, 1984.
47. Puckett CL, Wells HG: The gull wing incision in cleft lip rhinoplasty. *Cleft Palate J* 24:163, 1987.
48. Daniel R: Rhinoplasty: Creating an aesthetic tip. A preliminary report. *Plast Reconstr Surg* 80:775, 1987.
49. Wilson L: Correction of residual deformities of the lip and nose in repaired clefts of the primary palate (lip and alveolus). *Clin Plast Surg* 12:719, 1985.
50. Pruzansky S: Description, classification and analysis of unoperated clefts of the lip and palate. *Am J Orthod* 39:590, 1953.

30

Cleft Palate

Bruce S. Bauer, M.D., F.A.C.S. and Frank A. Vicari, M.D.

Under normal conditions, the palate functions in concert with the pharyngeal musculature to close the velopharyngeal valve. Clefting of the palate results in an absence of velopharyngeal closure and the inability to build up and sustain intraoral pressure. This has significant effects on both early feeding and the development of normal speech. In addition, the abnormal muscle anatomy present in cleft palate has an indirect effect on the function of the middle ear through the resultant anatomical disturbance present along the eustachian tube orifice from which the primary palatal muscles originate.

Before discussing the clinical aspects of cleft palate care and treatment, this chapter will review the normal and abnormal embryology, classification, possible etiologies, incidence, genetics, and palatal anatomy of the condition.

Embryology

The embryonic and fetal growth processes that are active in the development of the human face and cranium are of considerable interest with respect to both normal and abnormal development. Much of what we know and understand of these processes comes from study of non-mammalian species; the basic mechanisms active in the formation of the facial structures are similar, and much can be learned from the continued study of these models.

Normal development is dependent on mesodermal reinforcement of the two-layered ectodermal branchial membrane in the facial region (1, 2). This facial mesenchyme has its origin in neuroectoderm bordering the neural tube and migrates in three directions: anteriorly over the developing brain and around either side of the developing stomodeum (3).

While recent studies of human embryos have raised questions as to whether both the frontonasal process and neural crest cell migration exist in humans as we recognize them in other species (4–6), there is little doubt that facial development involves a complex interaction of cell proliferation, cell differentiation, cell movement, and cell death (2, 4). The ultimate product of this complex balance of processes is the development of normal facial structures. If the balance is disrupted, facial structures may be cleft, malpositioned, or even absent. Our understanding of the pathogenesis of clefting is still rudimentary, but it is best viewed in relation to the normal development of both primary and secondary palates.

Normal Development

PRIMARY PALATE

The cells of the anterior neural crest that give rise to the developing upper lip must arrive in their proper location at the appropriate time and in adequate numbers for the lip to develop normally. For the upper lip, these events are occurring between the 4th and 7th weeks of gestation (2, 7).

At the 4th week, the oral plate ruptures to establish continuity between the oral cavity and the foregut. At the same time, the nasal placodes appear cephalad to the oral cavity. As mesoderm is heaped up on either side of the paired nasal structures forming the medial and lateral nasal processes, the nasal pits begin to burrow deeper to create the nasal airways. Simultaneously, neuroectoderm is migrating anteriorly around the head in both directions to reinforce the maxillary processes. The migration continues medially until mesoderm streams into the intermaxillary (premaxillary) segment at the midline. The two medial nasal processes ultimately join to form the single definitive nose and contribute to the development of the nasal septum, columella, premaxilla, and philtrum. The lateral nasal process gives rise to the nasal alae (5).

In the upper lip, the mesoderm arrives to "fill out" the bilamellar branchial membrane first in the area of the incisive foramen. Additional mesoderm is then successively deposited, first anteriorly and then inferiorly, effecting closure of the nostril still followed by the lip, down to and including the vermilion (2).

Once the mesoderm has completed its migration and reinforcement of the entire primary palate (all structures anterior to the incisive foramen), the early facial structures are refined by a process of ectodermal sculpting wherein cells proliferate, move into areas, carve furrows, dig cavities, and hollow tunnels. This sculpting is accomplished through a sequence of cell polarization, followed by further differentiation (and alignment) of those cells close enough to the basement membrane to be nourished by transudate, and cell death of those farthest from the source of nourishment. This sculpting separates the dental lamina within the developing alveolus from the lip, thereby creating the alveolar-labial sulcus. It is also responsible for the deepening of the nasal pits and the lateral rupture of the buccal pharyngeal membrane.

Finally, at the 7th week, after all essential mesoderm has been deposited, additional "late-arriving" mesoderm migrates from each lateral side and piles up in the center of the prolabium and thickens to form the parallel philtral ridges (2).

SECONDARY PALATE

The formation of the secondary palate also involves a complex interaction of cell growth, differentiation, and movement. These processes occur during the 7th through 12th weeks of embryonic life and differ significantly from those that occur during earlier development of the lip.

The palatal shelves arise as outgrowths of the maxillary processes of the first branchial arch as migrating mesoderm bulges outward against the ectodermal surface. Initially, the palatal shelves lie caudally alongside the tongue (in the sagittal plane). This vertical orientation is maintained as long as the relatively large mass of developing tongue sits between the shelves in the small oral cavity.

With growth, the head begins to extend and the tongue drops downward, first posteriorly (at its base) and then progressively toward the tongue tip. As this occurs, the palatal shelves move toward the horizontal (axial) plane above the tongue. The posterior shelves reach the horizontal position first, followed by the middle and finally by the anterior portions adjacent to the incisive foramen (1, 3).

Once the palatal shelves reach the horizontal plane, they begin to fuse or merge in the midline. This occurs through a true process of fusion, unlike the mesodermal penetration process occurring in the primary palate. Contact of the opposing shelves is followed by adherence and then ectodermal degeneration at the contact points. A new ectodermal layer is formed over the fused palatal midline, and mesoderm merges beneath it.

Although fusion occurs primarily from anterior to posterior, it begins initially at a third of the way posterior, in the region of the hard palate, not at the incisive foramen. Fusion then proceeds up to the incisive foramen and back to the uvula. This may explain the rare findings of either a congenital fistula of the anterior hard palate or an epithelial cyst in a similar location.

Pathogenesis of Cleft Lip and Palate

PRIMARY PALATE

The normal development of the lip, as noted, is dependent on the maxillary processes and then progresses toward the midline, then overgrowing the medial nasal contribution of the intermaxillary/frontonasal process. This reinforcement of the central lip requires mesoderm of sufficient quantity, arriving at the appropriate time. When mesoderm is of insufficient quantity, the unreinforced bilamellar branchial membrane ruptures, and a cleft results. If there is total failure of mesodermal penetration, there is a complete cleft extending back to the incisive foramen (complete cleft of the primary palate). If mesoderm is present but insufficient, partial clefting occurs. Minimal deficiency in quantity may result in notching of the vermilion, a subcutaneous furrow, or an isolated thinning of the nostril still (2, 7).

Because mesoderm is programmed to arrive in the area of the incisive foramen prior to the nostril still, mid-lip, and vermilion, any event that slows mesodermal migration will affect the lower portions of the lip more than the area of the nostril floor. Failure of migration bilaterally will obviously result in a bilateral cleft, and asymmetrical clefts can be explained as a variable delay in medial migration of the reinforcing layer (2).

The fact that the fetal head is initially turned to the right and the left side is dependent may increase the time necessary to complete migration on the left side. This relative delay in left-sided migration may partially explain the increased incidence of left-sided clefts relative to right-sided clefts.

Finally, the process of ectodermal sculpting appears to be active late in the sequence of events leading to formation of a normal lip. Because it is dependent on the prior arrival of mesoderm, it will not occur in cases of complete clefting. Here, the mesodermal contribution to the premaxilla is absent. Therefore, in complete bilateral clefts, the refinement of an alveolar-labial sulcus and philtrum are absent.

SECONDARY PALATE

Formation of the normal secondary palate is also dependent on sufficient mesoderm and precise timing of its movement in the palatal shelf. Even in the presence of sufficient mesoderm, the palatal shelves will not reach one another in the midline if the tongue fails to move out of the way. This simple mechanical obstruction appears to explain those clefts associated with an abnormally small mandible and malpositioned tongue mass (e.g., Pierre Robin sequence) (1).

When no obvious obstruction exists to prevent palatal shelf movement from the vertical to the horizontal plane, it appears that clefting results from a failure of fusion alone. Total failure of adherence and fusion will result in a complete cleft from the incisive foramen back to the uvula, and a lesser degree of failure will result in an incomplete cleft. Because fusion is apparently preceded by a transient adherence of the palatal shelves, rupture occurring immediately after adherence may explain the occasional appearance of epithelial pearls in the cleft margin.

Finally, because adherence and fusion are followed by a merging of mesoderm from the opposing shelves, the concept of fusion of the shelves without mesodermal merging appears to explain the origin of a submucous cleft palate. This cleft variant may likewise be explained on the basis of fusion occurring in normal sequence but with mesenchyme in short supply.

Classification

On the basis of the distinctive embryological formation of the primary and secondary palate, clefts can be classi-

Table 30.1.
Classification of Cleft Palates

Clefts of first degree palate	Unilateral or bilateral, complete or incomplete
Clefts of second degree palate	Incomplete or complete
Clefts of first and second degree palate	Unilateral or bilateral, complete or incomplete

fied as shown in Table 30.1. Diagrammatically, for the simplification of record keeping, clefts can be represented by the striped-Y logo shown in Figure 30.1 (8).

Etiology of Cleft Lip and Palate

Various hypotheses have been advanced for the occurrence of facial clefting. In some 25% of cases, there is a family history, which does not follow either a normal recessive or dominant pattern. The condition appears to be multifactorial. It has been suggested that some cases of clefting are due to an overall reduction in the volume of the facial mesenchyme, which leads to clefting by virtue of failure of mesodermal penetration. In some cases, clefting appears associated with increased facial width, either alone or in association with encephalocele or with idiopathic hypertelorism or the presence of a teratoma. The characteristic U-shaped cleft of the Pierre Robin anomaly is thought to be dependent upon a persistent high position of the tongue, perhaps associated with a failure or delay of neck extension. This prevents descent of the tongue, which in turn, prevents elevation and a medial growth of the palatal shelves. Distortion of the facial processes or malposition resulting from oligohydramnios has been suggested as another possible etiological factor. The production of clefts of the secondary palate in experimental animals has frequently been accomplished by drug administration. The agents commonly used are steroids, anticonvulsants, diazepam, and aminopterin. There is some suggestion that phenytoin and diazepam may also be factors in causing clefting in humans. Infections during the first trimester of pregnancy, such as rubella or toxoplasmosis, have been associated with clefting.

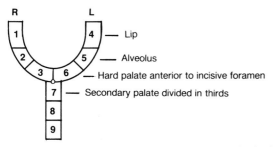

FIGURE 30.1. Classification of cleft lip and palate is depicted.

Incidence

It is difficult to determine the exact incidence of clefting because methods of obtaining data differ so markedly in different reports. It would appear that some degree of clefting occurs in approximately 1:600 to 1:1,000 live births in this country. Clefting is much more common in stillborns and abortuses (9, 10).

The incidence of clefting varies with race. It is estimated to be 1:750 in Caucasians, 1:2,000 in blacks, and 1:5,000 live births in orientals. Racial variation appears to be more marked in cleft lip with or without cleft palate (CL ± P) than in cleft palate (CP) alone.

Complete clefts of the primary and secondary palate are more common than isolated clefts of the primary palate alone in a ratio of 2:1. There are also significant differences in the incidence of CL ± P versus CP in the two sexes. CL ± P occurs twice as commonly in males as in females, whereas the exact reverse is true in clefts of the secondary palate, which occur twice as frequently in females as in males.

Complete clefts of the lip and palate are twice as common on the left side as on the right, although there is no known reason for this difference. The comparative frequency of unilateral clefts on the left versus unilateral clefts on the right versus bilateral clefts is 6:3:1. In a large cleft palate population, the distribution of types of clefting has been reported as 21% CL, 46% CL + P, and 33% CP.

Clefts may be considered as falling into one of three groups: genetic, environmental, and syndromic. A family history is twice as common in CL ± P as it is in CP. CP appears to be more commonly environmental than hereditary. Other associated congenital anomalies are seen in 29% of cases of clefting. More commonly, these other anomalies are associated with isolated CP rather than with CL ± P. As an isolated deformity, CP occurs slightly more frequently than CL ± P, but the majority of cases of CL ± P are isolated deformities. There are more than 150 syndromes described in which clefting may be a feature. CP alone is more commonly associated with a syndrome than is CL ± P.

The incidence of short stature in cleft patients has been noted to be 40 times that of the general population. Possibly, the midline clefting is associated with a disturbance in development of the anterior pituitary from Rathke's pouch.

Some association has been found between low socioeconomic status and an increased incidence of facial clefting, and it has been suggested that this is possibly related to less than adequate nutrition. However, isolated cleft cases environmentally appear to be significantly associated with higher socioeconomic status.

Inheritance

Once a child with a cleft is born into a family, the chances of clefting occurring increases significantly for subsequent siblings. It appears, therefore, that from the point of view of inheritance, CL ± P and CP follow different patterns (9–11). The figures for inheritance are given in Table 30.2.

Recent investigations suggest that, if the initial form of clefting in the family is of a severe extent, the chances of further clefts appearing in subsequent family members is greater than when the initial degree of clefting is minor (11).

Van der Woude's syndrome represents an important variation for the genetic guidelines listed in Table 30.2. It is an autosomal dominant disorder with lower lip pits in association with different degrees of lip and palatal clefting. There is a 70–80% risk of lip pits and a 40–50% chance for clefting of the lip and/or palate in families with this syndrome. Submucous clefting of the palate should be looked for in the absence of other signs of overt clefts when detailing the pedigree of a family with Van der Woude's syndrome.

Submucous cleft palate, nonsyndromal, has an incidence of approximately 1:1,200 live births. However, only about 10% of children with submucous clefts of the palate have speech problems; therefore, the condition may go undetected throughout life and the incidence could, in fact, be higher.

Table 30.2.
Cleft Lip and Cleft Palate Inheritance Risks

	Genetic Guidance
Cleft lip and palate (CL + P)	
Normal parents and 1 child with CL ± P	4% risk of another child with CL ± P
Normal parents and 1 affected child and positive family history	4% risk
Normal parents and affected child and child with additional anomaly	2% risk
Normal parents and 2 affected children	4% risk
Parent with CL ± P and no affected children	4% risk
Parent with CL ± P and child with CL ± P	14–17% risk
Cleft palate (CP)	
Normal parents and child with CP	2% risk of affected child
Normal parents and child with CP and positive family history	7% risk
Normal parents and child with CP and another anomaly	2% risk
Normal parents and 2 children with CP	1% risk
Parent with CP and no affected child	2–4% risk
Parent with CP and child with CP	15% risk

Anatomy of the Palate—Normal and in Clefting

The three muscles of the palate work in concert with the pharyngeal muscles to produce velopharyngeal closure. The tensor veli palatini muscles arise from the membranous wall of the eustachian tube. Their tendons pass around the hamular processes of the pterygoid and insert into the palatine aponeurosis. The levator veli palatini muscles also have their origin along the eustachian tube orifice. They meet in the midline in a sling-like fashion above and behind the aponeurosis. The musculus uvulae is a small midline muscle sitting above and behind the levator sling.

The vascular supply of the palate arises from the palatine vessels (greater and lesser) and from posterior septal contributions through the incisive foramen. Sensation is supplied by the maxillary division of the trigeminal nerve by way of the pterygopalatine and nasopalatine foramina. There is a dual motor innervation with motor branches of the trigeminal nerve to the tensor palatini and the vagus nerve through the pharyngeal plexus to the levator and musculus uvulae.

From a functional standpoint, the normal closure of the velopharyngeal valve is accomplished by the sphincteric action of the levator sling, which pulls the palate upward and backward toward the posterior pharyngeal wall. The palatopharyngeus muscles, which also form a sling, and the superior constrictor muscles help in this action. The musculus uvulae also contracts during speech, adding bulk to the area of convexity on the upper surface of the soft palate.

The most important point in the anatomy of the cleft palate is the fact that levator muscles, rather than running toward the midline, are directed anteriorly (longitudinally). They insert into the posterior border of the hard palate with their fibers parallel to the cleft margin. Several authors have emphasized this point (12–14). This abnormal orientation is also seen in submucous cleft palate; in these cases, the dehiscence of muscle in the midline can be seen clearly on transillumination through the nose. The triad of signs of submucous cleft palate is completed by the bony notch in the posterior border of the hard palate and a bifid uvula.

Early Considerations in Cleft Palate Care

Randall (15) stated that there are four points to be emphasized in the treatment of infants with clefts of the palate. These include: (*a*) feeding; (*b*) maintenance of an airway; (*c*) middle ear disease; and (*d*) the possibility of other abnormalities.

FEEDING

Although a child with a cleft palate may make sucking movements with the mouth, the cleft prevents the child from developing adequate suction. In general, however, swallowing mechanisms are normal; therefore, if the milk or formula can be delivered to the back of the child's throat, the infant will feed effectively.

While many specialized types of nipples have been recommended for the child with cleft palate, we have found the use of a standard disposable nipple with an enlarged hole to be successful in almost all cases. We strongly feel that this allows the mother to use the same type of bottle and nipple as she would with any other child and minimizes the feeling that the cleft child is different.

Breast feeding is usually not successful, unless milk production is very abundant. If the mother insists on breast feeding, one should monitor the infant's weight closely to assure sufficient intake.

AIRWAY

The infant with Pierre Robin anomaly or other conditions in which the cleft palate is seen in association with a micrognathia or retrognathic mandible may be particularly prone to upper airway obstruction. A discussion of treatment of these problems is beyond the scope of this chapter, but a logical management approach would be to attempt the simpler, more conservative techniques (e.g.,

prone positioning) before progressing to surgical intervention.

MIDDLE EAR DISEASE

As mentioned previously, the disturbance in anatomy associated with cleft palate also affects the function of the eustachian tube orifices. The parents should be aware of the increased possibility of middle ear infection so that the child will receive treatment promptly if symptoms arise. Careful follow-up in collaboration with an audiologist and an otolaryngologist, including examination, myringotomy, and tube placement when necessary, will prevent long-term hearing deficits.

ASSOCIATED DEFORMITIES

One must always keep in mind that the child with cleft palate may have other anomalies in as many as 29% of cases. These may be more common in association with isolated CP than with CL ± P, but the inclusion of Pierre Robin cases in these figures makes that difference more apparent than real. High among the associated anomalies are those affecting the cardiac and skeletal systems.

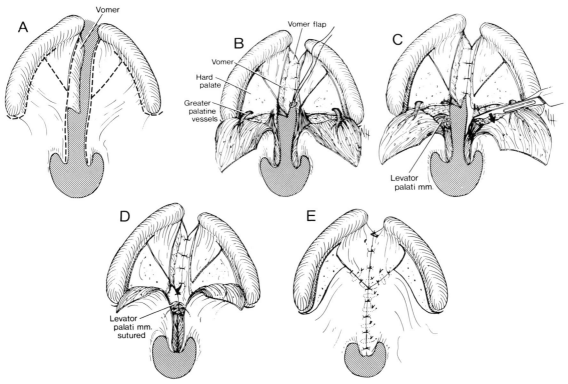

FIGURE 30.2.   The standard marking for the Wardill-Kilner V-Y palatal repair is shown. The palatal flaps are shown elevated. Notice that the vomer bone mucosa has been elevated and transferred laterally to create an anterior nasal floor closure. The palatine vessels can be further released from the flaps for greater movement of the flaps medially as needed in the wider palatal clefts. The levator muscles of the palate have been dis-

sected from their abnormal longitudinal attachments along the hard palate and rotated into a cross-sectional position. The levator musculature has now been sutured across the midline to construct the sling mechanism as in a normal palate. This is carried out after the closure of the palatal nasal mucosa. The palatal mucosa is shown in its new V-Y position closed with interrupted and mattress sutures of Dexon 3-0 or Vicryl 3-0.

Techniques of Palate Repair

The object of palate repair is the production of a competent velopharyngeal sphincter. It is not the purpose of this chapter to give a detailed description of all palate repair techniques. Instead, the more common techniques, the similarities and differences in technique, and some changing trends in repair will be described.

By and large, the standard techniques of palate repair have changed little in recent years. The two most common repairs are the V-Y (Veau-Wardill-Kilner) and the von Langenbeck repair. While various modifications can be combined with each of these repairs, the main difference between the two is that the V-Y repair, and its variations, involve elongation of the palate, whereas the von Langenbeck type repair does not.

The von Langenbeck repair consists essentially of a paring of the margins of the cleft and closure in the midline with the use of lateral relaxing incisions to relieve tension on the repair. Because the palatal flaps remain bipedicle, no elongation is accomplished. In the V-Y repair, elongation is accomplished, at least on the oral surface, by the well-known plastic surgery technique of V-to-Y advancement (Fig. 30.2).

A number of other techniques have been described to achieve palatal lengthening. Dorrance (16) placed a skin graft on the nasal side of the repair in order to increase the length of the palate without leaving a bare nasal surface. Cronin (17) released the nasal mucosa over the surface of the palate bone to gain length and to prevent the secondary contraction that may occur if the nasal side of the repair is left raw. Millard (18) devised an axial pattern

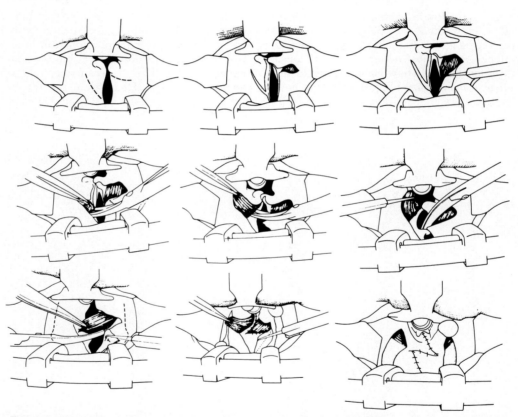

FIGURE 30.3. *Top left,* The posteriorly based limb of the Z-plasty in the oral mucosa includes the levator muscle on that side. *Top center,* The anteriorly based limb of the Z-plasty contains only oral mucosa and is cut closer to an 80° angle than a 60° angle to keep the transposed levator muscle from being inserted close to the posterior edge of the palatine bone. *Top right,* The anteriorly based oral mucosal flap is dissected off the levator muscle. *Center left,* The levator muscle is detached from its abnormal insertion into the posterior edge of the palatine bone. The plane of dissection between the levator muscle and the nasal mucosa is easily determined by lifting the nasal mucosa off the palatine bone with a small elevator (not shown). *Center,* This dissection between the levator muscle and the nasal mucosa is very difficult because the nasal mucosa is so thin. *Center right,* The Z-plasty in the nasal mucosa is reversed. Here the anteriorly based flap contains only nasal mucosa. *Bottom left,* The posteriorly based flap contains levator muscle and nasal mucosa. The muscle usually extends well beyond the mucosal flap as it inserts on the palatine bone. *Bottom center,* Closure of the nasal mucosa with the levator muscle from the right side allows shifting the muscle from its transverse orientation. Completion of the closure brings the left levator muscle into a transverse orientation overlapping the right levator muscle. *Bottom right,* Relaxing incisions may or may not be needed. Because width is sacrificed for length, in a very wide cleft the Z-plasty cannot be made very large, although the muscle flaps will extend well beyond the mucosal flaps. (From Randall P, LaRossa D, Solomon M, Cohen M: Experience with the Furlow double-reversing Z-plasty for cleft palate repair. *Plast Reconstr Surg* 77:569, 1986.)

flap of oral mucoperiosteum turned over and inserted in the nasal lining to accomplish the same objective. Manchester (19) carried out a wide division of the nasal mucosa; others have tried lengthening the nasal mucosa with a Z-plasty.

More recently, Furlow (20) then Randall et al. (21), using Furlow's technique, have gained additional soft palate length with a double reversing Z-plasty (Fig. 30.3). Although this procedure is gaining popularity, it is difficult to say if the speech results will be significantly better than the standard V-Y repair or von Langenbeck repair. As to the latter two repairs, the methods used to evaluate them and the reports of their speech results in the literature are difficult to interpret. Lindsay et al. (22) reviewed a large series of patients and showed that, in repair of isolated clefts of the secondary palate, there was no difference in speech results between the two procedures. Our own results, also based on the long-term follow-up of a large cleft population, confirm these findings. However, we observed significantly better results with the V-Y repair when clefts involved both the primary and the secondary palates.

Several brief comments are warranted about two other types of repair. First, although speech results may be very good after repairs incorporating a pharyngeal flap as a primary procedure, it would appear that most standard methods of palate repair achieve acceptable speech results in about 75% of cases with a single procedure carried out in infancy without a pharyngeal flap. Therefore, it seems that, in three of four cases, the primary pharyngeal flap is unnecessary. It may even be contraindicated in children with a limited nasopharyngeal airway. Second, there are those surgeons who still advocate delayed hard palate repair as described by Schweckendiek. In this repair, the soft palate is closed in the first year of life, but the hard palate repair is delayed with the hope of avoiding maxillary growth attenuation. Recent reports based on long-term follow-up indicate that neither the objective of good speech nor avoidance of maxillary collapse is achieved by the Schweckendiek procedure and it will probably be relegated to history (23).

Finally, with the increasing emphasis on a functional repair in cleft lip and palate surgery, attention has been directed recently toward reconstruction of the levator sling or intravelar veloplasty. By detaching the levator muscles from their abnormal attachment to the hard palate and repairing them in the midline with the muscle fibers oriented more normally, velopharyngeal closure may be accomplished more easily (24). An alternative approach to the levator reconstruction is that described by Furlow (20) and modified by Randall et al. (21). Any of the above approaches to muscle reconstruction can be used in combination with traditional techniques for closure of the hard palate cleft. The Furlow technique has the advantage of gaining additional soft palate length without the need for raising or shifting large mucoperiosteal flaps from the hard palate. It can also be used in combination with a primary pharyngeal flap if this is indicated and can be adapted for early soft palate closure (3–6 months) (21, 25).

A closer look at the relationship between age at time of palate repair and speech has led toward a trend of early repair. While the average age at palate repair today is 12–18 months, Dorf and Curtin (26) have pointed out that phoneme development is present by as early as 6 months. Based on these studies, they carried out repairs in the first few months of life and showed significantly improved speech results. Similarly, Randall et al. (25) have shown a remarkable reduction in the frequency with which pharyngeal flaps are needed to correct velopharyngeal incompetence when the palate repair was carried out at an earlier age.

Secondary Palatal Procedures

Secondary palatal surgery is directed at correction of two problem areas: the closure of palatal fistulas and the treatment of velopharyngeal incompetence. This requires close collaboration between a skilled speech pathologist and surgeon. Techniques for the evaluation of fistulas and velopharyngeal incompetence are discussed in Chapter 33.

PALATAL FISTULAS

Palatal fistulas may allow the troublesome leakage of fluid or food particles through the nose. They may cause chronic nasal irritation and, on occasion, may allow articulation distortion during speech. In general, the speech disturbance is only significant in the presence of a large fistula.

The closure of a palatal fistula can be among the most difficult of all surgical procedures, and in almost all cases, even small fistulas require the elevation of large palatal flaps. Without a completely tension-free repair, the recurrence rate is high. A greater number of previous attempts at closure is associated with a higher failure rate. If possible, a two-layer tension-free repair should be accomplished.

TREATMENT OF VELOPHARYNGEAL INCOMPETENCE

The most widely used secondary procedure for treatment of velopharyngeal incompetence is the pharyngeal flap, in which a flap of mucosa with underlying constrictor muscle is elevated from the posterior pharyngeal wall, either based above or below, turned forward, and inset into the soft palate. Although the superiorly based pharyngeal flap may be the most popular pharyngoplasty in the United States and Canada, there are, at least in theory, advantages of both superiorly and inferiorly based flaps. However, it is often difficult to tell the difference between the two, even on roentgenographic exam, once complete healing has occurred. Therefore, neither method appears to offer a definite advantage over the other (15).

The closure of the lateral ports after a pharyngeal flap is dependent on mesial movement of the lateral pharyngeal walls. A pharyngeal flap, therefore, may be unsuccessful in correcting velopharyngeal incompetence when it is placed below the point of lateral wall movement or when lateral wall movement is insufficient for the width of the flap (27). Some surgeons have applied techniques directed at tailoring the pharyngeal flap width to the amount of lateral wall movement (28).

Other techniques have been designed to decrease the anteroposterior dimension of the nasopharynx, thereby shortening the distance between the palate and the posterior pharyngeal wall. Small discrepancies may be obdurated by the insertion of retropharyngeal implants (i.e., shredded Teflon in glycerine, proplast), but pharyngoplasties such as those described by Hynes (29) and Orticochea (30) have been used with more success. The Hynes pharyngoplasty constructs a permanent and often contractile ridge on the posterior pharyngeal wall using transposed flaps of the salpingopharyngeus muscle. Orticochea's technique is a sphincter-type pharyngoplasty using two lateral flaps containing both posterior faucial pillars and the underlying palatopharyngeus muscle transposed beneath a pharyngeal flap, thereby creating a prominence on the posterior pharyngeal wall.

With increased emphasis on muscle function, both in palate repair and in pharyngeal wall motion, efforts have improved in localizing the ideal site of contact necessary to eliminate the persistent nasal escape. Recently, modifications of the Orticochea pharyngoplasty have been reported in which the site of lateral flap inset has been modified to maximize its function, and these efforts may significantly improve the results of pharyngoplasty (31, 32).

Finally, as discussed previously, it appears that one of the most important elements of palate repair may be in the reconstruction of the levator muscles (12, 20, 23). If the previous palate repair in a patient with persistent velopharyngeal incompetence has included neither palate lengthening nor levator reconstruction, these techniques, combined, may correct the incompetence while avoiding any pharyngeal surgery entirely (15).

References

1. Stark RB: Embryology of the oral cavity. In Stark RB (ed): *Plastic Surgery of the Head and Neck*. New York, Churchill Livingstone, 1986, vol 2, pp 1277–1279.
2. Stark RB: Embryology of the lips and chin. In Stark RB (ed): *Plastic Surgery of the Head and Neck*. New York, Churchill Livingstone, 1986, vol 2, pp 1167–1169.
3. Johnston MC: The neural crest in abnormalities of the face and brain. *Birth Defects* 11(7):1, 1975.
4. Vermeij-Keers CHR, Poelmann RE, Smits-Van Prooije AE, Van der Meulen JC: Hypertelorism and the median cleft face syndrome: An embryological analysis. *Ophthal Paediatr Genet (Amsterdam)* 4:97, 1984.
5. Sedano HO, Cohen MM Jr, Jirasek J, Gorlin RJ: Frontonasal dysplasia. *J Pediatr* 76:906, 1970.
6. Sulik KK: Craniofacial defects from genetic and teratogen-induced deficiencies in presomite embryos. *Birth Defects* 1(3):79, 1984.
7. Stark RB, Kaplan J: Development of the cleft lip and nose. *Plast Reconstr Surg* 51:413, 1973.
8. Kernahan DA, Stark RB: A new classification for cleft lip and cleft palate. *Plastic Reconstr Surg* 22:435, 1958.
9. Fogh-Anderson P: Vital statistics of cleft lip and palate—past, present and future. *Acta Chir Plast* 5:169, 1963.
10. Fogh-Anderson P: *Inheritance of Harelip and Cleft Palate*. Copenhagen, Nordisk Forlag-Arnold Busch, 1942.
11. Lynch HT, Kimberling WJ: Genetic counseling in cleft lip and cleft palate. *Plast Reconstr Surg* 68:800, 1981.
12. Kriens OB: Anatomy of the velopharyngeal area in cleft palate. *Clin Plast Surg* 2:261, 1975.
13. Latham RA, Long RE Jr, Latham EA: Cleft palate velopharyngeal musculature in a five-month-old infant: A three-dimensional histological reconstruction. *Cleft Palate J* 17:1, 1980.
14. Dickson DR, Dickson WM: Velopharyngeal anatomy. *J Speech Hear Res* 15:372, 1972.
15. Randall P: Cleft palate. In Grabb WC, Smith JW (eds): *Plastic Surgery*. Boston, Little, Brown & Company, 1979, p 205.
16. Dorrance GM: Lengthening of the soft palate operations. *Ann Surg* 82:208, 1925.
17. Cronin TD: Method of preventing raw area on the nasal surface of the hard palate in push-back surgery. *Plast Reconstr Surg* 20:474, 1957.
18. Millard DR Jr: The island flap in cleft palate surgery. *Surg Gynecol Obstet* 116:297, 1963.
19. Manchester WM: The repair of double cleft lip as part of an integrated program. *Plast Reconstr Surg* 45:207, 1970.
20. Furlow LT: Cleft palate repair by double opposing Z-plasty. *Plast Reconstr Surg* 78:724, 1986.
21. Randall P, LaRossa D, Solomon M, Cohen M: Experience with the Furlow double-reversing Z-plasty for cleft palate repair. *Plast Reconstr Surg* 77:569, 1986.
22. Lindsay WK, LeMesurier AB, Farmer AW: A study of speech results of a large series of cleft palate patients. *Plast Reconstr Surg* 29:273, 1962.
23. Jackson IT, McLennan G, Scheker LR: Primary veloplasty or primary palatoplasty: Some preliminary findings. *Plast Reconstr Surg* 72:153, 1983.
24. Braithwaite F: Cleft palate repair. In Gibson T (ed): *Modern Trends in Plastic Surgery*. London, Butterworth, 1964, pp 30–49.
25. Randall P, LaRossa DD, Fakhraee SM, et al: Cleft palate closure at 3 to 7 months of age: A preliminary report. *Plast Reconstr Surg* 71:624, 1983.
26. Dorf DS, Curtin JW: Early cleft palate repair and speech outcome. *Plast Reconstr Surg* 70:74, 1982.
27. Skolnick ML, McCall GN: Velopharyngeal competence and incompetence following pharyngeal flap surgery: Videofluoroscopic study in multiple projections. *Cleft Palate J* 9:1, 1972.
28. Shprintzen RJ, Lewin ML, Croft CB, et al: A comprehensive study of pharyngeal flap surgery: Tailor-made flaps. *Cleft Palate J* 16:46, 1979.
29. Hynes W: Pharyngoplasty by muscle transplantation. *Br J Plast Surg* 3:128, 1956.
30. Orticochea M: A review of 236 cleft palate patients treated with dynamic muscle sphincter. *Plast Reconstr Surg* 71:180, 1983.
31. Riski JR, Serafin D, Riefkohl R, et al: A rationale for modifying the site of insertion of the Orticochea pharyngoplasty. *Plast Reconstr Surg* 73:882, 1984.
32. Jackson IT: Sphincter pharyngoplasty. *Clin Plast Surg* 12:711, 1985.

31

Secondary Deformities of Cleft Lip and Palate

Joseph G. McCarthy, M.D., F.A.C.S. and Court B. Cutting, M.D.

The variety of secondary facial deformities after cleft lip and palate repair is unending and usually reflects the surgical techniques and principles employed at the time of the primary repair. It is essential that all infants with a cleft of the lip and/or palate be enrolled with a clinical team that can provide the judgment and clinical expertise to ensure the optimal result.

Secondary Lip Deformities

ANALYSIS OF THE PROBLEM

1. Full-thickness lip
   (a) Vertical excess
   (b) Vertical deficiency
   (c) Horizontal excess (including philtral)
   (d) Horizontal deficiency (including philtral)
2. Skin
   (a) Scars, stitch marks
   (b) Loss of philtral column
3. Vermilion–white line
   (a) Malalignment of white line
   (b) Loss of tubercle
   (c) Loss of Cupid's bow
   (d) Whistle deformity
4. Muscle
   (a) Incomplete union/malposition
5. Labiobuccal sulcus
   (a) Deficiency/obliteration

Full-Thickness Lip

The excessively long lip (*vertical excess*) (Fig. 31.1) is usually associated with certain types of primary lip repair. For example, the LeMesurier procedure has been generally abandoned because of this problem. Converse (1) described a technique of correcting this problem by excising the horizontal scar resulting from the closure. However, the excessively long lip is rarely seen after repair of a bilateral cleft lip.

Vertical deficiency (Fig. 31.2) in unilateral cleft lip is usually seen after a straight line or Rose-Thompson repair. In such a situation, if the vertical deficiency is severe, the cleft should be re-created by excising the surgical scar in a full-thickness fashion and lengthened using the procedure of Millard (2) or a Z-plasty technique. A vertical deficiency can also be temporarily observed at the level of the vermilion or labial mucosa in the first year after the Millard repair.

The short (vertical) lip after repair of a bilateral cleft poses more of a problem because lengthening of the lip is usually done at the expense of the horizontal lip dimension. For this reason, it is not uncommon to use an Abbé or cross-lip flap and re-create the entire philtrum. It is unlikely that simple Z-plasty techniques can correct this problem.

Horizontal excess is most commonly seen after bilateral cleft lip repair when there is gradual widening of the philtrum. Correction of this deficiency is relatively straightforward and usually involves resection of sufficient lip tissue so that the resulting scars simulate the philtral columns. The excess lip tissue can often be salvaged to lengthen the columella and elevate the nasal tip, as in the Millard forked-flap procedure (3; Fig. 31.3).

Horizontal deficiency (Fig. 31.4) is usually manifest as a tight upper lip resulting from excessive discarding of lip tissue at the time of the primary repair. On profile view, the lower lip usually projects more than the upper lip. The Abbé cross-lip flap is a satisfactory method of adding a significant amount of lip tissue to the midline of the upper lip and simulating the philtrum (Fig. 31.5). However, the appearance of the donor lower lip scar is not always satisfactory. In both the unilateral and bilateral cleft lip, it is preferable to place the Abbé flap in an upper midline incision (4). At a later date, the previous scars in the unilateral lip can be revised. In designing an Abbé flap, the surgeon should note that the width of the adult philtrum ranges from 8 to 12 mm at the vermilion border and from 6 to 9 mm at the columella. The maximum length of the normal adult philtrum is 17 mm. These dimensions must be followed in designing the Abbé flap.

Skin

If the full-thickness dimensions of the upper lip are satisfactory and there are only superficial cutaneous irregularities such as scars and suture marks, simple excision and revision can be performed. While dermabrasion can be a helpful technique for improving the appearance of superficial irregularities, it is generally disappointing in treating lip scars.

The presence of the philtrum is an absolute requirement for an aesthetically satisfactory upper lip and is the main advantage of the Millard repair (2) because the resulting scar simulates the philtral columns. Techniques

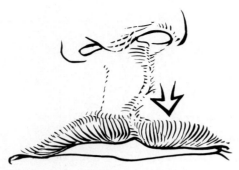

FIGURE 31.1. Vertical lip excess. (From Converse JM, et al: Secondary deformities of cleft lip, cleft lip and nose, and cleft palate. In Converse JM, McCarthy JG (eds): *Reconstructive Plastic Surgery*. Philadelphia, WB Saunders, 1977, vol 4, p 2165.)

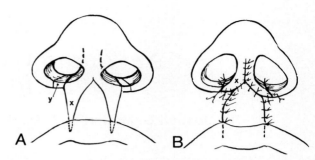

FIGURE 31.3. Forked flap technique of Millard (3). **A.** The outline of incisions and wedge excisions is shown from the nostril floor. **B.** Closure after advancement of the forehead flaps elevates the nasal tip and restores the Cupid's bow. (From Converse JM, et al: Secondary deformities of cleft lip, cleft lip and nose, and cleft palate. In Converse JM, McCarthy JG (eds): *Reconstructive Plastic Surgery*. Philadelphia, WB Saunders, 1977, vol 4, p 2165.)

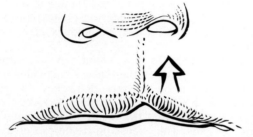

FIGURE 31.2. Vertical lip deficiency. (From Converse JM, et al: Secondary deformities of cleft lip, cleft lip and nose, and cleft palate. In Converse JM, McCarthy JG (eds): *Reconstructive Plastic Surgery*. Philadelphia, WB Saunders, 1977, vol 4, p 2165.)

FIGURE 31.4. Horizontal lip deficiency. (From Converse JM, et al: Secondary deformities of cleft lip, cleft lip and nose, and cleft palate. In Converse JM, McCarthy JG (eds): *Reconstructive Plastic Surgery*. Philadelphia, WB Saunders, 1977, vol 4, p 2165.)

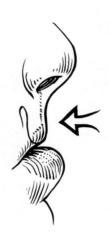

FIGURE 31.5. Cross-lip flap reconstruction of a horizontal and vertical lip deficiency. **A** and **B.** The lower lip donor flap and recipient incision are outlined. Note that the flap is placed in the midline to simulate the philtrum. The unilateral cleft lip scar can be revised at a later date. **C.** The flap is prepared by applying the principle of the muscle shelf. The shelf fits snugly under the columella, producing an elevation of the columella and facilitating skin-to-skin approximation in the repair of the subnasal area. **D.** Diagrammatic illustration shows the vascular supply. The flap is rotated on a small vascular pedicle, which includes a mucosal bridge. **E.** The shelving muscle flap is drawn under the columella by mattress sutures, which are tied over a small cotton bolster within the nostril. (From Converse JM, et al: Secondary deformities of cleft lip, cleft lip and nose, and cleft palate. In Converse JM, McCarthy JG (eds): *Reconstructive Plastic Surgery*. Philadelphia, WB Saunders, 1977, vol 4, p 2165.)

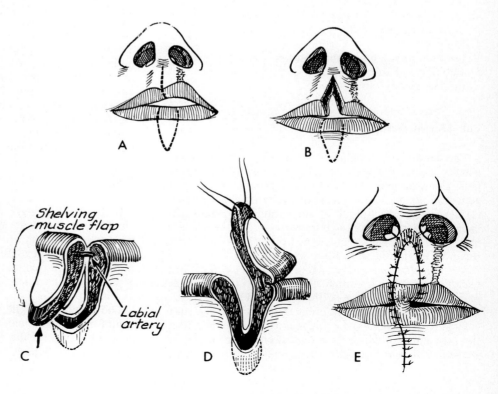

have been described for reconstructing the philtrum. The Abbé flap, when placed in the midline of the upper lip, simulates the philtrum (Fig. 31.5). Cutaneous rotation flaps have been described by O'Connor and McGregor (5), and Neuner (6) used auricular cartilage grafts, placed subcutaneously, to reconstruct the philtral columns and dimple.

Unfortunately, auricular cartilage reconstruction of the philtral column and dimple often looks satisfactory in a static photograph but appears stiff and unnatural during facial animation. A more satisfactory reconstruction of the philtral column and dimple may be accomplished by the technique illustrated in Figure 31.6. At the time of cleft lip revision, the medial skin edge is elevated away from the muscle of the lip. Care is taken not to dissect farther than the depth of the proposed philtral dimple. The muscle is then incised and overlapped over the medial muscle and sutured in place prior to skin repair. This type of "pants-over-vest" muscle repair exaggerates column projection and deepens the philtral dimple.

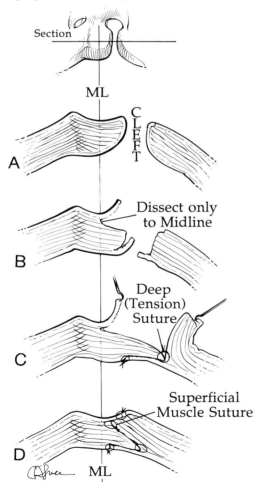

FIGURE 31.6. Pants-over-vest closure to simulate the philtral column. **A,** Unilateral cleft lip (ML, midline). **B,** Elevation of medial skin flap to ML. **C,** Posterior closure. **D,** Completion of closure. (From Converse JM, et al: Secondary deformities of cleft lip, cleft lip and nose, and cleft palate. In Converse JM, McCarthy JG (eds): *Reconstructive Plastic Surgery.* Philadelphia, WB Saunders, 1977, vol 4, p 2165.)

Vermilion–White Line

Malalignment at the level of the white line is not uncommon and has been referred to as the "red flare." It is usually corrected with an appropriately placed Z-plasty (Fig. 31.7).

The vermilion tubercle is also an essential aesthetic feature of the upper lip. Its absence is usually due to the fact that an excess of vermilion was sacrificed in the primary repair, or the orbicularis muscle was inadequately sutured at the cleft site. The correction usually requires that the inferior portion of the repair be reopened and flaps of vermilion and muscle advanced to the midline to simulate the tubercle.

The Cupid's bow is likewise a critical element of upper lip aesthetics. The advantage of the Millard unilateral lip repair is that it preserves the Cupid's bow. The triangular repair, however, tends to flatten the Cupid's bow, as shown in Figure 31.8.

The Cupid's bow can be excessively wide in the bilateral cleft lip, and the excess can be incorporated into skin flaps and used in lengthening of the columella (Fig. 31.3). If the lip scar is excised in a full-thickness fashion and the cleft re-created, the Millard rotation-advancement repair can be used, and a flap of orbicularis muscle from the lateral segment is advanced into a tunnel at the vermilion level of the medial portion of the lip.

The *whistle deformity* is characterized by a notching of the upper lip at the site of the lip repair. The incisors are usually exposed, and the patient lacks lip competence. The preferred repair includes the development of large bilateral rotation flaps with pedicles based on the vermilion border (Fig. 31.9). The flaps are then rotated toward the apex of the whistle deformity and closed in a V-Y

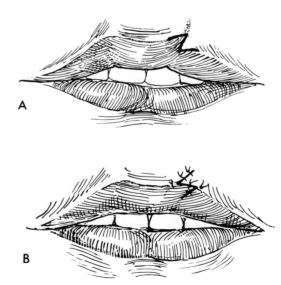

FIGURE 31.7. Malalignment at the level of the white line of the upper lip. **A.** The Z-plasty is outlined. **B.** Transposition of the flaps restores the white line. (From Converse JM, et al: Secondary deformities of cleft lip, cleft lip and nose, and cleft palate. In Converse JM, McCarthy JG (eds): *Reconstructive Plastic Surgery.* Philadelphia, WB Saunders, 1977, vol 4, p 2165.)

FIGURE 31.8. Flattening of the Cupid's bow as occurs with triangular cleft lip repair. (From Converse JM, et al: Secondary deformities of cleft lip, cleft lip and nose, and cleft palate. In Converse JM, McCarthy JG (eds): *Reconstructive Plastic Surgery.* Philadelphia, WB Saunders, 1977, vol 4, p 2165.)

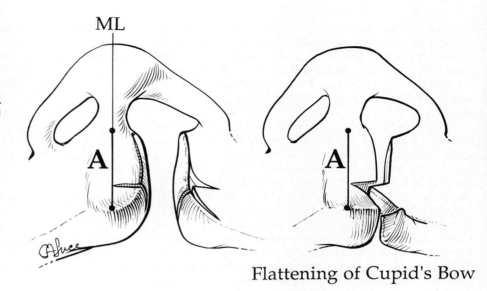

Flattening of Cupid's Bow

fashion. It is essential that the flaps be broadly based. For less severe whistle deformities, a Z-plasty can be performed at the level of the vermilion and labial mucosa. A useful technique is the "unequal" Z-plasty (Fig. 31.10), in which one flap contains some of the underlying orbicularis muscle (7; Fig. 31.8). Kapetansky (8) described double "pendulum" flaps of orbicularis muscle that are advanced into the whistle deformity defect.

Muscle

In recent years, particular emphasis has been placed on restoring the orbicularis sphincter (9). Failure to do so at the time of the primary repair results in persistent bulging of the ununited muscle bundles at the alar base in the lateral segment and the columella in the medial segment of the unilateral cleft lip and at both alar bases of the

bilateral cleft lip. Surgical correction (Fig. 31.11) involves full-thickness excision of the cleft lip scar, dissection of the muscle bundles, and division of the quadratus labii superioris muscle. The muscle flaps are then skeletonized and united at the cleft site in the unilateral cleft lip and in the prolabial segment of the bilateral cleft lip. The repair is completed by closure of the cutaneous, vermilion, and mucosal incisions.

Labiobuccal Sulcus

For severe *deficiencies* involving obliteration of the labiobuccal sulcus, the Esser inlay technique using either split-thickness skin graft or buccal mucosa has been employed. However, a prosthesis usually must be constructed to achieve satisfactory inset of the graft and also to prevent contracture of the sulcus in the year after sur-

FIGURE 31.9. Correction of the whistle deformity. **A.** At rest, the patient lacks complete lip competence, and the incisors are exposed. **B.** The bilateral labial mucosal rotation flaps are outlined. **C.** Rotation of the flaps lengthens the lip. **D.** The incisions are closed in a V-Y fashion. (From Converse JM, et al: Secondary deformities of cleft lip, cleft lip and nose, and cleft palate. In Converse JM, McCarthy JG (eds): *Reconstructive Plastic Surgery.* Philadelphia, WB Saunders, 1977, vol 4, p 2165.)

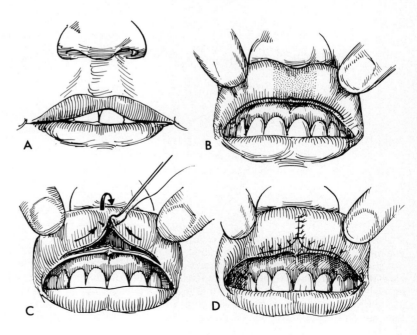

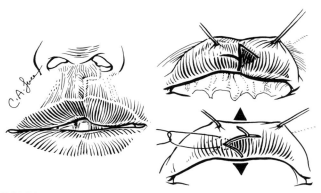

FIGURE 31.10. "Unequal" Z-plasty is performed for correction of a mild whistle deformity. *Left,* Lip incompetence with incisor exposure. *Right,* Flaps are outlined. The central limb is aligned at the whistle deformity. The cross-hatched flap contains underlying orbicularis muscle. The flaps are transposed. (From Converse JM, et al: Secondary deformities of cleft lip, cleft lip and nose, and cleft palate. In Converse JM, McCarthy JG (eds): *Reconstructive Plastic Surgery.* Philadelphia, WB Saunders, 1977, vol 4, p 2165.)

gery. The problem most often is seen at the junction of the prolabium and premaxilla after bilateral cleft lip repair. A variety of Z-plasty and V-Y advancement techniques have also been recommended for lesser deficiencies.

Deformities of the Alveolus, Maxilla, and Palate

ANALYSIS OF THE PROBLEM

1. Alveolus
   (a) Cleft, unilateral or bilateral ± lateral maxillary segment collapse
2. Maxilla
   (a) Pyriform aperture deficiency (Class I occlusion)
   (b) Maxillary hypoplasia (Class III malocclusion and anterior cross-bite)
3. Palate
   (a) Fistula
4. Combination of above

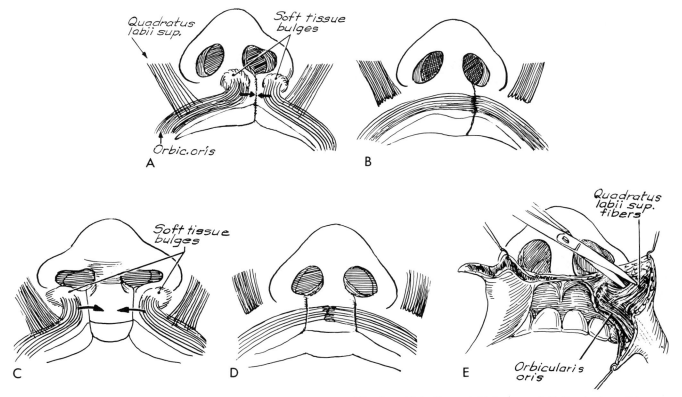

FIGURE 31.11. **A.** The orbicularis oris fibers are misdirected in the unilateral cleft lip, forming a bulge on each side of the cleft. **B.** After division of the fibers of the quadratus labii superioris muscle, the orbicularis oris muscle is redirected and sutured. **C.** A similar muscle malalignment is found in the complete bilateral cleft. **D.** The fibers of the orbicularis oris are redirected and introduced into the prolabial segment. **E.** Sectioning of the quadratus labii superioris muscle allows redirection of the orbicularis oris muscle. (From Converse JM, et al: Secondary deformities of cleft lip, cleft lip and nose, and cleft palate. In Converse JM, McCarthy JG (eds): *Reconstructive Plastic Surgery.* Philadelphia, WB Saunders, 1977, vol 4, p 2165.)

Alveolar Clefts

This discussion does not cover primary alveolar bone graft (performed as early as 3 months after the primary lip repair) but instead discusses secondary bone grafting of alveolar clefts performed before the eruption of the permanent canine teeth (7–12 years of age). There are numerous advantages associated with bone grafting of alveolar clefts at this age (10). If the erupting teeth can be brought into the bone-grafted space, the need for permanent dentures may be obviated. Moreover, the bone graft provides better periodontal support for teeth previously poorly encased in deficient alveolar bone at the site of the cleft. In addition, the bone grafts can also provide better support for the alar base and nasal platform. Bone grafting done in this region will also yield superior results in terms of simultaneous closure of associated oronasal fistulae.

In the repair of unilateral alveolar clefts, any lateral maxillary dentoalveolar segmental collapse is corrected orthodontically prior to the bone grafting procedure. It is imperative that, at the time of surgery, the bone grafts are covered by adequate soft tissue flaps on the nasal and oral sides (Fig. 31.12). In bilateral alveolar clefts, orthodontic therapy is usually required to expand the entire maxillary arch, and the orthodontic appliance must be kept in place at the time of surgery. Bone grafting in bilateral clefts requires careful attention to the maintenance of the blood supply to the premaxilla. A variety of bone graft donor sites are available, and the most commonly used sites are the calvaria (cranium) and ilium.

Maxilla

The maxillary hypoplasia observed in the cleft palate patient can take many forms. In some patients, the occlusion is satisfactory (class I), and the deficiency is restricted solely to the region of the pyriform aperture. In this situation, either autogenous septal cartilage (layered) or inner table iliac or outer table cranial bone grafts can be inserted through a buccal incision and carefully placed over the maxilla at the margin of the pyriform apparatus (Fig. 31.13). In addition to improving maxillary contour, the technique also provides better support to the nasal platform.

The other type of maxillary hypoplasia observed in the cleft palate patient is more generalized and involves the entire maxilla. An anterior cross bite and class III malocclusion are observed. Preoperative orthodontic therapy is employed in order to expand the maxillary arch and to exaggerate the anterior cross bite (11) in anticipation of a Le Fort I advancement osteotomy (Fig. 31.14). The latter is the ideal treatment for this type of maxillary hypoplasia. In addition to restoring the occlusion, the procedure affords considerable aesthetic improvement in lip posture and maxillary form. However, the patient with a repaired cleft palate is at risk for developing velopharyngeal incompetence after a Le Fort I advancement and must be forewarned preoperatively (12).

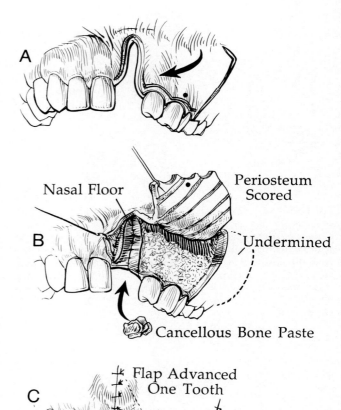

FIGURE 31.12. Closure and bone grafting of an alveolar cleft. **A,** Outline of gingival incisions. **B,** Elevation of anterior flaps and closure of posterior flap. **C,** Closure is complete. (From Converse JM, et al: Secondary deformities of cleft lip, cleft lip and nose, and cleft palate. In Converse JM, McCarthy JG (eds): *Reconstructive Plastic Surgery.* Philadelphia, WB Saunders, 1977, vol 4, p 2165.)

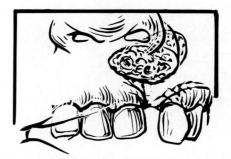

FIGURE 31.13. Bone or cartilage grafting of the maxilla in the region of the pyriform aperture. (From Converse JM, et al: Secondary deformities of cleft lip, cleft lip and nose, and cleft palate. In Converse JM, McCarthy JG (eds): *Reconstructive Plastic Surgery.* Philadelphia, WB Saunders, 1977, vol 4, p 2165.)

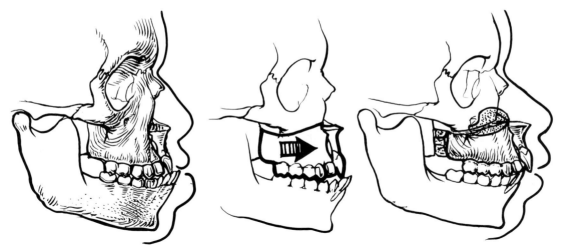

FIGURE 31.14.   Le Fort I advancement osteotomy. *Left,* Maxillary hypoplasia, anterior cross bite, and class III malocclusion are associated with repaired unilateral cleft lip/palate. *Center,* The osteotomy and direction of advancement are outlined. *Right,* After advancement, the bone grafts are placed in the retromaxillary space and over the anterior maxilla. (From Converse JM, et al: Secondary deformities of cleft lip, cleft lip and nose, and cleft palate. In Converse JM, McCarthy JG (eds): *Reconstructive Plastic Surgery.* Philadelphia, WB Saunders, 1977, vol 4, p 2165.)

Palate

Fistulae can be observed after cleft palate repair, usually in the region of the incisive foramen or at the junction of the hard and soft palate. Small oronasal fistulae are amenable to surgical correction provided that there is adequate vascularization of the surrounding soft tissue in order that mucoperiosteal flaps can provide coverage without tension (Fig. 31.12). A basic principle in the repair of palatal fistulae is that the flaps are designed to be relatively large in size. The lining flaps are usually obtained from the nasal cavity or vomer. Alternatively, turnover flaps (Fig. 31.15) can provide nasal coverage. The oral coverage flap is usually obtained from the palatal mucoperiosteum. Closure of large palatal fistulae poses a greater problem because of the paucity of local tissue for their reconstruction. Tongue flaps and even flaps from a distance have been reported for successful closure. However, an obturator constructed by a prosthodontist is a satisfactory alternative solution.

Combination of Above

The surgeon is often presented with the patient showing a combination of the above deformities: alveolar cleft, palatal fistula, deficiency in the region of the pyriform aperture, and unsatisfactory lip scar. In this situation, the technique illustrated in Figure 31.12 is indicated (13). In a single stage, the lip scar is excised and exposure of the alveolar cleft–oronasal fistula is gained. Nasal flaps in the region of the alveolus and turnover flaps are developed above the periphery of the oronasal (palatal) fistula in order to achieve nasal closure. Bone grafts, harvested either from the calvaria or ilium, are placed into the alveolar cleft and in the region of the pyriform aperture. A buccal vestibular flap is elevated and transposed across the alveolar flap in order to provide oral coverage in this area. Bilateral palatal mucoperiosteal flaps (Veau) are elevated in a subperiosteal plane and transposed over the palatal fistula. The lip revision is then accomplished as previously discussed.

Cleft Lip Nose Deformity

DESCRIPTION OF THE DEFORMITY

The surgical approach to the cleft nose deformity can be undertaken only after one gains an understanding of the anatomy and development of the deformity. The deformity may best be understood by reviewing Latham's (14) concept of cleft palate embryology. The premaxillary

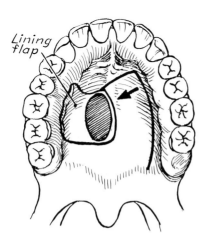

FIGURE 31.15.   Closure of a palatal fistula. The lining flap provides nasal closure, and a large palatal rotation flap is used for oral coverage. (From Converse JM, et al: Secondary deformities of cleft lip, cleft lip and nose, and cleft palate. In Converse JM, McCarthy JG (eds): *Reconstructive Plastic Surgery.* Philadelphia, WB Saunders, 1977, vol 4, p 2165.)

bony segment is connected to the base of the nasal septum by the "septo-premaxillary ligament." As the nasal septum grows anteriorly and inferiorly, it carries the premaxilla with it by virtue of the attachment of this ligament. If the mesodermal streaming from the lateral premaxilla penetrates the epithelial bilayer and the premaxilla is joined to the lateral palatal shelves, the premaxilla is held somewhat posterior by this attachment, and the lateral palatal shelves are drawn anterior and held somewhat separated from one another by the premaxilla.

The premaxilla is then drawn posteriorly along the base of the nasal septum. As this process continues, a nasal columella gradually forms, and the base of the ala of the nose is brought further anteriorly. However, if fusion fails to occur, the premaxilla is placed anteriorly along the base of the nasal septum and the base of the ala is posteriorly placed. This anatomical arrangement has adverse effects on the shape and development of the growing nose (15).

Because of the anterior displacement of the premaxilla, which is especially pronounced in a bilateral deformity, the columellar skin does not elongate properly. A retracted nasal tip is usually associated with the short columella. The posterior position of the alar base with respect to the columella tends to pull the alar cartilage (and nostril rim) laterally and inferiorly, thus obliterating the soft triangle of the nose, pulling domes apart, and producing a tendency to nasal tip bifidity. The posterior distraction of the alar cartilage results in flattening of the dome on the cleft side.

The effects on the nasal septum of this process have been described by Hogan and Converse (4) as a "tilted tripod" (Fig. 31.16). The lateral aspects of the nose may be considered to be leaves of a tent with the nasal septum forming the tent pole in the middle. If one side is displaced posteriorly, there is a tendency of the tent pole (septum) to buckle in the midportion and shift its base, resulting in nasal septal deviation.

Aside from the simple *positional* aspects of the cleft lip nasal deformity, one must also consider the mesodermal *deficiency* on the cleft side of the nose. Avery (16) studied the nasal capsule cartilage in the cleft deformity and documented a true deficiency in the nasal capsular cartilage. There is also an associated skeletal deficiency of the maxilla under the alar base and in the alveolus.

Because the cleft nasal deformity appears to arise from *malposition* and *deficiency* of tissue mass, surgical attempts to correct the problem must be tailored accordingly. Surgical efforts to correct the malposition alone are often inadequate. Grafting procedures under the alar base and in the nasal floor and pyriform aperture region are often required. It is the opinion of the authors that the deficient soft tissue matrix (i.e., nasal cutaneous and vestibular skin on the side of the cleft) poses the greatest challenge in the repair of the cleft lip nose deformity.

Huffman and Lierle (17) described the unilateral cleft lip nose on the basis of their extensive clinical experience as follows (Fig. 31.17). The nasal tip appears to be deviated to the noncleft side because of the flattening of the dome on the cleft side. The dorsally and caudally depressed dome on the cleft side obliterates the soft triangle of the nose and produces a flat dome. There is an obtuse angle between the medial and lateral groove of the cleft alar cartilage, and inward buckling of the cleft ala is also noted in the midposition of the lateral groove of the alar cartilage. There is usually a flattening or absence of the alar-facial groove. The bony platform under the cleft ala is deficient. Horizontal orientation of the nostril on the cleft side is present. It should also be noted that frequently the nostril is small. In association with the deviation of the septum, there is distortion of the columella, and the base of the columella is displaced to the noncleft side. The base of the medial crus is dorsally displaced on the cleft side. There is a vestibular web along the line of the upper edge of the lower lateral cartilage.

The above comments regarding the unilateral cleft

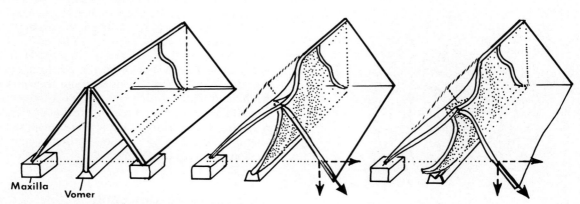

FIGURE 31.16. The tilted tripod. **Left.** Schematic representation of the nose illustrates the basic tripod nature of the nasal structures. The tripod consists of the dorsal portion of the septum and nasal bones and the two alar arms. **Middle.** The tilting effect results from maxillary hypoplasia with secondary deformity of the septum and cleft ala. **Right.** A more dramatic illustration of the convex deformity of the septum and the vertical bending of the septum posterior to the junction of the membranous and cartilaginous portions of the septum is evident. Restriction of the caudal border of the septum in its anterior thrust causes it to bend toward the normal nostril. If there is a more severe deformity of the vomer, the septum is displaced into the normal nostril. (After Hogan VM, Converse JM: Secondary deformities of unilateral cleft lip and nose. In Grabb WC, Rosenstein SE, Bzoch KR (eds): *Cleft Lip and Palate.* Boston, Little, Brown, 1971.)

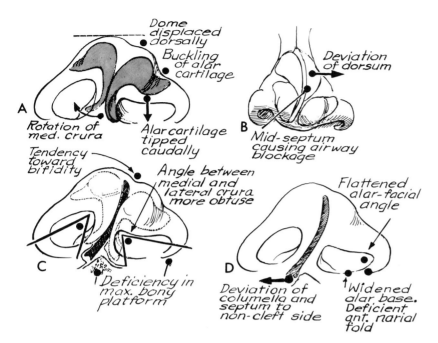

FIGURE 31.17. Deformities of the unilateral cleft lip nose. **A.** Deviation of the nasal tip is evident. **B.** Deviation of the nasal dorsum is shown. The alar cartilage is tipped caudally. **C.** The angle between the medial and lateral crura is more obtuse, and the dome is displaced dorsally. Note the buckling of the lateral crus and the deficiency of the maxillary bone platform. **D.** The columella and caudal septum are deviated to the noncleft side. The septum on the convex side causes varying degrees of obstruction and also accentuates the tendency to bifidity. (From Converse JM, et al: Secondary deformities of cleft lip, cleft lip and nose, and cleft palate. In Converse JM, McCarthy JG (eds): *Reconstructive Plastic Surgery.* Philadelphia, WB Saunders, 1977, vol 4, p 2165.)

nose deformity are generally applicable to the bilateral deformity with several modifications. Because the premaxilla is anteriorly positioned along the base of the septum in the bilateral cleft nose, the columella skin is reduced in size. The anteriorly posed premaxilla, in association with the posteriorly displaced alar bases, tends to produce tip bifidity as described by Stenstrom and Oberg (15). There is often severe flattening in the dome area with bilateral absence of the soft triangle. The absence of projection of the tip further accentuates the skin envelope deficiency in the bilateral cleft lip.

REPAIR OF THE UNILATERAL CLEFT NASAL DEFORMITY

Reconstruction of the Nasal Tip

An intranasal surgical approach is often taken in reconstruction of the tip as part of the cleft rhinoplasty. A rim incision provides maximal exposure to the nasal tip and usually obviates the need for external incisions. There are a number of suture suspension techniques that have been applied to the repositioning of the cleft ala to produce a more normal shape to the dome on the cleft side (Fig. 31.18). They usually involve suturing the surgically skeletonized ala to the upper lateral cartilages on the cleft and noncleft side as well as suturing the cleft dome to the dome on the noncleft side. These maneuvers mobilize the alar cartilage on the cleft side in a superior direction, reduce tip bifidity, and increase anterior projection of the cleft dome. Such a technique was described by Tajima and Maruyama (18). Potter (19) mobilized the entire cleft ala, including its mucosal lining, advanced it into the dome region, and sutured it to the dome on the opposite side. This was performed in conjunction with a modified Rethi incision for external approach to the nasal tip. Spira et al. (20) and Stenstrom (21) advocated similar suture

techniques. McIndoe and Rees (22) recommended mobilization of the cleft ala and suturing it to the upper lateral cartilage as well as the dome on the noncleft side. Similar sutures were used on the noncleft side to project the noncleft dome in a superior and anterior direction.

There are a large number of techniques that mobilize one or both lower lateral (alar) cartilages, split them, and rearrange them in such a way as to obtain a satisfactory nasal tip (Fig. 31.19). Kazanjian (23) advocated section-

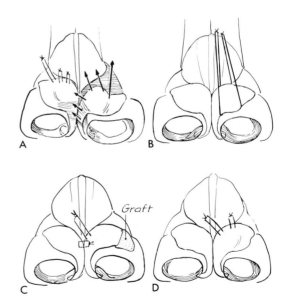

FIGURE 31.18. Suture fixation of the alar cartilage. **A.** The McIndoe and Rees (22) technique. **B.** The Stenstrom (21) technique. **C.** The method of repair by Rees et al. (37). **D.** The Reynolds and Horton (38) technique. (From Converse JM, et al: Secondary deformities of cleft lip, cleft lip and nose, and cleft palate. In Converse JM, McCarthy JG (eds): *Reconstructive Plastic Surgery.* Philadelphia, WB Saunders, 1977, vol 4, p 2165.)

FIGURE 31.19. Relocation of the alar cartilages. **A.** The Brown and McDowell (24) technique. **B.** The Erich (39) technique. **C.** The Humby (25) technique. **D.** Barsky's (26) method. **E.** The Whitlow and Constable (27) correction. (From Converse JM, et al: Secondary deformities of cleft lip, cleft lip and nose, and cleft palate. In Converse JM, McCarthy JG (eds): *Reconstructive Plastic Surgery.* Philadelphia, WB Saunders, 1977, vol 4, p 2165.)

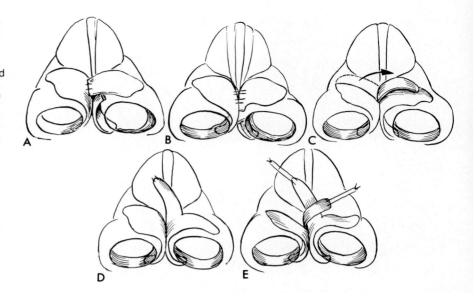

ing of both lower lateral cartilages at approximately the middle of the lateral crus. The alar segments were then mobilized medially and sutured together. Brown and McDowell (24) sectioned the junction between the medial and lateral crura on the cleft side and mobilized the lateral crus superiorly and medially such that it overlapped the tip of the noncleft dome to which it was sutured. Humby (25) divided the cephalic portion of the lateral crus on the noncleft side, leaving it attached on a medial pedicle. It was then mobilized and used to overlap the dome on the cleft side to gain tip projection. Barsky (26) divided the cephalic portion of the alar cartilage on the cleft side and mobilized it superiorly over the septum, suturing it in place. Whitlow and Constable (27) modified the above techniques in such a way that the cephalic scrolls overlapped one another in the dome region to add projection to the nasal tip.

Cartilage grafting techniques have also been applied to the cleft nose (Fig. 31.20). Fomon and associates (28) placed grafts under the base of the columella and over the cleft dome. Other authors have also placed auricular and septal cartilage grafts over the flattened cleft dome. Gorney and Falces (29) advocated placing a cartilage strut along the base of the septum to project the tip. Dibbell (30) sutured a rib cartilage graft in a pocket along the caudal border of the nasal septum from the anterior nasal spine area into the tip.

Shaping the Skin Envelope over the Tip

Thus far, the discussion has been restricted to techniques that are aimed at creating a cartilaginous skeleton to form a symmetrical nasal tip. While many of these techniques produce a satisfactory skeletal tip, the more difficult problem in cleft rhinoplasty involves the shape of the skin envelope that overlies the tip. The remainder of this section deals with various surgical techniques that have been used to address the problem of the deficiency of the skin envelope over the cleft nose.

Much attention has been directed at the inner vestibu-

lar web in cleft rhinoplasty. The mucosal shortage within the vestibule tends to pull the tip inferiorly and produces a small inner nostril. Potter (19) advocated a V-Y correction of the vestibular web, leaving the mucoperichondrium attached to the alar cartilage. The alar cartilage is then completely mobilized and transposed to create a skeletal support for the tip. Other authors have suggested that the vestibular web should simply be incised and a secondary defect created; this defect should be grafted with mucosa or split-thickness skin. Millard (31) suggested management of the vestibular web at the time of initial cleft lip repair by using an "L flap" from the lateral

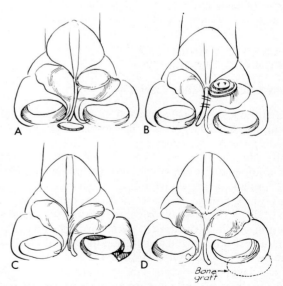

FIGURE 31.20. Graft augmentation. **A.** The revision by Fomon et al. (28). **B.** The Musgrave and Dupertuis (40) technique. **C.** Millard's (41) method. **D.** The approach described by Farrior (42), Longacre et al. (43), and Hogan and Converse (4). (From Converse JM, et al: Secondary deformities of cleft lip, cleft lip and nose, and cleft palate. In Converse JM, McCarthy JG (eds): *Reconstructive Plastic Surgery.* Philadelphia, WB Saunders, 1977, vol 4, p 2165.)

cleft segment and inserting it into the vestibular mucosa to correct the deficiency in this region.

Cutaneous hooding in the region of the soft triangle of the nose on the cleft side presents the most difficult problem in managing the skin envelope in the cleft nose. The flattening of the cartilaginous dome on the cleft side is accompanied by a cutaneous hood at the apex of the nostril. The lower edge of the deformed alar cartilage lies just within the flattened nostril margin. After mobilizing the alar cartilage with any of the methods previously described, the problem of the cutaneous hood must be addressed.

External (cutaneous) approaches to cleft rhinoplasty offer several advantages. Rim incisions coupled with an incision across the base of the columella allow complete unroofing of the dome. The complete exposure permits cartilaginous dome reconstruction under direct vision (delivery technique). The benefits of this approach must be balanced against the unfortunate necessity of an external scar. Bardach (7) recognized the shortage of skin of the columella and recommended the addition of a V-Y advancement of the excess skin from the lip on the cleft side (Fig. 31.21). This technique allows the surgeon to place the external scar within the lines of the cleft lip scar. Closure of the secondary defect in a V-Y fashion mobilizes the alar base on the cleft side medially. The tendency of the skin to "hood over" once again at the nostril apex may be reduced by suturing the rim incision at the nostril apex to the reconstructed nasal tip cartilage as just described.

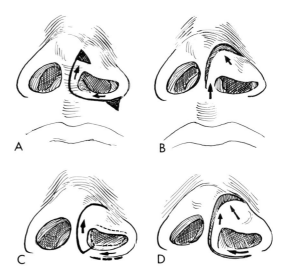

FIGURE 31.22. Alar unit rotations. **A.** The Blair (32) approach. **B.** Joseph's (33) technique. **C.** The Gillies and Kilner (34) method. **D.** Berkeley's (44) correction. (From Converse JM, et al: Secondary deformities of cleft lip, cleft lip and nose, and cleft palate. In Converse JM, McCarthy JG (eds): *Reconstructive Plastic Surgery.* Philadelphia, WB Saunders, 1977, vol 4, p 2165.)

If the skin on the cleft side of the columella is severely reduced in relation to that of the normal side, a more radical approach may be required. A vertical incision may be made in the columella between the medial crura. This incision is usually extended onto the dome to varying degrees and into the nostril floor. A superior advancement of the skin and the medial crus thus is achieved to augment the dome region and to increase the length of the columella skin. While the approach is often the most satisfactory, the scars in some patients may be disappointing. Blair (32) advocated such a procedure, including small Burrow's triangles in the region of the dome and the alar base on the cleft side (Fig. 31.22A). Using this incision, Joseph (33) excised ellipses of the skin in the dome region and advanced the flattened cleft dome superiorly and medially (Fig. 31.22B). Gillies and Kilner (34) advanced the columella-dome complex with a similar vertical incision along the length of the columella and mobilized a skin flap from the nasal floor to resurface the secondary defect created at the base of the columella (Fig. 31.22C). Berkeley (35) described what is probably the most widely used of these approaches (Fig. 31.22D). An incision is made around the base of the ala; it is extended along the nostril floor, between the medial crura, and onto the dome. The entire cleft-dome-nostril complex is then rotated to increase projection of the tip and lengthen the skin of the columella.

Repair of the Bilateral Cleft Lip Nasal Deformity

In the bilateral cleft lip nasal deformity, many of the findings previously discussed are observed on both sides. In addition, the extreme anterior position of the premax-

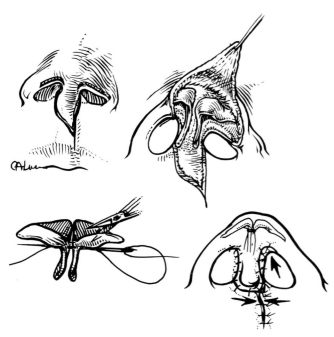

FIGURE 31.21. Bardach technique (7) of the cleft rhinoplasty. V-Y incision on the lip lengthens shortage of skin of columella. The external approach with complete mobilization of lateral crura allows precise control of tip shape. (From Converse JM, et al: Secondary deformities of cleft lip, cleft lip and nose, and cleft palate. In Converse JM, McCarthy JG (eds): *Reconstructive Plastic Surgery.* Philadelphia, WB Saunders, 1977, vol 4, p 2165.)

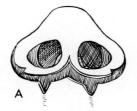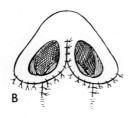

FIGURE 31.23. The columella is lengthened using the method of correcting the flat nasal tip with short columella. **A.** Bipedicle flaps of skin and subcutaneous tissue in the floor of the nostrils are based medially on the columella and laterally on the alae. A wedge of skin removed from the lower part of each ala diminishes the vertical length of the ala. **B.** Freely mobilized flaps are advanced medially and sutured together in the midline to provide the desired increase in the length of the columella. Triangles of skin on the upper lip, as shown in **A,** have been resected because redundant skin is present on the lip when the alae are transferred medially. (From Converse JM, et al: Secondary deformities of cleft lip, cleft lip and nose, and cleft palate. In Converse JM, McCarthy JG (eds): *Reconstructive Plastic Surgery.* Philadelphia, WB Saunders, 1977, vol 4, p 2165.)

illa at the base of the septum results in a columella that is often short or absent. The posterior position of the alar bases causes the domes to be splayed apart, producing tip bifidity.

Any of the cartilaginous skeletal tip reconstruction techniques discussed in the repair of the unilateral cleft lip nose may be applied to the bilateral cleft lip nose. The approach to the skin envelope problem and the short columella may be done in a number of ways and is the most difficult aspect of the correction of the bilateral cleft lip nasal deformity.

Columella lengthening is the most difficult aspect of correction of the bilateral cleft lip nasal deformity. A fork-flap technique has been advocated (Fig. 31.3) in which a bilateral V-Y advancement is accomplished. The excess tissue is derived from the wide prolabium along the lines of the previously created lip scar. The technique has the advantage that a new midline scar is not added to the lip. Furthermore, it allows the surgeon to revise the previous lip scars at the time of columella lengthening. However, closure of the fork-flap creates a midline scar at the base of the columella. Closure of the secondary deformities on the lip also tends to produce a slight weakening of the architecture of the Cupid's bow. Cronin (36) recommended lengthening the columella by extending an incision from the base of the columella just below the floor of the nose and onto the area around the alar base (Fig. 31.23). Rotation of the tissue anteriorly and medially is accomplished, producing a V-Y with the point of the Y being advanced to the middle of the columella. This technique has the added advantage of mobilizing the alar bases, which are often flared, toward the midline.

References

1. Converse JM: Correction of the dropping lateral portion of the cleft lip following the LeMesurier repair. *Plast Reconstr Surg* 55:501, 1975.
2. Millard DR: A primary camouflage in the unilateral harelip. In Skoog T (ed): *Transactions of the International Congress Plastic Surgery.* Baltimore, Williams & Wilkins Co, 1955, p 160.
3. Millard DR: Columella lengthening by a forked flap. *Plast Reconstr Surg* 22:454, 1958.
4. Hogan VM, Converse JM: Secondary deformities of unilateral cleft lip and nose. In Grabb WC, Rosenstein SE, Bzoch KR (eds): *Cleft Lip and Palate.* Boston, Little, Brown and Co, 1971, p 245.
5. O'Connor GB, McGregor MW: Surgical formation of the philtrum and the cutaneous upsweep. *Am J Surg* 95:227, 1958.
6. Neuner O: Secondary correction of cleft lip and palate. In Sanvenero-Rosselli G (ed): *Transactions of the Fourth International Congress of Plastic Surgery.* Amsterdam, Excerpta Medica, 1967, p 390.
7. Bardach J: Rozszczepy wargi gornej podniebienig. *Panstwowy Zaklad Wydawnictw Lekarskich* (in Polish). Warsaw, Poland, 1967.
8. Kapetansky DI: Double pendulum flaps for whistling deformities in bilateral cleft lips. *Plast Reconstr Surg* 47:321, 1971.
9. Randall P, Whitaker L, LaRossa D: The importance of muscle reconstruction in primary and secondary cleft lip repair. *Plast Reconstr Surg* 54:316, 1974.
10. Wolfe SA, Berkowitz S: The use of cranial bone grafts in the closure of alveolar and anterior palatal clefts. *Plast Reconstr Surg* 72:659, 1983.
11. McCarthy JG, Grayson B, Zide B: The relationship between the surgeon and orthodontist in orthognatic surgery. *Clin Plast Surg* 9:423, 1982.
12. McCarthy JG, Coccaro PJ, Schwartz M, et al: Velopharyngeal function following maxillary advancement. *Plast Reconstr Surg* 64:180, 1979.
13. Jackson IA, Munro IR, Salyer KE, et al (eds): Secondary problems in cleft lip and palate. In *Atlas of Craniomaxillofacial Surgery.* St. Louis, CV Mosby Co, 1982, p 590.
14. Latham RA: The pathogenesis of the skeletal deformity associated with unilateral cleft lip and palate. *Cleft Palate J* 6:404, 1969.
15. Stenstrom SJ, Oberg TRH: The nasal deformity in unilateral cleft lip. *Plast Reconstr Surg* 28:295, 1961.
16. Avery JK: The nasal capsule in cleft palate. *Anat Anz* 109:722, 1961.
17. Huffman WC, Lierle DM: Studies on the pathologic anatomy of the unilateral harelip nose. *Plast Reconstr Surg* 4:225, 1949.
18. Tajima S, Maruyama M: Reverse-U incision for secondary repair of the cleft lip nose. *Plast Reconstr Surg* 60:256, 1977.
19. Potter J: Some nasal tip deformities due to alar cartilage abnormalities. *Plast Reconstr Surg* 13:358, 1954.
20. Spira M, Hardy SB, Gerow FJ: Correction of nasal deformities accompanying unilateral cleft lip. *Cleft Palate J* 7:112, 1970.
21. Stenstrom SJ: The alar cartilage and the nasal deformity in unilateral cleft lip. *Plast Reconstr Surg* 38:223, 1966.
22. McIndoe AH, Rees TD: Synchronous repair of secondary deformities in cleft lip and nose. *Plast Reconstr Surg* 24:150, 1959.
23. Kazanjian VH: Secondary deformities in cleft palate patients. *Ann Surg* 109:442, 1939.
24. Brown JB, McDowell F: Secondary repair of cleft lips and their nasal deformities. *Ann Surg* 114:101, 1941.
25. Humby G: The nostril in secondary harelip. *Lancet* 1:1275, 1938.
26. Barsky AJ: *Principles and Practice of Plastic Surgery.* Baltimore, Williams & Wilkins Co, 1950, p 243.
27. Whitlow DR, Constable JD: Crossed alar wing procedure for correction of late deformity in the unilateral cleft lip nose. *Plast Reconstr Surg* 52:38, 1973.
28. Fomon S, Bell JW, Syracuse VR: Harelip-nose revision. *Arch Otolaryngol* 64:14, 1956.
29. Gorney M, Falces E: Repair of post cleft nasal deformities with gullwing cartilage graft. In *Abstracts of the Second International Congress on Cleft Palate,* Copenhagen, 1973, p 53.
30. Dibbell DG: A cartilaginous columellar strut in cleft lip rhinoplasties. *Br J Plast Surg* 29:247, 1976.
31. Millard DR: Earlier correction of the unilateral cleft lip nose. *Plast Reconstr Surg* 70:64, 1982.
32. Blair VP: Nasal deformities associated with congenital cleft of the lip. *JAMA* 84:185, 1925.

33. Joseph J: Nasenplastik und Sonstige Gesichtsplastik nebst einem anhang uber Mammaplastik. *Und Korperplastik*. Leipzig, Curt Kabitsch, 1931.
34. Gillies H, Kilner TP: Harelip: Operations for the correction of secondary deformities of cleft lip. *Lancet* 2:1369, 1932.
35. Berkeley WT: The cleft lip nose. *Plast Reconstr Surg* 23:567, 1959.
36. Cronin TD: Lengthening columella by use of skin from nasal floor and alae. *Plast Reconstr Surg* 21:417, 1958.
37. Rees TD, Guy CL, Converse JM: Repair of the cleft lip nose: Addendum to the synchronous technique with full thickness skin grafting of the nasal vestibule. *Plast Reconstr Surg* 37:47, 1966.
38. Reynolds JR, Horton CE: An alar lift in cleft lip rhinoplasty. *Plast Reconstr Surg* 35:377, 1965.
39. Erich JB: A technique for correcting a flat nostril in cases of repaired harelip. *Plast Reconstr Surg* 12:320, 1953.
40. Musgrave RH, Dupertuis SM: Revision of the unilateral cleft lip nostril. *Plast Reconstr Surg* 25:223, 1960.
41. Millard DR: The unilateral cleft lip nose. *Plast Reconstr Surg* 34:169, 1964.
42. Farrior RT: The problem of the unilateral cleft lip nose. *Laryngoscope* 72:289, 1962.
43. Longacre JJ, Halak DB, Munick LH, et al: A new approach to the correction of the nasal deformity following cleft lip repair. *Plast Reconstr Surg* 38:555, 1966.
44. Berkeley WT: Correction of secondary cleft-lip nasal deformities. *Plast Reconstr Surg* 44:234, 1969.

32

Orthodontics and Cephalometrics

Robert M. Mason, Ph.D., D.M.D.

Orthodontics is a specialty area of dentistry that is concerned primarily with diagnosing and treating abnormalities of the dental arches (1). Many malrelationships between the dental arches, or malocclusions, are intrinsic problems of tooth eruption or position. Other malocclusions, however, relate to malposition of the jaws. Such conditions are skeletal malocclusions, denoting that the underlying problem in tooth position relates to an abnormal position of the jaw(s).

The teeth provide lip support; that is, the position of the lips at rest is determined in part by support from the anterior dentition. In determining whether extractions would compromise the profile, many orthodontists use the guideline of the "esthetic line" (2). This is an imaginary line that connects the tip of the nose and the most prominent projection of the chin. For a well-balanced face, the lower lip should be within a few millimeters of approximating this line. The upper lip should be several millimeters behind this line. The diagnostic use of the esthetic line should be tempered with a range of differences in various racial or ethnic groups, as well as the patient's desires for facial appearance.

Orthodontics for the Patient with Cleft Lip and Palate

The interaction between orthodontist and plastic surgeon for patients with cleft lip and palate is an ongoing one that begins at birth and ends at the completion of all treatment in adulthood. In infancy, the orthodontist may be called upon to assist the surgeon in providing an environment wherein the cleft can be successfully closed after some retraction of a protrusive premaxillary segment. A protrusive premaxilla can be retracted with extraoral traction of some type, or by intraoral appliances that pit the palatal shelves against the premaxillary-vomerine complex. In such instances, the orthodontist serves at the pleasure of the surgeon in providing such retractions in those cases in which some appliance or headgear is needed.

There is considerable variation in the activities and philosophies of orthodontists regarding the disposition of the dental arches in the growing child with a repaired cleft lip or palate (3–5). In all patients, a hypoplastic situation is involved in that the cleft itself represents a loss of either soft tissue or bone to some extent.

Most children with a repaired cleft palate exhibit some form of collapse of the dental arch during development, especially between ages 3 and 8 years. Collapse of the upper dental arch results in a cross-bite condition, usually posterior to the cleft. A cross-bite is a condition in which one or a group of maxillary teeth are positioned lingual or palatal to their mandibular counterparts. In most children, whether clefted or not, a cross-bite represents a *condition* rather than a *problem*. Accordingly, it is now held that there is no need to correct a cross-bite just because it is there. A cross-bite corrected in the primary or mixed dentition period (when some baby and some permanent teeth are present) does not ensure that no treatment will be needed when the permanent teeth erupt.

Most orthodontists working with children with clefts do not treat many conditions in the primary dentition. Exceptions to this are badly rotated incisor teeth that either interfere with mastication or create a cosmetic or psychological problem for the child. The general guideline in treating a child with a cleft for orthodontic conditions before all permanent teeth have erupted is that, when indicated, work should be accomplished quickly and then be discontinued as expediently as possible. In this way, a child's cooperation is not severely compromised for the variety of orthodontic and surgical treatments that may be anticipated in the teenage years.

Expansion of the dental arch is an example of a procedure in orthodontics that may be considered from birth onward. Some infants may require expansion of the dental arch and palate to reposition the premaxilla properly before lip repair. Such expansion would be done with an acrylic appliance either pinned into the palate or affixed using the undercuts of the palatal shelves (4).

In the period of primary or mixed dentition, expansion may be indicated for those patients who need a maxillary or alveolar crestal bone graft. A maxillary bone graft is usually placed in the line of the primary palatal cleft up at the area of the nasal floor. Such grafts serve to stabilize the dental arch of the maxilla as well as provide an improved contour and support for the base of the nose (6).

Alveolar crestal bone grafts, by contrast, are placed on the crest of the alveolar ridge in many patients. Such grafts provide an adequate bony bed for permanent teeth to erupt through to find a normal place in the dental arch. A crestal graft also provides a more normal gingival contour to the maxillary dental arch. For mechanical support, a marrow graft seems most useful at the crest of the maxillary alveolus. The marrow is usually put through a bone mill and made into paste as used at the crest of the maxillary alveolus. This procedure provides a means for a permanent tooth to erupt through the graft, unlike a cortical bone graft, which forms an obstacle for tooth eruption.

The use of an alveolar crestal bone graft in a cleft patient is usually accomplished at 6 or 11 years of age. These age preferences relate to the development of the permanent lateral incisor and canine, respectively. The optimal time to place an alveolar crestal graft is before the permanent tooth in the area has erupted, and when the root of the tooth is half-formed (6).

Many children with clefts grow appropriately in the early school-age years, only to become midfacially retrusive as they approach the teenage range. It is very difficult to identify those children in the early years of development. Orthodontic treatment to prepare a child for midfacial surgery differs significantly from that designed simply to match the upper dental arch to the lower. Accordingly, the identification of potential cases of midfacial retrusion should be accomplished as soon as possible. Because there are no universally applicable principles or observations that would separate out potential jaw surgery cases at an early age, most orthodontists minimize therapy efforts until the full extent of the skeletal situation can be properly assessed (7).

Orthodontics for the Osteotomy Patient

Whether a patient has a history of cleft lip and palate or not, the appearance of a skeletal jaw dysplasia signals the need for treatment planning interactions between surgeon and orthodontist. It is uncommon for any patient to have surgery to reposition one of the jaws and dental arches without some orthodontic planning and treatment preoperatively and in the postsurgical stabilization period. Orthodontic treatment is a necessary part of the sequence of treatment for such patients because there are almost always dental compensations for the jaw variations seen. In the instance of a midfacial retrusion problem, for example, the upper incisor teeth usually flare forward, and the lower incisors are tipped lingually to maintain some contactual relationship in the presence of a skeletal malocclusion. Such positional changes of the teeth are not stable or desirable as the jaws are realigned surgically. Hence, orthodontic treatment preoperatively for the osteotomy patient involves *decompensating* the dentition; that is, realigning the teeth over each bone to which they are attached. The surgical correction of jaw position would then not only align the jaws but place the teeth in a stable relationship, one jaw to the other (8, 9).

An orthodontist working with an orthognathic surgery patient must know where the jaws are intended to be repositioned before planning any orthodontic treatment as a part of the total therapy. If the jaws are going to be tipped, impacted, rotated, or reduced in any way, the position of the teeth must be considered. One of the ways that the orthodontist prepares the patient for orthodontics is to mimic the surgery on stone models set up on a metal articulator. This laboratory procedure can change the jaw position in the laboratory and can guide the ortho-

dontist in determining the type and extent of orthodontic movement of the dentition before surgery.

Another role the orthodontist usually plays in planning for jaw surgery is constructing an acrylic splint that is wired between the teeth during surgery to stabilize the surgically created repositioning of the jaw(s). The use of such a splint ensures that there is no guesswork in surgery as to the desired position of the jaws and teeth, or the proper position of the skeletal and dental midlines. Work done preoperatively in the orthodontic laboratory can provide the surgeon with important, specific information as to the amount of bone to be removed or added and the direction of movement of the jaw(s) (8, 9).

For an optimal result from orthognathic surgery, a data base should include dental study models, facial and intraoral photographs, a Panorex radiograph of the teeth, and a frontal and lateral cephalogram. In addition, a careful clinical examination and history are necessary for adequate planning (10). Overall, osteotomy procedures to mobilize one jaw or the other, or both, involve the combined efforts of several specialty areas, especially orthodontics and surgery.

Because of the problems of moving bone and soft tissues in patients with clefts, there is a general guideline in surgery that any movements of the maxilla over 8 mm should probably involve both jaws. That is, it is usually better to accomplish some movement of the maxilla and some in the opposite direction of the mandible rather than to risk the vascular and other problems (such as relapse) inherent in attempting to move a cleft maxilla a greater distance than 8 mm. While it may be possible to advance a cleft maxilla safely more than 8 mm, most clinicians would tend to agree that the 8-mm figure is a reasonable cutoff point for deciding to do two-jaw surgery in a well-controlled osteotomy procedure associated with maxillary and mandibular dysplasias.

Orthodontics and Cephalometrics

Cephalometric x-ray films provide a means of evaluating the interrelationships of cranial, facial, and pharyngeal structures either on a longitudinal or on a serial basis. Speech clinicians have utilized lateral single-exposure (static) x-ray head films to study the functions of the velopharyngeal mechanism. Such films are obtained while the patient sustains a phonation of "ah," "ee," or "s." These tasks are thought to assess the *functional potential* of the velopharyngeal apparatus to achieve velopharyngeal closure as seen in the two dimensions of the lateral cephalogram (11).

The dynamics of speech are better appreciated by motion picture x-ray techniques, such as videofluoroscopy. Other techniques, such as magnetic resonance imaging, may provide a noninvasive means of obtaining baseline information currently being assessed by a host of radiographic instruments and techniques.

The orthodontist continues to rely primarily on the lateral and frontal static headplate for most diagnostic information. This is associated with the standardization of patient position and a fixed, 5-foot distance between the anode of the x-ray source and the midsagittal plane of the head. Radiographs so obtained can be measured, and the resultant data can be compared to normative information. Most of the cephalometric data base in orthodontics of interest to the plastic surgeon is associated with findings from the lateral, static x-ray film (12–14). Selected landmarks and normative data will be presented here (11).

UPPER FACE

The most common method of assessing the relative position of the maxilla is in relation to the cranial base. In the anteroposterior dimension, the angle formed by landmarks SNA provides this assessment (Fig. 32.1). The SN arm of the angle contributes the cranial component. The *nasion* (N) is the frontonasal suture, and *sella* (S) is the middle of the sella turcica. The line drawn from N to *point A* expresses the position of the maxilla. Point A is the most involuted portion of the anterior maxilla. This point is less variable than the *anterior nasal spine* (ANS), which is buried under the soft tissues of the nose.

A normal SNA is 82 ± 4°. Therefore, an SNA of 70° would indicate midface retrusion and an SNA of 90° would indicate maxillary protrusion. There are, of course, exceptions to such findings. A low position of S would affect this angle and would have to be corrected to obtain an accurate estimate of the SNA significance.

There are no well-established cephalometric norms for the vertical dimensions of the maxilla. *Upper facial height* is usually measured from N to the ANS, and *lower facial height* from the ANS to the *menton* (lowest point on the chin). The normative data for upper facial height (N-ANS) in adult males is 60 ± 4 mm, and for females, 56 ± 3 mm. Caution is urged in the use of these norms, however, because upper facial height should be viewed as a proportion of total facial height (45%) rather than as an isolated finding.

Useful information about facial height can also be obtained by identifying the location of the ANS and the PNS (the *posterior nasal spine*). The palatal plane, as determined by a line extending from ANS to PNS, is usually parallel with the SN line and should extend posteriorly to the anterior tubercle of the atlas.

If the ANS is higher or lower than the PNS, this may signal a vertical discrepancy in the position of the maxilla. A "canted" maxillary plane, such as with the PNS lower than the ANS, is often a sign of a skeletal dysplasia of the maxilla, such as posterior vertical maxillary excess. This situation would, incidentally, also create an anterior open-bite malocclusion.

LOWER FACE

The mandible is certainly an important structure to evaluate because it interrelates with the tongue, hyoid bone, and oropharyngeal area. The most frequently used measure of the horizontal position of the mandible is the angle SNB. *Point B* is the most involuted portion of the anterior mandible (Fig. 32.2). This area is above the chin and below the alveolus and is known as *supramentale*.

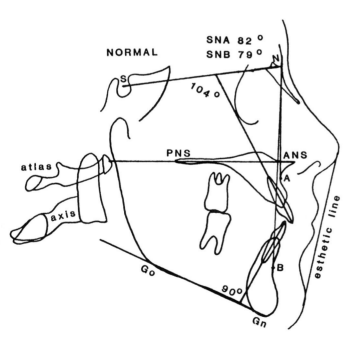

FIGURE 32.1. Selected radiographic landmarks and angles express the position of maxilla and mandible compared to the base of the skull. **SNA** expresses the horizontal position of the maxilla. **SNB** expresses the horizontal position of the mandible. **ANS-PNS** shows the palatal plane, which is typically at the same vertical level as the atlas. The upper incisor to the SN plane is shown, and the lower incisor to the mandibular plane (**Go-Gn**) is demonstrated.

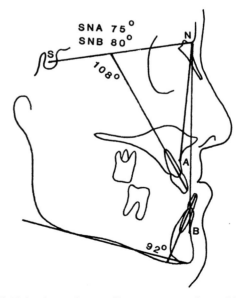

FIGURE 32.2. Lateral x-ray film traces a patient with pseudoprognathism. The cephalometric measures indicate a normal and a retruded maxilla in spite of the clinical appearance of a large mandible.

The measurement SNB expresses the horizontal position of the mandible with reference to the cranial base. The norm for SNB is 79 ± 3°. The SNB measurement, in comparison with SNA, provides the clinician with a basis for determining whether the patient has a true prognathism or a pseudoprognathism. As one might expect, a normal SNB in combination with a diminished SNA might give the appearance of mandibular prognathism rather than of midfacial retrusion, which is often the real cause of the jaw discrepancy.

While SNA and SNB relate the maxilla and mandible to the cranial base area, the measurement ANB relates maxilla to mandible. An ANB of 3° is normal, with a range of 0–5°.

DENTITION

Of the many dental measurements utilized in orthodontics and other areas of dentistry, the most useful for describing the position of the teeth relative to the bones to which they are attached involves the incisors. The angulation of the upper incisors is measured by extending a line from upper incisor tip, through the root of the incisor and extending to intersect a line from sella to nasion. The norm for upper incisor to NS is 104 ± 6°. For the lower incisor, the line from incisor tip through the root is extended to intersect a line that follows the mandibular plane. This is constructed by connecting a line from the mandibular angle (*gonion*) to the most anteroinferior point of the chin (*gnathion*). The norm for lower incisor to Go-Gn (the mandibular plane) is 95 ± 7°.

When the upper and lower incisor positions are considered, especially in comparison with the maxillary and mandibular positions (SNA and SNB), the clinician is provided with sufficient information to evaluate whether dental, skeletal, or a combination of variations is present.

CRANIAL BASE

Because the facial skeleton attaches onto the cranial base and is influenced in growth by the configuration of the base of the cranium, it is important to assess the cranial base area as part of a lateral cephalometric analysis. The landmarks nasion (N) and *basion* (Ba) serve to separate the neurocranium from the facial skeleton (Fig. 32.3). The basion is the most anterior projection of the foramen magnum. Unfortunately, a straight line drawn from nasion to basion does not reveal much of value about the configuration of the cranial base. The addition of another landmark, sella (S), permits an angular measure to be made as an expression of the cranial base area and its relationship with the facial skeleton.

The *cranial base angle* is formed by connecting lines between the nasion, the middle of the sella turcica, and the basion. Normal cranial base angle (N-S-Ba) is 130 ± 10°. That means that a cranial base angle less than 120° would indicate an acute cranial base, while one greater than 140° would be considered an obtuse cranial base.

Cranial base angle does not change greatly from childhood to adult form. Some fluctuation in the S-Ba arm of

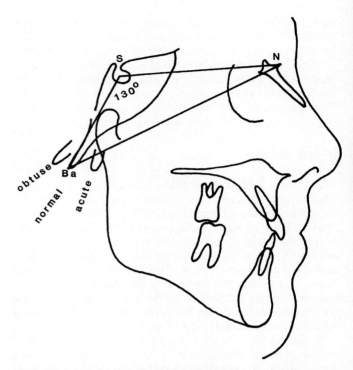

FIGURE 32.3. X-ray film traces the cranial base area from nasion (**N**) to basion (**Ba**). The configuration of the cranial base is expressed by cranial base angle from nasion (**N**) to sella turcica (**S**) to basion (**Ba**). Variations in cranial base angle are shown.

the angle does occur, however. Nonetheless, an individual with an acute cranial base early on maintains this pattern over time.

An acute cranial base could contribute to reduction of the nasopharyngeal airspace while also encouraging a *forward* growth tendency of the face. An obtuse cranial base angle, by contrast, would encourage a *downward* growth pattern of the face. This is because the temporomandibular joint area is positioned more posteriorly, as are other structures.

CERVICAL SPINE

The morphology of the cervical spine area is an important component of a lateral radiographic assessment. The upper vertebral column serves as an attachment for the muscles and soft tissues of the nasopharynx. If the cranial base angle is obtuse, for example, and the cervical spine is obliged to be positioned more posteriorly than normal because of the flexion of the cranial base, the bony or osseous depth of the nasopharynx is increased. This observation may be an especially important one if the patient is a candidate for adenoidectomy. Removal of the adenoid mass may lead to the development of hypernasal speech because of the increased osseous pharyngeal depth. In such situations, the adenoid mass is said to have *masked* a morphological problem that was there all along.

The upper three cervical vertebrae are most appropriate to examine because they are located in the area where

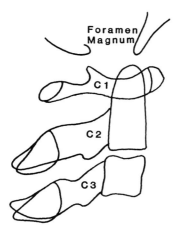

FIGURE 32.4. Right lateral view of a normal cervical spine shows C1, C2, and C3 in relationship to the foramen magnum.

velopharyngeal and lingual activity is prominent. It is quite common that the area of velopharyngeal and lingual activity is prominent. It is quite common that the area of velopharyngeal closure is adjacent to the first cervical vertebra (the atlas, or C1). The normal atlas, as seen in the lateral cephalometric projection (Fig. 32.4), has an anterior tubercle that extends about 2–3 mm anterior to the plane of the other cervical vertebrae. This is true whether the configuration of the cervical spine is straight (a "military" spine) or slightly curved (a *lordotic* cervical spine). In most adults, some normal lordosis is observed.

It is well known from cephalometric studies that a velopharyngeal gap of 3 mm is sufficient to create a hypernasal condition. Consequently, small variations in the configuration of the anterior tubercle of the atlas can potentially contribute in a significant way to the increased depth of the nasopharynx. The most common variations in the anterior tubercle of the atlas include flattening and superoposterior rotation (Fig. 32.5). These conditions are developmental variations that are *not* associated with any neurological deficit. Consequently, a radiologist may not attach any special significance to such findings. While they are morphological variations, they are common in the cleft palate population but not in a normal sample. Their appearance should alert the clinician to the possible deleterious consequences to normal nasal resonance balance (nasality) from a total adenoidectomy.

The atlas can be positioned in a superior location, above the usual area for velopharyngeal closure, if the

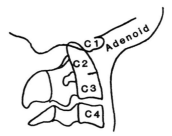

FIGURE 32.6. An anomalous cervical spine is shown in a patient with a submucous cleft palate deformity. The atlas is fused to the base of the skull (occipitalization of the atlas), and the spinous processes of C2 and C3 are fused. The odontoid process of C2 has invaginated into the foramen magnum, creating a potential hazard (see text for discussion).

occipital condyles are flattened or hypoplastic. The epitome of this situation is where the atlas is fused to the base of the skull (Fig. 32.6). *Occipitalization of the atlas,* as this condition is called, can be potentially dangerous to the patient's health because the second cervical vertebra is also positioned superiorly. If the odontoid process of C2 is positioned within the confines of the foramen magnum, the space for the spinal cord is compromised. This situation is referred to as *basilar invagination of the axis* (C2) into the foramen magnum. Any suspicious instances of the odontoid appearing to invade the space of the foramen magnum should be referred to a radiologist for a definitive evaluation. Such a patient needs to be positioned very carefully for intubation if surgery is undertaken. Hyperextension of the head for intubation serves to bring the *opisthion,* the posterior margin of the foramen magnum, forward. The spinal cord could potentially be damaged between the odontoid and opisthion.

Individuals with submucous cleft deformities have a relatively high incidence of cervical spine variations. In addition to the conditions mentioned above, fusion of the bodies or spinous processes of the second and third cervical vertebrae are common variations. Fusion of C1 and C2 is very rare. While cervical spine variations are more prominent in cleft than noncleft individuals, it appears that the frequency of occurrence in clefts increases as the severity of clefts decreases.

Cervical spine variations are also frequent in many syndromes, such as Klippel-Feil (short neck, low hairline, reduction in number of cervical vertebrae, or fusion of several vertebrae).

Altogether, the cervical spine area comprises one of the components of the osseous pharyngeal depth. Its configuration also contributes to the framework for the velopharyngeal portal. The anteroposterior location of the cervical spine is determined in large part by the configuration of the cranial base.

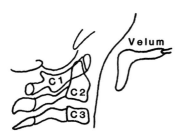

FIGURE 32.5. Flattening and superposterior rotation of the anterior tubercle of the atlas is shown. This minor variation can contribute to an increased depth of the pharynx.

References

1. Graber TM: *Orthodontics* 3rd ed. Philadelphia, WB Saunders Co, 1972.
2. Ricketts RM: Esthetics, environment, and the law of lip relation. *Am J Orthod* 54:272, 1968.

3. Ross RB, Johnston MC: The effect of early orthodontic treatment on a facial growth in cleft lip and palate. *Cleft Palate J* 4:157, 1967.
4. Georgiade NG, Mason RM, Riefkohl R, Georgiade G, Barwick W: Preoperative positioning of the protruding premaxilla in the bilateral cleft lip patient. *Plast Reconstr Surg* 83:1, 32, 1989.
5. Peat JH: Effects of presurgical oral orthopedics on bilateral complete clefts of the lip and palate. *Cleft Palate J* 19:100, 1982.
6. Waite DE, Kersten RB: Residual alveolar and palatal clefts. In Bell WH, Profitt WR, White RP (eds): *Surgical Correction of Dentofacial Deformities*. Philadelphia, WB Saunders Co, 1980, p 1329.
7. Profitt WR, Epker BN: Treatment planning for dentofacial deformities. In Bell WH, Profitt WR, White RP (eds): *Surgical Correction of Dentofacial Deformities*. Philadelphia, WB Saunders Co, 1980, p 155.
8. Bell WH, Proffit WR, White RP: *Surgical Correction of Dentofacial Deformities*. Philadelphia, WB Saunders Co, Vols I and II, 1980.
9. Epker BN, Woolford LM: *Dentofacial Deformities: Surgical-Orthodontic Correction*. St. Louis, CV Mosby Co, 1980.
10. Profitt WR, Epker BN, Ackerman JL: Systematic description of dentofacial deformities: The data base. In Bell WF, Profitt WR, White RP (eds): *Surgical Correction of Dentofacial Deformities*. Philadelphia, WB Saunders Co, 1980, p 105.
11. Bateman HE, Mason RM: *Applied Anatomy and Physiology of the Speech and Hearing Mechanism*. Springfield, IL, Charles C Thomas Co, 1984.
12. Broadbent BH, Broadbent BH Jr, Golden WH: *Bolton Standards of Dentofacial Developmental Growth*. St. Louis, CV Mosby Co, 1975.
13. Riolo ML, Moyers RE, McNamara JA Jr, et al: *An Atlas of Craniofacial Growth*. Monograph #2, Craniofacial Growth Series. Ann Arbor, Center for Human Growth and Development, University of Michigan, 1974.
14. Zide B, Grayson B, McCarthy JG: Cephalometric analysis: Part I. *Plast Reconstruc Surg* 68:5, 816, 1981.

33

Principles of Speech Pathology in the Child with Cleft Lip and Palate

John E. Riski, Ph.D. and Penny L. Mirrett, M.A.

The numerous problems found in the child born with cleft lip and palate necessitate attention from a team of professionals. The plastic surgeon is often the hub of this team and is the primary caregiver to the child. However, the plastic surgeon often depends on other members of the team for determining the necessity and timing of surgical procedures. The speech pathologist interacts with all members of the team but has unique interactions with the plastic surgeon because of the effect of surgical repair on speech function.

Role of Speech Pathologist

The role of the speech clinician varies as the child's oral-motor capabilities and linguistic system develop and as the surgical correction of the cleft proceeds. The role is variously one of counselor, evaluator, and treatment provider. Early in the child's life, the speech pathologist is a counselor to the parents about the development of communication skills. Informational pamphlets are often used as an adjunct to direct counseling. These pamphlets deal with problems associated with clefting, describe the professionals who will treat these problems, and list activities designed to stimulate speech and language skills (1). The speech pathologist is the team member who monitors emerging expressive language skills, which signal the ideal time for primary palate repair. As the child's expressive speech skills evolve, the speech pathologist will coordinate or provide treatment for the child's misarticulations and evaluate the competency of velopharyngeal function. With the plastic surgeon, any velopharyngeal incompetence is examined, and appropriate plans for secondary palatal surgery are made. Velopharyngeal function should also be carefully examined before a planned adenoidectomy or maxillary advancement to determine the effects of these procedures on speech quality.

BEFORE PALATAL CLOSURE

The parents are counseled regarding what to expect from their child's early speech attempts. Resonance will be hypernasal. The child will be able to say words with nasal sounds, such as "mama," correctly but will not say words with pressure sounds, such as "dada," correctly. The parents are instructed in techniques for stimulating speech and language development. This is achieved through frequent play activities that focus on verbal interaction between parent and child and appropriate modeling of speech and language by the parents.

AFTER PALATAL CLOSURE

Speech and language stimulation should continue with age-appropriate games, vocabulary, and syntax. The parents are now asked to focus on the sounds that the child makes. If there are no confounding developmental problems, we expect the child to begin making crisp, pressure consonants such as /p, b, t, d, k, and g/ between the ages of 18 months and 2 years. Often, the parents are asked to occlude the child's nose manually while playing "sound games," such as repeating the syllable "ba ba ba ba." Occluding the nose prevents any nasal air flow and directs the air stream to the oral cavity. The parents are also asked to observe any signs of velopharyngeal dysfunction such as nasal reflux while eating or drinking, or nasal air flow or facial grimacing while talking.

Assessment of Velopharyngeal Function

Normal velopharyngeal function provides adequate closure of the velopharyngeal portal for pressure speech sound production as well as adequate opening of the portal for nasal breathing and nasal speech sound production. Resonance should be neither hypernasal or hyponasal (2). Our understanding of normal velopharyngeal function has been aided by assessment of the portal using a variety of instruments, including multiview videofluoroscopy and nasal and oral endoscopy. Appreciation of the sphincteric nature of portal function during speech is somewhat recent (3).

Assessment of velopharyngeal dysfunction is one of the most frequently addressed topics in the cleft palate literature. It is necessarily important because velopharyngeal function reflects the success of surgical closure of the cleft and the need for secondary palatal surgery. A growing body of literature deals with the effectiveness of popular assessment tools, including radiography, cine- or videofluoroscopy (3–6), fiberoptic nasal (7, 8) or oral (9, 10) endoscopy, and pressure-flow transducers (11, 12). In addition to these most frequently used techniques, the literature also deals with sound pressure level instruments (13), accelerometers (14), and photodetectors (15).

Spirited discussion leads to only a few accepted tenets. Each of the techniques has its advantages and disadvantages. No one instrument provides all of the necessary information. Recently, an ad hoc committee of the American Cleft Palate Association suggested minimal standards for evaluation of velopharyngeal function. The standards included a perceptual evaluation of resonance and assessment using at least one instrument that provides evaluation during connected speech (i.e., fluoroscopy or pressure-flow instrumentation) (16).

Longitudinal study of velopharyngeal port function has demonstrated its instability in children as their phonological system develops and craniofacial growth and adenoid involution occur (17, 18). Some children develop velopharyngeal incompetency as the adenoids involute (19). Some children eventually resolve the hypernasality that is identified immediately following palatoplasty (20). These studies demonstrate the need for longitudinal assessment of velopharyngeal function and the need to exercise some caution before performing a pharyngoplasty.

Velopharyngeal function has an impact on speech proficiency. However, speech proficiency is not an adequate measure of velopharyngeal function. These two areas should be evaluated separately. It is possible to have severely defective speech and a competent velopharyngeal mechanism. In contrast, normal speech usually cannot be produced without a competent velopharyngeal mechanism.

NASAL AIRWAY PATENCY

The need for adequate nasal airway patency is also becoming more clearly understood. Aerodynamic assessment has demonstrated the requirements of adequate nasal airway patency (21). It has been suggested that nasal deformities decrease nasal patency in the cleft palate population (22). The pharyngeal flap pharyngoplasty further decreases nasal airway patency in children but not in adults (23). Recent investigations have revealed that both children and adults with cleft lip and palate demonstrate increased prevalence of mouth and mouth + nasal breathing (70%) when compared to the noncleft population (15–30%) (24).

EARLY INDICATORS OF FUNCTIONAL VELOPHARYNGEAL CLOSURE

The young child with limited speech, limited attention span, and a limited ability to cooperate presents a special problem for evaluation of velopharyngeal function. Patience and perseverance are necessary qualities of the examiner.

Observations made of a child's speech can provide important information when the child will not cooperate as an active participant in the evaluation. The appearance of accurately produced pressure sounds (especially "p" and "b") are good prognostic indicators of velopharyngeal competency (25). Additionally, observations of emerging language may alert the team and family members to concomitant language problems.

SCREENING VELOPHARYNGEAL CLOSURE

Numerous devices exist that can help determine whether or not the velopharyngeal port is opened or closed for speech. Generally, anything that is sensitive to air flow can be used. The advantage of these devices is that they are inexpensive, portable, noninvasive, and very accurate for determining the presence of nasal air flow. Examples of these devices include the See Scape (26) and nasal listening tube (27, 28). Other devices that are often used clinically are mirrors and paper paddles. The object of this screening is to monitor nasal air flow for a speech sample, such as "puppy, puppy," that should be devoid of nasal air flow. The presence of any air flow indicates some degree of velopharyngeal opening and also indicates that further objective testing is warranted.

OBJECTIVE ASSESSMENT OF VELOPHARYNGEAL FUNCTION

Formal assessment generally awaits the development of a mature, cooperative child. Although this usually happens around 4 years of age, sometimes a child can be tested formally as early as 2 or 3 or, at times, not until 5 or 6 years of age. Patience and persistence remain the watch words.

Pressure-Flow

Pressure-flow instrumentation measures of the oral-nasal pressure differential and the volume-velocity of nasal air flow provides quantifiable data about velopharyngeal port function for speech. The hydrokinetic equation ($A = \dot{V}/0.65\sqrt{[2(P_1 - P_2)/d]}$) has been modified by Warren and Dubois (11) for determining the area of the velopharyngeal port orifice. Recently, this modification of the hydrokinetic equation has stood the test of vigorous study (29, 30). Pressure-flow study is an objective and reliable method for serial, noninvasive measures of velopharyngeal port function. Pressure-flow instrumentation is now available on a commercial basis as Perci-PC (Palatal efficiency rating computed instantaneously; Microtronics Corp., Drawer 399, Carrboro, NC 27510). General application of pressure principles allows the assessment of velopharyngeal function, laryngeal airway resistance, and nasal airway patency (31).

Velopharyngeal competence is usually found when orifice size is less than 10 mm² and differential oral-nasal air pressure is greater than 3 cm H_2O. Borderline competence is usually related to an orifice size between 10 and 20 mm² and a differential pressure that is between 1 and 2.99 cm H_2O or a differential pressure that varies above and below 3.0 cm H_2O. Finally, an incompetent velopharyngeal mechanism is generally related to an orifice size greater than 20 mm² and a pressure differential less than 1 cm H_2O (32).

Radiography

Lateral still radiographs, cineradiography, and video-fluoroscopy have been used for some time to assess velopharyngeal function. The use of multiview video-fluoroscopy has been popularized by Skolnick and his colleagues (3, 4). These researchers have demonstrated the sphincteric nature of the velopharyngeal portal and the advantages of multiview assessment for surgical planning. Video- or cinefluoroscopy allows the assessment of velar function in its dynamic state for connected speech. Still radiographs often misrepresent velar function because of the limited speech sample that can be employed (6). In addition, shadows and the two-dimensional nature of the still radiograph can distort the true nature of velopharyngeal function.

Nasoendoscopy

Nasal endoscopes have been popularized as a tool for evaluating velopharyngeal function because there is no irradiation and because they allow direct observation of the portal during connected speech. There are rigid endoscopes and flexible endoscopes. Rigid scopes provide better optics, but flexible scopes are more comfortable to the patient. Each allows recording of the image using 35-mm or videotape formats. Each suffers from the disadvantage that younger patients are often difficult to scope successfully.

Endoscopy provides information similar to that obtained by base view videofluoroscopy. It provides information about the mesial movement of the lateral pharyngeal walls that cannot be provided by lateral radiography.

SPEECH ASSESSMENT

There have been numerous studies of articulation development in the cleft lip/palate population (33, 34). This research may be summarized by noting that children with clefts of the lip develop speech at normal rates, whereas children with clefts of the palate develop speech at a somewhat slower rate than normal. There is a positive relationship between the extent of clefting and the articulation deficiency. That is, children with clefts of the lip and palate have poorer articulation than children with clefts of the palate only. There is also a good deal of heterogeneity of articulation skills within any one type of cleft. For any one group of children with unilateral clefts of the lip and palate, there may be a number of children who will develop speech along normal developmental lines, and there will be other children who have extremely deficient or delayed articulation development (34).

The speech pathologist has a number of standardized articulation inventories at his or her disposal. However, no standardized test is useful without experienced clinical ears and eyes for transcribing a child's speech. Specific types of errors may indicate dysfunction of the velopharyngeal valve. These errors include hypernasal distortion, nasal air escape, glottal stops, and pharyngeal fricative sound substitutions. It has been suggested that the speech apparatus functions with the use of pressure-sensing regulators (35). Under normal valving conditions, a fairly constant pressure is maintained along the vocal tract during speech articulation. The unique misarticulations associated with velopharyngeal incompetence (VPI) may then be attempts to maintain a constant resistance in the presence of a loss of pressure through the velopharyngeal port.

The presence of some speech errors is normal in young children. Errors such as "tat/cat," "wabbit/rabbit," and "teef/teeth" are examples of normal developmental errors. Children are expected to outgrow these errors, although excessive errors (given the age of the child) should be treated with speech therapy.

The child with errors that reflect velopharyngeal dysfunction requires careful evaluation. These errors may persist after successful management of VPI. Because misarticulations are a learned behavior, they require unlearning (i.e., speech therapy). Recently, the identifiable repertoire of compensatory misarticulations used by children with cleft palate has been expanded to include pharyngeal stops, midpalatal stops, and nasal fricatives. These classifications have been added to the classic glottal stop and pharyngeal fricative substitutions (36).

When these errors are concomitant with VPI, the course of management is two-pronged. First, the VPI must be treated; second, the speech problem must be treated. In some cases, speech therapy can begin before the VPI is managed. In such cases, the nostrils can be occluded manually to direct the air stream orally. The child usually cannot employ newly learned sounds without holding his or her nose. Therapy before surgery can assist learning after surgery (37).

ORONASAL FISTULAS

The loss of air through an oronasal fistula can be detected and quantified with the assessment tools described previously. It is wise to repeat these measures once with the fistula open and a second time with the fistula temporarily occluded with dental wax (38) or chewing gum. With the fistula successfully occluded, the velopharyngeal port function can also be adequately tested.

Accurate assessment of air flow through the fistula is often confounded by obstructing turbinates or a deviated nasal septum. If the fistula is not patent, then certainly surgical intervention is not warranted for the time being.

A patent fistula will allow the loss of air for speech sounds produced anterior to its site. These are usually the /p, b, f, v, θ, and ð/ sounds, although others may be affected, depending on the location of the fistula and the placement of the tongue.

Fistulas should be managed when testing indicates air loss sufficient to undermine speech. Research suggests that only larger fistulas are capable of such air loss (39). Fistulas may be covered with a dental appliance or closed surgically. Surgical intervention should be delayed until after any planned maxillary arch expansion because this might reopen any fistula closed under tension.

Treatment Strategies

PALATOPLASTY

There is sufficient evidence to suggest that children who have their palate closed early (before 1 year of age) often develop normal speech earlier and more easily than children who have the palate closed later (40). This seems to be especially true for those consonant sounds that depend on oral air pressure (i.e., plosive and fricative sounds) (41). Because the palatoplasty is performed so that the child may develop normal speech, these factors are often important in planning the timing of the surgery.

The palatoplasty is usually successful in creating a competent velopharyngeal mechanism in 80% of children. This 80% success rate may or may not be influenced by the initial type of cleft (42, 43). Recent evidence has revealed, however, that the dimensions of the unoperated nasopharynx vary within each type of cleft. There is some discussion that the type and extent of palatoplasty should be tailored to the preoperative dimensions of the nasopharynx (44).

PHARYNGOPLASTY

A pharyngoplasty is recommended when a VPI has been documented and when it is determined that the situation will not resolve. The documentation of the VPI is often the responsibility of the speech pathologist on the cleft palate team. However, the plastic surgeon should be an active participant in this diagnosis, reviewing the pressure-flow and radiographic data and participating in the nasal endoscopic examination of velopharyngeal function. A pharyngoplasty should be performed as soon as the nontransient VPI can be documented. The speech pathologist should review the connected speech of young children in an effort to detect signs of oral pressure sounds, which indicate velopharyngeal competence, or nasal sounds or glottal stops, which may indicate VPI.

The most common form of pharyngoplasty performed today is the superiorly based pharyngeal flap. The morbidity after pharyngoplasty is low. However, pharyngoplasty has been demonstrated to increase nasal airway resistance (23), and at least one patient has developed anorexia nervosa (45). The flap itself is a static obturator. Velopharyngeal closure is achieved by mesial movement of the lateral pharyngeal walls around the flap. Pharyngeal flaps are most successful if placed at the point of maximal constriction of the lateral pharyngeal walls and made wide enough to fill the residual defect during attempted closure. This information can best be obtained through multiview videofluoroscopic examination with or without accompanying nasal endoscopy (46, 47).

Another form of pharyngoplasty that has been enjoying increasing success at several centers is the Orticochea or sphinctering pharyngoplasty (48, 49). The Orticochea is similar to the Hynes' pharyngoplasty in that it creates superiorly based flaps from the palatopharyngeus muscle. These flaps are then elevated and inserted into the posterior pharyngeal wall using either an inferiorly based or a superiorly based pharyngeal flap to line the lateral flaps. The success of this procedure has been increased by making the lateral flaps sufficiently large and placing them at the height of maximal velar elevation, as observed from lateral radiographic assessment (50).

COMBINED PRIMARY PHARYNGOPLASTY AND PALATOPLASTY

Because the initial palatoplasty may not be completely successful, a number of investigators have incorporated a primary pharyngoplasty. The procedure remains controversial. There is a reported increase in the number of patients with normal resonance by some investigators (51–53) but not by others (54). One study demonstrated that 54% of the children receiving the combined procedure did not require a pharyngoplasty (55). Additionally, although all patients demonstrated velopharyngeal competence, 27% still exhibited aberrant misarticulations that are usually associated with VPI. Thus, the combined procedure did not prevent the misarticulations it was designed to prevent. Although it is clear that some children will require a pharyngoplasty, we cannot accurately identify those children at the time of palatoplasty.

SUBMUCOUS CLEFT PALATE

Children with submucous cleft palate (SMCP) are unique in the cleft palate population. The frequency is reported to be between 1 : 10,000 and 1 : 20,000. About one half of individuals with SMCP present with VPI. Further, VPI is more common in the coronal type closure pattern (56).

READING DISABILITIES

It is accepted that children with cleft lip/palate (CLP) and cleft palate only (CPO) only have a higher prevalence of speech and language disorders. Recent investigation of reading abilities in these two groups revealed that the CLP group studied displayed a prevalence for reading disabilities similar to that of the general population (9%). In contrast, the CPO group demonstrated a much higher rate of reading disabilities (33%) (57).

SPEECH THERAPY

Speech therapy for the child with a cleft palate is similar to the therapy provided for any noncleft palate patient. The distinction is that the child with cleft palate may present with unique misarticulations not found in the noncleft population (36). The same speech therapy strategies and facilitating postures are used to correct misarticulations in the child with cleft lip/palate.

The practicing clinician should recognize that there is no evidence that demonstrates that speech therapy can improve soft palate function (58). That is, once a VPI is diagnosed as adversely affecting speech or speech development, it should be managed surgically or prosthetically.

FUNCTIONAL VPI

The practicing clinician should also recognize that there is a small number of noncleft children with normal soft palate function who use some form of nasal air emission as a sound substitution (59, 60). This is termed a "functional VPI" or a "sound-specific VPI." The characteristics include: normal resonance, sound-specific use of some form of nasal air escape (usually a posterior nasal fricative), normal velopharyngeal function for correctly produced sounds, and the ability to correctly produce the errored sound without nasal air escape. This patient presents a special challenge because the misarticulations mimic those associated with a VPI. In truth, this represents a maladaptive use of the velopharyngeal valve and can only be treated with appropriate speech therapy. The differential diagnosis of an organic VPI from a "functional" VPI is the key to correct management.

Summary

The child with a cleft lip/palate represents a special challenge. Successful management of the various problems requires special knowledge, special tools, and most importantly, close communication among professionals. A high success rate in providing normal speech should be achieved when these principles are employed by the experienced speech-language pathologist and team.

References

1. Brookshire BL, Lynch JI, Fox DR: *A Parent-Child Cleft Palate Curriculum: Developing Speech and Language.* Tigard, OR, CC Publications, Inc, 1980.
2. Riski JE, Hoke JA, Dolan EA: The role of pressure-flow and endoscopic assessment in successful palatal obturator revision. *Cleft Palate J* 26:1, 1989.
3. Skolnick ML: Videofluoroscopic examination of the velopharyngeal portal during phonation in lateral and base projections—a new technique for studying the mechanics of closure. *Cleft Palate J* 7:803, 1970.
4. Skolnick ML: Velopharyngeal function in cleft palate. *Clin Plast Surg* 2:285, 1975.
5. Williams WN: Radiological measures of abnormal speech physiology. In Bzoch KR (ed): *Communicative Disorders Related to Cleft Lip and Palate.* Boston, Little, Brown & Co, 1979, pp 249–262.
6. Williams WN, Eisenbach OR: Assessing VP function: The lateral still technique vs. cinefluorography. *Cleft Palate J* 18:45, 1981.
7. Pigott RW: The results of nasopharyngoscopic assessment of pharyngoplasty. *Scand J Plast Surg* 8:148, 1974.
8. Gilbert STJ, Pigott RW: The feasibility of nasal pharyngoscopy using the 70° Storz-Hopkins nasopharyngoscope. *Br J Plast Surg* 35:14, 1982.
9. Zwitman DH: Velopharyngeal physiology after pharyngeal flap surgery as assessed by oral endoscopy. *Cleft Palate J* 19:40, 1982.
10. Zwitman DH: Oral endoscopic comparison of velopharyngeal closure before and after pharyngeal flap. *Cleft Palate J* 19:40, 1982.
11. Warren DW, DuBois AB: A pressure flow technique for measuring velopharyngeal orifice area during continuous speech. *Cleft Palate J* 1:52, 1964.
12. Warren DW, Devereux JL: An analog study of cleft palate speech. *Cleft Palate J* 3:103, 1966.
13. Fletcher SC: *Diagnosing Speech Disorders from Cleft Palate.* New York, Grune & Stratton, Inc, 1978.
14. Horii Y, Lange JE: Distributional analyses of an index of nasal coupling (HONC) in simulated hypernasal speech. *Cleft Palate J* 18:279, 1981.
15. Dalston RM: Photodetector assessment of velopharyngeal activity. *Cleft Palate J* 19:1, 1982.
16. Dalston RM, Marsh JL, Vig KW, et al: Minimal standards for reporting the results of surgery on patients with cleft lip, cleft palate, or both: A proposal. *Cleft Palate J* 25:3, 1988.
17. Van Demark DR, Morris HL: Stability of velopharyngeal competency. *Cleft Palate J* 20:18, 1983.
18. Van Demark DR, Hardin MA, Morris HL: Assessment of velopharyngeal competence: A long-term process. *Cleft Palate J* 25:362, 1988.
19. Mason RM, Warren DW: Adenoid involution and developing hypernasality in cleft palate. *J Speech Hear Dis* 45:469, 1980.
20. Fox DR, Lynch JI, Cronin TD: Change in nasal resonance over time: A clinical study. *Cleft Palate J* 25:245, 1988.
21. Warren DW: A quantitative technique for assessing nasal airway impairment. *Am J Orthod* 86:306, 1984.
22. Warren DW, Duany LF, Fischer ND: Nasal pathway resistance in normal and cleft lip and cleft palate subjects. *Cleft Palate J* 6:134, 1969.
23. Warren DW, Trier WC, Bevin AG: Effect of restorative procedures on the nasopharyngeal airway in cleft palate. *Cleft Palate J* 11:367, 1974.
24. Hairfield WM, Warren DW, Seaton DL: Prevalence of mouthbreathing in cleft lip and palate. *Cleft Palate J* 25:135, 1988.
25. Van Demark DR: Predictability of velopharyngeal competency. *Cleft Palate J* 16:429, 1979.
26. See Scape. Pro-Ed, Austin, TX, 1988.
27. Blakeley RW: *The Practice of Speech Pathology: A Clinical Diary.* Springfield, IL, Charles C Thomas, 1972.
28. Riski JE, Millard RT: The process of speech evaluation and treatment. In Cooper HK, Harding RL, Krogman WM, Mazaheri M, Millard RT (eds): *Cleft Palate and Cleft Lip: A Team Approach to Clinical Management and Rehabilitation of the Patient.* Philadelphia, WB Saunders Co, 1979, pp 431–484.
29. Smith BE, Weinberg B: Prediction of velopharyngeal orifice size: A re-examination of model experimentation. *Cleft Palate J* 17:277, 1980.
30. Smith BE, Weinberg B: Prediction of modeled velopharyngeal orifice areas during steady flow conditions and during aerodynamic stimulation of voiceless stop consonants. *Cleft Palate J* 19:172, 1982.
31. Riski JE, Perci PC: *Computerized Pressure-Flow Assessment.* Scientific Exhibit, American Cleft Palate Association Meeting, New York, 1986.
32. Warren D: A method for rating palatal efficiency. *Cleft Palate J* 16:279, 1979.
33. Van Demark DR, Morris HL, VandeHaar C: Patterns of articulation abilities in speakers with cleft palate. *Cleft Palate J* 16:230, 1979.
34. Riski JE, DeLong E: Articulation development in children with cleft lip/palate. *Cleft Palate J* 21:57, 1984.
35. Warren DW: Compensatory speech behaviors in individuals with cleft palate: A regulation/control phenomenon? *Cleft Palate J* 23:251, 1986.
36. Trost JE: Articulatory additions to the classical description of the speech of persons with cleft palate. *Cleft Palate J* 18:193, 1981.
37. Riski JE, Kunze LH, Nailling KR, et al: Speech patterns and

disturbances associated with clefts and craniofacial anomalies. In Serafin D, Georgiade NG (eds): *Pediatric Plastic Surgery*. St. Louis, CV Mosby, 1984, p 246.

38. Bless DM, Ewanowski SJ, Dibbell DG: A technique for temporary obturation of fistulae—a clinical note. *Cleft Palate J* 17:297, 1980.

39. Shelton RL, Blank JL: Oronasal fistulas, intraoral air pressure, and nasal air flow during speech. *Cleft Palate J* 21:91, 1984.

40. Dorf DS, Curtin JW: Early cleft palate repair and speech outcome. *Plast Reconstr Surg* 70:74, 1982.

41. O'Gara MM, Logemann JA: Phonetic analyses of the speech development of babies with cleft palate. *Cleft Palate J* 25:122, 1988.

42. Riski JE: Articulation skills and oral-nasal resonance in children with pharyngeal flaps. *Cleft Palate J* 16:421, 1979.

43. Karnell MP, Van Demark DR: Longitudinal speech performance in patients with cleft palate: Comparisons based on secondary management. *Cleft Palate J* 23:278, 1986.

44. Komatsu Y, Genba R, Kohama G: Morphological studies of the velopharyngeal orifice in cleft palate. *Cleft Palate J* 19:275, 1982.

45. Zawarski RE: Anorexia nervosa following a pharyngeal flap operation. *Cleft Palate J* 18:223, 1981.

46. Skolnick ML, McCall GN: Velopharyngeal competence and incompetence following pharyngeal flap surgery: Video-fluoroscopic study in multiple projections. *Cleft Palate J* 9:1, 1972.

47. Sphrintzen RJ, Lewin ML, Croft CB, et al: A comprehensive study of pharyngeal flap surgery: Tailor-made flaps. *Cleft Palate J* 16:46, 1979.

48. Orticochea M: Construction of a dynamic muscle sphincter in cleft palates. *Plast Reconstr Surg* 41:323, 1968.

49. Orticochea M: A review of 236 cleft palate patients treated with dynamic muscle sphincter. *Plast Reconstr Surg* 71:180, 1983.

50. Riski JE, Serafin D, Riefkohl R, et al: A rationale for modifying the site of insertion of the Orticochea pharyngoplasty. *Plast Reconstr Surg* 73:882, 1984.

51. Bingham HG, Suthunyara P, Richards S, et al: Should the pharyngeal flap be used primarily with palatoplasty? *Cleft Palate J* 9:319, 1972.

52. Dalston RM, Stutteville OM: A clinical investigation of the efficacy of primary nasopalatal pharyngoplasty. *Cleft Palate J* 12:177, 1975.

53. Dorf DS, Curtin JW: Early cleft palate repair and speech outcome. *Plast Reconstr Surg* 70:74, 1982.

54. Morris HL: Velopharyngeal competence and primary cleft palate surgery, 1960–1971: A critical review. *Cleft Palate J* 10:62, 1973.

55. Riski JE, Georgiade NG, Serafin D, et al: The Orticochea pharyngoplasty and primary palatoplasty: An evaluation. *Ann Plast Surg* 18:303, 1987.

56. Velasco MG, Ysunza A, Hernandez X, et al: Diagnosis and treatment of submucous cleft palate: A review of 108 cases. *Cleft Palate J* 25:171, 1988.

57. Richman LC, Eliason MJ, Lindgren SD: Reading disability in children with clefts. *Cleft Palate J* 25:21, 1988.

58. Ruscello DM: A selected review of palatal training procedures. *Cleft Palate J* 19:181, 1982.

59. Peterson SJ: Nasal emission as a component of the misarticulation of sibilants and affricates. *J Speech Hear Disord* 40:106, 1975.

60. Riski JE: Functional velopharyngeal incompetence: Diagnoses and management. In Winitz H (ed): *Treating Articulation Disorders: For Clinicians by Clinicians*. Baltimore, University Park Press, 1984.

34

An Outline of Craniofacial Anomalies and Principles of Their Correction

Alexander C. Stratoudakis, M.D., F.A.C.S.

Although craniectomy for the correction of cranial deformities has been performed since the latter part of the 19th century with varying degrees of success, the correction of major facial deformities became possible much later. The earliest publication on this subject, by Gillies and Harrison in 1951 (1), was an isolated case report, followed by a long hiatus until Tessier's original publications in 1967 (2) describing the craniofacial osteotomies and marking the beginning of a new era in surgery with the creation of a new surgical specialty. Dr. Tessier's unique opportunity to see and operate on large numbers of patients from all over the world, along with his keen sense of observation and painstaking recordkeeping, have led to a better understanding and classification of craniofacial anomalies and to superior operative results.

Since the writing of this chapter for the first edition, there has been no major breakthrough in the field of craniofacial surgery. Interesting trends have included: (*a*) the increased use of miniplates and screws for rigid fixation of mobilized bone segments (this was popularized by Champy [3, 4], even though this method is being applied much more to maxillofacial as compared to orbitocranial procedures); (*b*) the clinical application of vascularized calvarial bone transfer to reconstruct defects around the orbit[a]; and (*c*) the further refinement and widespread use of three-dimensional tomography in the study and evaluation of the anomalies and in the planning of operative procedures.

Three-Dimensional Computed Tomographic

By means of specialized graphics programs, a spatial reconstruction of the craniofacial skeleton and soft tissues becomes possible from data gathered by conventional computed tomographic (CT) techniques. The images thus obtained are superior to conventional radiographs in that they are much clearer and more detailed. They can be manipulated on the monitor screen for study under any desired angle or section (enabling the detailed observation of any region of interest). Furthermore, they make possible the rapid and accurate measurement of angles and distances either in the conventional geometric way (i.e., point-to-point distance) or in a three-dimensional (3-D) mode (surface distance). In order for a 3-D study to be meaningful, it should be carried out according to a standardized protocol, such as the one proposed by Tessier and Hemmy (5). The entire head should always be scanned, dividing it into a zone of interest (1.5–2.0-mm slices) and zones of reference (3–4-mm slices). Naturally, young patients should be sedated because complete immobility is of paramount importance. We have not found general anesthesia to be necessary. The radiation dose administered is very small (on the order of 2.4 rads for a 2-mm slice and 2.2 rads for a 4-mm slice, with settings of 125 kVp, 230 mA, and a time of 3 sec on the Siemens DR 3 scanner) and is expressed in CTDI (Computerized Tomography Dose Index), which represents the total amount of radiation received by a slice of tissue (i.e., the sum of direct radiation to the particular slice along with the scattered radiation from adjacent slices) (6). We have performed CTDI measurements on multiple scanners with various settings and have made some interesting observations:

1. Radiation doses may vary significantly from scanner to scanner.
2. The CTDI difference is negligible between 2- and 4-mm cuts; therefore, the reason to obtain thicker cuts in the reference zones is to reduce the duration of the study and *not* the radiation dose.
3. Abutting and not overlapping cuts should be obtained, because in overlapping cuts, the CTDI increases precipitously (7).

For comparison purposes, it is mentioned that the lens, which is the most radiosensitive structure scanned, may receive as much as 23 rads during bilateral petrous bone tomography (8). The smallest single cataractogenic radiation dose is considered to be on the order of 200 rads (9, 10).

Custom-designed acrylic models or implants may be constructed by transferring the CT data to the CEMAX 1500 system. These may be used for record purposes, for "model" surgery, or for implantation, and although quite expensive, they may be of significant help in difficult cases (11–13).

---

[a] Tessier still prefers the use of free calvarial bone grafts, covered by muscle (personal communication, Boston, 1987).

Craniostenoses

"Craniostenosis" is a general term encompassing a variety of developmental disorders that are characterized by inadequate capacity of the cranium to accommodate the growing brain and resulting in compensatory deformities. The etiology of these disorders has not been elucidated yet, but the available information points to a pathological process in the cranial base. The term, however, does not accurately describe the milder forms, which are characterized by cranial deformities but in which there is no real restriction of the cranial capacity.

"Dyscephaly" is another term coined by Moss (14) for these conditions. Although accurate, it is not very elegant from an etymological point of view inasmuch as it means "bad head."

"Craniosynostosis" is also an inadequate term, in that it points to the premature closure of one or more cranial sutures. As indicated above, this is probably not the true pathogenetic factor. Dyscephaly may exist without premature sutural obliteration (14), and conversely, premature sutural obliteration may occur without deformation of the calvaria. This has been pointed out by A. Huxley (quoted in Bolk), and confirmed by Bolk (15) and Tessier (16).

Some cases of craniostenosis may be accompanied by facial deformities (namely, craniofacial dysostosis, Crouzon's, or Apert's disease), while similar facial deformities may occur without cranial involvement. Delaire (17) has used the term "facio-synostosis" for such conditions.

The dura mater (inner periosteum) is considered the guiding tissue in the morphogenesis of the calvaria. It is attached anteriorly to the crista galli, anterolaterally to the lesser sphenoidal wings, and posterolaterally to the petrous ridges. These sites of attachment correspond to the major dural reflections that conform to the early recesses in the developing brain. Thus, a longitudinal dural reflection develops between the cerebral hemispheres to become the falx cerebri; a band of dura reflects off the sphenoid wing into the early insular sulcus between the major frontal and parietotemporal regions of brain outgrowth to become the major anterolateral dural band. The dural reflections off the petrous ridges develop between the cerebrum and cerebellum to become the tentorium cerebelli, the major posterolateral dural band. Between 12 and 16 weeks, intramembranous ossification progresses in the central zones between the major reflective bands of the dura. From these central points, the mineralization spreads centrifugally toward the major bands within the dura. By 16 weeks, the radiating centers of ossification have almost reached the sites of reflective bands in the dura. These latter sites remain unossified as regions of connective tissue between outspreading islands of membranous bone. Biomechanical forces in the areas of major reflections of the dura apparently limit ossification in these regions (18).

Smith and Töndury (18) studied brain malformations in which abnormal dural reflections were found to conform to the nature of the aberrant brain. They observed the cranial sutures to be related directly to the unusual sites of dural reflections. This confirmed and extended the concepts of Moss that there is no genetic determination of the site of development of sutures, that there is no basic impetus for growth in the calvaria or its sutures, but that they respond in a compensatory fashion to the interior forces that normally consist of the outgrowth of the brain (18). Doubt has been cast upon this last point, however, by more recent experimental work (19, 20).

Separative motion of adjacent calvarial bones occurs in a direction perpendicular to the long axis of the intervening suture. Any functional ankylosis at a given sutural area will have two interrelated results: (*a*) inhibition of expansive, separative growth in directions normal (perpendicular) to the suture line; and (*b*) consequent redirection of the growth vector of the neural mass (14). This observation was first made by Virchow (21).

Redirection of the growth vector of the neural mass causes deformation either in the cranial vault (cranial dysmorphias), or in the weaker areas of the cranial base (greater sphenoidal wing and frontal bone—exorbitism, or ethmoid—prolapse of the cribriform plate and telorbitism) (16). Moss (22, 23) attributed premature sutural obliteration to dysmorphias of the cranial base, while Seeger and Gabrielsen (24) reminded us of Bertelsen's observation that the coronal suture, together with the frontosphenoidal and sphenoethmoidal sutures, form a continuous ring. They showed in a radiographic study that the process of premature closure of the coronal suture frequently extends into the base of the skull to involve the frontosphenoidal and perhaps other sutures. Finally, the postmortem studies by Stewart et al. (25), Kreiborg et al. (26), and Ousterhout and Melsen (27) further localize the pathology in Apert's disease in the cranial base. It appears to be a progressive disorder observed as an abnormality indicating decreased growth (short cranial base) in the bones of the cranial base in a 24- to 26-week-old embryo. An abnormality in the sutures and a histologically abnormal cranial base were observed at 22 months of age. In the 38-month-old specimen, there was synostosis of the spheno-occipital synchondrosis as well as synostosis of the vomer to the sphenoid and the maxilla.

Apart from the esthetic disfigurement, dyscephalies resulting in sutural fusions may cause functional disorders such as intracranial hypertension and hydrocephalus. This occurs frequently where multiple sutures are involved but occasionally also in single suture involvement (28, 29).

Signs of increased intracranial pressure include fundoscopic changes (papilledema, which may lead to visual loss), headaches, vomiting, or a beaten-silver appearance of the cranium on roentgenographic examination. Because these signs are frequently absent or difficult to detect in children, Marchac and Renier (30) believe that direct measurements should be carried out by means of an extradural strain gauge.

Deformities of the cranium are described by terms that are frequently very confusing. The terminology is presented here as clearly as possible.

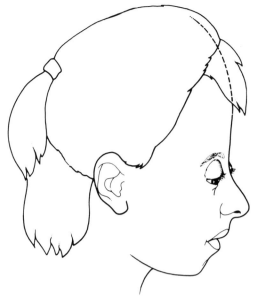

FIGURE 34.1. Acrocephaly (oxycephaly).

1. *Acrocephaly* is a term introduced by Lucea in 1847 as synonymous to the "tower skull" or oxycephaly of Virchow. It describes a cranium the anterior part of which is higher than the posterior, the vault slanting in a front-to-back direction (Figs. 34.1 and 34.2).

2. *Oxycephaly* is a term used by Virchow in 1852 to describe a deformity characterized by extreme upward growth with reduction of the lateral and the anteroposterior (AP) diameters. The nasofrontal angle is usually too obtuse or absent. This deformity is usually caused by dyscephalies resulting in fusion of the coronal sutures in which growth occurs in the interfrontal and interparietal lines (29).

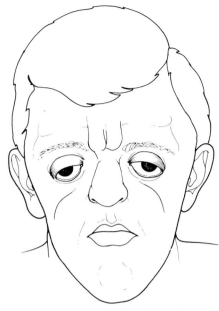

FIGURE 34.3. Acrocephalosyndactyly (Apert's syndrome) (turricephalic type).

3. *Turricephaly* describes a cranium with exaggerated upward growth caused by fusion of the frontoparietal sutures (Figs. 34.3 and 34.4).

4. *Scaphocephaly,* or hull-shaped cranium, is characterized by reduced cranial width with a compensatory increase in the AP length. It is seen with premature closure of the sagittal suture (Figs. 34.5 and 34.6).

5. *Trigonocephaly* is a cranial deformity in which the forehead is narrow and triangular, with a prominent ridge corresponding to the prematurely fused metopic suture (Fig. 34.7).

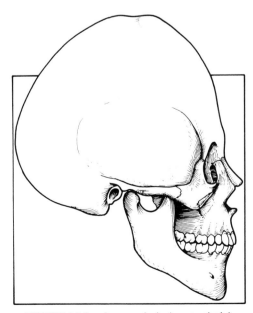

FIGURE 34.2. Acrocephaly (oxycephaly).

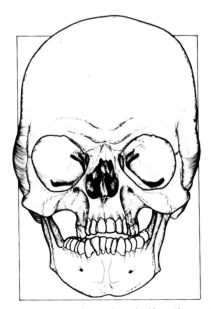

FIGURE 34.4. Acrocephalosyndactyly (Apert's syndrome) (turricephalic type).

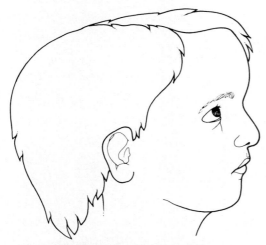

FIGURE 34.5. Scaphocephaly.

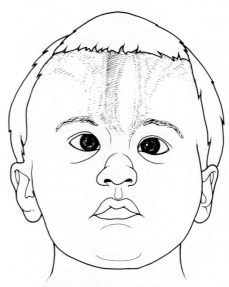

FIGURE 34.7. Trigonocephaly.

6. *Plagiocephaly* implies cranial asymmetry and may either be frontal, occipital, or hemicranial (31). Frontal plagiocephaly usually occurs with premature synostosis of the ipsilateral half of the coronal suture and frontosphenoidal suture and presents as a deformity involving both the cranium and the facial skeleton. The forehead is flattened on the affected side, with a backward and upward displacement of the affected orbit. The lesser sphenoidal wing has a more vertical orientation than normal, while the greater sphenoidal wing is retracted medially, altering the angle of the lateral orbital wall. The calvaria may also be deformed, bulging in the contralateral parietal area. The deformity becomes less pronounced at the level of the maxilla. Even less pronounced is the mandibular asymmetry. The mandible, even though asymmetrical, functions symmetrically, possibly because of a lower and more anterior position of the ipsilateral glenoid fossa (Tessier, unpublished data) (Figs. 34.8 and 34.9). Occipital plagiocephaly is a rare condition caused by "synostosis" of the lambdoid suture. It presents with significant flattening of the parieto-occipital region with compensatory bulging and projection of the opposite side. In fact, the suture is always open on radiographs and is accompanied by a sclerotic ridge adjacent to it. We have shown that, even though a suture might remain open radiographically, there is an important decrease in the number of structural "skeletoblasts" (osteoprogenitor cells) (32).

7. "Cloverleaf" or *Kleebattschädel* deformity is a term first used by Holtermueller and Wiedemann in 1960 (33). It seems to be a nonspecific consequence of multiple sutural fusions. A constriction ring develops in the lamboid-squamosal zone, allowing a disproportionate bulging of the frontal and temporal lobes, which gives the cranium a trilobar appearance (31).

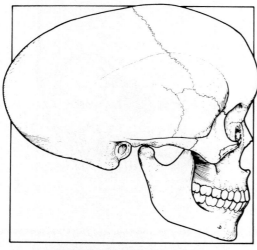

FIGURE 34.6. Scaphocephaly.

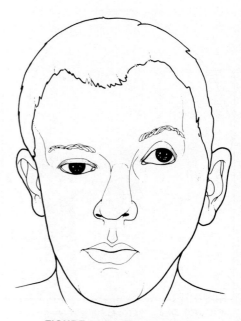

FIGURE 34.8. Plagiocephaly.

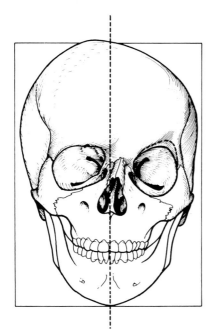

FIGURE 34.9. Plagiocephaly.

This deformity has been reported in association with multiple syndromes (Figs. 34.10 and 34.11). The heterogeneity of its pathogenesis and etiology has been discussed by Kokkich et al. (34) in the postmortem study of two neonatal human specimens.

Craniosynostosis Syndromes

A brief description follows of the more frequent syndromes affecting the cranium and face that, despite the significant variability in penetrance, are sufficiently well defined. The syndromes should not be classified on the basis of which sutures are synostosed because various sutures may be involved in different patients with the

same syndrome. Thus, the cranial malformation may be different in patients with the same disorder. The potential of mental retardation is probably present to some extent in all craniosynostosis syndromes. The incidence and severity of retardation, however, are more frequent in some syndromes than in others (35). The craniofacial syndromes display a definite pattern of Mendelian inheritance, making genetic counseling imperative.

CROUZON'S SYNDROME

This syndrome was reported in 1912 by M. O. Crouzon under the name "hereditary craniofacial dysostosis" in a paper describing the characteristic triad of anomalies: craniosynostosis, midfacial hypoplasia (which he, however, described as prognathism), and exophthalmos (36). Interestingly, Apert, who was present in that session, observed that the bony configuration was similar to that of individuals with premature synostosis of the sutures "of the cranial base and the posterior part of the cranium."

A variety of expressions is characteristic. The deformities may range from the very severe Kleebattschädel (Schiller, quoted in Cohen [35]) to the milder forms, which may go virtually unnoticed (31). Delaire (17) even suggested that certain instances of isolated "maxillary hypotrophy" may be part of the same pathological process of premature isolated faciosynostoses with the craniosynostosis remaining unnoticed.

The synostosis commonly begins during the first year of life, and it is usually complete by the third or fourth year of age. Synostosis may be evident at birth. Occasionally, no sutural involvement is noted (37).

The cranial vault is frequently brachycephalic or oxycephalic to a greater or lesser extent, even though dolichocephalic forms are noted (31). The lesser sphenoid wings are slanted in an upward direction, while the greater wings are displaced anteriorly by the protruding middle cranial fossa, contributing to the shortness of the orbital cavity (16). Midfacial retrusion results in class III

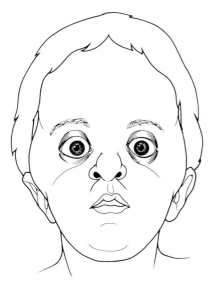

FIGURE 34.10. Kleebattschädel (cloverleaf).

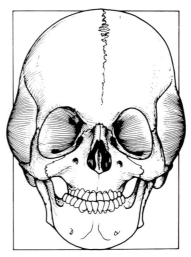

FIGURE 34.11. Kleebattschädel (cloverleaf).

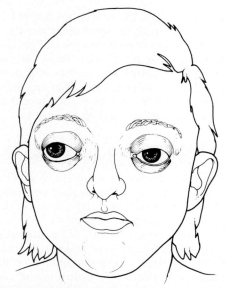

FIGURE 34.12. Craniofacial dysostosis (Crouzon's syndrome).

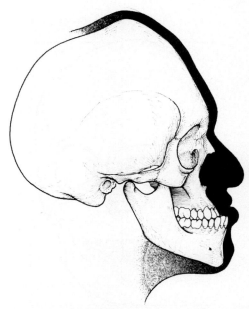

FIGURE 34.14. Craniofacial dysostosis (Crouzon's syndrome).

malocclusion and contributes to the shallowness of the orbits. The degree of exophthalmos ranges from mild to extreme. In more severe cases, eyelid closure may be impaired and jeopardize vision. The reduction in size of the midface in all three dimensions (maxillary atresia) may compromise nasal breathing (Figs. 34.12 through 34.14).

Raised intracranial pressure is frequent, making close monitoring of the affected child imperative. A search should be carried out for other congenital anomalies, skeletal or visceral.

APERT'S SYNDROME

The term "acrocephalosyndactyly" was proposed by Apert (38) in 1906 to describe "a teratologic type compatible with life and well characterized by the coexistence of the two following particularities: 1. High cranial vault flattened posteriorly and sometimes also on the sides, while bulging in an exaggerated fashion in the upper frontal region and, 2. syndactyly of the four extremities."

The calvaria is usually of the brachycephalic-turricephalic type with occipital flattening. The cranial base is foreshortened, particularly in the area of the sphenoid (i.e., the middle cranial fossa); the posterior cranial fossa, which is also short, bulges downward (Tessier, unpublished data). "The forehead is deformed in a peculiar fashion. The supraorbital margins protrude and above them is a transverse depression in the form of a concavity; above this concavity the superior part of the forehead forms a very prominent bulge, frequently more pronounced in the midline than laterally" (38). If telorbitism is present, it is generally of a mild degree. Midfacial retrusion is a constant feature, but the orbitostenosis and ocular proptosis are not as marked as in Crouzon's syndrome (31). The maxillary sinuses are underdeveloped in contrast to the overdevelopment of the ethmoid cells and frontal sinus. The maxilla is deficient, and the dentition is abnormal with crowded and impacted teeth. The incidence of cleft palate in this syndrome is reported to range from 11 to 30% (39). Low-set hairline, hypertrichosis of the eyebrows, and mild ptosis of the eyelids (particularly of their lateral aspect) may be present. The lower lip is well developed, while the oral commissures drop (Figs. 34.3 and 34.4).

Hydrocephalus has been reported, but the frequency of this finding is uncertain. Mental retardation is occasionally present. Whether it is primary or caused by

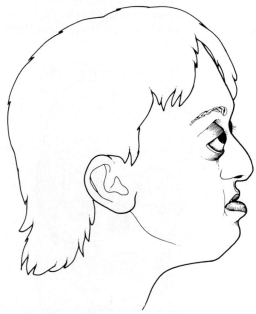

FIGURE 34.13. Craniofacial dysostosis (Crouzon's syndrome).

raised intracranial pressure is an unresolved question (31; Tessier, unpublished data).

Symmetrical syndactyly of all four limbs is characteristic, involving at least the three central digits, but frequently all five. The syndactyly involves the phalanges and nails as well as the soft tissues.

SAETHRE-CHOTZEN SYNDROME

This syndrome is characterized by a brachycephalic cranium with a variable degree of craniosynostosis, but not true craniostenosis, facial asymmetry, shallow orbits, telecanthus, nasal septal deviation, low-set hairline, and partial cutaneous syndactyly, which, however, is not a constant feature. Maxillary hypoplasia is not as pronounced as it is in Apert's or in Crouzon's syndromes (Figs. 34.15 through 34.17). Intelligence is frequently normal, but severe mental retardation has also been reported (31).

PFEIFFER SYNDROME

Described in 1964, this syndrome consists of craniosynostosis with cranial deformity of the brachy-turricephalic type, broad thumbs and great toes with deformed proximal phalanges, and occasionally partial soft tissue syndactyly. Other skeletal anomalies have also been described. Faciostenosis with maxillary retrusion and exorbitism, or telorbitism, may be present. Hydrocephalus and intracranial hypertension have been reported in association with this syndrome (Figs. 34.18 and 34.19). Intelligence is usually normal, but mental retardation is possible (31).

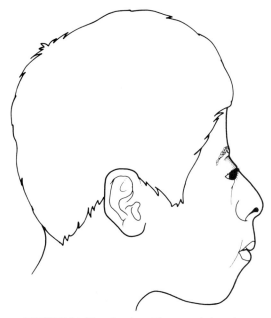

FIGURE 34.16. Saethre-Chotzen deformity.

CARPENTER SYNDROME

This syndrome was reported in 1901 and 1909 by Carpenter, a pediatrician, as a disorder of development in three (probably four) siblings. It consists of cranial malformations of variable shape (scapho- or acrocephalic) caused by various combinations of synostoses. The nasal bridge is flat, and the canthi are usually dystopic. There may be associated anomalies of the globe. The ears appear to be low set, and preauricular fistulas have been reported.

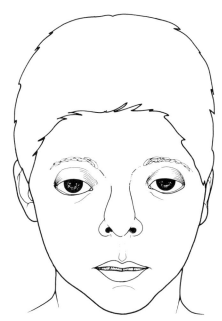

FIGURE 34.15. Saethre-Chotzen syndrome.

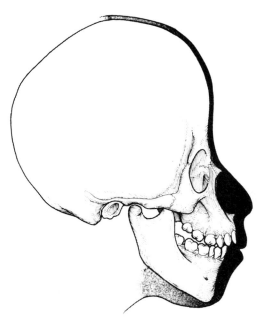

FIGURE 34.17. Saethre-Chotzen syndrome.

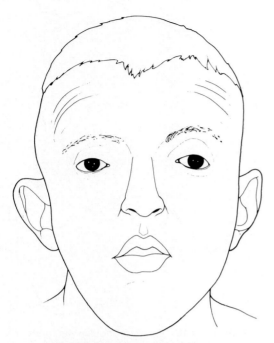

FIGURE 34.18. Pfeiffer syndrome.

Digital anomalies are an obligatory component of the syndrome. The hands are short with brachydactyly and variable soft tissue syndactyly. The feet show accessory preaxial digits and soft tissue syndactyly, which is usually extensive. Other skeletal findings have been reported.

Height is usually below the 25th percentile, but weight often above average. Other visceral congenital anomalies may be present. Inheritance is autosomal recessive (31, 35).

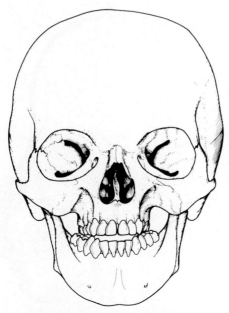

FIGURE 34.19. Pfeiffer syndrome.

Craniofacial Clefts

Facial clefting is a much rarer deformity than the common cleft lip or cleft lip and palate. The true incidence of such clefts is impossible to estimate. Kawamoto (40) in his excellent review gives rough figures ranging from 1.43 to 4.85/100,000 births but acknowledges that the true incidence is probably much higher. This is easily understood when one considers that: (*a*) conditions such as the Treacher Collins syndrome and hemifacial microsomia should be included among the clefting syndromes; (*b*) many conditions previously regarded as "hypoplasias" are, in reality, clefts (41); and (*c*) formes frustes and incomplete forms may go unnoticed.

There is no recognizable pattern of inheritance. Craniofacial clefts occur sporadically. Their etiology is unknown, and amniotic bands, which have been incriminated as being etiogenetic factors, can be blamed only in the rare case in which the cleft does not follow the "usual" pattern. Of the seven patients reported by Jones et al. (42), whose clefts were attributed to amniotic bands, six had encephaloceles of unusual pattern, and five (or six) had constriction rings or amputations of limbs.

Several different classifications of the major clefts have been proposed, but none gained universal acceptance. As a result of Tessier's unique opportunity to observe, examine, and operate on a large number of clefts throughout the world, coupled with his keen sense of observation and diligent recording of their anatomy, a simple, workable classification has evolved and seems to be gaining universal acceptance. The information that follows in this chapter has been drawn from his publications and from his teaching (41–45).

THE TESSIER CLASSIFICATION

This classification is based on the following observations: (*a*) a cleft may affect the facial or the cranial structures or both; (*b*) clefts occur along axes following constant patterns; and (*c*) the origin of even purely facial clefts probably lies in the cranial base (which may be profoundly affected in cases of facial clefting).

The orbit was selected as a point of reference because it belongs both to the cranial and to the facial skeleton; a numerical system was developed, numbering the axes of the various clefts around the orbit in a counterclockwise direction. Numbering starts from the "southbound" facial clefts and continues with the "northbound" cranial clefts (Figs. 34.20 and 34.21).

This numerical system is purely one of topographic description and describes neither the structures involved nor the severity of involvement of each structure. A cleft, for example, may spare the cheek and involve only the palpebral and labial structures.

Clefting does not imply involvement of all layers of tissue to the same extent. It seems that, from the midline to the infraorbital foramen, defects of the soft tissues are more severe than those of the bone, while from the infraorbital foramen to the temporal bone, the opposite holds

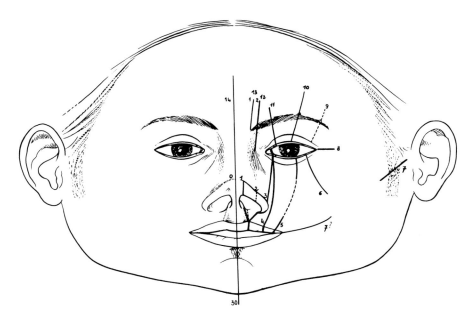

FIGURE 34.20. The Tessier classification of craniofacial clefts.

true. A "sclerodermic" patch of skin or an abnormal line of hair growth may be the only superficial indication of a cleft involving the deeper layers. Moore et al. have also reported the frequent occurrence of "hairline indicators," or markers in the hairline, in cases of "northbound" clefts, pointing in the direction of the cleft (46).

Whereas not all "hypoplasias" are clefts, all clefts have hypoplastic edges. Clefts do not course through foramina or grooves of neurovascular bundles. These may, however, be involved in the hypoplasia of the cleft margins.

"Northbound" and "southbound" clefts frequently coexist, and when they do, their axes frequently (but not always) follow the same direction. The cleft is then described by the dual number indicating each of the component clefts. Clefts may be bilateral, and when this is the case, they are frequently symmetrical (with regard to the axis of the cleft and not necessarily the severity of involvement of each side). Multiple clefts occasionally coexist, rendering the deformity even more complex and "unclassifiable."

The so-called clefts 0, 1, and 2 follow a course that is medial to the canthus and, therefore, do not pass through and do not disrupt the orbit itself. Equally, the so-called cleft 7 is a laterofacial cleft and does not have a course leading to or through the orbit. Clefts affecting the orbit frequently cause anomalies of the orbital contents (globe and extraocular muscles).

Cleft 0

Cleft 0, or median craniofacial dysrrhaphia, represents failure or delay in closure of the anterior neuropore. Its course is outlined from the anterior fontanelle through the frontal bone, crista galli, midline or the nose, columella, lip, and maxilla, and may actually involve the tongue, lower lip, and mandible. It may give rise to frontal, frontonasal, or frontoethmoidal encephaloceles, telorbitism, duplication of the nasal septum, and midline cleft of the lip. In its minor forms, it may present with minor telorbitism and a "flat" appearance in the area of

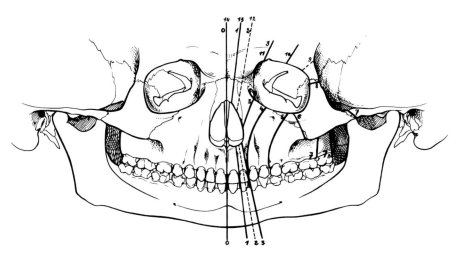

FIGURE 34.21. The Tessier classification of craniofacial clefts.

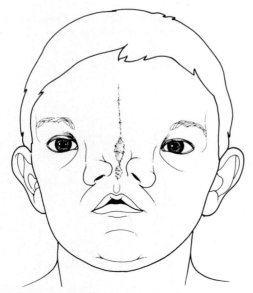

FIGURE 34.22. Cleft 0–14 (median craniofacial dysrrhaphia).

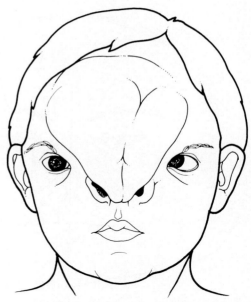

FIGURE 34.24. Cleft 1–13 (bilateral).

the glabella. Nasal gliomata are frequent, representing sequestration of glial tissue after obliteration of the anterior neuropore. Its cranial extension is cleft 14 (Figs. 34.22 and 34.23).

Cleft 1

Cleft 1, or paramedian craniofacial dysrrhaphia, courses through the frontal bone, the olfactory groove of the cribriform plate, between the nasal bone and the frontal process of the maxilla, and through the maxilla between the central and lateral incisors. It may cause telorbitism with a deep invagination of the dura in the area of the cribriform plate defect, naso-orbital encephalocele (which could also be caused by cleft 0), notching of the nostril in the area of the alar dome, and occasionally a cleft lip. Its cranial extension is cleft 13 (Figs. 34.24 and 34.25).

Cleft 2

Cleft 2, or paranasal cleft, is similar to cleft 1, but it is slightly more lateral. Its cranial extension is cleft 12.

Cleft 3

Cleft 3, or oculonasal cleft, is a medial orbitomaxillary cleft. Its course runs through the lacrimal bone, the frontal process of the maxilla, and into the alveolus between the lateral incisor and the canine. There is absence of the inferomedial wall of the orbit and lack of pneumatization of the maxillary antrum with absence of the septum sepa-

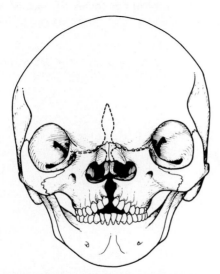

FIGURE 34.23. Cleft 0–14 (median craniofacial dyssrhaphia).

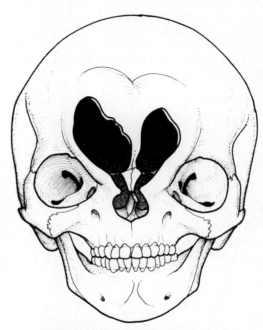

FIGURE 34.25. Cleft 1–13 (bilateral).

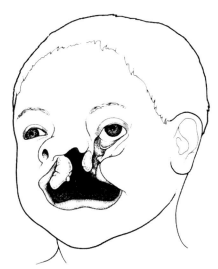

FIGURE 34.26. Cleft 3.

rating the nasal cavity from the antrum. With respect to the soft tissues, the medial canthus is displaced inferiorly. There is a coloboma of the lower eyelid, the conjunctiva and nasal mucosa being separated by a thin band of fibrous tissue. The lacrimal apparatus is invariably affected; the sac is either absent or present in the form of a mucocele. The lateral aspect of the nose is separated from the cheek, with considerable vertical shortness of the nose on the cleft side. The defect ends as a cleft lip. Its northbound continuation is cleft 11 (Figs. 34.26 and 34.27).

Cleft 4

Cleft 4, or oculofacial 1 cleft, is a central orbitomaxillary cleft. The upper portion of its course is similar to that of cleft 3. It courses medially to the infraorbital nerve and through the maxillary sinus, causing exstrophy of the an-

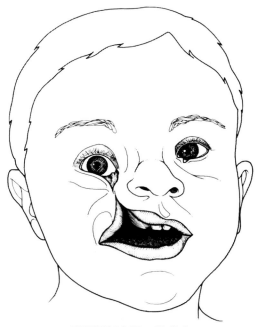

FIGURE 34.28. Cleft 4.

tral mucosa. However, the septum between the nasal cavity and the antrum is present. It ends, as in cleft 3, between the lateral incisor and the canine. With respect to the soft tissues, the medial canthal, palpebral, and lacrimal problems are similar to those of cleft 3, while the clefting between the nose and cheek occurs more laterally, sparing the nostril. The lip clefting takes place lateral to the philtral crest (Figs. 34.28 and 34.29). In its bilateral form, there is considerable shortness of the central part of the face.

Cleft 5

Cleft 5, or oculofacial 2 cleft, is a very rare lateral orbitomaxillary cleft, the course of which runs through

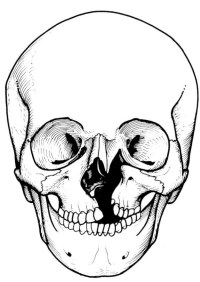

FIGURE 34.27. Cleft 3.

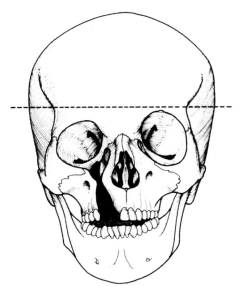

FIGURE 34.29. Cleft 4.

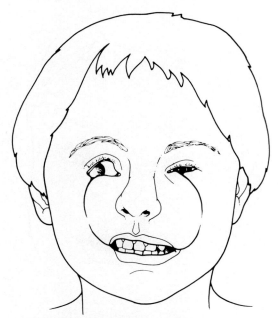

FIGURE 34.30. Cleft 5 (bilateral).

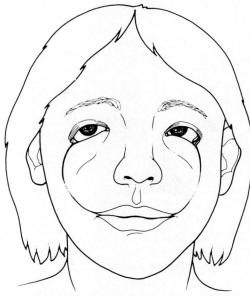

FIGURE 34.32. Cleft 6 (pure form, bilateral).

the orbital floor, lateral to the infraorbital nerve and the maxillary sinus, ending behind the canine in the premolar region. The soft tissue deformities consist of a coloboma of lateral third of the lower lid, ending as a cleft of the lip slightly medial to the commissure (Figs. 34.30 and 34.31).

Cleft 6

Cleft 6 separates the maxilla from the malar bone. The corresponding soft tissue deformities consist of a coloboma of the lower lid and a ''sclerodermic'' furrow of

skin from the coloboma to the angle of the mandible (Figs. 34.32 and 34.33).

Cleft 7

Cleft 7 courses between the malar and the temporal bones. The zygomatic arch is usually absent. The condyle, coronoid process, and mandibular ramus suffer various degrees of deformity. The temporal muscle is either absent or atrophic, forming a continuous temporomasseteric muscle. There may be an associated cleft of the scalp, or an abnormal pattern of hair growth may overlie the bony cleft. There are varying degrees of ear malformations. Cleft 7, however, may exist as pure macrostomia without any appreciable skeletal or ear deformity.

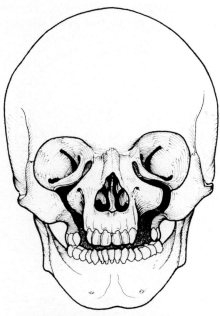

FIGURE 34.31. Cleft 5 (bilateral).

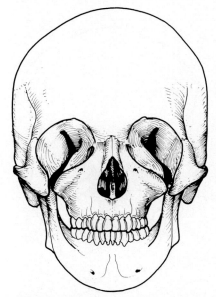

FIGURE 34.33. Cleft 6 (pure form, bilateral).

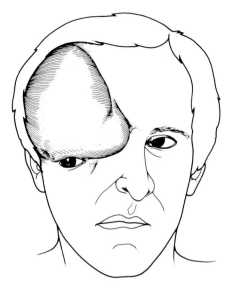

FIGURE 34.34. Cleft 10.

Cleft 8

Cleft 8 is a frontozygomatic cleft extending to the greater sphenoidal wing. In the soft tissues, there may either be a true cleft of the lateral canthus or a notch of the lower eyelid close to the canthus with a dermatocele.

Combinations of clefts 6, 7, and 8, in varying degrees of severity, constitute the Treacher Collins syndrome. With complete clefts 6, 7, and 8, the malar bone may be totally absent, or it may be present only as sesamoid-like bones in the temporomasseteric fascia.

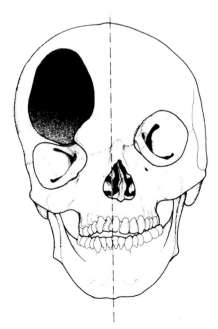

FIGURE 34.35. Cleft 10.

Cleft 9

Cleft 9 is an upper lateral orbital cleft of the superolateral orbital ridge-angle with a corresponding coloboma of the upper lid.

Cleft 10

Cleft 10 is an upper central orbital cleft of the frontal bone, supraorbital ridge, and orbital rod, which is lateral to the supraorbital neurovascular bundle, causing an encephalocele. It could be associated with a coloboma of the mid-third of the upper lid and/or eyebrow (Figs. 34.34 and 34.35).

Cleft 11

Cleft 11 is an upper medial orbital cleft through the frontal bone, frontal sinus, and lateral mass of the ethmoid, which is medial to the supraorbital neurovascular bundle. The corresponding soft tissue deformity is a coloboma of the medial third of the upper eyelid.

Telorbitism or Orbital Hypertelorism

The term "ocular hypertelorism" was first used by Greig (47) to describe a condition characterized by an abnormally wide distance between the orbits and hence, the eyes. The term "orbital hypertelorism" was proposed by Tessier (48) because the pathology lies in the orbits and not the eyes. Tessier (48) later proposed the term "telorbitism," which is the only etymologically correct term. All the above terms are still being used interchangeably.

Telorbitism is usually a congenital condition, with the exception of cases caused by fibrous dysplasia (49) and the few cases in which it has been argued that trauma has caused true telorbitism, rather than telecanthus. Tessier (41, 48–50) considers telorbitism always to be secondary either to a cleft or to craniostenosis (16, 48; Figs. 34.36 and 34.37). A differing opinion is expressed by Van der Meulen and Vaandrager (51), who pointed out that, at the time of their formation (7-mm crown-rump length [CRL]), the optic cups are widely apart, that the nasal capsule develops in a frontocaudal direction, and that 3 weeks later, at the 28-mm CRL stage, the interorbital distance has been reduced to normal. They make the statement that: "Hypertelorism is therefore due to a developmental arrest occurring between the fifth and eighth weeks of gestation. It may be associated with a cleft or craniosynostosis, but it is not due to these malformations" (51).

The interorbital distance is measured between the anterior lacrimal crests. According to Gunther (quoted in Tessier [48]), this distance varies in women from 18.5 to 29.5 mm, and in men from 19.5 to 30.7 mm. These measurements, however, may be misleading, as in cases of Crouzon's or Apert's syndromes with bulging medial orbital walls.

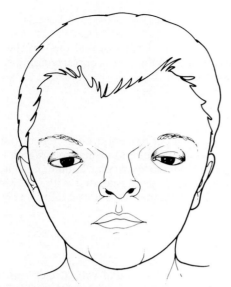

FIGURE 34.36. Telorbitism (with brachycephaly).

The classification into first-, second-, and third-degree hypertelorism is no longer in use because it has served no practical purpose. Up to 40 mm interorbital distance there is no true ocular malposition or deviation (except in cases associated with craniofacial dysostosis and exorbitism). In the more severe forms, at least in those compatible with life and normal intellect, the malformations spare the sphenoid bone, leaving the distance between the inner rims of the optic canals normal or near normal (2), making it possible for the "useful orbits" (15) to be brought closer together.

Severe forms of telorbitism are associated with lateralization of the orbits, that is, with a lateral tilting of the orbital plane. A foreshortened distance between the lateral canthus and the external auditory meatus (48), a wider than 90° angle between the lateral orbital walls on computed tomography (CT) scan cuts, or increased distance of the lateral orbital walls as compared to the values of Johr (52) and Laestadius et al. (53) characterize lateralized orbits. Munro (54) pointed out that true lateralization is always accompanied by displacement of the medial orbital walls.

Operative correction of telorbitism is undertaken both for functional reasons (restoration of binocular vision, if possible) and for obvious esthetic and psychological purposes.

Frontoethmoidal Encephalomeningoceles

Meningoceles represent failure of the neural tube to close, with herniation of central nervous system tissue. They occur in the midline of the head and spine from the region of the nose to the occiput and spinal column. Encephalomeningoceles of the anterior part of the head are rare in Western Europe, America, Australia, Japan, China, and Southern India. They are most frequent in Southeast Asia and Russia. Their incidence is reported to be 1 : 6,000 live births in Thailand (55).

Encephalomeningoceles may occur with a frontal bone defect in cleft 0–14 (Figs. 34.38 and 34.39) or 1–13 (Figs. 34.24 and 34.25), in which they are associated with telorbitism. When they are not associated with a cleft, the deformity may consist in a telecanthus with displacement of the medial orbital walls and deformation of the orbits rather than with true telorbitism.

The basic defect occurs between the frontal and ethmoid bones, and they are divided into: (*a*) *nasofrontal* when they project between the nasal and frontal bones into the arc of the glabella, pushing the nasal bones inferiorly and displacing the medial orbital walls laterally; (*b*) *nasoethmoidal,* in which the herniation protrudes *under* the nasal bones and *over* the upper lateral nasal cartilages, still remaining extranasal; and (*c*) *naso-orbital,* in which the herniation is located behind the nasal bones

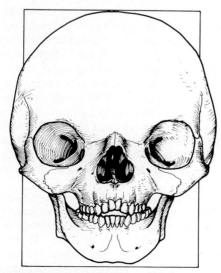

FIGURE 34.37. Telorbitism (with brachycephaly).

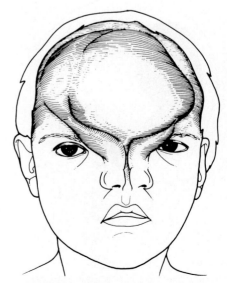

FIGURE 34.38. Encephalomeningocele (secondary to cleft 0–14) may be accompanied by telorbitism.

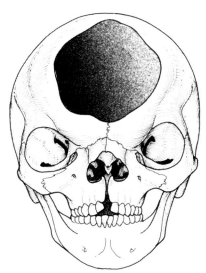

FIGURE 34.39. Encephalomeningocele (secondary to cleft 0–14).

and then deviates laterally, protruding through the medial orbital walls (56).

The dura is attached to the circumference of the bony defect, while beyond that it may be attenuated or absent, whereas the mass may contain atrophied parts of the frontal lobe or may be lined with ependyma and filled with cerebrospinal fluid (Tessier, unpublished data).

Early repair is advised in order to prevent the possibility of rupture and ulceration with ensuing meningitis and to prevent the secondary deformities, which increase in severity with age (55, 56).

Treatment generally consists of excision of the sac and its contents, obliteration of the dural and bony defects with pericranial and bone grafts, respectively, and in older individuals, correction of the secondary deformities as indicated.

There are other rare forms of meningoceles that exist through the base of the skull; however, the description of these is beyond the scope of this book (57, 58).

Oculomotor Disturbances in Craniofacial Malformation

Craniofacial malformations are characterized by the frequent occurrence of oculomotor disturbances. Abnormal ocular alignment can be explained on the basis of: (a) abnormal extraocular muscle vectors of action; (b) altered interorbital distance and angulation; (c) involvement of cranial nerves; or (d) structural abnormality or absence of specific extraocular muscles (59). Diamond and Whitaker (59) reported a 42% incidence of extraocular muscle anomalies in patients with strabismus due to craniofacial dysostosis, while it is pointed out that the true incidence is hard to estimate because only a small percentage of patients undergo exploration (59, 60).

The ocular deviation may occur in either the vertical or horizontal plane. Overall, Morax (60) has observed more vertical than horizontal imbalance. The V syndrome is the most classical (exotropia on upward gaze, esotropia on lower gaze), representing weakness of one or both superior obliques and hyperactivity of one or both inferior obliques (60). Ortiz-Monasterio et al. (61) attributed this phenomenon to increased arc of contact between the inferior muscles and the sclera in cases of exorbitism, whereas Morax (60) rejected this view because the V syndrome is not always reversed after correction of the exorbitism and because it can be observed with pure telorbitism (without exophthalmos) (60). Exotropia is also quite frequent in telorbitism (60) as well as in midfacial hypoplasia with exophthalmos (62).

The effect of correction of the craniofacial anomaly on the extraocular muscle balance is unpredictable. A preexisting deviation may remain unaffected by the procedure, or it may improve or be converted into a different type of imbalance (62).

Patients undergoing sagittal advancement show little tendency to change in their postoperative horizontal oculomotor deviation, in contrast to patients with telorbitism. Because orbital translocation in these patients is often delayed, correction of their strabismus should be considered before orbital translocation. In contrast, patients with telorbitism show a definite trend toward esodeviation after medial orbital translocation. The squint seems to stabilize about 6 months postoperatively, and Choy et al. (62) recommended that no orbital translocation be carried out in this group of patients until at least 6 months after the correction of telorbitism. Diamond and associates (59, 63) also recommended early alignment of the ocular axis, without distinction between sagittal and medial orbital translocation.

Surgical Correction of Craniofacial Anomalies

The earliest references in the literature on strip craniectomies for sutural synostosis are those of Lannelongue (64) and Lane (65). By the 1920s, the technique had found wide clinical acceptance in the United States (66). Strip craniectomies were performed by neurosurgeons employing the technique developed by Ingraham, Matson, and associates (67–69). Shillito and Matson (70) reviewed the results on 519 patients and found that only 52% had obtained an optimal aesthetic result (16).

Tessier (16) was the first to suggest detaching of the facial bones from the base of the cranium and moving them as required for the correction of deformities in Crouzon's and Apert's syndromes. He proposed advancing the orbitofrontal bandeau and stabilizing it in the advanced position. A variation of this method is used in the correction of plagiocephaly in infancy (Figs. 34.40 to 34.43).

Stricker et al. (71) were the first to mobilize and tilt the orbitofrontal bandeau in oxycephaly in young children with lateral bone grafts and transposition of bone flaps pedicled on the temporalis muscle.

In 1973, Marchac et al. (72) described a method of tilting the orbitofrontal bandeau with stabilization by means of a Z-plasty in the temporal region and simulta-

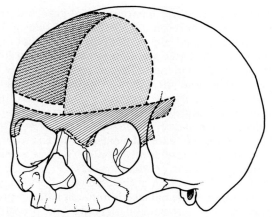

FIGURE 34.40. Correction of unilateral coronal synostosis (plagiocephaly) in infancy.

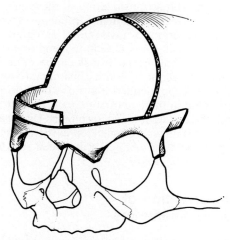

FIGURE 34.41. Correction of unilateral coronal synostosis (plagiocephaly) in infancy.

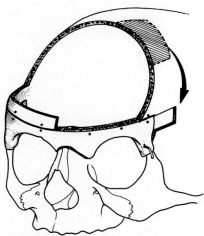

FIGURE 34.42. Correction of unilateral coronal synostosis (plagiocephaly) in infancy.

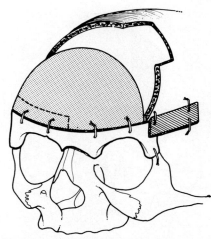

FIGURE 34.43. Correction of unilateral coronal synostosis (plagiocephaly) in infancy.

neous transposition of free bone "flaps" for fronto-orbital remodeling.

Hoffman and Mohr (73), recognizing the inadequacy of simple craniectomies to correct the facial deformities in coronal synostosis, suggested mobilization of the affected supraorbital rim in the infant (unilateral in hemicoronal synostosis and bilateral in synostosis of the entire coronal suture) by performing an osteotomy of the orbital roof, from the crista galli to the pterion, and extending the osteotomy laterally through the frontozygomatic process. The supraorbital rim is then advanced, creating a greenstick fracture at the nasion, and held in the advanced position by means of a cranial bone graft. They claimed excellent esthetic results in all cases operated. Similar osteotomies with some modifications are being used by Whitaker and associates (74, 75).

McCarthy et al. (76), with the insight provided by Seeger's and Gabrielsen's radiographic demonstration that the synostosis of the coronal suture extends into the cranial base (24), as well as by Tessier's description of the skeletal deformities in craniofacial dysostosis (16), extended the coronal craniectomy into the sphenozygomatic suture.

In 1979, Marchac and Renier (77) published the "floating forehead" procedure for treatment of brachycephaly. This procedure combines an advancement of the fronto-orbital bandeau with an extended coronal craniectomy, anchoring the bandeau only on the face (i.e., on the radix of the nose and the zygoma). Theoretically, the brain thrust will remain unopposed in pushing forward the frontofacial complex.

In cases of occipital plagiocephaly, we have performed an extensive bilateral parieto-occipital craniotomy, inverting and transposing the two parieto-occipital segments. The bone segment of the nonaffected side is applied over the cranial region of the affected side and gives it a satisfactory shape to which the dura adapts. At the same time, the deformed bony segment is fragmented as needed and applied to the contralateral side. A very satisfactory symmetry has been attained in these cases (Stratoudakis H. C., Gaines C., unpublished data).

The long-term effects of craniofacial surgery on infants are now becoming available. McCarthy et al. (78), reporting on a group of 50 patients, found that, while operated patients show a significant advantage over nonoperated patients and reconstructive surgery improves craniofacial form, surgery does not necessarily result in normal appearance. All patients with craniofacial dysostosis developed cross-bite (reflecting the fact that, despite earlier hopes, this surgery did not result in normal midfacial development), in contrast to the fronto-orbital region contour, which was generally satisfactory. Patients with bilateral coronal synostosis developed normal occlusal relationships. Refusion of sutures, associated with development of turricephaly, developed in three patients, all of whom were in the craniofacial dysostosis group. Calvarial contour irregularities were observed in eight patients, with or without defects, reflecting the unpredictability of calvarial bone regeneration (78). Morales and Whitaker (79), reviewing 49 patients with unilateral coronal synostosis, found that perfect symmetry was achieved in only 18%, while the majority of the others had a slight asymmetry that was obvious only to the trained eye.

In young children with midfacial retrusion, the procedure of choice remains the frontofacial monobloc advancement, which was described by Ortiz-Monasterio et al. (80) and modified by Raulo and Tessier (81). *As in every craniofacial procedure, the osteotomies are modified to fulfill the needs of the particular case.* The procedure is performed via an intracranial approach. The entire dissection is carried out through a coronal and a vestibular incision. The craniotomy is designed preserving a frontal bone bar between the frontal bone segment and the orbits. The frontal lobes are retracted, giving access to the orbital roofs. The temporal muscles are dissected from the temporal fossae, and the orbits and zygomata are dissected in a subperiosteal plane. A horizontal osteotomy is carried out through the lower frontal bone.

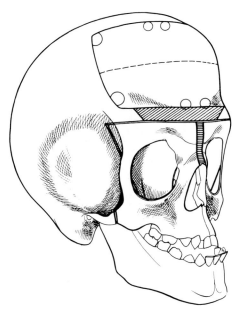

FIGURE 34.45. Frontofacial advancement (monoblock).

The orbital roofs are sectioned intracranially. The lateral and inferior orbital walls are sectioned starting in the sphenomaxillary (inferior orbital) fissure, and the medial orbital walls are sectioned behind the posterior lacrimal crest. The zygomatic arches are sectioned. Through the vestibular incision, the maxilla is dissected, and a pterygomaxillary disjunction carried out. At this point, the frontofacial mass is mobilized with Rowe forceps, and the posterior portion of the nasal septum is divided through the frontoethmoidal osteotomy. After advancement of the facial mass, the frontal bar is lengthened accordingly with a step osteotomy. Fixation is effected at the level of the forehead (to the frontal bar) and at the zygomatic arches with bone grafts, while bone blocks placed in the pterygomaxillary area maintain the maxilla in an advanced position. If the frontal bar is unsuitable or

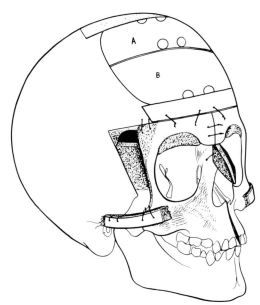

FIGURE 34.44. Frontofacial advancement (monoblock).

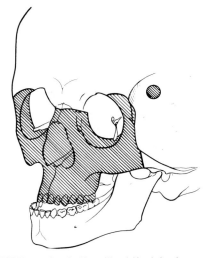

FIGURE 34.46. LeFort III midfacial advancement.

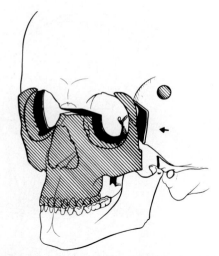

FIGURE 34.47. Le Fort III midfacial advancement.

weak, another one may be obtained from the biparietal area (Tessier, unpublished data) (Figs. 34.44 and 34.45).

A similar procedure has recently been described for infants suffering from severe airway obstruction, severe exophthalmia, and rapidly rising intracranial pressure. The entire frontofacial advancement is accomplished through the coronal incision. Experience so far with this procedure remains limited (82).

The monoblock frontofacial advancement is generally unsuitable for adults because the dead space created in the anterior cranial fossa by the advancement persists much longer than in children. This creates a real danger of sequestration or progressive resorption of the frontal bone "flap" (Tessier, unpublished data).

In adults, midfacial retrusion is corrected with a Le Fort III craniofacial disjunction. This procedure was pioneered by Tessier (83) and later modified by him. The transverse frontal crescent, the vertical frontal spur, and the semiopen method are all modifications of the same procedure designed to overcome specific problems (84) (Figs. 34.46 to 34.48).

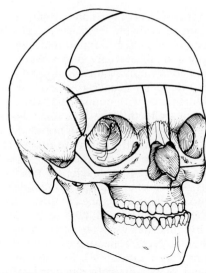

FIGURE 34.49. Orbital osteotomies for correction of telorbitism, and Le Fort I maxillary osteotomy.

Differential advancement of the orbital and maxillary complexes is also possible. To the Le Fort III osteotomies are added the osteotomies of a standard Le Fort I, and each complex is advanced as needed (84).

The late treatment of plagiocephaly in adults is a matter of considerably greater complexity than it is in the neonate. The procedure essentially consists in mobilizing the naso-orbital block in one unit, which is then tilted and advanced as needed. Tulasne and Tessier (85) have published an analysis of the anomaly and its correction.

The early attempts to correct telorbitism have been well outlined by Converse and associates (86, 87). In 1967, Tessier et al. (2) published their first paper on the subject, a scholarly study on the anatomy and surgical correction of this condition. The craniofacial approach was described for the first time.

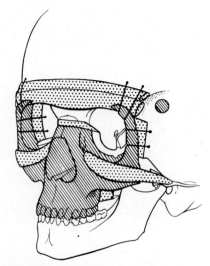

FIGURE 34.48. Le Fort III midfacial advancement.

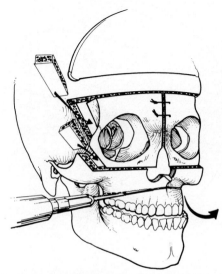

FIGURE 34.50. Orbital osteotomies for correction of telorbitism, and Le Fort I maxillary osteotomy.

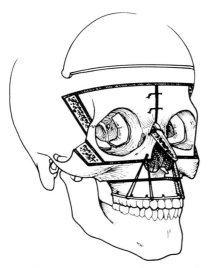

FIGURE 34.51. Orbital osteotomies for correction of telorbitism, and Le Fort I maxillary osteotomy.

Correction of telorbitism is based on the observation that the facial deformities stop at the level of the sphenoid and that the "useful orbits can be mobilized and approximated following resection of a central block of the floor of the anterior cranial fossa and frontal bone, including the ethmoid." Unfortunately, olfaction is sacrificed with resection of the ethmoid. Trying to overcome this drawback, Converse et al. (88) modified the osteotomies. Subsequent experience, however, showed that it is not always possible (48). Sailer and Landolt resect the cribriform plate using the operative microscope in an effort to preserve olfaction (89).

The various osteotomies separating the entire bony orbit from the cranium and adjacent facial bones are carried out. The orbits are mobilized and brought toward the midline, and a bilateral medial canthopexy is performed if the medial canthal tendons have been detached. The bony defects resulting from mobilization of the osteotomized segments are obliterated with bone grafts,

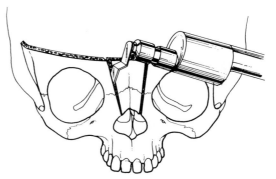

FIGURE 34.53. Facial bipartition.

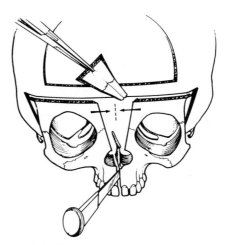

FIGURE 34.54. Facial bipartition.

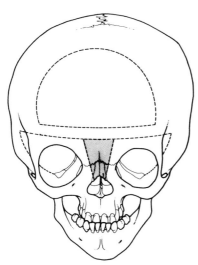

FIGURE 34.52. Facial bipartition.

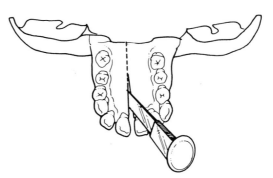

FIGURE 34.55. Facial bipartition.

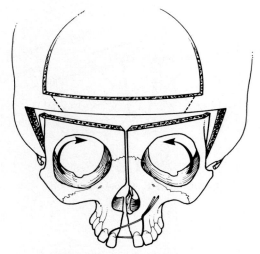

FIGURE 34.56. Facial bipartition.

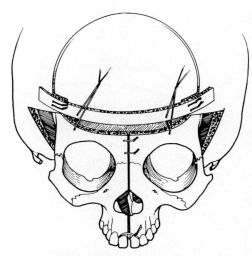

FIGURE 34.58. Facial bipartition.

while another bone graft is pegged into the frontal bone and wired to the frontal process of the maxilla to reconstruct and support the nasal bridge. A midline excision of skin eliminates the cutaneous redundancy approximating the eyebrows and canthi and provides a more pleasing appearance (Figs. 34.49 to 34.51).

The subcranial method of correction (2, 48) is no longer being used. Minor degrees of telorbitism can be camouflaged by burring the anterior lacrimal crests and performing a bilateral medial canthopexy (the intercanthal distance may be reduced up to 10 mm by this procedure). The intracranial route is used in all other cases.

The *facial bipartition* procedure is a derivative of the craniofacial approach to telorbitism, combining medial displacement of the orbits with maxillary expansion, where this is needed. It consists of mobilization of the frontofacial complex (as in the monoblock frontofacial advancement), and removal of a block of bone from the anterior cranial foss and the frontonasal area. The maxilla and hard palate are split in the midline, and the attach-

ments of the septum and vomer to the maxilla are severed. Medial displacement of the orbits results in maxillary expansion, with the hard palate–anterior nasal spine as pivoting point (Tessier, unpublished data) (Figs. 34.52 to 34.58).

Laterofacial Microsomias

Tessier has chosen this term to group together the following entities: Treacher Collins–Franceschetti complex, hemifacial microsomia, and the Goldenhar syndrome. He also includes Romberg's disease, which will not be discussed in this chapter (45).

For descriptive purposes, it seems logical to group these entities together because they may be considered as representing combinations of the same group of lateral facial clefts; namely, clefts 6, 7, and 8. Cleft 6 belongs specifically to the Treacher Collins and hemifacial microsomia, while cleft 8 belongs to both the Treacher Collins and the Goldenhar syndromes. It should be noted that these clefts can occur either singly or in any combination with each other, and that the phenotypes are varied and inconsistent (41).

TREACHER COLLINS–FRANCESCHETTI COMPLEX

The Treacher Collins–Franceschetti complex is referred to in the English literature as Treacher Collins or Berry syndrome, while in the French literature, it is called Franceschetti syndrome. it is also referred to as mandibulofacial dysostosis.

The first malformation of this type appears to have been published by Berry in 1889 (90). He described a notch occurring on the outer portion of the right lower lid of a 15-year-old girl but made no comment about the left eyelid. Her mother had the same deformity bilaterally. They displayed no other malformations. He commented on the possibility of hereditary transmission of the deformity. Treacher Collins (91) recorded two cases in

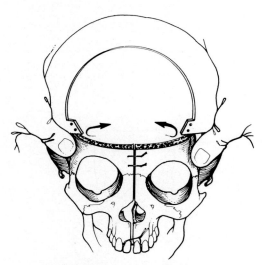

FIGURE 34.57. Facial bipartition.

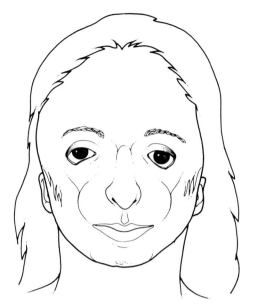

FIGURE 34.59.   Treacher Collins–Franceschetti syndrome.

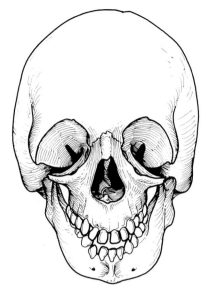

FIGURE 34.61.   *Treacher Collins–Franceschetti syndrome.*

1900, showing a more distinct development of this condition.

The first fully developed syndrome was described in two brothers in 1923 by De Lima and Monteiro, as quoted by Fischer in 1929 (92). Other authors followed.

In 1944, Franceschetti and Zwahlen (93) described two more cases. One of their patients, however, had microphthalmia and ectropia of the pupil, and because Tessier feels that the Treacher Collins–Franceschetti complex does not affect the eye (44), the question might be raised whether it was a true mandibulofacial dysostosis rather than a bilateral hemifacial microsomia or Goldenhar syndrome. In 1949, Franceschetti and Klein (94), in an extensive paper, reported four more cases, reviewed the previous publications, commented on the heredity

(dominant), and proposed a classification based on their observations. One of their cases, however, was unilateral, with orbital dystopia; therefore, one might question again whether it was a true case of mandibulofacial dysostosis, inasmuch as the consensus seems to be that the syndrome is always bilateral (44, 94).

Tessier's description of the Treacher Collins–Franceschetti complex, which follows here in detail (44; Figs. 34.59 to 34.64), is most meaningful because it is based on operative findings rather than on simple description of surface characteristics. He pointed out that the main characteristic of the complete forms is *a more or less total absence of the malar bone and of the zygomatic arch.* The bony deficits are between maxilla and zygoma (MZ), frontal bone and zygoma (FZ), or temporal bone and zygoma (TZ). The following malformations are observed.

Eye.   Frequent strabismus and amblyopia are evident.

Lower Eyelid.   There is a notch between the lateral and middle thirds; along the edges the eyelashes are absent, and the tarsus is atrophic.

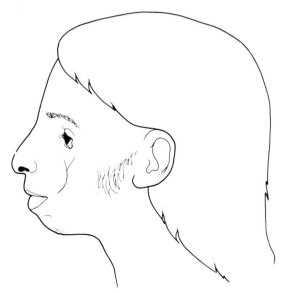

FIGURE 34.60.   A side view of deformities in the Treacher Collins–Franceschetti syndrome.

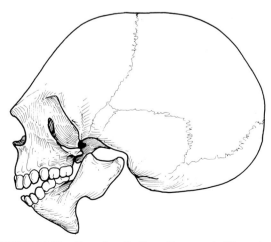

FIGURE 34.62.   Treacher Collins–Franceschetti syndrome.

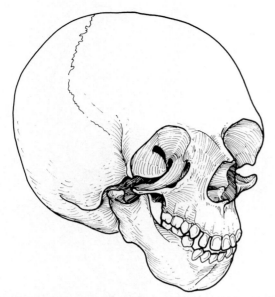

FIGURE 34.63.   Treacher Collins–Franceschetti syndrome.

Upper Eyelids.   There is occasional microform of a coloboma.

Eyebrow.   There is occasionally a notch or an ectropion of the lateral tail of the eyebrow.

Lacrimal Apparatus.   Frequent absence of the lower lacrimal punctum is apparent.

Lateral Canthus.   Deprived of a site of insertion, it is totally free, causing a brevity of the palpebral fissure.

Nose.   It may be narrow, deviated, hooked, or kyphotic. Frequent choanal atresia, which is rarely complete, is due to the vertical shortness of the maxilla and to the height of the palate.

Cheek.   A sclerodermic furrow extends from the lower eyelid notch toward the mandibular angle. On it are

occasionally observed hairs, which represent ectropic eyelashes.

Buccal Commissure.   It is frequently enlarged by a rudimentary macrostomia.

The Orbit in General.   The sphenomaxillary fissure (inferior orbital fissure) is open anteriorly because of the absence of the malar bone. The maxillary hypoplasia renders the infraorbital canal short. The infraorbital neurovascular pedicle may exit the orbital cavity without any bony trajectory. The orbital floor may have an inclination of up to 45° toward the sphenomaxillary fissure. The orbital contents are engaged in a large deficit, corresponding to a vertical increase of the orbit and, consequently, a decrease of the transverse diameter. The supraorbital ridge and superolateral angle and the lateral process of the frontal bone develop inferiorly and medially because of absence of the frontal process of the malar bone; the lateral canthus, therefore, is displaced inferiorly. There is no real lateral orbital ridge. The greater sphenoidal wing develops anteriorly because it does not encounter the zygomatic bone. The anterior portion of the greater wing is thin and irregular. It develops medially because the orbital contents sink in the inferolateral angle, which is widely open to the retromaxillary space.

Alveolar Bone and Palate.   The dental arch is narrow, the palate is high. The maxillary tuberosity is elevated, as is the palate, causing a vertical atresia of the choanae. The narrowing of the maxilla is responsible for their transverse atresia.

Maxilla and Maxillary Sinus.   The body of the maxilla is small, even though it appears normal, because of the absence of the malar bone.

Malar Bone.   The complete agenesis or severe hypoplasia of the malar bone is the characteristic malformation that explains all of the orbital anomalies. A rudimentary malar bone has been observed attached to the greater sphenoidal wing.

Temporal Region and Muscles.   In the majority of cases, one does not find even a small vestige of a zygomatic arch on the temporal bone. There might be one or more sesamoid bones in the normal course of the zygomatic arch. The absence of the zygomatic arch does not imply absence of the masseter because it inserts on the temporal fascia. This fascia belongs to both muscles, which become a common temporomasseteric muscle. The temporal muscle is usually atrophic.

Temporomandibular Joint.   The condyle and coronoid process are frequently hypoplastic.

Mandible.   The ascending ramus is short. There is a prominent antegonial notch. The lower border of the mandibular body is hypoplastic.

Chin.   Its retrusion and increase in height seem to be related to the vertical shortness of the ramus and to the cervical malformations.

Ear and Facial Nerve.   Microtia and cryptotia are frequent. In the pure form of Treacher Collins–Franceschetti syndrome, there is no facial nerve palsy.

Associated Malformations.   Cleft palate and vertebral malformations may accompany this complex. Franceschetti and Klein (94) pointed out that individuals afflicted by this condition have a strong, almost "familial" resemblance.

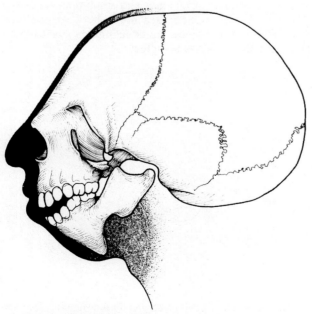

FIGURE 34.64.   Treacher Collins–Franceschetti syndrome.

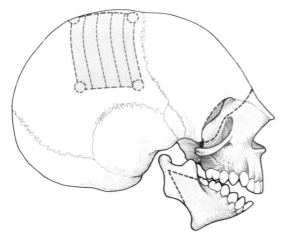

FIGURE 34.65. Integrate (midfacial and mandibular osteotomies for correction of severe forms of Treacher Collins–Franceschetti syndrome).

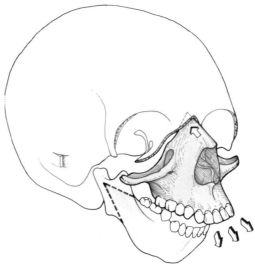

FIGURE 34.66. Integrate (midfacial and mandibular osteotomies for correction of severe forms of Treacher Collins–Franceschetti syndrome).

Treatment of the Treacher Collins–Franceschetti Syndrome

Operative correction of the Treacher Collins–Franceschetti deformities is aimed at reconstructing the missing or deficient elements of the facial skeleton, generally in three or four stages. The soft tissues are dealt with after the skeletal reconstruction, with the exception of the notches or colobomas of the lower lids. These are repaired first because, when at a later stage the orbits are dissected and bone grafts placed, the tension on the soft tissues might not allow their effective closure (Tessier, personal communication, 1983).

Minor procedures such as skin grafts, local flaps, and others carried out prematurely without being part of the overall treatment plan should by and large be avoided because they add scar tissue and render further dissection more difficult and less accurate.

The procedures to be carried out will depend on the degree of maxillomandibular deformities. If the deformities are not very severe, the first stage will consist in

reconstruction of the orbits and zygomatic arches with cranial and tibial bone grafts. Later, more appositional bone grafts may become necessary to build up further the areas of deficiency. Eventually, the maxillomandibular deformities are corrected as necessary. In cases with severe deformities, in which restriction of the airway is likely to exist because of a combination of maxillary atresia (restriction) and mandibular hypoplasia, Tessier has developed a procedure to which he has given the term "integrale" (integral—total procedure—indicating the performance simultaneously of midfacial and mandibular osteotomies). It consists in a midfacial osteotomy and forward "tilting" of the midface, with the area of the nasion as fulcrum, combined with a mandibular osteotomy to advance the mandible. The midfacial osteotomy is essentially a Le Fort II osteotomy because the zygomatic arches are absent and the sphenomaxillary (inferior orbital) fissures may be open anteriorly as a result of cleft 6.

FIGURE 34.67. Integrate (midfacial and mandibular osteotomies for correction of severe forms of Treacher Collins–Franceschetti syndrome).

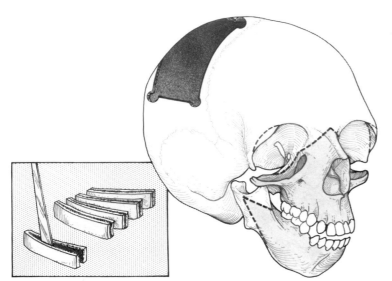

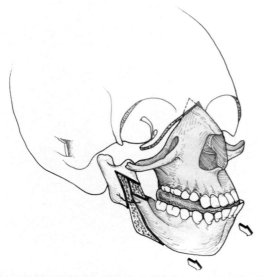

FIGURE 34.68. Integrate (midfacial and mandibular osteotomies for correction of severe forms of Treacher Collins–Franceschetti syndrome).

The mandibular osteotomy is of the C or inverted V type. The mobilized skeletal segments are stabilized with cranial and iliac bone grafts. Excellent midfacial stability is essential for this combination of procedures to be successful. If midfacial stability is not satisfactory, the mandibular osteotomy is deferred. The integrale is a difficult, lengthy procedure and involves hazardous dissection. A tracheostomy is always required for airway control (Figs. 34.65 to 34.69) (Tessier, personal communication, 1983). Complementary procedures such as lateral canthopexy adjustments, rhinoplasty, genioplasty, and/or lengthening of the suprahyoidal region with a Z-plasty are carried out after the major stages of reconstruction have been completed (44).

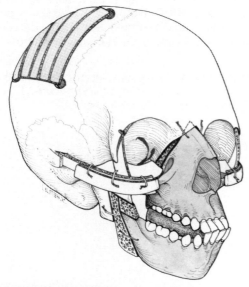

FIGURE 34.69. Integrate (midfacial and mandibular osteotomies for correction of severe forms of Treacher Collins–Franceschetti syndrome).

HEMIFACIAL MICROSOMIA

This term was first used by Gorlin and associates (95, 96) to refer to patients with unilateral microtia, macrostomia, and failure of formation of the mandibular ramus and condyle. Gorlin and associates (95, 96) have suggested that oculoauriculovertebral dysplasia (Goldenhar syndrome) is a variant of this complex characterized by vertebral anomalies, most often hemivertebras, and epibulbar dermoids. Several other terms have also been used in the international bibliography to designate this condition, such as first and second branchial arch syndrome (97), auriculobranchiogenic dysplasia (98), otomandibular dystosis (99), craniofacial microsomia (100), lateral facial dysplasia (101), otomandibular syndrome (which is the term used in the French literature) (44), and others. Furthermore, there have been several classifications into groups (97), types (102), and grades or types (103–105), which do not necessarily describe the same or similar phenotypes.

As previously mentioned, Tessier (41, 44) considers this malformation to be a clefting syndrome, among the most complex ones affecting the cranium, the upper part of the face, and the mandible. It is, in contradistinction to the Treacher Collins–Franceschetti complex, an *asymmetrical malformation* for which no genetic background has been identified (106). Its incidence is estimated to be between 1 : 3,500 (106) and 1 : 5,642 births (107). Although it is described as a unilateral deformity, bilateral forms are not infrequent (101, 102, 105, 107).

Skeletal Deformities

Even though the orbit, zygoma, temporal bone, maxilla, and nose may be involved (44, 107), the mandibular deformity is assumed to be the abnormal keystone. Asymmetrical mandibular growth is the earliest skeletal manifestation and seems to play a pivotal role in the progressive distortion of both ipsilateral and contralateral structures (107) with deviation toward the affected side. At birth, the defect often appears mild; with growth, asymmetry becomes more marked because of progressive development of the normal side. Only after full growth of the patient is the end-stage deformity evident (105; Figs. 34.70 to 34.73).

The Mandible. Pruzansky's classification of the mandibular deformity in hemifacial microsomia into grades (103) has been adopted by other authors (100, 105, 107, 108) because it provides a workable repository for cases with similar presentation. In *grade I,* the hypoplasia is minimal, and the difference with the assumed normal side is one of size. In *grade II,* there is a functioning but deformed temporomandibular joint that is usually displaced anteriorly and medially. The condyle, ramus, and sigmoid notch are distorted. In *grade III,* there is complete absence of the ramus and glenoid fossa. The mandibular body ends abruptly in the molar region.

The Maxilla. The maxilla is characterized by a transverse and vertical shortness. Its downward growth is im-

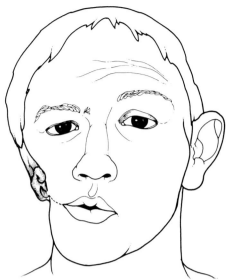

FIGURE 34.70.   Hemifacial microsomia.

peded by the vertical mandibular deficiency, causing an increasing obliquity of the occlusal plane.

The Malar Bone.   Variable degrees of hypoplasia are demonstrated (100). In severe cases, the temporal portion of the zygomatic arch is absent, while its malar portion is long with an inferior, posterior, and medial inclination toward the styloid. The orbit itself is retropositioned (44).

Soft Tissue Deformities

Facial soft tissues on the affected side may vary from normal to severely deficient. The skin, subcutaneous tissue, and facial musculature of expression may be affected. Hypoplasia of the parotid gland is not infrequent, placing the facial nerve in a vulnerable position (100).

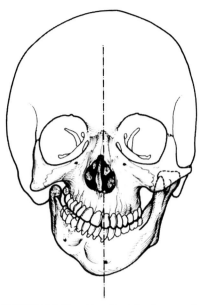

FIGURE 34.72.   Hemifacial microsomia.

The muscles of mastication may be underdeveloped or absent, especially in the grade III patient. In grade I defects, the muscles, although small, can usually be identified. Grade II patients exhibit combinations of these findings (105). Macrostomia (soft tissue component of cleft 7) of a variable degree may be present (44).

The external ear is characterized by a wide spectrum of anomalies, varying from a normal appearance to its total absence.

Anomalies of the Nervous System

A wide variety of central nervous system anomalies have been described in conjunction with hemifacial microsomia, such as agenesis of the corpus callosum, hy-

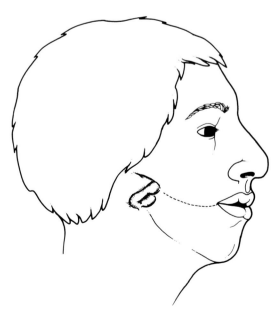

FIGURE 34.71.   Hemifacial microsomia.

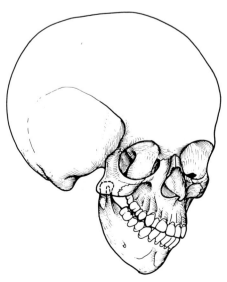

FIGURE 34.73.   Hemifacial microsomia.

drocephalus, unilateral hypoplasia of the brainstem and cerebellum, and others. Cranial nerve anomalies are also frequent. The most common cranial nerve anomaly is facial palsy. Converse and associates (100) provide an extensive bibliography on this subject.

GOLDENHAR SYNDROME

As in hemifacial microsomia, the Goldenhar syndrome consists of a cleft 7 but of lesser severity; it is also associated with a cleft 8 with oculopalpebral predominance that, contrary to the Treacher Collins–Franceschetti complex, affects only slightly the orbital cavity. The epibulbar dermoids are frequently in the inferolateral quadrant, along the axis of a cleft 6. It is frequently bilateral, but contrary to the Treacher Collins–Franceschetti complex, it is always very asymmetrical (44). Its anatomical characteristics are similar to those of hemifacial microsomia; however, characterization of this syndrome probably depends on the presence of oculopalpebral anomalies, particularly because Goldenhar's original paper (109) was focused on the association of anomalies of the eye and ear.

Treatment of Hemifacial Microsomia–Goldenhar Syndromes

The asymmetrical nature of these syndromes, their progressive character, the diminished growth potential of all tissues involved, and the three-dimensional distortion of anatomical structures accounts for the difficulties encountered in their treatment. It is evident that, because of the tremendous variability with which they present, their treatment will also vary greatly. For didactic purposes, general guidelines must be established as to the timing, rationale, and principles of the various procedures employed and the coordination of disciplines (jaw orthopaedics, surgery, and orthodontics) that have to be combined if the maximum benefit is to be obtained.

The goal of treatment in patients with hemifacial microsomia is improved function and optimal facial symmetry when growth is completed (110). The principles of treatment are: (*a*) stimulation of existing musculoskeletal units so that maximum growth may be achieved; (*b*) prevention of secondary underdevelopment of structures; (*c*) augmentation of deficient osseous structures and construction of missing portions of the skeleton with autogenous bone grafts; and (*d*) reconstruction of soft tissue defects when the skeletal procedures have been completed (ear reconstruction, facial reanimating in cases of facial nerve palsy, and others). It follows that treatment becomes more complex and the anticipated results less favorable as the deformity progresses from a grade (or type) I to a grade (or type) III.

The assessment and radiographic evaluation of patients with hemifacial microsomia and Goldenhar syndrome will not be discussed here. Detailed descriptions of this subject have been published, and the reader is referred to these sources (107, 111, 112).

Clinical observation has shown that the use of some orthopaedic orthodontic appliances can alter mandibular growth. This has been confirmed experimentally by Petrovic et al. (113). Any jaw orthopaedic appliance that elicits a forward positioning of the condylar process in a steady pattern will cause remodeling and bone apposition on the condylar head (114, 115).

When the temporomandibular joint is present, if only the condylar cartilage and disc are missing, and the joint functions without difficulty, the deficient growth may be successfully compensated with the use of an orthopaedic appliance (activator). If this fails to establish the required symmetry, a mandibular osteotomy of the ramus on the affected side to elongate and rotate the mandible is carried out generally during the age of mixed dentition (6–12 years). An open bite is created on the affected side, allowing for vertical maxillary growth and extrusion of the maxillary teeth in order to obtain a normal horizontal occlusal plane (105). The treatment becomes more complex if the patient is first seen as an adult. A compensatory osteotomy of the opposite ramus has to be performed because the nonaffected condyle cannot remodel and a Le Fort I osteotomy is necessary to level the occlusal plane.

In more severely affected temporomandibular joints that do not allow forward translation of the mandible either through the contraction of the lateral pterygoid muscle or with the help of an activator, severe growth restrictions must be anticipated (116). Treatment in these patients should still begin with the use of an activator because it may improve mobility and prevent further tipping of the occlusal plane (116). Furthermore, the stretching effort on the skin and muscles is beneficial (105). Early surgical correction aimed at correcting the mandibular asymmetry in three planes must be anticipated. If the existing temporomandibular joint is in a relatively normal anatomical location, it is maintained, and the mandible is osteotomized and elongated, rotated, and advanced. If the temporomandibular joint is displaced medially or anteriorly, it is excised, and a new joint is constructed at a site symmetrical with the opposite side. A compensatory osteotomy of the opposite side is almost always required. A posterior open bite, deliberately created, will allow vertical growth on the maxilla and eruption of maxillary teeth. In the adults, a Le Fort I osteotomy becomes necessary to achieve a horizontal occlusal plane (105).

If the temporomandibular joint is ankylosed, the preliminary orthopaedic treatment is eliminated because of the severe restriction of mobility, and surgical release becomes the first step of the treatment (117, 118).

When the mandibular ramus is missing (type III deformity), a ramus and glenoid fossa must be constructed, as symmetrically as possible to the opposite side. The surgical procedure is carried out when the child has a full complement of deciduous teeth (105). The mandibular ramus may be constructed either with rib grafts or with cranial bone grafts. When carried out early, an osteotomy of the opposite ramus is usually not necessary.

The desired position of the mandible is determined with bite registration splints, which are constructed on scale models preoperatively. Postoperatively, after the period of interdental fixation, the splint is wired to the maxilla, and the mandibular movements are controlled with rubber bands, which guide the mandible into proper occlusion in the splint. *A consistent pattern of jaw movements is considered essential for the strain distribution in the mandible and is a prerequisite for the remodeling of the bone graft.* Growth continues to be deficient on the affected side, and additional osteotomies are frequently necessary to reestablish symmetry (110).

Tessier (44) pointed out that not enough attention has been paid to the malformations of the orbit and the absence of the glenoid fossa and the zygomatic arch. The zygomatic arch is constructed, when absent, preferably with a cranial bone graft mortised into the temporal bone. The glenoid fossa may be constructed with iliac bone. The orbit is remodeled as needed. All these procedures are adapted, of course, to the patient's age.

Finally, on-lay bone grafts to improve skeletal contour, soft tissue augmentation, and reconstruction of the auricle (which is deferred until the skeletal reconstruction is completed and optimal symmetry attained) are carried out as needed.

Complications

The potential for complications in the domain of craniofacial surgery is significant. This is hardly surprising when one considers the extent and duration of craniofacial procedures, the multiple structures involved (cranium, orbits, maxilla, and occasionally the mandible), the close proximity of more or less septic cavities (nose, paranasal sinuses, oral cavity), the large amounts of grafted tissue, and the frequent creation of dead spaces (44).

A review of the largest published series substantiates the logical assumption that the majority of lethal complications follow procedures in which the intracranial route was used. Reported causes of death include:

1. Inadequate or excessive replacement of blood volume (44, 119, 120)
2. Cerebral edema (44, 119, 120)
3. Respiratory obstruction (44, 119, 120)
4. Infection (meningitis) (44, 119, 120)
5. Pneumomediastinum (44); an explanation of the pathogenesis of this complication is provided in another report (121)
6. Sagittal sinus thrombosis (120)
7. Epidural hematoma (29)
8. Tracheoesophageal fistula (44)
9. Erosion of the vena cava of a central line placed through the femoral vein (44)
10. Pulmonary embolism (44)

It becomes evident, therefore, that a large proportion of postoperative deaths can be traced back to a technical fault and that with increasing experience their frequency may be reduced.

Other nonlethal but nevertheless serious complications may also follow craniofacial procedures.

1. Infection may lead to soft tissue loss, osteomyelitis, localized abscesses, and sequestration of bone grafts. This appears to be the most frequent complication in all major reported series. The highest infection rate occurs in patients undergoing intracranial procedures, particularly where a communication of the cranial cavity with the nose, paranasal sinuses, and oral cavity is created (119, 120, 122). In an effort to reduce the incidence of infection, Jackson and coworkers have described the use of a galeal frontalis myofascial flap to eliminate communication of the nasopharynx with the anterior cranial fossa (123). The occurrence of bacterial contamination was shown to be directly proportional to the duration of the operative procedure (124).
2. Complications related to the orbital cavity and its contents include: (*a*) blindness, due to injury of the optic nerve (44, 119, 120); (*b*) hemianopsia (44); (*c*) diplopia (44, 119); (*d*) corneal ulceration (44); (*e*) neurogenic oculomotor palsy (119); and (*f*) obstruction of the lacrimal sac or nasolacrimal duct (44). A distinction must be made between true complications and sequelae of an operative procedure, which are more or less predictable, and the correction of which will be undertaken at a later stage, such as ptosis of the upper lid after correction of exophthalmia by midfacial advancement and enophthalmia after correction of telorbitism, caused by the increase in volume of the orbit (brought about by the orbital translocation).
3. Resorption of bone grafts, other than the true septic sequestrations, is another complication. The incidence and degree of resorption is difficult to quantify (44).
4. Cerebrospinal fluid leaks, frequently self-limiting, may require treatment by shunting or application of a dural patch (44, 119). When cerebrospinal fluid leakage occurred in conjunction with an intraoral procedure, the infection rate was 25% (20). Spontaneous subdural hygromas may occur after prolonged spinal drainage (125).
5. Velopharyngeal incompetence has been reported after facial advancement. Generally, however, the effect of such procedures on speech is beneficial because of improvement of the airway and of dental occlusion (44, 119).
6. Canthal drift and displacement of skeletal segments from their position of fixation may occur, comprising the esthetic result.
7. Inappropriate antidiuretic hormone secretion has been reported to follow craniofacial procedures (126) and after cleft palate surgery (127). If not recognized and treated immediately, this condition may have grave consequences. Serum electrolytes and osmolality must be monitored very closely.

Acknowledgment. This chapter is dedicated to Dr. Paul Tessier, who, in addition to being my teacher and respected friend, has graciously allowed me the publication of his valuable collection of illustrations.

References

1. Gillies H, Harrison SH: Operative correction by osteotomy of recessed malar maxillary compound in a case of oxycephaly. *Br J Plast Surg* 3:123, 1951.
2. Tessier P, Guiot G, Rougerie J, et al: Ostéotomies cranio-naso-orbito-faciales. Hypertélorisme. *Ann Chir Plast* 12:103, 1967.
3. Champy M, Lodde JP, Jaeger JH, Wilk H: Osterosyntheses mandibulaires selon la technique de michelet. 1. Bases biomechaniques. *Rev Stomat* 77:569, 1976.
4. Champy M, Lodde JP: Syntheses mandibulaires—localisationdes syntheses en fonction des contraintes mandibulaires. *Rev Stomat* 77:971, 1976.
5. Tessier PL, Hemmy DC: Protocol for CT scanning for three dimensional reformations, June 1985, 3rd Revision. Distributed to the participants of the First International Congress for Cranio-Maxillofacial Surgery, La Napoule, France, September 1985.
6. Johnson GC: CTDI, a clinical utility. Proceedings of the Conference of Radiation Control Directors, Inc, Frankfort, Kentucky, 1985.
7. Stratoudakis AC, Cox M: 30 imaging in the study of craniofacial anomalies. Read before the Symposium "3D Imaging in Medicine" sponsored by the Hospital of the University of Pennsylvania, Philadelphia, December 1987.
8. Dahlin H, Nylen O, Wilbrand H: Radiation dose distribution in temporal bone tomography. *Acta Radiol [Diagn] (Stockh)* 14:353, 1973.
9. Merraim GR, Focht EF: A clinical study of radiation cataracts and the relationship to the dose. *Am J Roentgenol* 77:759, 1957.
10. Focht EF, Merriam GR, Schwartz M, Velasquez AB, Mc Neill D: A method of radiation cataract analysis and its uses in experimental fractionation studies. *Radiology* 87:465, 1966.
11. Kaplan EN: 3D CT images for facial implant design and manufacture. *Clin Plast Surg* 14:663, 1987.
12. Toth BA, Ellis DS, Stewart WB: Computer designed prostheses for orbitocranial reconstruction. *Plast Reconstr Surg* 81:315, 1988.
13. Guyuron B, Ross RJ: Computer generated model surgery. *J Cranio-Maxillofac Surg* 17:101, 1989.
14. Moss M: Functional anatomy of cranial synostosis. *Child's Brain* 1:22, 1975.
15. Bolk L: On the premature obliteration of sutures in the human skull. *Am J Anat* 17:495, 1915.
16. Tessier P: Relationship of craniostenoses to craniofacial dysostoses and to faciostenoses. A study with therapeutic implications. *Plast Reconstr Surg* 48:224, 1971.
17. Delaire J: Considerations sur les synostoses prematures et leurs consequences au crane et a la face. *Rev Stomatol* 64:97, 1963.
18. Smith DW, Töndury G: Origin of the calvaria and its sutures. *Am J Dis Child* 132:662, 1978.
19. La Trenta GS, McCarthy JG, Cutting CB: The growth of vascularized onlay bone transfers. *Ann Plast Surg* 18:511, 1987.
20. Hirabayashi S, Harii K, Sakurai A, Takaki EK, Fukuda D: An experimental study of craniofacial growth in a heterotopic rat head transplant. *Plast Reconstr Surg* 82:236, 1988.
21. Virchow R: Ueber den cretinismus, nametlich in franken und über pathologischen schädelforamen. *Verhanl D Phys-Med Gesellschin Wurzborg* 2:230, 1851–2.
22. Moss ML: Premature synostosis of the frontal suture in the cleft palate skull. *Plast Reconstr Surg* 20:199, 1957.
23. Moss ML: The pathogenesis of premature cranial synostosis in man. *Acta Anat* 37:351, 1959.
24. Seeger JF, Gabrielsen TO: Premature closure of the frontosphenoidal suture in synostosis of the coronal suture. *Radiology* 101:631, 1971.
25. Stewart RE, Dixon G, Cohen A: The pathogenesis of premature craniosynostosis in acrocephalosyndactyly (Apert's syndrome). A reconsideration. *Plast Reconstr Surg* 59:699, 1977.
26. Kreiborg S, Prydsoe U, Dahl E, et al: Calvarium and cranial base in Apert's syndrome. An autopsy report. *Cleft Palate J* 13:296, 1976.
27. Ousterhout D, Melsen B: Cranial base deformity in Apert's syndrome. *Plast Reconstr Surg* 69:254, 1982.
28. Fishman MA, Hogan GR, Dodge PR: The concurrence of hydrocephalus and craniosynostosis. *J Neurosurg* 34:621, 1971.
29. Anderson B, Woodhall B: Visual loss in primary skull deformities. *Trans Am Acad Ophthalmol Otolaryngol* 57:497, 1953.
30. Marchac D, Renier D: *Chirurgie Cranio Faciale des Craniostenoses*. Paris, Médecine et Sciences Internationales, 1982, p 8.
31. David JD, Poswillo D, Simpson D: *The Craniosynostoses. Causes, Natural History, and Management*. New York, Springer-Verlag, 1982, p 153.
32. Stutzmann J, Petrovic A, Stratoudakis AC: Cytological features in craniosynostosis. Read Before the 67th Congress of the European Orthodontic Society, Copenhagen, June 1990.
33. Holtermueller K, Wiedemann HR: The clover leaf skull syndrome. *Med Monatsschr* 14:439, 1960.
34. Kokkich VG, Moffet BC, Cohen MM: The cloverleaf skull anomaly: An anatomic and histologic study of two specimens. *Cleft Palate J* 19:89, 1982.
35. Cohen MM: An etiologic and nosologic overview of craniosynostosis syndromes. *Birth Defects* 11:137, 1975.
36. Crouzon, MO: Dysostose cranio-faciale hereditaire. *Bull Mém Soc Méd Hôp Paris* 33:545, 1912.
37. Schiller JG: Craniofacial dysostosis of Crouzon: A case report and pedigree with emphasis on heredity. *Pediatrics* 23:107, 1959.
38. Apert EE: De l'Acrocéphalosyndactylie. *Bull Mém Soc Méd Hôp Paris* 23:1310, 1906.
39. Cohen MM: Craniosynostosis and syndromes with craniosynostosis: Incidence, genetics, penetrance, variability, and new syndrome updating. *Birth Defects* 15(5B):13, 1979.
40. Kawamoto HK: The kaleidoscopic world of rare craniofacial clefts: Order out of chaos (Tessier classification). *Clin Plast Surg* 3:529, 1976.
41. Tessier P: Anatomical classification of facial, craniofacial and laterofacial clefts. In Tessier P, Callahan A, Mustarde JC, Salyer K (eds): *Symposium on Plastic Surgery in the Orbital Region*. St. Louis, CV Mosby Co, 1976, Vol 12, p 189.
42. Jones KL, Smith DW, Hall BD, et al: A pattern of craniofacial and limb defects secondary to abberant tissue bands. *J Pediatr* 84:90, 1974.
43. Tessier P: Colobomas: Vertical and oblique complete facial clefts. *Panminerva Med* 11:95, 1969.
44. Tessier P: Fentes orbito-faciales verticales et obliques (Colobomas) complètes et frustes. *Ann Chir Plast* 14:301, 1969.
45. Tessier P: In Rougier J, Tessier P, Hervouet F, Woillez M, Lekieffre M, Derome P (eds): *Chirugie Plastique Orbito-Palpebrale*. Paris, Masson, 1977, p 223.
46. Moore MH, David JD, Cooter RD: Hairline indicators of craniofacial clefts. *Plast Reconstr Surg* 82:589, 1988.
47. Greig DM: Hypertelorism: A hitherto undifferentiated congenital craniofacial deformity. *Edinburgh Med J* 31:560, 1924.
48. Tessier P: Orbital hypertelorism. In Tessier P, Callahan A, Mustardé JC, Salyer K (eds): *Symposium on Plastic Surgery in the Orbital Region*. St. Louis, CV Mosby Co, 1976, Vol 12, p 255.
49. Derome PJ, Visot A: La dysplasie fibreuse cranienne. *Neuro Chirurg* 29(Suppl 1):5, 1983, p 67.
50. Tessier P, Guiot G, Derome P: Orbital hypertelorism. Definitive treatment of orbital hypertelorism (ORH) by craniofacial or by extracranial osteotomies. *Scand J Plast Reconstr Surg* 7:39, 1973.
51. Van der Meulen JCH, Vaandrager JM: Surgery related to the correction of hypertelorism. *Plast Reconstr Surg* 71:6, 1983.
52. Johr P: Valeurs moyennes et limites normales en fonction de l'âge, de quelques mesures de la tête et de la région orbitaire. *J Génét Hum* 2:247, 1953.
53. Laestadius ND, Aase JM, Smith DW: Normal inner canthal and outer orbital dimensions. *J Pediatr* 74:465, 1969.
54. Munro IR: Discussion of: Surgery related to the correction of hypertelorism by Van der Meulen JCH, Vaandrager JM (reference 34). *Plast Reconstr Surg* 71:18, 1982.
55. Charoonsmith T: Review of 310 patients with frontoethmoidal

encephalomeningocele with reference to plastic reconstruction. In Williams B (ed): *Transactions of the 8th International Congress of Plastic Surgery*. Montreal, Canadian Society of Plastic Surgeons, 1983, p 314.

56. David JD, Simpson D, White J: Fronto-nasal encephaloceles: Morphology and treatment. In Williams B (ed): *Transactions of the 8th International Congress of Plastic Surgery*. Montreal, Canadian Society of Plastic Surgeons, 1983, p 311.

57. Suwanwela CN, Suwanwela A: A morphological classification of sincipital encephalomeningoceles. *J Neurosurg* 36:201, 1972.

58. Morris WMM, Locksen W, Le Roux PAJ: Spheno-maxillary meningoencephalocele. *J Cranio-Maxillofac Surg* 17:359, 1989.

59. Diamond GR, Whitaker L: Ocular motility in craniofacial reconstruction. *Plast Reconstr Surg* 73:31, 1984.

60. Morax S: Oculo-motor disorders in craniofacial malformations. *J Maxillofac Surg* 12:1, 1984.

61. Ortiz-Monasterio F, Fuente del Campo A, Limon-Brown E: Mechanism and correction of V syndrome in craniofacial dysostosis. In Tessier P, Callahan A, Mustardé JC, Salyer K (eds): *Symposium on Plastic Surgery in the Orbital Region*. St. Louis, CV Mosby Co, 1976, Vol 12, p 246.

62. Choy AE, Margolis S, Breinin GM, et al: Analysis of preoperative and postoperative extraocular muscle function in surgical translocation of bony orbits: A preliminary report. In Converse JM, McCarthy J, Wood-Smith D (eds): *Symposium on Diagnosis and Treatment of Craniofacial Anomalies*. St. Louis, CV Mosby Co, 1979, Vol 20, p 128.

63. Diamond G, Katowitz JA, Whitaker LH, et al: Ocular alignment after craniofacial reconstruction. *Am J Ophthalmol* 90:248, 1980.

64. Lannelongue J: De la craniectomie dans la microcephalie. *CR Acad Sci* 110:1382, 1890.

65. Lane LC: Pioneer craniectomy for relief of mental imbecility due to premature sutural closure and microcephalus. *JAMA* 18:49, 1892.

66. McCarthy JG: New concepts in the surgical treatment of the craniofacial synostosis syndromes in the infant. *Clin Plast Surg* 6:201, 1979.

67. Ingraham FD, Alexander E Jr, Matson DD: Clinical studies in craniosynostosis, analysis of fifty cases and description of a method of surgical treatment. *Surgery* 24:518, 1948.

68. McLaurin RL, Matson DD: Importance of early surgical treatment of craniosynostosis: Review of 36 cases treated during the first six months of life. *Pediatrics* 10:637, 1952.

69. Ingraham FD, Matson DD: *Neurosurgery of infancy and childhood*. Springfield, IL, Charles C Thomas Co, 1954, p 83.

70. Shillito J, Matson DD: Craniosynostosis: A review of 519 surgical patients. *Pediatrics* 41:829, 1968.

71. Stricker M, Montaut J, Hepner H, et al: Les ostéotomies du crane et de la face. *Ann Chir Plast* 17:233, 1972.

72. Marchac D, Cophignon J, Van der Meulen J, et al: A propos des ostéotomies d'Advancement due crane et de la face. *Ann Chir Plast* 19:311, 1974.

73. Hoffman H, Mohr G: Lateral canthal advancement of the supraorbital margin. A new corrective technique in the treatment of coronal synostosis. *J Neurosurg* 45:376, 1976.

74. Whitaker LA, Schut L, Ker LP: Early surgery for isolated craniofacial dysostosis. *Plast Reconstr Surg* 60:575, 1977.

75. Whitaker LA, Schut L, Rosen HM: Congenital craniofacial asymmetry: Early treatment. *Scand J Plast Reconstr Surg* 15:227, 1981.

76. McCarthy J, Coccaro PJ, Epstein F, et al: Early release in the infant with craniofacial dysostosis. The role of the sphenozygomatic suture. *Plast Reconstr Surg* 62:335, 1978.

77. Marchac D, Renier D: Le Front flottant, traitement précoce des facio-craniosténoses. *Ann Chir Plast* 24:121, 1979.

78. McCarthy J, Epstein F, Sadove M, et al: Early surgery for craniofacial synostosis: An 8-year experience. *Plast Reconstr Surg* 73:521, 1984.

79. Morales L, Whitaker L: Coronal synostosis: Asymmetrical manifestations and treatment in infancy. In Williams B (ed): *Transactions of the 8th International Congress of Plastic Sur-gery*. Montreal, Canadian Society of Plastic Surgeons, 1983, p 288.

80. Ortiz-Monasterio F, Fuenta del Campo A, Carillo A: Advancement of the orbits and the midface in one piece, combined with frontal repositioning of correction of Crouzon's deformities. *Plast Reconstr Surg* 61:507, 1978.

81. Raulo Y, Tessier P: Fronto-facial advancement for Crouzon's and Apert's syndromes. *Scand J Plast Reconstr Surg* 15:245, 1981.

82. Muhlbauer W, Anderl H, Marchac D: Complete fronto-facial advancement in infants with craniofacial dysostosis. In Williams B (ed): *Transactions of the 8th International Congress of Plastic Surgery*. Montreal, Canadian Society of Plastic Surgeons, 1983, p 318.

83. Tessier P: Ostéotomies totales de la face. Syndrome de Crouzon. Syndrome d'Apert. Oxycéphalies Scaphocéphalies Turricéphalies. *Ann Chir Plast* 12:273, 1967.

84. Tessier P: Recent improvements in treatment of facial and cranial deformities of Crouzon's disease and Apert's syndrome. In Tessier P, Callahan A, Mustardé JC, Salyer K (eds): *Symposium on Plastic Surgery in the Orbital Region*. St. Louis, CV Mosby Co, 1976, Vol 12, p 271.

85. Tulasne JF, Tessier P: Analysis and late treatment of plagiocephaly. Unilateral coronal synostosis. *Scand J Plast Reconstr Surg* 15:257, 1981.

86. Converse JM, McCarthy J, Wood-Smith D: Reconstructive plastic surgery for orbital hypertelorism. In Converse JM, McCarthy J, Wood-Smith D (eds): *Symposium on Diagnosis and Treatment of Craniofacial Anomalies*. St. Louis, CV Mosby Co, 1979, p 207.

87. Converse JM, McCarthy J: Orbital hypertelorism. *Scand J Plast Reconstr Surg* 15:265, 1981.

88. Converse JM, Ransohoff J, Matthews ES, et al: Ocular hypertelorism and pseudohypertelorism. Advances in surgical treatment. *Plast Reconstr Surg* 45:1, 1970.

89. Sailer RF, Landolt RM: A new method for the correction of hypertelorism with preservation of the olfactory nerve filaments. *J Cranio-Maxillofac Surg* 15:122, 1987.

90. Berry GA: Note on a congenital defect (?coloboma) of the lower lid. *Ophthal Hosp Rep* 12:255, 1889.

91. Collins ET: Case with symmetrical congenital notches in the outer part of each lower lid and defective development of the malar bones. *Trans Ophthal Soc UK* 20:190, 1900.

92. Fischer H: *Les Dysmorphies Congénitales Craniofaciales du Rachis et Leurs Syndromes Cliniques*. Paris, Vigot Frères, 1929.

93. Franceschetti A, Zwahlen P: Un syndrome nouveau: La dysostose mandibulo-faciale. *Bull Acad Suisse Sci Méd* 1:60, 1944.

94. Franceschetti A, Klein D: The mandibulo-facial dysostosis. A new hereditary syndrome. *Acta Ophthalmol* 27:143, 1949.

95. Gorlin RJ, Jue KL, Jacobsen U, Goldschmidt E: Oculoauriculovertebral dysplasia. *J Pediatr* 63:991, 1963.

96. Gorlin RJ, Pindborg JJ, Cohen MM: *Syndromes of the Head and Neck*. New York, McGraw-Hill, 1976.

97. Grabb WC: The first and second branchial arch syndrome. *Plast Reconstr Surg* 36:485, 1965.

98. Caronni EP: Embryogenesis and classification of branchial auricular dysplasia. In: *Transactions of the 5th International Congress of Plastic Surgery*. Melbourne, Butterworth, 1971.

99. Obwegeser HL: Correction of the skeletal anomalies of otomandibular dysostosis. *J Maxillofac Surg* 2:73, 1974.

100. Converse JM, McCarthy JG, Wood-Smith D, et al: Craniofacial microsomia. In Converse JM (ed): *Reconstructive Plastic Surgery*. Philadelphia, WB Saunders Co, 1977, Vol IV, pp 2359–2400.

101. Ross RB: Lateral facial dysplasia (first and second branchial arch syndrome, hemifacial microsomia). *Birth Defects* 11:51, 1975.

102. Tenconi R, Hall BD: Hemifacial microsomia: Phenotypic classification, clinical implications and genetic aspects. In Harvold EP (ed): *Treatment of Hemifacial Microsomia*. New York, Alan R. Liss, 1983, pp 39–50.

103. Pruzansky S: Not all dwarfed mandibles are alike. *Birth Defects* 5:120, 1969.
104. Swanson LT, Murray JE: Asymmetries of the lower part of the face. In Whitaker LA, Randall P (eds): *Symposium on Reconstruction of Jaw Deformities.* St. Louis, CV Mosby Co, 1978, pp 171–211.
105. Murray JE, Kaban LB, Mulliken JB: Analysis and treatment of hemifacial microsomia. *Plast Reconstr Surg* 74:186, 1984.
106. Poswillo D: Otomandibular deformity: Pathogenesis as a guide to reconstruction. *J Maxillofac Surg* 2:64, 1974.
107. Kaban LB, Mulliken JB, Murray JE: Three dimensional approach to analysis and treatment of hemifacial microsomia. *Cleft Palate J* 18:90, 1981.
108. McCarthy JG: Craniofacial microsomia. In Serafin D, Georgiade N (eds): *Pediatric Plastic Surgery.* St. Louis, CV Mosby Co, 1984, Vol 1, pp 499–517.
109. Goldenhar M: Associations malformations de l'oeil et de l'oreille, en particulier le syndrome dermoide épibulbaire—Appendices auriculaires—fistula auris congenita et ses relations avec la dysostose mandibulo-faciale. *J Génet Hum* 1:243, 1952.
110. Vargervik K: Sequence and timing of treatment phases in hemifacial microsomia. In Harvold EP (ed): *Treatment of Hemifacial Microsomia.* New York, Alan R. Liss, 1983, pp 133–138.
111. Chierici, G: Radiologic assessment of facial asymmetry. In Harvold EP (ed): *Treatment of Hemifacial Microsomia.* New York, Alan R. Liss, 1983, pp 57–88.
112. Vargervik K, Miller A: Assessment of facial and masticatory muscles in hemifacial microsomia. In Harvold EP (ed): *Treatment of Hemifacial Microsomia.* New York, Alan R. Liss, 1983, 113–132.
113. Petrovic AG, Stutzmann JJ, Gasson N: The final length of the mandible: Is it genetically predetermined? In Carlson DS (ed): *Craniofacial Biology, Monograph No. 10, Craniofacial Growth Series,* Ann Arbor, Center for Human Growth and Development, University of Michigan, 1981.
114. Harvold EP: The theoretical basis for the treatment of hemifacial microsomia. In Harvold EP (ed): *Treatment of Hemifacial Microsomia.* New York, Alan R. Liss, 1983, pp 1–38.
115. McNamara JA: Neuromuscular and skeletal adaptations to altered function in the orofacial region. *Am J Orthod* 64:578, 1973.
116. Vargervik K: Treatment of hemifacial microsomia in patients with abnormal but functioning temporomandibular articulation. In Harvold EP (ed): *Treatment of Hemifacial Microsomia.* New York, Alan R. Liss, 1983, pp 179–206.
117. Ousterhout DK, Owsley JQ: Skeletal surgery in hemifacial microsomia. In Harvold EP (ed): *Treatment of Hemifacial Microsomia.* New York, Alan R. Liss, 1983, pp 155–168.
118. Vargervik K: Treatment of hemifacial microsomia in patients without a functioning temporomandibular articulation. In Harvold EP (ed): *Treatment of Hemifacial Microsomia.* New York, Alan R. Liss, 1983, pp 207–242.
119. Whitaker LW, Munro IR, Salyer KE et al: Combined report of problems and complications in 793 craniofacial operations. *Plast Reconstr Surg* 64:198, 1979.
120. Sabatier RE, Munro IR, Lauritzen CG: A review of two thousand craniomaxillofacial operations. In Williams B (ed): *Transactions of the 8th International Congress of Plastic Surgery.* Montreal, Canadian Society of Plastic Surgeons, 1983, p 318.
121. Diaz JH, Henling CE: Pneumoperitoneum and cardiac arrest during craniofacial reconstruction. *Anesth Analg* 61:146, 1982.
122. David DJ, Cooter RD: Craniofacial infection in 10 years of transcranial surgery. *Plast Reconstr Surg* 80:513, 1987.
123. Jackson IT, Adham MN, March RW: Use of the galea frontalis myofascial flap in craniofacial surgery. *Plast Reconstr Surg* 77:905, 1986.
124. Cerisola JA, Rohwedder R: Bacteriological contamination of the operating field in craniofacial surgery. A new schedule of antibiotic prophylaxis. In Williams B (ed): *Transactions of the 8th International Congress of Plastic Surgery.* Montreal, Canadian Society of Plastic Surgeons, 1983, p 283.
125. Rosen HM, Simeone FR: Spontaneous subdural hygromas: A complication following cranofacial surgery. *Ann Plast Surg* 18:245, 1987.
126. Brones MF, Kawamoto HK, Renaudin J: Inappropriate antidiuretic hormone syndrome in craniofacial surgery. *Plast Reconstr Surg* 71:1, 1983.
127. Coleman JC III: The syndrome of inappropriate secretion of antidiuretic hormone associated with cleft palate: Report of a case and review of the literature. *Ann Plast Surg* 12:207, 1984.

35

Facial Osteotomies

S. Anthony Wolfe, M.D., F.A.C.S.

Webster defines the face as the front part of the human head, including the chin, mouth, nose, cheeks, eyes, and usually the forehead. Osteotomies of the facial skeleton can alter the form and function of all of these structures.

Osteotomies That Alter Neither Form Nor Function

Osteotomies that do not alter form or function are *osteotomies for access,* and most of the earliest osteotomies performed on the facial skeleton fell into this category (1, 2). They are still of great usefulness and should not be forgotten when a difficult problem in surgical exposure presents itself.

A frontal craniotomy is the most commonly used osteotomy for access and is the first part of every neurosurgical intracranial intervention. Craniofacial surgery, a joint enterprise by a neurosurgeon and a plastic surgeon, has done a great deal to acquaint the two specialties with each other. For neurosurgeons who have not had the opportunity to take part on a craniofacial team, the plastic surgeon puts forward the following gentle pleas:

1. Use the coronal (i.e., ear-to-ear) incision whenever possible. (There are coronal incisions and hemicoronal incisions, but to say "bicoronal" is redundant and incorrect.) The incision should be 4–5 cm behind the anterior hairline, not at the scalp-hairline junction. It should stop just above the attachment of the ear, not anterior to this.
2. The temporal muscle should be respected and preserved. It has innumerable uses to the reconstructive surgeon.
3. The frontal bone segment (it is not a "flap" unless it has preserved soft tissue attachments providing blood supply) should be rigidly fixed in place, and gaps in osteotomy lines should be filled in with bone slivers or bone paste from the craniotomy perforator. A "cookie cutter" can take a plug of inner table bone to fit precisely into the burr holes (GL Lovass, personal communication).
4. Whenever possible, as much of the skull should be preserved as possible. Craniotomy by rongeur, with discarding of the bone removed, creates a defect and is probably not often necessary, although this must be a neurosurgical decision. Rongeuring away bone for exposure creates a defect that may require subsequent

correction and discards a valuable bone graft donor source.
5. Subsequent operations should use the same coronal incision and not make another incision several centimeters or inches away.

Osteotomies for access to the orbital contents include the superior, lateral, and inferior marginotomies, in which the segment is removed and replaced after the intraorbital work is done (3–5; Fig. 35.1) (Case 35.1).

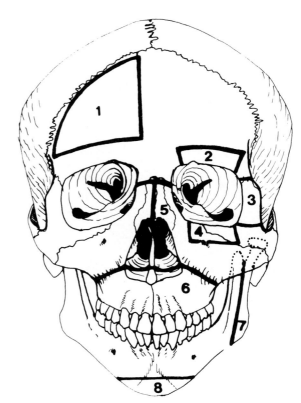

FIGURE 35.1. Access osteotomies: **1,** frontal craniotomy; **2,** supraorbital marginotomy; **3,** lateral orbitotomy (Krönlein); **4,** inferior marginotomy; **5,** midfacial split, which can be associated with Le Fort III osteotomy for access to central cranial base tumors; **6,** Le Fort I osteotomy, used on occasion to provide access to the posterior pharynx and cranial base; **7,** ramus osteotomy, providing access to the pterygopalatine fossa; and **8,** horizontal osteotomy of the symphysis, providing intraoral access to the sublingual gland region. In addition to these, midline symphyseal osteotomies and numerous variations on the depicted osteotomy lines can be devised.

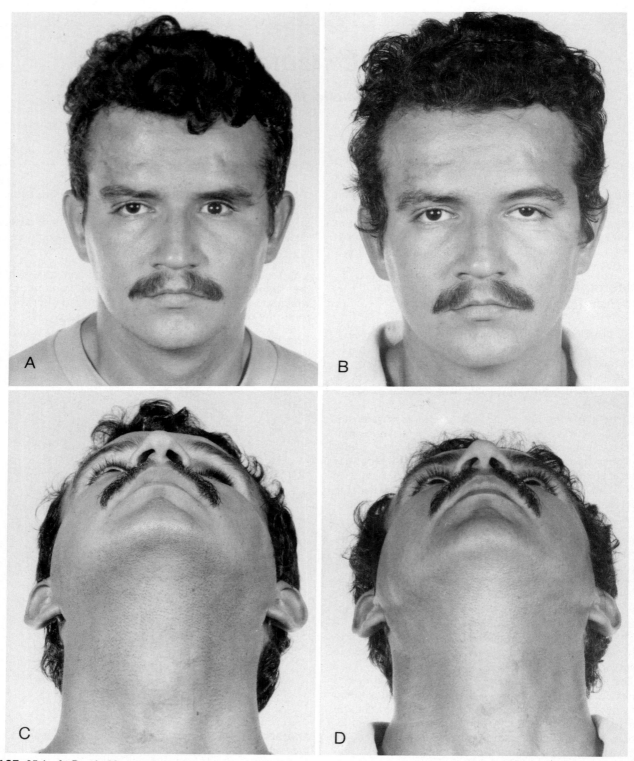

CASE 35.1. A–D. A 29-year-old patient with posttraumatic enophthalmos of the left eye due to a defect of the orbital floor. A circumferential orbital dissection was carried out along with an inferior marginotomy. The marginotomy is a useful procedure in certain cases because it facilitates the retrieval of orbital contents that are prolapsed into the maxillary sinus. The drawings (Case 35.1**E** and **F**) indicate osteotomy lines for the inferior marginotomy, which preserves the infraorbital nerve in both its orbital and maxillary positions. After the orbital contents are replaced in the orbit, the inferior segment is replaced and fixed with either wires or miniplates. An autogenous bone graft is used to correct the orbital floor defect. In virtually all cases of enophthalmos associated with a seeing eye, correction can be obtained using this or related procedures. The inferior marginotomy is an example of an osteotomy for access.

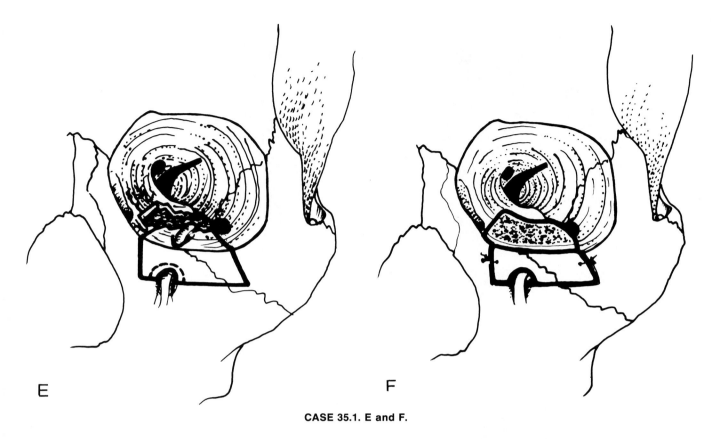

E

F

CASE 35.1. E and F.

Another type of osteotomy that, if not done for access, is at least for passage would be the temporary removal of the zygomatic arch and a portion of the malar bone. It is performed for temporalis muscle transfers for maxillary reconstruction and in other cases in which the temporal muscle or a portion of the temporal muscle is transferred to the lower midface. If the muscle is brought over the zygomatic arch, it makes a fairly noticeable bulge, and the arc of rotation is limited. Removal of the zygoma takes care of both of these problems, and after the muscle has been taken to the place where it is needed, the zygomatic arch/malar bone segment is replaced with a miniplate anteriorly and one single wire posteriorly (Case 35.2).

Luhr (6) has described the removal of the lateral cortical plate of the mandible to give access to difficult impacted third molars. The segment is plated back in place after tooth removal (Case 35.3).

Le Fort I and III osteotomies coupled with midpalatal splits provide access to the nasopharynx for complex tumor removal (7).

The mandible can be split in the midline or through the ramus to provide access to the pterygopalatine fossa and floor of the mouth (8). When marginotomies are done on irradiated tissues or on the mandible, soft tissue attachments should be maintained for blood supply. At the termination of an exposure marginotomy, the removed or displaced segment is rigidly fixed in place with wire osteosyntheses or miniplates that can be left in place (titanium or Vitallium).

When tumors involving the facial skeleton—particularly tumors of limited or no malignant potential, such as meningioma or fibrous dysplasia—are removed, form and function are, of course, often altered. Whenever possible, immediate reconstruction using autogenous bone grafts, usually cranial in origin, is performed with rigid fixation.

Osteotomies That Alter Form but Not Function

This type of "aesthetic facial sculpting" includes genioplasty, correction of masseteric hypertrophy, reduction of frontal bossing by osteotomy and recession of the anterior wall of the frontal sinus, and osteotomies of the malar bone to increase the malar prominence.

GENIOPLASTY

Genioplasty is the simplest and most commonly performed lower facial osteotomy and should be part of every plastic surgeon's repertoire. Chin implants are acceptable treatment for cases involving minor degrees of retrogenia in which there are neither alterations in the

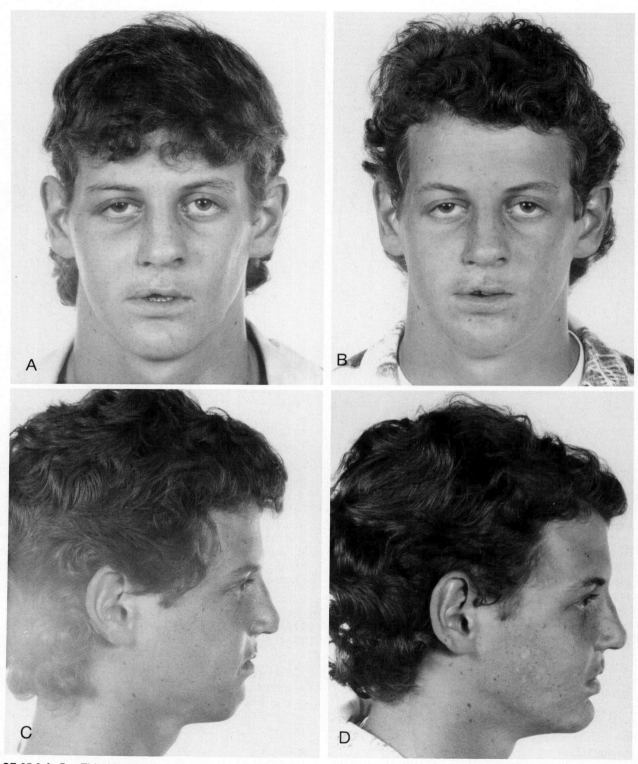

CASE 35.2 A–D. This 18-year-old patient had a cleft lip repair in infancy followed by a palatal island flap to provide nasal tissue for maintenance of the push-back type of palatal repair. In his midteens, he was operated on elsewhere and underwent a Le Fort I osteotomy. Unfortunately, the circulation through and beyond the donor area of the island flap was inadequate, and he lost a portion of his anterior palate. Correction was obtained by performing another Le Fort I osteotomy and transposing temporal muscle down to the defect. Cranial bone grafting was used at the same time to fill in the alveolar defect. The patient also underwent a genioplasty at the same surgery. The temporal muscle is a very useful tool in facial reconstructive surgery. When it is transposed to the lower face, removing the zygomatic arch temporarily permits the muscle to be brought below rather than over the arch, which has in the past been associated with an unsightly bulge. After the muscle transposition, the zygomatic arch is put back in place.

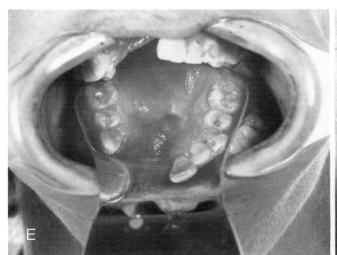
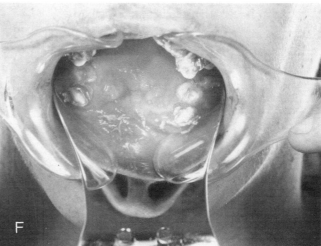

CASE 35.2. E and F.

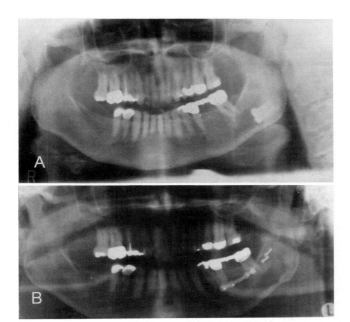

CASE 35.3 A and B. A 70-year-old patient with a low impacted third molar tooth. It had formed a dentigerous cyst, which then went on to become infected. The lateral cortex of the mandible was removed by a modified sagittal split; both of the cuts were through the outer cortex, one midway up the ascending ramus and the other between the tooth space between the bicuspid and the remaining molar. The lateral cortical segment was maintained with some of the masseteric fibers attached and retracted laterally. This provided exposure to remove the tooth and the entire cyst wall, and to visualize and preserve the infraorbital nerve over a distance of almost 5 cm. The lateral cortical segments were replaced with one miniplate and several small screws, and the patient went on to make an uneventful recovery. This is another example of an osteotomy for access.

vertical dimension of the chin nor lateral asymmetry. All other types of chin deformity require the ability to deal directly with the osseous malformation. The following types of genioplasty are commonly used.

Sliding Advancement

In a sliding advancement a lower labial sulcus incision is made, sparing the frenulum and developing a superior cuff that contains a small amount of muscle to aid in subsequent closure of the incision. A subperiosteal dissection of the symphysis is performed, and the mental nerves, located at the base of the first bicuspid or between the first and second bicuspids, may or may not be visualized. A horizontal osteotomy is performed with an oscillating saw 7–10 mm above the lower border of the symphysis. The entire osteotomy should be performed with the saw, and in some cases, a reciprocating saw is required to cut the posterior cortex laterally. If the basilar segment is downfractured, a small lip of bone usually comes with it and needs to be burred down to allow a proper advancement. If the osteotomy is carried laterally beyond the mental foramen, it must remain 4–5 mm below the foramen because the mental nerve is lower in the mandible before it ascends to emerge through the mental foramen. The basilar segment with its muscular attachments (geniohyoid, genioglossus, anterior belly of the digastric, and possibly some of the myelohyoid) is then advanced and fixed in its desired new position. I still prefer to perform this osteosynthesis with wires passed through the anterior cortex of the upper segment and the posterior cortex of the basilar segment. This can provide 4–10 mm of advancement, depending upon where the drill holes are placed in the basilar segment and the angle at which the osteotomy was performed.

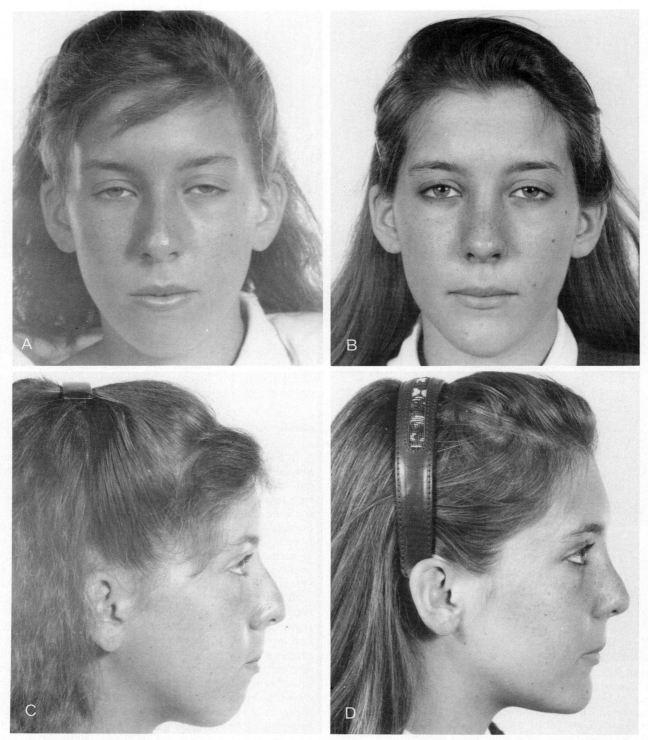

CASE 35.4. A–D. A 15-year-old girl shown before and after a rhinoplasty and reduction/advancement genioplasty.

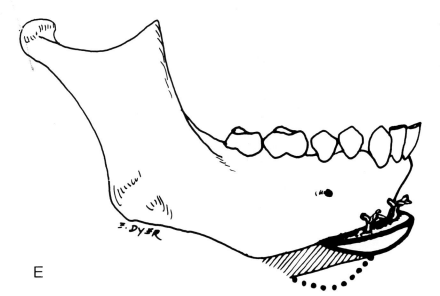

E

Centering Genioplasty

In a centering genioplasty the basilar segment can be shifted side to side, or cut obliquely and a triangular wedge of bone removed from the prominent side to be used as a bone graft on the deficient side.

Reduction Genioplasty

Reduction genioplasty is done when one wishes to reduce the vertical height of the chin (Case 35.4). A second horizontal osteotomy is performed parallel to the first osteotomy, and a segment of bone is removed. In cleft lip and palate patients, who often appear to have large chins, this bone segment can be used for maxillary needs (on-lay bone graft beneath a deficient alar base, or over the osteotomy lines of a Le Fort I osteotomy). The basilar segment is often slightly advanced to maintain a labiomental fold. One should not strip the muscles from the basilar segment and burr down or resect the lower border to reduce a prominent chin; this will often result in a flat-appearing chin with a sac of redundant skin hanging down beneath it.

Jumping Genioplasty

In a jumping genioplasty the basilar segment is elevated on top of the upper symphysis. This both increases chin projection (by 10–15 mm) and shortens the vertical dimension by the height of the basilar segment. Fixation is best performed by countersunk Kirschner wires or screws because there is a tendency for the attached muscles to tilt the basilar segment downward.

Lengthening Genioplasty

In lengthening genioplasty, after the horizontal osteotomy, three outer table cranial grafts are taken and fixed together with a miniscrew. Grafts are preferred to any alloplastic material. The bone graft is fixed to the upper symphysis with several miniplates, and the basilar segment is then fixed to the now stable bone graft, in an advanced position if desired. The soft tissue closure must be done with particular care when free bone grafts are inserted, and antibiotics are obligatory.

Staged Serial Genioplasty

Patients with particularly severe microgenia may appear not to have any chin at all, but rather a straight line that runs from lower lip to hyoid. These patients must all have mandibular retrognathia (class II malocclusion) as well, and associated premaxillary protrusion is often present. A staged procedure might include a premaxillary setback (Wassmund) and a jumping or lengthening genioplasty at the first stage and then, 6 months later, a mandibular advancement and a sliding advancement genioplasty through the old genioplasty.

The genioplasty is often a complementary procedure performed along with other reconstructive or aesthetic procedures, and it can often add substantially to the overall result.

MASSETERIC HYPERTROPHY

Masseteric hypertrophy condition usually has two components: an increase in the bulk of the masseter mus-

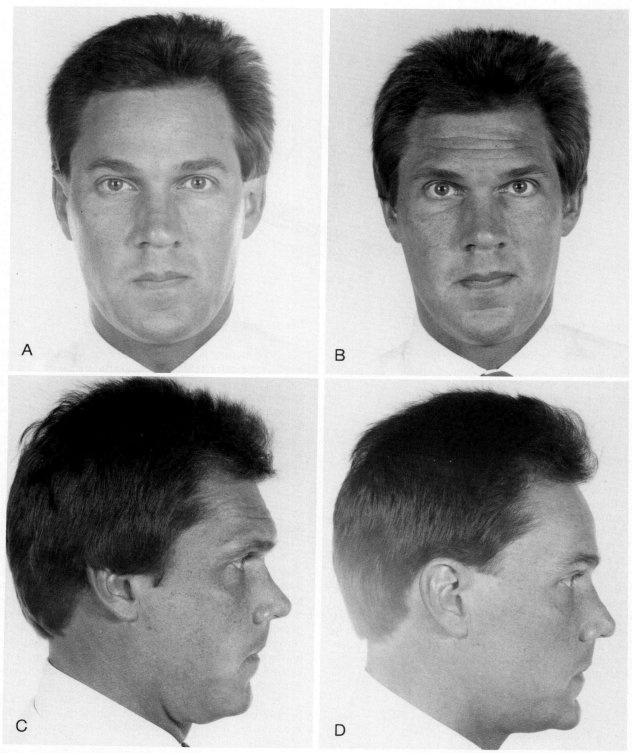

CASE 35.5. A–D. A 34-year-old male dissatisfied with the appearance of his forehead and brow region. Radiographs showed a giant hyperpneumatization of the frontal sinus. Through a coronal approach, the anterior wall of the frontal sinus was recessed posteriorly. Portions of the frontalis muscle were removed, and a standard forehead lift was performed along with a reduction genioplasty.

cle and visible exostoses at the gonial angle. Dental occlusion is usually normal. Treatment consists of a trimming of the thickened muscle and removal of the excessive bone from the mandibular angle through an intraoral approach. Here the instrumentation used in the sagittal split procedure is indispensable.

REDUCTION OF FRONTAL BOSSING

Excessive frontal bossing is usually seen in men, and for this reason, examination of the frontal region is one of the methods used by physical anthropologists and forensic pathologists to determine the sex of a skull. Thus, transsexual patients may seek to change a normal male frontal pattern to a softer, more female configuration. In milder cases, it is sufficient to burr down the bony excess, stopping short of entering the frontal sinus. More pronounced cases are often associated with a hyperpneumatization of the frontal sinus, and the lateral extent of the sinus should be determined beforehand by radiographs (Case 35.5). An upper orbital dissection is carried out, and osteotomies are made into the frontal sinus near its uppermost extent and across the orbital roof, avoiding intracranial penetration. The anterior wall of the frontal sinus is removed, and vertical supporting septae in the sinus are burred down until the anterior wall can be adequately recessed. The sinus is irrigated free of debris, and the anterior wall is replaced with a rigid osteosynthesis. If overdone, this procedure can be feminizing.

ANTERIOR MALAR OSTEOTOMY

Most malar augmentations are performed with alloplastic material (9), and osteotomies to increase malar prominence are relatively unexplored, although malar reduction is a common procedure in the Orient. On-lay bone grafts, even when rigidly fixed, can undergo varying degrees of resorption, and they must be completely symmetrical to be successful. An oblique osteotomy, via a combined coronal and intraoral approach, can be carried beneath the malar prominence, avoiding the orbit and the infraorbital nerve. Most of the masseteric attachment is left in place. An interpositional cranial bone graft is placed beneath the osteotomized segment, and several screws are used for rigid fixation. This procedure can be combined with the long-performed "mask lift" or subperiosteal facelift and lateral canthopexy, which was reemphasized by Tessier (10).

Osteotomies That Affect Form and Function

IN INFANCY

Fronto-orbital Advancement

Fronto-orbital advancement is performed as a unilateral procedure for plagiocephaly (unilateral coronal synostosis) or bilaterally for brachycephaly (bilateral coronal synostosis) or the craniofacial dysostoses (Crouzon's, Apert's, and a variety of other syndromes) (Cases 35.6 and 35.7). These deformities, in which there is a premature sutural closure or lack of growth potential of the suture, are associated with inadequate skull growth, and increased intracranial pressure and ventricular distortion have been observed in many untreated patients, even with unilateral conditions (11).

Monobloc Frontofacial Advancement

A monobloc frontofacial advancement is a Le Fort III advancement that includes the orbital roof and frontal bone. It is a major surgical undertaking and can give excellent functional results from the substantial increase in intracranial orbital and airway capacity. However, it has considerable risk in infancy and should be performed only when there are compelling functional reasons, such as severe exorbitism threatening vision or airway inadequacy with documented oxygen desaturation and a likely need for tracheostomy. This procedure should be performed only by the most experienced craniofacial surgeons in a limited number of centers. In the 4–10-year-old age group, it is the procedure of choice for Crouzon's, Apert's, and other craniofacial dysostoses (Case 35.8).

Orbital Dystopias

Orbital dystopias, either transverse (hypertelorism, hypotelorism) or vertical, can be corrected near the age of 2 years with satisfactory results, but further surgery on the nose can be anticipated in these cases if an early nasal reconstruction has been done.

Osteotomies on the upper portion of the face (orbitocranial) can be performed in infancy and childhood with satisfactory, stable results. The brain and eyes, as they enlarge, exert a "growth force" on the surrounding osseous structures. Tooth-bearing structures may be shifted along with the orbitocranial structures, as in the monobloc frontofacial advancement; these early craniofacial procedures are *not* intended to effect a permanent correction of malocclusion. Instead, they provide functional relief in other areas, such as an increase in cranial and orbital capacity and an enlargement of the nasopharyngeal airway. Subsequent maxillofacial surgery on the lower tooth-bearing structures will almost certainly be required in the teens to provide satisfactory dental occlusion. In essence, a craniomaxillofacial deformity is converted to a simpler maxillofacial deformity, which is dealt with like other maxillofacial deformities. Growth of the orbital and cranial areas is largely completed by age 6 years, but the tooth-bearing structures of the lower maxilla and mandible do not reach their final growth, irrespective of what growth potential is present, until the midteens (Case 35.9).

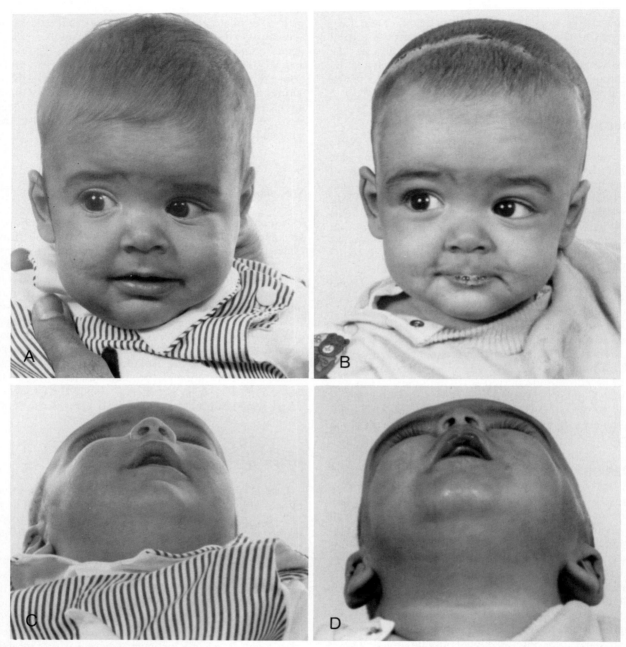

CASE 35.6 A–D. A 5-month-old infant with right unilateral coronal synostosis (plagiocephaly). Postoperatively, she is shown after a right fronto-orbital advancement, as depicted in Case 35.6 **E** and **F.**

AFTER REACHING DENTAL MATURITY

Most maxillary growth is complete by the age of 10–12 years, and the mandible continues growing until 14–15 years in a female (onset of menarche) and 16–18 years in a male, under normal circumstances (12). Patients with various types of skeletal dysplasias, of course, can exhibit markedly abnormal growth patterns. It is acceptable in particularly severe malformations to operate earlier than one might normally, and to accept the fact that the correction obtained will not be permanent and that further surgery will be required at a later age to provide an adequate final result. For less severe deformities, however, it is better to wait and perform the correction once.

Malocclusion

Malocclusion is defined as an abnormal relationship of the maxillary to the mandibular teeth. In certain types of

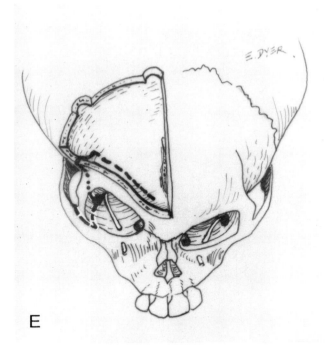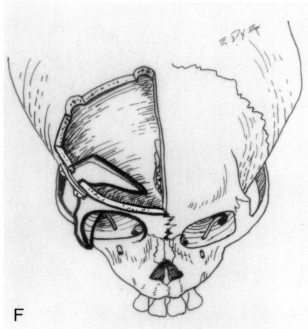

CASE 35.6. E–F.

malocclusion, the skeletal "platforms" of the maxilla and mandible are in good relationship to one another, and the malocclusion can be corrected by orthodontic means alone, sometimes with extraction of teeth. In other situations, the skeletal platforms are *not* in a good relationship, and the jaws themselves will need to be moved before a good dental occlusion can be obtained. The following steps will allow the determination of where the problem lies, what will be appropriate treatment, and when treatment should be undertaken.

Clinical Examination

Very frequently, a diagnosis can be made by careful examination of the patient alone. Does the midface appear retrusive? Is the chin long? Are the gonial angles flat? How do the two jaws relate to the upper facial structures of the forehead, nose, and orbital cavities?

Dental Examination

How does the upper dental arch relate to the lower dental arch? How are the individual teeth related? Edward Angle, considered to be the father of orthodontics, provided a classification of dental relationships that is used throughout the world (12; Fig. 35.2).

Case I: (a "normal" occlusal relationship): the mesiobuccal cusp of the first maxillary molar falls into the buccal groove of the first mandibular molar. The maxillary cuspid falls between the mandibular cuspid and first bicuspid. There is a normal overjet and overbite of the maxillary incisors in front of the mandibular incisors.

Class II: the maxillary teeth lie mesial (anterior, or toward the dental midline) to the class I relationship.

Class III: the maxillary teeth lie distal (posterior, or toward the end of the dental arch) to the class I relationship.

This occlusal classification tells one only about the relationship of the teeth. A patient can be in class I and have both arches in an abnormal position relative to the skull base, as in bimaxillary protrusion, bimaxillary retrusion, or a vertical maxillary excess or deficiency. A patient can be in class II because of overdevelopment of the maxilla or underdevelopment of the mandible. A class III relationship can be due to underdevelopment of the maxilla or overdevelopment of the mandible.

Clinical examination gives a good indication of where the problem lies. Confirmation is obtained by roentgenological examination.

Cephalometric Evaluation

A lateral cephalometric film is obtained with the patient's head in a headholder with a prong in the external auditory meatus and another at the nasofrontal angle. The film is behind and parallel to the head, and the x-ray source is positioned 60 inches away from the midplane of the patient's head.

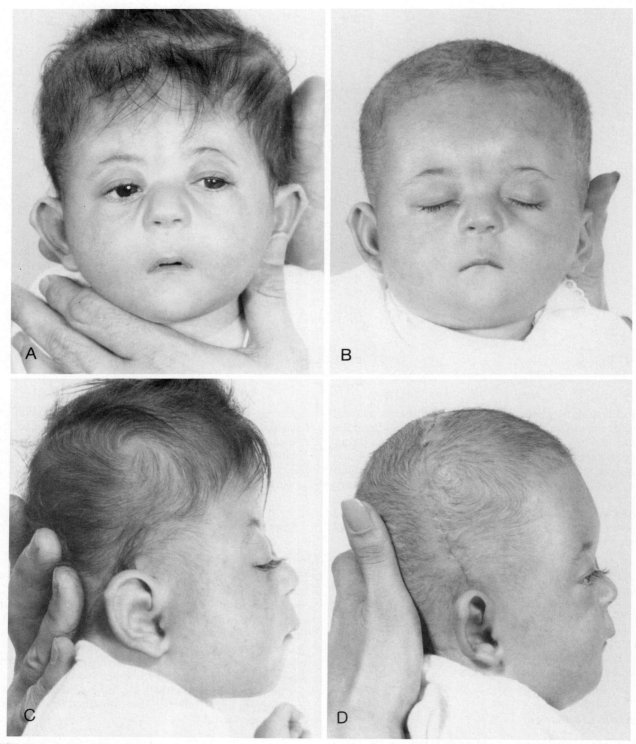

CASE 35.7. A–D. A 7-month-old child with bilateral coronal synostosis shown before and after a bilateral frontoorbital advancement. In cases with a synostosis confirmed to the coronal sutures, this release should be corrective and allow for normal head and facial growth. It is sometimes difficult to distinguish this type of patient from one with Crouzon's disease, in which there is lower facial synostosis as well. In the case of the Crouzon's dysostosis, subsequent lower facial surgery will be necessary.

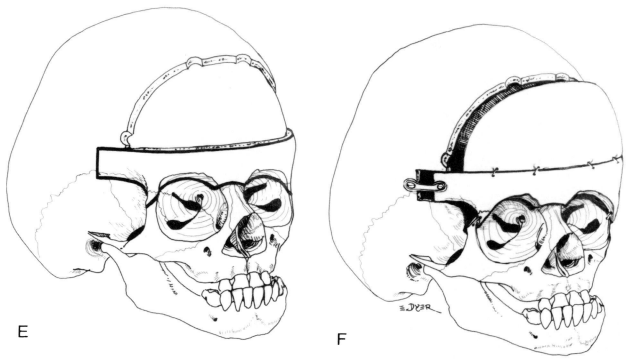

E

F

CASE 35.7. E and F.

A number of methods of cephalometric analysis are available (13–18), and each orthodontist has his or her own preferred method or methods. Identifiable landmarks are found at the midpoint of the sella (point S), the nasofrontal suture or nasion (point N), on the maxilla above the apices of the central incisors (point A), and at the level of the apices of the mandibular central incisors (point B). These points, plus numerous others, establish angular measurements, which are compared to normative data that are largely developed from the Bolton standards. (It must be recognized that the Bolton standards were developed from serial films taken of faculty children at the University of Michigan; therefore, they are representative only of a Caucasian population.) Cephalometric analysis is of value in confirming one's clinical impression and determining which jaw structures need to be moved in order to bring the patient to "normal values." It should be stressed that treatment planning is *not* done from cephalometric examination alone; clinical and dental examination are of at least equal importance. Cephalometric analysis is of even more limited value in patients with major craniofacial malformations, in which there may be an abnormality of the cranial base or an absent or asymmetrical ear canal. Perhaps the greatest value of cephalometry is in following the growth of patients with various abnormalities and in evaluating the stability or relapse of altered jaw structures following surgery.

Orthognathic Surgery

All surgical procedures moving tooth-bearing structures in order to provide improved dental occlusion and better jaw/facial relationships *must* be coordinated with an orthodontist. A surgeon working without orthodontic input may end up with a patient who "looks good" but who has a disastrous occlusal result. Conversely, an orthodontist who is ignorant of the possibilities and indications for surgery may end up with a patient who *does not* look good, but whose teeth have, by long and laborious orthodontic treatment, a reasonably satisfactory occlusal result. Unfortunately, this result is often obtained by inducing abnormal axial inclinations of the teeth; therefore, the dental results in fact may not be so satisfactory.

Surgery and Orthodontics Versus Orthodontics Alone

Certain conditions, such as premaxillary or bimaxillary protrusion, can be treated satisfactorily by dental extractions and orthodontics alone. However, moving teeth through bone is a slow process, requiring 12–18 months or more until completion of the case. A surgical procedure such as a segmental maxillary osteotomy (Wassmund), in which several bicuspids are extracted and bone is removed to permit the premaxillary segment to be moved back surgically, may shorten the overall treatment time markedly. Intermaxillary fixation is not required, and only relatively minor orthodontic adjustments are required to bring the case to completion. The decision as to which route to take can be made only by the patient.

Once a diagnosis has been made that establishes the need for surgery to alter the position of the jaw bases (maxilla, mandible, or both) in the anteroposterior, vertical, or horizontal planes (or all of the above), the orthodontist comes into play first.

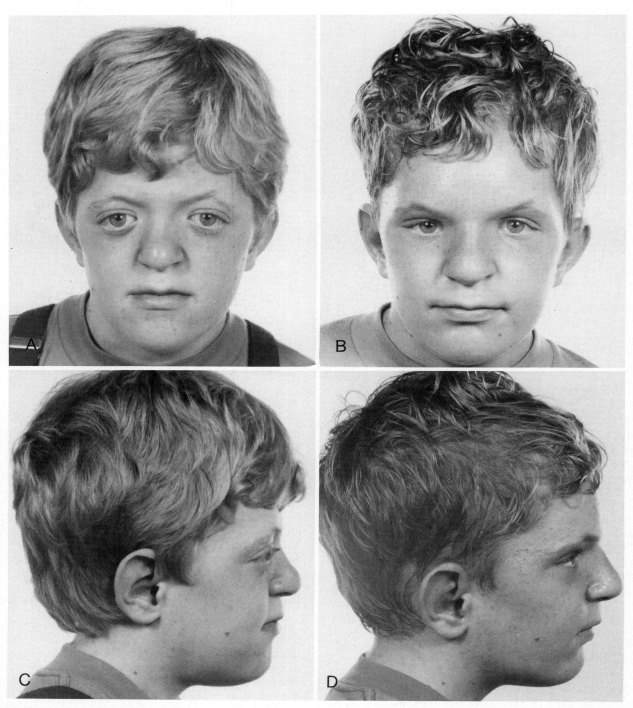

CASE 35.8. A–D. An 11-year-old boy with Apert's syndrome shown before and after an intracranial monobloc frontofacial advancement. This is a major operative undertaking, but in my opinion, it provides the best results for the craniofacial dysostoses of Apert and Crouzon. The monobloc procedure is ideally done between the ages of 4 and 12, although it can be done earlier if there are compelling functional reasons such as airway obstruction. After the early teens, the complication rate increases because of the inability of the brain to expand into the retrofrontal dead space. For this reason, the monobloc is contraindicated in patients who have had ventricular decompressive shunts (22).

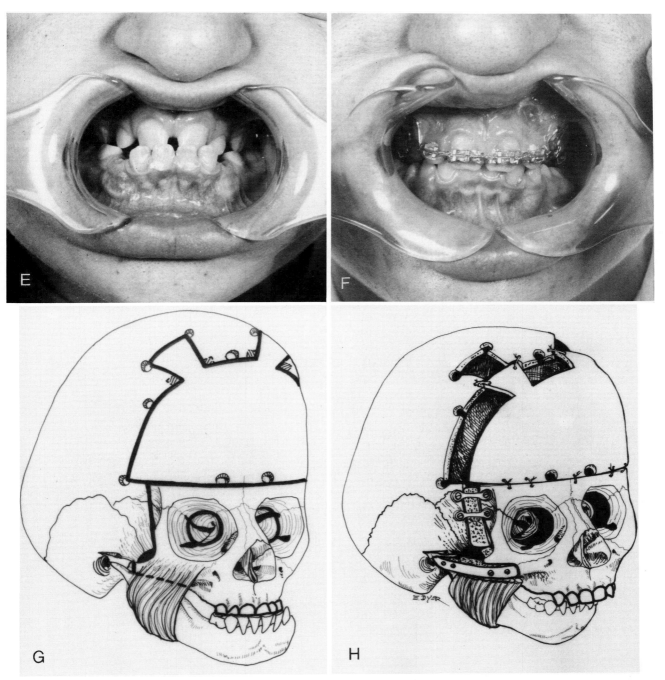

CASE 35.8. E–H.

Involvement of the Orthodontist in Orthognathic Surgery

1. The orthodontist aids in establishing the diagnosis and a treatment plan.
2. The orthodontist supervises dental treatment of caries and periodontal disease.
3. The orthodontist bands teeth and begins preliminary orthodontic treatment to remove dental interferences. These are nature's compensation to the deformity,

and they must be corrected before surgery. For example, dental compensations in a patient with mandibular prognathism may have partly compensated for the abnormal jaw position by labial tilting of the maxillary incisors and lingual tilting of the mandibular incisors. As a result, a discrepancy of only a few millimeters at the incisor level may exist. Surgery to move the jaw back only these few millimeters would be ill-advised, and the orthodontist should first bring the incisors into a proper axial relationship with supporting basal bone.

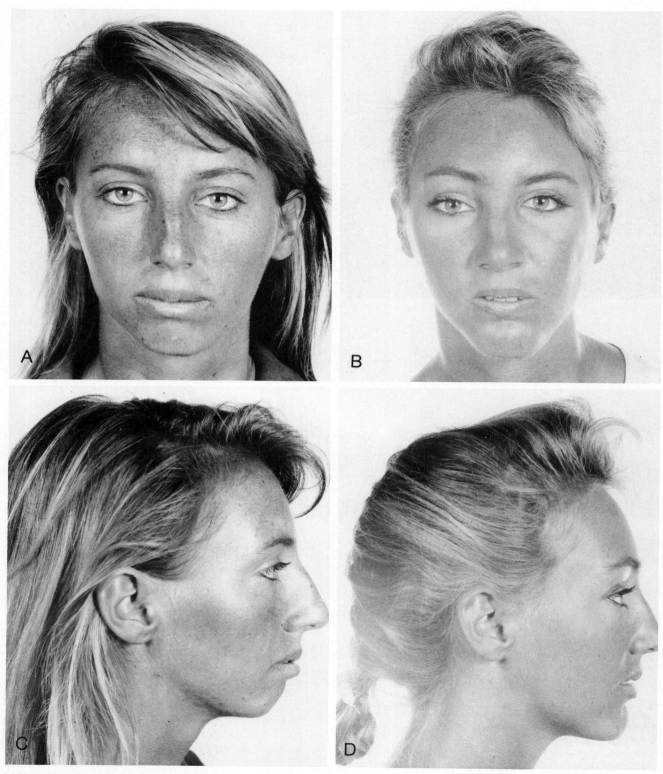

CASE 35.9. A–D. A 23-year-old patient shown before and after a transcranial elevation of the left orbital cavity to correct a left orbital dystopia (probably due to torticollis). At the same time, a Le Fort I maxillary advancement, bilateral sagittal splits, and an advancement/lengthening genioplasty were performed. This was a one-stage procedure involving virtually all the areas of the facial skeleton. The drawings in Case 35.9 **I–L** show one-stage correction of facial scoliosis by transcranial elevation of left orbit, Le Fort I osteotomy and horizontalization of the maxillary occlusal plane, bilateral sagittal splitting to allow shifting of the mandible to the new midline, and horizontal osteotomy of the mandibular symphysis with an interpositional cranial bone graft.

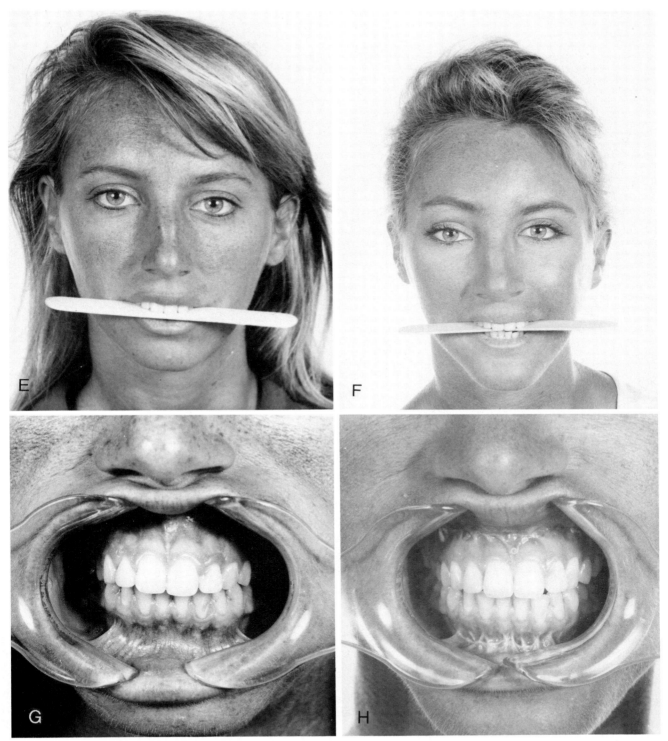

CASE 35.9.   E–H.

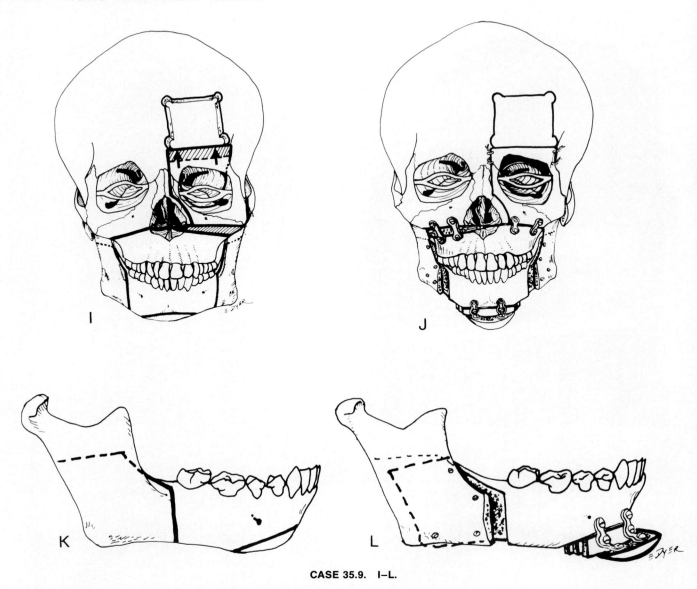

CASE 35.9. I–L.

This might increase the incisal gap to 8–10 mm, at which time surgery would be carried out.

4. Orthodontic treatment should provide two coherent dental arches that fit together. If the bulk of the required orthodontic treatment is done before surgery and the final arch form is obtained, the teeth may intercuspidate so well that a surgical occlusal splint is not required. Postoperative orthodontic treatment under these circumstances may be minimal. This approach, however, makes no allowance for postoperative relapse. Alternatively, the orthodontist may opt to only remove the gross dental interferences beforehand, and to make a splint that indicates to the surgeon where the jaw should be positioned. With the jaw in its desired new position, the orthodontist can then do most of the orthodontic dental alignment after surgery. Which approach to take depends on the preferences of the individual team.

5. In two-jaw surgery, the orthodontist should take a face bow transfer to an articulated dental model, so that the occlusal plane and condylar position can be controlled (19). During the stages of model surgery, an intermediate splint is made to establish the new position of the first jaw to be moved relative to the old position of the other jaw. The first-moved jaw is then rigidly fixed in its new position, and the other jaw is then moved in relation to it to give the final result.

6. Immediately following surgery, the orthodontist or the surgeon should check an orthopantomograph (Panorex) to be certain that the condyles are properly seated in the glenoid fossae if the patient is in intermaxillary fixation. The use of rigid internal fixation without intermaxillary blockage has simplified this; one can be more certain about condylar position at the time of surgery by simply inspecting passive jaw opening and closing.

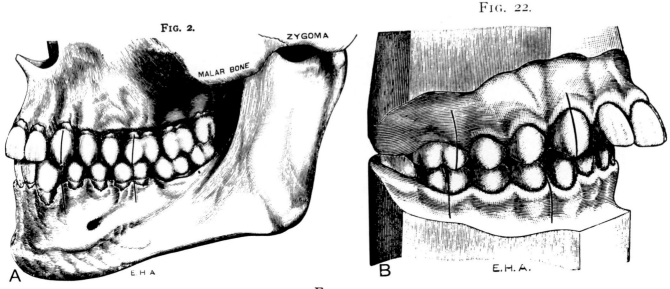

FIG. 2.

ZYGOMA

MALAR BONE

E.H.A

A

FIG. 22.

B E.H.A.

FIG. 30.

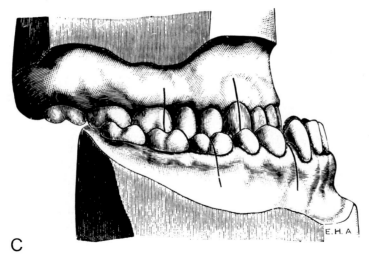

E.H.A

C

FIGURE 35.2. Etchings made by Edward Hartley Angle, M.D., D.D.S., who is widely recognized as the father of American (and international) orthodontics. **A,** Figure 2 represents normal occlusion (Angle class I) in which the mesiobuccal cusp of the maxillary first molar occludes into the buccal groove of the mandibular first molar. The maxillary cuspid falls on a line between the mandibular cuspid and first bicuspid. **B,** Figure 22 shows class II malocclusion in which the mesiobuccal cusp of the maxillary first molar occludes medial (more anterior) to the buccal groove. Note also the abnormal position of the maxillary cuspid in relation to the mandibular teeth. **C,** Figure 30 shows class III malocclusion with the reverse situation, the mesiobuccal cusp of the maxillary first molar occluding distal (more posterior) to the buccal groove of the mandibular first molar. (From Angle EH: *Treatment of Malocclusion of the Teeth and Fractures of the Maxillae. Angle's System.* Philadelphia, SS White Dental Manufacturing System, 1900.)

7. After a short delay following surgery, the orthodontist can begin the final orthodontic alignment.
8. The orthodontist follows the patient postoperatively for signs of relapse. In some instances, if this is picked up early, it can be overcome by traction devices such as the Delaire headframe (20).

Surgical Procedures on the Jaws to Correct Malocclusion

Once a proper diagnosis has been made and presurgical orthodontic preparation of the patient completed, most forms of malocclusion that do not involve the orbitocra-

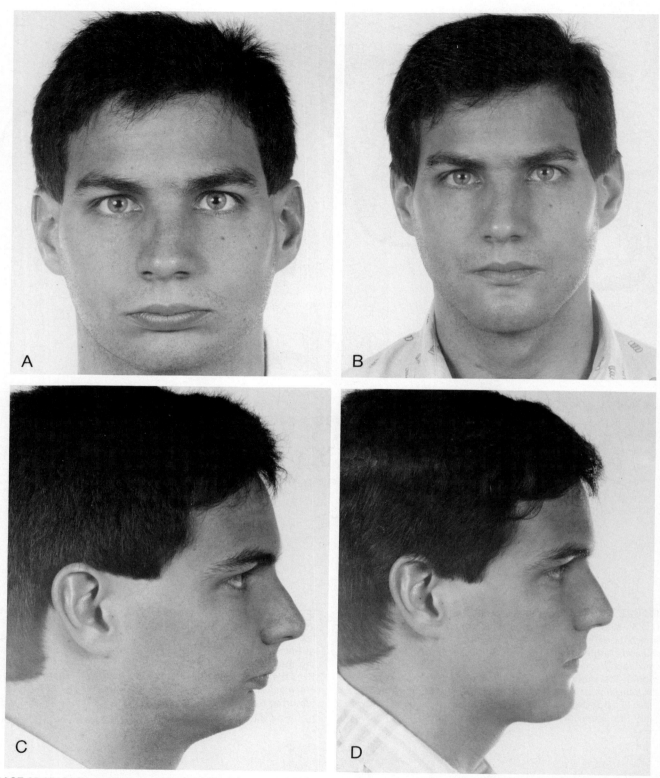

CASE 35.10. A–D. A 25-year-old male shown before and after mandibular advancement by sagittal splitting and a lengthening genioplasty. Intermaxillary fixation was not employed. Note the improvement in the deep labiomental fold, which is obtained both by giving better dental support for the lower lip and by lengthening the chin.

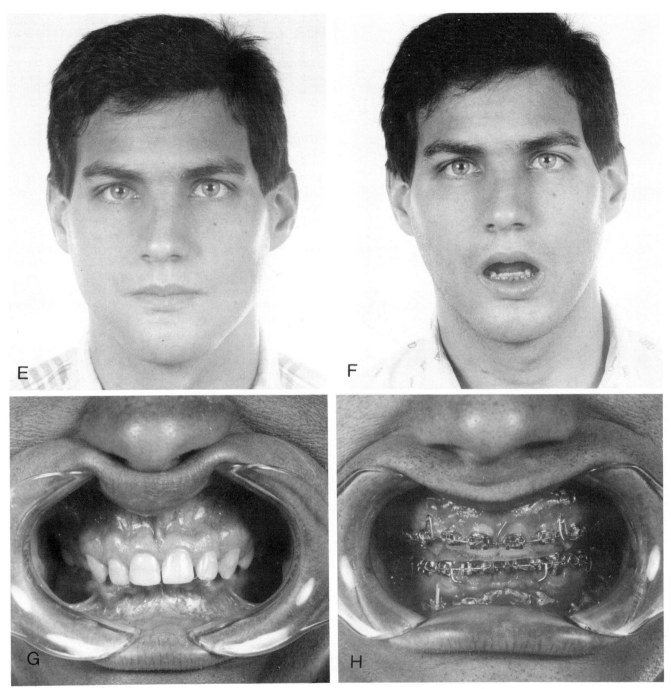

CASE 35.10. E–H.

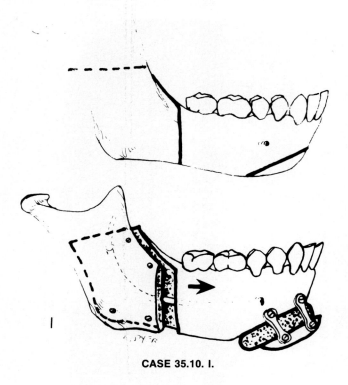

CASE 35.10. I.

nial portion of the face can be corrected by using one or more of a relatively limited number of surgical procedures. With the capability to skillfully perform a sagittal splitting procedure for the mandible and a Le Fort I osteotomy with its variations for the maxilla, a surgeon could likely deal with 80% of patients who require orthognathic surgery.

Technique, indubitably, is important for good results, but even the most flawlessly performed procedure will give a poor result if it is the wrong operation. Diagnosis, planning, and proper orthodontic preparation of the patient far overshadow technical considerations of exactly how a cut is made.

Mandibular Osteotomies

Segmental Osteotomies. The Köle procedure is used to correct an open bite due to a downward curve of the mandibular occlusal plane (curve of Spee). If dental considerations permit, the two first bicuspids are removed, and a vertical osteotomy is carried down from the extraction sites to a level below the apices of the teeth. If dental extractions are not to be done, the orthodontist should open up a space of 3–4 mm between the teeth to permit the osteotomy to be done without injury to the dental roots. The two vertical osteotomies are connected by a horizontal osteotomy, and care is taken not to damage the posterior mucoperiosteum, which provides blood supply to the dentoalveolar segment. The tooth-bearing segment is then elevated to its desired position. An acrylic splint, which has been previously prepared on a sectioned dental model, is used both as a guide to the surgeon as to the proper position for the dentoalveolar segment and as a means of stabilization of the segment. The splint is wired to stable posterior teeth: intermaxillary fixation is not required. A genioplasty can be performed at the same time, but care should be taken to maintain an intact strut of mandible between the horizontal osteotomy of the Köle procedure and the horizontal osteotomy of the genioplasty.

FIGURE 35.3. The sagittal split procedure, in my opinion, is the procedure of choice for most mandibular orthognathic surgery. The operation is performed entirely intraorally. It can be used both for retrognathia **(A)** and prognathia **(B)**. With the use of rigid internal fixation by small titanium screws (which can be placed either through a very small trocar or, in some cases, entirely transorally) intermaxillary fixation can be dispensed with in most cases. Two technically difficult parts of the operation are avoiding damage to the inferior alveolar nerve and properly positioning the condylar segment.

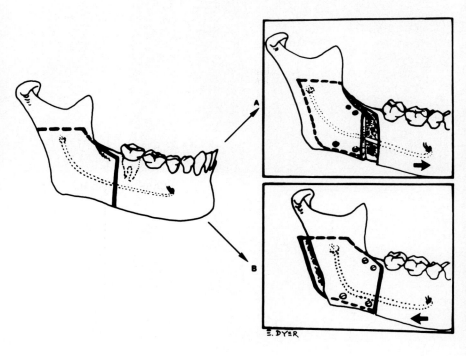

Sagittal Split Procedure. With the increasing use of rigid screw fixation, this has become the procedure of choice for movements of the entire tooth-bearing portion of the mandible. The other acceptable procedure for mandibular prognathism, the intraoral vertical osteotomy, has been largely supplanted by the sagittal split because intermaxillary fixation can be avoided with the rigidly fixed sagittal split (Case 35.10). The extraoral vertical or oblique osteotomy should, in my opinion, be considered extinct because it makes an avoidable facial scar. The sagittal split is also the only procedure that can be used for correction of both mandibular prognathism and mandibular retrognathia (Fig. 35.3).

Incisions are made intraorally from the first molar and extend up the lateral aspect of the ascending ramus. This procedure cannot be performed without special instruments based on those designed specifically for this purpose by Hugo Obwegeser. After subperiosteal dissection of the lateral aspect of the ramus and posterior border (stripping off the pterygomasseteric sling), the sigmoid notch is identified. A medial dissection is performed about 15 mm below the sigmoid notch (above the entry of the inferior alveolar nerve into the medial aspect of the ramus). With protective channel retractors in place, a medial osteotomy is performed with a reciprocating saw or Lindemann side-cutting burr. It should extend through the medial cortex and a bit more. A lateral osteotomy is performed just through the cortex at about the level of the second molar. A series of drill holes are then made just inside the external oblique ridge of the mandible, connecting the two previously made osteotomies. These holes are connected with a fissure burr that is carried just into bleeding cancellous bone. Then, thin, slightly curved Dautrey osteotomies are driven through the ramus, staying just beneath the lateral cortex to avoid injury to the inferior alveolar nerve.

When the split is completed, the lateral (condylar) segment should be freely mobile. The inferior alveolar nerve can often be seen coursing through the cancellous bone of the medial (tooth-bearing) segment. Once both osteotomies are completed, the tooth-bearing segment is then either advanced or moved back, depending upon whether one is treating retrognathia or prognathia. One good way to be sure the splits are complete is to move the jaw posteriorly beyond its original position. When the desired occlusal relationship of the tooth-bearing segment with the maxilla is established, usually by an occlusal splint, intermaxillary fixation is temporarily established. The condylar segments are pushed gently backward and upward to seat the condyles in the glenoid fossae. In prognathism, a segment of the condylar segment just behind the lateral cut is resected, and in retrognathia, a gap will open up in this area corresponding to the extent of the mandibular advancement. Most surgeons now prefer rigid screw fixation, which can be done with oblique screws placed intraorally along the upper border of the ramus, or screws placed perpendicularly through the split fragments using a percutaneous transbuccal guarded trochar. After completion of the osteosyntheses, intermaxil-

lary fixation is released, and the occlusion is checked. The intraoral incisions are closed with a running absorbable suture.

The sagittal split is an ingenious and versatile procedure that requires special instrumentation and surgical precision and gentleness. The most frequent complication is a temporary parasthesia of the lip, but return of sensation should occur within a few months if the nerve has been maintained intact. The sagittal split is not recommended for patients with small, malformed ascending rami, or for the correction of an open bite. It is good for straight forward or backward movements of the tooth-bearing mandible. For advancement of a mandible with a small ramus, an inverted-L osteotomy through an external cervical incision with an interpositional bone graft is preferred. Other mandibular osteotomies, such as body osteotomy or subapical osteotomy, are rarely performed.

Anterior open bites are best dealt with by a maxillary osteotomy.

Maxillary Osteotomies

Segmental Osteotomies. The premaxillary osteotomy, or Wassmund procedure, usually involves the extraction of the two first bicuspids. A vertical osteotomy is made from the extraction site to the level of the piriform rim, and a horizontal osteotomy is made through the premaxilla below the nasal spine. Submucoperiosteal tunnels are dissected across the palate from the dental extraction sites, and with one finger on the palatal mucosa to protect the vital blood supply, bone across the palate is removed with a burr. The premaxilla can then be downfractured, and further removal of bone is carried out under direct vision until the premaxillary segment can be moved back to its desired position. A splint wired to the posterior teeth provides fixation. Again, intermaxillary fixation is not required (Case 35.11).

The Schuchardt procedure is a segmental posterior maxillary osteotomy used to intrude the maxillary molar segments to close an anterior open bite, but it has been largely supplanted for this purpose by the Le Fort I osteotomy.

Le Fort I Osteotomy. All Le Fort osteotomies receive their name from the Le Fort fractures (I, II, and III), which were described at the turn of the century by the French anatomist René Le Fort (21). The osteotomies differ from the fractures in that the pterygoid plates are kept intact, and therefore, strictly speaking, they should be called Le Fort *type* osteotomies.

The Le Fort I osteotomy is the workhorse of maxillary surgery (Fig. 35.4). After completion of the osteotomy and mobilization of the maxilla, the tooth-bearing segment can be moved upward, forward, down, backward (to a limited extent), or side-to-side, or it may be tilted and yawed in a variety of planes. Dental extractions can be combined with segmentation osteotomies to shift multiple maxillary segments independently.

A vertical measurement is taken at the beginning of the operation from a tattoo mark on the medial canthal ten-

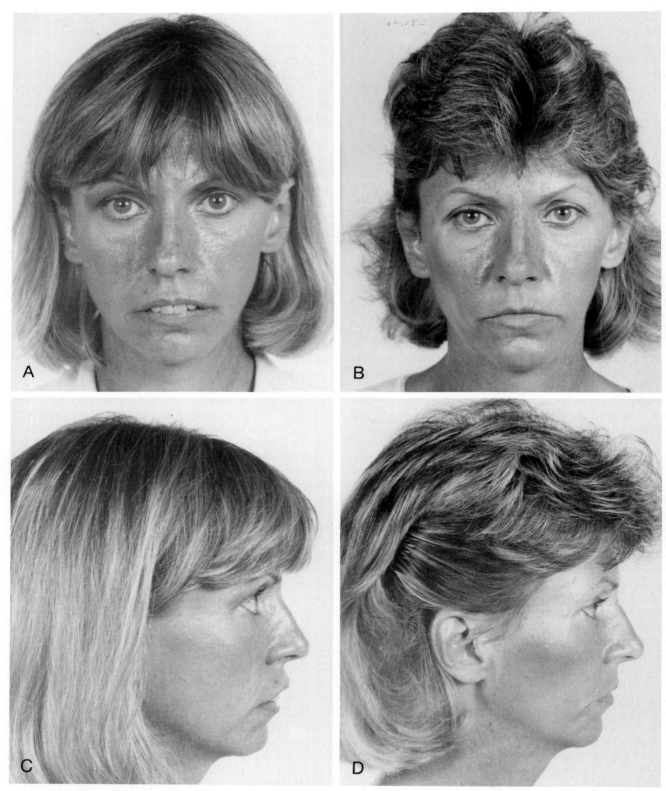

CASE 35.11. A–D. A 39-year-old patient shown before and after an anterior maxillary osteotomy (Wassmund), associated with the extraction of two first bicuspids. This type of anterior premaxillary setback requires a splint wired to the remaining maxillary teeth but does not require intermaxillary fixation.

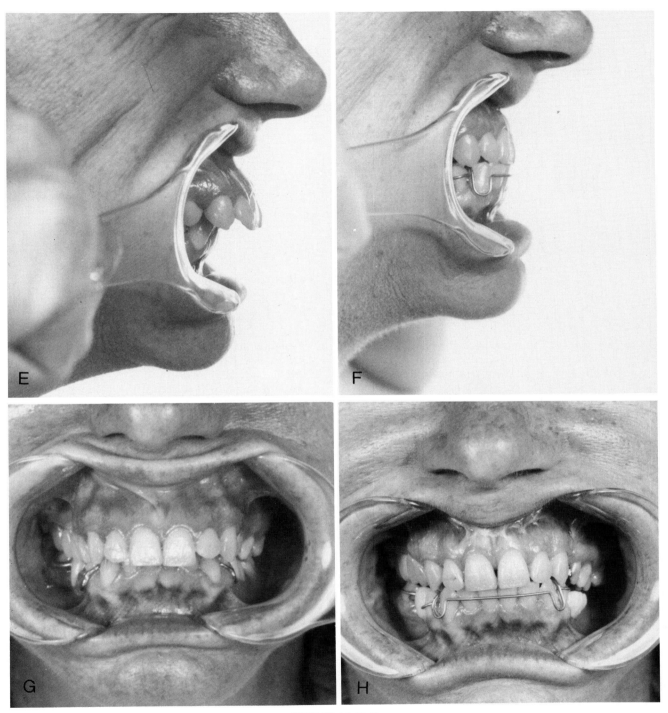

CASE 35.11. E–H.

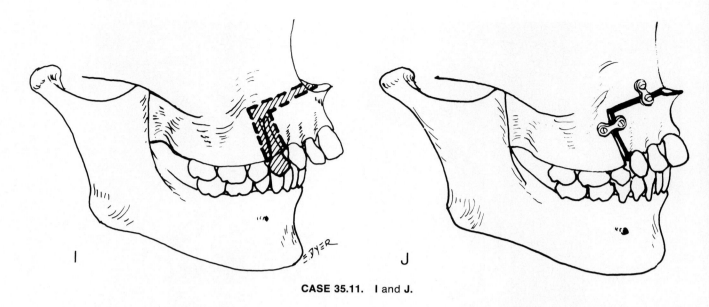

CASE 35.11. I and J.

don to the edge of the lateral incisor. The amount of central incisor show should also be recorded preoperatively with the lips in the open rest position. Normally, one should see 2–3 mm of tooth below the vermilion border of the upper lip.

An upper buccal sulcus incision is made, preserving an adequate cuff inferiorly for subsequent closure, and a subperiosteal dissection of the anterior maxilla is performed, exposing the infraorbital nerves. The dissection is carried posteriorly into the pterygomaxillary space, and a dissection of the nasal mucosa is carried out. The horizontal osteotomy is then carried medially above the level of the piriform rim (to avoid the high root of the cuspid) and extends posteriorly beneath the malar prominence. The medial maxillary walls are cut with the saw, and the septum is divided from the palate with a guarded osteotome. The final step of a Le Fort I–type osteotomy is the insertion of a curved osteotome between the maxillary tuberosity and the pterygoid plates and the cutting of the palatine bone, which is their only connection. The maxilla is then downfractured by downward finger pressure alone; in rare instances, the Rowe disimpaction forceps are required. Further mobilization of the maxilla is done with a blunt instrument behind the maxillary tuberosity to lever the maxilla forward. In cleft palate patients with persistent alveolar clefts, the maxilla will be in two segments at this stage.

After the maxilla has been completely mobilized (to the point that it can be easily moved in all directions with a tissue forceps), it can be placed in its new desired position. Various possibilities are:

1. Resecting a portion of the superior maxilla and moving the maxilla upward, to correct a vertical maxillary excess (long face).

2. Lengthening the maxilla with an interpositional bone graft (short face).
3. Advancing the maxilla.
4. Moving the maxilla posteriorly, which will require removal of teeth if movement of more than 2–3 mm is required.
5. Tilting the maxilla up posteriorly (correction of an open bite) or tilting one side down or up (to straighten a canted occlusal plane).
6. Performing further segmentation, either a palatal split, for palatal expansion, or dental extractions with multiple maxillary osteotomies, for complex maxillary deformities.

After the maxilla or the maxillary segments are fixed into the splint, the splint is brought into occlusion with the mandibular teeth, and the entire maxillomandibular complex is brought into its proper vertical relationship by using measurements from the tattoo mark on the medial canthal tendon. Miniplates fix the maxilla to stable upper portions of the maxilla and the malar buttress (Case 35.12).

Autogenous bone grafts, usually cranial in origin, are placed in gaps such as those seen in lengthened or expanded maxillae or in cleft patients. Bone grafts are generally placed over the anterior maxillary osteotomy lines in cleft patients and in patients who are having an advancement of more than 8 mm. In two-jaw surgery, the maxilla is usually done first. Sometimes, all of the sagittal split will be done beforehand except the actual splitting itself. The maxilla is moved to its desired position with the mandible in its old position, using a prefabricated occlusal splint. After the maxilla is stabilized, the mandibular osteotomies are completed, and the mandible is

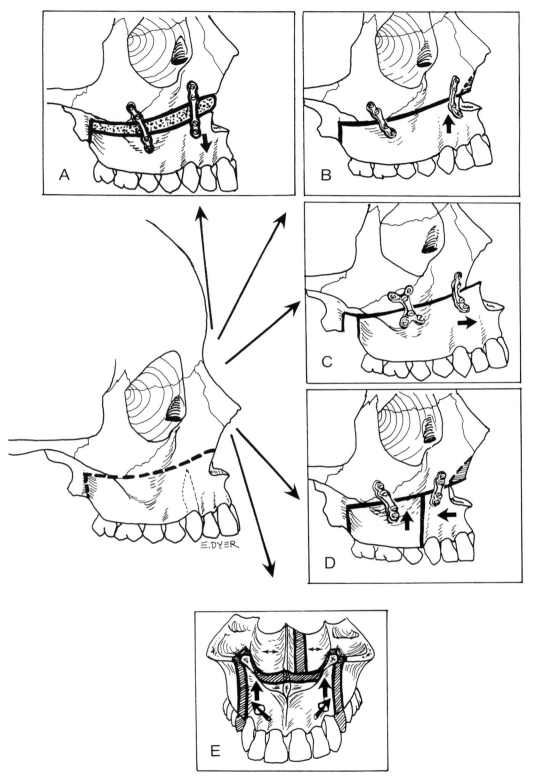

FIGURE 35.4. The Le Fort I osteotomy is the workhorse of maxillary orthognathic surgery. The maxilla can be lengthened with an interpositional bone graft **(A),** elevated for correction of vertical maxillary excess **(B),** advanced for correction of maxillary hypoplasia or class III malocclusion **(C),** or segmented with removal of teeth in three- or four-part maxillary osteotomies **(D** and **E).** With the use of rigid internal fixation, the majority of patients having any of these osteotomies, even when combined with mandibular osteotomies, do not require intermaxillary fixation. (From Wolfe SA: In Aston, Smith (eds): *Plastic Surgery.* Boston, Little, Brown, & Co, 1991, p 227.)

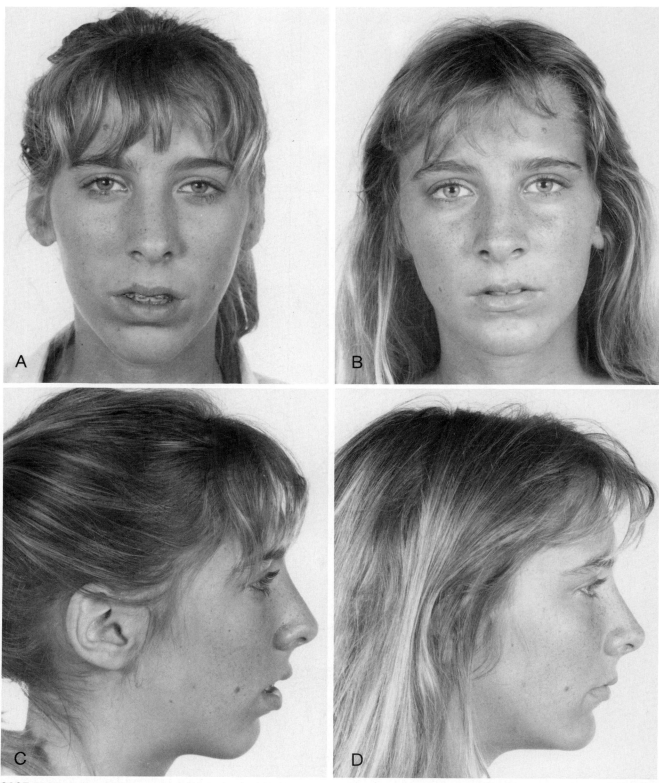

CASE 35.12. A–D. A 17-year-old patient who had had a long course of orthodontic treatment and had a slight residual anterior open bite. She had an excessive show of the maxillary incisors with her mouth in the rest position (2–3 mm of tooth should normally show) and on a smile showed gingiva above the tooth. She is shown after a Le Fort I osteotomy, maxillary impaction, and advancement genioplasty.

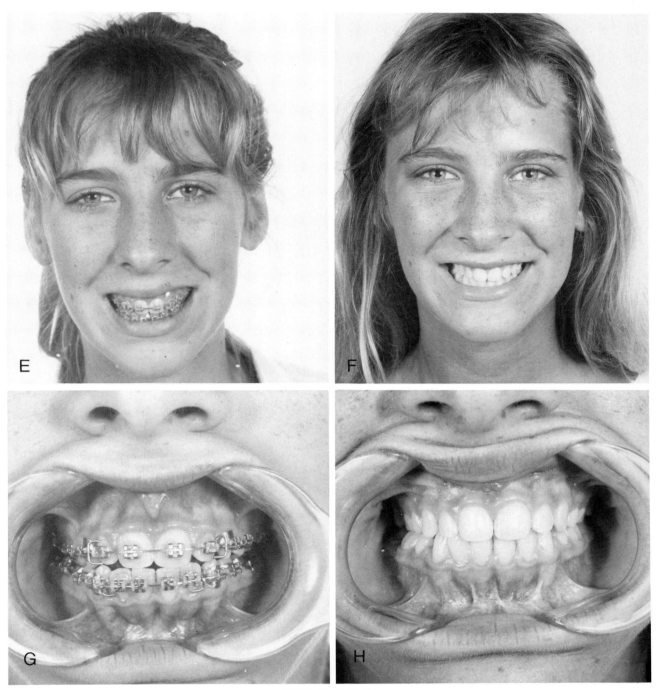

CASE 35.12. E–H.

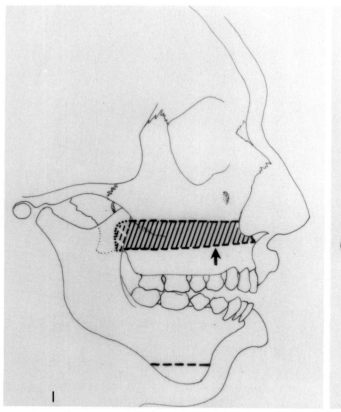 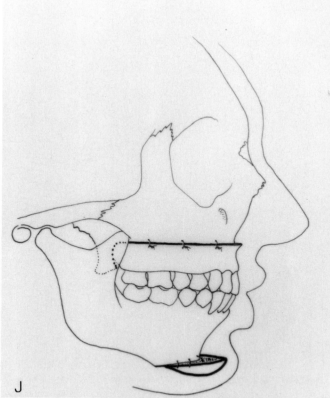

CASE 35.12. I and J.

moved to its final position with the use of a second, final splint.

Two-jaw surgery is indicated when:

1. There is a major occlusal gap (12 mm or more), and particularly when cephalometric analysis shows that the deformity is shared by both the maxilla and the mandible.
2. There are horizontal abnormalities with a canted occlusal plane, such as in hemifacial microsomia.
3. A mandibular deformity is associated with an open bite.

Internal Rigid Fixation. The advantages of internal rigid fixation are that:

1. The occlusion can be checked on the operating table with functional opening and closing, even if two-jaw surgery is done.
2. Most often, intermaxillary fixation can be dispensed with altogether, or the period of intermaxillary fixation can be shortened (Case 35.13).
3. With bones held by rigid osteosyntheses, there seems to be less swelling.

There are no disadvantages that I know of for the use of rigid fixation in the maxilla other than the cost of the plates and screws; in the mandible, the condyle may be torqued in the fossa, or the inferior alveolar nerve may be overly compressed. Both of these possibilities are probably avoidable with experience and a light touch.

If intermaxillary fixation is not used, the patient's occlusion must be followed carefully because small shifts can occur even with the use of rigid internal fixation. Particular attention should be paid to midlines. If a slight shift is noticed, several weeks of elastics in intermaxillary fixation usually will remedy the situation.

Miniplate Systems. An acceptable miniplate system should be:

1. Relatively inexpensive.
2. Made of a metal that is soft enough that it can be bent, but hard enough to maintain rigid fixation (titanium and Vitallium are acceptable).
3. Corrosion-proof (titanium and Vitallium are acceptable; stainless steel is not).
4. Small enough, with flat screw heads, that plates cannot be felt through the skin.
5. Provided with self-tapping (not requiring preliminary thread drilling) screws.

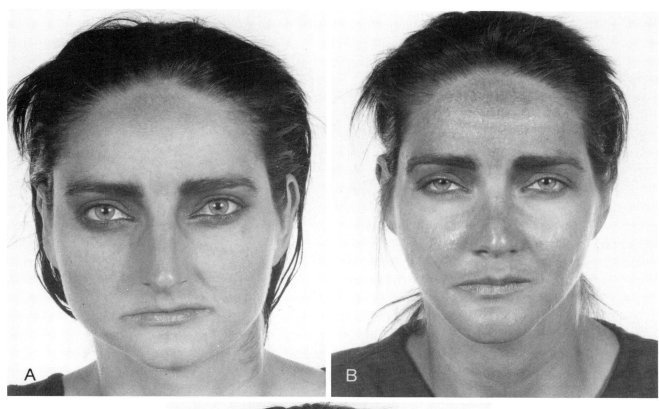

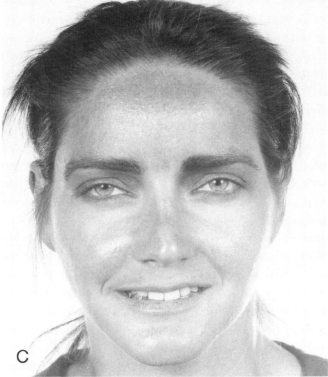

CASE 35.13. A–C. A 27-year-old patient with maxillary and mandibular deformities involving both the upper and lower jaw. She underwent a one-stage procedure consisting of a Le Fort I osteotomy, maxillary lengthening and advancement, a sagittal split with mandibular advancement, and a lengthening genioplasty with an interpositional bone graft. Rigid internal fixation obviated the need for intermaxillary fixation. In her postoperative photograph, she is shown recovering from a mild sunburn.

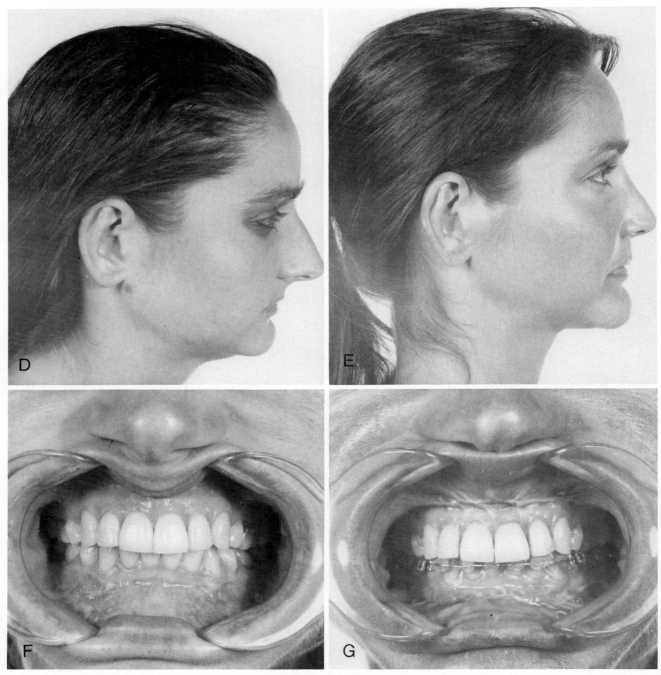

CASE 35.13. D–G.

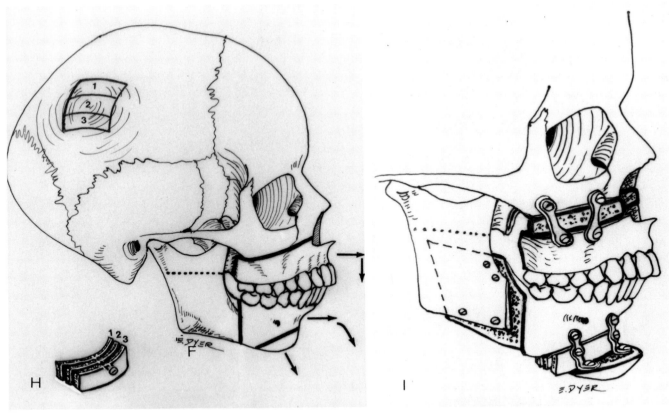

CASE 35.13.   H and I.

6. Provided with easy-to-load screwdrivers that hold the screws themselves.

Most of the commercially available systems fulfill these criteria, with the possible exception of number 1.

Higher Maxillary Osteotomies Requiring Extraoral Approaches

Le Fort II Osteotomy. The indications for a Le Fort II osteotomy are fairly limited. It should be used in a severe midface retrusion without exorbitism, such as a severe cleft lip and palate deformity, a Crouzon's dysostosis without exorbitism, or a hemifacial microsomia with a shift of the nasoethmoid. The osteotomy is made across the nasal root through a coronal approach and carried either medial or lateral to the infraorbital foramen and then down the maxilla obliquely to continue posteriorly along the path of a Le Fort I osteotomy.

Le Fort III Osteotomy. The subcranial Le Fort III osteotomy is indicated in patients who have major midface retrusion and exorbitism, such as a Crouzon's dysostosis. In younger patients (less than 12–13 years old) with Crouzon's, Apert's, or other craniofacial dysostoses, the monobloc frontofacial advancement is preferred. Older patients do not seem to be able to handle the retrofrontal dead space as well as younger ones, and they have a higher complication rate, with infection and loss of frontal bone. Patients with ventricular shunts in place also have higher complication rates after the monobloc advancement, and they should probably all be treated by extracranial procedure, irrespective of age (22).

The subcranial Le Fort III osteotomy is performed through coronal and vestibular incisions alone. A transverse frontal crescent gives the best orbital contour, and it is carried down to separate the lateral orbital rim from the cranial base. The osteotomy goes into the inferior orbital fissure and nearly connects with the medial osteotomy extending down from the nasofrontal osteotomy. The nasofrontal osteotomy should be continued for a distance along the cranial base with an osteotome to section the vomer and prevent an avulsion of the cribriform plate. The zygomatic arches are sectioned, and a pterygomaxillary disjunction is done as in a Le Fort I osteotomy. Frequently, however, more of the posterior maxilla needs to be separated from the pterygoid. The septum is sectioned down to the posterior hard palate with a guarded osteotome (avoiding the nasotracheal tube), and the midface is mobilized with Rowe disimpaction forceps. If there is a disproportion between the extent of the exorbitism and the retromaxillism, it is an easy matter to section the already mobilized maxilla at the Le Fort I level to regulate the occlusion after the exorbitism has been corrected. The maxillary segments are fixed in their proper positions with miniplates, and cranial bone grafts are used in all bone gaps (Case 35.14).

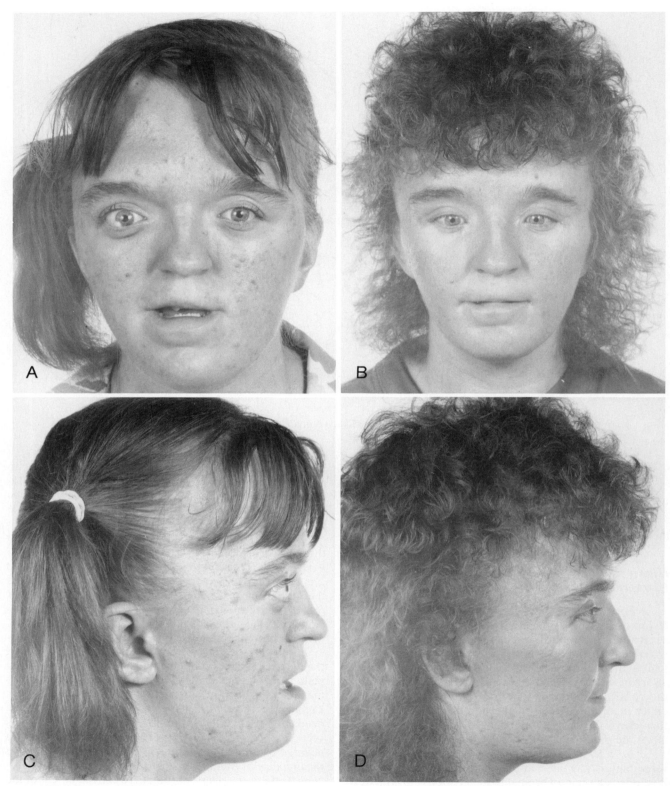

CASE 35.14. A–D. A 17-year-old patient with Apert's syndrome who underwent a one-stage extracranial Le Fort III maxillary advancement, genioplasty, and removal of a right epibulbar dermoid. The extracranial Le Fort III is preferred to the intracranial monobloc procedure in patients over the age of 12–14 for reasons mentioned in the text.

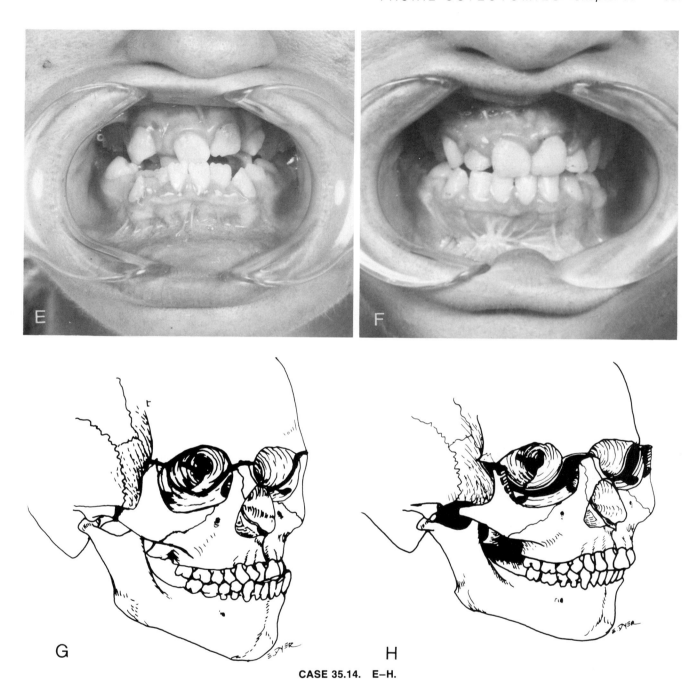

CASE 35.14.   E–H.

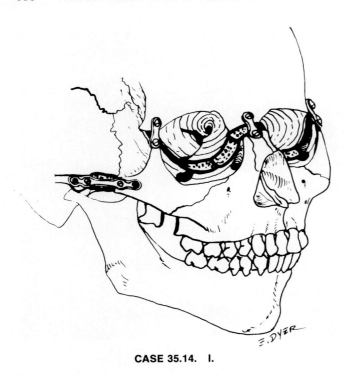

CASE 35.14. I.

Conclusion

The facial skeleton, in spite of the complexity of the soft tissue structures of the face, is easily approached through coronal and intraoral incisions, and a large variety of osteotomies can be performed. Planning of operations often involves the collaboration of a neurosurgeon, ophthalmologist, or orthodontist, depending on the area. The facial bones are covered by substantial well-vascularized soft tissues, and if proper osteosyntheses are performed, they heal solidly and rapidly. Over the past decade, the increasing use of rigid internal fixation and the harvesting of required bone grafts from the cranium have led to simpler operations, shorter operating times, improved results, and fewer complications.

References

1. Von Langenbeck B: *Deutsch Klin* 1861, p 281.
2. Cheever DW: Displacement of the upper jaw. *Med Surg Rep Boston City Hosp* 1:156, 1870.
3. Tessier P: Inferior orbitotomy: A new approach to the orbital floor. *Clin Plast Surg* 9:569, 1982.
4. Sullivan W, Kawamoto HK: Periorbital marginotomies: Anatomy and Applications. *J Cran Maxillofac Surg* 17:206, 1989.
5. Wolfe SA: A rationale for the surgical treatment of exophthalmos and exorbitism. *J Maxillofac Surg* 5:249, 1977.
6. Luhr HG: Miniplates for the prevention of fractures in problem cases of dento-alveolar surgery. Presented at Symposium on Rigid Fixation of the Craniomaxillofacial Skeleton, Toronto, Canada, September 10, 1989.
7. Derome PT: The transbasal approach to tumors involving the base of the skull. In Schmidek HP, Sweet WH (Eds): *Current Techniques in Operative Neurosurgery*. New York, Grune & Stratton, 1977, p 223.
8. Loré JM: *Atlas of Head & Neck Surgery*. Philadelphia, WB Saunders Co, 1988.
9. Whitaker LA, Pertschuk M: Facial skeletal contouring for aesthetic purposes. *Plast Reconstr Surg* 69:248, 1982.
10. Tessier P: Face lifting and frontal rhytidectomy. In *Transactions of the Seventh International Congress of Plastic & Reconstructive Surgery*. Cartgraf, Sao Paulo, Brazil, 1979, p 393.
11. Marchac D, et al: Intracranial pressure in craniostenosis: 302 recordings. In Marchac D (ed): *Craniofacial Surgery*. New York, Springer-Verlag, 1987, p 110.
12. Angle EW: *Treatment of Malocclusion of the Teeth and Fractures of the Maxilla, Angle's System*. Philadelphia, S.S. White Publications, 1898.
13. Burstone DJ, James RB, Legan H, Murphy GA, Horton LA: Cephalometrics for orthognathic surgery. *J Oral Maxillofac Surg* 36:269, 1978.
14. Downs UB: Variation in facial relationships: Their significance in treatment and prognosis. *Am J Orthod Dentofacial Orthop* 34:812, 1948.
15. Steiner CC: The use of cephalometrics as an aid to planning and assessing orthodontic treatment. *Am J Orthod Dentofac Orthop* 46:721, 1960.
16. Ricketts RM, Bench RW, et al: *Bioprogressive Therapy*. Rocky Mountain Publications, Denver, 1979.
17. Jacobsen A: Re "WITS" appraisal of jaw disharmony. *Am J Orthod Dentofacial Orthop* 67:125, 1975.
18. Wolford LM, Hilliard FW, Dugan DJ: *Surgical Treatment Objectives*. St. Louis, CV Mosby Co, 1985.
19. Berkowitz S: Analysis and treatment planning in patients with craniofacial anomalies. In Wolfe SA, Berkowitz S (eds): *Plastic Surgery of the Facial Skeleton*. Boston, Little, Brown & Co, 1989, p 39.
20. Delaire J: Ziele und Ergebnisse extraoraler Zuege in postero-anterorer Richtung in Anwendung eine Orthopaedischen Moske bei der Behandlung von Faellen der Klasse III. *Fortschr Kieferorthop* 37:247, 1976.
21. Le Fort R: Étude expérimental sur les fractures de la machoire supérieure. *Rev Chir Paris* 23:214, 1901.
22. Kawamoto HK Jr: Complication following monobloc frontofacial advancement. Presented at the Annual Meeting of the American Association of Plastic Surgeons, Palm Beach, May 3, 1988.

Suggested Readings

Bell WH, Profitt WR, White RP: *Surgical Correction of Dentofacial Deformities*. Philadelphia, WB Saunders, 1980.

Epker BN, Fish LC: *Dentofacial Deformities, Integrated Orthodontic and Surgical Correction*. St. Louis, CV Mosby Co, 1986.

Epker BN, Wolford LM: *Dentofacial Deformities, Surgical-Orthodontic Correction*. St. Louis, CV Mosby Co, 1980.

Wolfe SA: (translation of Tessier P): *Plastic Surgery of the Orbit and Eyelids*. New York, Masson, 1981.

Wolfe SA, Berkowitz S: *Plastic Surgery of the Facial Skeleton*. Boston, Little, Brown & Co, 1989.

36

Basic Principles in Management of Facial Injuries

Richard Carlton Schultz, M.D., F.A.C.S.

An important concept in the treatment of facial injuries is their placement in the context of total patient management, including other injuries. Attention of the highest professional quality should always be given to injuries of the face. However, they are almost never fatal and usually can be assigned lower treatment priority (1). Any neglect of facial trauma can be unfortunate, but more serious outcomes may be realized if immediate attention is not directed to more obscure but possibly life-threatening injuries. Definitive treatment of most facial injuries when properly cleansed and dressed may be deferred up to 24 hr without jeopardizing functional and esthetic results (2). Animal bites, close range shotgun injuries, and accidental tattoos are exceptions.

Treatment Priorities

In treating patients with extensive facial injuries, the order of priorities is consistent: airway clearance, control of hemorrhage, management of shock, treatment of associated injuries, and triage of facial injuries.

AIRWAY CLEARANCE

Facial injuries in themselves are seldom an indication for tracheostomy unless there are associated injuries of the cranium, neck, or chest. Blood, dentures, or vomitus may obstruct the upper airway, but these can usually be cleared quickly by sweeping a finger deep into the mouth and oral pharynx. Aspiration or tracheostomy can never be as prompt or informative as the use of a finger in such circumstances. Tracheostomy, when indicated, should be performed in the operating room whenever possible, with an assistant. The operation (Fig. 36.1) should be planned with the future function and appearance of the patient in mind. Vertical neck incisions should be avoided for all but the most emergent tracheostomy.

The condition of the patient with an airway problem stemming from uncontrolled facial hemorrhage or grossly displaced facial tissue can often be dramatically improved simply by sitting him upright. When such a patient makes a violent effort to sit up or thrust his head forward, he should be allowed to do so because he is almost invariably exhibiting a protective reflex to maintain the upper airway. Strapping or forcibly holding prone a patient with extensive facial injuries could result in asphyxiation.

The reader is referred to Chapter 37 for additional information on airway clearance.

HEMORRHAGE CONTROL

Although alarming in appearance, bleeding from facial wounds is rarely responsible for systemic shock. It is seldom of such magnitude as to require emergency blood transfusion. Extensive arterial hemorrhage usually results from injury to the external maxillary artery, the superficial temporal artery, or the angular artery, and it almost always can be controlled by direct pressure. Ligation of the vessel can be done directly through the wound. The most dangerous aspect of facial hemorrhage is the possibility of its obstructing the upper airway. Swallowing large amounts of blood will usually cause gastric irritation and lead to vomiting, thus further complicating management of the patient.

SHOCK

Shock is rarely caused by facial injury alone. Extensive facial injuries, including facial bone fractures, seldom cause great pain. When a patient with facial injuries is found in shock, associated injuries should be suspected and evaluated as the cause. The cardiopulmonary, neuromuscular, and gastrointestinal systems all have a bearing on decisions concerning facial injury treatment.

FACIAL INJURY DIAGNOSIS

Three basic techniques are used to diagnose facial injuries. *Observation* logically begins with soft tissue injury. Symmetry is important because imbalance can be an indication of underlying facial bone fracture and displacement. *Palpation* of the bony prominences bilaterally reinforces observations. Landmarks can sometimes be obscured by overlying hematoma or edema. Systematic palpation, even in the presence of obvious injury, helps in the detection of more subtle defects (Fig. 36.2). Tenderness can usually be elicited at the site of facial bone fracture, but discomfort is seldom exquisite.

Radiographic examination is another diagnostic technique. Gross facial bone fractures usually can be diagnosed without radiographic confirmation, and some grossly displaced facial bone fractures will not be visualized well on radiographs. Despite this, radiographic stud-

FIGURE 36.1. An operative technique for tracheostomy.

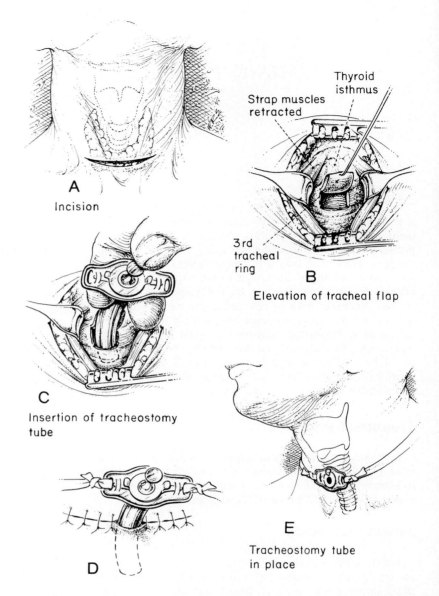

A

Incision

B

Strap muscles retracted

Thyroid isthmus

3rd tracheal ring

Elevation of tracheal flap

C

Insertion of tracheostomy tube

D

E

Tracheostomy tube in place

ies are of value in the evaluation of facial injury. The single most informative view is the Waters (occipitomental) view. This is taken with the patient in the prone position and the neck somewhat extended (Fig. 36.3). A complete series of facial bone radiographs includes special views of the nasal bones, the mandible, the mandibular condyles, the maxilla, and the zygomatic arch. More precise or additional information can often be obtained from special radiographic techniques, including laminographic studies, panoramic scanography (Panorex), and computed tomography (CT scans), the latter being the most definitive study.

TRIAGE OF FACIAL INJURIES

After life-threatening problems have been resolved, soft tissue injuries amenable to repair under local anesthesia are usually treated first. Complex facial injuries with tissue loss and extensive fractures can seldom be treated immediately because patients with such injuries are usually poor candidates for a general anesthetic (Fig. 36.4). When definitive care must be postponed, the simplest type of accurate tissue approximation will help promote a better end result. If necessary, repair of soft tissue injuries can be delayed without compromising the final outcome, provided bleeding has been controlled and wounds have been properly cleansed and dressed. Systemic antibiotics are advisable when significant delay in soft tissue repair is anticipated.

Reduction and fixation of facial bone fractures almost never need be considered an emergency. For best results, conditions should be as nearly ideal as possible before attempting any but the simplest type of reduction. Facial bone fractures become more difficult to reduce once healing has begun between fracture fragments. Although healing actually begins immediately, most facial bone fractures can be readily reduced within a 2-week period after injury. Because facial bones are membranous in origin, the healing that takes place begins with fibrous

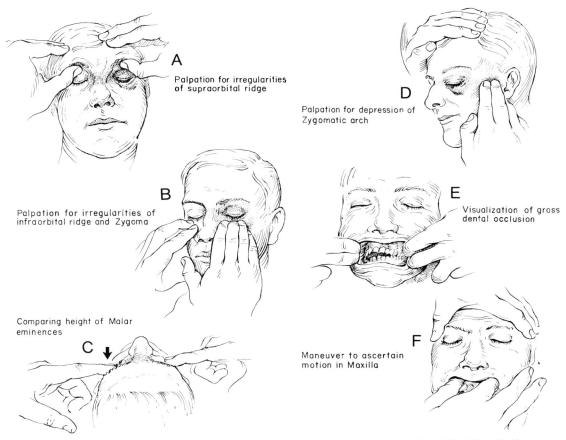

FIGURE 36.2. A technique for physical examination of the facial bones using bilateral palpation.

A Palpation for irregularities of supraorbital ridge

B Palpation for irregularities of infraorbital ridge and Zygoma

C Comparing height of Malar eminences

D Palpation for depression of Zygomatic arch

E Visualization of gross dental occlusion

F Maneuver to ascertain motion in Maxilla

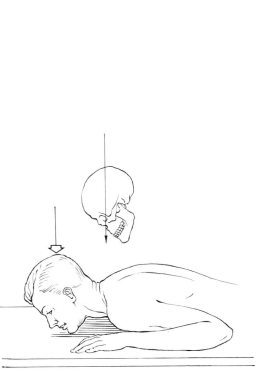

FIGURE 36.3. The position assumed for a Waters (occipito-mental) radiographic view.

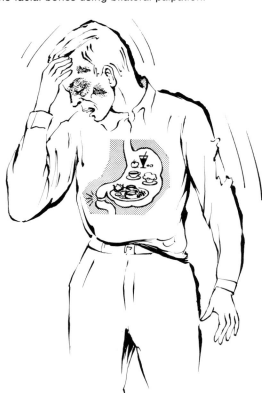

FIGURE 36.4. Facial injury patients are often poor candidates for general anesthesia.

union, and this can usually be overcome by manipulation and sharp dissection. Healing is accelerated in children; therefore, reduction of fractures should be attempted within 5–7 days of injury whenever possible.

DOCUMENTATION OF INJURY

The nature of facial injury care is such that the physician is frequently called upon by insurance companies, personal injury attorneys, and the courts to describe succinctly the extent of the original injury. This can be facilitated by maintaining a proper record of injury from the time of first examination. Appropriate records of facial injuries should include diagnosis of type of injury, anatomical location, and measurements of soft tissue injuries. In addition, a photograph of each extensive facial injury should be taken before definitive treatment begins. This record can subsequently prove invaluable in understanding and explaining secondary problems and the nature of final healing. A simplified outline organizing the facial bone skeleton into thirds can be useful in systematically diagnosing and recording facial bone fractures (Fig. 36.5).

Anesthesia

Treatment is directed at achieving functional and cosmetically acceptable healing of all injured tissue in the shortest possible time. In planning both emergency and definitive treatment, the issue of anesthesia must be addressed. Anesthesia serves only two purposes: (*a*) it prevents the patient from experiencing pain during surgery; and (*b*) it allows the surgeon greater ease in operating by ensuring him or her a quiet, accessible patient. Given a reasonably cooperative patient and a suitable injury, local anesthesia is preferable from the standpoint of safety and ultimate comfort for the patient. This is particularly true in emergency situations, in which patients are not good candidates for general anesthesia because they often arrive in the emergency room with blood, food, or alcohol in their stomachs.

Repair of deep structures and open reduction of most major facial bone fractures are best performed under general endotracheal anesthesia. When possible, these should be planned as elective procedures, allowing the patient to come to surgery with an empty stomach. With a skilled anesthesiologist and surgeon, tracheostomy solely for the purpose of treating facial injuries is seldom indicated.

Treatment of Soft Tissue Injuries

Once the patient is anesthetized, the wound is cleansed. Surrounding skin should be washed with soap or an antiseptic preparation (Betadine, Phisohex, or Hibiclens), taking care to avoid soaking the wound itself with solution. The wound should be irrigated with saline solution using a bulb syringe or jet lavage, which incorporates a pulsating water stream. Any solution except normal saline can be injurious to wounds, and other preparations do not provide any significant antibacterial effect.

TYPES OF WOUNDS

Soft tissue trauma may vary in degree of severity, but it can generally be categorized as: contusion, abrasion, puncture, laceration, avulsion flap, avulsion defect, or accidental tattoo. Contusions, abrasions, and puncture wounds can usually be managed by cleansing and a protective dressing. When such wounds are complicated by hematoma, the blood should be evacuated rather than allowed to resorb. During the early stage (the first 7–10 days), a hematoma can be evacuated through a small surgical incision. A more conservative approach to treatment is needle aspiration, usually performed successfully after 10–14 days. Retained foreign bodies and accidental tattoo require removal of the embedded foreign bodies. The exception to this is metal fragments from missiles. Bullets or missile fragments are usually sterile as they enter the face and commonly penetrate deeply. If there is minimum reaction, more harm is often done by attempted removal than by leaving them in place. Glass, ornamental metal, wood splinters, and dental fragments are foreign bodies that require removal. The treatment of accidental tattoo usually requires scrubbing with a stiff scrub brush. Care must be exercised to avoid overzealous scrubbing so as to prevent conversion of a partial-thickness injury into a full-thickness dermal defect requiring skin grafting. Once these small foreign particles have become fixed in the tissues, a formal surgical abrasion is necessary, and this procedure should be planned under general anesthesia with the use of power equipment.

After appropriate cleansing and wound irrigation, simple lacerations are treated by primary closure. When wound edges are beveled or "feathered" or when there is

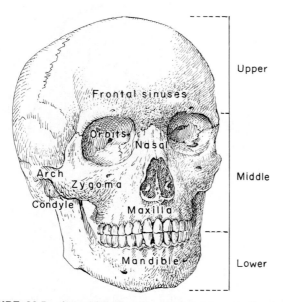

FIGURE 36.5. Area identification of facial bones; the facial skeleton can be divided into upper, middle, and lower zones for diagnosis and treatment of facial fractures.

obvious devitalized tissue, appropriate débridement is performed. Most facial wounds should be managed with very conservative débridement. Questionable viable facial tissue will often survive because of its excellent blood supply. Overly aggressive débridement may result in the loss of vital bits of soft tissue needed for later reconstruction. Lacerations are closed in layers, using a minimum but adequate number of sutures. Buried sutures are a potential nidus of infection, but so is dead space filled with blood or serum.

Soft tissue wounds are repaired with attention to symmetry of facial features. Tissue is always returned to its position of origin.

An avulsion flap is an undermined laceration in which the flap's nourishment is essentially restricted to its pedicle. Because the broad, tangentially located scar tissue in the dermis and subcutaneous tissue interferes with free circulation of venous blood and lymph, there is often a resulting venous engorgement and lymphedema. This causes swelling of the flap and partially contributes to spreading and subsequent depression of the peripheral scar. Furthermore, as the scar contracts, the central avulsion flap tissue assumes a heaped-up appearance. It is important, therefore, to minimize the thin, beveled portion of these flaps. If the flap is small and fortuitously located, it can be totally excised and the problem resolved. When avulsion flaps are large or involve features, a more conservative approach to repair must be taken. The thinnest peripheral portions of the flap should be cut away to form perpendicular edges of skin closure (Fig. 36.6).

When anatomical approximation is not possible because of missing tissue, coverage by local flaps or skin grafts is performed as a primary surgical procedure. Flaps used for this purpose can be: (*a*) rotation advancement, (*b*) transposition, (*c*) direct pedicle, (*d*) tubed pedicle, (*e*) island pedicle, and (*f*) free direct transfer (microvascular anastomosis).

Either full-thickness or split-thickness free skin grafts can be employed. When a defect is relatively small and the base is clean, a full-thickness graft provides a superior cover with elastic properties, thickness, and color

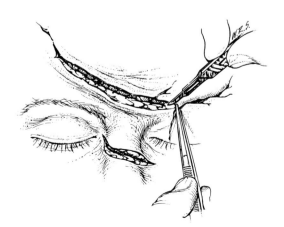

FIGURE 36.6. Excision of beveled edge of avulsion flaps helps create a perpendicular surface for better skin closure and healing.

more closely resembling adjacent skin. Full-thickness grafts are usually taken from areas where the donor site can be closed primarily. Such donor sites include the postauricular area, upper eyelid, supraclavicular area, and antecubital fossa. In general, donor sites as close as possible to the defect should be selected so as to achieve the best possible match of color and texture. Split-thickness skin grafts can be cut either thick or thin. For defects that are less than ideal recipient sites, thin grafts tend to vascularize more readily. Thick split-thickness skin grafts are ideal and often provide a definitive repair for large, clean defects. These grafts are usually best taken with a drum-type, hand-operated dermatome (Padget dermatome). Soft tissue defects should be covered by skin as promptly as the patient's general condition permits, even if the procedure must be performed under local anesthesia. A fresh, uncontaminated wound is the best possible bed for accepting a skin graft.

FACIAL NERVE AND PAROTID GLAND INJURY

Facial nerve injury is diagnosed on the basis of physical examination and anatomical landmarks. An uncooperative patient, an extensive soft tissue injury, or extensive edema may make the physical examination inconclusive. Under ordinary circumstances, muscular paralysis on the involved side of the face indicates nerve injury.

Division of branches of the facial nerve medial to the midpupillary line does not usually require repair because the branching cross-nerve supply tends to reinnervate the appropriate muscle spontaneously. Lateral to this point, nerve repair should be attempted in order to guide the advancing axons to the motor endplate in the muscle. The most severe functional deficit from division of a single nerve branch is that of the temporal branch. This causes paralysis of the eyelid and subsequent exposure of the cornea. The temporal nerve branch courses superiorly at a point halfway between the tragus and the lateral canthus, becoming superficial at this point.

The mandibular branch of the facial nerve is also commonly injured. This branch is always deep to the platysma muscle when posterior to the facial artery. It then courses near the lower border of the mandible, although it may be found 1 cm below the mandible. Anterior to the facial artery, the nerve becomes more superficial and is nearly always found above the lower border of the mandible.

When proximal laceration of the branch of the facial nerve is suspected, exploration should be undertaken to identify the nerve ends. The epineurium is best reapproximated with fine suture material under magnification. Injury to a major nerve trunk should be repaired with fascicular sutures using an operating microscope.

The parotid duct can be divided by a deep laceration posterior to the anterior border of the masseter muscle. The parotid duct courses along a line from the tragus of the ear to the midportion of the upper lip. It lies deep near the anterior border of the masseter muscle, emptying into the oral cavity adjacent to the first maxillary molar tooth.

Laceration of the parotid duct will frequently damage the buccal branch of the facial nerve. When there is complete laceration of the parotid duct, an end-to-end anastomosis over a small Silastic catheter can be performed. As an alternate procedure, the proximal cut end of the duct can be sutured to the oral mucosa to maintain parotid duct function.

When clear fluid is seen leaking from a wound in the parotid region, injury to the gland should be suspected. The gland itself need not be sutured. Salivary fistula is a common complication after skin repair of an underlying glandular laceration. This usually closes without treatment in about 3 weeks.

EYELID INJURY

Injuries to thin eyelid skin may result in small avulsion flaps that appear questionably viable. Such flaps usually survive if replaced anatomically. Divided muscle and tarsal plate should be identified and repaired separately with fine absorbable suture. The tarsal plate is adherent to the conjunctiva and can be repaired with the conjunctiva. Lacerations of the thin orbital septum usually do not require separate closure, provided the orbicularis oculi muscle is repaired.

Lacerations of the lacrimal apparatus must be recognized and repaired to prevent epiphora and dacryocystitis postoperatively. The divided lacrimal duct may be cannulated with a heavy nylon suture and then reapproximated with fine absorbable sutures. After a week, the nylon stent is removed. Fine, soft polyethylene catheters can be used for cannulization. When injury to the lacrimal system is severe, primary dacryorhinocystostomy should be considered.

EAR INJURY

Lacerations through the full thickness of the ear are best repaired by cutaneous-perichondrial sutures. The cartilage margins may require conservative trimming to facilitate skin closure, but cartilage itself need not be sutured. Hematoma of the ear from blunt trauma may be potentially disfiguring if left untreated. Aspiration or incision and drainage will evacuate the hematoma in the early stages. If untreated, the hematoma undergoes organization and fibrosis, leading to the classical "cauliflower ear."

NASAL INJURY

Lacerations through the nostrils are repaired by closure of the mucous membrane with absorbable sutures and approximation of the skin using fine nonabsorbable sutures. Special care should be taken to align the nostril border accurately. Suturing the alar or upper lateral cartilages is not ordinarily necessary. Nasal fracture, of course, should be suspected, and can often be diagnosed clinically and treated at the same time soft tissue repair is undertaken. Techniques of closed reduction of displaced nasal fractures are discussed below.

Facial Bone Fractures

DIAGNOSIS

The patient suffering extensive facial fractures can present an awesome appearance. Forces sufficient to fracture the bony facial structure may also cause disfiguring soft tissue injury. Displacement of the bony fragments further distorts the facial contour. The severity of a facial wound must not draw the examiner's attention away from potentially more severe visceral injuries. Similarly, the severity of soft tissue destruction should not distract the examiner from a complete examination of the facial skeleton. Diagnosis of bony injuries must sometimes rest on clinical evaluation alone. Initial radiographs may not always demonstrate facial fractures, or the severity of the injuries may preclude the patient's undergoing a complete radiographic examination.

Poor dental occlusion may be the first clue of mandibular or maxillary fracture. Diplopia may also be the only positive finding of a fractured orbital floor. Personal observation can disclose depressed frontal sinuses, a deviated nasal complex, a depressed zygoma, enophthalmos, an asymmetrical mandible, or a malaligned dental arch. Systematic bimanual palpation will help the physician avoid missing less obvious fractures (Fig. 36.2). Palpation of the bony parts can usually elicit tenderness and sometimes motion and crepitus at the fracture sites.

FRACTURES OF UPPER THIRD OF FACE

Fractures of the upper one third of the face are less common than those of the lower two thirds of the face because of the protection afforded by an energy-absorbing projecting part, the nose. Fractures of the frontal area usually involve the thinner bones of the frontal sinuses or the supraorbital ridges. Because of their close proximity to the brain, injuries in this area are likely to have a higher morbidity and to be more life-threatening than other facial fractures.

Positive physical findings usually appear in the ocular region as a result of extravasation of blood into the orbital area. Periorbital ecchymosis is observed in nearly all cases; diplopia is inconstant. Diplopia is seen with depressed supraorbital fractures, but it is not commonly found with glabellar fractures. Nasal fractures and overlying lacerations of the forehead are commonly found in association with fractures of the upper one third of the face.

Treatment of supraorbital fractures involves reduction of the bony fragments by either direct or indirect approach with interosseous fixation when required for stabilization (Fig. 36.7). Appropriate débridement of avascular or pulped sinus mucosa, accurate replacement of soft tissue, and systemic antibiotic therapy should accompany the bony reduction. Although advocated by some, removal of comminuted bone fragments and extirpation of the sinus results in gross deformity and requires extensive secondary reconstruction. Cranialization of the frontal sinuses should be avoided if other methods of contour restoration are available. Primary bone recon-

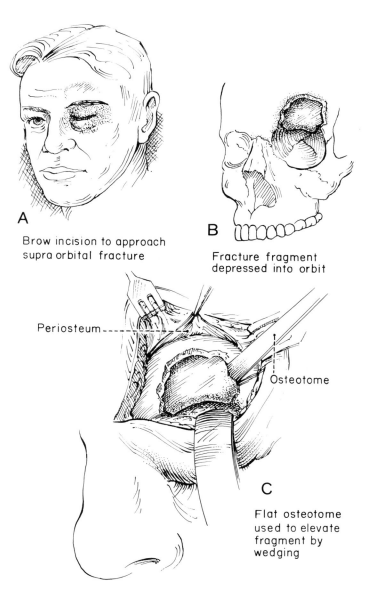

FIGURE 36.7. The operative technique for reduction of depressed superorbital fractures by wedging maneuver; segments sometimes require interosseous wire fixation.

A
Brow incision to approach supra orbital fracture

B
Fracture fragment depressed into orbit

Periosteum

Osteotome

C
Flat osteotome used to elevate fragment by wedging

struction (with or without bone grafting), as outlined above, gives excellent functional and esthetic results without complications.

Many techniques developed for craniofacial surgery can be used for both primary and secondary management of fractures of the upper one third of the face (3, 4). Among these are the bitemporal forehead flap approach to the fractures, rigid interfragment wiring, and primary as well as secondary bone grafting using rib, calvarial, or cancellous bone (Fig. 36.8).

FACIAL FRACTURES IN CHILDREN

In general, the mechanism of injury, the diagnosis, and the management of facial bone fractures in children do not differ greatly from that in the adult, although a few differences do exist (5). Lack of cooperation in children

may require that diagnosis rely more on radiographic findings than clinical examination.

Because of greater resiliency in the facial bones of children, greenstick fractures, rather than completely displaced fractures, are more common. Because bony union may occur early in children, fractures should be reduced within the first week after injury whenever possible. Condylar fractures in children may cause a potential growth problem as a result of involvement of the epiphyseal growth center. Although retardation of growth on the involved side can occur, it is only seen rarely. This usually results from intracapsular injuries. As with adults, closed treatment is the preferred method of management, even in instances of a medially displaced condyle. Intermaxillary fixation is more difficult in children because of the instability of deciduous teeth; this occasionally precludes using the teeth to maintain occlusion. Mixed or absent dentition may complicate the stability of arch bars

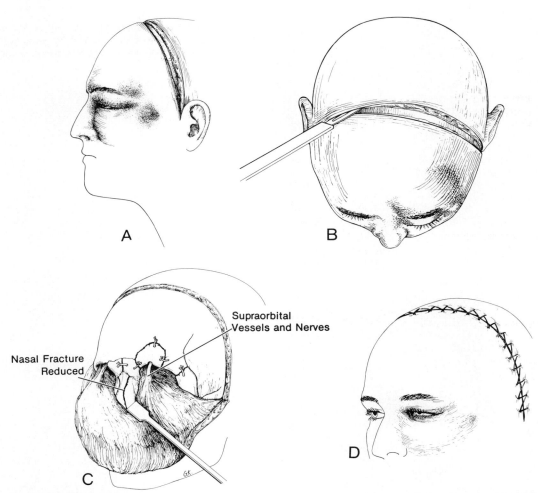

FIGURE 36.8.   The craniofacial approach to the management of fractures of the upper and middle face. **A and B,** Development of the bitemporal coronal forehead flap. **C,** Fractures of the upper and middle face or rigid interosseous wire fixation are exposed. **D,** A forehead flap is replaced and closed with resulting scar concealed.

or ligatures about the teeth. Acrylic splints and supplementary direct osseous fixation of the arch bars may be required (Fig. 36.9).

Treatment of displaced fractures of the body of the mandible is influenced by the lack of nondental bony substance for direct interosseous wire fixation. During the period of mixed dentition, deciduous teeth may be exfoliating and permanent teeth just erupting. This may interfere with the use of interdental wires and arch bars. When such fractures make the conventional methods of management inappropriate, a custom fabricated acrylic splint can be used. Such splints can be held in position by circum-mandibular wiring (Fig. 36.10).

The sequelae of facial fractures in infants and young children can be very significant. The seriousness is compounded by the effects of the fractures on future facial growth and development. Therefore, the initial examination must be precise and should be repeated at frequent intervals as the swelling resorbs. This will guide reduction as early as possible to avoid malunion and subsequent growth deformities.

Gunshot Wounds of the Face

Gunshot wounds of the face typically involve soft tissue and bone. They can either appear trivial or be among the most severe injuries, depending on the range, velocity, and caliber of the shot (6). Therapeutic hazards exist at both extremes. A small-caliber entrance wound may appear inconsequential, but the damage created along its course cannot be assumed to be insignificant. An exit wound, when it occurs, is often of substantially greater dimension. At the other extreme, point-blank shotgun wounds inflict extensive damage to facial bones and soft tissue. Survival may appear doubtful and lead to therapeutic apathy. Unless death is immediate, the injuries are usually survivable, despite the grotesque destruction of facial features. An organized, disciplined approach to patient management will overcome initial feelings of futility and inertia.

Only shotgun wounds fired at close range (i.e., less than 10 feet) are usually serious. When fired from greater distances, the shot may penetrate the skin and deep fas-

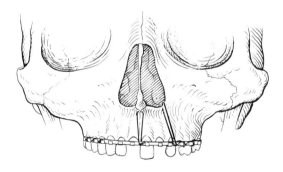

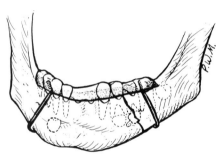

FIGURE 36.10. Acrylic cap splints can be stabilized by circummandibular wires, with deciduous teeth and multiple tooth buds.

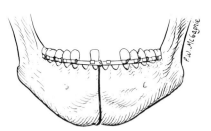

FIGURE 36.9. Maxillary and mandibular arch bars can be stabilized by supplementary fixation wires passed through the anterior nasal spine or the piriform aperture or circumferentially about the mandible.

cia. However, tissue avulsion or pulping does not occur. Embedded shot should be removed if it is accessible or interferes with function (e.g., if it is in the eye or eyelid, tongue, or temporomandibular joint). Nonsymptomatic, deeply embedded metallic missiles are best left unexplored to avoid the possibility of further damage.

The person who intends to commit suicide with a 30-inch barrel gun typically places the muzzle beneath the chin (Fig. 36.11) or in the mouth. In pulling the trigger, a jerk may result in reflex extension of the head or turning away from the muzzle when it is in the mouth. This reflex action alters the intended course of the shot and saves the victim's life. The charge then explodes into the chin or cheeks, depositing gunpowder, wadding and shot into the soft tissues and ripping away mucous membrane, bone, cartilage, and skin along its path.

Destruction caused by such shotgun wounds can be extensive, completely distorting and avulsing the regional anatomy. As would be expected, many structural components that lie along the trajectory are endangered (mandible, tongue, teeth, parotid gland and Stensen's duct, palate, maxilla, zygoma, nasal structures, maxillary and ethmoidal sinuses, orbital bones, lower and upper eyelids, and brow). In addition, damage to the eyes, ears, branches of the facial nerve, cervical spine, and intracranial contents may occur. It is surprising how often the eyes, frontal sinuses, and central nervous system are not

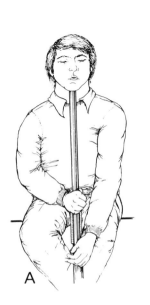

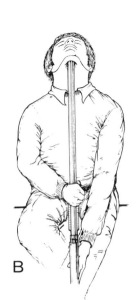

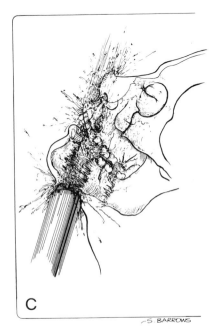

FIGURE 36.11. Mechanism of facial injuries in attempting suicide with a shotgun placed beneath the mandible (see text).

injured. Frequently, there is severe damage to the naso-pharynx, but the oral pharynx can escape sufficiently to permit the victim to maintain an airway in the upright position unless massive edema occurs. For these reasons, a person with massive destruction can arrive in the hospital emergency room in a sitting position, alert, and in possession of his faculties. Body position is often the key to survival. Having the patient assume the supine position, particularly for a prolonged ambulance ride, may result in death. Treatment is determined by the time that has elapsed since the moment of injury.

IMMEDIATE CARE

The upper airway must be guaranteed. Aspiration of blood and removal of broken teeth and dentures or obstructing bone and soft tissue from the oral pharynx must be accomplished at once. The tongue, when fragmented and unsupported, must be controlled with heavy sutures. The most common complication of surviving victims is aspiration pneumonia. When surgery is anticipated, the easiest way to maintain the airway is by an awake orotracheal intubation using a cuffed endotracheal tube of the largest appropriate size. An immediate emergency tracheostomy may be necessary but can be extremely difficult when there is massive bleeding and the patient is thrashing about in a semirecumbent position. Tracheostomy is best done over an endotracheal tube at the end of the initial operative procedure.

Goals of the first operative procedure are: (*a*) life-saving measures (removal of debris from the airway, tracheostomy if indicated, and hemostasis); (*b*) protection of the eyes, central nervous system, and facial nerves; (*c*) preservation of as much viable bone and soft tissue as possible; (*d*) removal of cartridge packing and wadding and accessible portions of the metallic missile(s); (*e*) débridement of obviously nonviable tissue, excising the wound of entrance if possible; (*f*) stabilization of the bony framework of the face if feasible; and (*g*) provision of soft tissue cover and lining of the oral cavity and nose to the extent that the condition of the patient will allow.

These goals can ordinarily be accomplished by a careful unfolding of the injury, conservative débridement, and gentle, accurate replacement and suturing of remaining parts. Repair of oral and nasal mucosa should be as accurate as possible, but where large segments of soft tissue are missing, closure of mucous membrane to the skin may be the best temporary alternative. Wounds are left open where the viability of tissue is uncertain.

Eyelid coverage must be provided; tarsorrhaphies are performed when lid closure is doubtful. Unless damage to the globe is severe, enucleation can be postponed because sympathetic ophthalmia does not occur before 10 days and more usually not before 31 days.

Only gross realignment of bony parts, particularly the mandible, may be possible initially. Stabilization of upper and lower dental arches by intermaxillary fixation is ideal, but the simplest form of obtaining bone contact may have to suffice. Because of massive fragmentation, repair of the periosteum with absorbable sutures may be all that is indicated at first.

Tight primary closure is contraindicated when the wound is grossly contaminated, old, or massively edematous. The decision to introduce direct distant pedicle flaps, free microvascular flaps, or bone grafts into this wound at the time of the initial procedure varies with the patient. Although the benefits of early reconstruction are undeniable, the possible loss of unique replacement tissue as a result of avascular necrosis and infection can prove disastrous.

Summary

Because of their functional and esthetic significance, facial injuries dictate special attention. Although logically divided into soft tissue injuries and facial bone fractures, each type of injury interrelates and bears on the management approach of the other. The preceding discussion has outlined the important early management of these injuries. Specific types of injuries and principles of treatment are discussed. Occasionally, extensive facial trauma requires secondary reconstructive procedures to maximize results.

Although facial fractures are relatively uncommon and sequelae rare in children, there may be long-term consequences. Conditions secondary to such injuries may include interruption in facial growth and the potential for permanent functional impairment. Therefore, it is incumbent upon the surgeon to be familiar with these possible occurrences and execute an appropriate management plan. Prevention lies in an aggressive approach to diagnosis and incisive timing in definitive treatment.

References

1. Schultz RC: The nature of facial injury emergencies. *Surg Clin North Am* 52:99, 1972.
2. Schultz RC, Oldham RJ: An overview of facial injuries. *Surg Clin North Am* 57:987, 1977.
3. Jackson IT, Munro IR, Salyer KE, et al: Traumatic deformities: Primary and secondary treatment. In *Atlas of Craniomaxillofacial Surgery*. St. Louis, CV Mosby Co, 1982, p 647.
4. Jones WD III, Whitaker LA, Murtagh F: Applications of reconstructive craniofacial techniques to acute craniofacial trauma. *J Trauma* 17:339, 1977.
5. Schultz RC: Pediatric facial fractures. In Kernahan DA, Thomson HG (eds): *Symposium on Pediatric Plastic Surgery*. St. Louis, CV Mosby Co, 1982, p 249.
6. Schultz RC: Gunshot wounds of the face. In Schultz RC (ed): *Facial Injuries*, ed. 3. Chicago, Year Book Medical Publishers, 1988.

37

Management of Midfacial Fractures

Paul N. Manson, M.D., F.A.C.S.

The frontal cranium and the face are frequently injured because of their exposed position. In our society, sophisticated transportation and increased mobility contribute to facial injury. The automobile and motorcycle, industrial accidents, fights, and falls account for the majority of etiological factors in facial trauma. The management of frontal cranial and facial injuries requires the simultaneous ability to reconstruct both soft tissue and bone injury.

Complete Evaluation

Two thirds of the patients with significant maxillofacial injury will sustain injury to other organ systems (1, 2). Brain injury and cervical spine injury often coexist with facial fractures. The efforts of a specialty team should be coordinated with the activities of general surgeons specializing in trauma who supervise the care of the patient and integrate the activities of all specialists. All organ systems must be evaluated systematically and monitored continuously during the initial resuscitation and operative management of the multiply injured patient. Such observations rely on the placement of arterial and venous monitoring lines; urethral catheterization; diagnostic peritoneal lavage; radiographs of the pelvis, extremities, chest, and spine; and the placement of devices for monitoring intracranial pressure in those patients with reduced Glascow Coma Scale scores or abnormal computed tomography (CT) scans.

A systematic evaluation is important as a means of ensuring a complete examination. It also enables the examiner to determine the priority of treatment when multiple injuries are present. Individual treatment plans must receive prioritization. Emergency treatment is directed toward life-threatening events such as airway obstruction, aspiration, hemorrhage, cervical spine and spinal cord injury, and intracranial injury.

Emergency Treatment of Maxillofacial Injuries

There are three ways in which maxillofacial injuries may result in death: via airway obstruction, aspiration, or hemorrhage.

AIRWAY OBSTRUCTION

Airway obstruction demands immediate attention and may be corrected with maneuvers as simple as repositioning the jaw or tongue or removal of obstructions such as fractured teeth, bridgework, or denture segments. Intubation is a secure method of controlling the airway. A tracheostomy may be advisable in some patients with maxillofacial injuries who would be difficult to reintubate or who demonstrate impending respiratory obstruction (stridor, retraction, drooling, inability to swallow).

With the advent of rigid internal skeletal fixation, the patient may often have intermaxillary fixation (IMF) released at an early time following operative treatment. If intermaxillary fixation is to be employed on a prolonged basis postoperatively, a tracheostomy should be considered in the following patients:

1. Patients with a head injury who are comatose and require prolonged intermaxillary fixation as a component of treatment for a jaw fracture.
2. Head injury (spastic, semipurposeful, or rigid) patients who require intermaxillary fixation as a component of treatment for a jaw fracture.
3. Patients with combined maxillary, mandibular, and nasal fractures (panfacial injury).
4. Patients with combined maxillary and nasal or mandibular and nasal fractures in which unstable occlusal relationships make prolonged IMF desirable in the face of an inadequate airway (nasopharyngeal or neck swelling).
5. Patients with massive head and neck soft tissue swelling, which would make reintubation difficult.
6. Patients with pulmonary injury that requires prolonged intubation. Early extubation is unlikely in these patients, and it is difficult to observe proper occlusal relationships in patients with endotracheal tubes.
7. Patients with pharyngeal, laryngeal, or tracheal injury.

A tracheostomy may be omitted when rigid fixation of facial fractures is employed, IMF is discontinued postoperatively, and the occlusion is easily observed.

ASPIRATION

Pulmonary aspiration is a common finding in patients presenting with maxillofacial trauma. Fractures of the jaws frequently make it difficult for a patient to control and swallow secretions. Nasopharyngeal hemorrhage may be aspirated. Aspirated material may otherwise represent gastric contents or nasal and oral secretions. Patients who have aspirated should be managed initially by positioning and tracheal suctioning. Inability to control aspiration with these maneuvers will require intubation. If aspiration has resulted in hypoxia, intubation, positive end-expiratory pressure (PEEP), bronchodilators, antibiotics, and bronchoscopy may be advisable. Because pulmonary compliance is severely altered following significant aspiration, operative procedures should be of limited duration.

HEMORRHAGE

Major hemorrhage from head and neck injury represents a life-threatening event. Hemorrhage may occur from cutaneous lacerations that involve arteries. Hemorrhage may usually be controlled by bandages, direct pressure, or hemostat clamp occlusion. The partially transected artery often continues to bleed beneath a bandage. When applying hemostats, care should be exercised to avoid facial nerve injury. When the source of the bleeding is from the nose or mouth, the hemorrhage may not be controlled directly. Nasopharyngeal hemorrhage may accompany any fracture of the midface or orbit; hemorrhage presenting from the nose may even be from a cranial base source with lacerations of the dural venous sinuses or the carotid arterial system.

Profuse nasopharyngeal bleeding usually accompanies LeFort maxillary fractures. Nasal bleeding occurs with fractures of the nose, the orbit, and the maxilla. Usually, nasopharyngeal bleeding ceases spontaneously. Nasopharyngeal bleeding that requires control is best managed with the following techniques:

1. *Anterior/posterior nasal packing.* A gauze pack or Foley balloon is placed in the posterior pharynx. The Foley balloon is placed in the pharynx by passing it through the nose, inflating it, and then drawing it against the posterior choanae. Terramycin-soaked Adaptic packing or antibiotic-impregnated gauze packing is then used to pack the anterior portion of the nose, utilizing the posterior pack as an obturator.
2. *Maxillary fracture reduction.* Placing the teeth in intermaxillary fixation generally reduces sinus fractures and reduces bleeding by providing stability and reduced traction on veins.
3. *External compression.* A multilayer (Barton type) bandage may be wrapped around the face to provide external pressure.
4. *Bilateral external carotid and superficial temporal artery ligation.* Persistent hemorrhage that does not respond to the above maneuvers requires an angiogram to identify the source of bleeding. Usually, bleeding

occurs from fractures involving arteries and veins in the walls of the sinuses and in the pterygoid areas. Such hemorrhage is best controlled by ligating the two large source arteries. Such ligations, however, rarely are required.

Coagulopathies may contribute to hemorrhage. Coagulopathies are often observed early following injury to the central nervous system. Coagulation factors should be monitored hourly and replacement provided (3).

Cervical Spine and Spinal Cord Injuries

Injuries to the cervical spine occur in 10% of patients with maxillofacial trauma. Conversely, 18% of patients with cervical spine injuries have a maxillofacial injury (4). There is an association between injuries to the frontal bone and midface and cervical hyperextension injuries. There is also an association between injuries of the upper portion of the cervical spine and the mandible; therefore, mandibular fractures should prompt a careful examination of the cervical area. Injuries in the upper and lower areas of the cervical spine are the most difficult to demonstrate. Carefully taken cervical spine films with inferior traction on the shoulders will usually demonstrate the entire cervical skeleton. The most commonly missed lesions occur at C1, C2, and C7, which are difficult to visualize. Flexion-extension films and a cervical CT scan should be obtained to confirm the presence of injury in specific cases. Pain is a reliable indication of cervical injury. A neurological examination is an essential part of any head and neck evaluation.

Head Injury

Patients with head injury (5) are identified on the basis of a Glasgow Coma Scale evaluation, neurological examination, and CT scan. The prognosis of head injury is generally better for patients who are under 40 years of age. Patients who are in shock, who have abnormal posturing, who have pulmonary injury, and whose Glasgow Coma Scale scores are less than 10 generally have a poor prognosis (6–9). The Glasgow Coma Scale (Table 37.1) evaluates eye opening response, the ability to talk, the ability to move the extremities, and the ability to follow commands. A graded scale evaluates responses for each criterion. A total score less than 10 should be taken as a grave prognostic sign.

The presence of coma in itself does not represent justification for postponing maxillofacial injury treatment (10). Often, simple maneuvers may accomplish satisfactory reduction in a timely fashion; one such maneuver is intermaxillary fixation. Many patients in coma will survive, improve, and ultimately be able to work and provide for their own needs. One half of patients who are in coma for a period longer than 1 week are able to return to useful work (7, 9, 10). However, the presence of even short periods of unconsciousness may herald some disability following minor head injury. Many patients with "mi-

Table 37.1.
Glasgow Coma Scale

Criteria	Points
Eyes open	5
Spontaneously	4
To speech	3
To pain	2
None	1
Best verbal response	
Oriented	5
Confused	4
Inappropriate	3
Incomprehensible	2
None	1
Best motor response	
Obey commands	5
Localized pain	4
Flexion to pain	3
Extension to pain	2
None	1

nor'' head injuries demonstrate difficulty with interpersonal relationships, memory, and irritability. The use of the Glasgow Coma Scale and the CT scan identifies patients who require intracranial pressure monitoring during anesthesia. This technique allows comatose patients to be safely monitored during prolonged operations. Blood loss and shock must be avoided because they reduce cerebral circulation and contribute to increased cerebral edema through ischemia and anoxia.

Intracranial pressures in excess of 25 mm Hg are accompanied by at least a 30% mortality rate. All but emergent injury management is postponed in the face of intracranial pressures in excess of 15 mm Hg. The performance of intracranial neurosurgery and the necessity for removal of cerebral cortex do not represent contraindications to maxillofacial injury repair. Many patients have a good prognosis despite their neurological injury.

Evaluation of Maxillofacial Injuries

The maxillofacial injury evaluation consists (ideally) of an accurate history, a complete physical examination, and radiographs. In many trauma cases, an accurate history of the accident cannot be obtained. The patient's past medical history must be integrated into the care plan. This information is obtained during the initial clinical examination. A complete examination of the cranium, the face, and the neck is performed in a systematic manner. The examination should progress from either superior to inferior or inferior to superior. This evaluation includes the assessment of symmetry and palpation of all bony surfaces to detect irregularities, bony crepitus, level discrepancy of bony structure, lacerations, bruises, and areas of tenderness. A sensory nerve evaluation detects sensory deficits. An evaluation of motor function should be completed. A full examination of the cranial nerves is required. A thorough search for occult lacerations of the

ear, including the ear canal, the scalp, the nasal and oral cavities, and the pharynx, should be completed. An evaluation of the patient's occlusion, the excursion of the mandible, the symmetry of the dental arches, the presence of broken or fractured teeth, and the ability to bring the teeth into full intercuspation in proper occlusion should be noted. The presence of intraoral lacerations, fractured or missing teeth, intraoral (especially gingival) lacerations, level discrepancies, or gaps in the dentition should suggest the possibility of a fracture involving the upper or lower jaw. Bruising or ecchymoses in the palate, buccal sulcus, or lips should suggest an underlying fracture. The visual acuity and pupillary responses should be noted in the record. Abnormal extraocular motion, double vision, and abnormalities of the globe and fundus should be searched for and identified.

Once the initial resuscitation and clinical evaluation have been completed, additional records and studies should be obtained contingent upon the patient's condition and treatment priority.

Old photographs from the family are sometimes helpful in demonstrating the preinjury structure of the patient's face. Preexisting facial asymmetry is sometimes not easily perceived from an examination. Study of preinjury photographs allows the surgeon to visualize the result to be obtained by surgical reconstruction. Plain radiographs may be obtained in the emergency department. These supplement the clinical evaluation and are most useful in the evaluation of mandibular fractures. They provide significant information in cases that require early operative intervention. The multiply injured patient should not be sent unaccompanied or unmonitored to the radiology department for extensive examinations. The combination of plain films and a physical examination sufficiently identifies most injuries requiring emergency treatment. Reversed Waters, Townes, anterior, posterior, and lateral skull films, and anterior-posterior and lateral oblique mandibular films may be obtained with portable techniques in the emergency departments. These films may be obtained even in patients with cervical spine injuries by proper positioning.

The craniofacial CT scan is an essential component of evaluation of any midface injury (11). Treatment should not proceed without it. It should be obtained following the initial examination of the patient, stabilization of vital signs, and confirmation that the patient is stable. The examination requires transportation to a CT scanner. Many patients will require observation or monitoring during this evaluation. The evaluation includes axial and coronal views to visualize the entire midface. In patients unable to be suitably positioned for coronal examinations, reconstructions from the axial images may be performed in the CT console. Patients with head injuries should have facial injury CTs completed at the time of cranial CT evaluations. CT scans are required on any frontal, basilar skull, frontal sinus, nasoethmoidal, orbital, zygomatic, or maxillary fracture. CT scans are also helpful even in nasal fractures to confirm the direction and degree of displacement and to exclude other injuries.

An arteriogram may rarely be necessary for the identification of a source of bleeding. In penetrating or ballistic injuries of the midface, arteriograms may be required to exclude damage to the internal carotid artery.

DENTAL MODELS

Dental models provide an essential record of the occlusion. They may be helpful in the construction of acrylic splints or positioning devices to assist management of fractures involving the occlusion (12). Alveolar fractures or sagittal fractures of the maxilla are injuries that may benefit from this management. Previous dental or orthodontic records may be helpful in determining preinjury occlusion. Patients who are partially dentulous sometimes have obscure occlusal relationships. Edentulous patients should have their dentures present for fracture reduction. Fractured dentures may be repaired with acrylic.

Management of Midfacial Fractures

Most facial injuries may be managed early after the injury. Early or immediate operative treatment is not associated with increased morbidity or mortality in the absence of other injuries. Significant injuries must be excluded by an orderly examination of all other organ systems. The early or immediate management of facial injuries is recommended for all cranial, nasoethmoidal, and frontal sinus fractures, as well as for open fractures, fractures with gross comminution or significant soft tissue lacerations, and gunshot and shotgun wounds. Highly comminuted injuries must have early stabilization. Patients with combined injuries of the frontal and midfacial skeleton benefit from early definitive fracture reduction. Early fracture reduction allows the soft tissue to heal over an anatomically reconstructed skeleton, and the patient's final appearance often benefits from early treatment (12–14). Delayed treatment requires increased dissection and soft tissue mobilization to be able to reposition fractured bones properly. Soft tissue contracture begins within 48 hr and impedes bone repositioning. All facial injuries have a component of soft tissue injury. Deferred treatment of facial injuries requires soft tissue incisions and dissection during the vulnerable period in which soft tissue is recovering from the initial injury. Soft tissue healing and contracture respond unfavorably to further surgical manipulation. Therefore, the appearance of the patient will be improved by early definitive fracture reduction because the soft tissue then undergoes a single healing period from the injury and the simultaneous reconstruction.

CEREBROSPINAL FLUID RHINORRHEA

The presence of cerebrospinal fluid (CSF) rhinorrhea is encountered in high maxillary and nasoethmoidal fractures. One fourth of the patients with Le Fort II and Le Fort III fractures demonstrate cerebrospinal fluid rhinorrhea, in which CSF leaks into the nose as the result of a dural and arachnoid laceration (15). Fifty to 75% of fron-

tal basilar and nasoethmoidal fractures are accompanied by CSF rhinorrhea. It may be difficult to identify CSF in the presence of bloody nasal secretions. The double ring sign, in which nasal discharge is absorbed onto a white paper towel, is sometimes helpful. A clear ring extending from a central blood-tinged spot is suggestive of blood-tinged CSF. Dural fistulas in the presence of displaced fractures are usually managed with direct operative repair.

In some cases, CSF fistulas are not associated with displaced fractures. These may or may not require definitive repair. Many CSF fistulas (in the absence of displaced fractures) will close within a 2-week period of observation (15). In fact, most (75%) seal within several days.

Antibiotics are of limited effectiveness in the sterilization of CSF when employed over a prolonged period (16–18). An antibiotic selectively inhibits the growth of susceptible organisms. Antibiotics are only effective in preventing meningitis from susceptible organisms. Given prolonged drainage of CSF, any antibiotics will eventually select resistant microorganisms as the colonizing agents. These organisms are more difficult to treat. The prolonged treatment of a CSF leak with antibiotics is thus not justified. Prophylactic "antibiotics" are often employed for a short (48–72-hr) period around the time of fracture reduction, especially if fracture reduction is performed immediately. Nasal packing and nasogastric tubes are generally avoided in patients with CSF fistulas because the presence of intranasal packing or tubes contributes to nasal obstruction and bacterial growth (19–21).

Patients who have Le Fort fractures and CSF fistulas should be initially placed in intermaxillary fixation. As a general principle, placing every patient with a maxillary fracture in intermaxillary fixation through the period of rigid fixation and fracture reduction is desirable. It immediately positions the occlusion and provides stability for facial fracture fragments. Surprisingly accurate reduction of a midfacial fracture may be provided merely by placing a patient in intermaxillary fixation.

All soft tissue injuries should be repaired as early as possible following the injury. Repair of soft tissue injuries and placing the jaws in intermaxillary fixation represent two desirable goals of midfacial injury treatment that can be accomplished in spite of the condition of the patient. They should always be accomplished.

Determining the Amount of Definitive Treatment to be Performed at the Time of the Injury

The amount of treatment to be administered on an early or immediate basis should be determined. The patient's other injuries are evaluated, and a conversation with the general surgeon is completed (4). As much treatment as possible should be completed as early after the injury as the patient's condition permits. Patients with multisystem injuries commonly suffer a number of septic complications, which begin about 1 week after the injury

(1, 4, 10). These include systemic sepsis, pulmonary failure, and deterioration of liver and renal function. Such complications preclude an early return to the operating room for definitive management of facial fractures. The multiply injured patient is often in the best condition that will be observed for a 2–3-week period immediately after the injury. The immediate postinjury period thus represents a desirable time for definitive maxillofacial fracture treatment in the face of multiple injuries.

Regional Management of Facial Fractures

NASAL FRACTURES

The nose, because of its prominent position, is one of the most commonly fractured bones of the facial skeleton. Additionally, its low resistance to impact makes it vulnerable to fracture.

In nasal fractures, displacement is generally lateral and posterior. Combinations are the routine. Fractures with lateral displacement are frequently the result of an altercation or a sporting accident. Injuries resulting from such insults vary from minimally depressed fractures isolated to the distal portion of the nasal skeleton to completely comminuted disruptions of all of the bony and cartilaginous components of the nose. The degree and type of displacement are confirmed both by physical analysis and by radiographs or CT scans. Patients who demonstrate posterior displacement have widening of the nasal bridge. Edema, crepitus, ecchymosis, and epistaxis are present. External or internal lacerations may be observed. A septal hematoma may accumulate around a septal fracture. Tenderness and swelling indicate the position of the nasal fracture. Partial or total airway obstruction may result from displaced bone, hematoma, or swelling. The nasal bones may be unstable either unilaterally or bilaterally.

Laterally dislocated nasal fractures are managed by a closed reduction under general or local anesthesia. The external nose is anesthetized by regional block, and the internal nose is anesthetized by cocaine on adrenalin-soaked pledgets. The fractures are first completed; then, the pyramid and septal fractures are repositioned by digital manipulation and instrumentation. An Asch forceps is used to position the septum, and an elevator or the back

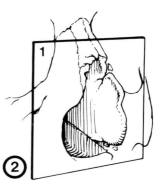

FIGURE 37.2. The pattern of disruption in plane 1 frontal impact nasal injuries. (Redrawn from Stranc MF, Robertson GA: A classification of internal injuries of the nasal skeleton. *Ann Plast Surg* 2:468, 1979.)

of a scalpel handle is used to reposition the fractured nasal bones from within the nose. Intranasal manipulation is alternated with external (finger) manipulation to reposition nasal bone fragments. Palpation and visualization confirm fracture reduction. It may be difficult to confirm fracture reduction when edema is severe; some surgeons prefer to wait until edema has resolved to allow improved perception of proper fracture reduction. An external splint and intranasal packing are used to support the fracture reduction. Any significant septal hematoma is drained to prevent cartilage necrosis.

Frontal impact nasal injuries are characterized by posterior displacement (Fig. 37.1). Stranc and Robertson (22) categorized nasal fractures by separately identifying lateral and posterior displacement. Frontal impact nasal fractures are divided into categories based on the degree of comminution and posterior displacement. Plane 1, plane 2, and plane 3 injuries exist, and vary with the force, comminution, and extent of fracture involvement of the nasal skeleton (Fig. 37.1). Plane 1 injuries present with edema and ecchymosis in the area of the distal nasal bridge and tip (Fig. 37.2). The force is concentrated primarily on the cartilage structures, and little comminution of the nasal bones is identified. The injury to the septum may be more severe and result in some irregularity of the

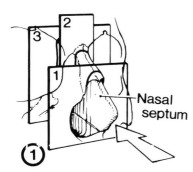

Nasal septum

FIGURE 37.1. Frontal impact nasal injury in planes 1, 2, and 3. (Redrawn from Stranc MF, Robertson GA: A classification of internal injuries of the nasal skeleton. *Ann Plast Surg* 2:468, 1979.)

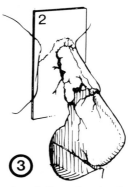

FIGURE 37.3. The site of disruption in plane 2 frontal impact nasal injuries. The nasal bones are comminuted. (Redrawn from Stranc MF, Robertson GA: A classification of internal injuries of the nasal skeleton. *Ann Plast Surg* 2:468, 1979.)

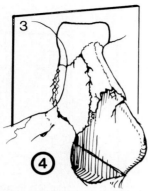

FIGURE 37.4. The site of disruption in plane 3 injuries. The frontal process of the maxilla (medial orbital rim) is comminuted. (Redrawn from Stranc MF, Robertson GA: A classification of internal injuries of the nasal skeleton. *Ann Plast Surg* 2:468, 1979.)

distal nose and some saddling of the distal bridge. Plane 1 injuries are treated by closed reduction.

Plane 2 injuries (Fig. 37.3) demonstrate increased comminution. The fracture is usually bilateral, and there is moderate edema, ecchymosis, and widening of the nasal bridge. Dorsal depression is easily identified. Most plane 2 fractures are managed by closed reduction. When the fracture involvement is severe, significant saddling of the dorsum may persist despite closed reduction manipulation. Such patients may be managed with early or delayed bone or cartilage grafting to augment the height of the nose. When septal fractures are severe, initial repositioning may not guarantee nasal airway patency. Patients with nasal fractures should be advised that they may require a nasal septal reconstruction some months after the injury, depending on the direction of cartilage deformation with healing.

Plane 3 nasal fractures (Fig. 37.4) result from severe injury forces. They demonstrate fractures extending outside the nasal skeleton and into the medial orbits. These injuries are characterized by fractures of the frontal process of the maxilla and are in fact nasoethmoidal-orbital fractures. Abnormal intracranial findings and other midfacial fractures typically accompany these injuries. Marked loss of nasal skeletal support and extreme comminution of the nasal bones are detected on physical examination. Unilateral or bilateral telecanthus characterize these injuries. Plane 3 injuries require open reduction and internal fixation with immediate bone grafting. This open reduction may be performed through lacerations if appropriate. Otherwise, the coronal incision is preferred. In unusual cases, local incisions (the midline, frontal nasal, or horizontal limb of an open sky incision) may be employed for plane 3 (nasoethmoidal-orbital) fracture reduction. Precise repositioning of all existing bone and cartilage is performed with direct exposure of all fractured bone fragments. Shortening and contracture of the nasal skeleton are reduced if immediate bone and cartilage grafting supplement the repair of existing supporting structures.

In the treatment of the common nasal fracture, the most frequent mistake is to fail to thoroughly complete the fracture. After reduction, the nasal bones must be easily deviated in either direction if postoperative stability is to be assured. Occasionally, osteotomy is necessary to complete a "greenstick" fracture. Thorough completion of septal fractures by instrumentation with an Asch forceps allows replacement of the septum in a normal position. If the attachments of the upper or lower lateral cartilages are torn, the dislocated cartilages should be replaced by direct suturing techniques. Generally, such avulsion is accompanied by an external laceration. All patients with nasal fractures should be warned that revisional procedures are frequently required. These may include procedures to reposition the nasal pyramid, reposition the nasal septum, or improve the airway. The healing of fractures involving cartilage is unpredictable. The mucoperichondrium exerts tension as the area heals and may cause the cartilage to warp during the period of healing, resulting in deviation.

Certain nasal fractures exhibit depression of the nasal dorsum. These represent Stranc plane 2 or 3 nasal injuries with comminution of the distal nose and result in loss of the height, projection, and length of the nose. Isolated plane 2 or 3 nasal fractures may require dorsal nasal bone or cartilage grafting, and nasal fractures that are open through lacerations tend to benefit from open reduction, which is accomplished either with fine plates and screws or small (#30) wires. The provision of a dorsal nasal bone graft (utilizing either calvarial or rib sources) and the provision of a caudal cartilage strut are sometimes required to reestablish the normal skeletal dimensions of the original nasal architecture in plane 2 or 3 injuries.

NASOETHMOID FRACTURES

Nasoethmoid fractures are in reality plane 3 nasal fractures. The sine qua non of the nasoethmoidal injury is a fracture involving the medial orbital rim (Fig. 37.5). The lower two thirds of the orbital rim contains the area for attachment of the canthal ligament (23). Once this section of bone is fractured, the potential for canthal ligament displacement exists (24). In recent schemes of classification of nasoethmoidal-orbital injuries (23, 25), this area represents the "central fragment" of more complicated nasoethmoidal-orbital injuries. Mobility of this fragment may be assessed with direct digital pressure over the canthal ligament. Displacement or a "click" indicates mobility. Alternatively, a bimanual examination (26) may be performed with a clamp inside the nose underneath the canthal ligament and an index fingertip palpating deeply over the medial orbital rim externally. Simultaneous internal and external pressure by clamp and digital manipulation allows the central fragment to move between the index finger and the clamp. Mobility or displacement indicates the need for an open reduction.

A high index of suspicion should be present to identify minimally displaced nasoethmoidal-orbital fractures (11). About one third of nasoethmoidal fractures are unilateral

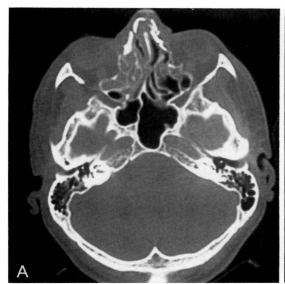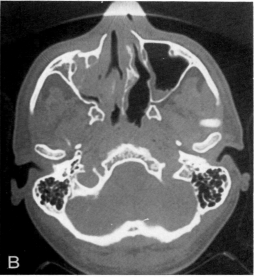

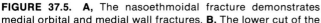

FIGURE 37.5. A, The nasoethmoidal fracture demonstrates medial orbital and medial wall fractures. **B,** The lower cut of the axial CT scan demonstrates the inferior orbital rim fracture. Illustrated is a unilateral nasoethmoidal-orbital fracture.

(Fig. 37.5), and many are only slightly displaced or impacted. The presence of lacerations in the forehead or nasal area, ''spectacle'' hematoma, and the presence of a moderately displaced frontal impact nasal fracture with depression of the bridge and shortening of the nose should indicate the possibility of a nasoethmoidal-orbital injury. Both the CT scan and a thorough clinical evaluation should be performed to confirm the diagnosis. In frontal impact nasal fractures, the nose appears foreshortened and has a dorsal depression and an obtuse nasolabial angle. Nasoethmoidal fractures commonly are accompanied by nasal bleeding, and a CSF leak may be present. In the acute injury, the CSF leak may not be identifiable because of the presence of bloody nasal secretion. Telecanthus is absolute evidence of a nasoethmoidal-orbital fracture. The degree of telecanthus depends on the degree of comminution of the fractures and the presence of intact periosteal attachments. Initially, the intercanthal distance may not appear increased, but it may increase with time from the initial injury.

The radiographic diagnosis of the nasoethmoidal-orbital injury is indicated by fractures surrounding the central fragment on a CT scan (11). Fractures should involve the nose, the junction of the frontal process of the maxilla with the glabella, the inferior orbital rim, and the medial (ethmoidal) orbital wall. These four fractures define the central fragment as ''free'' and potentially able to displace. Medial orbital wall and floor fractures are seen universally with nasoethmoidal-orbital injuries. There are fluid levels present in the ethmoid and maxillary sinuses.

Plain radiographs do not accurately confirm the nasoethmoidal-orbital fracture. Axial and coronal CT scans provide precise capability for definition of the injury and for planning the reconstruction. Isolated ethmoidal fractures (medial orbital wall) are not nasoethmoidal injuries and frequently do not require treatment if the extent of displacement is minimal.

CT scans should be taken in the axial and coronal planes, and the interval of section should be reduced 1.5–2.0 mm for reconstruction. The areas of the brain, frontal bone, and frontal sinus as well as the entire maxilla must be assessed. The examination must be complete in order to define extensions of nasoethmoidal fractures that may occur unilaterally or bilaterally. Nasoethmoidal fractures commonly accompany unilateral orbital injuries such as the supraorbital fracture or fracture dislocation of the zygoma. Bilateral injuries are often seen in craniofacial and Le Fort fractures.

Nasoethmoidal fractures are generally seen in four fracture patterns (23):

1. Localized central midface injury. This is an isolated nasoethmoidal fracture and is usually observed bilaterally. The fracture may be confined to the nasoethmoidal-orbital area, or it may extend into the zygomatic or frontal sinus region.
2. Lateral orbital nasal injuries: These fractures are unilateral and extend either superiorly into the frontal bone or inferiorly into the inferior orbital rim. Nasal fractures occur with this injury.
3. High Le Fort (II or III) fractures: These may be either unilateral or bilateral. They are either comminuted or noncomminuted.
4. Craniofacial fractures: The common pattern of a craniofacial injury includes a Le Fort III fracture on one side and a Le Fort IV fracture with frontal bone involvement on the contralateral side.

The central fracture fragment of the nasoethmoidal-orbital injury consists of the lower two thirds of the medial orbital rim, which includes the attached canthal ligament and the lacrimal fossa. Medial orbital rim fractures and fractures of the orbital floor, medial orbital wall, nose, frontal sinus, medial supraorbital rim, and medial maxilla are also present with varying degree of comminution.

The timing of treatment of nasoethmoidal-orbital fractures is important because improved aesthetic results are more easily achieved when early open reduction is performed. Fractures are ideally treated soon after the injury, and it has been our experience that it becomes more difficult to obtain a good aesthetic result when reductions occur more than 2–3 days after the fracture.

Closed treatment is not appropriate for nasoethmoidal-orbital fractures that are mobile or displaced. Open reduction must be performed (Fig. 37.6) and should include the following:

1. A thorough exposure of all fractured areas.
2. Initial linking of the fragments with interfragment wires.
3. Replacement of bone gaps in the medial orbital wall, floor, and nose with autogenous bone graft material.
4. Junctional (frontal bone and inferior orbital rim) plate and screw fixation performed following tightening of the interfragment wires.

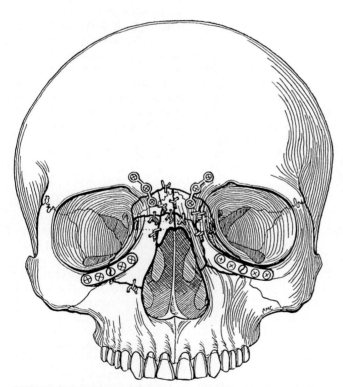

FIGURE 37.6. Open reduction of nasoethmoidal-orbital fracture. After adequate exposure, all orbital rim and nasal bone fragments are linked with interfragment wires. The transnasal reduction of the medial orbital rims is the most important step in nasoethmoidal-orbital fracture treatment and is performed posterior and superior to the medial canthal ligament. Dislocation of the central (canthal tendon–bearing) bone fragment anteriorly and laterally allows placement of drill holes posterior to the ligament. The wires are passed, then tightened. The assembled bone fragments are stabilized by junctional plate and screw fixation to the frontal bone and to the inferior orbital rims.

5. A wired transnasal reduction of the medial orbital rim. This is the most essential component of nasoethmoidal-orbital fracture treatment. It should be performed posterior and superior to the lacrimal fossa. The canthal ligament should not be detached in the reduction because this step avoids the step of canthal reattachment.

Surgical Exposure

Occasionally, an overlying laceration is suitable for exposure of a localized fracture. Lacerations should not be significantly extended; this generally results in additional deformity. Local incisions are only appropriate for localized fractures. The vertical midline incision over the root of the nose may be used in Caucasians, or the horizontal limb only of the open sky approach may be preferred for direct exposure. In bald patients, a local incision may be preferred over a coronal incision for localized fractures.

The standard surgical exposure of a nasoethmoidal-orbital fracture involves a coronal incision to expose the superior orbit, the use of subciliary incisions (skin-muscle flap) to expose the inferior orbit, and the use of a gingival-buccal sulcus incision to expose the pyriform aperture and the nasomaxillary buttresses.

Technique of Open Reduction

Fracture fragments are exposed, mobilized, and linked with interfragment wires. The entire orbital rim should be initially reconstituted with interfragment wiring. Holes are drilled posterior and superior to the lacrimal fossa in the central fragment of the medial orbital rim. Several sets of wires are passed transnasally at this level to reattach a detached canthus, to provide wires for an external soft tissue bolster, and, most importantly, for the transnasal reduction of the medial orbital rims.

The interfragment wires and the transnasal reduction wires are tightened. Junctional plate and screw fixation is then used to stabilize the nasoethmoidal complex superiorly to the frontal bone and inferiorly to the remainder of the inferior orbital rim. At this point, inspection of the medial and inferior internal orbit reveals any need for bone grafts. A bone graft is often used on the nasal dorsum to augment height, to correct projection, or simply to smooth dorsal nasal contour.

Ideally, the canthal ligament should not be detached in the reduction. If the canthal ligament requires reattachment, it should be connected to an additional set of transnasal reduction wires that are passed posterior and superior to the lacrimal fossa. This reattachment is the final step in tightening soft tissue to the bony skeleton prior to closing the coronal incision. Medial orbital bone grafting should be completed before the canthal ligament reattachment is performed. If detached, the lateral aspect of the canthal ligament is generally exposed with a 1–2-mm incision adjacent to the medial commissure of the eyelids. A braided suture is passed two times through the canthal ligament, avoiding the lacrimal system (27). This suture is then passed internally to the inner aspect of the coronal incision and connected to the transnasal reduction wires. Tightening the wires allows for an accurate reapproximation of the canthal ligament to the bony skeleton.

It is virtually impossible to overcorrect the intercanthal distance. The bony intercanthal distance in Caucasians should be 16–23 mm, and an additional 5–7 mm per side of "soft tissue distance" should be added. When required, the transnasal canthopexy should be completed after the initial bone reduction, and the remainder of the incisions then closed.

Soft tissue bolsters may be used to approximate skin to the bony skeleton. They help reestablish the "nasoorbital valley" and prevent the accumulation of soft tissue swelling or hematoma between the reconstructed skeleton and the skin. Any bolsters used should be padded with orthopaedic felt wrapped with Xeroform gauze. They are removed 1–3 weeks after the surgery. These "compression bolsters" have no function in the maintenance of the intercanthal distance, which must be achieved with an internal open reduction.

Dorsal nasal bone grafts are often best positioned with the use of a small maxillary adaption plate attached from the frontal bone to the posterior-superior aspect of the nasal bone graft. This allows for adjustment of the projection of the dorsum of the nose. A patient treated with open reduction and bone grafting is seen in Figure 37.7.

Occasionally, a caudal cartilage graft should be added to re-create soft tissue support for the caudal aspect of the nose.

INTERNAL ORBIT

The internal orbit is reconstructed by (*a*) repositioning fragments of the rim, (*b*) identifying the location of intact bone in the back of the orbit, and (*c*) laying bone graft between these landmarks. In the floor, an intact orbital bone "ledge" is usually present 30–38 mm behind the anterior rim. Bone grafts may be positioned between the reconstructed anterior rim and the posterior ledge following identification of an intact bony margin all around the defect. Medially, the ledge of intact bone is usually present at or before the posterior ethmoidal foramen. Bone grafts should be positioned from this area extending anteriorly to the lacrimal system to reproduce the normal contour of the ethmoidal sinuses.

The lacrimal system is usually injured in the canalicular portion by direct lacerations or by medial canthal ligament avulsion; both are infrequent. The "bony" lacrimal system is the most frequently compromised area; repositioning the bone fragments allows for the best function of the system. Exploration of the lacrimal system is not performed at the time of the facial fracture repair except in

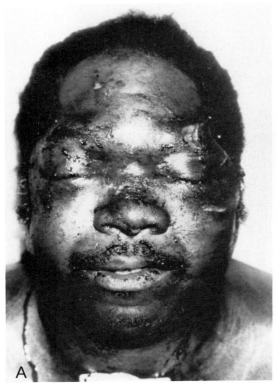 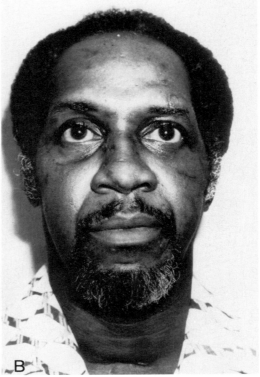

FIGURE 37.7.   A, A patient with Le Fort III, nasoethmoid, bilateral subcondylar, and mandibular body fractures is seen following injury. **B,** Postoperative result obtained following a single operation that included complete open reduction and bone grafting.

instances of direct laceration or ligament avulsion (27). Several studies have shown that the lacrimal system functions best when the bone fragments are precisely reduced.

FRACTURES OF THE ZYGOMA

Fractures of the zygomatic area represent the second most frequent midfacial injury. The prominent position of the malar eminence accounts for the frequency of fracture dislocation. Zygomatic fractures may occur either as an isolated injury or in combination with other fractures, such as Le Fort fractures (11). There are certain clinical findings that should suggest the presence of a zygomatic fracture. The most sensitive are the combination of pe-

riorbital ecchymosis and subconjunctival hemorrhage. If the zygomatic bone is depressed, there may be depression of the lateral canthus by virtue of the fact that the lateral canthus attaches to Whitnall's tubercle, which is on the internal surface of the frontal process of the zygoma. Depression of the cheek may be observed following resolution of the swelling. There may be palpable "step" deformities of the lateral and inferior orbital rim. Unilateral epistaxis is often present because of the maxillary sinus fracture. If extraocular muscles are contused or entrapped, diplopia may result. If the floor of the orbit is significantly depressed, the globe may sink backward and downward, producing enophthalmos and ocular dystopia. A hematoma may be observed in the upper buccal sulcus. If the zygomatic arch is depressed medially, it may impinge on the coronoid process of the mandible,

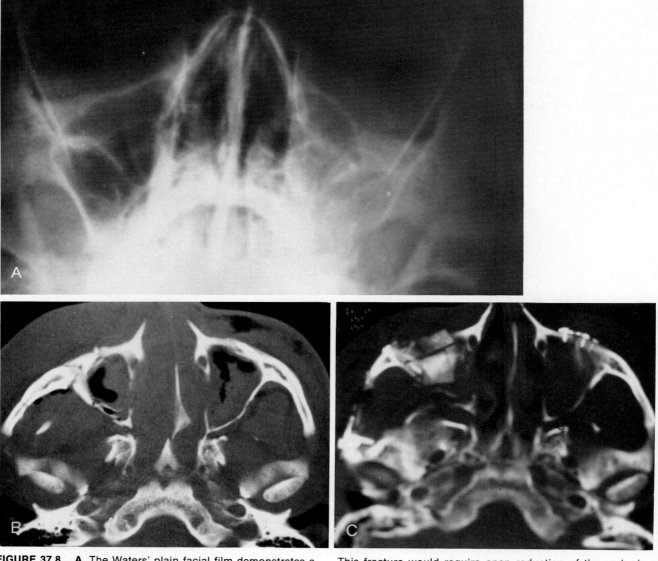

FIGURE 37.8. **A,** The Waters' plain facial film demonstrates a zygomatic fracture. **B and C,** CT scans demonstrate a more complex zygomatic fracture with lateral displacement of the arch.

This fracture would require open reduction of the arch via a coronal incision, combined with standard anterior approaches (lower eyelid and gingival sulcus exposures).

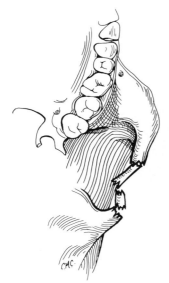

FIGURE 37.9. An isolated zygomatic arch fracture is depicted; medial displacement in a "W"-shaped form is common.

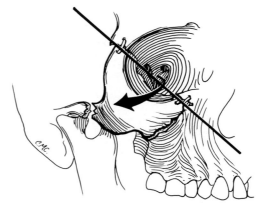

FIGURE 37.11. Wire interfragment fixation of the zygoma at the orbital rim merely creates an axis about which rotation can occur. Wires should be used for initial positioning. The reduction should then be adjusted by forcep traction and stabilized by plate and screw fixation. In noncomminuted fractures, the zygomaticofrontal suture and inferior orbital rim are used for stabilization. In comminuted injuries, the zygomaticofrontal suture, the inferior orbital rim, and the zygomaticomaxillary buttress are utilized. If lateral displacement of the zygomatic arch is identified on the CT scan, an open reduction of the zygomatic arch by a coronal incision is required by a medial displacement is managed through anterior approach.

restricting mandibular function. Numbness in the distribution of the infraorbital nerve is a reliable sign of zygomatic or orbital floor fracture. Anesthesia or hypesthesia may involve the upper anterior maxillary teeth alone or the soft tissues of the ipsilateral upper lip, cheek, and nose. Difficulty chewing and a minor occlusal disturbance may accompany zygomatic fractures in the presence of swelling involving the temporal region, depression of the arch, or posterior displacement of the malar eminence by virtue of interference with the coronoid process.

Radiographic evaluation must include a CT scan. Plain films (unnecessary if a CT scan is taken) also demonstrate the injury (28), and Waters', Caldwell's, and submen-

tovertex views are those usually obtained. The Waters' view (Fig. 37.8**A**) identifies the lateral wall of the maxillary antrum, the inferior orbital rim, and the orbital floor. The submentovertex view identifies depression of the zygomatic arch and the anterior prominence of the malar eminence. The Caldwell's view demonstrates distraction at the zygomaticofrontal suture. A CT scan most accurately demonstrates the injury (Fig. 37.8**B**).

Isolated fractures of the zygomatic arch generally demonstrate only medial displacement (29; Fig. 37.9). Frequently, a W-shaped deformity with depression of the lateral cheek is identified. If the medial displacement is

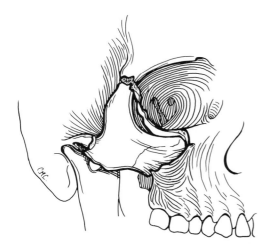

FIGURE 37.10. A zygomatic fracture that demonstrates complete dislocation at all anterior buttress articulations. Open reduction would be required through anterior approaches. Anterior approaches consist of **(a)** a lower eyelid incision and **(b)** an exposure through the gingival-buccal sulcus. The zygomaticofrontal suture is exposed by detaching the lateral canthal ligament and retracting the incision superiorly.

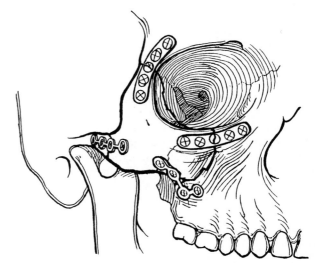

FIGURE 37.12. Fixation of the zygoma is performed at its buttress articulations by initial interfragment wire reduction, which is then stabilized by plate and screw fixation.

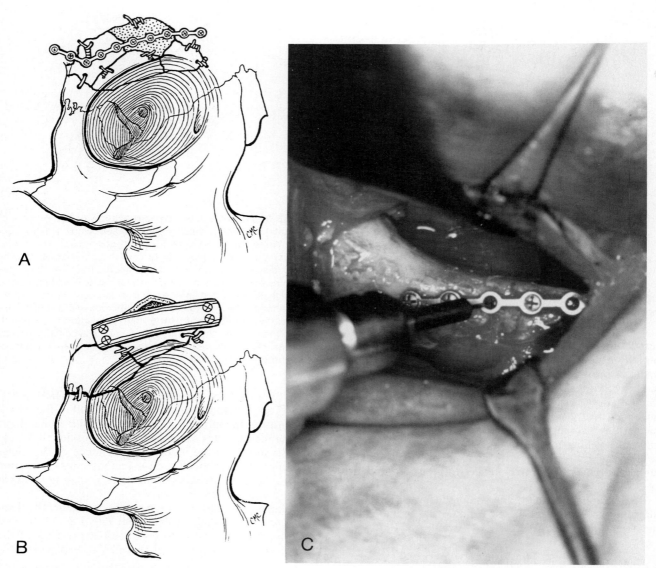

FIGURE 37.13. A, Fragments of the superior orbital rim are reassembled by interfragment wires. **B,** Autogenous bone grafts (such as rib or calvarial bone) are used for bone defects. Lag screw fixation of the bone graft is seen. The assembled fragments are stabilized with plate and screw fixation to improve projection and contour. **C,** The microsystem is used at the inferior orbital rim.

sufficient, the arch impinges on the coronoid process of the mandible and restricts motion. Isolated fractures of the zygomatic arch may be reduced through a Gillie's approach. An incision is made in the temporal region through the temporal fascia to expose the temporalis muscle (29). An elevator is passed underneath the arch, and by pressing the arch laterally, the arch is reduced. Usually, further support is not required because the arch is stable. Occasionally, an arch requires support by means of an open reduction, K wire fixation, or packing beneath the arch. Some surgeons place a protective guard over the arch and tape it to the skin to prevent postoperative displacement.

All zygomatic fractures should be evaluated with an axial and a coronal CT scan. In patients who are not able to have true coronal images, the axial images should be reconstructed coronally. Zygomatic fractures should be analyzed by CT scan for confirmation of both displacement and fragmentation. Displaced fractures should be treated with an open reduction. Anterior approaches (the subciliary and gingival-buccal sulcus incisions) may be utilized for fractures that do not demonstrate lateral displacement or comminution of the zygomatic arch (Fig. 37.10). Fractures that show extreme displacement of the malar eminence and shattering of the greater wing of the sphenoid are usually accompanied by lateral displacement of the zygomatic arch, and all of these deformities benefit from the coronal approach (Fig. 37.11). They can be visualized and anatomically reduced only with the full approach of the anterior incisions (gingival-buccal sulcus and lower lid skin-muscle flap with detachment of the lateral canthus for exposure of the zygomaticofrontal suture) and the addition of a coronal incision for arch and lateral orbital exposure. Most zygoma fractures (and 95% of isolated zygoma fractures are included in this group) may be satisfactorily reduced through anterior incisions alone. The zygomaticofrontal suture, infraorbital rim, greater wing of the sphenoid, and zygomaticomaxillary buttress are visualized, and interfragment wires are placed to provide initial alignment (Fig. 37.12). Final adjustments of bone position are made, and a five-hole maxillary adaption plate is placed at the zygomaticofrontal suture. The microsystem is used for the infraorbital rim (Fig. 37.13**A**), and an ''L'' plate from the 2.0 mm system is used at the zygomaticomaxillary buttress adjacent to the maxillary alveolus.

Some zygomatic fractures are minimally displaced and theoretically amenable to a closed reduction. For a closed reduction to be stable, the fracture should be ''greensticked'' or incomplete at the zygomaticofrontal suture (the incomplete component provides stability) (29). The displaced portion of the fracture is then pushed back into position by a variety of reduction maneuvers that employ force either within the maxillary sinus or beneath the malar eminence. The ''greenstick'' component renders the fracture stable. Closed reductions may also be rendered stable by ''wedging'' or ''interlocking'' of fracture edges. Closed reduction methods have their disadvantages. Studies have shown that open reductions provide more consistent and accurate alignment and provide better stability. Fractures treated by closed reduction should be carefully selected; they must be nondisplaced at the zygomaticofrontal suture, should be treated early, and should be completely noncomminuted. In practice, I utilize closed reductions only for zygomatic arch fractures.

The number of sites of fixation for a zygomatic fracture reduction is open to question (30). For minimally comminuted fractures, one plate at the zygomaticofrontal suture is probably sufficient. My practice is always to additionally place a small (microsystem) (Fig. 37.13**B**) plate at the inferior orbital rim, which is a guide to alignment. For any comminuted injuries, it is helpful to provide both alignment and fixation at at least three anterior sites: the zygomaticofrontal suture, the inferior orbital rim, and the zygomaticomaxillary buttress. Exposure of all three of these areas is obtained through two incisions; the lower lid subciliary skin flap (31) and the gingival buccal sulcus. The conjunctival incision with lateral canthotomy may substitute for the lower lid skin-muscle flap. The lateral canthus is routinely detached and then reattached after completing the fracture reduction. It should be reattached toward the level of the zygomaticofrontal suture.

If the arch is laterally displaced, an open reduction through a coronal incision is required. The arch should be reconstructed as flat as possible to enhance malar projection. As the arch is brought into a flat reduction, the greater wing of the sphenoid comes into alignment with the oribtal process of the zygoma. This is a sensitive guide to both proper malar projection and proper arch reduction.

FRONTAL BONE AND FRONTOBASILAR FRACTURES

Trauma to the forehead may result in fractures of the frontal bone. The bone fracture often includes the supraorbital and temporal area and the frontal sinus. Often, two areas of the frontal skull, a lateral area and a central (frontal sinus) region, are involved in an injury. Patients with forehead lacerations and ecchymoses should be thoroughly examined to exclude frontal fractures. The neurological status may be normal or may be altered as the result of a cerebral contusion. A high index of suspicion should be present so that all fractures may be identified. The occult fracture of the posterior wall of the frontal sinus is especially important to identify because it implies possible brain injury. A CT scan is the best diagnostic evaluation of the frontal sinus and the anterior cranial fossa frontal bone (32).

Occasionally, frontal bone injuries may be treated through existing lacerations. Usually, it is wiser to expose the area with a coronal incision.

Fractures of the frontal sinus may involve the anterior wall alone, the anterior and posterior wall, the posterior wall alone, or both walls and the nasal frontal duct. Fractures of the anterior wall may be treated by localized mucosal débridement and replacement of anterior wall fragments (33–37). It is essential that the nasal frontal duct be functioning to utilize this limited reconstructive technique.

When frontal sinus fractures involve the anterior and the posterior walls and most of the posterior wall is to be preserved, there are several treatment chocies: (*a*) limited débridement, (*b*) obliteration by either osteoneogenesis or bone grafting, and (*c*) cranialization.

One choice is débridement of all mucosa and obliteration by plugging the duct and filling the cavity with bone grafts. Reconstruction of the anterior wall is completed. When excessive comminution of posterior wall bone exists, cranialization is preferred. Always, mucosal fragments are débrided, and any CSF leak is closed. The success of reconstructive treatment methods depends on proper function of the nasal frontal duct (38), which cannot be guaranteed. Studies have shown that the nasal frontal duct may not remain open following even moderate injury. It is my preference to manage most frontal sinus injuries by obliteration. Following repair of the CSF leak and débridement of any loose posterior wall fragments, all sinus mucosa is removed, and the walls of the sinus are lightly burred with an abrasive bit to eliminate invaginated areas of mucosa. The nasal frontal duct is then covered with several layers of calvarial bone graft. The first layer is impacted into the duct. The remainder of the frontal sinus may be filled with calvarial bone shavings (39) or allowed to auto-obliterate.

For years, I routinely plugged the nasal frontal duct but did not obliterate the remainder of the frontal sinus cavity. The frontal sinus cavity then fills slowly with a combination of scar tissue and bone over time, a process called osteoneogenesis. The procedure by which the cavity is obliterated with calvarial bone shavings is a better procedure in my opinion. It does require meticulous mucosal removal or abscess formation will rapidly follow.

When the entire posterior sinus wall has been destroyed it is removed, and frontal sinus should be "cranialized." This is performed by removing all remaining fragments of mucosa, burring the existing walls with an abrasive bit, and reconstructing the anterior cranial fossa floor with calvarial bone grafts. Several layers of bone graft are used, and the initial layer is impacted into the duct. The procedure essentially converts the frontal sinus into a portion of the cranial cavity, hence "cranialization."

Frontal bone fractures often include a linear fracture extension along the anterior cranial fossa. The fracture extends along the roof of the orbit and back through the base of the skull (32). Often, frontal fractures exist with nasoethmoidal, upper orbital, and Le Fort fractures. These upper Le Fort fractures may produce a CSF leak even in the absence of a frontal vault fracture. Such symptoms occur by fracture extension along the base of the anterior cranial fossa. Fractures that comminute the vault of the frontal bone are managed by reduction, initial positioning with interosseous wiring, and plate and screw fixation, following the appropriate neurosurgical procedure. Plate and screw fixation stabilizes projection of bone fragments initially linked with wires (40, 41). The frontal bone fragments provide an abundant source of calvarial bone graft by harvest of the inner table. The use of small (1.5-mm or microsystem) plates in the frontal area makes reconstruction materials less palpable and visible.

Success in primary bone replacement in frontal basilar fractures requires proper management of involved frontal and ethmoidal sinuses. In the absence of definitive management as described, with elimination of the sinus mucosa and bone grafting, an incidence of major complications of 20–30% follows central midface and frontal crush fractures. Major complications may result in meningitis, brain abscess, and death.

Treatment should now be oriented toward primary reconstruction of the frontal bone with existing fragments almost irrespective of the degree of injury. In rare cases, the patient's condition may be such that the skin is simply closed following neurosurgery and a delayed cranioplasty is performed.

In the event of infection, the usual etiology is obstruction of the frontal and ethmoidal sinuses. Infections require drainage and débridement of devitalized bone, and may require abandoning the reconstruction if the infection persists. Localized infections often respond to drainage and local débridement without dismantling the bone reconstruction (42).

SAGITTAL FRACTURES OF THE MAXILLA AND PALATE

Sagittal fractures of the maxilla and palate are less common than other types of Le Fort and maxillary fractures (43). They may exist either as an isolated alveolar fracture, separating a hemialveolus from the remainder of the maxilla, or as a segment of a more complicated Le Fort injury, which extends superiorly within the midfacial skeleton. Patients with a maxillary fracture that includes sagittal division of the palate present with abnormal lateral mobility of the segments of the maxillary dentition. The fracture line usually exits anteriorly between the first bicuspids and extends along the midline of the palate. Anterior, lateral, and superior displacement of the unstable segment are typical; the palatal mucosa, gingiva, and lip are frequently lacerated. Vertical lacerations of the lip and the gingival mucosa should suggest the possibility of a sagittal fracture of the maxilla.

These fractures require stabilization either with open reduction (Fig. 37.14) or a dental acrylic splint (Fig. 37.15). Internal fixation involves stabilization in the roof of the mouth with plates and screws (Fig. 37.14**A**). Either a longitudinal incision over the fracture or the palatal laceration serves as access to the fracture. The fracture should be stabilized by open reduction with plate and screw fixation at the pyriform aperture (Fig. 37.14**B**). The Le Fort I level buttresses, nasomaxillary, and zygomaticomaxillary buttresses should also be stabilized with internal fixation and bone grafting. Bone grafts should be employed if bone gaps exceed 5 mm. The use of a dental acrylic splint is sometimes necessary to provide fine occlusal alignment of the dentition. A dental splint is placed on the palatal surface of the maxillary teeth and covers a portion of the roof of the mouth. It prevents rotation of the maxillary dental segments. The dental splint is made from dental models that are sectioned at the areas of the fracture and reassembled into a proper occlusal relationship. The dental splint is either ligated to the molar and bicuspid teeth or fixed by the use of a circumpalatal wire that extends up over the floor of the nose on each side (Fig. 37.15). Occasionally, a smaller segment of the maxilla, representing the posterolateral alveolar segment containing the molar teeth, will be fractured. This segment usually is displaced laterally, superiorly, and posteriorly. This fracture is treated with a dental acrylic splint and perhaps by open reduction. Alveolar fractures of the maxilla may require 12–16 weeks to fully consolidate; constant observation of the occlusion is indicated through the period of healing.

Le Fort Fractures

The classification of maxillary fractures was developed by René Le Fort (44) on the basis of cadaver experiments performed in the early portion of this century (Fig. 37.16). Le Fort used the superior level where the facial bones were sectioned from the upper facial or cranial skeleton as the designation of the Le Fort fracture level. The fracture levels represent weak areas of the midfacial skeleton that are predisposed to fracture (44, 45).

A Le Fort I level fracture is a transverse or horizontal fracture that separates the lower maxillary alveolus from the superior midfacial skeleton. The fracture line runs above the base above the roots of the maxillary teeth from the pyriform aperture to the pterygoid plate area.

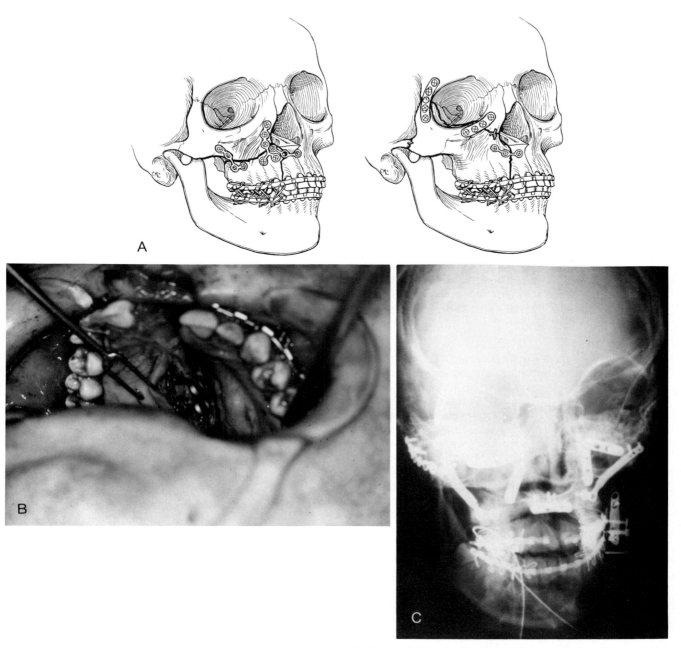

FIGURE 37.14. **A,** Sagittal fractures of the maxilla require precise open reduction spanning fractures anteriorly. Two fracture variations are seen. **B,** Exposure of the fracture in the roof of the mouth allows stabilization with plate and screw reduction. Open reduction and internal fixation are additionally performed at the pyriform aperture **(A–C)** and the zygomaticomaxillary buttress **(A, C)** to stabilize the fracture to the remainder of the maxilla. Plate and screw fixation is utilized. For fractures extending higher in the facial skeleton, plate and screw fixation extends to stabilize each fracture site. (**A** from Manson PN, Shack RB, Leonard LG, Su CT, Hoopes JE: Sagittal fractures of the maxilla and palate. *Plast Reconstr Surg* 72:484, 1983.)

The Le Fort II fracture is a pyramidal fracture of the maxilla. It separates a central nasomaxillary segment from the zygomatic and upper lateral orbital portions of the midfacial skeleton. The Le Fort II level fracture may travel over the distal nose through its cartilaginous portion, enter the opposite orbit, and cross the inferior orbital rims to separate the lateral zygoma from the medial maxilla as the fracture travels toward the pterygoid plate region. Upper Le Fort II level fractures separate the frontal processes of the maxilla and the nasal bones from the glabellar region of the frontal bone. The remainder of the fracture line is as previously described.

The Le Fort III level fracture represents the true craniofacial dysjunction (46, 47), by which the cranium is com-

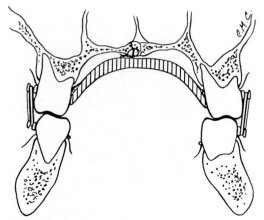

FIGURE 37.15. The use of an acrylic palatal splint is helpful in some cases of dentoalveolar fractures to stabilize the dentition. The acrylic splint, placed on the palatal surface of the teeth, stabilizes the teeth against rotation in the face of intermaxillary elastic traction. (From Manson PN, Shack RB, Leonard LG, Su CT, Hoopes JE: Sagittal fractures of the maxilla and palate. *Plast Reconstr Surg* 72:484, 1983.)

pletely separated from the facial bones. The fracture begins at the zygomaticofrontal junction and traverses the lateral, inferior, and medial orbit to travel between the frontal processes of the maxilla, the nasal bones, and the glabella. A Le Fort III superior level fracture is commonly present unilaterally with a Le Fort II superior level fracture on the opposite side. Analysis of the facial bone fragments in the usual Le Fort III fracture case generally reveals comminuted facial fractures below the superior level of the fracture on each side. The Le Fort III level fracture thus often consists of a separate zygomatic segment, and Le Fort I and II maxillary segments. Occasion-

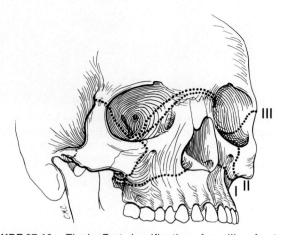

FIGURE 37.16. The Le Fort classification of maxillary fractures. The Le Fort I fracture is a horizontal fracture sectioning the maxillary alveolus from the upper craniofacial skeleton. The Le Fort II fracture separates a pyramidally shaped nasomaxillary fragment from the upper craniofacial skeleton. The Le Fort III fractu⎯ is a craniofacial dysjunction, separating all the facial bones from the cranium. Generally, combinations of fractures exist in the same injury. Comminution is the rule, rather than the pure patterns illustrated.

ally, a high Le Fort II or III level fracture will exist as a single fragment and demonstrate little or no maxillary mobility. These fractures are minimally displaced and present with only slight occlusal disturbance. Bilateral eyelid ecchymoses are invariably present. Air-fluid levels are seen in the maxillary and ethmoidal sinuses on CT scan.

The Le Fort IV fracture level was not described by Le Fort (32). The designation of "Le Fort IV" level refers to the frontal basilar region, which consists of the frontal bone, frontal sinus, superior orbital rims, and anterior cranial base. Many Le Fort maxillary fractures extend into the frontal area, and these are designated as Le Fort IV level fractures.

The usual symptoms of a maxillary fracture are maxillary mobility and malocclusion. In Le Fort II and III level fractures, bilateral eyelid ecchymoses will be present. Nasopharyngeal bleeding may be profuse, depending on the severity of the fracture. Facial edema is present. A CSF fistula occurs in 25–50% of upper (Le Fort II and III) fractures. The patients often demonstrate an elongated and retruded midface with an anterior open bite in untreated injuries (48). Signs of zygomatic, nasal, nasoethmoidal and orbital floor, and medial orbital fractures may be present. Occasionally, a Le Fort fracture is displaced but not mobile (49).

Intermaxillary fixation is the principle treatment utilized to restore the projection of the lower midface by placing the patient into proper occlusion. Intermaxillary fixation should be applied as soon as possible after the injury, and the use of intermaxillary fixation minimizes further fracture displacement. Intermaxillary fixation to an intact mandible restores the projection of the lower midfacial segment by aligning it with a normally positioned mandible. The stability and projection of the upper midface must be restored by open reduction and rigid internal fixation, using bone grafts where appropriate. Exposure of the lower portion of the Le Fort fracture is obtained through a bilateral gingival-buccal sulcus incision, which exposes the entire Le Fort I level. In Le Fort II, III, and IV fractures, subciliary skin-muscle flap incisions and the bicoronal incision (50) provide exposure to the superior portion of the midfacial skeleton (12–14, 34, 51–54). The nasomaxillary and the zygomaticomaxillary buttress segments are stabilized using plate and screw fixation, and bone grafts are added when bone gaps exceed 5 mm. The coronal incision provides exposure for the zygomaticofrontal suture, orbital roof, frontal bone, frontal sinus and nasoethmoidal area. The lower portion of the orbit and zygoma are visualized through the subciliary skin-muscle flap incisions. The zygomatic arch is visualized by a coronal incision after dissecting under the temporalis fascia (55; Fig. 37.17**A** and **B**).

Patients managed with rigid fixation may have the intermaxillary fixation discontinued after fracture reduction if sufficient stability is obtained. In comminuted fractures, intermaxillary fixation is best maintained for a 1–2-week period, and the patient is then allowed to function and take a soft diet. The length of intermaxillary fixation is determined by the comminution of the fracture and the stability obtained by the open reduction. Con-

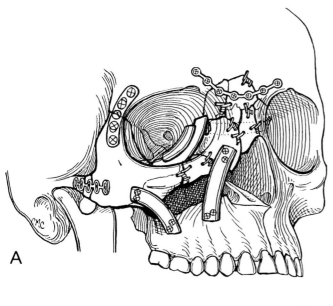

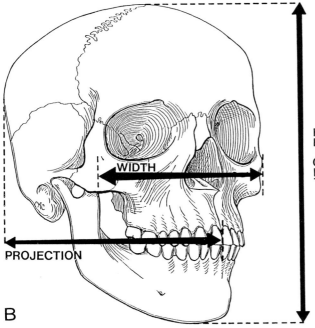

FIGURE 37.17. **A,** The buttresses of the facial skeleton are reassembled utilizing bone grafts where required. The initial interfragment wiring is stabilized with rigid fixation. **B,** The face must be reassembled and stabilized in its three dimensions of height, width, and projection. Conceptually, control of facial width is the most important concept. Stabilizing width often reciprocally restores projection. Facial height is the last dimension to be addressed. (© JHU Art as Applied to Medicine.)

stant (biweekly) observation of the occlusion is necessary in all patients who have undergone Le Fort fracture treatment. Displacement may be observed in spite of the performance of open reduction and rigid internal fixation because maxillary bone is thin. Brief elastic traction generally restores occlusion in these cases.

Late treatment of Le Fort fractures requires mobilization of the fracture segments and repositioning the fracture fragments into proper anatomical relationships. Early treatment is preferred because it necessitates less manipulation and dissection. In edentulous Le Fort fractures, buttress bone grafting should be utilized in addition to rigid internal fixation; dental splints or dentures are modified to provide intermaxillary fixation and are utilized intraoperatively as the key to maxillary projection. Intermaxillary fixation and perhaps the splints may be discontinued after application of rigid internal fixation. The dentures are initially secured either with screws to the aveolus or by the use of wires that extend from the dental splint up over a stable point such as the maxillary alveolus, zygomatic arch, a hole in the pyriform aperture, or the inferior orbital rim.

When comminuted fractures involve the maxilla and the mandible, it is necessary to stabilize the mandible (56) in both its vertical and horizontal components as a stable base for maxillary fracture reduction. The midface reduction cannot support a fractured mandible. When fractures of the frontal bone exist with comminuted midfacial fractures, the frontal bone stabilization and any intracranial neurosurgery are first completed. Segments of the orbital rims are linked with wires and then stabilized with plate and screw fixation. In stabilizing the zygoma, it is necessary to correct midfacial width, which tends to be wide in patients with high-energy zygomatic fractures. The zygomatic arch should be reconstructed as flat as possible and should represent the first point of rigid fixation of the zygoma after linking the fragment with wires. The remainder of the zygoma is then stabilized. Rigid fixation as a treatment for midface fractures has eliminated the use of suspension wires (57) and head frames (5, 21, 58, 59; Figs. 37.18 and 37.19).

ORBITAL FRACTURES

The symptoms of an orbital floor or wall fracture are periorbital ecchymosis and subconjunctival hemorrhage (60). Frequently, hypesthesia or anesthesia are present in the distribution of the infraorbital nerve in floor fractures. Depending on the extent of fracture and the damage to eye muscles, horizontal or vertical eye muscle imbalances and ocular dystopia may be present. If the fractures involve the medial orbit and the orbital floor, ipsilateral epistaxis may be present. Enophthalmos (recession of the globe into the orbit) is present if the fracture expands the bony orbital volume ("blow-out" fracture). If the fracture contracts the orbital volume ("blow-in" fracture), the orbit will be constricted, and the globe may be displaced forward. Fractures may be confined only to the thin middle section of the internal orbit ("pure" orbital fracture), or they may be "impure," involving both the rim and the internal portions of the orbit. Commonly, pure orbital fractures involve the lower medial orbital wall and the floor of the orbit simultaneously. Isolated fractures of the medial wall, which produce subcutaneous emphysema, epistaxis, horizontal diplopia, and enoph-

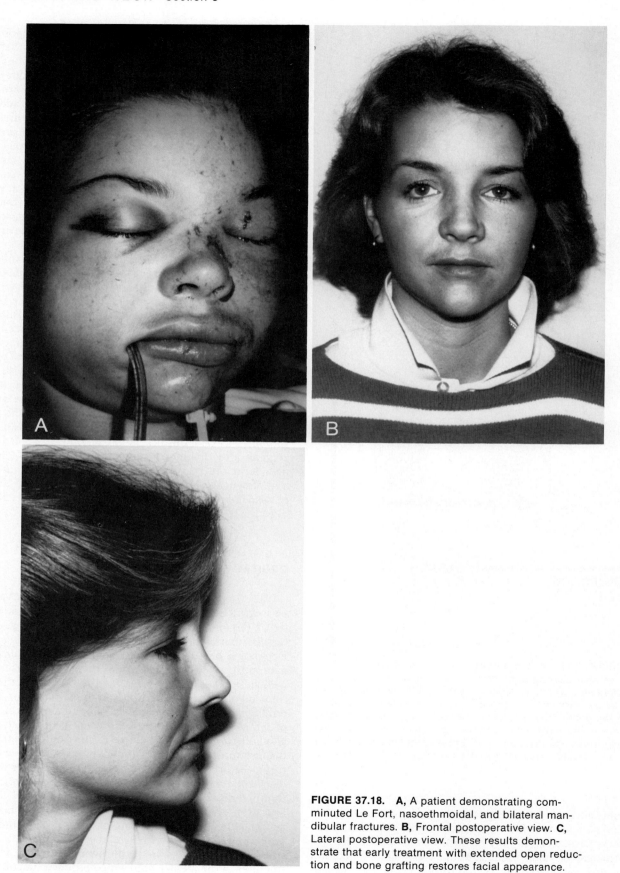

FIGURE 37.18. **A,** A patient demonstrating comminuted Le Fort, nasoethmoidal, and bilateral mandibular fractures. **B,** Frontal postoperative view. **C,** Lateral postoperative view. These results demonstrate that early treatment with extended open reduction and bone grafting restores facial appearance.

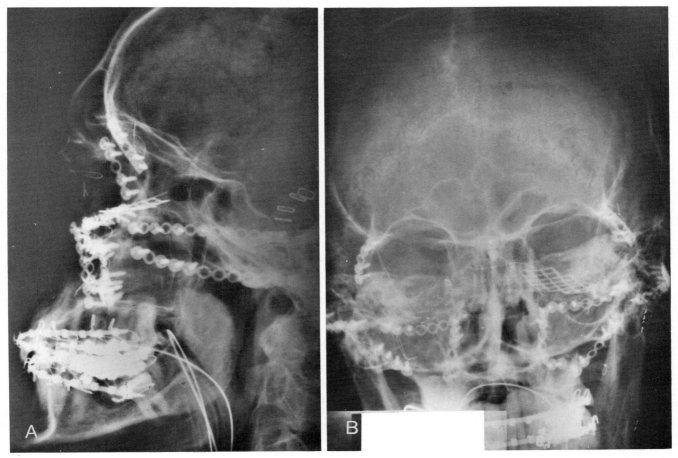

FIGURE 37.19. Postoperative radiographs of a pan-facial fracture reduction demonstrate stabilization of the facial buttresses by titanium plate and screw fixation.

thalmos, also exist. Rarely do medial wall orbital fractures incarcerate extraocular muscles.

The mechanism of orbital fractures involves both hydraulic force from soft tissue compression and a blow to the orbital rim with a "buckling force" displacement of the orbital floor. Displacement of the rim causes a "buckling" to occur in the thin orbital floor, and if sufficient, this buckling causes a fracture to occur (61). The rim may not be fractured, despite displacement, because of its stronger structure. Soft tissue pressure then forces extraocular fat (and perhaps an extraocular muscle) into the fracture site and this may result in incarceration of orbital movement. Manson et al. have described the fine system of ligaments that extends throughout all orbital soft tissue (62). The ligament system accounts for the tethering of extraocular structures to each other. When periorbital fat is incarcerated in an orbital fracture, the excursion of an eye muscle may be tethered because of these diffuse ligament connections, despite the fact that it is not physically incarcerated. The fine ligament system explains how this limitation of movement occurs by diffuse interconnections.

All patients with orbital fractures deserve a careful clinical evaluation of the globe. Visual acuity and the speed and symmetry of pupillary reactivity provide evidence of optic nerve integrity. Confrontation fields, intraocular pressure, and funduscopic examination are also performed.

Orbital fractures are evaluated by axial and coronal CT scan sections. In patients unable to cooperate for coronal sections, the axial sections are reconstructed into a coronal format. Although orbital fractures may be visualized on plain films, the diagnostic detail required for visualization of soft tissue, bone, and the extraocular muscles is only obtained with CT. Bone and soft tissue windows and diagnosis of muscle incarceration versus muscle contusion.

The need for surgery is based on the volume change of the orbit and the position of the fracture segments in relation to the muscle involved with diplopia. There are therefore two general indications for surgery: volume correction and release of incarcerated orbital tissues. The following are indications for operations:

1. Entrapment of an extraocular muscle or orbital fat that produces muscle movement restriction in the presence of a positive forced duction examination and diplopia in a functional field of gaze.
2. Enophthalmos or exophthalmos exceeding 2–3 mm as

a result of fracture displacement (more than 2–3 ml of volume change will begin to produce globe positional change).

3. Vertical or horizontal globe positional change that is aesthetically undesirable.
4. Infraorbital sensory deficit in the face of an orbital rim fracture, especially if fragments compress the inferior orbital nerve foramen.

Entrapment of the movement of an extraocular muscle or of adjacent fat, which tethers the muscle excursion by virtue of its ligament connections, is an indication for open reduction. The CT scan should demonstrate the fracture and its relation to the muscle involved. If the muscle or the fat appears to be trapped in the fracture, operation is indicated in the face of diplopia within a functional field of gaze and a positive forced duction examination. The forced duction test is applied by grasping the insertion of an extraocular muscle just peripheral to the corneal limbus. The application of a drop of local anesthetic agent provides comfort. The globe is rotated; the absence of full rotation indicates possible muscle incarceration. The force generation test is performed by grasping the insertion of a muscle and asking the patient to voluntarily rotate the globe, noting the force generated. Saccadic velocities (63) differentiate the rate of acceleration of ocular movement and often differentiate muscle entrapment, paralysis, and contusion. Contusion may produce a positive forced duction examination by production of edema. Most muscle deficits are due to contusion or paralysis and many resolve almost completely and spontaneously. Therefore, many internal orbital fractures that will not result in significant enophthalmos will not benefit from reduction. Superior and inferior muscle imbalance and double vision are more often due to muscle contusion than fat and fascial entrapment. Actual muscle incarceration is quite uncommon. The functional goal of treatment is to obtain orthophoric vision in the primary field of gaze and not necessarily full normal movement without any diplopia. This goal can be accomplished with nonoperative treatment in many limited orbital floor fractures, a fact that was emphasized by Putterman et al. (64).

Surgical treatment is indicated for muscle incarceration that produces visually handicapping diplopia. Likewise, when orbital volume changes will result in cosmetically deforming enophthalmos or exophthalmos, surgery is indicated (Fig. 37.20). It is my opinion that early surgery in the face of dense muscle incarceration improves final range of motion. Vertical dystopia of the globe is corrected by orbital reconstruction. The sensory deficit accompanying orbital floor fractures usually spontaneously resolves almost completely unless the rim is involved, compressing the foramen. When rim fractures compress the infraorbital nerve, this compression should be specifically released. This situation may be documented on CT scan. Patients with sensory deficits following orbital fractures are rarely improved by late nerve decompression or neurolysis. The most disabling double vision is that present inferiorly in the down gaze or reading position. Paralysis of the superior rectus muscle may mimic a trapped inferior rectus. A careful evaluation of the entire orbit with CT scan is mandatory, and formal visual fields are suggested (40, 41).

Supraorbital fractures involve the supraorbital rim and orbital roof. They are usually displaced inferiorly and posteriorly and create a downward and outward projection of the globe. Lid closure may be incomplete, and, if so, corneal exposure is common (65). Early fracture reduction should be considered in these patients. Frontal sinus fractures and dural fistulas often coexist with supraorbital fractures and should be managed appropriately.

The lateral orbit (greater wing of the sphenoid) is often fractured in fractures of the zygoma. This fracture may represent only a linear fracture of the junction of the orbital process of the zygoma and the greater wing of the sphenoid, or the fracture may be comminuted, extending into the greater wing of the sphenoid and enlarging the orbit in this location.

The weakest area of the orbital wall is the medial wall of the orbit over the ethmoid sinuses, the lamina papyracea. The next weakest area is the orbital floor. The floor is often fractured in its medial section, where it is inclined at a 30° angle as it extends posteriorly. The plane of the orbital floor also inclines medially at a 45° angle to reach the ethmoidal region. It is this inclined inferomedial section that is the usual area that is "blown out" in internal orbital fractures. The area is located medial to the groove and canal for the infraorbital nerve. In inferomedial orbital fractures, the postbulbar orbital constriction is lost and the orbital volume increases, allowing the globe to sink downward, backward, and medially.

Fractures of the orbital floor are exposed through a subciliary skin-muscle flap (31) or conjunctival incision with a lateral canthotomy. The lower half of the medial orbital wall may be explored by retraction of the globe through this incision. If the fracture extends into the upper portion of the medial orbit, a coronal incision or a local incision over the lateral aspect of the nose is required.

The lateral orbit may be explored through a subciliary incision by detaching the canthal ligament. If the greater wing of the sphenoid is fractured, exposure through a coronal approach is preferred. The orbital roof and superior orbital rim are explored through either a laceration or a coronal incision.

Safe exploration of the orbit is performed only with the knowledge of the location of the superior and inferior orbital fissures and their contents. The exact location of the optic nerve should be kept in mind. The optic foramen is located 40–45 mm posterior to the inferior orbital rim and is superior and medial to the usual floor dissection even if it extends 35–38 mm posteriorly. The entire area of the bone deficit should be visualized, and a ledge of intact bone should be identified all around the orbit to be used as a guide to reconstruction (Fig. 37.21). If the orbital rim is intact, the defect is spanned with bone grafts or alloplastic material. Currently, Medpor is my preferred material for small defects because it can be contoured similarly to bone. Both the bone graft and the artificial material should be secured by wiring to the rim

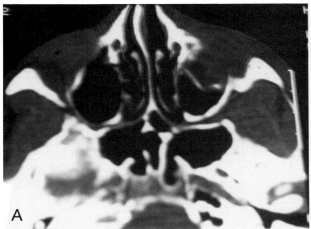
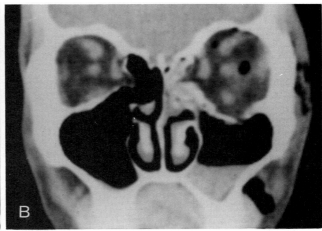
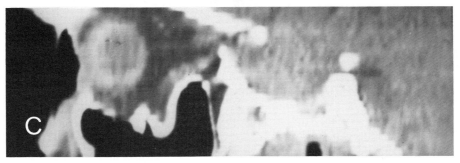

FIGURE 37.20. **A,** A "blow-out" fracture of the orbital floor demonstrated on an axial CT scan. A fragment of bone is seen depressed in the right maxillary antrum. Little precise evaluation of fracture displacement is possible. **B,** The coronal CT scan allows precise determination of the extent of displacement. Additionally, the relation of the inferior and medial rectus muscles to the fracture site is identified. The amount of soft tissue incarcerated in the fracture may be quantified. There is a relationship between the volume of displaced tissue and the subsequent development of enophthalmos. The CT scan therefore permits accurate prediction of patients who would benefit from operation for either release of muscle incarceration (diplopia) or volume correction (enophthalmos). **C,** The CT scan taken in the longitudinal orbital projection demonstrates a "blow-out" fracture. Inferior displacement of the floor of the orbit is noted. The orbital contents are herniated downward into the maxillary sinus. An intact "ledge" of bone is seen in the orbit posteriorly.

or by using a screw to affix the graft to stable orbital bone. A forced duction examination should be performed before dissection, again after dissection, and finally after artificial material or bone grafts are inserted to document that the reconstruction has not impinged an extraocular muscle. If orbital rim fractures coexist with the fracture of the internal orbit, the orbital rim fragments are initially linked with wires and stabilized in anatomical position with plate and screw fixation. The entire orbital defect should have been dissected to identify intact posterior, medial, and lateral bone. Bone grafts or alloplastic materials are then used to span the area of the defect.

In simple internal orbital fractures, alloplastic material is often employed despite open communication with the sinus. Either 0.8-mm Supramid or 1.5-mm Medpor is utilized. In placing bone grafts or orbital implants, the location of the optic nerve must be recalled, and the bone graft must be designed to avoid any pressure. In the reconstruction of medical orbital wall defects, the optic nerve is often directly posterior to the intact bone, which is usually in the area of the posterior ethmoidal foramen. Care must be taken not to have a bone graft or implant impinge on the optic nerve in this location because it is directly posterior in line with the medial orbital wall.

Sources for bone grafts include split calvarium, rib, and iliac crest.

Complications from orbital surgery occur in 10–15% of cases. The most common include eyelid deformities such as scleral show and ectropion. Careful attention to hemostasis and accurate dissection planes minimize these problems. Blindness following the reduction of orbital floor or zygomatic fractures has been associated with blind packing of the maxillary antrum, the use of large orbital floor implants, vigorous zygomatic fracture mobilization with extension of fractures to the orbital apex, trauma to the globe, retrobulbar hemorrhage, and retinal detachment. Late evolution of an ocular injury may also be responsible for visual loss. It is important that the visual acuity be documented before the surgery and that pupillary activity be noted, because these findings provide clues to preexisting optic nerve impairment postoperatively. Significant postoperative hematoma should be evacuated. In fractures sectioning the posterior orbit, the superior orbital fissure syndrome (66) may occur. It consists of ophthalmoplegia (paralysis of cranial nerves IV, V, and VI), anesthesia in V-1, ptosis, and proptosis. When blindness is present, the syndrome is called the orbital apex syndrome.

FIGURE 37.21. A, A medial orbital wall fracture is managed by split rib or calvarial bone grafting. The intact bone posteriorly is frequently at the level of the posterior ethmoidal foramen. The optic nerve is 5 mm posterior to this area, is directly behind it, and must be precisely protected. **B,** The usual location of an inferomedial "blow-out" fracture. The area has been dissected, and intact bone is identified around the edges of the entire orbital defect. Bone grafts may then be placed to cover the defect. **C,** An inferolateral defect managed with split rib or calvarial bone grafts. (© JHU Art as Applied to Medicine.)

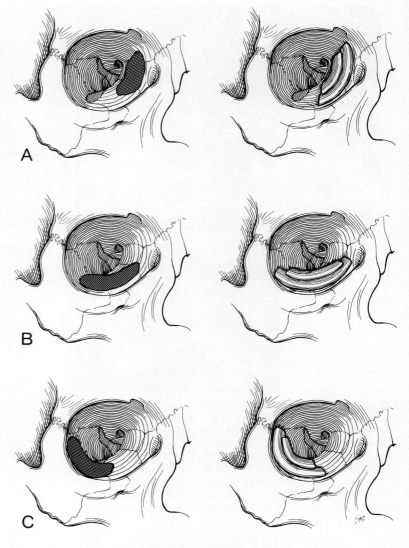

Orbital fractures benefit from early surgical intervention when specific indications are present. Contraindications include globe rupture, retinal detachment, and internal globe injury. In patients with significant orbital volume change, who would develop enophthalmos if their fractures were untreated, better aesthetic and functional results are achieved with primary management.

References

1. Gwyn PP, Carraway JH, Horton CE, et al: Facial fractures—associated injuries and complications. *Plast Reconstr Surg* 47:225, 1971.
2. Schultz RC: Facial injuries from automobile accidents: A study of 400 consecutive cases. *Plast Reconstr Surg* 40:415, 1967.
3. Kaufman HH, Hui KS, Mattson JC, et al: Clinicopathological correlations of disseminated intravascular coagulation in patients with head injury. *Neurosurgery* 15:34, 1984.
4. Dunham C, Cowley RA: *Shock Trauma/Critical Care Manual*. Baltimore, University Park Press, 1982.
5. Georgiade N, Nash T: An external cranial fixation apparatus for severe maxillofacial injuries. *Plast Reconstr Surg* 38:142, 1966.
6. Becker DP, Miller JD, Ward JD, et al: The outcome from severe head injury with early diagnosis and intensive management. *J Neurosurg* 47:491, 1977.
7. Lewin W, Marshall TF, Roberts AH: Long-term outcome after severe head injury. *Br Med J* 2:1533, 1979.
8. Klauber MR, Marchall LE, Barrett-Conner E, et al: Prospective study of patients hospitalized with head injury in San Diego County, 1978. *Neurosurgery* 9:236, 1981.
9. McDonald JV: The surgical management of severe open brain injuries with consideration of the long-term results. *J Trauma* 20:842, 1980.
10. Mektubjian SR: Operative policy in severe facial trauma in combination with other severe injuries. *J Maxillofacial Surg* 10:14, 1982.
11. Markowitz B, Manson PN, Mirvis S: Toward CT based facial fracture treatment. *Plast Reconstr Surg* 85:202, 1990.
12. Manson PN: Management of facial fractures. *Perspect Plastic Surg* 1:1, 1988.
13. Manson, PN: The fourth dimension in facial injury treatment. In *Proceedings of the Walter Reed Bone Symposium*. Washington, DC, U.S. Government Printing Office, 1989.
14. Manson PN, Crawley WA, Yaremchuk, MJ, Rochman GM, Hoopes JE, French JE: Midface fractures: Advantages of extended open reduction and immediate bone grafting. *Plast Reconstr Surg* 76:1, 1985.
15. Leech P, Patterson A: Conservative and operative management for cerebrospinal leakage after closed head injury. *Lancet* 1:1013, 1973.
16. Haines SJ: Systemic antibiotic prophylaxis in neurological surgery. *Neurosurgery* 6:355, 1980.

17. Hoff JT, Brewin AU: Antibiotics for basilar skull fractures. *J Neurosurg* 44:649, 1976.

18. Klastersky J, Sadeghi M, Brihaye J: Antimicrobial prophylaxis in patient with rhinorrhea and otorrhea: A double blind study. *Surg Neurol* 6:111, 1976.

19. Gruss JS, MacKinnon SE: Complex maxillary fractures: The role of buttress stabilization and immediate bone grafting. *Plast Reconstr Surg* 75:303, 1985.

20. Gruss JE, MacKinnon SE, Kassek E, Cooper, PW: The role of primary bone grafting in complex craniomaxillofacial trauma. *Plast Reconstr Surg* 75:17, 1985.

21. Irby WB, Rast WC: Extracranial fixation of the facial skeleton: Review and report of case. *J Oral Surg* 27:900, 1969.

22. Stranc MF, Robertson GA: A classification of internal injuries of the nasal skeleton. *Ann Plast Surg* 2:468, 1979.

23. Markowitz B, Manson PN, Sargent L, et al: Management of the medial canthal tendon is nasoethmoid-orbital fractures: The importance of the central fragment in treatment and classification. *Plast Reconstr Surg* 87:843, 1991.

24. Zide B, McCarthy J: The medial canthus revisited: An anatomical basis for canthopexy. *Ann Plast Surg* 9:1, 1983.

25. Gruss JS: Naso-ethmoid-orbital fractures: Classification and role of primary bone grafting. *Plast Reconstr Surg* 75:303, 1985.

26. Paskert JP, Manson PN: The bimanual examination for assessing instability in naso-ethmoidal orbital injuries. *Plast Reconstr Surg* 83:165, 1989.

27. Gruss JS, Hurwitz JJ, Nik NA, et al: The pattern and incidence of nasolacrimal injury in naso-orbito-ethmoid fractures: The role of delayed assessment and dacryocystorhinostomy. *Br J Plast Surg* 38:116, 1985.

28. Gillies HD, Kilner TP, Stone D: Fractures of the malar-zygomatic compound: With a description of a new x-ray position. *Br J Surg* 14:651, 1927.

29. Knight JS, North JF: The classification of malar fractures: An analysis of displacement as a guide to treatment. *Br J Plast Surg* 13:325, 1961.

30. Yanagisawa E: Pitfalls in the management of zygomatic fractures. *Laryngoscope* 83:527, 1973.

31. Manson PN, Ruas E, Iliff N, Yaremchuk M: Single lower eyelid incision for exposure of the zygomatic bone and orbital reconstruction. *Plast Reconstr Surg* 79:120, 1987.

32. Manson PN: Frontobasilar fractures: I. Experimental mechanism and classification. II. Clinical management. (Submitted for publication.)

33. Heckler FR. Discussion of Luce EA: Frontal sinus fractures: Guidelines to management. *Plast Reconstr Surg* 80:509, 1987.

34. Merville LC, Derome P: Concomitant dislocations of the face and skull. *J Maxillofacial Surg* 6:2, 1978.

35. Newman MH, Travis LW: Frontal sinus fractures. *Laryngoscope* 83:1281, 1973.

36. Pollak K, Payne E: Fractures of the frontal sinus. *Otolaryngol Clin North Am* 9:517, 1976.

37. Stanley R: Fractures of the frontal sinus. *Clin Plast Surg* 16:115, 1989.

38. Schenck NL: Frontal sinus disease: III. Experimental and clinical factors in failure of the frontal osteoplastic operation. *Laryngoscope* 85:76, 1975.

39. Wolfe SA, Johnson P: Frontal sinus injuries: Primary care and management of late complications. *Plast Reconstr Surg* 92:78, 1988.

40. Nadell J, Kline DG: Primary reconstruction of depressed frontal skull fractures including those involving the sinus, orbit and cribriform plate. *J Neurosurg* 41:200, 1974.

41. Schultz RC: Supraorbital and glabellar fractures. Presented to American College of Surgeons, Chicago, 1982.

42. Larrabee WF, Travis LW, Tabb HG: Frontal sinus fractures—their suppurative complications and surgical management. *Laryngoscope* 90:1810, 1980.

43. Manson PN, Shack RB, Leonard LG, Su CT, Hoopes JE: Sagittal fractures of the maxilla and palate. *Plast Reconstr Surg* 72:484, 1983.

44. LeFort R: Étude experimentale sur les fracturs de la Machoire supérieure, Parts I, II, III. *Rev Chir Paris* 23:208, 360, 479, 1901.

45. Manson PN: Some thoughts on the classification and treatment of LeFort fractures. *Ann Plast Surg* 17:356, 1986.

46. Nahum AM: Biomechanics of maxillofacial trauma. *Clin Plast Surg* 2:59, 1975.

47. Sturla F, Absi D, Buquet J: Anatomic and mechanical considerations of craniofacial fractures: An experimental study. *Plast Reconstr Surg* 66:815, 1980.

48. Stanley RB Jr: Reconstruction of midface vertical dimension following LeFort fractures. *Arch Otorhinolaryngol* 110:571, 1984.

49. Manson PN, Romano J, Crawley W, Mirvis S, et al: Incomplete LeFort fractures. *Plast Reconstr Surg* 85:355, 1990.

50. Salyer R, Jackson I, Whittaker L, Monasterio F, Munro I: *Atlas of Cranial-maxillofacial Surgery*. St. Louis, CV Mosby & Company, 1980.

51. Manson PN, Hoopes JE, Su CT: Structural pillars of the facial skeleton: An approach to the management of LeFort fractures. *Plast Reconstr Surg* 64:54, 1980.

52. Markowitz B, Manson PN: Organization of treatment for a panfacial fracture. *Plast Surg Clin* 16:105, 1989.

53. Sofferman RA, Danielson PA, Quatela V, Reed RR: Retrospective analysis of surgically treated LeFort fractures. *Arch Otolaryngol* 109:446, 1983.

54. Stanley RB, Nowak GM: Midfacial fractures: The importance of angle of impact to horizontal craniofacial buttresses. *Otolaryngol Head Neck Surg* 93:186, 1985.

55. Rowe LD, Brandt-Zawadski M: Spacial analysis of midfacial fractures with multidirectional and computed tomography: Clinipathologic correlates in 44 cases. *Otolaryngol Head Neck Surg* 90:651, 1982.

56. Hagan EH, Huelke DF: An analysis of 319 case reports of mandibular fractures. *J Oral Surg* 19:93, 1961.

57. Adams WM: Internal wiring fixation of facial fractures. *Surgery* 12:523, 1942.

58. Butow KW, Roos AW: External craniofacial fixation treatment for midfacial fractures, Parts I, III, III. *J Dent Assoc South Africa* September, 590, 1986.

59. Irby W: *Facial Trauma and Concomitant Problems,* ed 2. St. Louis, CV Mosby & Company, 1984.

60. Converse JM, Smith B, O'Bear MF, et al: Orbital blowout fractures: A ten year survey. *Plast Reconstr Surg* 39:20, 1967.

61. Fujino T, Makino K: Entrapment mechanism and ocular injury in orbital blowout fracture. *Plast Reconstr Surg* 65:571, 1980.

62. Manson PN, Clifford CM, Su CT, et al: Mechanisms of global support and post-traumatic enophthalmos: (I) anatomy of the ligament sling and its relation to intramuscular cone orbital fat. *Plast Reconstr Surg* 77:193, 1985.

63. Metz HS, Scott WE, Madson E: Saccadic velocity and active force studies in blowout fractures of the orbit. *Am J Ophthalmol* 78:665, 1975.

64. Putterman AM, Stevens T, Vrist MF: Nonsurgical management of blowout fractures of the orbital floor. *Am J Ophthalmol* 77:232, 1974.

65. Schultz RC: Supraorbital and glabellar fractures. *Plast Reconstr Surg* 45:227, 1970.

66. Hedstrom J, Parsons J, Maloney J, Doku HC: Superior orbital fissure syndrome: Report of a case. *J Oral Surg* 32:198, 1974.

Suggested Readings

Andreasen JO: *Traumatic Injuries of the Teeth,* ed 2. Philadelphia, WB Saunders Co, 1981.

Archer WH: *Oral and Maxillofacial Surgery*. Philadelphia, WB Saunders Co, 1975.

Aston SJ, Hornblass A, Meltzer MA, et al: *Third International Symposium of Plastic and Reconstructive Surgery of the Eye and Adnexa*. Baltimore, Williams & Wilkins Co, 1982.

Converse JM: *Surgical Treatment of Facial Injuries*. Baltimore, Williams & Wilkins, 1974.

Dingman R, Natvig P: *Surgery of Facial Fractures*. Philadelphia, WB Saunders Co, 1964.

DuBrul EL: *Sicher's Oral Anatomy*. St. Louis, CV Mosby Co, 1980.

Georgiade NG: *Plastic and Maxillofacial Trauma Symposium*. St. Louis, CV Mosby Co, 1969.

Irby WB: *Facial Trauma and Concomitant Problems*. St. Louis, CV Mosby Co, 1979.

Jackson IT: Management of acute craniofacial injuries. In Caronni EP (ed): *Craniofacial Surgery*. Boston, Little, Brown, 1985, p 441.

Kawamoto HK Jr, Wolfe SA: Maxillofacial surgery. In Kawamoto KH Jr, Wolfe SA (eds): *Clinics in Plastic Surgery*. Philadelphia, WB Saunders Co, October, 1982.

Kelly J: *Management of War Injuries to the Jaws and Related Structures*. Document no. 008-045-0018-6. Washington, DC, U.S. Government Printing Office, 1900.

Kruger GO: *Oral Surgery*. St. Louis, CV Mosby Co, 1979.

Rowe NL, Killey HC: *Fractures of the Facial Skeleton,* London, E & S Livingstone, 1968.

Tessier P, et al: *Symposium on Plastic Surgery in the Orbital Region*. St. Louis, CV Mosby Co, 1976.

38

Mandibular Fractures

Mark A. Anton, M.D. and Jonathan S. Jacobs, D.M.D., M.D. F.A.C.S.

The multifunctional and cosmetic importance of the mandible is unmatched by any bone in the body. Stability, motion, and form must be fully restored after injury so that eating, speaking, breathing, and facial balance may be maintained.

Etiology

Mandibular fractures account for about 10–25% of all facial fractures, but these percentages can vary significantly, depending on the cause of the trauma (1, 2). In the past, the majority of fractured mandibles reportedly resulted from motor vehicle accidents, but the more frequent use of seat belts has decreased these numbers. More recent studies from large urban medical centers show that interpersonal assaults were the primary cause of mandibular fractures (3; DP Sinn, unpublished data from Parkland Memorial Hospital, Dallas, 1985). Other less common causes include athletic injuries, falls, gunshot wounds, and pathological fractures. In children, the most common cause of fractured mandibles is a fall from a bicycle or steps (4).

Anatomy

MANDIBULAR ANATOMY

The mandible is unique in that it is the only U-shaped bone in the human skeleton and has the only ginglymoarthrodial joints in the body, which allow for rotational and translational movement.

The mandible is divided into several anatomical regions, and fracture sites are generally classified into one of these areas (Fig. 38.1). In 1964, Dingman and Natvig reported the incidence of fractures in these different regions (5), and data from other authors yield similar results (6, 7). A more recent study, in which more mandibular fractures resulted from physical violence than from motor vehicle accidents, revealed relatively more fractures occurring in the regions of the symphysis, parasymphysis, and angle and fewer in the condylar process (Fig. 38.1). The incidence of fractures in the ramus, coronoid process, and alveolar process is relatively small in all the studies.

The mandibular foramen, on the medial aspect of the ramus, is situated below the sigmoid/mandibular notch on a line continuous with the occlusal plane (Fig. 38.2**A**). A spicule of bone, the lingula, is situated anterior and inferior to this foramen. The inferior alveolar artery, vein, and nerve pass through the mandibular foramen into the mandibular canal to supply blood and sensation to each of the teeth (Fig. 38.2**B**). This nerve continues through the mental foramen as the mental nerve and supplies sensation to the lower lip. The mental foramen is located laterally below the first and second premolars. Blood supply to the mandible is partially provided by the inferior alveolar artery, but much of it is provided through muscle and gingival attachments, particularly on the lingual side.

The mylohyoid muscle attaches to the mylohyoid line (Fig. 38.3) on the medial surface of the mandible, and the muscles join in the midline at the mylohyoid raphe. This muscle functions as an elevator of the tongue. Anterosuperior and posteroinferior to this mylohyoid line are the sublingual and submandibular fossae, respectively, in which lay the glands of the same name. The mylohyoid artery and nerve lie in the mylohyoid groove, which extends inferiorly from the mandibular foramen.

The geniohyoid muscles originate from the hyoid bone and insert onto the genial tubercles (mental spines), which are located on the lingual midline of the mandible (Figs. 38.2**A** and 38.3). The anterior bellies of the digastric muscles insert into the digastric fossae just lateral to the mental spines. These two pairs of muscles form an anterior group of muscles that serve to depress and retract the mandible.

The posterior group of muscles that generally serve to elevate or protrude the mandible consist of the temporalis, masseter, and medial and lateral pterygoid muscles (Fig. 38.4). The temporalis muscle originates in the temporal fossa and inserts onto the coronoid process and the superior aspect of the external oblique line. The masseter originates in two heads from the zygoma and zygomatic arch and inserts onto the lateral aspect of the mandibular angle. The medial pterygoid muscle originates from the fossa between the pterygoid plates and inserts onto the medial aspect of the angle. The masseter and medial pterygoid muscles form an effective sling around the inferior margin of the mandible, and with the temporalis muscle, they can generate 50 lb/in^2 of pressure during mastication.

The lateral pterygoid muscle consists of two muscle bellies (Fig. 38.5). The inferior lateral pterygoid origi-

FIGURE 38.1. Anatomical regions of the mandible with percentages of reported fractures.

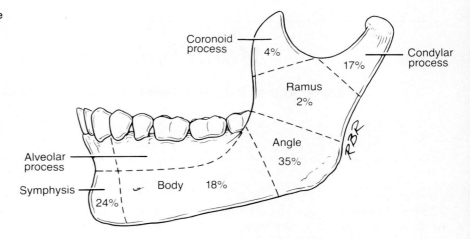

nates from the lateral pterygoid plate and inserts onto the neck of the condyle, producing protrusion of the mandible when contracting. The superior lateral pterygoid originates from the sphenoid bone and inserts on the fibrous capsule and meniscus of the temporomandibular joint (TMJ). This muscle stabilizes the meniscus during jaw movement. The TMJ consists of a fibrous articular disc sandwiched between two synovial joints. This is the only joint in the body with rotational movement (early in jaw opening) and translational movement (with wide opening of the jaw). The lateral pterygoid muscles produce this translational movement either unilaterally or bilaterally to allow mandibular deviation to the side opposite the contraction.

FIGURE 38.2. Mandibular anatomy (see text).

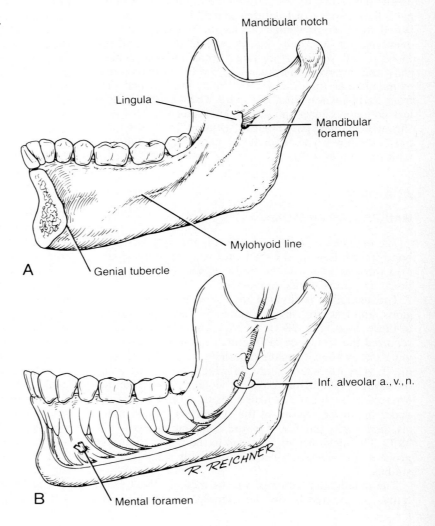

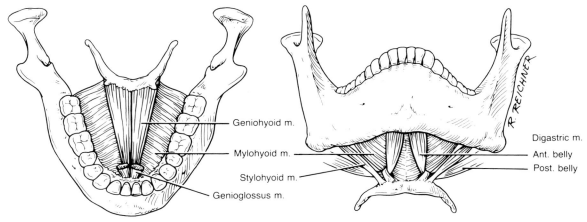

FIGURE 38.3. Muscles of the floor of the mouth and suprahyoid region; depressors of the anterior mandible.

It is important to understand the direction of pull of these masticatory muscles so that the forces acting on a fracture site are anticipated and accounted for when it is reduced and fixed. Some orientations of fractures are termed "favorable" or "unfavorable," depending on whether the attached muscles reduce or distract the fracture site.

In subcondylar fractures, the condyle tends to be displaced medially and anteriorly by the lateral pterygoid muscle (Fig. 38.6). The fate of the articular disc in most cases is unclear. The superiorly directed force of the medial pterygoid, masseter, and temporalis muscles (closing muscles) may then cause a decrease in height of the posterior mandible and an anterior bite deformity. When the line of the fracture goes through the mandibular angle, there may be enough of the masseter–medial pterygoid muscle sling on each side of the fracture site to keep it reduced. If the fracture site is in the anterior portion of this sling, it may act like the vertically unfavorable body fracture, as described below.

Fractures in the body of the mandible may be classified as vertically and horizontally favorable or unfavorable. If the vertical orientation of the fracture is from posterosuperior to anteroinferior (Fig. 38.7**A**), the pull of the closing muscles will reduce the fracture (vertically favorable fracture). If vertical orientation of the fracture is in the other direction (Fig. 38.7**B**), the fracture site will be distracted (vertically unfavorable fracture) by the superior

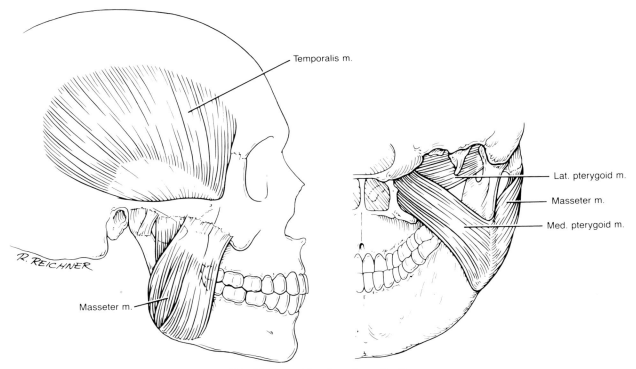

FIGURE 38.4. Muscles of mastication.

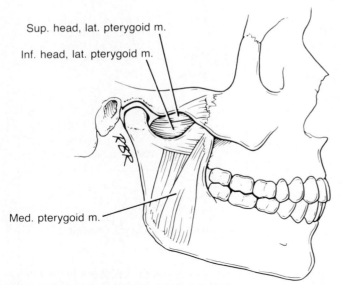

FIGURE 38.5. Internal anatomy of the temporomandibular joint; insertion of the lateral pterygoid muscle into both the articular disc and condylar neck. The medial pterygoid forms the medial portion of the muscle sling around the ramus.

pull of the closing muscles on the posterior segment and the inferior pull of the suprahyoid muscles on the anterior segment.

In a horizontal plane, if the fracture occurs as depicted in Figure 38.8**A**, pull from the pterygoid and masseter muscle should help reduce the proximal segment laterally (horizontally favorable fracture). If the fracture occurs in the opposite direction (Fig. 38.8**B**), the unopposed pull of the pterygoid muscles will cause displacement of the fracture (horizontally unfavorable fracture).

Segmental fractures of the body may be medially displaced by tension from the mylohyoid muscles (Fig. 38.9), and in a bilateral parasymphyseal fracture, the anterior mandible may be posteriorly displaced by the geniohyoid and digastric muscles (Fig. 38.10).

DENTAL ANATOMY

The horizontal portion of the mandible is comprised of corticocancellous bone with a thick, compact inferior border. The alveolar process is based on this foundation and provides the supporting matrix for the teeth. Basic dental anatomy is outlined in Figure 38.11. Each tooth socket is lined with a sheath of dense bone, called the lamina dura, and the tooth is secured and suspended in this socket via radially arranged, collagenous periodontal ligament fibers. There are also strong groups of fibers running between adjacent teeth and to the overlying mucosa. The roots of the teeth are approximately twice the length of the crown. This relationship is important when using screw-plate fixation because the root tips must be avoided.

Tooth fractures are classified by the proximity of the fracture line to the pulp cavity (Fig. 38.12). Even teeth with class III fractures (i.e., exposure of the pulp) may be salvaged with endodontic therapy. Teeth with fractures extending through the root may not be salvaged. If a permanent tooth is avulsed from the socket, it is best to replace and stabilize the tooth after minimal irrigation to remove any debris. If this is accomplished within 30 min from the time of avulsion, the chances of tooth survival are good. The chance of survival decreases about 1% for every minute after that time (8). Deciduous teeth generally do not need to be reimplanted.

Each tooth has a dual blood supply with anastomoses outside the root in the periapical area (Fig. 38.11). One blood supply enters the tooth through the apical foramen and supplies the pulp and dentin. The other is a network of vessels entering through the periodontal ligament to the cementum. Because of this dual blood supply, a tooth that has lost its apical supply may still be retained.

The presence or absence of teeth greatly influences the type of mandibular fracture that may occur. Impacted third molars weaken the mandible at the angle and increase the likelihood of fractures occurring in this region. The anterior mandibular body is another frequent site of fracture because of the weakness caused by the long ca-

FIGURE 38.6. Displacement of the condyle due to anteromedial pull of the lateral pterygoid muscle.

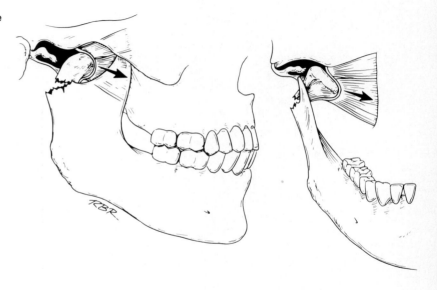

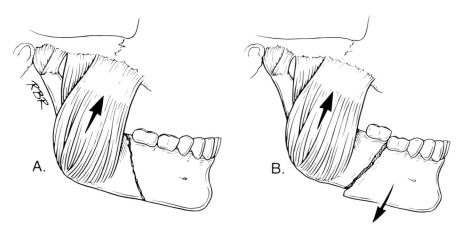

FIGURE 38.7. **A,** Favorably oriented fracture of the posterior body of the mandible. The masseter tends to reduce the fracture in this orientation (rare). **B,** Unfavorably displaced fracture of the posterior body of the mandible. The masseter–internal pterygoid muscle sling tends to disrupt this fracture line. A tooth that remains firm in the proximal fragment will act as a stop to this displacement if there is opposing occlusion.

nine tooth and the mental foramen. Any fractures that extend through a tooth socket should be considered open fractures and treated accordingly.

The mandible is weakened in early childhood with numerous unerupted and permanent teeth, but fractures are usually incomplete and minimally displaced. The pediatric mandible is more malleable; therefore, fractures are less frequent. In older patients, when permanent teeth are lost, the alveolar ridge is resorbed, and the mandible is weakened at those points. The edentulous mandible is weakest of all.

Diagnosis

CLINICAL EXAMINATION

Because mandibular fractures most often result from assaults and motor vehicle accidents, it is not uncommon to find associated injuries of the head, spine, thorax, or abdomen. These injuries may be life-threatening and must be immediately evaluated, as must any threat of

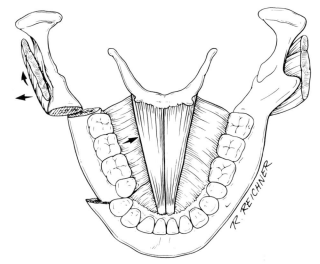

FIGURE 38.9. Segmental fractures of the mandibular body displaced medially by the action of the floor musculature.

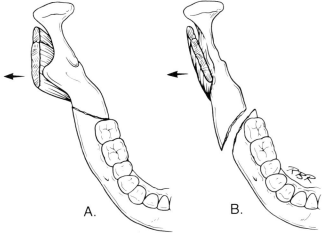

FIGURE 38.8. **A,** Favorably oriented fracture. Pull of the masseter on the mandibular angle tends to displace the proximal fragment laterally. The condylar head acts as a fulcrum. **B,** Unfavorably oriented fracture. Sagittal angulation in the dimension allows displacement laterally.

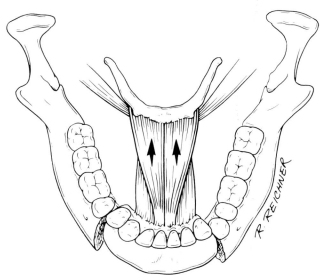

FIGURE 38.10. Bilateral body or parasymphseal fractures allow for inferior displacement of the distal fragment through the action of the suprahyoid musculature.

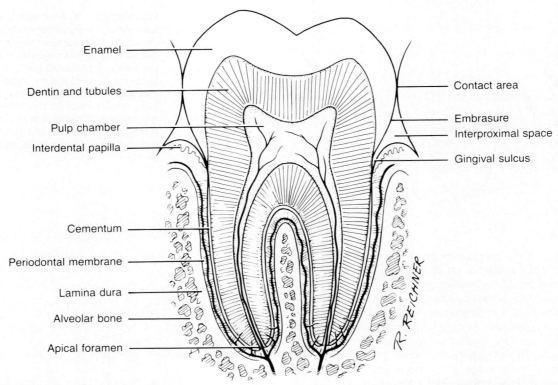

FIGURE 38.11. Anatomy of a molar tooth and the surrounding alveolar bone. Note blood supply to the pulp chamber through racemosing vessels at the root tip.

FIGURE 38.12. Dental fractures. The extent of exposure of the pulp is related to the possibility for salvage. In general, root fractures are not salvagable.

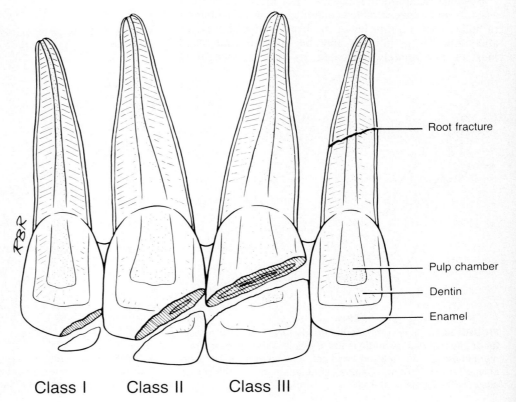

Class I   Class II   Class III

airway interference from a mandibular fracture. Bilateral condylar and symphysis fractures will result in a ''flail'' mandible, allowing posterior displacement of the tongue and soft tissues and possible upper airway obstruction. Oral bleeding dentures, or broken teeth can also compromise the airway.

A thorough history should, of course, be obtained with attention to dental hygiene, tooth or periodontal disease, preinjury malocclusion, previous maxillary or mandibular fractures, and any TMJ symptoms. The most common complaints in patients with acute mandibular fractures are pain and malocclusion. Other symptoms include trismus, swelling, numbness, and ecchymosis.

Visual inspection should be done both externally and intraorally for asymmetry, malocclusion, lacerations, ecchymosis, fractured or displaced teeth, and restrictions or deviations in opening, closing, or protrusion. Intraoral ecchymosis or hematoma are usually indicative of an underlying fracture. Careful external and internal palpation of the mandible will reveal areas of tenderness and step-offs. The condylar region may be palpated in the preauricular area and by placing one's fingers in the external auditory canals. If a fracture interrupts or violates the inferior alveolar or mental nerve, there will be numbness of the lower lip and other tissues served by those nerves.

RADIOLOGICAL EXAMINATION

If a mandibular fracture is suspected, the patient should undergo a radiographic examination that should include a ''mandibular series'' and Panorex (Fig. 38.13). The mandibular series usually includes a posterior-anterior (PA) view, Townes view, and right and left lateral oblique views. The PA view should be extended to demonstrate the condylar necks. These views may be modified for the severely injured patient who must remain supine.

Different parts of the mandible may be seen better in each of these radiographic views, but it is the additional panoramic view (Panorex) that is the most informative because it shows the entire mandible. However, the symphyseal and parasymphyseal regions may lack definition, and a fracture in this area may go undetected. An intraoral occlusal projection of the mandibular parasymphysis will augment the Panorex in this region. When routine radiographs fail to adequately demonstrate subcondylar fractures, tomography may be used to provide better detail. Coronal computed tomography (CT) may also be used to furnish more information about the fragments.

Principles of Treatment

Basic principles and goals of the treatment of mandibular fractures are directed toward restoring a normal functional relationship between the jaws and teeth, ensuring adequate union of the fracture segments, maintaining facial symmetry and balance, and preventing infection or other untoward sequelae.

After confirming that no other serious injuries exist, a definitive diagnosis should be made, and expedient treatment should be carried out. The essential operative principles have not changed since they were introduced many centuries ago—that is, adequate reduction of the fractured segments and immobilization of the parts to allow healing of the bone. The simplest and most effective treatment that accomplishes this goal is always the most desirable approach.

New patients with mandibular fractures will benefit from antibiotic therapy because the majority of such fractures are classified as open fractures (9). Exceptions to this statement include those fractures in the region of the condyle and coronoid. It may also be prudent to prescribe antibiotics when concomitant injuries indicate their use.

For a day or so after the injury, inadequate oral fluid intake is not unusual. Appropriate intravenous fluids may be necessary to ensure fluid and electrolyte requirements. Thereafter, clear liquids and pureed foods by mouth are consumed with little difficulty. It is not unusual for patients in maxillomandibular fixation for 6 weeks to lose 10 pounds or more; therefore, counseling for a ''wired jaw'' diet is necessary.

Maintaining good oral hygiene with immobilized jaws is extremely important. This is especially true in patients with compound oral wounds or intraoral lacerations. Small, soft pediatric toothbrushes, mouthwashes, hydrogen peroxide, and, in selected cases, a Water Pik may be helpful.

Methods of Fixation

The management of mandibular fractures can be a simple or a complex task. Some undisplaced fractures may be immobilized with a Barton bandage, but most will require interdental fixation, maxillomandibular fixation, and/or interosseous fixation with wires or screws and/or plates. The use of a dental splint, made from preoperative dental models, may also be indicated.

BANDAGE FIXATION

A Barton bandage is a type of maxillomandibular fixation that may be utilized if an undisplaced fracture needs immobilization and other methods are not available. The bandage can be reinforced with tape but will still need to be replaced periodically as it loosens.

INTERDENTAL FIXATION

Fractures of the alveolar process alone, in which the teeth are securely in their sockets, can be treated by reduction and fixation with an arch bar (Fig. 38.14), but it is difficult to orient the teeth into their precise preinjury occlusion without maxillomandibular fixation. If individual teeth are loose, then a lingual splint (made preoperatively) may add stability and help to prevent any vertical extrusion of the teeth. This method will also allow approximation of the preinjury occlusion in the most controlled fashion. Many types of intradental fixation are available, but the arch bar is most commonly used.

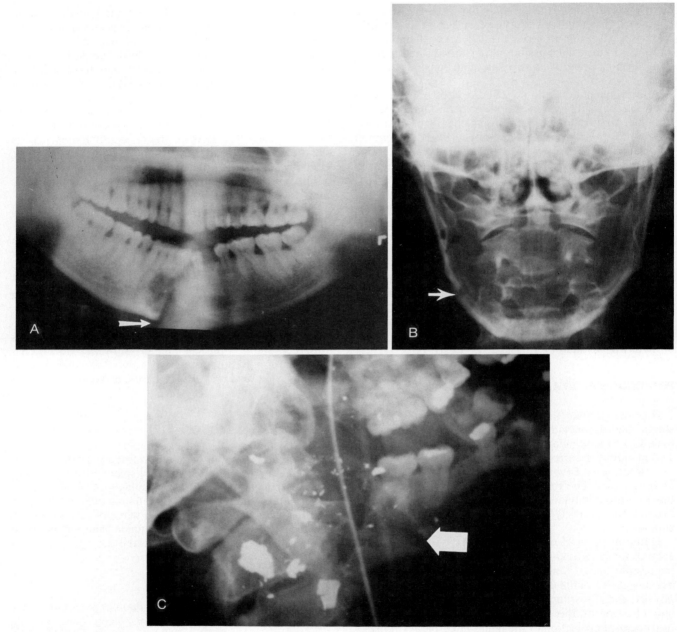

FIGURE 38.13.   A, Panorex; arrow marks site of parasymphy-seal fracture. **B,** PA radiograph of mandible; arrow marks site of angle fracture in an edentulous patient. **C,** Lateral radiograph of mandible; arrow marks site of angle fracture caused by gunshot.

MAXILLOMANDIBULAR (INTERMAXILLARY) FIXATION

In the past, almost all mandibular fractures needed some form of maxillomandibular fixation (MMF), whether treated with closed or open reduction, in order to immobilize the mandible and allow healing to occur. When the techniques of internal rigid plate and screw fixation are used, MMF is required to place the teeth in proper occlusion prior to application of the plates. The MMF may then be released either at the completion of surgery or soon thereafter.

Arch Bar Fixation

Placement of a secure, comfortable arch bar is an essential technique to master. The Erich dental arch bar is the most frequently used of all those available and is depicted in the figures in this chapter. If the arch bar is not properly secured, this improper immobilization may lead to malocclusion and/or malunion.

The arch bar is bent to conform to the teeth of the mandible, and the center of the bar is aligned with the midline. Any part of the arch bar that extends beyond the first molar may usually be trimmed, unless further stabili-

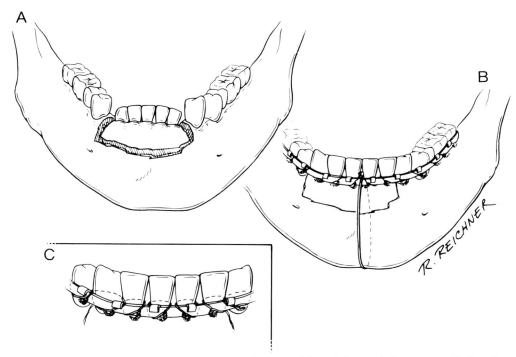

FIGURE 38.14. Fixation of mandibular aveolar fracture with arch bar and circum-mandibular wires.

zation is needed from the more posterior molars (Fig. 38.15). The lugs on the mandibular arch bar should open inferiorly, and those on the maxillary arch bar should be pointed in the opposite direction. The bar is then secured to the canine, premolars, and first molar on each side with 24- or 25-gauge stainless steel wire. One should try to avoid including any gingival tissue within the circumdental wire, and constant tension should be directed toward the roots of the teeth when tightening these wires. The twisted ends are then bent in toward the gingiva. Care should also be taken to hold the wire, with a dental instrument or elevator, below the cingulum of the canine when twisting this wire tightly. Generally, the arch bar should not be in contact with or ligated to the incisor teeth. The immobility of the arch bar should then be tested, and the circumdental wires tightened further, if necessary. If the lugs on the arch bar are blocked by the circumdental wires, the lugs may be slightly bent out so they may readily receive the maxillomandibular wires or elastics. After the maxillary arch bar is applied in the same fashion, the teeth may be put into occlusion, and the mandibular and maxillary arch bars are stabilized in position with dental elastics or 25- or 26-gauge wire. These elastics or wires may be oriented in a direction to produce traction in the desired vector.

Many modifications and additions to this description of arch bar application exist. The placement of wires around the central and lateral incisors should be avoided, if possible, because extrusion of these teeth can easily occur. If an incisor does require a circumdental wire, 26- or 28-gauge wire should be used, and all of the incisors should be wired in order to distribute the force evenly. When incisors are attached to the arch bars, maxillomandibular

elastics or wires between incisors are avoided because they can also inadvertently extrude teeth. Circumferential wiring of the mandible may be needed for added stability of the lower arch bar if there is an insufficient number of teeth to which to attach the arch bar (Fig. 38.14**B**).

When the arch bar is placed across a fracture line, it may be utilized to help compress and fixate the fracture (a tension band). This is achieved by first wiring the arch bar to the teeth on the opposing segment in such a way that the circumdental wires are tightened around an arch bar lug located farther from the stable segment. Tightening the wires will therefore compress and fixate the fracture along the interdental plane. Care should be taken not to apply this force to teeth immediately adjacent to the fracture because they may be forced from their sockets.

One may also use a continuous arch bar when multiple segments of the mandible are fractured, but the teeth should be placed into occlusion when doing the final tightening of the circumdental wires, so that preinjury occlusion is correctly reconstructed. A less preferred approach entails dividing the arch bar at the multiple fracture sites so that the fractured mandibular segments may be brought into occlusion with the teeth of the maxillary arch, preferably with a dental splint (10). This will ensure optimal occlusion.

Noncontinuous Loop Fixation

Maxillomandibular fixation with Ivy loops on the first two molars of each jaw is rarely used but is a simple and effective method of immobilization for condylar fractures. The Kazanjian button can provide similar immobi-

FIGURE 38.15. **A,** The arch bar is trimmed to conform to the length of the dental arch. **B,** It is contoured distally to allow it to exactly conform to the dentition and prevent extrusion into the soft tissues of the cheek. **C,** In the pediatric situation, the primary molars and canine are used for fixation. **D,** The conical shape of the canine tooth sometimes necessitates a special loop over the bar to allow for securing the wire below the crest of contour of the tooth's cingulum. **E,** The arch bar when completed is most often secured to the first molar tooth but may be extended as necessary. In addition, the arch bar is kept from contact on the incisor teeth, and ligatures around the incisors are usually avoided.

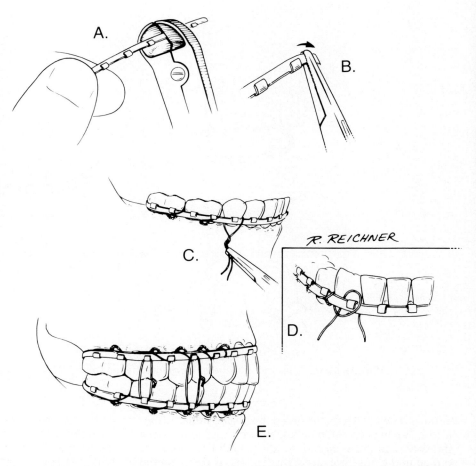

lization (Fig. 38.16). Although each button is usually based on two teeth, it may be formed with one circumdental wire. These methods lack the stability of the arch bar technique, but they may be quickly applied at the bedside.

Continuous Loop Fixation

Stout and Obwegeser have described a continuous wire loop method for producing MMF (11; Fig. 38.17). This loop of 25-gauge wire should extend from canine to first molar, and the twisted loops in the interdental space

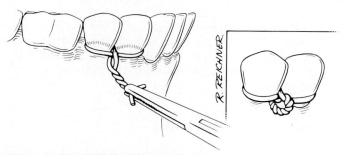

FIGURE 38.16. A Kazanjian button is placed by using 22- or 24-gauge wire secured as depicted through the premolar/molar region onto the adjacent teeth. The twist is tightened down on the labial loop.

are kept short. Maxillomandibular fixation may then be produced by twist tightening a 26-gauge wire between the opposing loops on the maxilla and mandible.

Maxillomandibular fixation of any type may be complete with wires or elastics, but the former may be better in the uncooperative patient who is constantly trying to open his or her mouth for talking or chewing. Maxillomandibular fixation with wires provides better stability than elastics and may therefore be preferred when rigid internal fixation is not used. Elastics have the advantage of being more easily adjusted or removed.

Patients with jaw fractures that are repaired with rigid screw-plate fixation may be released from MMF at the end of the fixation. This approach minimizes the risk of airway compromise and aspiration in the immediate postoperative period and therefore decreases the need for intensive care unit monitoring. Some surgeons release the MMF after a week postoperatively in order to minimize stress at the fracture sites and take advantage of the "settling" of the occlusion that occurs with MMF. The hardware is kept on the jaws in case it is needed at some time during the healing period for MMF. Also, the arch bar may serve as a tension band across the fracture site. In those patients without rigid fixation, the MMF is usually maintained for about 6 weeks, except in the cases of condyle fractures, in which motion needs to be resumed early. If the fracture site seems solid and nontender after 6 weeks of MMF, the jaws may be released from each other. If there is no pain or motion at the fracture site

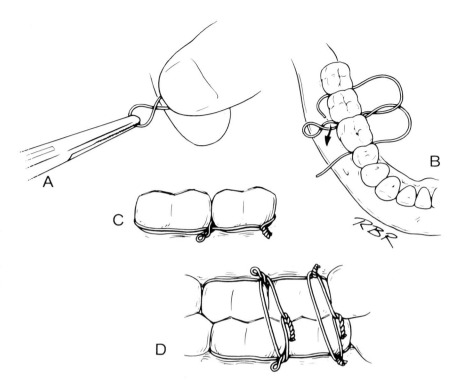

FIGURE 38.17. Technique of continuous loop wire fixation.

after a week or two of a soft diet and the occlusion is maintained, the hardware may be removed.

INTEROSSEOUS FIXATION

Many mandibular fractures are unstable with MMF alone and require open reduction and interosseous fixation. Interosseous fixation may be achieved with wiring, plate and screws, or external fixators. Kirschner wires are seldom used because superior methods are available.

Exposure may be obtained through external or intraoral incisions, but with percutaneous drilling and screwing and right-angle drills and screwdrivers, the intraoral approach can frequently be used. External approaches should especially be contemplated when complex, comminuted fractures are present. Inferior buccal sulcus incisions will allow exposure of most mandibular fractures, but with more anterior incisions, injury to the mental nerve by traction or cutting must be avoided. A cuff of mucosa should be left attached to the gingiva to allow easy closure, and the very superficial course of the mental nerve under the mucosa should be noted.

A submental incision will provide excellent exposure of midline and parasymphyseal fractures without the attendant risks of working around the mental nerve and intraoral bacterial contamination. Posterior body and angle fractures may also be exposed through submandibular incisions, but care should be taken to avoid the subplatysmal course of the marginal mandibular nerve. If it is possible, it is best to place the patient in MMF prior to interosseous fixation, in order to ensure that the occlusion is correct. Stabilization of the bony fragments while drilling may be done with bone-grasping forceps, but at times this is quite difficult because of the angle of the bones to the

wound. The fracture site should be débrided of any bone chips and old blood to allow direct, close approximation of the bone segments. Closure of the wounds should be in layers so that optimal coverage of the hardware is obtained. The use of suction drainage is up to the discretion of the surgeon.

Interosseous Wire Fixation

A variety of wiring patterns are possible, and two of the more common ones are described here. Once exposure is obtained and the fracture reduced, two holes should be drilled on one side of the fracture line, and 24-gauge wire is threaded in a simple fashion (Fig. 38.18). The patient must be in MMF when final twists are placed. Once tightened, the twisted wire ends may be inserted back into one of the drill holes. Another method entails drilling one hole on each side of the fracture and threading a 24-gauge wire through these holes and then in a crisscross fashion under the inferior margin of the mandible. Because micromotion is still possible along the fracture line when utilizing interosseous wire fixation, the mandible still needs immobilization with MMF for 6 weeks, as described above.

Metal Plate and Screw Fixation

Anatomical reduction and compression of mandibular fractures with rigid plate and screw fixation technique allows faster bone healing and immediate restoration of mandibular motion. Studies have shown that tight cortex-to-cortex contact results in primary bone healing by direct bone deposition and Haversian remodeling (12, 13).

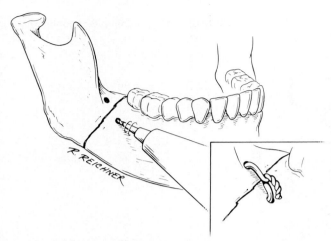

FIGURE 38.18. Technique of simple wire fixation placed through an intraoral approach at the mandibular angle. *Note:* The patient must be in intermaxillary fixation prior to tightening this wire fixator.

This bypasses the characteristics of secondary bone healing found in fracture sites that still have a small gap or motion remaining. This secondary process entails granulation tissue deposition, followed by callous and cartilaginous tissue before true bone bridging occurs (14).

There are many mandibular plate and screw fixation systems commercially available, but they all follow similar principles. The systems made of titanium or Vitallium have such excellent tissue compatibility that the hardware does not need to be removed unless placed in a child or across a defect that has been bone grafted. It is advised to remove plates in children (4–5 weeks postoperatively) so that potential growth is not impaired, and in bone grafted defects (3–4 months postoperatively) so that functional stress may be reestablished through the bone graft.

It should be noted that the various systems should not be used together in the same wound because the metals may interact and cause demineralization secondary to galvanic currents. It is sometimes necessary to use stainless steel wire to approximate smaller fragments of bone prior to rigid plate fixation of the larger segments. This should not produce any significant electrical interaction with the plates, especially if they are not in contact with each other.

One practical difference between the systems is that some have self-tapping screws, whereas others require pretapping of the holes. One should document the type of system used in a case, so that the correct screwdriver is available if the hardware ever needs to be removed. Whatever system is used, it is imperative to run the drill at a slow speed and with plenty of cooling irrigation in order to minimize the heat of friction and maximize bone viability. Mandibular plates and screws are bigger and sturdier than those used for facial or hand fractures in order to handle the stronger forces exerted through the lower jaw.

To achieve this functional stability, the compression plate must be perfectly conformed to the surface of the reduced fractured area, while maintaining perfect prein-

jury occlusion. If the plate is not conformed well, then when the screws are tightened, the bone will move to fit the plate and not vice versa (Fig. 38.19**A**). The plate may be slightly overbent, as depicted in Figure 38.19**B**, so that compressive forces are also applied to the opposite (lingual) cortex when the bicortical screws are applied.

The plates are usually applied along the lateral-inferior border of the mandible because this is where the thickest stress-absorbing bone is located, and it avoids the mandibular canal and roots of the teeth. The distance between the mandibular canal and the inferior border of the mandible varies, but a Panorex may reveal the course of the canal more precisely. The inner holes of the plate also need to be far enough away from the fracture line (of both cotices) so that the area is not further fractured with the application of the screws. The relationship of the fracture lines in the lingual cortex and labial-buccal cortex may be determined by direct inspection and evaluation of the radiographs and computed tomograms.

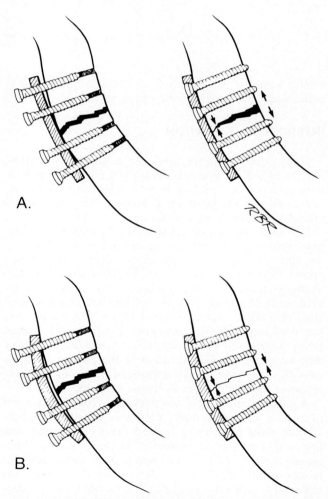

FIGURE 38.19. Application of compression plates to the mandible. **A,** It is important that the plate be well adapted to the fracture site because a straight plate will cause distraction at the lingual cortex. **B,** Overbending of the plate as depicted will allow for compression at the lingual cortex.

It is important to have applied tension across the fracture line in the alveolar process in the form of an arch bar, wires, or small plate prior to application of the inferior border plate. This is necessary so that compression along the inferior border does not alter the occlusion. Placing the patient in MMF will also help maintain this relationship.

Once the interdental and possibly maxillomandibular fixations are applied, the fracture is reduced, and the compression plate is appropriately conformed, the drilling of holes may proceed (Fig. 38.20). One of the holes closest to the fracture should be drilled first, and the depth of the hole is then measured. The appropriate length screw is then screwed in, but not tightly. The plate is then adjusted so that this screw is eccentrically positioned in the plate hole, and drilling is then commenced in the closest hole on the opposite side of the fracture. This second bone hole is also eccentrically positioned within the plate hole, and then the appropriate length screw is applied. Both of these screws are then alternately tightened a little at a time until full compression of the fracture is attained. The last two holes, further away from the fracture line, are then drilled in neutral positions, and screws are applied. If the fracture line is already closely approximated before application of the plate and screws, the eccentric positioning of the first two screws should not be overdone because it can lead to fracture of the bone around the screw, and the head will not be well seated.

The use of internal rigid fixation allows MMF to be released at the end of surgery or soon thereafter, and this has many advantages. With concomitant fractures in the condylar region, early mobilization and physiotherapy may be instituted to optimize treatment in that area. It can prevent life-threatening complications in patients with multiple trauma, seizures, or other mental disabilities and perhaps prevent the need of a tracheostomy. The weight loss usually associated with 6 weeks of MMF may also be avoided.

Multiple investigators have shown that the incidence of infection is directly related to the mobility of the bone fragments and that rigid immobilization decreases this incidence. In fact, the increased risk or presence of infection in mandibular fractures, which are amenable to internal rigid fixation, is an indication for the use of compression plates or screws (15, 16).

Compression (Lag) Screw Fixation

Lag screws may also be used for rigid internal fixation in horizontally oblique fractures of the lateral and anterior mandible. The principle of placing lag screws entails overdrilling the diameter of the hole in the proximal cortex so that the threads of the screw only take hold of the distal cortex. When the screw is tightened, the head of the screw compresses the proximal fragment against the distal fragment, which is gripped by the screw threads. A lag or compression screw placed perpendicular to the fracture plane provides the best compression, but the fragments may slide on one another. Placing the screw perpendicular to the long axis (surface) of the bone minimizes displacement, but it does not provide very good compression. Thus, the optimal orientation of the lag screw is along a line that bisects the angle produced by the two above orientations (Fig. 38.21). One lag screw is frequently insufficient to immobilize a fracture. It is often used with a second lag screw, a plate, or MMF.

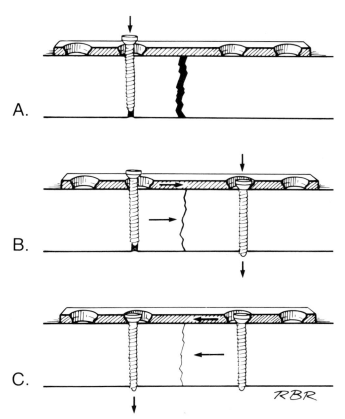

FIGURE 38.20. Order of holes drilled for compression plating. See text for explanation.

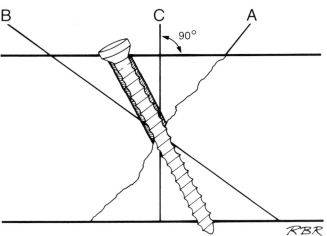

FIGURE 38.21. Principles of lag screw fixation (see text for explanation).

EXTERNAL FIXATION

External fixation of mandibular fractures is indicated when secondary healing does not occur after débridement of an infected fracture that was originally treated with internal rigid fixation. It may also be used when there has been significant soft tissue damage and segmental loss of bone secondary to the initial trauma or subsequent infection. This approach allows soft tissues to heal without the impedance of foreign bodies and avoids the necessity of MMF so that motion may be resumed in the immediate postoperative period. Disadvantages include scarring at the pin holes, potential infection via the pin tracts, and the cumbersome nature of the appliance.

Both monophasic and biphasic methods for application of an external fixator have been described (17, 18). As the latter name implies, there are two phases to this technique. The first phase entails placing two screws into stable bone on each side of the fracture. This is accomplished by making small stab incisions over the lateral inferior border of the mandible and bluntly dissecting down to bone. An obturator may be used for exposure and to prevent damage to the soft tissues. Appropriately sized drill holes are then created below the mandibular canal, and the pins are screwed through both cortices. The external ends of the pins should be roughly on the same plane, and a slight amount of divergence is preferable. Fixation clamps and rods are then placed on at least

one pin on either side of the fracture and then tightened with the exposed fracture segments reduced or aligned as well as possible. The second phase entails preparing a quick-drying acrylic and pouring it into a long, rectangular metal splint (Fig. 38.22). When the acrylic is doughy to the touch, it is transferred to the ends of the four pins, and then the nuts are screwed on the ends. The acrylic is held in position while it hardens so that it is far enough away from the skin to allow cleaning of the pins. Once it is hard, the fixation clamps and rods may be removed.

The monophase method is simpler because it obviates the need for fixation clamps and rods. With this technique, one may use the same pins as described above or use 3.6- or 4.0-mm threaded Steinmann pins, which are usually easily available. Once the pins are in place, a no. 10 or 11 plastic endotracheal tube is prepared by cutting holes in the tube to go over the end of each pin. Once the tube is in place, the fracture is held in a reduced and/or well-aligned position, and the mixed acrylic is injected into the end of the tube with a sterile 50-ml catheter-tip syringe. The tube is held in place until the acrylic hardens. The pins and tube may be coated with petroleum ointment before injecting the acrylic so that excess acrylic may be easily removed from these areas when it is in the doughy stage. Antibacterial ointment is placed around the pins at the skin. Daily care of these pin sites is needed. Removal of these external fixators is a simple task.

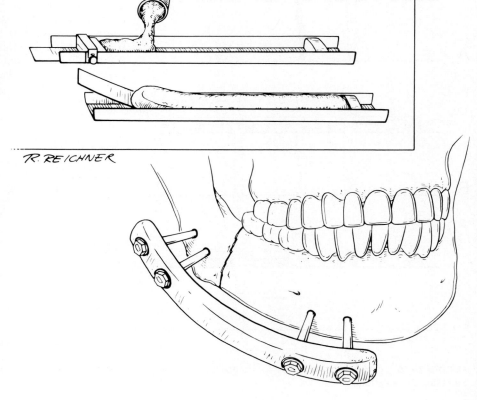

FIGURE 38.22. Placement of external pin fixation. Note fabrication of acrylic splint in the provided forming device (inset). This acrylic is transferred to the external fixation pins when it is of doughy consistency. At least two pins are necessary for stabilization on either side of the fracture. First phase fixation device is not shown.

R. REICHNER

DENTAL SPLINTS

Dental splints are useful and sometimes necessary to restore preinjury occlusion when trauma has resulted in loss of teeth or multiple alveolar ridge fractures. These splints are classified as either occlusal, lingual, or Gunning. The Gunning splints or the patient's modified dentures have application in edentulous patients.

The making of acrylic splints entails routine dental techniques, and the help of a general dentist, prosthodontist, or dental technician may be of great value in this regard. The process entails taking impressions of the maxillary and mandibular arches with alginate. Dental stone or plaster is poured into these impressions to create models of the dental arches. Cuts may then be made in the models of patients with multiple fractures that correspond to the fracture lines. The individual segments are fixed into position for proper occlusion with dental or sticky wax, as judged by the occlusion with the maxillary arch. With the models on a dental articulator, a minimal opening space is set, and the occlusal surfaces lubricated. Partially cured acrylic is then placed in the occlusal plane, and the articulator is closed to produce a dental occlusal splint. The splint is then trimmed, and holes may be made along its edge to allow for the passage of wires. A second type of splint is fabricated along the lingual border of the mandible with holes placed for circumdental wires. Gunning splints are made for the edentulous patient in a manner approximating the construction of full dentures.

The taking of impressions in the patient with multiple alveolar fractures will often need to be done under a general anesthetic because of the pain it can produce. Once the splint is prepared, the patient may be taken back to surgery and placed into maxillomandibular occlusion with the splint guiding the teeth into their proper positions.

Each of the cuspid and incisor teeth have only one cusp and therefore no vertical stops from opposing teeth, unlike the premolars and molars. When these teeth are loose within their sockets or in a fragment of bone that is loose, they require MMF with a dental splint in order to produce this vertical stop and proper orientation.

In the patient with previous or traumatic loss of key teeth, a partial denture may be altered by the attachment of arch bar–type lugs. This partial denture may then be secured to the mandible with circum-mandibular wires, and a second splint, if needed, can be secured to the maxillary arch with circumzygomatic, infraorbital rim, piriform margin, and/or anterior nasal spine suspensory wires.

In edentulous patients, their own dentures may be modified and secured to both arches for MMF. Modifications may entail placing hooks or holes in the lateral surfaces for the passage of maxillomandibular wires. The anterior teeth may also be removed to permit eating and drinking (Fig. 38.23). If the dentures are not available or the patient does not desire alteration of them, a Gunning-type splint may be constructed.

Regional Considerations in Fracture Management

Many of the techniques involved in the management of mandibular fractures have been discussed in the above section, but certain regional considerations need attention.

ALVEOLAR PROCESS AND TEETH

Fractures of the alveolar process will often leave enough mucosal attachments to segments to maintain via-

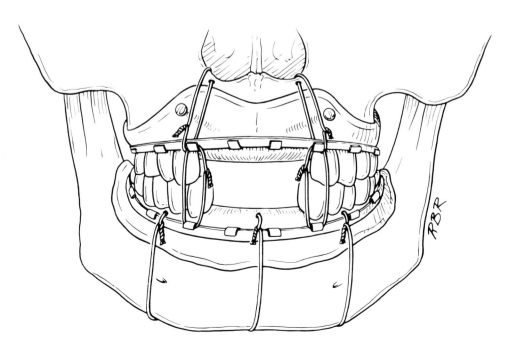

FIGURE 38.23. Dentures modified as Gunning splints. *Note:* Fixation is by circum-mandibular wires for the lower splint and by pyriform aperture and/or transalveolar screws for the maxillary splint. The incisor teeth have been removed to allow for function.

bility. These fractured segments should be reduced and immobilized with interdental fixation and possibly the use of a dental splint, as previously described. Some of these teeth may require endodontic treatment or extraction at a later date if they prove to be devitalized. If a segment of alveolar process has been avulsed to the point of being assuredly devitalized, removal of this bone and closure with local soft tissue is indicated. Completely avulsed teeth should be placed back into their sockets and may well need restorative dentistry at a later time.

Teeth in the line of fracture should not be routinely extracted; they may still be viable and may help to stabilize the fracture. However, teeth with dental or periodontal disease, which may increase the risk of infection, should be removed. Teeth in this category include impacted third molars and those with severe caries and no effective crown, periapical infections in the line of fracture, significant periodontal disease in the line of fracture, and/or fractured roots.

Extraction of a tooth requires a pulling force with gentle rocking motion so that it is removed without further fracturing. The dental socket should be thoroughly débrided with a bone curette and irrigated to remove any root fragments or dental follicular tissue. Any protruding bone spicules around the socket may then be removed to allow loose closure of the gingiva.

SYMPHYSIS AND PARASYMPHYSIS

Fractures of the mandibular midline are uncommon but, when present, they are likely to be associated with condylar fractures. It is sometimes difficult to see these fractures on the Panorex; therefore, occlusal radiographs should be obtained. These fractures are best treated with open reduction through a submental or inferior buccal incision and fixation with interosseous wires and arch bar or rigid plate and screws. When associated with condylar fractures, rigid internal fixation will allow early mobilization of the lower jaw. The relationship between the fracture lines through the lingual and labial/buccal cortices should be thoroughly evaluated so that all screws engage both cortices without causing fragmentation near either fracture line.

Fractures in the parasymphyseal region are more common and, like those in the midline, may be hard to anatomically reduce because of the considerable muscular forces pulling on the fragments. These fractures are not uncommonly associated with other fractures of the contralateral mandible. Treatment options are the same as those described for midline fractures. The approach is more frequently extraoral to avoid damage to the mental nerve.

BODY

A nondisplaced, vertically and horizontally favorable fracture of the mandibular body may be treated with closed reduction and MMF, but this decision depends on the specifics of each case. It is most often optimal to openly reduce these fractures and apply internal rigid fixation to the lower border of the mandible, with MMF as needed. It should be noted that, if severe mandibular trauma results in the loss of bone, one should consider the use of a long mandibular reconstruction plate, with 4 or 5 screws on each end, to span the defect. After soft tissue healing has occurred, secondary bone grafting may be accomplished with iliac crest or cranial bone grafts.

ANGLE

The presence of a third molar makes the mandibular angle particularly prone to fracture, especially from a lateral impact. The fracture line often extends through the socket of this molar, making it an open fracture. If the third molar has roots that make it difficult to apply a rigid plate and screws, is impacted, and/or is partially covered with an operculum of gingiva harboring bacteria, it should be extracted. If the third molar is not diseased and assists in the stability of the reduced fracture, it may be best to retain the tooth. With the tooth removed, this fracture is amenable to superior border reduction and unicortical plate fixation from an intraoral approach.

Patients with nondisplaced fractures may be treated with closed reduction and MMF, but posterior angle fractures, behind the last tooth, frequently require internal rigid fixation. These fractures may also be approached through intraoral incisions, which reduces the risk of facial nerve damage seen with external incisions. Contralateral mandibular fractures, especially at the condylar neck, are often associated.

VERTICAL RAMUS

Fractures of the ramus are uncommon and rarely displaced because of the splinting effect of the masseter–medial pterygoid muscle sling. Unless displacement causes vertical shortening, these fractures are generally immobilized with MMF. If open reduction and internal rigid fixation are needed, an intraoral approach may be used with the help of percutaneous drilling and screwing or right-angled instruments. An external incision may be needed if further exposure is needed.

CORONOID PROCESS

Isolated fractures of the coronoid process are rare, and the possibility of concomitant fractures should be investigated. These fractures may be caused by severe contraction of the temporalis muscle. Distraction of the fractured coronoid is seldom found because the tendinous attachments from the temporalis muscle extend onto the anterior border of the vertical ramus. These isolated fractures are usually treated without any type of fixation, and the patient is placed on a soft diet until the pain resolves. Patients with complaints of severe pain may benefit from short-term MMF in order to alleviate this problem.

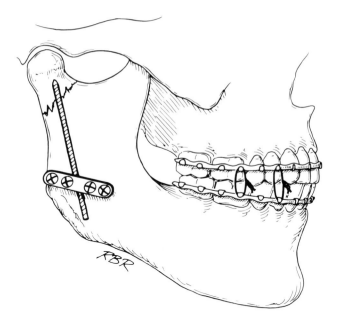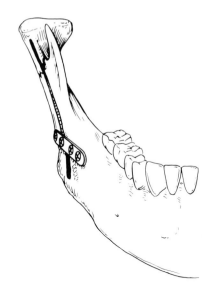

FIGURE 38.24. Preferred method for fixation of condylar fractures. A threaded K wire is used to skewer the condylar neck. A trough is cut in the ramus for the placement of the pin, and the pin is secured with a bone plate. *Note:* A stainless steel plate is necessary because it will be in contact with the pin made of the same material.

CONDYLE

Subcondylar fractures are relatively common because the neck is structurally weak. The condyle is usually displaced medially by the pull from the lateral pterygoid muscle, and secondary vertical shortening of the posterior mandible with an open bite deformity may occur from the pull of the closing muscles. The exact position of the condyle may be determined with plain or computed tomograms.

The proper management of these fractures is still controversial, but animal and clinical studies (19–21) tend to support conservative treatment with closed reduction and MMF for 2–3 weeks. This is especially true when the condylar head is still in the articular fossa. This period of MMF would be followed by progressive physical therapy to maximize opening and protrusion of the mandible.

Open reduction of condylar fractures is indicated if: (*a*) the condyle is displaced into the middle cranial fossa; (*b*) there is lateral extracapsular displacement of the condyle; (*c*) the displaced condyle still functionally blocks opening or closing of the mandible after a 2-week trial period of MMF; and (*d*) a posterior vertical shortening of the mandible with an open bite deformity persists after a 2-week trial period of MMF. Relative indications include bilateral condylar fractures associated with comminuted, unstable midfacial fractures; and bilateral condylar fractures in an edentulous patient when a splint is unavailable or impossible because of alveolar ridge atrophy (20).

Many methods of stabilization have been described, including rigid plating, interosseous wiring, K wire or pin fixation, and replacement of the condyle with a prosthesis. The placement of a threaded Steinman pin from below into the fractured condylar neck and its fixation into a trough cut into the vertical ramus and angle, is the preferred means of alignment (Fig. 38.24).

Exposure of the condylar region may require a submandibular and/or preauricular approach, depending on the exact position of the fracture. Percutaneous drilling and screwing may be needed to fix the plate. Care should be taken to minimally strip the condyle of its periosteal blood supply and only drill the holes necessary, in order to minimize the chance of avascular necrosis of the condylar head. Depending on the stability of the repair, mandibular motion may begin in the immediate postoperative period or after 2–3 weeks of MMF. If necessary, the condylar head may be removed in order to apply appropriate screws and plates and then replaced as a bone graft with rigid fixation.

Fractures extending through the condylar head should be treated with MMF for 10–14 days, followed by progressive physical therapy. Late sequelae of closed and open reductions include avascular necrosis of the condylar head, TMJ pain, arthritic changes in the TMJ, and decreased motion.

Fractures in Children

Fractures of the mandible in children are rare. In addition to their protected environment, a child's facial skeleton is soft and resilient and can sustain considerable insult without fracture. When a fracture does occur, it is often incomplete ("greenstick" fracture). In Rowe's study (22) of 500 facial fractures, there was only a 1.2% incidence of mandibular fractures in children 5 years old and younger and a 4.4% incidence in the 6–12-year-old group. Most of these fractures resulted from a bicycle or car accident or a fall from various heights.

Management of mandibular fractures in children must take into account their fast healing capacity and the growth potential of bone. Therefore, these fractures should be reduced as soon as possible to avoid malunion, and immobilization only needs to be maintained for 2 weeks postoperatively.

The deciduous teeth have a bell or cone shape, and this makes application of wires and arch bars difficult. The numerous developing tooth buds in the pediatric mandible make internal fixation difficult; therefore, it is only used when absolutely necessary. When indicated, interosseous wires or microplates and screws may be carefully placed along the very inferior margin of the mandible. Some surgeons believe that monocortical screws may be used in children in order to avoid the tooth buds. Plates and screws in pediatric mandibular fractures should be removed 4–5 weeks postoperatively in order to minimize any adverse affects on growth.

Mandibular fractures in children are usually treated with closed reduction and immobilization with some type of splint. If a full complement of firm, noncarious primary teeth or a sufficient number of erupted permanent teeth are present, arch bars may be secured with 28-gauge circumdental wires and supplemented with circum-mandibular wires. The patient is then placed into maxillomandibular fixation with elastics. If there is not a sufficient number of erupted teeth for arch bar fixation, an acrylic lingual splint may be made and secured to the mandible with circum-mandibular wires. This single arch splint will sufficiently immobilize the mandible and allow for mandibular motion if a concomitant condylar fracture is present. Unilateral subcondylar fractures are treated in the same fashion, but the period of immobilization is reduced to about 1 week.

Bilaterally displaced subcondylar fractures with posterior vertical shortening and open bite deformity in the pediatric patient require closed reduction and MMF for 3–4 weeks. Open reduction should be avoided at all costs because the procedure may result in some degree of arthrosis and growth disturbance. Also, children's condyles have tremendous potential for remodeling.

In the first 3 years of life, the condylar head consists of a delicate vascular "sponge" and thin cortical bone, and it is a center for mandibular growth. A significant blow during this age can result in severe compression and crushing of this structure, with secondary hemorrhage and hemarthrosis of the joint. This can then lead to ankylosis of the joint and growth disturbances. These intracapsular condylar head fractures should not be immobilized and may be additionally treated with aspiration of the joint.

Fractures in the Edentulous Patient

Fractures of the edentulous mandible can be difficult to manage. After the loss of teeth, there is resorption of the alveolar bone, and the vertical height of the denture-bearing area is significantly reduced. The atrophied, edentulous mandible is weaker with thin cortical plates, and the blood supply is essentially from periosteal vessels. These factors contribute to a decreased healing potential, resulting in a 20% incidence of nonunion (23).

Simple, undisplaced fractures can often be managed with pureed diet and observation. Unstable fractures may be openly reduced and immobilized with interosseous wires or, preferably, with rigid plate and screw fixation. In the severely atrophied jaw, the periosteum may be left on the bone to maximize blood supply, and the plate is placed over the periosteum.

Many edentulous patients with fractured mandibles may also be treated by splinting of the fracture with the patient's own dentures or a Gunning-type splint, as previously described. These are secured to the mandible on each side of the fracture with circum-mandibular wires. Adequate immobilization is sometimes difficult with this method because the denture or splint may not sit well on the mobile tissue that is usually present and cannot be secured too tightly to the mandible without causing soft tissue necrosis. Primary bone grafting and external fixation are other options to consider.

Postoperative Care

It is critical in the immediate postoperative period to have good airway control in the patient with MMF. While in the operating room, the stomach contents should be aspirated with a nasogastric tube. The tube may be left in overnight. The patient should not be extubated until he or she is alert enough to control his or her own airway. Upon extubation, a nasal trumpet airway may be inserted to assist air exchange. Suction and wire cutters should be kept at the bedside at all times. Patients treated with internal rigid fixation and release of MMF at the end of the case have less risk of developing any airway problems.

Feedings should progress from a clear liquid diet for 1–2 days to a nutritious "wired jaw" diet. Dietary counseling is often helpful. Good oral hygiene is encouraged with frequent mouth rinsing and the use of a Water Pik. Perioperative antibiotics are ordered, and perioperative steroids may be used to ostensibly decrease swelling.

Complications

Malocclusion is the most obvious complication resulting from mandibular fractures and their treatment. This may be secondary to malunion or nonunion, which in turn can result from infection.

Infection is treated by débridement of all nonviable tissue and any loose screws or plates. Plates and screws that are secure may be left intact, and in most cases, the wound should heal without difficulty.

Minor malocclusions can often be corrected by selective grinding of teeth or orthodontia. When nonunion or malunion occurs, secondary surgery is required at a later date to excise the fibrous malunion and bone graft any remaining defect. This bone graft should be rigidly fixed to the remaining bone, if possible. Iliac crest bone grafts have the advantage of providing cancellous bone and some cortical bone if needed for rigidity, but the donor site is painful. Split cranial bone grafts do not provide cancellous bone that may be needed to fill in irregularities in the recipient site, but they do provide an excellent thin on-lay of strong bone, which may be more easily immobilized with rigid fixation. The donor site is also relatively pain-free.

Temporomandibular joint symptoms of pain and clicking may occur with mandibular trauma and treatment of the fractures. These may resolve with physiotherapy and bite blocks, but if this conservative therapy continues to be ineffective, surgical intervention may become necessary.

Conclusion

The mandible remains the most difficult of facial bones to treat when fractured. New methods of plate and screw fixation have improved treatment modalities in a variety of situations. Continued evolution of these techniques, with improvements in patient care, is expected.

References

1. Rowe NL, Williams JLL: *Maxillofacial Injuries*. Edinburgh, Churchill Livingstone, 1985.
2. Schultz RC: *Facial Injuries,* ed 3. Year Book Medical Publishers, 1988.
3. Busuito MJ, Smith DJ Jr, Robson MC: Mandibular fractures in an urban trauma center. *J Trauma* 26:826, 1986.
4. Reil B, Kranz S: Traumatology of the maxillofacial region in childhood. *J Maxillofac Surg* 4:197, 1976.
5. Dingman RO, Natvig P: *Surgery of Facial Fractures*. Philadelphia, WB Saunders, 1964.
6. Hagan EH, Huelke DF: An analysis of 319 case reports of mandibular fractures. *J Oral Surg* 19:93, 1961.
7. Larsen OD, Nielsen A: Mandibular fractures—an analysis of their etiology and location in 286 patients. *Scand J Plast Reconstr Surg* 10:213, 1976.
8. Coccia CT: A clinical investigation of root resorption rates and reimplanted permanent incisors: A five year study. *J Endodontics* 6:413, 1980.
9. Zallen RD, Curry JT: A study of antibiotic usage in compound mandibular fractures. *J Oral Surg* 33:431, 1975.
10. Magee WP Jr: Dental principles applied to management of mandibular fractures. In Schultz RC (ed): *Facial Injuries,* ed 3. Year Book Medical Publishers, 1988.
11. Parker D: *Synopsis of Traumatic Injuries of the Face and Jaw.* St. Louis, CV Mosby, 1942, p 154.
12. Perren SM, Huggler A, Russenberger M, Straummer F, Muller ME, Allgower M: A method of measuring the change in compression applied to living cortical bone. *Acta Orthop Scand [Suppl]* 7:125, 1969.
13. Schenk RK, Willenegger H: Morphological findings in primary fracture healing. *Symp Biol Hung* 7:75, 1967.
14. Reitzik M, Schoorl W: Bone repair in the mandible. *J Oral Maxillofac Surg* 41:215, 1983.
15. Becker HL: Treatment of initially infected mandibular fractures with bone plates. *J Oral Surg* 37:310, 1979.
16. Tu HK, Tenhulzen D: Compression osteosynthesis of mandibular fractures: A retrospective study. *J Oral Maxillofac Surg* 43:585, 1985.
17. Waite DE: External biphase pin method for fixation of mandible. *Mayo Clin Proc* 42:294, 1967.
18. Wessberg GA, Schendel S, Epker BN: Monophase extraskeletal fixation. *J Oral Surg* 37:892, 1979.
19. Beekler DM, Walker RV: Condyle fractures. *J Oral Surg* 27:563, 1969.
20. Zide MF, Kent JN: Indication for open reduction of mandibular condyle fractures. *J Oral Maxillofac Surg* 41:89, 1983.
21. Russell D, Nosti JC, Reavis C: Treatment of fractures of the mandibular condyle. *J Trauma* 12:704, 1972.
22. Rowe NL: Fractures of the jaws in children. *J Oral Surg* 27:497, 1969.
23. Bruce RA, Strachan DS: Fractures of the edentulous mandible. The Chalmers J. Lyons Academy Study. *J Oral Surg* 34:973, 1976.

39

Benign and Malignant Tumors of the Oral Cavity

**Mark S. Granick, M.D., F.A.C.S., Mark P. Solomon, M.D., F.A.C.S.,
Dwight C. Hanna, M.D., F.A.C.S. and E. Douglas Newton, M.D., F.A.C.S.**

Anatomy

Tumors of the oral cavity are classified according to their size and location within the oral cavity. The classification and staging of these lesions aid in determining the proper treatment program and in prognosis. Consequently, a clear understanding of the various anatomical zones within the oral cavity is necessary in order to precisely define the extent and location of tumor growth. In addition, it is important to understand the anatomy of the remaining portions of the upper aerodigestive tract because some tumors extend beyond the oral cavity and, in some instances, there are synchronous or metachronous tumors.

The oral cavity (Fig. 39.1) begins at the cutaneous-vermilion border and extends to the level of the tonsillar pillars. Included within the oral cavity are the lips, the buccal surfaces, the buccal sulci, the alveolus and teeth, the hard palate, the floor of the mouth, the mobile portion of the tongue (anterior two thirds of the tongue, anterior to the circumvallate papillae), the retromolar trigone.

Other areas of relevance include the oropharynx, the hypopharynx, and the larynx. The nasopharynx is also an area that needs to be examined. The nasopharynx includes the nasal side of the soft palate and the area posterior to the choana, extending to the level of the posterior pharyngeal wall where the soft palate makes contact. The oropharynx includes the tonsils, the posterior tonsillar pillars, and the lateral and posterior pharyngeal walls to the level of the hyoid. Also included within the oropharynx is the sessile portion of the tongue posterior to the circumvallate papillae, known as the base of the tongue, and the valleculae. The hypopharynx is the area inferior to the hyoid to the level of the esophageal inlet. This includes the pyriform sinuses and the pharyngeal walls. The larynx includes the epiglottis and all of the structures leading into the larynx, as well as the glottis and the area immediately below the glottis and above the trachea. The larynx is subclassified into the supraglottic, glottic, and subglottic regions.

Examination

Patients who have tumors of the oral cavity require complete head and neck examinations. This examination is relatively simple to perform, but it should be done systematically each time to avoid overlooking pathology.

The first portion of the examination consists of a gross inspection of the patient's habitus, including personal hygiene, nutritional status, and affect. Personal factors are very important in deciding the appropriate course of therapy in patients with head and neck cancer. The next area of concern is inspection of the skin, including the scalp. Close inspection of the external ears, the external auditory canal, and the tympanic membranes is then required. Tumors of the external auditory canal can metastasize to the neck, and alterations in middle ear physiology can actually represent lesions obstructing the eustachian orifice in the nasopharynx. Many patients with oral tumors will present with ear pain, and it is important to rule out otological pathology in their evaluation.

The examination then proceeds to the nose, and an intranasal examination is performed. In order to do this examination properly, a coaxial light source is required. This will allow direct visualization of all of the areas of the nasal cavity. The nondominant hand should hold the nasal speculum, which is placed in the nostril and opened in a longitudinal direction to avoid impact on the nasal septum. When the nasal speculum is opened against the nasal septum, it is quite irritating for the patient. Care must be taken not to overlook evaluation of the nasal vestibule, which can easily be covered by the nasal speculum during the intranasal examination. If the patient has congested nasal mucosa, it is necessary to spray the nasal membranes with a vasoconstrictor.

Examination of the oral cavity commences with a look at the lips. Then, using two tongue depressors, the lips are retracted, and the buccal sulci and membranes are directly viewed. The teeth and alveolus are examined. Loose teeth without evidence of periodontal disease or infection are early warning signs of cancer. The floor of the mouth is next examined, and it is necessary to retract the tongue using a tongue blade to fully view the floor of the mouth. Function of the submandibular gland is assessed by milking the submandibular gland and observing the orifice of Wharton's duct. The entire tongue is then checked, starting at the root, where the frenulum attaches to the floor of the mouth, then the lateral surfaces, and finally the dorsal portion of the tongue. The retromolar trigone is then inspected by retracting the tongue medially and looking at the inner surface of the mandible inferior and posterior to the level of the molars. This mucosally lined surface is easily overlooked unless it is directly examined. The hard and soft palates are then visualized. After completion of this thorough visual in-

FIGURE 39.1. Anatomy of the oral cavity. From Granick MS, Larson DL: Management of head and neck cancer. In Russell R (ed): *PSEF: Instructional Courses*, vol II. St. Louis, CV Mosby, 1989.)

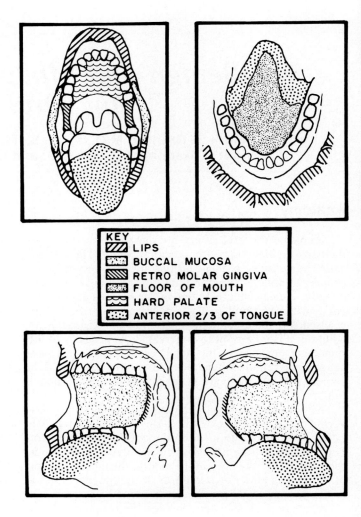

KEY
- LIPS
- BUCCAL MUCOSA
- RETRO MOLAR GINGIVA
- FLOOR OF MOUTH
- HARD PALATE
- ANTERIOR 2/3 OF TONGUE

spection of the oral cavity, the oropharynx is similarly examined. The tonsils, soft palate, sessile tongue, and pharyngeal walls are checked. After completion of the visual examination, it is necessary to palpate the mucosal surfaces and the teeth. This is done with a glove-lined finger in the mouth and a hand placed externally to bimanually palpate the structures in the floor of the mouth and cheek.

An indirect laryngoscopy is then performed on all patients. This consists of retracting the tongue in one hand and using the coaxial light source to illuminate the larynx indirectly by means of a laryngeal mirror. This technique is used to visualize the laryngeal structures. In patients with pathology involving any of the upper aerodigestive tract, fiberoptic laryngoscopy is then performed.

The examination is completed by a thorough palpation of the neck. Each of the different areas of the neck is palpated individually and gently. A light touch is more effective in discerning subcutaneous and deeper lesions than the heavy hand. It is easiest to stand behind the seated patient and palpate the neck by starting cephalad, gradually working downward using both hands on either side of the neck so that the two sides can be compared to each other. The thyroid is then palpated by having the patient swallow while the examiner feels the thyroid lobes.

It is necessary to carefully document any and all abnormal findings on a pictorial record. Anatomical charts of the head and neck are available through The American Cancer Society and through many publishers. On one of these charts, the size and precise location of each lesion should be carefully documented. This information is critical in staging the patient and as an accurate record for comparison in the future.

At this time, any suspicious lesions in the oral cavity should be biopsied. Normally, biopsy can be performed under local anesthesia or without anesthesia in the office with a simple biopsy punch. In patients who are extremely anxious or who have a hyperactive gag reflex, it may be necessary to perform a more thorough examination and biopsy under anesthesia. Certainly, if there are any lesions elsewhere in the upper aerodigestive tract, it is necessary to perform a direct laryngoscopy under general anesthesia.

Benign Lesions

SALIVARY GLAND LESIONS

Minor salivary glands are found throughout the oral mucosa. These glands produce a seromucinous secretion. Obstruction or rupture of the ducts of these glands can lead to formation of a mucous cyst (mucocele) (Fig. 39.2). The cystic lesions involving the sublingual or submandibular gland are called ranulas (Fig. 39.3). A ranula can occupy a large area in the floor of the mouth and can plunge deep into the anterior neck structures. Treatment of these lesions consists of simple excision or marsupialization of larger cysts.

Salivary duct stones can be found in Wharton's duct and can be palpated as hard submucosal masses in the floor of the mouth. Frequently, the presence of sialolithiasis causes symptoms of swelling and pain in the submandibular gland associated with eating. Stones can be removed transorally if they are in the distal portions of the duct. Stones located in the hilar area of the gland need to be removed through an external approach in the neck in conjunction with removal of the submandibular gland. Attempted removal of hilar stones through the floor of the mouth can lead to injury of the lingual artery and nerve.

Benign tumors of the minor salivary glands can occur anywhere that minor salivary glands are present. The most common of these lesions is a benign mixed tumor (pleomorphic adenoma). These are typically firm, slow growing, mobile, and submucosal. Approximately 50% of minor salivary gland tumors are malignant. Malignant tumors may be clinically indistinguishable from benign tumors. This necessitates a local excision with a margin of normal tissue of any small salivary gland tumor in the oral cavity. Larger lesions that cannot be simply removed should undergo an incisional biopsy.

Necrotizing sialometaplasia is a benign tumor that is most commonly present on the palate. It usually occurs as a spontaneously forming mass with ulceration. It can also be present secondary to surgery, trauma, or infection and can occur anywhere within the oral cavity. This tumor is benign but can be mistaken for a malignancy (see Chapter 21).

OTHER BENIGN LESIONS

Dermoid cysts can occur in the floor of the mouth near the midline. They can also occur at the base of the tongue. They are slow growing and generally present with swelling in the submental area and floor of the mouth. Dermoid cysts require excision of the cyst and cyst wall and are unlikely to recur.

Bony exostoses of the mandible or palate are bony masses attached to the skeletal structures and covered by a thin layer of mucosa. They present functional problems in patients who need to be fitted for prostheses or dentures. In those settings, they can be removed by simple excision (Fig. 39.4).

Reparative giant cell granulomas (epulides) are reddish-brown, friable tumors that occur along the alveolar ridge. They are frequently present between incisor and canine teeth (Fig. 39.5). Histologically, they resemble the brown tumor associated with hyperparathyroidism. Consequently, patients who have these lesions should have their serum calcium level evaluated. Treatment of giant cell granulomas consists of wide local excision.

Granular cell myoblastomas are well-circumscribed, firm lesions that are frequently found within the muscle of the tongue but that can be present anywhere in the oral cavity. These lesions are derived from the neural crest cells, are benign, and are adequately treated by local excision.

Vascular malformations, including hemangiomas and lymphangiomas, can occur in the oral cavity and are most frequent in children. In the absence of ulceration, bleeding, or functional disabilities associated with these tumors, no treatment is necessary. When these tumors are growing rapidly or are symptomatic, they can be treated

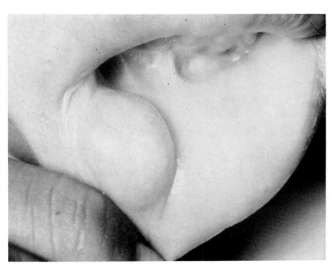

FIGURE 39.2. A mucocele of the lower lip.

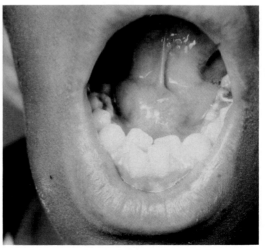

FIGURE 39.3. A ranula in the floor of the mouth.

FIGURE 39.4. Bony exostoses of the palate (**A**) and mandible (**B**).

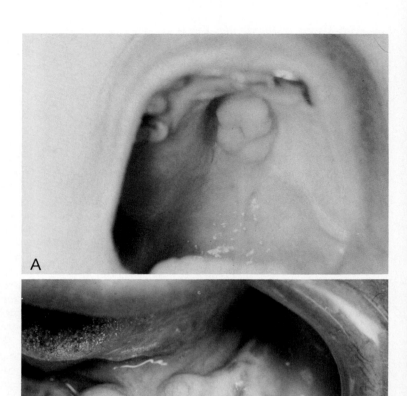

by local excision, high-dose short-term steroids, laser vaporization, or low-dose external beam irradiation (Fig. 39.6). Mucosal polyps and fibromas can occur in areas of mucosal trauma. These are usually found on the buccal mucosa along the bite plane where mucosa can be caught between the teeth. Median rhomboid glossitis is a raised reddish area usually on the central raphe of the dorsal surface of the tongue; it is another benign condition that can be treated with local excision or simply observed.

Aphthous ulcers (canker sores) are painful ulcerations that occur in the oral cavity. These are generally of short duration. They can occur in a cyclical fashion in some

FIGURE 39.5. A reparative granuloma (epulis) on the lower jaw.

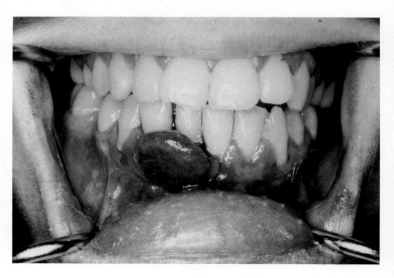

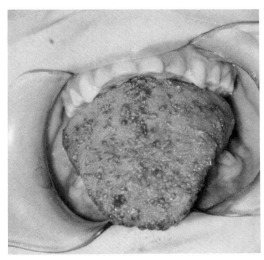

FIGURE 39.6. The tongue is infiltrated with hemangioma.

patients. In general, these lesions have a white base and an erythematous rim. They resolve without treatment.

Tuberculous granulomas can occur in the oral cavity and can appear quite similar to squamous cell carcinoma. These need to be distinguished from squamous cell carcinoma by histological examination of a biopsy specimen. Treatment consists of standard antituberculous medications using established protocols over prolonged periods of time.

Premalignant Tumors

Leukoplakia (Fig. 39.7) refers to any white patch on the oral mucosa. Leukoplakia is generally associated with hyperkeratosis. Most leukoplakias are found in patients who smoke. They can be directly related to the type of smoking. For instance, patients who use chewing

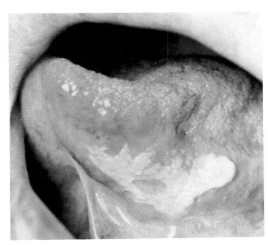

FIGURE 39.7. Leukoplakia of the tongue is seen as a white patch.

tobacco will frequently have leukoplakia in the buccal sulcus, whereas patients who smoke cheroots (small cigars with square-cut ends) are predisposed to developing leukoplakia on the ventral surface of the tongue. There is considerable disagreement in the literature with regard to the degree of malignant transformation in oral leukoplakia (1). This is a result of the fact that many studies are based on the appearance of the lesions rather than their histological evaluation. The best indicator for likely malignant degeneration of a white oral lesion is the presence of dysplasia or carcinoma in situ on histological evaluation.

The treatment of oral leukoplakia involves histological confirmation of the nature of the lesion, followed by removal of the etiological factor responsible for its formation. The most effective means to resolve leukoplakia is cessation of smoking. In lesions that demonstrate dysplasia or carcinoma in situ, surgical excision is necessary.

Erythroplakia is a bright red, velvety lesion that occurs anywhere in the oral cavity. This is a dangerous lesion because it is almost always associated with dysplasia, carcinoma in situ, or invasive carcinoma (2). Any red lesion of the oral cavity requires histological evaluation. Treatment generally consists of excision. Patients must be warned about the risk of continued tobacco and alcohol use.

Malignant Tumors

The vast majority of the malignancies occurring in the oral cavity are squamous cell carcinomas (SCCs). Most of the remaining tumors are of salivary gland origin and are discussed in detail in Chapter 21. Consequently, this chapter will focus entirely on SCCs.

Chronic exposure to a variety of irritants in susceptible people initiates the development of SCC. Tobacco use in any form is the major irritant responsible for its development. The effect of tobacco works synergistically with alcohol, although alcohol alone does not appear to be carcinogenic. A variety of other environmental irritants, including occupational exposure to chemicals and nutritional factors, appear to influence the development of SCC. Several potentially premalignant conditions have been identified and are thought to sensitize individuals to become more susceptible to carcinogenic agents. These disorders include Plummer-Vinson syndrome, lichen planus, tertiary syphilis, and discoid lupus erythematosus (1). In addition, there are several hereditary syndromes associated with the development of SCC, such as basal cell nevus syndrome and xeroderma pigmentosum. There has been an association between the Epstein-Barr virus and carcinoma of the nasopharynx, as well as an association between herpes simplex virus and carcinoma of the oral cavity. Finally, poor oral hygiene with chronic gingivitis, peridontitis, and poor dental care is a frequent associated factor in patients who present with SCC of the oral cavity. Another known etiological factor is the effect of ultraviolet radiation from sunlight influencing the development of SCC on the vermilion portion of the lip.

HISTOPATHOLOGY

Squamous cell carcinoma consists of a tumor with nests and columns of malignant epithelial cells that infiltrate into the subepithelial layers. Nuclear pleomorphism is typical. Tumors can be graded from well differentiated to poorly differentiated. In the well-differentiated tumors, the malignant cells produce keratin, and keratin pearls can be identified. Under oil-immersion views, intercellular bridging can be seen. As the tumors become less well differentiated, the nuclear differentiation degenerates, and the density of mitotic figures increases. The histological pattern of SCC can usually be reliably identified on frozen section analysis. This enables the pathologist to perform an accurate intraoperative assessment of the excised tissue.

TUMOR CLASSIFICATION

Classification of SCC is currently based on a TNM system, which considers several descriptors in characterizing the tumor. The first descriptor is T, which refers to two-dimensional tumor size. The N descriptor refers to the nodal status in the cervical region. The final descriptor, M, refers to metastatic disease beyond the cervical lymph nodes (Table 39.1). The TNM classification is based on the clinical evaluation of the patient, not the pathological evaluation. Once a TNM status is derived, the patient can then be placed into a tumor stage (Fig. 39.8).

The widely used TNM system allows the surgeon to classify a patient in such a way that appropriate therapy for a given tumor can be selected and prognosis of outcome can be made fairly accurately. The system does have some limitations. The primary limitation is the use of two-dimensional tumor size as the basis for the T classification. Recently, attempts have been made to modify

Table 39.1.
TNM Classification of Head and Neck Tumors

TIS	Tumor in situ
T 1	0.1–2.0 cm
T 2	2.1–4.0 cm
T 3	4.1–6.0 cm
T 4	> 6.1 cm or invading adjacent structures
N 0	No regional adenopathy
N 1	Ipsilateral adenopathy
N 2	Single ipsilateral node 3–6 cm or multiple ipsilateral nodes < 6 cm
N 3	Massive ipsilateral or contralateral nodes
M 0	No evidence of metastases
M I	Metastases beyond the cervical lymph nodes
M X	Metastases not assessed

the classification system by examining tumor depth as a variable in oral carcinoma. In fact, tumor depth beyond 1.5 mm has been shown to be associated with a highly increased risk of loco-regional failure and cervical metastases (3). As studies of this nature emerge, the classification system of oral cancer will undoubtedly be modified.

PATIENT CONSIDERATIONS

Once a patient has been diagnosed as having SCC of the oral cavity, a variety of considerations of the patient's habits, social setting, and physiological state need to be reviewed before developing a comprehensive treatment plan. There are numerous ways to treat any of these tumors, and the goal of therapy is to benefit the patient. Consequently, therapy needs to be adapted to the individual patient.

The first important aspect of the evaluation is to determine whether or not the index tumor site is, in fact, the only involved area of the upper aerodigestive tract. In approximately 10% of these patients, there is a synchro-

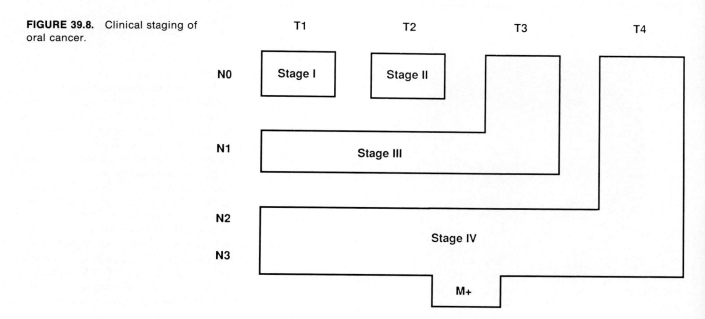

FIGURE 39.8. Clinical staging of oral cancer.

nous second primary tumor (4). It is imperative to thoroughly examine the patient to rule out the possibility of a second primary. This assessment requires a detailed physical examination and, usually, a laryngoscopy under anesthesia. A laryngoscopy can be combined with the initial diagnostic biopsy if a patient is unable to cooperate with an office biopsy technique. Otherwise, if a second lesion is suspected or a suspicious area is noted, the laryngoscopy can be performed as a separate procedure. If the patient has been thoroughly evaluated in the office with a fiberoptic endoscope and an indirect examination and there is no evidence of a second primary, a laryngoscopy can be performed prior to definitive surgery at the same setting.

In addition to evaluating the patient for a second primary, the examiner should realize that the possibility of metastatic disease also exists. In general, SCC metastasizes first to the lymph nodes of the neck. Beyond that point, it tends to spread to the lung. An extensive metastatic workup is not indicated. A plain chest radiograph and liver function studies are the only tests required. If additional studies are needed to develop a treatment plan or to further evaluate an abnormal result on the basic screen, they can be ordered as indicated. Arteriography is useful in patients who have vascular tumors, but it is rarely necessary in patients with squamous cell carcinoma. Radionuclide scanning also has little use in these patients. In the head and neck, radionuclide scanning is primarily useful in evaluating thyroid tumors. Fine-needle aspiration has a role in evaluating an undiagnosed mass in the neck that is not associated with any evident oral tumor. The accuracy of a fine-needle aspiration is largely dependent on the pathologist's experience with cytological interpretation.

The patient's dental status is critical to the outcome of treatment. Patients who have poor oral hygiene are more prone to complications of infection and wound healing after surgery. During the course of treatment with radiotherapy, dental caries and periodontitis will increase the risk of osteoradionecrosis of the mandible and maxilla. Therefore, each patient, before undergoing any treatment for oral cancer, needs a dental evaluation and prophylactic treatment.

The patient's nutritional needs must also be addressed. Many patients have sustained significant weight loss and are malnourished at the time of presentation. Dietary supplementation, either orally, by nasogastric tube, or by percutaneous endoscopic gastrostomy, is indicated prior to initiating a definitive treatment plan in most patients with oral tumors.

Certain patient habits, such as smoking and alcohol abuse, function as critical factors in terms of the patient's survival outcome. Patients who continue to smoke and drink have a 40% risk of developing a second primary SCC in the upper aerodigestive tract after treatment of their first lesion. This very high risk level can be considerably reduced by cessation of smoking. Alcoholic patients are difficult to treat by any modality. However, radiation therapy requires long-term compliance. Outside of a protected setting, patients who are alcoholic are unlikely to adequately participate in the full course of the radiation therapy. Consequently, we find that definitive surgery is the preferred treatment modality in alcoholics.

The patient's physiological status is also a critical factor. In this regard, age is a consideration. Young patients who develop SCC tend to have more aggressive tumors and a worse prognosis than middle-aged or older patients. The metabolic status of the patient who presents with SCC is often poor because of personal abuse and nutritional deficiencies. The metabolic status of patients should be corrected with nutritional supplementation and metabolic support prior to surgery. Most unfavorable metabolic states can be reversed prior to surgery with proper medical care.

TREATMENT OF ORAL SCC

Surgery

Surgery is still the preferred method of treatment for most cancers of the oral cavity. Surgical therapy consists of precise removal of the tumor and a margin of normal-appearing tissue around the tumor. Frozen section analysis at the time of surgery is used to confirm that the tumor has been removed with adequate margins. Patients who are in good metabolic shape generally tolerate these surgical procedures well. In most instances, surgical therapy provides the best opportunity for the cure of the tumor.

There are disadvantages to the surgical approach to these tumors. A primary disadvantage is the functional problems with speech and swallowing that can result from ablation of structures in the oral cavity. In addition, surgery leads to aesthetic alterations, which can be devastating to a patient. Reconstructive options that can minimize these problems are currently available. Another disadvantage of surgery is its inability to precisely eliminate foci of microscopic disease. For this reason, adjuvant radiotherapy and, potentially, chemotherapy are useful adjuncts in the treatment of patients with advanced disease. Finally, surgical procedures in the oral cavity have a relatively high incidence of complications. In the head and neck region, problems with postoperative infection and the development of orocutaneous fistulas are always worrisome and problematic; however, these complications are rarely fatal.

Radiotherapy

Radiation therapy offers the distinct advantage of minimal aesthetic and functional alterations following treatment. Radiation also has the ability to sterilize microscopic tumor deposits. The limitations of radiation therapy are the considerable acute and progressive chronic morbidity, as well as the ineffectiveness of radiation to ablate large tumor volumes. Acute morbidity associated with radiation therapy consists of mucositis, odynophagia, swelling, and a general feeding of malaise. The long-term effects of radiation therapy leave the patient with loss of taste, a chronically irritated and dry mouth, the risk of osteonecrosis of the mandible and temporal bone (which can be a disastrous occurrence), and permanent alteration in the healing abilities of the tissues that have been treated.

Additional Treatment Modalities

Chemotherapy at this time is an unreliable adjunct in the treatment of head and neck cancer. Some patients respond dramatically to chemotherapy treatments, but the effects are usually short lived, and regrowth of the tumor usually occurs in 3–6 months.

As an adjuvant in treating massive or potentially unresectable tumors, there is a definite place for chemotherapy in today's treatment armamentarium. If a patient is pretreated with chemotherapy, tumor size is often reduced to the point where surgical ablation of the tumor is feasible. The appropriate extent of surgery after a tumor has been pretreated is an issue that is presently unresolved. A variety of multicenter protocols are currently evaluating the impact that chemotherapy pretreatment has on the extent of surgical ablation.

Heat has been considered a potentially worthwhile adjunct to chemotherapy and radiation. By heating a tumor to 43°C, the effect of the chemotherapy and radiation seems to be potentiated. Difficulties with these methods include the techniques available for delivery of the heat and the level of discomfort to the patient during the treatment.

Cryotherapy and electrocautery have been used as destructive techniques to palliate massive tumors, and to that extent they are acceptable therapies. Photodynamic therapy consists of laser activation of a photosensitizing dye, which concentrates in the tumor. As of this time, it does not have a clear role in tumor management.

TUMORS BY SITE

Lip

Lip cancers are the most common form of oral SCC. Approximately 95% of lip cancers are SCC, and most of these appear on the lower lip. A history of smoking and sun exposure are typical. Basal cell carcinomas occur less frequently and usually appear on the upper lip, often as a direct extension of a cutaneous lesion.

Lip cancer usually presents as an ulceration (Fig. 39.9). Induration around the base of the tumor is a common clinical finding and helps to delineate the extent of tumor infiltration. Leukoplakia often is present adjacent to the tumor.

While most of the patients with lip cancer have a relatively benign course, approximately 10% of these tumors become extremely aggressive and are lethal. Ominous clinical findings are the presence of cervical lymphadenopathy and evidence of perineural invasion. Nerve involvement is noted by anesthesia in the distribution of the mental nerve and by an enlarged mental foramen on Panorex.

The treatment of lip cancer is surgical. A margin of 1 cm circumferentially around the tumor should be obtained. All specimens should be checked by frozen sec-

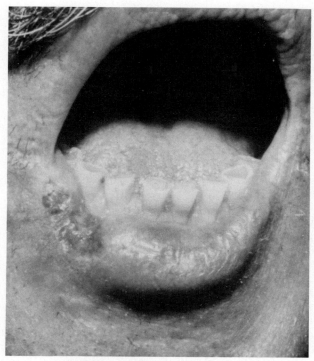

FIGURE 39.9.   A SCC on the lower lip.

tion prior to reconstructing the defect. Adjacent leukoplakia needs to be removed with a lip shave procedure. Tumors that present with anesthesia along the mental nerve should be carefully checked for adequacy of margins. Squamous cell carcinoma can spread perineurally, and cancers of the lip can involve the mental nerve, which travels through the mandible. Tumors of the lip usually do not present with clinically positive cervical nodes; however, these tumors can metastasize to the neck. Neck dissection is reserved for patients with clinically evident disease in the neck or those with very advanced tumors of the lip.

Reconstruction of the ablative lip defect depends on the size and location of the wound. Tumors measuring less than one quarter of the lip length can be closed primarily after removing them as a wedge. Larger tumor defects require flap closure. There are a number of flaps available for closing the lip, and these are described in Chapter 44.

Survival of patients with lip carcinoma is approximately 95% at 5 years. These patients clearly do better than patients with other oral tumors; however, this can be a fatal disease, and they must be monitored regularly during the 5 years after initial treatment.

Oral Tongue

The oral tongue consists of the mobile portion of the tongue distal to the circumvallate papillae. This is the next most frequent site of oral carcinoma. The vast majority of tongue tumors are SCC (Fig. 39.10). The lateral surface of the tongue is the most common location of

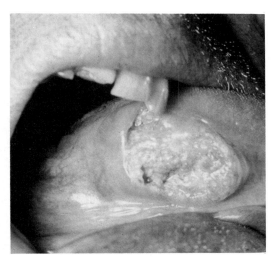

FIGURE 39.10. This SCC is located on the lateral mobile tongue.

primary tongue cancer. Tumors are detected earlier in the oral tongue than in the base of the tongue because the base is more posterior and hidden from easy examination. Patients with tongue tumors present with either exophytic or invasive tumors. Palpation of the tumor is an accurate means of assessing the extent of the lesion. Tongue tumors tend to be painful and can interfere with eating. Advanced tumors of the tongue are usually associated with severe nutritional deficits. Referred otalgia is a common presenting symptom. Tongue cancers tend to metastasize and commonly spread to the upper and mid-jugular nodal chains.

Treatment of tongue tumors consists of a partial glossectomy that includes the hemitongue distal to the circumvallate papillae (5–8). T1 lesions can be removed by wedge resection. Treatment of the neck is a controversial issue. Clearly, in patients with clinically evident nodal disease, lymphadenectomy is appropriate. In patients with clinically negative necks, elective neck dissection reveals histological evidence of tumor in 25% of patients. Consequently, in patients with T2 or greater lesions, elective neck dissection is appropriate. Radiation treatment of tongue lesions, including external beam or implantation, yields survival rates comparable to those following surgery. The long-term and short-term complications of irradiation, however, are much more severe than those of surgery, and we prefer to use radiation therapy as an adjunctive treatment in more advanced tumors.

Floor of The Mouth

Carcinoma of the floor of the mouth (Fig. 39.11) is a disease of older patients. This is a relatively quiet area of the mouth, and symptoms are generally present only with advanced disease. The usual complaints are local or referred pain to the ear caused by involvement of the lingual nerve. The pattern of nodal metastases is to the submental and submandibular lymph nodes.

Treatment of these lesions (9) consists of local excision with a skin graft or local flap reconstruction in T1 lesions. T2 lesions require more aggressive resection. A close inspection of the status of the mandible is important (10, 11). Mandibular involvement can usually be treated by marginal mandibulectomy if the tumor encroaches on the alveolar aspect of the mandible (12, 13). For very large advanced tumors with gross mandibular involvement, composite resection is necessary. Resulting surgical defects require elaborate reconstructive procedures. Treatment of the neck necessitates lymphadenectomy in clinically positive necks (14). Tumor thickness is found to be highly predictive of neck metastases in floor-of-the-mouth tumors (3, 15). For lesions thicker than 1.5 mm, there is a 60% risk of neck metastases, and cervical lymphadenectomy is appropriate (16). Radiation therapy plays a distinct role in these tumors, particularly as a postsurgical adjunct.

Buccal Mucosa

Buccal carcinomas are primarily associated with the use of oral tobacco (1). These tumors account for less than 10% of oral tumors. With the increasing incidence of snuff dipping in the United States, a higher incidence of these tumors has been present in the past several years, with an increasing occurrence of these lesions in younger patients (17). Buccal carcinomas are frequently of a verrucous nature, and these have a slightly better prognosis than other forms of SCC found in the oral cavity. However, approximately 20% of the verrucous carcinomas have foci of SCC, and these have a more aggressive course, like the usual SCC (18). Metastases to the submandibular and jugular lymph nodes are typical, and the incidence of cervical metastases is 40%.

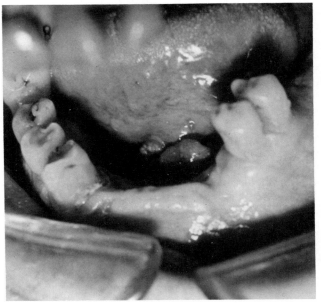

FIGURE 39.11. The floor of this mouth contains a SCC.

Surgical treatment of buccal carcinoma is more effective than primary radiation treatment (18, 19). For improved local control of tumors, postoperative adjuvant radiation therapy is advantageous, particularly in advanced tumors and in those hybrid tumors with foci of SCC. Because of the high incidence of metastases to the neck, elective neck dissection is appropriate. Reconstruction of the defect depends on the extent of excision. Split-thickness skin grafts are appropriate for mucosal defects. Musculocutaneous or microvascular flaps are better suited for repairing composite tissue losses.

Palate

Carcinomas of the superior alveolus and hard palate are unusual tumors in the United States. They are more common in other areas of the world, where reverse smoking is a common practice. This consists of smoking with the lit end of the cigarette in the mouth. In the United States, the majority of palatal tumors arise from the minor salivary glands (see Chapter 21). Treatment of tumors of the palate consists of local excision with removal of bone where indicated. Reconstruction of this area can be performed by using distant pedicle flaps or microvascular tissue transfers. It is not always necessary to replace bone that has been removed from the palate. The primary goal of reconstruction is to achieve oronasal separation to allow speech and eating to continue with minimal disruption.

Unknown Primary

Unknown primary tumors in the neck are SCC that appear as metastatic disease in the neck with no known source of primary tumor. An adult patient who presents with a mass (Fig. 39.12) in the upper two thirds of the neck should be assumed to have metastatic SCC until proven otherwise. The evaluation of a neck mass consists of a thorough endoscopic examination, random biopsies of the common sites for small primary tumors (Waldeyer's ring structures), aspiration needle biopsy of the tumor mass, and open biopsy of the tumor mass, if necessary. Tumors presenting in the posterior area of the neck usually spread from areas of the head and neck outside the oral cavity. Oral lesions usually metastasize to the submental, submandibular, and upper and midjugular regions (20). Once a thorough investigation has been undertaken and no primary tumor can be identified, definitive treatment should be instituted. This consists of a cervical lymphadenectomy followed by postoperative irradiation of the neck and the usual sites of hidden primary tumors. These sites include the nasopharynx and all of the Waldeyer's ring structures. In patients with N1 neck tumors, irradiation alone yields results comparable to those of surgery and offers the additional option of treating a presumed primary site.

NECK DISSECTION

Crile described the basic technique of radical neck dissection in 1906 (21). His operation consisted of an en bloc

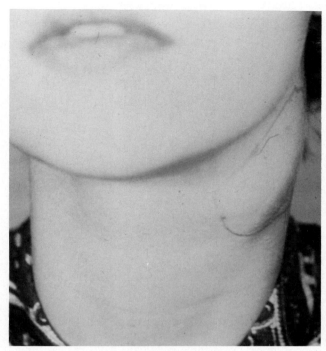

FIGURE 39.12.   Any unexplained neck mass in an adult is cancer until proven otherwise.

removal of all of the contents of the lateral neck, including the cervical lymphatics, jugular vein, sternocleidomastoid muscle, and any nerves that were present. In 1951, Martin et al. (22) outlined the indications, technique, and complications of radical neck dissection, and this has remained the oncological standard to this time. In the 1960s, various forms of less radical neck dissections were introduced. Functional (modified or conservative) neck dissections have proven to be comparable to radical neck dissections in terms of outcome. Survival outcome following functional neck dissection is similar to that of the classic radical neck dissection. In addition, some function is preserved by removing simply the lymph nodal groups at risk and not the remaining structures of the neck (23).

The approach to treatment of SCC metastatic to the neck is controversial to this day. It is fairly well agreed that patients who have clinically positive neck disease at or subsequent to the time of presentation with their tumor require cervical lymphadenectomy. The issue of elective or "prophylactic" neck dissection is where the controversy exists. One approach is to perform elective neck dissections in patients who have tumors that are at high risk for having occult metastases or for developing metastatic disease at some future date (24). The alternative approach is to perform a staging neck dissection; the first echelon of lymphatic tissue is removed, and if this is pathologically negative, the lymphadenectomy is halted at that time. Alternatively, if the first echelon nodes are histologically involved, additional extension of the lymphadenectomy can be performed. The next option is to observe the patient without performing lymphadenectomy and to operate on the neck only if clinically evident disease appears at some future time (25). There is a real

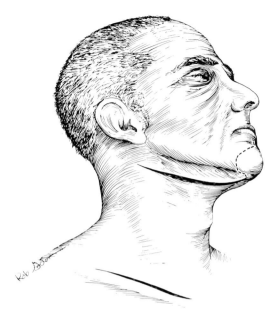

FIGURE 39.13.   A MacFee incision for cervical lymphadenectomy.

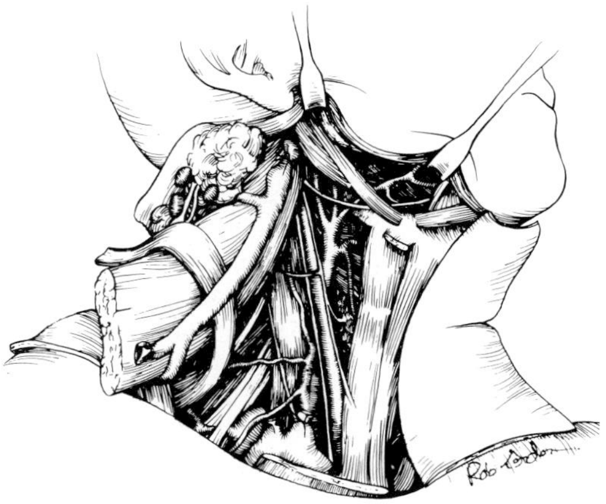

FIGURE 39.14.   The classical radical neck dissection includes removal of the sternocleidomastoid muscle, jugular vein, submandibular gland, and remaining lymphatic contents of the neck.

FIGURE 39.15.   The outline of a pectoralis flap. Note the arc of rotation possible with this flap.

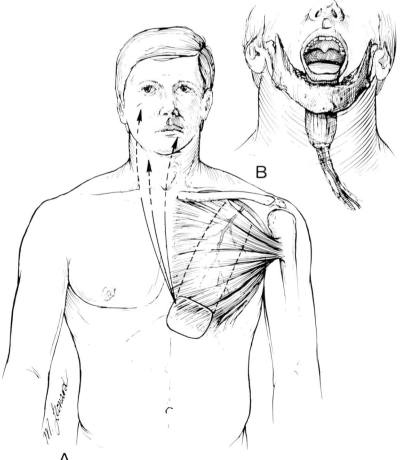

risk of poor follow-up in some of these patients, but patients who have late lymph node dissections do comparably well. One final option is to irradiate clinically negative necks in patients with high-risk primary tumors. Because aggressive, high-risk primary tumors are generally treated with adjunctive radiation, it is a relatively straightforward matter to include the ipsilateral neck within the treatment portal at little additional morbidity or risk to the patient. Occasionally, there are midline tumors in the oral cavity with metastatic disease to both sides of the neck. In these cases, it is best either to stage the neck dissections, if the internal jugular is to be removed, or to perform bilateral simultaneous neck dissections using the functional jugular vein preservation techniques.

Access to the neck is best obtained with a MacFee incision (Fig. 39.13). There are many options for gaining access to the neck structures, but the MacFee incision affords consistent wound healing with minimal risk of exposure to the underlying vessels of the neck (26). The upper incision is made from the mastoid tip to the contralateral submental area. It is carried approximately 2.5 cm below the mandibular border. The lower incision is made approximately 3.0 cm above the clavicle in a curvilinear fashion from the midline anteriorly to the border of the trapezius posteriorly. The incisions are carried through skin and subcutaneous tissue and then through the platysma. The superior flap is raised carefully, and the marginal mandibular branch of the facial nerve is identified and preserved. The nerve is usually found immediately below the platysma, crossing the posterior facial vein. This is retracted along with the cheek flap superiorly. The inferior incision is raised below the level of the platysma. Both flaps are sutured back for retraction during the remainder of the procedure. The central skin flap is raised in the subplatysmal plane. A 1-in Penrose drain is then passed around the central flap and used for retraction of this tissue during various parts of the neck dissection.

The classical radical neck dissection involves removal of the sternocleidomastoid muscle, the internal jugular vein, the spinal accessory nerve, and all of the remaining tissue (Fig. 39.14). Borders of the dissection are the trapezius posteriorly, the clavicle inferiorly, the midline of the neck medially, and the marginal rim of the mandible superiorly. First, the inferior heads of the sternocleidomastoid muscle are divided at their insertions. The individual structures of the carotid sheath are identified and cleaned of fascia. The internal jugular vein is divided and suture ligated. The fascial carpet of the neck is identified and left intact, and the posterior triangle contents are divided to the level of the trapezius muscle. The contents of the neck are then swept superiorly and medially, dividing the cervical nerves along the way. Care is taken to prevent injury to the vagus, phrenic, and brachial plexus structures. The omohyoid muscle is divided as it crosses the scalene muscles. The central skin flap is carefully retracted during this procedure, and the contents of the neck can be brought out through the upper pole of the incision for better exposure once the inferior attachments are divided.

As the dissection proceeds superiorly, the hypoglossal

nerve, which is located deep to the posterior belly of the digastric muscle crossing above the carotid bifurcation, is carefully preserved. The omohyoid muscle is divided. The insertion of the sternocleidomastoid muscle is divided. The tail of the parotid is divided from the remaining portion of the parotid gland. The underlying digastric and stylohyoid muscles are divided as well. The contents of the submandibular triangle are then dissected with care to preserve the lingual nerve as well as the previously identified and protected branch of the facial nerve. The jugular vein is divided below the skull base and suture ligated. After assuring complete hemostasis and checking for the absence of chylous leakage, two suction catheters are introduced through inferior stab incisions placed in the wound, and the skin flaps are closed in layers.

In the years following Martin's standardization of the classic radical neck dissection (22), little variation took place until the 1960s. At that time, Bocca et al. (23) popu-

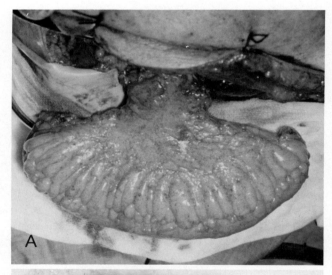

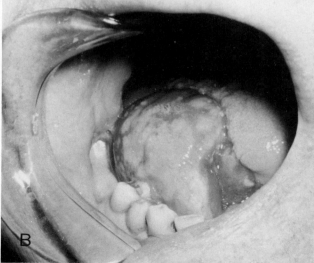

FIGURE 39.16. **A,** A jejunal segment has been connected to the neck by microvascular anastomoses. **B,** The flap is used to reconstruct a hemiglossectomy defect.

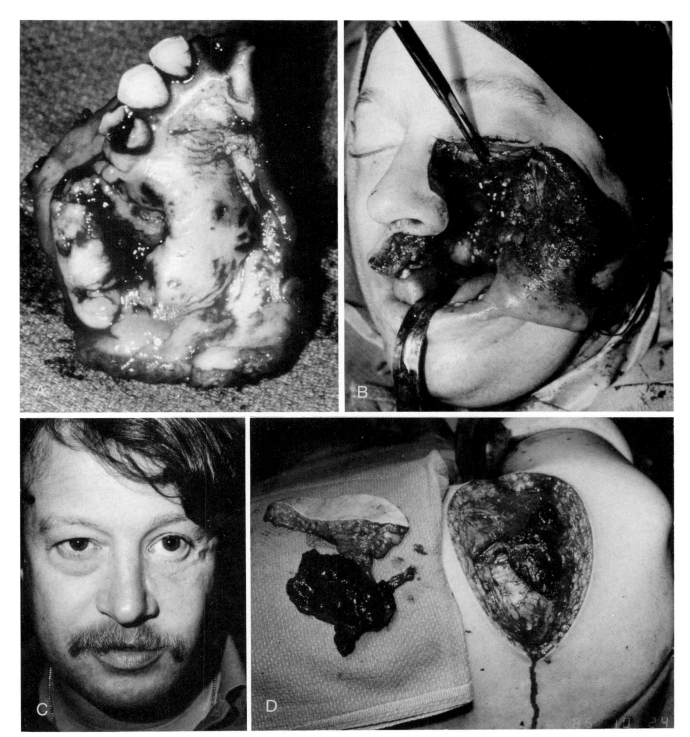

FIGURE 39.17. **A**, A total maxillectomy specimen. **B**, The maxillectomy defect consists of loss of bony support of the eye and full-thickness hard palate. **C**, A composite scapula free flap is harvested. The bone segment will support the eye and facial tissues. The skin will line the palate. The fat will obliterate the sinus. **D**, The patient is shown 1 year postoperatively.

larized a variation of the classical radical neck dissection by removing the fascial envelope containing the lymphatics of the neck and preserving the contents of the submandibular triangle and the spinal accessory nerve. As the literature began to support the oncological validity of this approach, many variations were performed. The most universally accepted aspect of functional neck dissection is the preservation of the spinal accessory nerve in cases in which this nerve is not directly involved with tumor. The most widely performed functional neck dissection preserves not only the spinal accessory nerve but the cervical roots, the sternocleidomastoid muscle, and the internal jugular vein as well. All of the areolar tissue surrounding the carotid sheath, as well as all of the lymphatic-bearing tissue of the neck from the rim of the mandible down to the clavicle, is removed. In recent years, limited regional dissections of the neck have been popularized. The concept behind regional neck resection is the fact that tumors of the oral cavity generally spread in a predictable fashion (20). Thus, by removing the first echelon of involved nodes, a reliable prediction can be made as to the risk of involvement of more distal lymphatics. If the tumor can be arrested at the first echelon of nodes, it is necessary only to extend the dissection to the next echelon of nodes without risking incomplete removal of involved lymphatics.

RECONSTRUCTION

The principles of reconstructive surgery in the head and neck region are identical to those elsewhere in the body. The difficulty with head and neck reconstructive surgery is the need for improvement in the patient's function, structure, and appearance. Failure to provide satisfactory improvements in any of these areas yields a poor result. Many defects can be closed by simply reapproximating tissues or by applying a simple skin graft, such as the resection of a lesion of the floor of the mouth. Occasionally, skin grafts can be used in conjunction with a prosthesis to achieve a satisfactory result for the patient with minimal reconstructive effort. The complexity arises when the need for composite tissue restoration or restoration of the integrity of the oral cavity is needed.

Skin grafts are easily applied to the intraoral structures. The grafts are usually meshed at 1.5 to 1 and are then sutured in place with chromic catgut sutures. The graft is quilted to the underlying bed to prevent it from shearing during the motion of the residual oral tissues. A bolster consisting of a single piece of cotton gauze immersed in balsam Peru is applied over the graft. This mixture has the unique ability to not adhere to the underlying skin graft and to suppress bacterial growth within the bolster. After 1 week, the bolster is removed, and a program of local hygiene is instituted.

Larger defects require more sophisticated reconstruction using a variety of local, regional, or distant flaps, depending on the specific needs of the patient. The major workhorse flaps for the head and neck remain the pectoralis myocutaneous flap (27), latissimus dorsi myocutaneous flap (28), and the trapezius myocutaneous flap (29, 30). Each of these three flaps has a consistent and dependable vascular pedicle, is easily accessed, and is easily dissected. The donor sites can usually be closed primarily, and the functional losses from the rotation of the donor muscles are minimal. The advantage of the use of the pectoralis muscle over the trapezius and latissimus muscles is the availability of this flap on the anterior chest wall, which eliminates the need to reposition the patient intraoperatively (Fig. 39.15). The advent of a diverse group of microvascular tissue transfers that are reliable and particularly well suited for head and neck reconstruction has largely supplanted the classic forms of head and

neck reconstruction. Free bowel transfers are well suited for lining the pharynx, oral cavity, or cervical esophagus with mucosal tissue (31; Fig. 39.16). Radial forearm (32), dorsalis pedis (33), and scapular (34, 35) flaps have become the standard for lining the oral cavity with thin, hairless tissue. The vascularized bone accompanying the iliac crest and groin flap combination (36), the scapular flap, the dorsalis pedis flap along with the metatarsal bone, the fibula, the radial bone in association with skin islands, and other composite tissues have vastly improved the options for reconstructing extensive mandibular and maxillary defects (Fig. 39.17). All of these flaps can be revascularized by anastomoses either directly to the remaining vessels in the neck or via vein grafts to the contralateral neck. When properly designed and executed, these flaps are robust and withstand irradiation postoperatively quite satisfactorily. The level of sophistication in reconstructing head and neck tumor defects continues to improve. The available donor tissues must be individualized for the specific needs of the patient before selecting a reconstructive technique.

It is important to approach a patient with oral cancer with the concept of eliminating the tumor as the first objective. A variety of reconstructive options must be kept in mind, but the final choice of the reconstructive technique must wait until the tumor is adequately removed. One final caution is to avoid predetermining the reconstruction prior to the completion of the ablation. The primary goal in operating on patients with head and neck cancer is to cure the cancer. While the reconstructive aspect of head and neck surgery is challenging and gratifying, it plays a secondary role to the management of the cancer. The vast array of reconstructive options should act as a support to the oncological surgeon and allow an aggressive, complete tumor resection with the knowledge that residual defects can almost always be satisfactorily restored.

References

1. Pindborg JJ: Premalignant and malignant lesions of the oral mucosa. In Ariyan SE (ed): *Cancer of the Head and Neck.* St. Louis, CV Mosby, 1987, p 163.
2. Shafer WG, Waldron CA: Erythroplakias of the oral cavity. *Cancer* 36:1021, 1975.
3. Spiro RH, Huvos AG, Wong GY, et al: Predictive value of tumor thickness in SCC confined to the tongue and floor of the mouth. *Am J Surg* 152:345, 1986.
4. Leipzig B, Zellmer JE, Klug D: The role of endoscopy in evaluating patients with head and neck cancer. *Arch Otolaryngol* 111:589, 1985.
5. Callery CD, Spiro RH, Strong EW: Changing trends in the management of squamous cell carcinoma of the tongue. *Am J Surg* 148:449, 1984.
6. Ferraro J, Beaver BL, Young D, et al: Primary procedure in carcinoma of the tongue: Local resection versus combined local resection and radical neck dissection. *J Surg Oncol* 21:245, 1982.
7. Ildstad ST, Bigelow ME, Rememsnyder JP: Squamous cell carcinoma of the mobile tongue. *Am J Surg* 145:443, 1983.
8. Leipzig B, Cummings CW, Chung CT, et al: Carcinoma of the anterior tongue. *Ann Otol* 91:94, 1982.
9. Applebaum EL, Collins WL, Bytell DE: Carcinoma of the floor of the mouth. *Arch Otolaryngol* 106:419, 1980.

10. O'Brien CJ, Carter RL, Soo K-C, et al: Invasion of the mandible by squamous carcinoma of the oral cavity and oropharynx. *Head Neck Surg* 8:247, 1986.
11. Gilbert S, Tzadik A, Leonard G: Mandibular involvement by oral squamous cell carcinoma. *Laryngoscope* 96:96, 1986.
12. Wald RM Jr, Calcaterra TC: Lower alveolar carcinoma: Segmental versus marginal resection. *Arch Otolaryngol* 109:578, 1983.
13. Marchetta FC, Sako K, Murphy JB: The periosteum of the mandible and intraoral carcinoma. *Am J Surg* 122:711, 1971.
14. Patterson HC, Dobie RA, Cummings GW: Treatment of clinically negative necks in floor of mouth carcinoma. *Laryngoscope* 94:820, 1984.
15. Crossman JD, Gluckman J, Whiteley J, et al: Squamous cell carcinoma of the floor of the mouth. *Head Neck Surg* 3:2, 1980.
16. Mohit-Tabatabi MA, Sobel HJ, Rush BF, et al: Relation of thickness of floor of mouth stage I and stage II cancers to regional metastases. *Am J Surg* 152:351, 1986.
17. Greer RO, Poulson TC: Oral tissue alterations associated with the use of smokeless tobacco by teenagers I. Clinical findings. *Oral Surg* 56:275, 1983.
18. Medina JE, Dichtel W, Luna MA: Verrucous-squamous carcinomas of the oral cavity: Clinicopathologic study of 104 cases. *Arch Otolaryngol* 110:437, 1984.
19. Ildstad ST, Bigelow ME, Remensnyder JP: Clinical behavior and results of current therapeutic modalities for squamous cell carcinoma of the buccal mucosa. *Surg Gynecol Obstet* 160:254, 1985.
20. Lindberg R: Distribution of cervical lymph node metastases from squamous cell carcinoma of the upper respiratory and digestive tracts. *Cancer* 29:1446, 1972.
21. Crile G Sr: Excision of cancer of the head and neck with special reference to the plan of dissection based on 132 operations. *JAMA* 47:1780, 1906.
22. Martin H, DelValle B, Ehrlich H, et al: Neck dissection. *Cancer* 4:441, 1951.
23. Bocca E, Pignataro O, Oldini C, et al: Functional neck dissection: Evaluation and review of 843 cases. *Laryngoscope* 94:942, 1984.
24. Jesse RH: The philosophy of treatment of neck nodes. *Ear Nose Throat J* 56:125, 1977.
25. Vandenbrouck G, Sancho-Garmer H, Chassagne D, et al: Elective versus therapeutic neck dissection in epidermoid carcinoma of the oral cavity: Results of a randomized clinical trial. *Cancer* 46:386, 1980.
26. Daniell CH, Fee WE Jr: MacFee incisions: Dispelling the myth of cervical flap vascular inadequacy. *Head Neck Surg* 9:167, 1987.
27. Ariyan S: The pectoralis major myocutaneous flap: A versatile flap for reconstruction in the head and neck. *Plast Reconstr Surg* 63:73, 1979.
28. Quillen CG: Latissimus dorsi myocutaneous flaps in head and neck reconstruction. *Plast Reconstr Surg* 63:664, 1979.
29. Demergasso F, Piazza MV: Trapezius myocutaneous flap in reconstructive surgery for head and neck cancer: An original technique. *Am J Surg* 138:533, 1979.
30. Nichter LS, Morgan RF, Harman DM, et al: The trapezius musculocutaneous flap in head and neck reconstruction: Potential pitfalls. *Head Neck Surg* 7:129, 1984.
31. Hester JR, McConnell FMS, Nahai F, et al: Reconstruction of cervical esophagus, hypopharynx, and oral cavity using the free jejunal transfer. *Am J Surg* 140:487, 1980.
32. Soutar DS, Scheker LR, Tanner NSB, et al: The radial forearm flap: A versatile method for intraoral reconstruction. *Br J Plast Surg* 36:1, 1983.
33. Man D, Acland RD: The microarterial anatomy of the dorsalis pedis flap and its clinical applications. *Plast Reconstr Surg* 64:419, 1980.
34. Silverberg B, Banis JC, Acland RD: Mandibular reconstruction with bone transfer. *Am J Surg* 150:440, 1985.
35. Granick MS, Newton ED, Hanna DC: Scapular free flap for repair of massive lower facial defects. *Head Neck Surg* 8:436, 1986.
36. Taylor GI: Reconstruction of the mandible with free composite iliac bone grafts. *Ann Plast Surg* 9:361, 1982.

40

Chemotherapy of Head and Neck Cancer

Timothy J. Panella, M.D. and Andrew T. Huang, M.D.

With the standard combination of surgical and radiation treatment, the 5-year survival rate of patients with advanced head and neck cancer is approximately 30% (1). Of the 70% of patients who do poorly, one half of them develop locally recurrent disease (2) and the other half develop distant metastases (3). Many of these patients are also left with debilitating functional and cosmetic deformities from their disease and its treatment. The use of chemotherapy for treating cancer of the head and neck began early in the 1950s. When it was first tested in patients having recurrent disease, chemotherapy showed limited benefits. Later, trials involving patients with previously untreated tumors demonstrated better responses. Chemotherapy was therefore subsequently included as an adjunct to surgery and radiation with the intention of improving survival and quality of life in patients with more advanced cancer (4).

There are four settings in which antineoplastic drugs are employed for patients with head and neck cancer. The most commonly accepted use of chemotherapy is in the palliation of advanced, recurrent, or refractory disease. Three other uses of chemotherapy have been tested in newly diagnosed patients with more advanced stages III and IV cancer. Chemotherapy given before primary surgery or irradiation is called "neoadjuvant" or "induction" adjuvant therapy. When adjuvant therapy temporally overlaps the primary management, the terms "concurrent" or "simultaneous" are used. The administration of antineoplastic agents after primary treatment is termed "consolidation" or "maintenance." For this chapter, we use the terms "induction," "concurrent," and "consolidation" for these three types of adjuvant chemotherapy. The usefulness of adjuvant chemotherapy as part of the standard care for head and neck cancer patients has not yet been unequivocally proven outside of well-defined clinical trials.

In this chapter, the use of chemotherapy in head and neck cancer is explored, followed by a discussion of the most active single agents. Recent data from many clinical trials of combination chemotherapy also are reviewed.

Chemotherapy Fundamentals

Squamous cell carcinoma of the head and neck region biologically resembles squamous cell carcinoma of other regions of the body. It tends to begin mucosally and extend to locoregional nodes before metastasizing to distant organs. The localized nature of stages I and II disease permits successful surgery and radiotherapy. Larger tumors of stages III and IV are more difficult to manage with primary surgery or radiation, and they are frequently associated with distant metastatic foci (3, 5). The size of the primary tumor and lymph nodes correlates inversely with the response to radiation or chemotherapy (6–10). These observations form the basis of support for the multimodality approach of therapy.

PROGNOSTIC FACTORS FOR CHEMOTHERAPY RESPONSE

In head and neck cancer, several factors influence the response to chemotherapy. Bulky primary tumors and lymph nodes give a less favorable response to treatment. Poor performance status of the patient (11, 12) also is associated with a decreased response to chemotherapy, possibly due to low tolerance of full-dose chemotherapy, malnutrition, and abnormal drug metabolism from liver or renal dysfunction. Most chemotherapy trials only accept patients of higher performance status. Thus, the effect of chemotherapy on the ill patients may not be fully represented in the published reports. Poor response or recurrence of disease after chemotherapy or radiotherapy is associated with a decreased response to later treatments (13).

A correlation between tumor differentiation and prognosis has been reported (14–16). Crissman et al. noted an improved survival rate in patients whose tumors contained less keratin (17). Responses to chemotherapy and radiotherapy (17, 18) have been shown by some investigators to be higher in poorly differentiated tumors. Ensley et al. (18) observed that, while poorly differentiated tumors responded better to chemotherapy, they recurred more readily. Patients with well-differentiated tumors that have responded to chemotherapy survive longer. A statistically significant correlation between differentiation and chemotherapy response or overall survival has not been observed (19–22).

The anatomical location of the primary tumor has a lesser effect on the response to chemotherapy in most trials (21–23), except in oral and nasopharygeal carcinomas (6, 7, 24). Response to induction adjuvant chemotherapy frequently predicts improved survival. This topic is discussed later under "Induction Therapy."

COMBINATION CHEMOTHERAPY

Several principles of chemotherapy common to the treatment of all solid tumors have been specifically tested in head and neck cancer. Goldie and Coldman hypothesized that two effective drugs administered simultaneously will kill a larger number of tumor cells than each drug given sequentially because of a decrease in the development of resistance (25, 26). As the treatment of many malignancies evolves on the basis of this hypothesis, so does the treatment of head and neck cancer.

Initially, single-drug treatments were tested in recurrent head and neck cancer. Methotrexate, bleomycin, 5-fluorouracil (5-FU), and cisplatin were found to be the most active single agents (2, 27). Several combinations of these active agents have shown surprisingly high response rates (28). However, many published prospective randomized trials failed to show improved survival following treatments with various combinations of these agents in comparison to no treatment (29).

CHEMOTHERAPY DOSE INTENSITY

Questions concerning chemotherapy dose intensity have been examined in several experimental tumor systems. Some in vivo evidence has been presented supporting the hypothesis that higher doses of chemotherapy increase the effectiveness of the active agents in treating experimental tumors (30). If this reasoning is true, the higher the doses of drug administered the better the tumor kill. While doses of chemotherapy sufficiently high to require bone marrow support have not been tested in head and neck cancer, several trials have evaluated this hypothesis at a more conventional dose range. Veronesi et al. compared 60 and 120 mg/m^2 of cisplatin and found no difference in the tumor response rate (31). Two separate studies that used cisplatin at 200 mg/m^2 (4, 32) found response rates (46% and 73%) no higher than those at standard doses. While one of these trials (32) found a slight benefit with the higher dose, the responses were short and toxicity was high. Four randomized trials comparing standard and high-dose methotrexate have also failed to show improvement in response rates (33). Other drugs have not been studied in a manner addressing the dose-response question in head and neck cancer.

The issue of dose intensity also needs consideration when comparing different clinical trials. In most, if not all, studies the amount of chemotherapy received by the patients is less than the full dose intended for them. The degree of dosage diminution is rarely specified in the published reports. Patients with head and neck cancer have a poor record of completing therapy. In a recent Northern California Oncology Group (NCOG) trial using bleomycin and methotrexate (22), none of the patients received the full treatment intended. Compliance was almost as poor in the final report of a study by the Head and Neck Cancer Contracts Program (20). Patients are unable to complete their treatment principally because of toxicity, tumor progression, patient refusal to continue, noncom-

pliance, and poor social support (34). It is rarely meaningful to evaluate the effect of chemotherapy from trials with such frequent protocol violations.

Active Single Agents

METHOTREXATE

Methotrexate was the first drug used in head and neck cancer chemotherapy (35). It is an antimetabolite that irreversibly inhibits dihydrofolate reductase (DHFR), resulting in decreased formation of tetrahydrofolic acid from folic acid. Consequently, thymidylate formation, and therefore DNA synthesis, is inhibited. The tetrahydrofolic acid derivative leucovorin, which is available commercially, can be administered to rescue the inhibition of methotrexate and reduce or prevent toxicity to rapidly proliferating normal tissues such as the bone marrow, skin, and gastrointestinal tract.

In trials using conventional doses, methotrexate has been given both weekly (36) and monthly (37, 38). In these studies, the highest response rates were seen with weekly therapy; thus, a weekly dose between 30 and 60 mg/m^2 is frequently the standard to which newer treatments are compared. The length of response averages 3 months in most of these studies. Randomized trials have failed to show a benefit for different dose regimens of methotrexate (39). High-dose methotrexate with leucovorin rescue (40, 41) offers similar response rates at considerably higher cost and toxicity to the patients.

CISPLATIN

Cisplatin (*cis*-diaminodichloroplatinum) is an alkylating agent that binds to DNA, producing intra- and interstrand cross-linking. The drug is excreted by the kidneys and is nephrotoxic. Pretreatment hydration and mannitol diuresis lessen the risk of renal damage. Other effects are severe nausea and vomiting, ototoxicity, mild myelotoxicity, peripheral neuropathy, hypozincemia (42), and hypomagnesemia.

As a single agent, cisplatin is given every 3–4 weeks intravenously. At the usual doses of 60–120 mg/m^2, its toxicity is acceptable. Whether the drug is infused over 24 hr (43), given as a bolus (44), or divided over 5 days (45), the response averages 30%. In patients who have not had prior chemotherapy or radiation, the response rate can be as high as 70% (44). As with methotrexate, the duration of response is measured in months. Two randomized trials comparing methotrexate to cisplatin found no difference in overall response in recurrent or advanced disease (46, 47). Cisplatin can also be given as a 5-day continuous infusion. There is evidence that this may lead to increased exposure of tumor to the active, non-protein-bound drug (48). While there is no improvement of response with this treatment schedule (49), trials testing its use in combination with other drugs (e.g., 5-FU) show promise (50).

BLEOMYCIN

Bleomycin is an antineoplastic antibiotic isolated from a strain of *Streptomyces*. Its main mode of action is probably inhibition of DNA synthesis and chromosomal fragmentation. The dose-limiting toxic effect is pulmonary fibrosis, which occurs most frequently in those patients receiving over 200 units/m^2. Fever and chills after administration are common, and rare anaphylaxis can occur. A one-unit test dose may be used prior to administration of treatment. Bleomycin induces little or no myelotoxicity and frequently is used in combination with other myelotoxic drugs. The standard dose of bleomycin is 5–15 units/m^2 intravenously (IV) or intramuscularly (IM). It is associated with a response rate of 20% (51, 52) and a short (1–2-month) duration of response. To avoid pulmonary toxicity (19), alternate scheduling, such as continuous infusions (20, 24), has been used in combination regimens.

5-FLUOROURACIL

5-Fluorouracil is a fluorinated pyrimidine antimetabolite. Its deoxyribosyl intermediate is a competitive inhibitor of thymidylate synthetase in the conversion of deoxyuridylate to thymidylate; therefore, it blocks DNA synthesis. The dose-limiting effect is mucositis and myelotoxicity. The standard method of administration is an IV bolus or continuous infusion (53). The overall response rate is 15% (27, 54). 5-FU is frequently combined with cisplatin and is also used concurrently with radiation therapy. Whereas leucovorin is often used to moderate the toxicity of methotrexate, conversely, it potentiates the effect of 5-FU. Leucovorin increases the inhibition of thymidylate synthetase by favoring the binding of deoxyribosylated 5-FU to the enzyme. It is unclear whether the combination of 5-FU and leucovorin offers better therapeutic benefit than 5-FU alone given at higher doses.

OTHER SINGLE AGENTS

Other single agents also used in head and neck cancer are the lipid-soluble antifolate trimetrexate (response rate, 26%) (55, 56), mitoquazone (MGBG) (22%) (57), the cisplatin derivative carboplatin (25%) (58), hydroxyurea (39%), cyclophosphamide (36%), vinblastine (29%), adriamycin (23%) (59), and nitrosoureas (33%) (60). As with most single agents, these are associated with short response durations.

Inoperable, Recurrent, and Refractory Disease

Chemotherapy has been demonstrated to offer some degree of palliation for head and neck cancer patients with inoperable disease from the onset, recurrent disease

not amenable to further surgery or radiation, or persistent disease after primary treatment. Many single agents are tested in this patient population. Palliative chemotherapy is frequently attempted for pain control, ulcerating lesions, esophageal or tracheal obstruction, and control of distant metastases. Patients with hypercalcemia, bone involvement, tumor resistance to prior chemoradiotherapy (11), or inadequate family and social support are poor candidates for consideration of chemotherapy.

Single agents and multiagent combinations have been used as palliative treatment for patients with poor prognoses. Many of the multiagent trials have been reviewed (61). An improvement in overall response rate with multiagent combinations over single agents of approximately 10% is generally observed. The best combination seems to be 5-FU with cisplatin given every 3 weeks. A randomized comparison of patients treated with cisplatin in combination with either 5-day continuous infusion or 5 daily boluses of 5-FU (1000 mg/m^2/day) showed a significant improvement in the group receiving prolonged infusion (62). The combination of cisplatin and infusional 5-FU can be given IV or intra-arterially, and the results from intra-arterial administration (response rate, 43%) are similar to those from trials using the IV route (63).

Some recent trials are summarized in Table 40.1. As can be seen, treatments with new agents, different schedules, and other methods to enhance the effectiveness of old agents have been evaluated. The differences in response rates and survival are due to differences in therapy and patient selection criteria.

There have been eight recent randomized trials comparing single agents to combinations (5, 68–74), three of which reported significantly improved response with combination agents as compared to the single regimens (69, 73, 74). However, there was no significant improvement in survival using multiple agents. Toxicity was higher in the combination treatment arms. Two of these studies included the highly active combination of cisplatin and 5-FU, which was compared to methotrexate alone and methotrexate with cisplatin.

In the most recent study (73), Forastiere et al. compared cisplatin plus 4-day continuous infusion of 5-FU versus carboplatin plus 5-FU versus weekly IV methotrexate. With 202 patients evaluated for response, they obtained a 30% overall response rate with the cisplatin combination, an 18% response rate with the carboplatin combination, and a significantly lower 11% response rate with methotrexate alone. The response duration was 4 months. Survival was not different in any of the three treatment arms. Jacobs et al. obtained similar results showing increased response rates with cisplatin and 5-FU (31%) when compared with 5-FU (14%) or cisplatin (14%) alone (74). No improvement in response duration or survival was observed, however.

In metastatic, inoperable, or recurrent cancer, the goal of treatment is to improve quality of life. A weekly treatment, in modest doses, of methotrexate as a single agent is a reasonable standard treatment and shows the lowest toxicity. The regimen containing cisplatin with continuous-infusion 5-FU is also useful.

Table 40.1.
Recent Trials in Inoperable, Recurrent, and Advanced Head and Neck Cancer

| Investigators | Treatment | No. of Patients | Response Rate (%)[a] | | Median Survival |
			CR	CR + PR	
Tapazoglou et al. (53)	5-FU continuous IV daily × 5	11	0	72	nr[b]
Deitmer and Urbanitz (64)	Cisplatin, bleomycin, methotrexate with rescue	63	21	73	nr
Robert (56)	Trimetrexate IVP[c] daily × 5	38	0	26	17.3 weeks
Choksi et al. (65)	Cisplatin over 24 hr, 5-FU over 5 days	20	10	25	36 weeks
Vokes et al. (66)	Cisplatin, 5-FU continuous with leucovorin rescue	18	5	56	26 weeks
Mackintosh et al. (67)	5-FU IVP, methotrexate with rescue	107	6.8	46	30 weeks
Forastiere et al. (57)	Guanylhydrazone (MGBG) IV weekly	17	0	6	nr

[a] CR, complete response; PR, partial response.
[b] Not reported.
[c] Intravenous push.

Induction Chemotherapy

Radiation and surgery are capable of curing early-stage tumors and are the standard treatments responsible for current cancer treatment success. However, in patients with advanced disease, radiation and surgery are not as successful and often cause excessive toxicity or unacceptable mutilation. Induction adjunctive chemotherapy is therefore attempted; it is given prior to standard treatments as a cytoreductive measure to improve the treatment outcome in these patients.

Induction chemotherapy trials in head and neck cancer have generated some new ideas in oncology. Induction chemotherapy does reduce tumor burden and many potentially render radiation or surgery more effective. Furthermore, it is also possible that early chemotherapy may provide additional control of distant occult micrometastases, which are more frequently associated with advanced stages of disease.

Response to induction chemotherapy may also be predictive of later response and final survival. Several studies have shown better survival in the group of patients who achieve complete response initially to induction chemotherapy and a poorer survival for those who do not (1, 7, 24, 75). This reported survival advantage, which has not been completely accepted, may be a truthful observation or may result from a selection bias of a good-prognosis group. Either way, the most important benefit in induction chemotherapy is an initial high complete response rate. Because there is no other method for discerning good from poor prognostic groups, the response to induction chemotherapy is currently viewed as a reasonable predictor for favorable outcome and has been utilized to alter treatment.

Studies have also been designed to examine whether surgery may be circumvented in some head and neck cancers. In a recent report, surgery was replaced by curative radiotherapy given to 12 patients who attained a complete response to induction chemotherapy. These patients maintained a better overall survival rate than those who had surgery alone (70% versus 53%) (10). This finding has special significance for patients whose tumors are not easily accessible or amenable to surgery—for example, tumor of the nasopharynx (76), larynx, tongue, and paranasal sinuses. The first prospective trial of this approach was recently presented (77). Patients with stages III or IV laryngeal cancer were randomized to either induction chemotherapy followed by radiation, or surgery and postoperative radiation. After two cycles of chemotherapy, patients with partial or complete response were given one more cycle before radiation. Patients who did not respond to chemotherapy or those whose disease persisted after radiation underwent "salvage" laryngectomy. In a rather large series of 275 patients, preservation of the larynx was achieved in 61% of patients randomized to the induction chemotherapy arm. At 2 years of follow-up, the survival was not inferior in the patients on the larynx-preserving arm. Other trials of organ-sparing induction chemotherapy are being planned.

For patients in whom radiation is not feasible (e.g., because of prior radiation to the area of tumor involvement, tumor growth near vital organs, or patient refusal), there is preliminary evidence that chemotherapy may substitute for radiation. Spaulding et al. (79) reported on patients with operable stage III or IV disease who were given induction chemotherapy. In those patients in whom treatment caused a tumor regression (to stage I or II), radical surgery was performed. Radiation was added only if tumor was found at surgical margins, extended through the capsule of lymph nodes, involved muscle, or was in the farthest level of lymph node groups. Ninety-one percent of the patients were spared radiotherapy. While this approach has been followed in other more recent studies, it is as yet too early to evaluate the degree of local control or the survival of these patients (8, 50, 78, 79).

Initially, there were concerns that induction chemotherapy might render subsequent therapy much more toxic. Corey et al. (80) reported an increase in postoperative complications from 39% to 52% in patients pretreated with high-dose methotrexate. The interval between chemotherapy and surgery in this study was rather short, and complications consisted of increased incidence of pneumonia, sepsis, mucositis, thrombocytopenia, and leukopenia. In the case of surgery performed after bleomycin, a lower intraoperative fractional inspired oxygen level may decrease the incidence of pulmonary toxicity. While patients receiving induction therapy must be monitored for increased toxicity, most major randomized trials found minimal change in early or late complications following subsequent radical surgery or full-dose radiation (19, 24, 76, 78, 81).

Recurrent disease after initial treatment of advanced head and neck cancer is often local. Clinically evident distant metastasis occurs in 6–15% of patients (82). In autopsy series (3), however, the incidence of metastasis is as high as 50%. One proposed benefit of induction chemotherapy is a decrease in the incidence of distant metastasis. It is presumed that, at the time of initial presentation, patients with stages III and IV disease have occult micrometastatic disease. Chemotherapy is, in theory, effective when there is a low tumor burden and fewer hypoxic or resistant cells. To date, however, induction chemotherapy has failed to show any significant reduction of subsequent metastatic cancer (7, 19, 20, 22, 83). In head and neck cancer, induction chemotherapy is an effective debulking treatment, but it is incapable of securing ultimate complete tumor eradication.

The development of regimens for induction chemotherapy began with methotrexate (84), and although complete responses were low (1), tumor regression observed in responders induced continuing interest (83). Initial chemotherapy with various cisplatin, bleomycin, methotrexate, and vinca alkaloid combinations increased the complete response rate to the 20% range (33). As cisplatin and 5-FU combinations were developed, the number of complete responses increased to 54% (1). Combined results of 13 studies using cisplatin and 5-FU give an average complete response rate of 35% and an overall response rate of 86% (1, 50, 85). As combinations of drugs with superior complete response rates are designed, prolongation of survival may become more likely.

Table 40.2 presents the results of six prospective randomized trials comparing treatment of advanced head and neck cancer with and without induction chemotherapy. This table illustrates the high degree of variability in response rates from report to report in many prospective randomized trials. Several other studies combined induction and consolidation chemotherapy together. These studies are discussed in the next section.

Recent single-arm studies showing high response rates are listed in Table 40.3. Two studies have shown impressive pathological complete responses. Krasnow et al. (90) used five antineoplastic agents in their study. In their trial, the second course of treatment was given to coincide with maximal red blood cell membrane fluidity (90). Bernal et al. gave cisplatin by infusion over 4 days (50). Infusion of cisplatin is believed to increase tissue exposure to the active non–protein-bound drug (91). With a follow-up of 22 months, none of Bernal et al.'s patients with a complete response to chemotherapy has relapsed (50). In these studies as well as others, patients who did not complete their treatment regimen relapsed quickly. Patients who tolerated induction chemotherapy without delays or reductions of drug dosage tended to do well. Definitive surgery and/or radiation are, however, necessary for these patients.

Consolidation Chemotherapy

The rationale for giving consolidation adjuvant chemotherapy after primary surgery or radiation differs from that of palliative chemotherapy for recurrent disease or induction chemotherapy. The presence of locoregional or distant recurrence after primary treatment with surgery and/or radiation implies that viable local microscopic and metastatic tumors still exist. The assumption that effective chemotherapy has a greater impact when tumor burden is small (93) offers a rationale for treating breast or head and neck cancer in the immediate period after definitive therapy with surgery and radiation. Consolidation chemotherapy given temporally after definitive therapy also avoids the problem of patients refusing subsequent primary treatment after an initial good response to induc-

Table 40.2.
Response Rates from Randomized Trials Using Induction Chemotherapy

Investigators	Treatment[a]	No. of Patients Randomized	Response Rate (%)[b]	
			CR	CR + PR
Schuller et al. (19)	Cisplatin, bleomycin, VCR vs. none	158	19	70
Martin et al. (86)	Cisplatin, bleomycin, MTX, 5-FU vs. none	107	6	49
Toohill et al. (87)	Cisplatin, 5-FU vs. none	60	19	85
H + N Contracts (20)	Cisplatin, bleomycin × 1 cycle vs. none	462	3	37
Carugati et al. (88)	Cisplatin, bleomycin	120	nr[c]	44
	Cisplatin, bleomycin, MTX vs. none		nr	59
Kun et al. (89)	Bleomycin, CTX, MTX, 5-FU vs. none	83	5	63

[a] VCR, vincristine; MTX, methotrexate, CTX, cyclophosphamide.
[b] CR, complete response; PR, partial response.
[c] Not reported.

Table 40.3.
Recent, Promising, Single-arm Induction Chemotherapy Trials

Investigators	Treatment[a]	No. of Patients	Response Rate (%)[b]		CR + PR	Median Survival
			CR	pCR		
Ensley et al. (34)	5-FU infusion × 5 days + cisplatin, alt. with MTX with rescue + 5-FU	46	46	28	85	nr
Cheung et al. (92)	Cisplatin intra-arterial infusion × 5 days + MTX	18	35	0	94	>156 weeks
Forastiere et al. (75)	Cisplatin, mitoquazone weekly	26	27	19	65	70 weeks
Dasmahapatra et al. (81)	Cisplatin, MTX with rescue, bleomycin	25	48	nr[c]	84	nr
Krasnow et al. (90)	Vinblastine, bleomycin, MTX, 5-FU cisplatin	25	36	36	68	42% 3 years
Bernal et al. (50)	Cisplatin + 5-FU both as infusion	37	46	36	86	80% 2 years

[a] MTX, methotrexate.
[b] CR, pathological complete response; PR, partial response.
[c] Not reported.

tion therapy. Some chemotherapy trials combine induction and consolidation chemotherapy in the form of a "sandwiched" schedule.

The benefit of consolidation chemotherapy reported in several single-arm studies (24, 94) has been difficult to confirm in randomized trials. A single-agent trial by Rentschler et al. randomized patients who underwent standard surgery and radiation plus methotrexate chemotherapy against those who received standard treatment without chemotherapy. No significant difference in disease-free or overall survival could be demonstrated (95). As with induction chemotherapy, there is evidence suggesting that patients with chemosensitive tumors may benefit from consolidation chemotherapy. Ervin et al. (24) randomized 46 patients, who were free of disease after responding to induction chemotherapy and primary treatment with radiation or surgery, to three additional cycles of cisplatin, bleomycin, and methotrexate or to no further therapy. In this subgroup of patients with chemosensitive tumors, those who received consolidation therapy had significantly fewer locoregional failures and better disease-free survival rates. This trial provides evidence to suggest that, in chemosensitive tumors, antineoplastic agents may alter the natural history of the disease. Furthermore, it suggests that additional exposure to these agents may be beneficial.

Five known prospective randomized trials compared standard surgery/radiation with and without multiagent consolidation chemotherapy (20–23, 51). In these five studies, cisplatin was not administered in combination with 5-FU, and the patient compliance rate was extremely low in the three trials describing compliance (20, 22, 51). Based on these studies, it is difficult to draw firm conclusions concerning the merit of consolidation chemotherapy. Trials that adopt agents that induce a high complete response rate and treat patients who are appropriately chosen and are highly compliant are necessary for determining the efficacy of induction and consolidation chemotherapy.

Concurrent Chemotherapy and Radiotherapy

Concurrent treatment with radiation and chemotherapy for head and neck cancer began in 1959 (96). The major reason for combining these two different modalities of treatment was to seek synergism. The first agent used was 5-FU.

Evidence of therapeutic enhancement by concurrent radiation and chemotherapy came from the work of Heidelberger and colleagues, who showed that noncurative doses of radiation could be made curative by combining them with noncurative doses of 5-FU in mice (97). In 1971, Vietti et al. studied the timing of bolus 5-FU in relation to radiotherapy (XRT) and found synergism when 5-FU was given 5–8 hr after XRT (98). Byfield et al. confirmed that synergism only occurred when bolus 5-FU was given after XRT. In in vitro experiments varying the incubation time of 5-FU, synergism was associated with exposure to the drug lasting longer than 48 hr after XRT (99). The drug levels associated with in vitro synergy were similar to levels found in patients receiving 48–120-hour infusions (0.5 μg/ml). On the basis of their data, Byfield et al. suggested that, in human trials, the best synergistic effect of chemotherapy with radiation could be obtained by infusing 5-FU for at least 48 hr. Cisplatin and XRT interactions have also been studied. The evidence supports an additive effect rather than synergism (100). The major benefit of concurrent cisplatin may be in the enhancement of radiosensitivity in tumor hypoxic areas. There are in vivo data supporting its use 30 min prior to radiotherapy (100).

Concurrent chemoradiation therapy may be employed as curative treatment for advanced-stage disease or palliation for advanced/recurrent disease (101, 102). Early trials combined single-agent hydroxyurea, methotrexate, or bleomycin with radiation (27). Randomized trials (103, 104) comparing the use of these single agents with or without radiation failed to show improved survival except in oral cavity cancers. Concurrent 5-FU chemotherapy was later found to offer better survival in three studies (96, 105, 106). Subsequent studies of concurrent radiation and cisplatin with and without 5-FU reported complete response rates ranging from 52% to 75% (1, 107). Wendt et al. (108) later used cisplatin, continuous-infusion 5-FU, and leucovorin; they observed an extraordinary 87% complete response rate. This combination was an improvement over the use of cisplatin and higher doses of infusional 5-FU without leucovorin (complete response rate, 60%) as reported elsewhere (109, 110). Preliminary studies investigating the use of carboplatin with irradiation indicate no improvement in response rates (111).

Two recent prospective, randomized trials of concurrent therapy compared simultaneous and sequential administration of cisplatin and 5-FU (112, 113). A superior complete remission rate was demonstrated in the simultaneous arm in one study (112).

Knowledge of radiobiological interaction of radiation and chemotherapy is quickly accumulating. Proper scheduling between these two treatment options will be an important research topic for the near future.

Salivary Gland Carcinoma

Cancer of the salivary gland represents 5–10% of head and neck malignancies (114). The most common histologies are mucoepidermoid, adenoid cystic, adenocarcinoma, and malignant mixed. Except for adenocarcinoma, these tumors tend to grow slowly, even when metastatic (115). Unlike squamous cell carcinoma, distant metastasis from adenoidcystic carcinoma occurs in approximately 41% of patients (116), and locoregional lymph nodes are involved only 10% of the time. The primary treatment for adenoid cystic carcinoma has been surgery; however, the tumor spreads deep into surrounding tissue, and it is often difficult to obtain meaningful tumor-free margins (116). In select cases, radiation will decrease the incidence of locoregional failure that occurs in over 50% of patients with salivary gland carcinoma (117, 118). Because of the rarity of salivary gland tumors, chemotherapy trials are usually single arm and small and encompass many years of follow-up. Although adjuvant trials have been conducted (119, 120), the use of antineoplastic agents is usually in the metastatic or recurrent setting.

The most active single agents for salivary gland tumors are cisplatin, adriamycin, and 5-FU, with overall response rates between 46% and 50% (121). Responsiveness to these agents varies according to histological subtypes (119); however, Kaplan et al. (121) found that nearly all types of tumors responded to cisplatin and 5-FU. Adenoid cystic carcinoma, adenocarcinoma, and malignant mixed carcinoma also responded to adriamycin. Mucoepidermoid carcinoma, similarly to squamous cell carcinoma, responds to methotrexate. The overall response rates are similar for all types of carcinomas, averaging 10% complete response and 44% overall response.

Various combinations of the above single agents and other less active drugs have been tested. The response rates are higher with combination than with single (115, 122) agents. The response duration ranges from 5 to 10 months. Although survival does not appear to improve with chemotherapy (115, 119–122), significant palliation is frequently observed, and the toxicity is tolerable. Chemotherapy is thus primarily used for palliation and in clinical trials.

Chemotherapy in Head and Neck Cancer

In the treatment of head and neck cancer, surgery and radiation are responsible for the current level of cures, predominantly in early stages of disease. Chemotherapy by itself clearly reduces tumor burden in the majority of trials thus far reported, but it has not been shown to offer significant improvement in survival. This lack of correlation between tumor regression and survival is disappointing. The coexistence of many intercurrent problems, such as uncorrected nutritional imbalance, immunological deficiencies, involvement of areas that circumvent effective treatment delivery, and the presence of resistant tumor cells, are determining factors that influence survival. The only hope of success in advanced disease in the future is to understand tumor biology in relation to chemotherapy, radiation, and surgery and to employ these three effective treatment modalities by proper scheduling.

The observation of remarkable complete responses noted in concurrent chemoirradiation trials for advanced stage disease sheds new light on the direction of future treatment research of head and neck cancer.

References

1. Choksi AJ, DImery IW, Hong WK: Adjuvant chemotherapy of head and neck cancer: The past, the present, and the future. *Semin Oncol* 15(Suppl 3):45, 1988.
2. Hong WK, Bromer R: Medical intelligence. Current concepts: Chemotherapy in head and neck cancer. *N Engl J Med* 308:75, 1983
3. Kotwall C, Sako K, Razack MS, et al: Metastatic patterns in squamous cell cancer of the head and neck. *Am J Surg* 154:439, 1987.
4. Havlin KA, Kuhn JG, Myers WJ: High-dose cisplatin for locally advanced or metastatic head and neck cancer. *Cancer* 63:423, 1989.
5. Slotman GJ, Mohit T, Raina S: The incidence of metastasis after multimodal therapy for cancer of the head and neck. *Cancer* 54:2009, 1984.
6. Wolf GT, Makuch RW, Baker SR: Predictive factors for tumor response to preoperative chemotherapy in patients with head and neck squamous carcinoma: The Head and Neck Contracts Program. *Cancer* 54:2869, 1984.
7. Fazekas JT, Sommer C, Kramer S: Tumor regression and other prognosticators in advanced head and neck cancers: A sequel to the RTOG methotrexate study. *Int J Radiat Oncol Biol Phys* 9:957, 1983.
8. Spaulding MB, Lore JM, Sundquist N: Long-term follow-up of chemotherapy in advanced head and neck cancer. *Arch Otolaryngol Head Neck Surg* 115:68, 1989.
9. Kies MS, Pecaro BC, Bordon LI: Preoperative combination chemotherapy for advanced stage head and neck cancer. *Am J Surg* 148:367, 1984.

10. Jacobs C, Goffinet DR, Goffinet L: Chemotherapy as a substitute for surgery in the treatment of advanced resectable head and neck cancer. *Cancer* 60:1178, 1987.

11. Amer MH, Al-Sarraf M, Vaitkevicius VK: Factors that affect response to chemotherapy and survival of patients with advanced head and neck cancer. *Cancer* 43:2202, 1979.

12. Jacobs C, Meyers F, Hendrickson C, et al. A randomized phase II study of cisplatin with or without methotrexate for recurrent squamous cell carcinoma of the head and neck: A Northern California Oncology Group study. *Cancer* 52:1563, 1983.

13. Ensley JF, Jacobs JR, Weaver A: Correlation between response to cisplatinum-combination chemotherapy and subsequent radiotherapy in previously untreated patients with advanced squamous cell cancers of the head and neck. *Cancer* 54:811, 1984.

14. Mc Gavran MH, Bauer WC, Ogura JH: The incidence of cervical lymph node metastases from epidermoid carcinoma of the larynx and their relationship to certain characteristics of the primary tumor. *Cancer* 14:55, 1961.

15. Shear M, Hawkins DM, Farr HW: The prediction of lymph node metastasis from oral squamous carcinoma. *Cancer* 37:1701, 1976.

16. Platz H, Fries R, Hudec M, et al: The prognostic relevance of various factors at the time of the first admission of the patient; Retrospective DOSAK study on carcinoma of the oral cavity. *J Maxillofac Surg* 11:3, 1983.

17. Crissman JD, Pajak TF, Zarbo RJ, et al: Improved response and survival to combined cisplatin and radiation in non-keratinizing squamous cell carcinomas of the head and neck. *Cancer* 59:1391, 1987.

18. Ensley J, Crissman J, Kish J: The impact of conventional morphologic analysis on response rates and survival in patients with advanced head and neck cancers treated initially with cisplatin-containing combination chemotherapy. *Cancer* 57:711, 1986.

19. Schuller DE, Metch B, Stein DW: Preoperative chemotherapy in advanced resectable head and neck cancer: Final report of the Southwest Oncology Group. *Laryngoscope* 98:1205, 1988.

20. Head and Neck Contracts Program: Adjuvant chemotherapy for advanced head and neck squamous carcinoma (final report). *Cancer* 60:301, 1987.

21. Taylor SG, Applebaum E, Showel JL: A randomized trial of adjuvant chemotherapy in head and neck cancer. *J Clin Oncol* 3:672, 1985.

22. Fu KK, Phillips TL, Silverberg IJ: Combined radiotherapy and chemotherapy with bleomycin and methotrexate for advanced inoperable head and neck cancer: Update of a Northern California Oncology Group randomized trial. *J Clin Oncol* 5:1410, 1987.

23. Holoye PY, Grossman TW, Toohill RJ: Randomized study of adjuvant chemotherapy for head and neck cancer. *Otolaryngol Head Neck Surg* 93:712, 1985.

24. Ervin TJ, Clark JR, Weichselbaum RR, et al: An analysis of induction and adjuvant chemotherapy in the multidisciplinary treatment of squamous-cell carcinoma of the head and neck. *J Clin Oncol* 5:10, 1987.

25. Goldie JH, Coldman AJ: A mathematical model for relating the drug sensitivity of tumors to their spontaneous mutation rate. *Cancer Treat Rep* 63:1727, 1973.

26. Goldie JH, Coldman AJ, Gudquskas GA: Rationale for the use of alternating non-cross resistant chemotherapy. *Cancer Treat Rep* 66:439, 1984.

27. Al-Sarraf M: Chemotherapy strategies in squamous cell carcinoma of the head and neck. *CRC Crit Rev Oncol Hematol* 1:323, 1984.

28. Greenberg B, Ahmann F, Garewal H, et al: Neoadjuvant therapy for advanced head and neck cancer with allopurinol-modulated high-dose 5-fluorouracil and cisplatin. A phase I-II study. *Cancer* 59:1860, 1987.

29. Al-Sarraf: Head and neck cancer: Chemotherapy concepts. *Semin Oncol* 15:70, 1988.

30. Frei E, Canellos GP: Dose: A critical factor in cancer therapy. *Am J Med* 69:585, 1980.

31. Veronesi A, Zagonel V, Tirelli U, et al: High-dose versus low-dose cisplatin in advanced head and neck squamous carcinoma: A randomized study. *J Clin Oncol* 3:1105, 1985.

32. Forasteire AA, Takasugi BJ, Baker SR, et al: High-dose cisplatin in advanced head and neck cancer. *Cancer Chemother Pharmacol* 19:155, 1987.

33. Mead GM, Jacobs C: Changing role of chemotherapy in treatment of head and neck cancer. *Am J Med* 73:582, 1982.

34. Ensley J, Tapazoglou KE, Jacobs A, et al: An intensive five course, alternating combination chemotherapy induction regimen used in patients with advanced unresectable head and neck cancer. *J Clin Oncol* 6:1147, 1988.

35. Carter SK: The chemotherapy of head and neck cancer. *Semin Oncol* 4:413, 1977.

36. Leone LA, Albala MM, Rege VB: Treatment of carcinoma of the head and neck with intravenous methotrexate. *Cancer* 21:828, 1968.

37. Papac RJ, Jacobs EM, Foye LV, Donohue DM: Systemic therapy with amthopterin in squamous carcinoma of the head and neck. *Cancer Chemother Rep* 32:47, 1963.

38. Lane M, Moore JE III, Levin H, Smith FE: Methotrexate therapy for squamous cell carcinoma of the head and neck. *JAMA* 204:561, 1968.

39. Taylor SG, McGuire WP, Hauck WW, Showel JL, Lad TE: A randomized comparison of high-dose infusion methotrexate versus standard-dose weekly therapy in head and neck squamous cancer. *J Clin Oncol* 2:1006, 1984.

40. Levitt M, Mosher MB, DeConti RC, et al: Improved therapeutic index of methotrexate with leucovorin rescue. *Cancer Res* 33:1729, 1973.

41. Frei E III, Blum RH, Pitman SW, et al: High dose methotrexate with leucovorin rescue. Rationale and spectrum of antitumor activity. *Am J Med* 68:370, 1980.

42. Sweeney JD, Ziegler P, Pruet C, Spaulding MB: Hyperzincuria and hypozincemia in patients treated with cisplatin. *Cancer* 63:2093, 1989.

43. Jacobs C, Bertino JR, Goffinet DR, Fee WE, Goode RL: 24-hour infusion of cis-platinum in head and neck cancers. *Cancer* 42:2135, 1978.

44. Wittes R, Heller K, Randolph V, et al: *Cis*-dichlorodiamineplatinum (II)-based chemotherapy as initial treatment of advanced head and neck cancer. *Cancer Treat Rep* 63:1533, 1979.

45. Mechl Z, Kerpel-Fronius S, Decker A, et al: Comparative evaluation of two administration schedules of *cis*-dichlorodiamineplatinum in ovarian and head and neck cancers: A CMEA chemotherapy group study. *Neoplasma* 34:37, 1987.

46. Hong WK, Schaifer S, Issell B, et al: A prospective, randomized trial of methotrexate versus cisplatin in the treatment of recurrent squamous cell carcinoma of the head and neck. *Cancer* 52:206, 1983.

47. Grose WE, Lehane DE, Dixon DO, et al: Comparison of methotrexate and cisplatin for patients with advanced squamous cell carcinoma of the head and neck region: A Southwest Oncology Group Study. *Cancer Treat Rep* 69:577, 1985.

48. Belliveau JF, Posner MR, Ferrari L, et al: Cisplatin administered as a continuous 5-day infusion. Plasma platinum levels and urine platinum excretion. *Cancer Treat Rep* 70:1215, 1986.

49. Posner MR, Ferrari L, Belliveau JF, et al: A phase I trial of continuous infusion cisplatin. *Cancer* 59:15, 1987.

50. Bernal AG, Cruz JJ, Sanchez P, et al: Four-day continuous infusion of cisplatin and 5-fluorouracil in head and neck cancer. *Cancer* 63:1927, 1989.

51. Stell PM, Dalby JE, Strickland P, et al: Sequential chemotherapy and radiotherapy in advanced head and neck cancer. *Clin Radiol* 34:463, 1983.

52. Durkin WJ, Pugh RP, Jacobe E, et al: Bleomycin (NSC-125066) therapy of responsive solid tumors. *Oncology* 33:260, 1976.

53. Tapazoglou E, Kish J, Ensley J, et al: The activity of a single-agent 5-fluorouracil infusion in advanced and recurrent head and neck cancer. *Cancer* 57:1105, 1986.

54. Ansfield F, Schroeder J, Curreri A: A five-year clinical experience with 5-fluorouracil. *JAMA* 181:295, 1962.

55. Lin JT, Cashmore AR, Baker M, et al: Phase I studies with

trimetrexate: Clinical pharmacology, analytical methodology, and pharmacokinetics. *Cancer Res* 47:609, 1987.

56. Robert F: Trimetrexate as a single agent in patients with advanced head and neck cancer. *Semin Oncol* 15(Suppl 2):22, 1988.

57. Forastiere AA, Natale RB, Wheeler RR: Phase II trial of methylglyoxal bis (guanylhydrazone) (MGBG) in advanced head and neck cancer. *Cancer* 58:2585, 1986.

58. Eisenberger M, Hornedo J, Silva H, Donehower R, Spaulding M, Ban Echo D: Carboplatin (NSC-211-140): An active platinum analogue for the treatment of squamous cell carcinoma of the head and neck. *J Clin Oncol* 4:1506, 1986.

59. Forastiere AA: Review: Management of advanced stage squamous cell carcinoma of the head and neck. *Am J Med Sci* 291:405, 1986.

60. Huang AT, Lucas VS, Baughn SG: A trial of outpatient chemotherapy for recurrent head and neck tumors. *Cancer* 45:2038, 1980.

61. Al-Sarraf M: Head and neck cancer: Chemotherapy concepts. *Semin Oncol* 15:70, 1988.

62. Kish JA, Ensley JF, Jacobs J, et al: A randomized trial of cisplatin (CACP) and 5-fluorouracil infusion and CACP + 5-FU bolus for recurrent and advanced squamous cell carcinoma of the head and neck. *Cancer* 56:2740, 1985.

63. Baker SR, Forastiere AA, Wheeler R, et al: Intra-arterial chemotherapy for head and neck cancer. *Arch Otolaryngol Head Neck Surg* 113:183, 1987.

64. Deitmer T, Urbanitz D: Chemotherapy in head and neck cancer with bleomycin, cisplatinum, and methotrexate. *J Cancer Res Clin Oncol* 114:644, 1988.

65. Choksi AJ, Hong WK, Dimery IW, et al: Continuous cisplatin and 5-fluorouracil infusion in recurrent head and neck squamous cell carcinoma. *Cancer* 61:909, 1988.

66. Vokes EE, Schilsky RL, Weichselbaum RR, et al: Cisplatin 5-fluorouracil, and high-dose oral leucovorin for advanced head and neck cancer. *Cancer* 63:1048, 1989.

67. Mackintosh JF, Coates AS, Tattersall MHN, et al: Chemotherapy of advanced head and neck cancer: Updated results of a randomized trial of the order of administration of sequential methotrexate and 5-fluorouracil. *Med Pediatr Oncol* 16:304, 1988.

68. Drelichman A, Cumming G, Al-Sarraf M: A randomized trial of the combination of cis-platinum, Oncovin, and bleomycin (COB) versus methotrexate in patients with advanced squamous cell carcinoma of the head and neck. *Cancer* 52:399, 1983.

69. Vogl SE, Schoenfeld DA, Kaplan BH, et al: A randomized prospective comparison of methotrexate with a combination of methotrexate, bleomycin, and cisplatin in head and neck cancer. *Cancer* 56:432, 1985.

70. Williams SD, Velez-Garcia C, Essessee I, et al: Chemotherapy for head and neck cancer: Comparison of cisplatin, vinblastine, and bleomycin versus methotrexate. *Cancer* 57(Adv I):18, 1986.

71. Campbell JB, Dorman EB, McCormick M, et al: A randomized phase III trial of cisplatinum, methotrexate, cisplatinum + methotrexate, and cisplatinum + 5-fluorouracil in end-stage head and neck cancer. *Acta Otolaryngol* 103:519, 1987.

72. Eisenberger M, Krasnow S, Ellenberg S, et al: A comparison of carboblatin and methotrexate versus methotrexate in recurrent squamous cell cancer of the head and neck. *Proc Am Soc Clin Oncol* 7(A594):153, 1988.

73. Forastiere A, Metch B, Keppen M, Schuller D, Ensley J, Coltman C: Randomized comparison of cisplatin + 5-fluorouracil versus carboplatin + 5-FU versus methotrexate in advanced squamous cell carcinoma of the head and neck. *Proc Am Soc Clin Oncol* 8(A655):168, 1989.

74. Jacobs C, Lyman G, Velez-Garcia E, et al: Comparison of infusional 5-fluorouracil and cisplatin in combination and as single agents for recurrent and metastatic head and neck cancer. *Proc Am Soc Clin Oncol* 7(A595):154, 1988.

75. Forastiere AA, Perry DJ, Wolf GT, et al: Cisplatin and mitoquazone: An induction chemotherapy regimen in advanced head and neck cancer. *Cancer* 62:2304, 1988.

76. Zidan J, Kuten A, Cohen Y, et al: Multidrug chemotherapy using bleomycin, methotrexate, and cisplatin combined with radical radiotherapy in advanced head and neck cancer. *Cancer* 59:24, 1987.

77. Hong WK, Wolf GT, Fisher S, et al: Laryngeal preservation with induction chemotherapy and radiotherapy in the treatment for advanced laryngeal cancer: Interim survival data of BACSP #268. *Proc Am Soc Clin Oncol* 8(A650):167, 1989.

78. Clark JR, Ervin TJ, Tuttle SA, et al: Pathology of surgery after induction chemotherapy: An analysis of resectability and locoregional control. *Laryngoscope* 96:292, 1986.

79. Spaulding M, Ziegler P, Sundquist N, et al: Induction therapy in head and neck cancer. *Cancer* 57:1110, 1986.

80. Corey JP, Caldarelli DD, Hutchinson JC, et al: Surgical complications in patients with head and neck cancer receiving chemotherapy. *Arch Otolaryngol Head Neck Surg* 112:437, 1986.

81. Dasmahapatra KS, Mohit-tabatabai MA, Rush BF, et al: Cancer of the tonsil: Improved survival with combination therapy. *Cancer* 57:451, 1986.

82. Slotman GJ, Mohit T, Raina S, et al: The incidence of metastasis after multimodal therapy for cancer of the head and neck. *Cancer* 54:2009, 1984.

83. Ervin TJ, Kirkwood J, Weichselbaum RR, et al: Improved survival for patients with advanced carcinoma of the head and neck treated with methotrexate-leucovorin prior to definitive radiotherapy or surgery. *Laryngoscope* 91:1181, 1981.

84. Tarpley JL, Chaetien PB, Alexander JC, et al: High dose methotrexate as a preoperative adjuvant treatment of epidermoid carcinoma of the head and neck. *Am J Surg* 136:481, 1975.

85. Jacobs JR, Pajak TF, Kinzie J, et al: Induction chemotherapy in advanced head and neck cancer. *Arch Otolaryngol Head Neck Surg* 113:193, 1987.

86. Martin M, Mazeron JJ, Brun B, et al: Neo-adjuvant polychemotherapy of head and neck cancer. *Proc Am Soc Clin Oncol* 7(A590):152, 1988.

87. Toohill RJ, Anderson T, Byhardt RW, et al: Cisplatin and fluorouracil as neoadjuvant therapy in head and neck cancer: A preliminary report. *Arch Otolaryngol Head Neck Surg* 113:758, 1987.

88. Carugati A, Pradier R, de la Torre A, Roffo AH: Combination chemotherapy pre radical treatment for head and neck squamous cell carcinoma. *Proc Am Soc Clin Oncol* 7(A589):152, 1988.

89. Kun LE, Toohill RJ, Holoye PY, et al: A randomized study of chemotherapy for cancer of the upper aerodigestive tract. *Int J Radiat Oncol Biol Phys* 12:173, 1986.

90. Krasnow SH, Cohen MH, Johnston-Early A, et al: Combined therapy for stage III-IV head and neck cancer: Preliminary results. *J Clin Oncol* 7:804, 1984.

91. Belliveau JF, Posner MR, Ferrari L, et al: Cisplatin administered as a continuous 5-day infusion. Plasma platinum levels and urine platinum excretion. *Cancer Treat Rep* 70:1215, 1986.

92. Cheung DK, Regan J, Savin M: A pilot study of intraarterial chemotherapy with cisplatin in locally advanced head and neck cancers. *Cancer* 61:903, 1988.

93. Goldie JH, Coldman AJ: A mathematical model for relating the drug sensitivity of tumors to their spontaneous mutation rate. *Cancer Treat Rep* 63:1727, 1979.

94. Johnson JT, Myers EN, Schramm VL, et al: Adjuvant chemotherapy for high-risk squamous-cell carcinoma of the head and neck. *J Clin Oncol* 5:546, 1987.

95. Rentschler RE, Wilbur DW, Petti GH, et al: Adjuvant methotrexate escalated to toxicity for resectable stage III and IV squamous head and neck carcinomas–A prospective randomized study. *J Clin Oncol* 5:278, 1987.

96. Gollin FF, Ansfield FJ, Brandenburg JH, et al: Combined therapy in advanced head and neck cancer: A randomized study. *Rad Ther Nucl Med* 114:83, 1972.

97. Heidelberger C, Griesbach L, Montag BJ, et al: Studies on fluorinated pyrimidines. II. Effects of transplanted tumors. *Cancer Res* 18:305, 1958.

98. Vietti T, Eggerding F, Valeriote F, et al: Combined effect of X

radiation and 5-fluorouracil on survival of transplanted leukemic cells. *J Natl Cancer Inst* 47:865, 1971.

99. Byfield JE, Calabro-Jones P, Klisak I, et al: Pharmacologic requirements for obtaining sensitization of human tumor cells in vitro to combined 5-fluorouracil or ftorafur and x rays. *Int J Rad Oncol Biol Phys* 8:1923, 1982.

100. Dewit L: Combined treatment of radiation and *cis*-diamminedichloroplatinum (II): A review of experimental and clinical data. *Int J Rad Oncol Biol Phys* 13:403, 1986.

101. Al-Sarraf M, Pajak TF, Marcial VA, et al: Concurrent radiotherapy and chemotherapy with cisplatin in inoperable squamous cell carcinoma of the head and neck: An RTOG study. *Cancer* 59:259, 1987.

102. Vokes EE, Panje WR, Schilsky RL, et al: Hydroxyurea, fluorouracil, and concomitant radiotherapy in poor-prognosis head and neck cancer: A phase I-II study. *J Clin Oncol* 7:761, 1989.

103. Fu KK, Theodore PL, Silverberg IJ, et al: Combined radiotherapy and chemotherapy with bleomycin and methotrexate for advanced inoperable head and neck cancer: Update of a Northern California Oncology Group randomized trial. *J Clin Oncol* 5:1410, 1987.

104. Million RR, Cassisi NJ, Wittes RE: Cancer of the head and neck. In Devita VT, Hellman S, Rosenberg SA (eds): *Cancer, Principles and Practice of Oncology*, ed 2. Philadelphia, JB Lippincott Co, 1985, p 428.

105. Lo TC, Wiley AL, Ansfield FJ, et al: Combined radiation therapy and 5-fluorouracil for advanced squamous cell carcinoma of the oral cavity and oropharynx: A randomized study. *Radiat Ther Nucl Med* 126:229, 1976.

106. Ansfield FJ, Ramirex G, Davis HL Jr, et al: Treatment of advanced cancer of the head and neck. *Cancer* 25:78, 1970.

107. Giri PG, Taylor SA: Concurrent chemotherapy and radiation therapy in advanced head and neck cancer. *Am J Clin Oncol* 10:417, 1987.

108. Wendt TG, Wustrow TPU, Hartenstein RC: Accelerated split-course radiotherapy and simultaneous *cis*-dichlorodiammine-platinum and 5-fluorouracil chemotherapy with folinic acid enhancement for unresectable carcinoma of the head and neck. *Radiother Oncol* 10:277, 1987.

109. Adelstein DJ, Sharan VM, Earle S, et al: Chemoradiotherapy as initial management in patients with squamous cell carcinoma of the head and neck. *Cancer Treat Rep* 70:761, 1986.

110. Murthy AK, Taylor SG, Showel J: Treatment of advanced head and neck cancer with concomitant radiation and chemotherapy. *Int J Rad Oncol Biol Phys* 13:1807, 1987.

111. Sinibaldi V, Eisinberger M, Jacobs M, et al: Treatment of advanced unresectable stage IV squamous cell carcinoma of the head and neck with combined carboplatin and radiotherapy. *Proc Am Soc Clin Oncol* 8(A659):169, 1989.

112. Adelstein DJ, Sharan VM, Earl AS, et al: A prospective randomized trial of simultaneous versus sequential chemoradiotherapy for squamous cell head and neck cancer. *Proc Am Soc Clin Oncol* 8(A648):167, 1989.

113. Cognetti F, Carlini P, Pinnard P, et al: Preliminary results of a randomized trial of sequential versus simultaneous chemo and radiotherapy in patients with locally advanced unresectable squamous cell carcinoma of the head and neck. *Proc Am Soc Clin Oncol* 8(A661):170, 1989.

114. Rentschler R, Burgess MA, Byers R: Chemotherapy of malignant salivary gland neoplasms: A 25 year review of M.D. Anderson Hospital experience. *Cancer* 40:619, 1977.

115. Creagan ET, Woods JE, Rubin J, et al: Cisplatin-based chemotherapy for neoplasms arising from salivary glands and contiguous structures in the head and neck. *Cancer* 62:2313, 1988.

116. Shingaki S, Saito R, Kawasaki T, et al: Adenoid cystic carcinoma of the major and minor salivary glands. *J Maxillofac Surg* 14:53, 1984.

117. Matsuba HM, Thawley SE, Mauney M: Improved treatment of salivary adenocarcinomas: Planned combined surgery and irradiation. *Laryngoscope* 96:904, 1986.

118. Fu KK, Leibel SA, Levine ML, et al: Carcinoma of the major and minor salivary glands: Analysis of treatment results and sites and causes of failure. *Cancer* 40:2882, 1977.

119. Venook AP, Tseng A, Meyers FJ, et al: Cisplatin, doxorubicin, and 5-fluorouracil chemotherapy for salivary gland malignancies: A pilot study of the Northern California Oncology Group. *J Clin Oncol* 5:951, 1987.

120. Triozzi PL, Brantley A, Fisher S, et al: 5-Fluorouracil, cyclophosphamide, and vincristine for adenoid cystic carcinoma of the head and neck. *Cancer* 59:887, 1987.

121. Kaplan MJ, Johns ME, Cantrell RW: Chemotherapy for salivary gland cancer. *Otolaryngol Head Neck Surg* 95:165, 1986.

122. Dryfuss AI, Clark JR, Fallon BG: Cyclophosphamide, doxorubicin, and cisplatin combination chemotherapy for advanced carcinomas of salivary gland origin. *Cancer* 60:2869, 1987.

41

Basic Principles of Radiation Oncology

Kenneth A. Leopold, M.D. and Leonard R. Prosnitz, M.D.

The field of radiation oncology has undergone rapid growth since entering the "supervoltage" era in the early 1960s. The specialty, then referred to as therapeutic radiology, formally separated from radiology in 1974. Because of its increasing involvement with cancer patients, the specialty was formally renamed radiation oncology in 1986.

The previous three decades have brought increasing levels of sophistication in radiobiology, radiophysics, and treatment-related equipment. These factors, combined with expanding clinical experience in the use of radiation, both by itself and combined with other therapeutic modalities, has led the specialty into a prominent position in the care of patients with cancer.

The estimated incidence of cancer in the United States is 1 million new cases (excluding nonmelanoma skin cancers and carcinoma in situ) in 1989 (1). Radiation is used in 50–60% of these patients (2). Because radiation is increasingly being employed earlier in patients' therapy and often with curative intent, and because patients often live longer after being treated with radiation, there are increasing numbers of patients who have undergone treatment with radiation being seen by other specialists. This is especially true of the plastic surgeon, who might be called on to assist in the care of the chronic or delayed soft tissue complications and other possible problems of long-term survivors who have been irradiated for their cancer. This chapter provides an overview of the field of radiation oncology, emphasizing aspects potentially important to the plastic surgeon.

Radiotherapy Equipment

Treatment of tumors with x-rays was first performed only 1 month after the discovery of x-rays by Roentgen in January, 1896 (3). Treatment with radium was used shortly after its discovery by the Curies in 1898 (3). Advances followed slowly in the next several decades; these included more reliable x-ray tubes (Coolidge, 1913), the ionization chamber for output measurement (Szilard, 1914), and the use of fractionated radiation (Regaud, Coutard, Baclesse, the 1920s) (4).

Major and rapid advances in radiotherapy were largely a result of the development of radioactive cobalt (^{60}Co) machines and linear accelerators in the decades following World War II. These machines produced "megavoltage" (or "supervoltage") radiation and yielded greater penetration into tissue and relative skin sparing (see "Radiation Physics" section). High photon output was obtained from this equipment, and this allowed for the placement of energy sources at a much greater distance than was previously possible (80–100 cm from the patient, typically). This further aided delivery of relatively higher radiation doses at depth (see "Radiation Physics" section) as well as allowed for placement of the machine on a gantry that could rotate 360° around the patient. These factors combined to allow relatively good delivery of radiation energy well inside the patient (where tumors are generally located), as well as timely, accurate, and reproducible patient setup and treatment (multifield treatments typically take 10–15 min per patient). Over the years, linear accelerators (linacs) have largely replaced ^{60}Co machines because of their improved delivery of radiation at depth and sharper field edges (i.e., less radiation given to tissues outside of the desired target), radiation safety concerns, and the ability of linacs to produce electrons (see "Radiation Physics" section).

Modern radiation oncology departments have a number of other essential pieces of equipment. The vast majority of patients presently undergo a treatment simulation. The treatment simulator is a diagnostic/fluoroscopic x-ray machine designed with the same geometry as a linear accelerator. This allows for appropriate radiation field placement because diagnostic quality radiographs may be taken to verify field placement. Simulator films are also used as templates for customized radiation blocks that allow field shaping to minimize radiation to normal tissues. Specialized immobilization devices are frequently used to enhance reproducibility of field setup from treatment to treatment.

Most patients undergo computerized treatment planning to determine the best field arrangement in order to deliver a homogeneous dose to the tumor and minimize the normal tissue dose. Newer treatment planning techniques offer the potential for viewing dose distribution in three dimensions and from varying angles.

All radiation oncology departments have or have available to them a variety of radioisotopes useful in "implant" or brachytherapy. This technique has the advantage of concentrating the radiation dose in the tumor to a much greater extent than is possible with external beam therapy (treatment from a linac). In this setting, material emitting radiation is placed on or within a tumor. Commonly used isotopes include cesium-137, iridium-192, gold-198, and iodine-125.

Modern radiation oncology facilities are set up for a variety of clinical situations, including head and neck and gynecological examinations. Fiberoptic instruments and advanced, sophisticated photographic equipment are available.

Radiobiological Principles

The fundamental radiobiological principles that underlie clinical radiation therapy were largely elucidated after basic clinical radiotherapeutic practices were established on an empirical basis. Nevertheless, an understanding of these principles is of considerable importance for both the radiation oncologist and the surgeon. It provides a rational basis on which to select radiotherapy or alternate treatments in particular clinical situations. It enables one to plan combinations of radiation therapy, surgery, and chemotherapy on a scientific basis. Finally, knowledge of radiation biology enables the oncologist to undertake new investigative approaches to improve the current management techniques for carcinoma.

The essence of cancer therapy is to deprive tumor cells of their clonogenicity—that is, their ability to replicate. This can be accomplished by their removal (surgery) or by cellular damage in situ. Radiation deprives cells of their clonogenicity via DNA damage. This comes about as a result of the ionizing effect of high-energy radiation. Interaction of any particular photon or particle of radiation with the material at which it is aimed is an all-or-none phenomenon. If there is an interaction, high-energy radiation (e.g., x-rays) has the ability to displace electrons from their normal orbits. These energetic electrons may interact directly with DNA, or they may interact with nearby molecules (such as water) to create highly reactive free radicals that may subsequently damage DNA. The type and extent of DNA damage is variable, ranging from nucleoside base changes to double-strand chain breaks. The ability of the cell to repair damage is dependent on the type and extent of changes as well as the integrity of repair mechanisms (5).

Attempts to understand the cellular effects of radiation have led investigators to irradiate cells in vitro. A typical radiation cell survival curve is shown in Figure 41.1 (6). These data are derived from exposing cells in tissue culture to single doses of radiation. The logarithm of the fraction of cells that survive irradiation is plotted on the *y*-axis against the dose of radiation, which is plotted linearly on the *x*-axis. The curve consists of two portions: an initial "shoulder," which is thought to represent a dose range in which repair of sublethal injury takes place, and a straight line portion in which a given dose of radiation kills a constant proportion of the cells. The shoulder portion of the curve implies that more than one target must be inactivated within the cell before lethality occurs. The slope of the exponential portion of the curve is $-1/D_0$, where D_0 is that dose of radiation required to reduce the surviving fraction of cells to 37% of its former value. The straight line portion of the curve may be extrapolated back to the *y*-axis, and a certain whole number value (*n*), called the extrapolation number, is obtained.

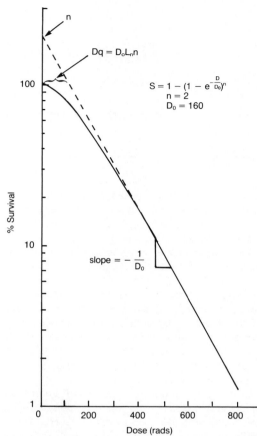

FIGURE 41.1.   Radiation cell survival curve for a single dose of radiation. In the example shown, $D_0 = 160$ rad and $n = 2$. See text for additional explanation.

This quantity is roughly a measure of the ability of the cell to repair radiation damage. A high value for *n*, such as has been seen in malignant melanoma (7), implies a large capacity for repair of radiation damage and provides an explanation for the clinical radioresistance of this tumor.

Data obtained from the construction of radiation cell survival curves for a variety of cells in tissue culture have provided for the first time a precise and meaningful definition of radiosensitivity. For many years, this term was used in a rather loose way to describe simply whether or not a tumor regressed when treated with radiotherapy. (Such a regression response might better be termed "radioresponsiveness.") It provided a very crude measure at best as to whether tumors had been permanently controlled. Radiosensitivity is better defined in terms of the D_0. The great majority of epidermoid and adenocarcinomas have similar D_0 values, as do most normal tissues, although some nonepithelial malignancies such as seminomas or lymphomas are much more sensitive to radiation and have smaller D_0 values. Therefore, other concepts must be explored to explain the variations of response of different tumors to radiation, as well as to explain how one can destroy the tumor cells without destroying the functional integrity of normal tissue within the field of radiation.

A number of clinically relevant conclusions can be made based on a consideration of the cell survival curve. Because cell killing is proportional to the logarithm of the number of cells irradiated, smaller numbers of cells require a lesser dose of radiation. This has led to the so-called shrinking field technique and the concept of subclinical disease, in which doses in the range of 4500–5000 cGy are adequate to control potential microscopic foci of disease, but doses in the neighborhood of 6500–7000 cGy will be required for the control of gross disease (8). Conversely, one can appreciate that a reduction in tumor volume by approximately 90% by some surgical procedure is only a one-log reduction in the number of cells being irradiated and has very little influence on the overall radiation dose necessary for tumor control.

Cell survival curve considerations lend further insight into the meaning of clinical response. The average tumor contains approximately 10^9 cells/cm^3; thus, a tumor containing 10^{11} cells would be a rather large tumor indeed. A reduction by any treatment from 10^{11} to 10^8 cells would constitute a very impressive partial response but would fall far short of the kind of tumor cell kill required for local control. It is generally accepted that tumors containing 10^7 or fewer cells are not clinically detectable; therefore, a "complete response" might involve death of all the tumor cells in question but could also involve a reduction to 10^7 or 10^6 viable cells. Thus, complete response as a measure of tumor cure is a very primitive kind of test, and at the present time it is no substitute for long-term observation.

OXYGEN EFFECT

We have indicated that the inherent radiosensitivity of most tumors and normal tissues, as defined by the D_0 on the radiation cell survival curve, is nearly the same for well-oxygenated tissues. The situation is substantially altered, however, when oxygen in the tissues is lacking. Hypoxic cells in tissue culture, as well as in animal tumors, are 2.5–3.0 times more resistant to the lethal effects of radiation than well-oxygenated cells. The presence of hypoxic cells within human tumors is thought to have a major influence on the effectiveness of radiation therapy (9).

The problem of hypoxic cells has had a major impact on the thinking of radiation oncologists and the entire direction of radiation oncological research. Many major research efforts in the field have been directed toward overcoming this problem. Attempts to overcome the hypoxic cell problem have included the use of hyperbaric oxygen, compounds with electron affinity that selectively sensitize hypoxic cells, or densely ionizing or high linear energy transfer radiation, such as neutrons or *pi* mesons, whose biological effect is not influenced by the lack of oxygen. Also, radiation dose fractionation schedules can be altered in order to facilitate reoxygenation between radiation fractions. Finally, the use of hyperthermia, which is known to sensitize cells to the action of radiation and which is thought to act selectively on hypoxic cells

and tissues, has been tried in an attempt to eliminate the effects of hypoxia (10).

ALTERATIONS IN RADIATION DOSE FRACTIONATION SCHEDULES

The cell survival curve shown in Figure 41.1 is derived from examining the lethal effect of graded single doses of irradiation. If two doses of radiation are given, spaced at least 6 hr apart, a curve of the type shown in Figure 41.2 is obtained. The shoulder portion of the curve is repeated before the curve again becomes exponential. It can readily be seen from an examination of Figure 41.2 that a larger dose of radiation is required to produce the same biological effect if it is given in two increments rather than one. A certain amount of repair of radiation damage has taken place between fractions.

Long before this phenomenon was quantitatively explored by radiation biologists, fractionated radiation was used by clinicians because empirically this seemed to be the best way of delivering a tumoricidal dose without excessive damage to normal tissues. All radiation dose schedules must be described in terms of the total number of rads or grays (1 Gy = 100 rad) delivered, the number of grays per fraction, and the overall treatment time. It is clear that longer treatment times and smaller sized fractions require a greater total dose in grays for the same biological effect. There is no simple formula, however, to relate different fractionation schedules. A variety of different fractionation schedules have been tried empirically; the "traditional" schedule is 2 Gy/day, five fractions per week. The optimal schedule, however, remains unresolved for the great majority of human tumors (6).

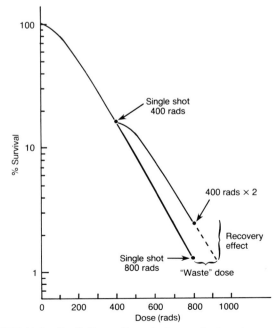

FIGURE 41.2. Radiation cell survival curve for two doses of 400 rad each illustrating repair of radiation damage in the interval between the two treatments.

TUMOR REGRESSION

The rate of growth of a tumor depends on numerous factors, including cell cycle time, the fraction of cells that are actively proliferating (growth fraction), and the rate at which dead cells or their breakdown products are removed from the tumor (cell loss factor) (11). These factors also affect the rate at which a tumor regresses after irradiation. Volume changes in an irradiated tumor eventually reflect the extent of tumor cell kill but may proceed with a very variable rate.

The cellular target of ionizing radiation is believed to be DNA, and the meaningful biological endpoint is the loss of cellular reproductive capabilities. Although the molecular effects of radiation are very rapid, occurring within seconds, the time to cell death is quite variable. Cell death occurs during mitosis (11), and there may be a number of cycles before a faulty division takes place. The time to mitosis depends on cell cycle time and growth fraction. Once the cells are dead, their breakdown products must be removed from the tumor, and this time course can vary considerably. These factors make it difficult to base clinical decisions on the observed rate of the tumor response to irradiation (12, 13). The only reliable guide to determining treatment parameters remains observations of long-term results in large numbers of patients.

The rationale for avoiding treatment decisions for a given patient based largely on the clinical response also applies to decision making based on histopathological response. For the reasons cited above, histopathological response to radiation may be delayed by weeks (and sometimes months), especially if the tissue in question has a long cell cycle time or small growth fraction. Conversely, the absence of microscopic evidence of intact tumor cells in a biopsy specimen does not preclude the presence of intact tumor cells in situ.

Radiation Physics

A few basic concepts in radiation physics must be understood to adequately appreciate radiation therapy. In most situations, high-energy photons (x-rays) are used in radiation treatments. High-energy photons are produced for clinical use in two ways. In the first, electrons are accelerated in linear accelerators and are directed to impinge upon metallic targets. This interaction produces x-ray photons (by "bremsstrahlung" interaction). The photons have a range of energies, the highest corresponding to the incident electrons' energy. By convention, the beam's energy is referred to by this peak energy. Most linear accelerators in clinical use today range in energy from 4 to 20 million electron volts (MeV). High-energy photons have alternatively been obtained from the nuclear decay of ^{60}Co. This decay yields two "gamma ray" photons with energies of 1.17 and 1.33 MeV. Whichever photon production method is used, the photon beams are subsequently filtered (to give a homogeneous dose throughout the field) and collimated (to give a well-defined field).

Photons can interact with matter in a number of ways, depending on the energy of the photons. In the range of energies used for therapy, absorption is largely dependent on the electron density of the irradiated material, as opposed to diagnostic x-rays, in which absorption is dependent on the cube of the atomic number and thus provides the well-recognized contrast patterns. This allows for more homogeneous distribution and less bone absorption, unlike the older "ortho"- or "kilo"-voltage machines. When ionizing photons interact with matter, they give up their energy to electrons. These secondary electrons then interact with surrounding tissue to produce the biological effects of radiation. At low photon energies (i.e., kilovoltage and orthovoltage), these electrons are emitted through 360°, and the skin therefore receives a full dose. With increasing energies (i.e., megavoltage), electrons tend to be emitted in more forward directions. Accordingly, the skin receives relatively less dose with increasing photon energies. This skin-sparing effect is an important advantage of megavoltage radiation over kilo- or orthovoltage.

The probability of high-energy photon interaction with matter decreases with increasing energy. This translates into higher dose at depth (better penetration) for higher energy beams (Fig. 41.3). Greater depth dose is another important advantage of megavoltage radiation.

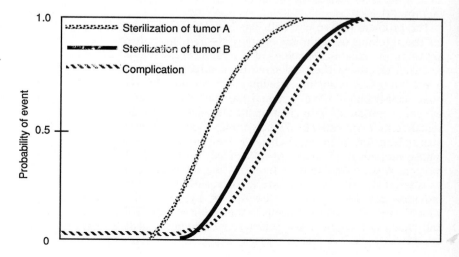

FIGURE 41.3. Probability of tumor sterilization and normal tissue complication versus radiation dose. Tumor A represents a radiosensitive tumor (such as seminoma). Tumor sterilization is likely with a low risk of a complication. Tumor B represents a radiosensitive tumor (such as glioblastom multiforma). Tumor sterilization is unlikely unless a high risk of a complication (e.g., brain necrosis) is accepted.

Sterilization of tumor A
Sterilization of tumor B
Complication

Probability of event

Attempts are generally made to keep doses at various points inside the tumor to within 10% (i.e., <10% inhomogeneity). This can rarely be done with a single radiation field, and hence two or more fields are generally employed. The dose at any point is found by summing the contributions from each field. Today, this is done almost exclusively by computers (computerized dosimetry). Customized field shaping can be performed by inserting individually cut, lead-based blocks in the path of the beam. Wedge-shaped blocks and tissue compensation blocks can also be used to improve the homogeneity of dose.

Electrons are often used to treat skin or superficial lesions. Electrons have the advantage of relatively higher skin and superficial dose and more abrupt decrease in dose at depth than high-energy photons.

The discussion up until now has concerned radiation beams generated at 80–100 cm from the patient. By being at a relatively long distance, these "external" beam treatments are able to deliver greater dose at depth. This is related to the $1/r^2$ phenomenon. The number of rays passing through any region at a distance r_1 from a source is related to the number of rays at distance r_2 by the inverse of the ratio of the squares of the distance $[1/(r_2^2/r_1^2)]$. In other words, the dose declines by the square of the distance from the source. Thus, without taking into account weakening of the beam in tissue by absorption (i.e., attenuation), the beam would be weaker at a depth because of the increased distance from the beam's origin.

Although the $1/r^2$ effect is an obstacle to be overcome in external beam treatment, this effect can be used to advantage in brachytherapy. In brachytherapy, radioactive material is placed on (with plaques or intracavitary devices) or in (with catheters or needles) tumors. If the entire tumor can be adequately covered with such devices, there is a much higher dose of radiation delivered to the tumor than to surrounding tissue, predominantly as a result of the $1/r^2$ effect.

General Clinical Principles

Radiation therapy, like surgery, is in general a locoregional treatment modality. As such, its curative potential for any disease is limited by the incidence of distant metastases. The importance of locoregional control cannot be overemphasized, however (14). The morbidity from locoregional tumor extension in a variety of sites is well known to medical personnel who deal with cancer patients. Cure obviously is impossible without locoregional control, and systemic therapies (e.g., chemotherapy) are least effective at sites of bulk disease (15). Finally, as systemic therapies become more effective and patients live longer, morbidity from locoregional tumor extension will increase.

As with surgery, radiation therapy has its attendant risks and complications. It is incumbent on the radiation oncologist to weigh the potential risks and benefits of irradiation, to devise a treatment plan that yields the best therapeutic ratio, and to know when other modalities are more appropriate than radiotherapy. The radiation oncologist must decide how much tissue volume to treat, what

dose to use, and what physical parameters to use. Tumor site and extent, patterns of spread, and the patient's tolerance of treatment and the possible side effects (as influenced by age and nutritional status, for example) must be considered. The impact of therapy upon psychosocial factors (e.g., sexual function, voice quality) also must be weighed.

As a simplification, the probability of both tumor sterilization and complications rise with dose. The risk of these events occurring for a given dose is generally considered to follow a bell-shaped curve. If the cumulative probability of these events is thus plotted against dose, the result is a sigmoid-shaped curve (Fig. 41.3). It can be seen that, in the steep portion of the curve, small increases in dose can lead to large increases in both tumor control and complications. The optimum situation occurs when the probability of tumor sterilization is high with low doses (such as with small tumors or very radiosensitive tumors) and the probability of unacceptable complication is low with high doses (such as with small irradiated volumes or volumes devoid of vital structures).

A number of different strategies have been developed in attempts to improve the therapeutic gain ratio (TGR). The most important of these is the shrinking field concept popularized in the 1950s by Fletcher and colleagues at the M.D. Anderson Hospital (8). Both in theory and in practice, higher doses of radiation are needed to sterilize regions of greater tumor infestation. Accordingly, regions of clinically detectable disease should receive a higher dose than regions of presumed microscopic or occult disease. Fletcher advocated initial fields encompassing both known disease and suspected regions of extension, followed by smaller fields (boost or "cone-down" fields) taken to higher doses to regions of greater tumor involvement.

Doses prescribed will vary from case to case. In general, for solid tumors in patients treated with curative intent, doses for subclinical disease will range from 40 to 60 Gy (4000–6000 rad) and for gross disease from 60 to 80 Gy, given in "conventional" fractionation (i.e., 2 Gy to fraction, five fractions per week). It can theoretically be shown that, if one part of the tumor receives less dose than the rest, the probability of sterilization rapidly becomes dependent on the dose to this point. Accordingly, the dose is usually prescribed to the portion of tumor that will receive the smallest dose (i.e., tumor minimum dose).

At times, in order to cover all points of tumor involvement, overlying critical structures may receive an unacceptably high dose. This dilemma can often be rectified by the use of angled or multiple fields. Such fields effectively lower the dose to any nontarget tissues.

HYPERFRACTIONATION

Another method of improving TGR is the use of smaller doses per fraction to higher total doses (hyperfractionation). This exploits the radiobiological differences between tissues that react rapidly and those that respond over long periods following radiation (16). Acutely reacting tissues have steeper cell survival shoulders than tissues that respond more slowly to radiation. By giving smaller doses per fraction, therefore, slowly responding tissues will have a relatively greater ability to repair sublethal damage. Most tumors are rapidly dividing, while tissues involved with long-term complications (e.g., small blood vessels, soft tissue) are slowly responding. In order to avoid loss of treatment efficacy secondary to tumor repopulation during a course of therapy, multiple (usually two) doses per day are often given when hyperfractionated schemes are used (16).

HYPOXIC CELL SENSITIZERS

A number of compounds with electron affinity have been developed that appear to mimic the effect of oxygen and therefore to sensitize poorly oxygenated cells to irradiation. They do so by interacting with the radiation-damaged molecules containing free electrons to fix these molecules in a damaged chemical state. These drugs tend to be more slowly excreted in hypoxic regions as compared to well oxygenated regions; therefore, they accumulate more readily in areas of limited vascular permeability. Misonidazole is the most widely studied of this class of compounds. Preliminary results in brain tumors and head and neck cancers have been mildly encouraging, but the usefulness of this drug has been limited to date by the neurotoxicity observed at the high drug concentrations required for radiosensitization. Nevertheless, investigations are continuing in an attempt to develop effective analogs that will be less toxic (17).

HIGH LINEAR ENERGY TRANSFER RADIATION

High linear energy transfer (LET) radiation beams include neutrons, *pi* mesons, and a variety of other heavy particles, all of which are densely ionizing. This type of radiation alters the shape of the survival curve; the shoulder region is either reduced or absent, presumably because densely ionizing beams result in DNA damage that cannot be repaired. Because of the high density of the damage produced by this type of radiation, there is relatively little influence of oxygen on the process. This has been the impetus for the development of high LET radiation sources for use in clinical radiotherapy. To date, such efforts have been hampered by technical complexity and the expense of developing equipment. The most commonly studied type is the neutron radiation beam. There is as yet limited clinical evidence, and trials in the United States and elsewhere in this important area continue (18).

Multimodality Therapy

In many situations, tumors are so extensive that attempts at cure with one treatment modality have a very low likelihood of success. However, by combining modalities, each with their own toxicities, greater probability of tumor control can be achieved with lower probability of prohibitive toxicity. The added "cost" of such

regimens is generally more acute toxicity or additional types of non–life-threatening morbidities. For instance, attempted cure of an advanced head and neck cancer can be undertaken with either radiation or surgery alone, resulting in a high probability of radionecrosis or functional deficit, respectively. Alternatively, a higher probability of tumor control might be obtainable using both approaches together. In this case, the patient will be left with some xerostomia and radiation fibrosis, and some functional impairment from resection.

SURGERY AND RADIATION THERAPY

Large tumors often necessitate unacceptably high doses of radiation or unacceptably extensive surgery for reasonable chances of locoregional control. In this setting, resection may be used for removal of gross disease, followed by radiation for treatment of microscopic extension. In general, however, debulking surgery that does not remove all gross tumor is not advisable because it has little impact on the dose of radiation required. Combination radiation and surgery is widely accepted in numerous situations, including head and neck cancers, breast cancer, rectal cancer, gynecological cancers, and soft tissue sarcomas.

Proponents exist for both pre- and postoperative radiation. Preoperative radiation offers the advantage of undisturbed vasculature (presumably leading to less hypoxia in regions of microscopic extension), initial treatment of all presumed sites of disease, treatment of smaller volumes (because postoperatively all surgically manipulated tissue is at risk for tumor dissemination), and theoretically decreased risk of intraoperative tumor seeding of viable cells. The advantages of postoperative treatment include a lower risk of healing problems, avoiding inadequate resection secondary to tumor regression, and unnecessary radiation in patients with very early or disseminated disease detected at the time of surgery.

CHEMOTHERAPY AND RADIATION THERAPY

Although surgery and radiotherapy are both local treatments, the use of chemotherapy and radiotherapy in combination may convey systemic as well as local benefits. Frequently, all three modalities may be used in combination. Two general approaches to the interdigitation of chemotherapy and radiation therapy have been used. One is sequential treatment, which allows for full doses of each modality. The hope is that the additive effects will render the patient disease free. The negative aspects to this approach are the possibility that cells that are resistant to chemotherapy might repopulate the tumor before radiation is given and that the patient will experience full long-term toxicities. Alternatively, simultaneous chemotherapy and radiation can be used. Here, repopulation is less of an issue, and the two modalities might act synergistically within the irradiated volume. Also, because the doses needed of each modality might be less, long-term toxicities might be lower. The negative aspects of concurrent therapy are increased acute morbidity and perhaps lower tolerable doses of chemotherapy with accompanying lesser impact on occult distant disease (11).

HYPERTHERMIA AND RADIATION THERAPY

Heat has been shown to be a potent cytotoxic agent, especially when combined with radiation (19). Radiation kill will be increased by several orders of magnitude when combined with tumor temperatures of at least 42.5°C for around 1 hr. The combination of radiation and heat is theoretically appealing because heat is most effective in tumor populations in which radiation is least effective (i.e., in hypoxic regions) (19). Heat is also more effective against cells in the synthesis phase of the cell cycle, whereas radiation is most effective on cells in mitosis. Furthermore, studies have shown that heat can potentiate radiation damage, probably by interfering with repair mechanisms. Most tumors are less able to dissipate heat than normal tissues because of abnormal tumor vasculature (most notably the absence of arterioles, which can vasodilate); this allows for the preferential heating of tumors. The actual heating of human tumors in situ, particularly those at a distance from the body surface, remains a formidable problem. Equipment is still very much in the developmental stage. Optimal thermal dose remains to be defined. This is an area of extensive research activity at present (19).

Radiation Complications

Radiation complications are generally divided into three temporal categories: acute, subacute, and chronic. In large part, this is a function of the cellular turnover rate of a given tissue or organ because radiation damage generally is not expressed until cells attempt to replicate. Tissues falling into the acutely reacting category include mucosa, hematopoietic lines, and germ cells. Late-reacting tissues include nerves, muscle, and endothelium.

Radiation-induced skin changes (20) vary with respect to time as a function of the turnover rates of the various skin tissues. In general, the latency period (time from completion of irradiation to effect) and degree of changes are dose/fraction dependent. With conventionally fractionated, moderate-dose radiation, the first reaction is erythema of the skin surface, followed by flaking or peeling (dry desquamation). These changes are consequences of radiation effects on the epithelial stem cells. With higher doses to the skin, enough basal cells might be killed to cause denudation (moist desquamation). These acute reactions generally begin 10–20 days after initiation of therapy and spontaneously heal 10–20 days after completion.

With modern supervoltage radiotherapy, late skin changes are unusual unless a deliberate effort is made to treat the skin or the skin receives high doses from "tangential" beams. Skin at high risk for tumor involvement includes areas involved with tumor, surgical scars at risk for seeding, and areas of possible dermal lymphatic involvement (as in skin over the chest wall following mastectomy in patients with multiple nodal involvement or lymphatic vessel involvement). When the skin receives high radiation doses, epidermal atrophy and telangiectasias (from loss of small blood vessels in the dermis), alopecia (hair follicle loss), dryness (sebaceous and sweat gland loss), and hypopigmentation (melanocyte loss) occur. Wounds heal poorly, and infections occur more readily and are harder to control secondary to poorer vasculature. These changes generally are first noticeable 6–12 months after treatment and are progressive with time.

Radiation fibrosis of the subcutaneous layer follows a similar temporal pattern. This is seen to some degree in practically all irradiated patients.

Surgery Following Radiation Therapy

Surgical procedures must be performed with caution in previously irradiated tissue (21). Tissues will be harder to manipulate secondary to subcutaneous fibrosis. Wound healing and infectious complications will be more prevalent because of depletion of the microvasculature (endarteritis). Not infrequently, myocutaneous or pedicle grafts are required to adequately cover these regions.

In patients who have undergone surgical procedures, attempts should be made to avoid radiation to the wound for at least 6–10 days. During this proliferative stage of healing, the wound has a large number of macrophages and replicating fibroblasts that are quite sensitive to radiation. Loss of these elements will delay healing and, together with the loss of polymorphonuclear leukocytes, will predispose to infection (22). When immediate tumor regression is required to alleviate morbid or life-threatening situations (e.g., tracheal compression or spinal cord compression), however, radiation therapy should be begun immediately, and appropriate wound care should be given as needed.

Specific Disease Sites

HEAD AND NECK CANCER

Radiation or surgery alone is sufficient for many very early tumors without nodal involvement. As a general rule, surgery alone should not be used in large tumors (T4 and many T3s) (23), in any size tumor showing aggressive tendencies (high grade, lymphatic and/or blood vessel invasion) (24), or in situations in which more than one lymph node is involved with cancer or there is extracapsular extension of disease (23, 25).

Heroic efforts using surgical procedures that are excessively functionally debilitating in patients with extensive cancers are usually rewarded with tumor recurrence in addition to debilitating surgical defects (23). Such patients are almost invariably better treated primarily with radiation, possibly with concurrent chemotherapy and/or hyperfractionation.

BREAST CANCER

Numerous studies, both prospective and retrospective, support the contention that locoregional control and overall cure of breast cancer with excisional biopsy and radiation are at least as good as with mastectomy (modified radical or radical) (26, 27). Few women with early-stage (I-II) breast cancer should be advised to undergo mastectomy because it is "better cancer treatment," "safer," or "more likely to get rid of the cancer." Additionally, many effective ways exist to interdigitate radiation with chemotherapy (28), and this should not be used as an argument against excisional biopsy and radiation. It is also worth noting that patients with multiple nodal involvement, extensive blood vessel and/or lymphatic vessel involvement, or involvement of the pectoral fascia should generally be treated with a course of postmastectomy radiation requiring nearly the same time commitment (approximately 6 weeks) as primary radiation therapy (29).

With reasonable radiation techniques, breast cosmesis is largely dependent on the operative procedure performed. Although negative tumor margins should be sought, the removal of large portions of the breast (including quadrantectomies) is frowned on. Most radiation oncologists will boost doses to the tumor bed to a level that should be sufficient to sterilize microscopic disease. The placement of radiopaque clips in the tumor bed will facilitate such boost treatments. Curvilinear incisions directly over the lesion generally lead to best results. Axillary lymph node dissections should be performed through a separate incision (28).

The entire breast is included in the first course of radiation in order to treat occult separate foci of disease. The dose to the breast is generally 45–50 Gy, often with a boost dose to the tumor bed to bring the total dose to 60–64 Gy (28). Lymph node–bearing regions are variably treated, depending on the clinical situation. After axillary lymph node dissection, consideration should be given to irradiating levels I and II only if numerous involved nodes are found or extracapsular extension is noted (28).

SKIN CANCERS

Nonmelanoma skin cancers can usually be effectively treated with a number of methods, including simple excision or cryosurgery. The use of the Mohs technique also has a strong theoretical and clinical basis. Radiation therapy is another very effective treatment modality for basal cell and squamous cell carcinomas of the skin. It should be strongly considered in areas where resection would entail extensive reconstruction, such as the nose, periorbital regions, and ears. Similar arguments pertain to squamous cell carcinomas of the lip when lesions are over 1.5–2.0 cm or involve a commissure. Should lesions involve cartilage, however, surgery is usually the preferred treatment because radionecrosis of the cartilage is a distinct possibility. Using appropriately fractionated treatment, long-term cosmesis is excellent, and local control is over 90% (30, 31).

References

1. *American Cancer Society Facts and Figures*. New York, American Cancer Society, 1989.
2. *Radiation Oncology in Integrated Cancer Management*. Report of the Inter-Society Council for Radiation Oncology, 1986.
3. Glasser O: *Wilhelm Conrad Roentgen and the Early History of the Roentgen Ray*. London, John Bale, Sons, & Danielsson, Ltd, 1933.
4. Coutard H: Principles of x-ray therapy of malignant disease. *Lancet* 2:1, 1934.
5. Stewart FA: Modification of normal tissue response to radiotherapy and chemotherapy. *Int J Radiat Oncol Biol Phys* 16:1195, 1989.
6. Peschel RE, Fischer JJ: Optimization of the time dose relationship. *Semin Oncol* 8:38, 1981.
7. Barranco SC, Romsdahl MM, Humphrey RM: The radiation response of human malignant melanoma cells grown in vitro. *Cancer Res* 31:830, 1971.
8. Fletcher GH: The evolution of the basic concepts underlying the practice of radiotherapy from 1949–1977. *Radiology* 127:3, 1978.
9. Andrews JR: *The Radiobiology of Human Cancer Radiotherapy*, ed 2. Baltimore, University Park Press, 1978.
10. Guichard M: Chemical manipulations of tissue oxygenation for therapeutic benefit. *Int J Radiat Oncol Biol Phys* 16:1125, 1989.
11. Suit HD: Radiation biology: The conceptual and practical impact on radiation therapy. *Radiat Res* 94:10, 1983.
12. Suit HD, Walker AM: Assessment of the response of tumors to radiation: Clinical and experimental studies. *Br J Cancer* 41(Suppl 4):1, 1980.
13. Dische S, Bennett MH, Saunders MI, et al: Tumor regression as a guide to prognosis: A clinical study. *Br J Radiol* 53:454, 1980.
14. Suit HD, Westgate SJ: Impact of local control on survival. *Int J Radiat Oncol Biol Phys* 12:453, 1986.
15. DeVita VT Jr: Principles of chemotherapy. In DeVita VT Jr, Hellman S, Rosenberg SA (eds): *Principles and Practice of Oncology*. Philadelphia, JB Lippincott Co, 1989.
16. Withers HR, Taylor LMJ, Maciejewski B: The hazard of accelerated tumor clonogen repopulation during radiotherapy. *Acta Oncol* 27:131, 1988.
17. Coleman N, Bump EA, Kramer RA: Chemical modifiers of cancer treatment. *J Clin Oncol* 6:709, 1988.
18. Zink S, Antoine J, Mahoney FJ: Fast neutron trials in the United States. *Am J Clin Oncol* 12:277, 1989.
19. Oleson JR, Calderwood SK, Coughlin CT, et al: Biological and clinical aspects of hyperthermia in cancer therapy. *Am J Clin Oncol* 11:368, 1988.
20. Hall EJ: Dose-response relationships for normal tissues. In *Radiobiology for the Radiobiologist*, ed 3. Philadelphia, JB Lippincott Co, 1989.
21. Robinson DW: The hazards of surgery in irradiated tissue. *Ann Plastic Surg* 11:74, 1983.
22. Shamberger R: Effect of chemotherapy and radiotherapy on wound healing: Experimental studies. *Recent Results Cancer Res* 98:17, 1985.
23. Million RM, Cassisi NJ: General principles for treatment of cancers in the head and neck: Combining surgery and radiation therapy. In *Management of Head and Neck Cancer: A Multidisciplinary Approach*. Philadelphia, JB Lippincott Co, 1984.
24. Soo K-C, Carter R, Berr L, O'Brien C, Bliss J, Shaw H: Prognostic implications of perineural spread in squamous carcinomas of the head and neck. *Laryngoscope* 96:1145, 1986.
25. Carter R, Bliss J, Soo K-C, O'Brien C: Radical neck dissections for squamous cell carcinomas: Pathological findings and their clinical implications with particular reference to transcapsular spread. *Int J Radiat Oncol Biol Phys* 13:825, 1987.

26. Fisher B, Redmond C, Poisson R, et al: Eight-year results of a randomized clinical trial comparing total mastectomy and lumpectomy with or without irradiation in the treatment of breast cancer. *N Engl J Med* 320:822, 1989.
27. Kurtz J, Amalric R, Brandone H, et al: Local recurrence after breast-conserving surgery and radiotherapy: Frequency, time course, and prognosis. *Cancer* 63:1912, 1989.
28. Recht A, Connolly JL, Schnitt SJ, et al: Conservative surgery and radiation therapy for early breast cancer: Results, controversies and unsolved problems. *Semin Oncol* 13:434, 1986.

29. Edland RW: Presidential address: Does adjuvant radiotherapy have a role in the postmastectomy management of patients with operable breast cancer—revisited. *Int J Radiat Oncol Biol Phys* 15:519, 1988.
30. Million RM, Cassisi NJ: Oral cavity. In *Management of Head and Neck Cancer: A Multidisciplinary Approach*. Philadelphia, JB Lippincott Co, 1984.
31. Brady LW, Binnick SA, Fitzpatrick PJ: Skin cancer. In Perez CA, Brady LW (eds): *Principles and Practice of Radiation Oncology*. Philadelphia, JB Lippincott Co, 1987.

42

Solid and Cystic Tumors of the Jaw

Nicholas G. Georgiade, D.D.S., M.D., F.A.C.S., Gregory S. Georgiade, M.D., F.A.C.S., and Thomas Benedict Harter, M.D.

A diversity of tumors of the mandible and maxilla are presented in this chapter from a broad frame of reference. They include cystic, inflammatory, developmental, and posttraumatic masses that should be considered in any differential diagnosis. Radiological evaluation encompasses tumor tissues that are radiopaque, radiolucent, and/or combinations of varying densities. The final diagnosis of a presenting mass will most often require histological interpretation. Characteristically, benign cysts and tumors expand the bone, but they do not invade the cortex.

Cysts

CYSTS OF ODONTOGENIC ORIGIN

Cysts of the mandible and maxilla of odontogenic origin arise from an alteration of the enamel organ and include those discussed below.

Dentigerous

The dentigerous cyst is the second most frequently occurring odontogenic cyst and is seen surrounding the crown of an unerupted tooth (Fig. 42.1). It is thought to arise as a result of reduction in the enamel-forming epithelium after the crown is completely formed. Typically, the cyst will have an epithelial lining and may vary from 2 cm in diameter to extensive expansion of the jaw. Dentigerous cysts are not usually painful in the absence of infection and rarely will expand so rapidly that discomfort results from pressure on a sensory nerve. The posterior area of the mandible is the most common site of dentigerous cysts, and the third molar is the tooth most frequently involved. Signs and symptoms include delayed eruption of a tooth, swelling, and asymmetry. Smaller cysts may be managed successfully with enucleation and primary closure. When the dentigerous cyst is large, treatment alternatives (e.g., decompression, marsupialization) may be used to advantage, particularly in tooth-bearing areas of children when the tooth is not impacted and is ready to erupt once it is relieved of the cyst. These pericoronal lesions may recur as a cyst or as an ameloblastoma.

Radicular

The radicular cyst occurs at the apex of a nonvital tooth (Fig. 42.2). It is associated with degeneration of the pulp and may result in low-grade apical infection, appearing as a well-circumscribed periapical radiolucency. Because this process is thought to initiate the growth of the epithelial component, radicular cysts may be classified as inflammatory. These cysts may also be referred to as apical, periodontal, radiculodental, and/or root cysts. Like other odontogenic cysts, this variant may have cholesterol crystals in the liquid aspirant. Management of small periapical cysts is usually conservative, with nonsurgical root canal therapy. Radicular cysts with radiolucencies over 2 cm in diameter may indicate the need for apical curettage and more extensive root resection. In cases in which restoration of dentition is not facilitated, extraction of the offending tooth may be the alternative of choice.

Follicular (Primordial)

A follicular cyst is a relatively rare type of odontogenic cyst that develops before calcified enamel or dentine is formed (Fig. 42.3). It is found in place of a tooth and is characterized by the absence of any dentition within the cyst. Such cysts usually occur as an abnormal formation of the enamel organ and present as a well-circumscribed, radiolucent area with a multilocular appearance. On microscopic examination, about one half have proven to be filled with keratin, resulting in a radiolucent, hazy appearance. Primordial cysts are found most frequently between the ages of 10 and 30 years, and the mandibular molar region represents the most common site of development. Management is similar to that of other odontogenic cysts, although the high rate of recurrence of follicular cysts requires more vigorous curettement and postsurgical follow-up with radiographs to ensure resolution.

FIGURE 42.1. Dentigerous cyst. Note the presence of a tooth partially developed in the large cystic cavity of the mandible body and ramus. The smooth walls are characteristic of this slowly expanding cyst.

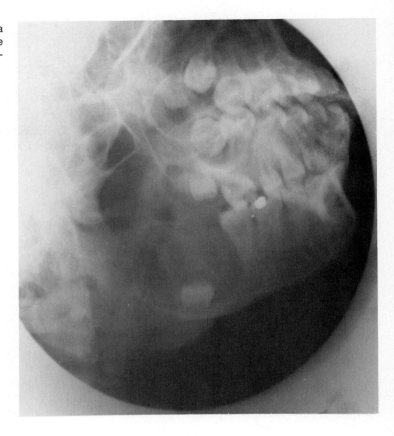

FIGURE 42.2. Radicular cyst at the apex of the central incisor tooth. Note the thickened periodontal membrane and irregular walls of this low-grade inflammatory cyst.

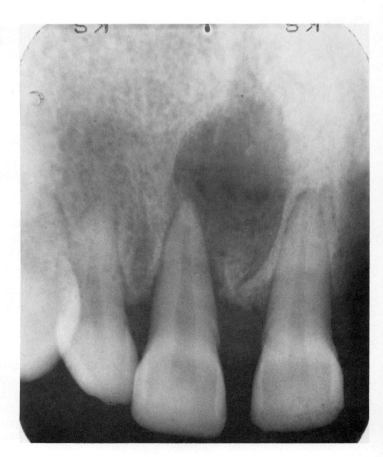

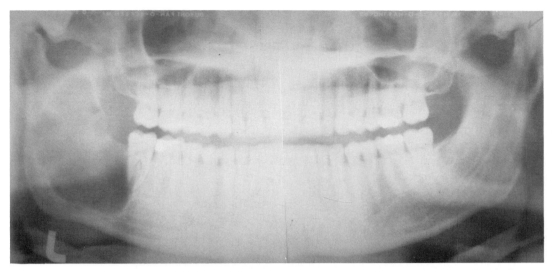

FIGURE 42.3. Follicular (primordial) cyst is characterized by absence of embedded dentition; it is otherwise similar to a dentigerous cyst on the radiograph.

Ameloblastic Fibroma (Soft Mixed Odontoma)

In ameloblastic fibromas, the radiolucent area on the radiograph is seen to be encapsulated and well defined and may be unilocular or multilocular (Fig. 42.4). This cystic mass is related to an abnormality of the dental follicle. It contains both odontogenic and ameloblastic epithelium in dental connective tissue that is primitive and papilla-like. The ameloblastic fibroma is usually found during the erupting stage of the dentition and may spread the roots of adjacent teeth. A majority occur in the posterior mandible, although either jaw may be affected. It is most often seen in individuals under 20 years of age. The incidence is highest in the premolar-molar region, and expansion is usually slow. Treatment is conservative enucleation, and few recurrences are observed because

the connective tissue capsule is not usually invaded by ameloblastic cells.

CYSTS OF NONODONTOGENIC ORIGIN

Cysts of nonodontogenic origin of the mandible and maxilla include globulomaxillary cysts and median (naso-) palatine cysts.

Globulomaxillary

The globulomaxillary cyst is a fissural cyst arising at the junction of the globular portion of the medial nasal process and the maxillary process, usually between the maxillary lateral incisor and the canine tooth, with no

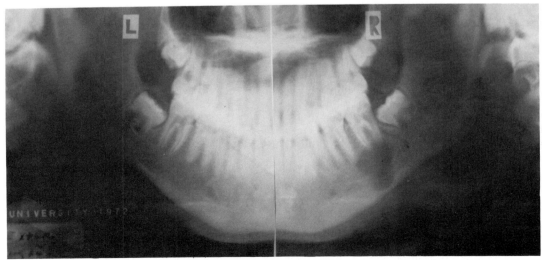

FIGURE 42.4. Ameloblastic fibroma (soft mixed odontoma) appears as an irregular radiolucent area composed of solid substance and originates from both epithelial and mesenchymal tissue. (This expanding cyst was diagnosed in a young child.)

FIGURE 42.5. A globulomaxillary cyst in its typical location between the lateral and canine tooth. Note the marked divergence of the root apices.

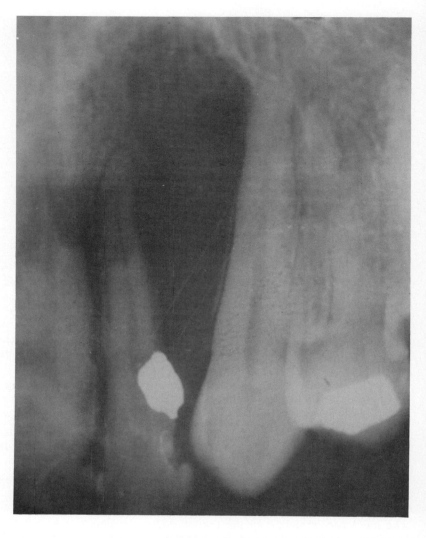

loss of pulp vitality (Fig. 42.5). On the radiograph, it appears as a well-defined radiolucency between the roots and is shaped like an inverted tear. The amber-colored fluid on aspiration is a useful sign in differential diagnosis. It is probable that such cysts form as a result of entrapment of epithelial remnants in the region of the incisive suture; however, the origin of the epithelial nests is yet a matter of dispute. Globulomaxillary cysts are often asymptomatic until they become enlarged or expand, at which time complaints of swelling and pain may be reported. The latter are usually indicative of secondary infection. Surgical excision is the treatment modality, and care must be taken not to devitalize the adjacent teeth during the procedure. Radiographic follow-up is important to assure that the defect has resolved and there is no recurrence.

Median (Naso-) Palatine

The median cyst is formed as a result of "trapping" of tissue during fusion of the palatine process with the pre-maxilla and is an uncommon bony cyst (Fig. 42.6). The type of epithelium found in the cyst will vary depending on its location. Cysts in the incisive canal area contain stratified squamous epithelium, whereas the posteriorly located cysts have cuboidal or respiratory epithelium. With increasing cyst size, patients may report a painless bulging in the roof of the mouth, and on inspection, the mucosa may appear more glossy than usual. Unilocular radiolucency is seen in the midline of the palate. After surgical excision (with a mucoperiosteal flap raised from the anterior to ensure good access and permit total removal), clinical and radiographic follow-up is essential.

NONEPITHELIAL CYSTS

Aneurysmal Bone Cyst

An aneurysmal bone cyst is characterized by numerous capillaries intermixed with prominent vascular spaces and the presence of multinucleated giant cells. It is sometimes referred to as a false cyst because it does not have an epithelial lining. In most instances, it expands the cortical plates but does not destroy them. Radiographs occasionally will reveal an irregular area of destruction of the cortical plate of the mandible and "scalloping." The histological picture of the tissue reveals a cellular, fibrous

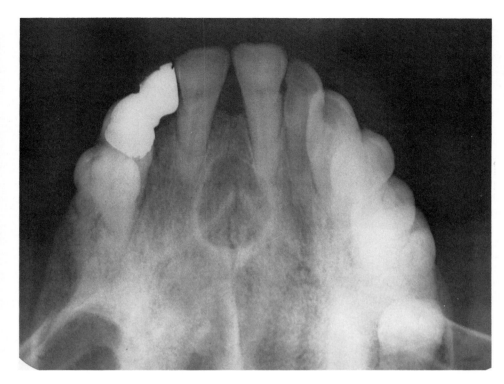

FIGURE 42.6. Nasopalatine cyst. An incisive canal lesion is shown in the characteristic palatal mid-line area. Typically, these cysts do not increase remarkably; note the well-circumscribed cortical prominence of the cyst wall.

pattern. Cysts of this variety are slow-growing and affect the mandible considerably more often than the maxilla. These entities usually develop in young people under the age of 20 years. Aneurysmal bone cysts may be somewhat tender, and teeth may be displaced or missing (Fig. 42.7). On inspection, the cyst is reddish-brown in color owing to its rich blood supply, and resembles a sponge. Management consists of aspiration to avoid the unexpected and dangerous entrance into a hemangioma or arteriovenous shunt. Treatment is then by surgical curettement; hemorrhage is moderate and easily arrested. The recurrence of an aneurysmal bone cyst is rare.

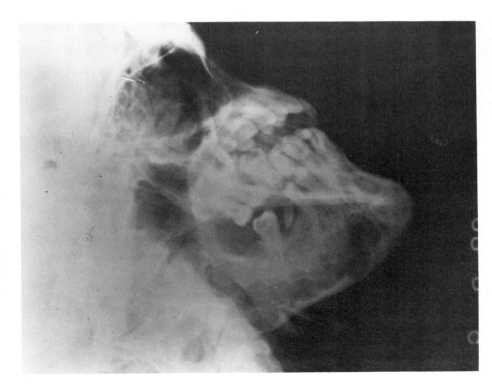

FIGURE 42.7. An aneurysmal bone cyst (nonepithelial) simulates a developmental cyst but displays a sparse connective tissue lining (rather than an epithelial one). It is seen as a solid area of radiolucency with an irregular outline of the cyst wall.

TRAUMATIC BONE CYST

In cases of traumatic bone cyst, the "cystic" area in the mandible results from a traumatic episode and is devoid of an epithelial lining, although it usually will have a thin area of connective tissue (Fig. 42.8). It is often found unexpectedly on routine radiographs and appears round to oval with a scalloped superior margin produced by its molding around the roots of mandibular premolars or molars. As with cementoma, the tooth pulp is usually vital. The maxilla is seldom involved, and traumatic bone cyst is uncommon in those over the age of 25 years. Infrequently, the jaw will reveal regional expansion, and typically, there is no aspirant. Management includes surgical exploration to ensure a correct diagnosis (radiographic imaging and the usual clinical features cannot be relied upon alone). Subsequent enucleation and curettage, which produce hemorrhage into the cavity, will typically provide regression and obliteration by bone. During the healing period, close radiographic observation is recommended.

Tumors

TUMORS OF ODONTOGENIC ORIGIN

Tumors of the jaw having to do with the origin and formation of the teeth include those discussed below.

Dentinoma

This is an aberrant formation of dentine and connective tissue in association with an unerupted tooth. On the ra- diograph, it is seen as an irregular, opaque mass attached to the crown of an unerupted tooth.

Complex, Compound, and Mixed Odontoma

Complex Odontoma

A complex odontomas is composed of aberrant tissue of all the dental elements. On the radiograph, there is an irregular, opaque mass usually in close proximity to a mandibular molar or premolar tooth. The calcified dental tissues have no morphological similarity even to rudimentary teeth.

Compound Odontoma

A compound odontoma develops independently of a tooth follicle but contains normal enamel, dentine, and cementum relationships (i.e., normal composition of a tooth-like structure). It is observed more frequently than the complex odontoma. As a congregation of misshapen small teeth, the compound odontoma is easily recognized on radiographs as a radiopaque, irregular formation with varying numbers of small conical teeth present (Fig. 42.9). The maxilla is the most common site of this odontoma (although it may occur in the mandible), with a predilection for the incisor-canine region.

Mixed Odontoma

Some tumors are a combination of both types discussed above. The mixed odontoma is constituted of calcified masses of dental tissue in random arrangement as well as multiple tooth-like structures.

FIGURE 42.8. A traumatic bone cyst is characterized by the absence of epithelial tissue, a scalloped superior margin molding around the roots of the premolars and molars, and regional expansion of the jaw (*R*).

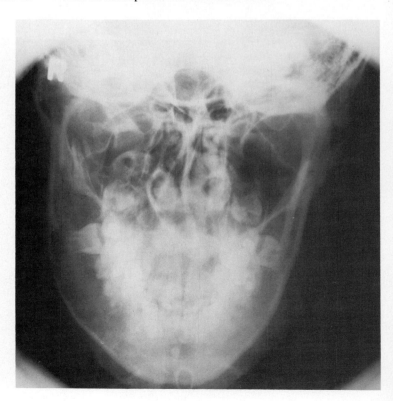

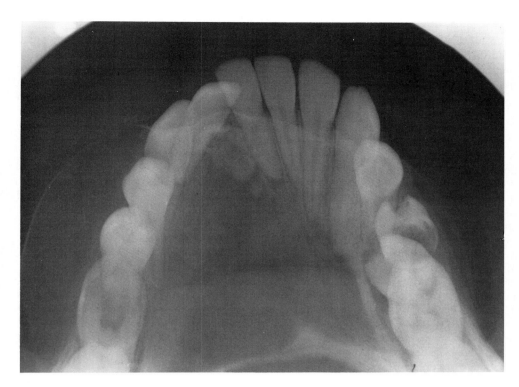

FIGURE 42.9. Compound odontoma is characterized by abnormal tissue of the dental element and usually appears in the canine area.

Cementoma

The cementoma has its origin from the periodontal ligament of an erupted tooth. It undergoes a transformation from an initial appearance of replacing the medullary bone to that of a fibrous matrix, resembling an ossifying fibroma. This tumor occurs as a continuation of the peri-odontal membrane, usually of a mandibular premolar or molar tooth. The area is gradually replaced with scattered spicules of bone, and in the mature phase, the entire original area of radiolucency will become calcified and appear as a well-defined, radiopaque lesion with fibrous tissue at the periphery (Fig. 42.10). The transformation requires at least 6 years. During this entire process, the involved

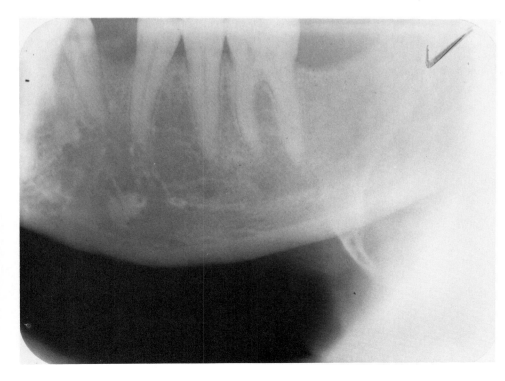

FIGURE 42.10. Cementoma presents with a characteristic area of calcification shown surrounded by an irregular area of radiolucency.

tooth or teeth remain vital, and no resorption of tooth apices occurs, as opposed to the tooth with a radicular cyst or granuloma. A biopsy is performed to establish the diagnosis, followed by excision and curettement. Benign fibroosseous lesions originating in a periodontal ligament tend not to recur.

Ameloblastoma

The ameloblastoma originates from ectodermal epithelium with differentiation into ameloblasts, the enamel-forming cells. It may develop from any of the epithelial elements, such as dentigerous cysts, enamel organ, or periodontal membranes. The picture will vary on the radiograph; it may closely resemble a dentigerous cyst, or it may present as a multilocular cyst with a bubble-like or honeycomb appearance. The predominant site is the posterior mandible. Destruction of the cortex and root apices is a usual finding in larger cystic masses. Ameloblastomas have their onset in adulthood, usually between the ages of 20 and 50 years.

Because of the propensity of ameloblastomas to recur, fairly radical surgical management may be chosen, followed by regular reexamination. However, treatment modalities may range from conservative incision to wide block resection and bone graft. The latter approach has been most effective in precluding recurrence.

Microscopically, a true ameloblastoma may be one of several histological types. The *acanthomatous* histological type is more aggressive, and metastases have been seen in our series of patients with this cytological pattern (Fig. 42.11). The acanthomatous histological picture is characteristic of squamous metaplasia with islands of keratinizing squamous epithelium. The most common histological finding is the *follicular* ameloblastoma, which has the typical tall, columnar, deep-staining cells (the ameloblasts) that resemble stellate reticulum of the enamel organ (Fig. 42.12). The *plexiform* type of ameloblastoma will have irregular strands of epithelial cells interspaced with ameloblastoma cells (Fig. 42.13).

The *ameloblastic fibroma* may mimic the ameloblastoma, and care must be taken to differentiate this asymptomatic, slowly expanding benign tumor. Histologically, it is characterized by proliferation of epithelial cells and mesenchymal elements with cords and islands of epithelial cells. This is a tumor of the young and responds well to conservative currettage (Fig. 42.14).

TUMORS OF NONODONTOGENIC ORIGIN

Nonodontogenic tumors of the mandible and maxilla encompass a large variety of benign and malignant lesions. This section presents those tumors most likely to be seen; however, many are not covered because of their infrequent occurrence.

Bony Exostoses

The most common of the benign tumors are the bony exostoses usually found in the palate (torus platinus), in the mandible (torus mandibularis), or on the buccal surfaces of either mandibular or maxillary dentition. They are thought to be hereditary in origin. Bony exostoses are slow-growing, painless, bony protrusions and cause me-

FIGURE 42.11. Mixed acanthoma and follicular ameloblastoma. Note irregular resorption of the mandible with expansion and destruction of the lingual and buccal cortical plates.

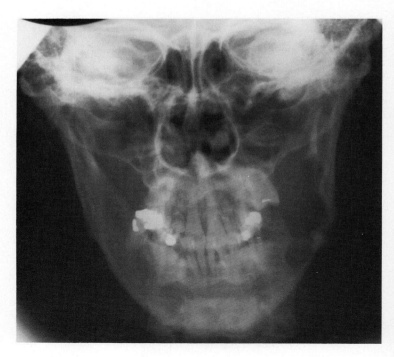

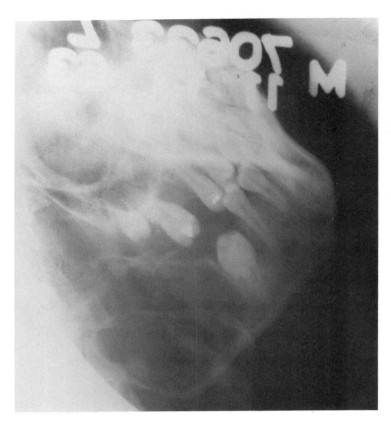

FIGURE 42.12. Cystic ameloblastoma (follicular) revealed as a large multilocular cystic area of the mandible.

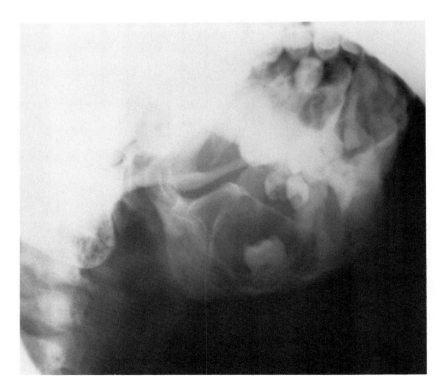

FIGURE 42.13. Cystic ameloblastoma (plexiform). It is difficult to differentiate between this and a dentigerous cyst, as is evident in this radiographic image.

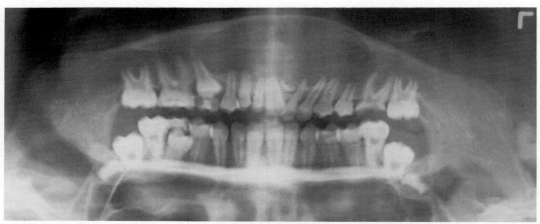

FIGURE 42.14. Ameloblastic fibroma. A large, soft, radiolucent mass is shown in a 9-year-old child; the regular outline of this expanded mass extends from a mandibular molar to the opposite side.

chanical and oral problems because of their progressive enlargement. Treatment is surgical removal.

Osteomas

These bony tumors are found in the mandible, the maxilla, or other facial bones. They are derived from osteoblastic activity and may be single or multiple. On the radiograph, they characteristically appear as irregular, very radiopaque masses (Figs. 42.15 and 42.16). Multiple osteomas, but no pigmented macules, occur in Gardner's syndrome, which is a familial condition. This syndrome is manifested by multiple osteomas and by the presence of multiple polyps in the colon, epidermoid cysts, and desmoid tumors (1, 2).

Osteoid Osteoma

The osteoid osteoma is a small mass occurring in the mandible or maxilla that is characterized by its often painful presence. Radiographically, it is seen as a circumscribed, radiopaque area surrounded by an irregular area of decreased density. Histologically, this represents a dense area of osteoid tissue and new bone surrounded by a well-vascularized area of osteogenic connective tissue (3).

FIGURE 42.15. Osteomas are characterized by the presence of very dense bone with extensive radiopaque appearance.

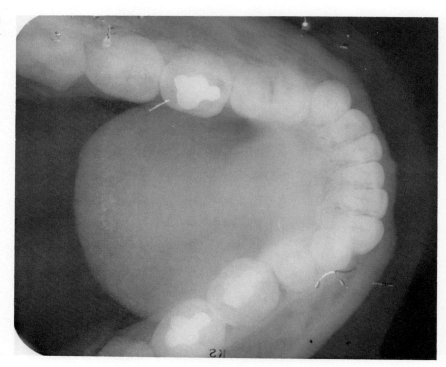

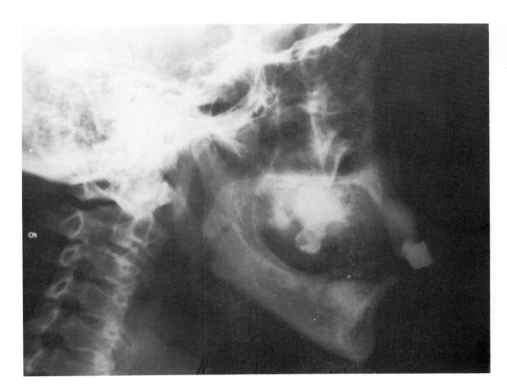

FIGURE 42.16. Condensing osteitis. The lesion shown is the result of chronic periapical infection.

Giant Cell Reparative Granuloma

Clinically, the giant cell reparative granuloma is characterized by a slowly expanding mass, with the most usual site of involvement in the mandible anterior to the second molar teeth. It usually occurs in children or teenagers and is frequently noticed when there is displacement of the dentition. Radiographs reveal an irregular, osteolytic area with migration of teeth (Figs. 42.17 and 42.18). There may also be an area that can be multilocular in character. The differential diagnosis may be obscured because of the similarity in appearance between this lesion and a benign cyst or ameloblastoma. Treatment is conservative, and curettage of the involved area is usually sufficient to yield a favorable response.

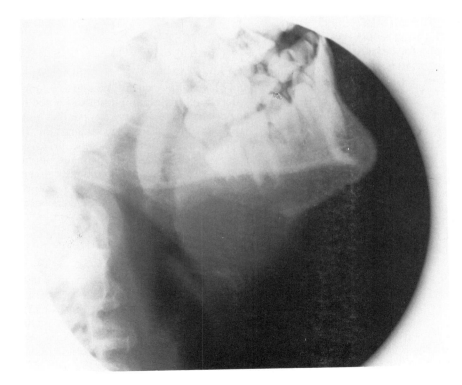

FIGURE 42.17. Giant cell tumor. Irregular expanding translucent area at the angle of mandible is shown in a 9-year-old child; haziness typical of this semisolid tumor mass can be seen.

FIGURE 42.18. Giant cell tumor. Expanding osteolytic area is revealed in the posterior mandibular area of 5-year-old patient.

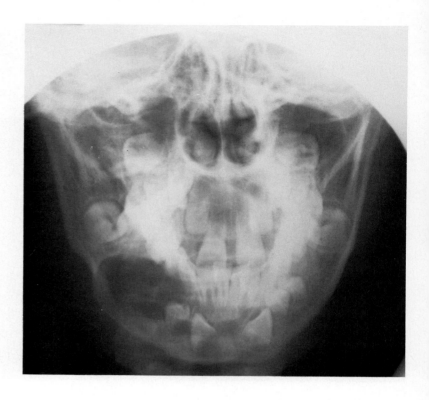

Hemangioma

An infrequent occurrence in the mandible and even less frequent in the maxilla, the hemangioma may be of congenital or traumatic origin. It is composed of various-sized thin-walled vessels scattered throughout the bony trabeculae. Clinical findings are of a firm, painless mass increasing in size. On the radiograph, a honeycomb, multiple cystic area is seen. The first clinical sign may be loosening of dentition or gingival bleeding. Treatment of a hemangioma may be by surgery, by sclerosing solutions, or both. Angiograms are advantageous for determining the size before treatment, because what is observed radiographically may only be a minor portion of the lesion.

TUMORS OF MESODERMAL ORIGIN

Fibromyxoma

Fibromyxoma is characterized by its slow growth with expanding cortex (Fig. 42.19). It is found in both the maxilla and the mandible. On the radiograph, it is seen as a well-circumscribed, radiolucent area that histologically resembles the stellate reticulum found in early tooth formation. Currettage and local resection is the treatment of choice.

TUMORS OF BONY ORIGIN

Osteogenic Sarcoma

Osteogenic sarcoma is a highly malignant mass of the bone originating from connective tissue, forming osteoid

and bone. It occurs in younger people (10–40 years, peaking at about age 27), and appears in the mandible more often than in the maxilla. The radiological appearance will vary from an irregular, poorly defined lytic lesion to one with a preponderance of bony formation with characteristic bony spicules described as a "sun ray" appearance (Fig. 42.20). The prognosis is better in the mandible. Resection and radiation therapy is the treatment of choice.

Multiple Myeloma

This bony tumor often involves the mandible or maxilla and arises from plasma-like cells in the marrow (Fig. 42.21). The presence of multiple bone lesions is noted in older individuals. An early myeloma may appear as multiple osteolytic, radiolucent areas on the radiograph. In the latest stages, larger and more widespread areas of bony destruction are observed. Diagnosis is made on the basis of the presence of hyperglobulinemia with a reversal of the serum albumin-globulin ratio and the presence of Bence Jones protein in the urine. Treatment includes the use of steroids, cytotoxic drugs, and radiation.

RARELY OCCURRING TUMORS

Other tumors found in the mandible or maxilla that rarely occur include *Ewing's sarcoma*, which originates in the maturing reticulum cell bone marrow (Fig. 42.22). Extensive bone destruction is seen on radiological evaluation. This tumor is rarely found in the maxilla. *Angiosarcoma* is another malignant tumor of vascular origin manifested by multiple areas of radiolucency in the mandible

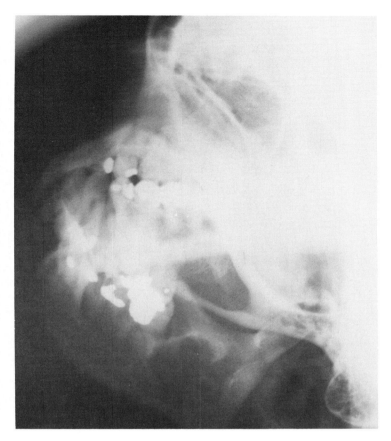

FIGURE 42.19. Fibromyxoma. A fairly well-circumscribed radiolucent area with some trabeculation noticed throughout in a 30-year-old patient.

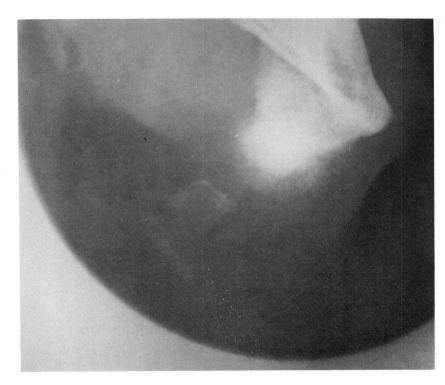

FIGURE 42.20. Osteogenic sarcoma. The typical ''sun ray'' appearance can be seen in rapidly progressive tumor at the right angle of the mandible.

FIGURE 42.21. Myeloma. Large radiolucent area at the angle and ramus of the mandible is at the typical site; multiple radiolucent ("punched out") areas are not uncommon.

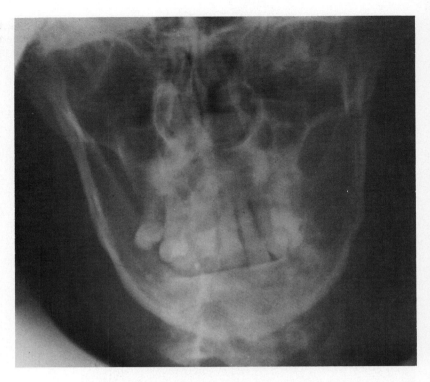

(Fig. 42.23). *Fibrosarcoma* of the jaw occurs as an osteolytic lesion in the mandible or maxilla.

METASTATIC TUMORS

Metastatic tumors involving the mandible and maxilla are more commonly from squamous cell carcinoma of the

FIGURE 42.22. Ewing's sarcoma. Extensive irregular destruction of the mandible with apical tooth resorption and cortical bone loss in a 12-year-old patient.

surrounding oral tissue (e.g., the lip, tongue, buccal, and alveolar areas). The mandible is the most common site of metastasis, and older people tend to be affected most often. However, some metastatic tumors of the jaw have a high incidence in children. Primary tumors of the breast, uterus, lung, and thyroid will metastasize to the mandible. Radiographic evaluation reveals a singular os-

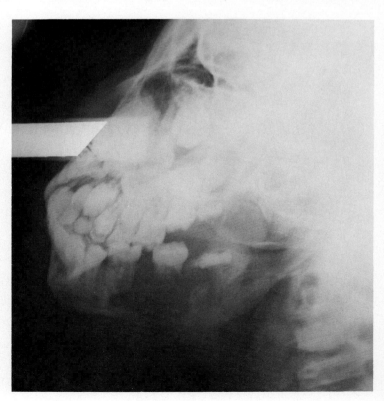

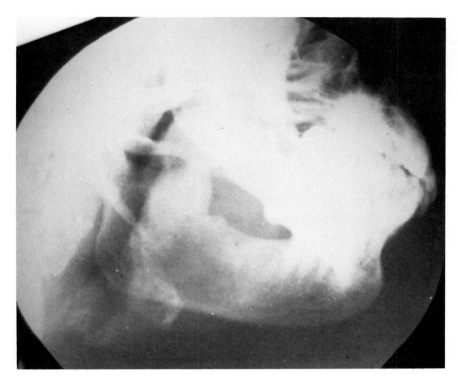

FIGURE 42.23. Angiosarcoma. The scattered granular radiolucent lesion affects large areas of the mandible; areas of irregularly dispersed calcification are visualized.

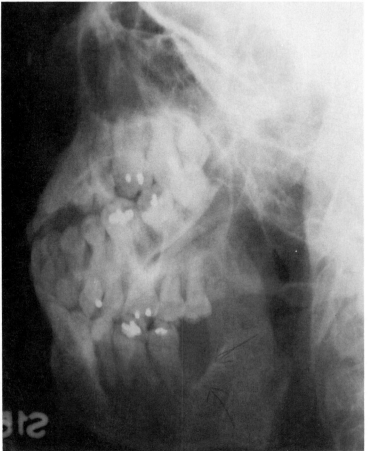

FIGURE 42.24. Metastatic carcinoma. The irregular area of cortical loss shown in the retromolar area of the mandible represents metastasis of a uterine carcinoma in a 42-year-old female.

FIGURE 42.25. Metastatic cancer. Moderately radiopaque, large diffuse mass in the mandible of a 70-year-old male with metastases from the prostate.

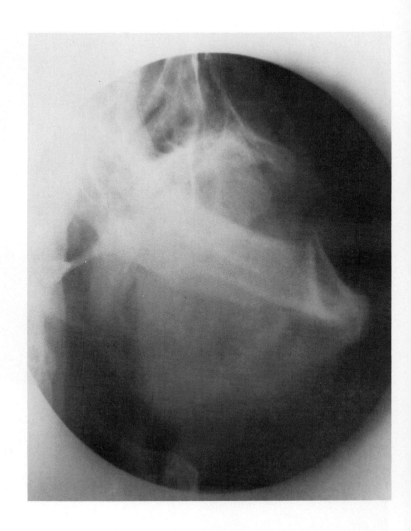

FIGURE 42.26. Ossifying fibroma. A large radiopaque mass involving the right maxilla, orbital floor, and zygoma can be seen; the "ground glass" appearance is characteristic of mixed fibrous and osseous elements seen with fibrous dysplasia.

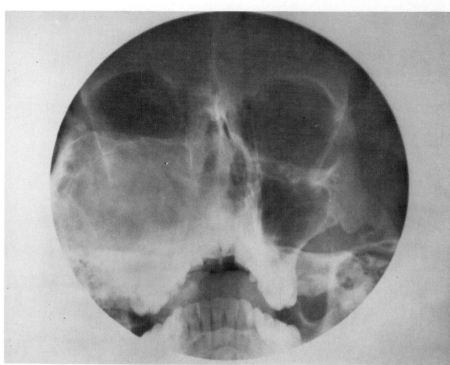

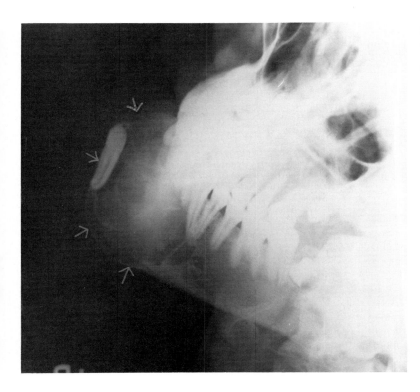

FIGURE 42.27. Ossifying fibroma. A larger osseous lesion with fibrous elements expands the anterior mandible; marked displacement of the canine tooth with irregular erosion of the inferior cortical plate can be seen.

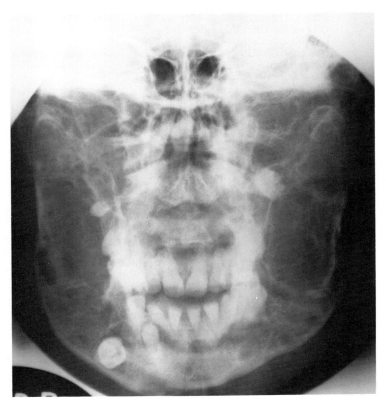

FIGURE 42.28. Familial fibrous dysplasia (cherubism). Extensive multiloculated, slightly radiopaque cystic expansile areas are shown throughout the mandible and other facial bones; disrupted dentition can be seen surrounding these areas in a 14-year-old with painless masses that have been increasing gradually over a 10-year period. Notice the thinning of the cortex with irregular fine septa.

teolytic lesion centrally located in the mandible (Figs. 42.24 and 42.25). The varying areas of bone destruction may resemble osteomyelitis. In many instances, the differential diagnosis can only be made by tissue diagnosis.

FIBROUS DYSPLASIA

Fibrous dysplasia is found in the membranous facial bones of younger individuals and usually becomes less active with maturity. In this group, the proportion of fibrous tissue to osseous metaplasia is greater. The characteristic clinical picture is one of an increasing firm mass, presenting in either the maxilla or mandible. The area of fibrous dysplasia can manifest as a single fibroosseous mass, or it may have multiple areas of involvement most commonly occurring in the maxilla (Fig. 42.26).

The radiographic appearance will vary, depending on the amount of fibrous tissue in relation to osseous tissue. The radiograph may be one of a cystic-like appearance. However, magnification will usually reveal a pattern of diffuse areas of calcification (Fig. 42.27). A preponderance of osseous tissue will be seen in more mature tumors, often being referred to as ossifying fibromas at this stage. Larger bony tumors should be evaluated with a computed tomography (CT) scan because of possible involvement of the orbital areas and base of the skull. Conservative surgical curettement via an intraoral approach will usually be sufficient in managing the tumor. There may be surges in growth during hormonal changes that require close clinical and radiographic observation. However, if growth continues, it is not uncommon to repeat this procedure a few years later. Radiation therapy is not generally recommended because it may induce sarcoma.

PAGET'S DISEASE (OSTEITIS DEFORMANS)

Paget's disease resembles an ossifying fibroma on radiographic and histological evaluation. However, it occurs in the older age group and appears in multiple areas of the mandible and maxilla. The maxilla is the predominant jaw of involvement. In contrast, fibrous dysplasia occurs as a single lesion and is seen more frequently in younger individuals. Paget's will also appear in other areas of the skull and skeleton. An elevated serum phosphatase level is another distinguishing feature.

FAMILIAL FIBROUS DYSPLASIA (CHERUBISM)

Familial fibrous dysplasia is characterized by multiple areas of fibrous dysplasia in the maxilla and mandible, occurring as early as 1 year of age (Fig. 42.28). As a variant of fibrous dysplasia, this is an inherited genetic disorder. The usual period of rapid growth is until puberty. Radiographic appearance reveals multiple cystic

areas in all regions of the mandible and maxilla with expansion of the bones. Treatment is conservative via an intraoral approach with multiple curettement procedures spaced as indicated over a number of years.

References

1. Gardner EJ, Richards RC: Multiple cutaneous and subcutaneous lesions occurring simultaneously with hereditary polyposis and osteomatosis. *Am J Hum Genet* 5:139, 1953.
2. Halse A, Roed-Peterson B, Lund K: Gardner's syndrome. *J Oral Surg* 33:673, 1975.
3. Lichtenstein L: *Bone Tumors*, ed 5. St. Louis, CV Mosby Co, 1977.

Suggested Readings

Baden E: Terminology of the ameloblastoma: History and current usage. *J Oral Surg* 23:40, 1965.

Barros RE, Dominguez FV, Cabrini RL: Myxoma of the jaws. *Oral Surg* 27:225, 1969.

Block RM, Bushell A, Rodriques H, et al: A histopathologic, histobacteriologic, and radiographic study of periapical endodontic surgical specimens. *Oral Surg Oral Med Oral Pathol* 42:656, 1976.

Borghelli RF, Barros RE, Zampieri J: Ewing sarcoma of the mandible: Report of case. *J Oral Surg* 36:473, 1978.

Bruce KW, Royer RQ: Multiple myeloma occurring in the jaws. *Oral Surg Oral Med Oral Pathol* 6:729, 1953.

Cornyn J: Fibro-calcific lesions to the jaws. Presentation to American Academy of Dental Radiology, Chicago, October 24, 1975.

Eversol ELR, Sabes WR, Rovin S: Fibrous dysplasia: A nosologic problem in the diagnosis of fibro-osseous lesions of the jaw. *J Oral Pathol* 1:189, 1972.

Fung EH: Ameloblastomas. *Int J Oral Surg* 7:305, 1978.

Geschichter CF, Copeland MM: *Tumors of Bone*. Philadelphia, JB Lippincott Co, 1949.

Gorlin RJ, Chaudhry AP, Pindborg JJ: Odontogenic tumors: Classification, histopathology and clinical behavior in man and domesticated animals. *Cancer* 14:73, 1961.

Hager RC, Taylor CG, Allen PM: Ameloblastic fibroma: Report of case. *J Oral Surg* 36:66, 1978.

Harder F: Myxomas of the jaws. *Int J Oral Surg* 7:148, 1978.

High CL, Frew AL, Glass RT: Osteosarcoma of the mandible. *Oral Surg Oral Med Oral Pathol* 45:678, 1978.

King DR, Moore GE: An analysis of torus palatinus in a transatlantic study. *J Oral Med* 31:44, 1976.

Kuepper RC, Harrigan WF: Treatment of mandibular cherubism. *J Oral Surg* 36:638, 1978.

Lichtenstein L, Jaffe H: Fibrous dysplasia of bone. *Arch Pathol* 33:777, 1942.

Lund BA, Dahlin DC: Hemangiomas of the mandible and maxilla. *J Oral Surg* 22:234, 1964.

Minderjahn A: Incidence and clinical differentiation of odontogenic tumors. *J Maxillofac Surg* 7:142, 1979.

Minkow B, Laufer D, Gutman D: Treatment of oral hemangiomas with local sclerosing agents. *Int J Oral Surg* 8:18, 1979.

Mourshed F: A roentgenographic study of dentigerous cysts. I. Incidence in a population sample. *Oral Surg Oral Med Oral Pathol* 18:47, 1964.

Nordin BEC: *Metabolic Bone and Stone Disease*. Baltimore, Williams & Wilkins Co, 1973, p 17.

Rapoport A, Sobrinho JD, DeCarvalho MB, et al: Ewing's sarcoma of the mandible. *Oral Surg Oral Med Oral Pathol* 44:89, 1977.

Regezi JA, Kerr DA, Courtney, RM: Odontogenic tumors: Analysis of 706 cases. *J Oral Surg* 36:771, 1978.

Reyneke JP: Aneurysmal bone cyst of the maxilla. *Oral Surg* 45:441, 1978.

Roca AN, Smith JL, MacComb WS, et al: Ewing's sarcoma of the maxilla and mandible. *Oral Surg* 25:194, 1968.

Shafer WG: Ameloblastic fibroma. *J Oral Surg* 13:317, 1955.

Shafer WG: Presentation to American College of Stomatologic Surgeons, Maywood, IL, 1978.

Steidler NE, Cook RM, Reade PC: Aneurysmal bone cysts of the jaws: A case report and review of the literature. *Br J Oral Surg* 16:254, 1979.

Taicher S, Azaz B: Lesions resembling globulomaxillary cysts. *Oral Surg Oral Med Oral Pathol* 44:25, 1977.

Toretti EF, Miller AS, Peezick B: Odontomas: An analysis of 167 cases. *J Periodontol* 8:282, 1984.

Trodahl JN: Ameloblastic fibroma, a survey of cases from the Armed Forces Institute of Pathology. *Oral Surg Oral Med Oral Pathol* 33:547, 1972.

Willis RA: *Pathology of Tumors,* ed 4. London, Butterworth & Co, Ltd, 1967.

Wood NK, Goaz PW: *Differential Diagnosis of Oral Lesions*. St. Louis, CV Mosby Co, 1980.

Zegarelli E, Zishin D: Cementomas. *Am J Orthod* 29:285, 1943.

43

Craniofacial Tumors

Ian T. Jackson, M.D., F.R.C.S., F.A.C.S., F.R.A.C.S. (Hon.)

Craniofacial tumors are tumors of the base of the skull. In the past, because of difficulties in exposure, they have frequently been excised piecemeal or incompletely, if at all. Recurrences have been frequent. Attempts at resection have been associated with significant complications, especially extradural abscesses and meningitis (1, 2). Application of techniques used for the correction of congenital craniofacial anomalies has given surgeons excellent ways of access and has allowed more en bloc resections with greatly decreased morbidity. There are indications in our own series that the cure rate will also be improved with this more aggressive approach.

Craniofacial tumors may be untreated at the time of referral, but many are recurrent after surgery, radiotherapy, or chemotherapy. The pathology varies from nonmalignant to malignant; the latter are carcinoma and frequently, in younger patients, sarcoma (Table 43.1). In the vast majority of cases, excisional surgery is the therapeutic modality of choice, followed by radiotherapy and/or chemotherapy as indicated. It is only in rhabdomyosarcoma of the orbit in children that this regimen is not used. In these cases, the lesion is biopsied to confirm the diagnosis, and the definitive treatment is radiotherapy and chemotherapy. The consensus of opinion is that this therapeutic regimen gives cure rates superior to those of surgical resection (3–6).

Anatomical Division of the Skull Base

Previously, there has been no attempt to systematize the surgical treatment of skull base tumors. It is useful to divide the cranial base into segments and to use this segmentation to provide accurate tumor location (7, 8; Table 43.2).

The basic division is into an *anterior area* and a *posterior area*. The former is the anterior cranial fossa, and the latter is a composite of the middle and posterior cranial fossae. The posterior area can be further subdivided into an *anterior*, a *central*, and a *posterior* segment. The anterior segment lies between the orbit and the anterior surface of the petrous bone; the central segment is the petrous bone itself; and the posterior segment is bounded by the posterior face of the petrous bone anteriorly and the midline posteriorly (i.e., the posterior cranial fossa).

These areas contain foramina, which are important because they allow escape of intracranial tumors from and entry of extracranial tumors into the cranial cavity (Table 43.3). Knowledge of the contents and position of these

Table 43.1.
Tumors Involving Anterior Cranial Fossa

Malignant
  Squamous carcinoma
  Basal cell carcinoma
  Melanoma
  Adenocystic carcinoma
  Chondrosarcoma
  Osteogenic sarcoma
  Neuroblastoma
  Neurofibrosarcoma
  Liposarcoma
  Malignant hemangiopericytoma
  Adenocarcinoma
  Mucoepidermoid carcinoma
  Esthesioneuroblastoma

Nonmalignant
  Neurofibroma
  Osteoma
  Meningioma
  Pleomorphic salivary adenoma
  Intradiploic dermoid

foramina is mandatory in skull base surgery. It should also be appreciated that the intracranial end of the foramen may lie in a different position from the extracranial end. This fact is important, particularly in the resection of tumors involving the petrous bone, through which the tortuous carotid canal courses.

Anterior Area (Anterior Cranial Fossa)

Any tumors involving the frontal bone, frontal or ethmoid sinuses, orbit or its contents, or nasopharynx can

Table 43.2.
Classification of Skull Base for Tumor Resection

Anterior area	Anterior cranial fossa
Posterior area	Middle and posterior cranial fossa, subdivided as follows:
	Anterior segment: anterior wall of middle cranial fossa to anterior border of petrous temporal bone
	Central segment: petrous temporal bone
	Posterior segment: posterior border of petrous temporal bone to midline of posterior cranial fossa

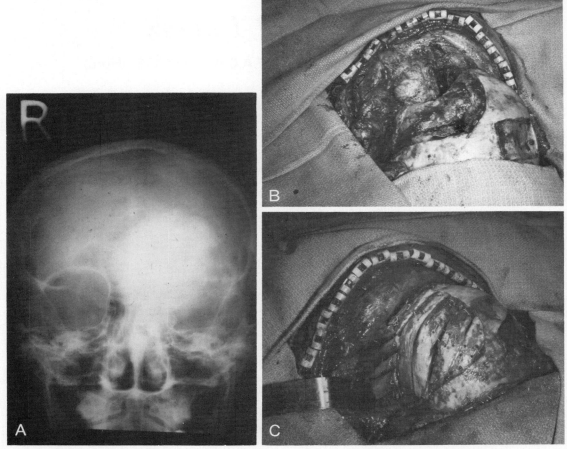

FIGURE 43.1. **A**, Radiograph showing left frontonasoorbital fibrous dysplasia. **B**, Resection of left orbit to the floor together with the involved frontal and nasal regions. **C**, Reconstruction is performed with split-skull and split-rib grafts.

directly invade the anterior cranial fossa. Tumors arising in the brain or meninges can similarly involve the skull base. Indirect involvement may result from skin, maxilla, or muscle; this invasion uses the structures mentioned above as avenues for entry into the cranium.

If this is appreciated, intracranial involvement will be more frequently suspected and looked for using computed tomography (CT) scans. Any suggestion of this occurrence calls for a neurosurgical consultation before surgery. As a result of this, the neurosurgeon may plan to be involved or, if the invasion is not definite, he or she can be on call at the time of surgery.

NONMALIGNANT TUMORS

The nonmalignant tumors are mainly neurofibroma, osteoma, and intradiploic dermoid. The meningioma can be recurrent and may eventually be responsible for the patient's death. The best example, albeit not pathologically a true tumor, is fibrous dysplasia. It behaves as a tumor and is treated the same, using total resection and, because it is nonmalignant, performing immediate reconstruction (9, 10). The presenting problems are deformity and, occasionally, decreasing visual acuity as a result of involvement of the optic foramen.

The frontoorbital region is affected most frequently; therefore, the coronal flap approach is used. If possible, a complete intracranial and extracranial resection is performed with removal of all affected bone (Fig. 43.1). This frequently means resection of frontal bone, orbital roof, and medial and lateral orbital walls. Reconstruction is performed using split-skull grafts and split-rib grafts. The former are a spin-off from the surgery of congenital de-

Table 43.3.
Foramina of the Posterior Area of the Skull Base

Anterior segment	Foramen rotundum—maxillary nerve
	Foramen ovale—mandibular nerve
	Foramen lacerum—internal carotid artery
	Foramen spinosum—middle meningeal artery
Central segment	Internal acoustic meatus
	Internal carotid canal
Posterior segment	Jugular foramen—internal jugular vein
	Foramen magnum

fects and are now the most frequently used bone grafts in the upper facial area (11, 12). After this procedure, there is little or no tendency for recurrence; the cosmetic defect is corrected, and if it has been necessary to decompress the optic nerve, deterioration of visual acuity may be halted.

Complications should be few if the appropriate antibiotics are given and the surgery is performed with due care. A lesson learned from congenital craniofacial procedures is the importance of closing any connections between the extradural space and the nasopharynx. Failure to do this will result in possible extradural abscess and meningitis. Closure of this area can be effected in various ways, and these are presented in the relevant sections. The most useful technique in the situation described here is the galeal-frontalis muscle flap (13). This flap is raised

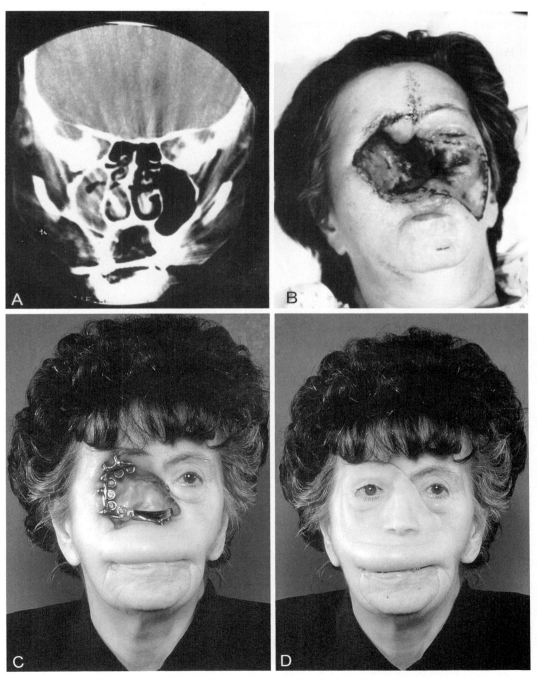

FIGURE 43.2.   **A**, Recurrent midface basal cell carcinoma was present for 30 years after 60 operative procedures. **B**, Extensive craniofacial resection with ablation of orbit, excision of anterior cranial fossa to posterior wall of sphenoid sinus, and excision of affected cheek; extended glabellar flap was developed to reconstruct the cranial base. Prosthesis base was secured with osseointegrated titanium implants. **C and D**, The prosthesis was held in place with magnets.

based on the supraorbital and supratrochlear vessels, and it can be made as long as necessary. After being elevated, it can be turned down and packed and sutured into the defect. This has proven to be most effective in dealing with this potentially disastrous situation.

MALIGNANT TUMORS

Frequently, malignant tumors recur after surgery, radiotherapy, and chemotherapy (this group makes up 75% of our cases), or they have a potential for recurrence. Therefore, often only limited reconstruction is performed. Covering up such a situation with a complex reconstruction may lead to a lethal delay in the diagnosis

of recurrence. This is discussed in more detail later. All resections are performed with frozen section control.

Penetrating Midface Tumors

Penetrating midface tumors (Fig. 43.2) are usually recurrent basal cell carcinomas, occasionally squamous cell carcinoma (SCC), and much less frequently adenocystic or mucoepidermoid carcinomas, adenocarcinomas, sarcomas, or esthesioneuroblastomas. Resection is performed with frozen section control. This involves removal of all involved facial areas: the nose or its remnant; varying parts of the orbit (perhaps exenteration); the palate; a varying amount of the nasopharynx; the central

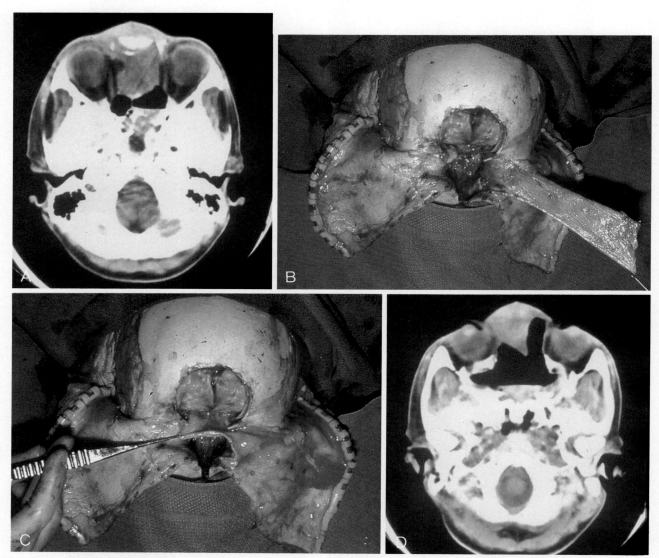

FIGURE 43.3. Recurrent adenocarcinoma of right ethmoid sinus and nasopharynx treated with radiation therapy. **A,** CT scan showing the adenocarcinoma of the right ethmoid sinus. **B,** Wide resection of tumor through anterior craniostomy, with ga- leal-frontalis flap elevated. *C,* Galeal-frontalis flap sutured to the base of the anterior cranial fossa to separate it from the naso- pharynx. **D,** Postoperative result on 18 months' followup.

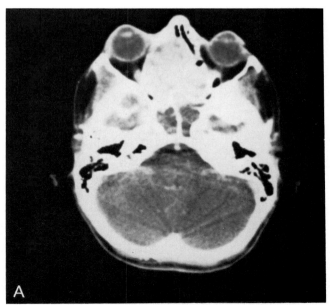

FIGURE 43.4. **A**, A young patient presents with nasal septal and anterior cranial base chondrosarcoma seen on the axial CT scan. **B**, Midface osteotomy was performed to obtain tumor exposure.

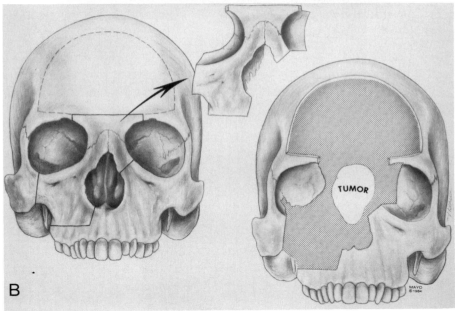

anterior cranial fossa base and the overlying dura, if involved; and the ethmoid and sphenoid sinuses. A dural repair is performed using stored dura, fascia, or periosteum. This is exposed to the nasopharynx and must be protected by viable tissue. This can be effected by suturing an extended glabellar flap (14), a midline forehead flap (15, 16), or a galeal frontalis flap (17) to the skull base and the posterior wall of the sphenoid sinus through drill holes. In the past, skin flaps were favored in cases with previous heavy doses of radiotherapy; galea from the frontal or temporal area or temporalis muscle is now used almost exclusively.

Reconstruction is often provided by an external prosthesis. These patients must be followed up with frequent visits, at least annual CT scans, and biopsies if any suspi-cious area appears in the field of resection. Using this regimen, we have had three local recurrences in 30 cases over a period of 10 years.

Ethmoid Carcinoma

Any tumor arising in or invading the ethmoids should be treated as an anterior cranial base tumor (Fig. 43.3). It should be approached using a coronal scalp flap and a frontal bone flap. The ethmoid block is outlined intracranially and extracranially and is resected. If skin is involved, this is included in the resection. Orbital involvement calls for orbitectomy, and maxillary involvement requires maxillectomy. The ethmoid, orbit, and maxilla

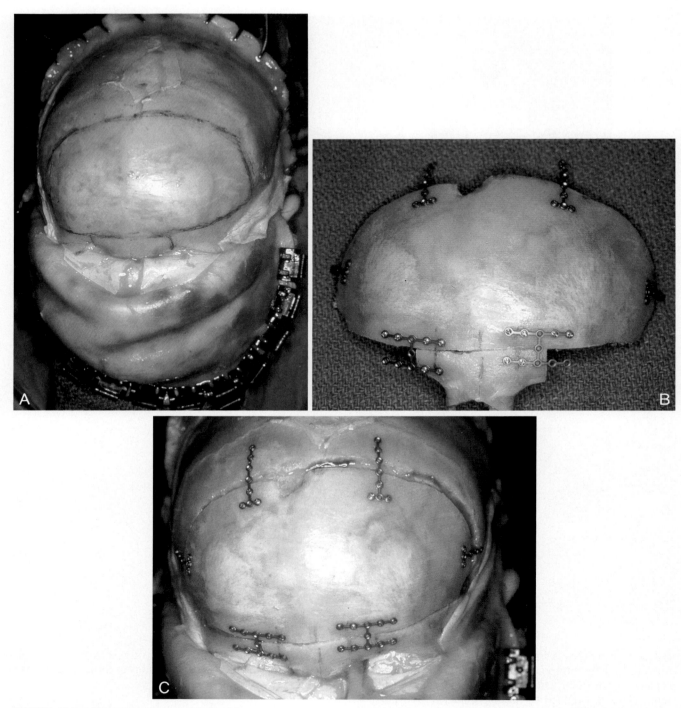

FIGURE 43.5. Side table reassembly of craniofacial segments. **A,** Planned osteotomies, frontal and glabellonasal. **B,** Side table reassembly of osteotomies using microplates. Note microplates protruding from edge of osteotomies. **C,** Reinsertion of reassembled osteotomies.

should be removed as a single block of tissue, if possible, with clean margins. Again, it is important to close the defect down into the nasopharynx with a galeal-frontalis flap or an extended glabellar flap. If there has been skin involvement, the skin defect is usually not reconstructed and is handled with a combination of intraoral and extraoral prostheses. Reconstruction can be undertaken at a later date.

Midface Sarcoma

Midface sarcomas (Fig. 43.4) frequently arise in the nasal septum; if they are far posterior, they defy early diagnosis because their main symptoms are nasal airway obstruction and anosmia, which are not uncommon in the general population. The nasal mucosa may be congested, and the patient is treated for allergy. The diagnosis is made on tomography, CT scan, and nasendoscopy. Because of the difficulty in early diagnosis, the tumors are frequently advanced when they present. In the past, these gave great problems in exposure; consequently, complete resection was difficult, if not impossible, in some cases.

The preferred approach is through a coronal flap and frontal bone flap with a face-splitting incision. A new concept in craniofacial approaches has been that of osteotomy for exposure with subsequent replacement (18). The term used for this technique is "exposure osteotomy" or "facial disassembly." Any combination of osteotomies may be used with removal of bone or maintenance of a soft tissue pedicle. With this tumor, this approach makes all the difference to exposure after the frontal craniotomy. The bony midface [e.g., glabella, nasal bones, orbit, and maxilla (sparing the teeth)], is removed as a block, as required. This exposes the base of the skull and the tumor. It is now possible to resect the tumor in one piece with good margins. This may not be possible in some cases; however, that state of affairs has rarely been encountered.

The bony segment is reassembled on a side table, using mini or microplates, and replaced; however, it is now exposed to the nasopharynx (Fig. 43.5). This can again be covered with a galeal-frontalis flap. A split-skin graft is applied to this and held in place with sutures and a pack. The pack can be withdrawn through the nose in a few days' time. In this way, primary healing is achieved, and the area can be observed for recurrence using the nasendoscope.

ORBITAL TUMORS

Craniofacial Osteotomy and En Bloc Resection

Nonmalignant orbital tumors (Fig. 43.6) can be exposed through a craniofacial approach. This is chosen for the tumors lying in the superior and posterior orbital area. A coronal scalp flap and a frontal bone flap are used. The orbital roof and supraorbital rim are osteotomized as a block and removed. Exposure of the tumor is excellent. It can be removed en bloc under direct vision, and afterward the osteotomy is wired back into place. This resection can be accomplished without causing any cosmetic deformity or external facial scars.

An approach such as this is also used for malignant tumors that are localized and can be resected with a margin of soft tissue. It is also favored for sphenoid wing meningiomas.

Partial Orbitectomy

When the tumor involves the orbital wall, a partial orbitectomy and exenteration may be necessary. The necessity for an intracranial approach is judged by tumor position. Any malignant osteoinvasive tumor in the posterosuperior position should be approached in this way. These may be tumors arising in the orbit and invading the bone from within, or extraorbital tumors that invade from

without. Enough of the orbit should be removed to assure total tumor removal.

Total Orbitectomy

Very rarely, extensive tumors (Fig. 43.7) or tumors known to be aggressive occurring in or around the orbit will require total resection of the orbit and its contents. The osteotomy is the same as that used for hypertelorism; bony cuts are made across the orbital roof, down the lateral wall, horizontally across the maxilla below the infraorbital nerve, and vertically up the medial wall. In cases in which the tumor is situated far posteriorly in the orbit, the optic nerve is divided within the dura to allow for complete resection. The nasopharynx is closed off with a galeal-frontalis flap and/or temporalis galea based on the superficial temporal vessels or the temporalis mus-

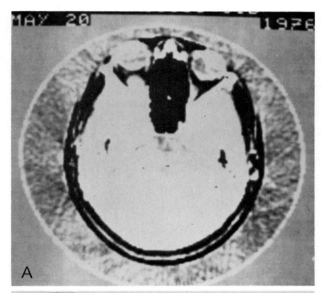

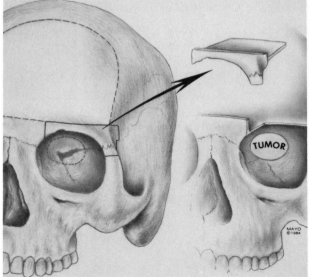

FIGURE 43.6. **A,** Neurofibroma deep in the orbit well is seen on axial CT scan. **B,** Osteotomy is performed for exposure.

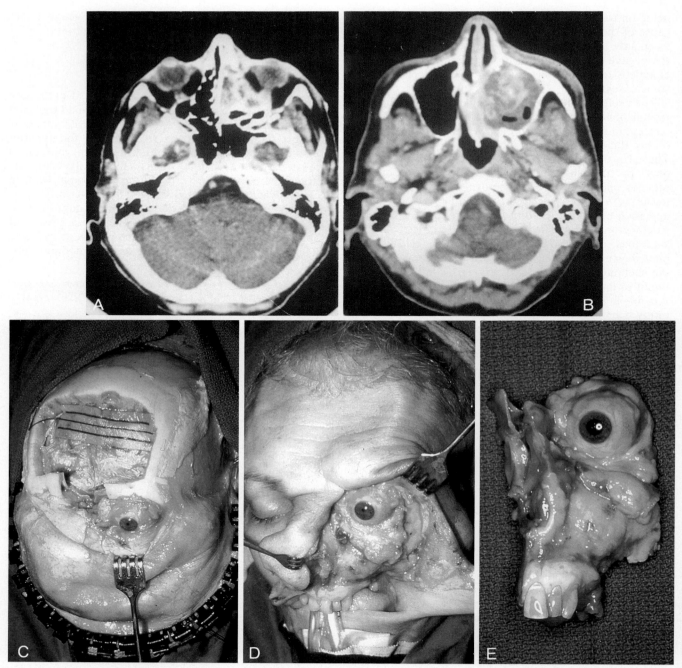

FIGURE 43.7. A malignant melanoma of the maxillary sinus, nasopharynx, ethmoid sinus, and orbit. **A and B**, Axial CT scans showing the extent of the tumor. **C**, Frontoglabellar approach to skull base and orbit. **D**, Approach to maxilla, lower orbit, and anterior nasopharynx through Weber-Ferguson incision. **E**, Block resection of region with wide clearance of melanoma.

cle with application of a split-skin graft. Skin cover is achieved with a forehead or chest flap (e.g., pectoralis major, deltopectoral).

Middle Cranial Fossa (Posterior Area, Anterior Segment)

NONMALIGNANT TUMORS

The two most commonly encountered tumors in this category are partly orbital, partly middle fossa tumors. These are orbital neurofibroma and fibrous dysplasia.

Neurofibroma

Only the advanced cases (Fig. 43.8) are considered. The less severe cases call for surgery to the eyelid, recession of the still-functioning globe, and reconstruction of any bony defects (19, 20).

The problem case is the one that presents with eyelid involvement so gross that the lids appear very edematous and cannot open; they may hang down onto the cheek. The eye pulsates and is proptotic and blind. There is neurofibroma present in the temple. Pain and epiphora are present, and the patient usually wears a patch over the eye.

Radiological examination and CT scans show the orbit to be enlarged and egg shaped, with an absence of the greater wing of the sphenoid. This, in turn, causes a large defect in the posterior wall of the orbit (anterior wall of the middle cranial fossa) through which the temporal lobe herniates. This accounts for the eye protrusion and pulsation.

The approach to this problem is varied. It has been suggested that the bone defect be reconstructed, the orbit enlarged by an osteotomy, and some debulking of the neurofibroma undertaken to achieve recession of the globe. The eyelids are then trimmed to thin them and leave the fissure permanently open. The usual result obtained using this technique is poor.

It has been found more satisfactory to remove the orbital contents completely, together with the involved temporal area. The eyelid skin is preserved inasmuch as this is never involved by the neurofibroma. The bony posterior orbital defect is reconstructed with split-rib grafts or split-skull grafts, and these are wired into position to give a solid closure of the defect. The orbit is then reduced in size using an ostectomy and osteotomies; any contour defects are made up with bone grafts (21).

The whole area is now covered with the eyelids. The edges are sutured together, and the skin is pushed into the orbital cavity and held there with a pack. Once healing is achieved, the patient is fitted with an external prosthesis of eye and lids, masked by spectacles.

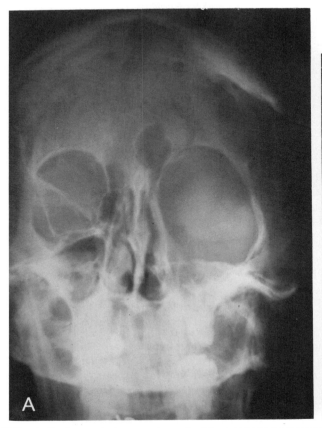
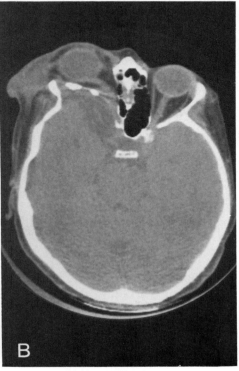

FIGURE 43.8. **A**, Radiograph shows enlarged orbit and absence of greater sphenoid wing caused by neurofibroma. **B**, Axial CT scan shows protrusion of the temporal lobe.

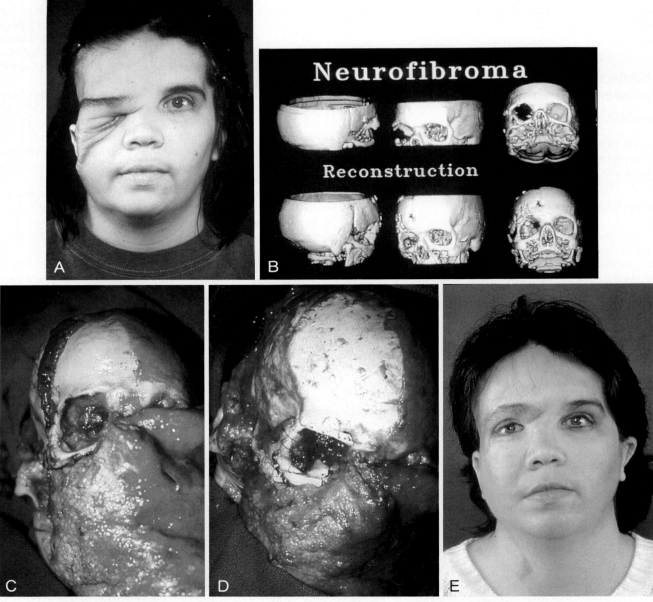

FIGURE 43.9. Neurofibroma of the right orbitotemporal region. **A**, Preoperative appearance. **B**, Three-dimensional reconstruction showing the size and shape of the right orbit together with the bony defect. **C**, Exposure of the deformed orbit. **D**, Orbital osteotomies completed. **E**, Postoperative result. In addition to the osteotomies, a rectus abdominis free flap was used to replace the facial soft tissue defect following excision.

This technique may seem an admission of surgical defeat, but it has resulted in satisfied patients with a good aesthetic result and complete relief of symptoms (Fig. 43.9).

It is sometimes possible to preserve the eyelids and reconstruct them in such a fashion that only an ocular prosthesis is necessary.

Fibrous Dysplasia

Fibrous dysplasia (Fig. 43.10) may involve the posterolateral area of the orbit and the middle cranial fossa. The main reason for operating is proptosis and occasionally progressive diminution of visual acuity.

The area is approached using a coronal flap and a frontotemporal bone flap. The orbital contents and the temporalis muscle are dissected subperiosteally to expose the tumor in the temporal fossa and the orbit. An orbitomaxillary osteotomy is performed to give further enhancement of exposure. The frontal and temporal lobes are elevated, and the involved area is resected with a margin of nonaffected bone. If the latter is not possible, a subtotal resection is effected. Reconstruction is achieved using split-skull grafts plated in position. The osteotomies and craniotomies are replaced, and the scalp is sutured.

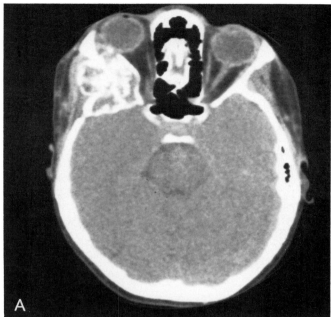

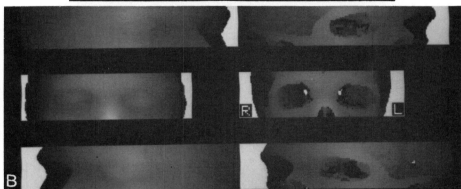

FIGURE 43.10. **A**, A patient showed fibrous dysplasia of right orbit and middle cranial fossa on axial CT scan. **B**, A three-dimensional scan gives a good idea of the size and position of the tumor. **C**, Orbitozygomatic osteotomy is performed for exposure and resection of the involved area. **D**, Postoperative result is shown with postoperative axial CT scan.

SUPERIOR INFRATEMPORAL FOSSA TUMORS

Superior infratemporal fossa tumors are frequently meningiomas that appear in the orbit and the temporal area. This causes proptosis of the involved eye and bulging above the zygomatic arch. There is often blindness or severe diminution of visual acuity. CT scan shows the position of the lesion and the very considerable stretching of the optic nerve and extraocular muscles. The extent of the meningioma within the sphenoid bone and in the middle cranial fossa also is clearly seen.

The surgical approach is similar to that described for fibrous dysplasia (Fig. 43.11); however, the osteotomy frequently must be more extensive. Inclusion of the supraorbital rim and roof, lateral orbital wall, a portion of the zygoma, and the zygomatic arch in the osteotomy will give adequate exposure for removal of the extracranial portion of the tumor. The intracranial resection proceeds as indicated by the size and position of the tumor. Reconstruction is performed using split-skull grafts. The exposure osteotomy segments and craniotomy bone flap are replaced.

It must be realized that many of these meningiomas are recurrent and the chances of total resection are not high. However, even with subtotal removal, one can buy considerable time for the patient and improve the deformity to a varying degree.

LOW INFRATEMPORAL FOSSA TUMORS

Again, low infratemporal fossa tumors may be meningiomas, but they may also be neurofibromas. Extracranial tumors invading this area are squamous carcinomas, adenocarcinomas, adenocystic carcinomas, and various types of sarcomas.

There are two main approaches to this region: the microdrilling technique of Fisch et al. (22) and the combined intracranial and extracranial technique (23, 24). The former method is largely used by otolaryngologists, and experience is limited to facial nerve exposure within the temporal bone. It is the combined intracranial and extracranial approach that is described here (Fig. 43.12).

FIGURE 43.10C and D.

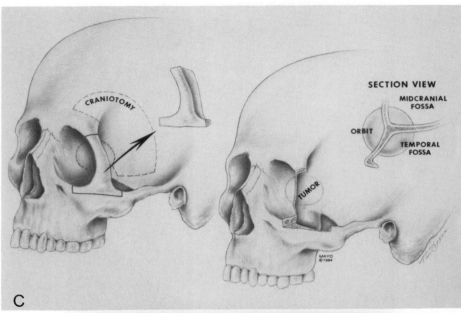

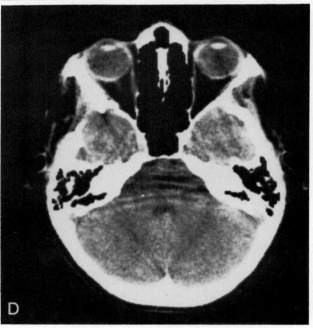

The skin incision begins in the scalp. It is taken down in front of the ear, as for a face lift, and continues into the neck as indicated. This large scalp, face, and neck flap is elevated to give exposure to the frontotemporal, zygomatic, and mandibular areas. A temporal craniotomy is performed, and the temporal lobe is elevated until the tumor comes into view. The chances of excision can be assessed at this point. If resection is considered possible, the operation proceeds. If the tumor is extensive and there is displacement or suggested involvement of the carotid, or if there are palpable neck nodes, a neck dissection is performed. This has a twofold advantage: involved nodes are removed, and the external carotid artery and the internal jugular vein are identified and can be followed up to the skull base, which makes the skull base resection much easier and safer.

In order to clear the exposure to the base of the middle cranial fossa, certain structures must be removed: the total parotid (with facial nerve preservation) (25), the zygomatic arch (26), and sometimes the ascending ramus of the mandible. A dissection is performed extracranially to visualize the dimensions of the tumor. The skull base is now resected until the involved foramen is reached. The tumor can now be dissected out and removed under direct vision, with or without bone as indicated.

The temporal bone flap is replaced, and the skull base

is reconstructed with a split-skull graft (27). The zygomatic arch and, occasionally, the ascending ramus are replaced and plated. The problem with this latter procedure is its potential for causing trismus. The skin incision is closed with drainage.

Occasionally, in extensive tumors, an orbital osteotomy may be necessary. In tumors situated medially behind the maxilla, an anterior approach using the Weber-Ferguson incision and incorporating a partial maxillectomy in the procedure may be indicated.

Posterior Area, Central Segment

Tumors of the central segment include squamous or basal cell carcinomas of the external ear that involve the petrous bone, and parotid tumors that have extended deeply into the ear cleft following surgery and radiation therapy or recurrence. These are adenocystic, mucoepidermoid, squamous, and undifferentiated carcinomas. The third variety are squamous carcinomas arising in the middle ear.

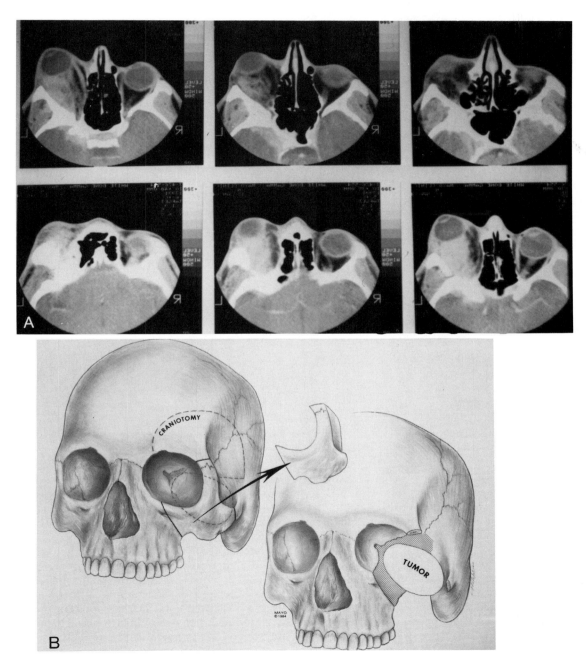

FIGURE 43.11. **A**, Recurrent meningioma of left middle cranial fossa invading the orbit and upper infratemporal fossa shows well on axial CT scans. **B**, Orbitozygomatic osteotomy is performed for exposure and resection of the involved area.

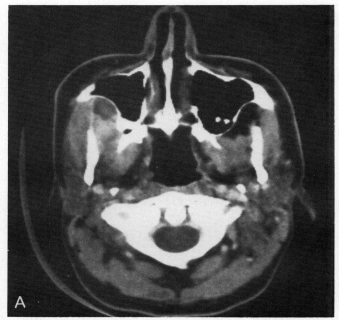

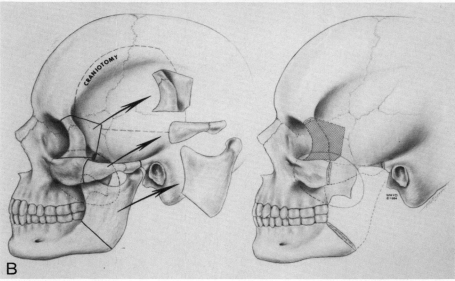

FIGURE 43.12. **A**, Liposarcoma of the left infratemporal fossa area that involves the skull base and posterior maxilla is seen on the axial CT scan. **B**, Osteotomies are used for exposure.

Partial petrosectomy does not involve entry into the cranial cavity and is not considered in this chapter. It is sufficient to say that, in these cases, cover is obtained with a temporal muscle transposition and a split-skin graft. The operation of radical petrosectomy is presented here (23, 28, 29).

The incision curves over the temporoparietal area down in front of the ear. The incision may be taken around the ear if the ear is to be included in the resection. It continues in a vertical curvilinear fashion to give exposure in the neck. The external ear may, in some cases, be preserved; in these cases, it is lifted with the posterior flap, and the ear canal is transected. A temporal craniotomy is performed, and the cranial aspect of the petrous bone is exposed. This is necessary in order to assess

resectability. Frequently, there may be tumor extension into the temporal lobe dura. This is an ominous prognostic sign in middle ear cancer. The apex of the petrous bone is inspected because, if the tumor has spread beyond this into the cavernous sinus, curative resection may be impossible.

If the tumor is judged to be resectable, exposure from the neck is begun. Primary or recurrent parotid tumors necessitate total parotidectomy. A total or partial neck dissection is used to locate the important structures, particularly the internal carotid artery as it enters the base of the skull. Care is taken to preserve the internal jugular vein intact. If this is tied off early in the procedure, it results in considerable distention of the lateral sinus. This increases the technical difficulties of the procedure because of increased venous oozing and can result in severe bleeding if the sinus is broached. As the soft tissue is dissected from the skull anterior and posterior to the meatus, further extension of tumor may be noted, and a wider resection should be executed. It is not unusual to remove the ascending ramus of the mandible and a portion of the zygomatic arch. No attempt is made to preserve the facial nerve because it will be sacrificed in the resection.

Osteotomies are now made downward from the temporal craniotomy to reach to the skull base behind and in front of the ear canal. The position of the osteotomies is determined by the extent of the tumor. The temporal lobe is retracted, and the osteotomies are continued medially in the skull base. These extend until the most medial part of the tumor has been passed. Using an air drill from above and below, the carotid artery is freed from its bony canal. It should now be possible to free the petrous bone medially and, by a series of gentle rocking movements, to loosen and remove it. At this point, the main fear is that the internal carotid artery may be disrupted. If possible, some indication of cross-flow should be obtained before surgery. This can be done by compression during angiography, cross-clamping, electroencephalographic evaluation over a time period, or blood flow estimation using radioactive tracers during surgery with occlusion of the internal carotid on the side of surgery. Although these methods are not absolutely accurate, they can be help to

determine whether the vessel can be safely sacrificed without disrupting the patient's neurological status.

If dura has been sacrificed, a repair is performed. There may be no skin defect, and the ear is returned to its former position and sutured. If a defect is present, it may be closed with a scalp rotation flap or, if it is more extensive, a pectoralis myocutaneous flap (30). Latissimus dorsi and trapezius myocutaneous flaps have been used, but these involve turning the patient and are not recommended. More recently, free tissue transfer of latissimus, scapular, or rectus abdominis flaps have been used (31–33).

This is technically a very difficult procedure, and unfortunately, the results are not always satisfactory. In penetrating external basal cell carcinomas and SCC, the results are usually good if the resection is adequate. Middle ear carcinomas are rarely cured even with postoperative radiotherapy. Recurrent parotid tumors give mixed results, particularly types of adenocystic carcinoma, which may recur several years after the original resection. The complications of this procedure are deafness, facial palsy, a potential for severe hemorrhage during surgery, and hemiplegia. Entry into the cavernous sinus may cause blindness or, at least, an immobile eye. Perhaps the most troublesome postoperative problem is vertigo; fortunately, it tends to resolve with time. Postoperative radiotherapy will aggravate this problem and make it more long lasting.

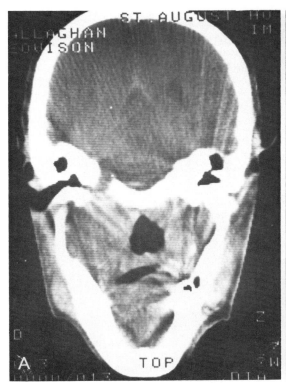
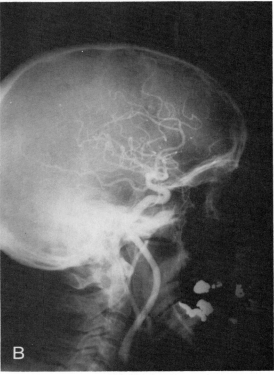

FIGURE 43.13. **A**, Neurofibroma of the posteiror cranial fossa exits into the neck through the jugular foramen, producing "parotid" swelling and wasting of trapezius and sternocleido-mastoid muscles. Coronal CT scan shows enlarged jugular foramen. **B**, Carotid angiogram illustrates anterior displacement of the vessels by the tumor in the neck.

Posterior Cranial Fossa (Posterior Area, Posterior Segment)

Tumors of the posterior cranial fossa rarely involve the plastic surgeon. These are usually acoustic neuromas, neurofibromas, or meningioma; fibrous dysplasia may also occur in this region. Extracranial sarcomas of various cell types arising in the posterior neck may involve this region.

Fortunately, these will usually cause intracranial symptoms such as headache or dizziness; therefore, the patient is directed to the neurologist or neurosurgeon. Because of the tumor position in relation to the cerebellar pontine region, the last four cranial nerves are compressed, resulting in some typical signs. There is wasting and weakness of the trapezius and sternocleidomastoid muscles, wasting of the tongue, hoarseness, and occasionally, dysphagia. The tumor escapes from the jugular foramen and can present as a deep lobe of parotid tumor. On basal tomography and CT scans, the jugular foramen is often much enlarged as compared to the noninvolved side (Fig. 43.13). There may be anterior displacement of the carotid vessels when the tumor extends into the neck.

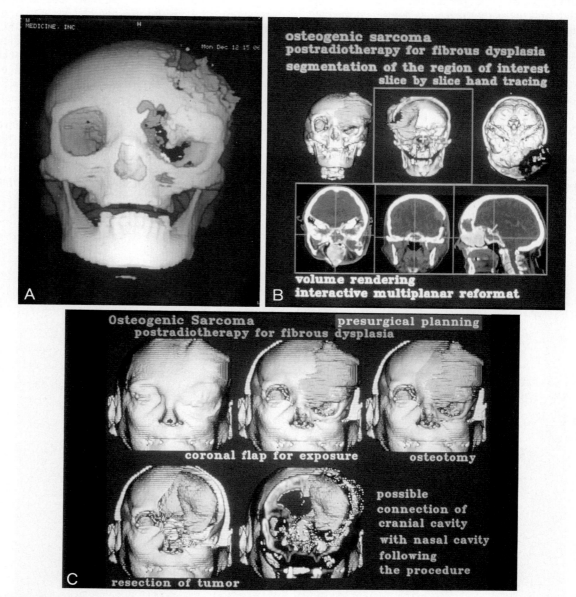

FIGURE 43.14. Three-dimension CT scan imaging. **A**, Commercial three-dimensional CT scan showing right frontoorbital osteogenic sarcoma following radiation therapy for fibrous dysplasia. **B**, New generation of three-dimensional CT scan using Analyze (Department of Biodynamics, Mayo Clinic, Rochester, MN) software. The upper three images show the reformatted CT scan with the tumor in green and the eye in lilac. The lower images are axial, coronal, and sagittal scans taken from the three-dimensional reformatting. **C**, Images produced by Analyze showing the facial soft tissue appearance, the tumor, the planned resection in purple, the anterior part of the planned resection, and the posterior part of the planned resection. These images are useful in giving an approximate idea of what the postresection anatomical defect will be.

Exposure is by a posterior scalp flap based inferiorly; on the side of the tumor, the anterior edge of the incision is carried forward and downward to deal with any tumor extension into the neck. The scalp flap is tedious to raise. Several layers of muscle must be stripped off the skull in the occipital area. The transverse processes of the atlas and axis are reached, and the vertebral artery is preserved.

The jugular foramen is isolated by dissection from the neck. The facial nerve may have to be dissected away from the tumor. An occipital craniotomy is performed to view the intracranial aspect of the tumor. It is now usually possible to perform the resection under good vision. No reconstructive measures are necessary apart from a dural repair if there has been dural damage or involvement.

Conclusion

The adaptation of techniques used in craniofacial deformity correction to skull base tumor resection has greatly improved the lots of the patient and the surgeon. Resections are carried out under good vision with good exposure; therefore, one hopes that the results may be improved. Areas of bone are removed for exposure and subsequently replaced, thus minimizing the eventual deformity. This makes the decision to proceed with surgery somewhat easier for surgeon and patient.

New methods of external prosthesis fitting make life more tolerable after these large procedures. Osseointegrated titanium implants allow the establishment of an external framework onto which the prosthesis may be clipped using magnets (Fig. 43.2**C** and **D**). The use of skull bone grafts and fixation of grafts and bony segments with lag screws and mini and microplates has improved and accelerated such surgery (34).

Preoperative assessment is more sophisticated. All patients have CT scans and many have angiography. It is unwise to attempt to excise a basal skull tumor without knowing the position of the carotid vessels. In some cases, three-dimensional imaging is used (Fig. 43.14), and this may be utilized more frequently in the future. Magnetic resonance imaging is excellent for the delineation of soft tissue and is being used more and more in skull base tumor assessment. With the advent of free tissue transfer using microvascular techniques, reconstruction has become and will become even more sophisticated in time. However, enthusiasm must be tempered by knowledge of tumor biology. In many cases, immediate reconstruction may be performed, but in those cases with multiple recurrences of highly aggressive tumors after multimodality treatment, sophisticated reconstruction should probably be postponed. To have a method available is not a reason for using it! In patients with a dismal prognosis, the very best reconstruction should be performed in order to make the remainder of their lives tolerable (32).

Above all, this type of surgery is a cooperative team effort. Neurosurgeon, plastic surgeon, anesthesiologist, oncologist, and radiotherapist must work together in an integrated fashion. If this is done, the surgery should have a low mortality and, it is hoped, an improved cure rate.

References

1. Ketcham AS, Wilkins RH, Van Buren JM, et al: A combined intracranial facial approach to the paranasal sinuses. *Am J Surg* 106:698, 1963.
2. Ketcham AS, Hoye RC, Van Buren JM, et al: Complications of intracranial facial resection of tumors of the paranasal sinuses. *Am J Surg* 112:591, 1966.
3. Schuller DE, Lawrence TL, Newton WA Jr: Childhood rhabdomyosarcomas of the head and neck. *Arch Otolaryngol* 105:689, 1979.
4. Heyn RM, Holland R, Newton WA Jr, et al: The role of combined chemotherapy in the treatment of rhabdomyosarcoma in children. *Cancer* 34:2128, 1974.
5. Ghavimi F, Exelby PR, D'Angio GJ, et al: Multidisciplinary treatment of embryonal rhabdomyosarcoma in children. *Cancer* 35:677, 1975.
6. Healy GB, Jaffe N, Cassady JR: Rhabdomyosarcoma of the head and neck: Diagnosis and management. *Head Neck Surg* 1:334, 1979.
7. Jackson IT, Hide TAH: Further extensions of craniofacial surgery. *Rec Adv Plast Surg* 2:241, 1981.
8. Jackson IT, Hide TAH: A systematic approach to tumors of the base of the skull. *J Maxillofac Surg* 10:92, 1982.
9. Jackson IT, Hide TAH, Gomuwka PK, et al: Treatment of cranioorbital fibrous dysplasia. *J Maxillofac Surg* 10:138, 1982.
10. Munro IT, Chen YR: Radical treatment for frontoorbital fibrous dysplasia: The chain-link fence. *Plast Reconstr Surg* 67:719, 1981.
11. Tessier P: Autogenous bone grafts from the calvarium for facial and cranial applications. *Clin Plast Surg* 9:531, 1982.
12. Jackson IT, Pellett CC, Smith JM: The skull as a bone graft donor site. *Ann Plast Surg* 11:527, 1983.
13. Jackson IT, Marsh WR, Hide TAH: Treatment of tumors involving the anterior cranial fossa. *Head Neck Surg* 6:901, 1984.
14. Jackson IT, Laws ER, Martin RD: A craniofacial approach to advanced recurrent cancer of the central face. *Head Neck Surg* 5:474, 1983.
15. Ketcham AS, Chretien PB, Schour L, Herdt JR, Ommaya AK, Van Buren JM: Surgical treatment of patients with advanced cancer of the paranasal sinuses. In *Neoplasia of the Head and Neck*. Chicago, Year Book Medical Publishers, 1974, p 187.
16. Ousterhout DK, Tessier P: Closure of large cribriform defects with a forehead flap. *J Maxillofac Surg* 9:7, 1981.
17. Bridger GP: Radical surgery for ethmoid cancer. *Arch Otolaryngol* 106:630, 1980.
18. Jackson IT, Marsh WR, Bite U, et al: Craniofacial osteotomies to facilitate skull base tumour resection. *Br J Plast Surg* 39:153, 1986.
19. van der Meulen JC, Moscona AR, Vandrachen M, et al: Management of orbitofacial neurofibromatosis. *Ann Plast Surg* 8:213, 1982.
20. Marchac D: Intracranial management of the orbital cavity and palpebra remodeling for orbitopalpebral neurofibromatosis. *Plast Reconstr Surg* 73:534, 1981.
21. Jackson IT, Laws ER Jr, Martin RD: The surgical management of orbital neurofibromatosis. *Plast Reconstr Surg* 71:751, 1983.
22. Fisch U, Pillsbury HC, Sasaki CT: Infratemporal approach to the skull base. In Sasaki CT, McCabe BF, Kirchner JA (eds): *Surgery of the Skull Base*. Philadelphia, JB Lippincott Co, 1984, p 141.
23. Jackson IT, Munro IR, Salyer KE, et al: *Atlas of Craniomaxillofacial Surgery*. St. Louis, CV Mosby Co, 1982.
24. Donald RJ: Infratemporal fossa and skull base. In Donald PG (ed): *Head and Neck Cancer. Management of the Difficult Case*. Philadelphia, WB Saunders Co, 1984, p 277.
25. McCabe BF, Work WP: Parotidectomy with special reference to the facial nerve. In English GM (ed): *Otolaryngology*, New York, Harper & Row, 1984, vol 3, chpt 63.

26. Fisch U, Pillsbury HC: Infratemporal fossa approach to lesions in the temporal bone and base of the skull. *Arch Otolaryngol* 105:99, 1979.
27. Jackson IT, Smith J, Mixter RC: Nasal bone grafting using split skull grafts. *Ann Plast Surg* 11:533, 1983.
28. Campbell E, Volk BM, Burklund CW: Total resection of the temporal bone for malignancy of the middle ear. *Ann Surg* 134:397, 1951.
29. Parsons H, Lewis JS: Subtotal resection of the temporal bone for cancer of the ear. *Cancer* 7:995, 1954.
30. Baker SR: Surgical reconstruction after extensive skull base surgery. *Otolaryngol Clin North Am* 17:591, 1984.
31. Jones NF, Sekhar LN, Schramm VL: Free rectus abdominis muscle flap reconstruction of the middle and posterior cranial base. *Plast Reconstr Surg* 78:471, 1986.
32. Jones NF, Hardesty RA, Swartz WM, et al: Extensive and complex defects of the scalp, middle third of the face and palate: The role of microsurgical reconstruction. *Plast Reconstr Surg* 82:937, 1988.
33. Jackson IT, Tolman DE, Desjardins RP, et al: A new method for fixation of external prostheses. *Plast Reconstr Surg* 77:668, 1986.
34. French DJ, Jackson IT, Tolman DE: A system of osseointegrated implants and its application to dental and facial rehabilitation. *Eur J Plast Surg* 11(1):14, 1988.

44

Basic Principles of Reconstruction of the Lip, Oral Commissure, and Cheek

Norman Hugo, M.D., F.A.C.S.

The face and notably the lips and cheeks are important structures not only of aesthetic value but also for expression vibrancy, and vitality. As such, both functional and aesthetic restoration of deformed parts receive high priority. The aims of reconstruction in the lips and cheeks are the restoration of appearance and reinstitution of function. Often, this involves the repair of several layers of missing tissues, and these need to be supplied in order to attain a superior result. This chapter deals sequentially with deformities of the lips and then deformities of the cheeks. With the advent of newer approaches, many of the older procedures are not presently used. Such advances as musculocutaneous flaps have allowed greater imagination and magnitude in reconstruction and as a consequence surgeons have achieved superior results.

It is axiomatic in the repair of cheek and lip defects that the best source of donor material is similar tissue. If the lip can be reconstructed with lip tissue, this is the better way. Similarly, if one can use tissues from the head and neck area in juxtaposition to the cheek for its reconstruction, the results are usually better. Although this is not always possible, the surgeon should think of these donor areas primarily. While free flaps are more dramatic, their color and thickness often are unsuitable for repair in those areas.

Lips

LIP SHAVE WITH MUCOSAL ADVANCEMENT

For patients with severe leukoplakia or multiple superficial carcinomas from prolonged smoking and exposure to the elements, the procedure of choice is a lip shave. This is done by excising the mucosa from the vermilion border backward until the unaffected area is reached. It is excised down to the muscle. Bilateral relaxing incisions are made laterally at each corner of the mouth downward into the deep sulcus and the entire mucosa is elevated and advanced forward to cover the area (1). The mucosa will become keratinized after exposure (Fig. 44.1). The cosmetic result is quite acceptable and the recurrence rate minimal in properly selected patients (2).

COMMISSURE REPAIR

After a surgical or traumatic insult, such as an electrical burn, to the commissure in which the vermilion and a portion of the skin and muscle are destroyed, the resul-

tant cicatricial healing obliterates the normal sharp angle of the mouth as well as reduces the aperture. Previous methods of repair have employed creation of small flaps in which either the upper or the lower lip is repaired and then mucosa is advanced to cover the donor defect (3, 4). This has resulted in adequate repair but usually a rounded commissure. A simpler method with better results is incision to restore the oral aperture and a hook to prevent reapproximation of the raw surfaces (5). With subsequent epithelialization and maintenance of the hook until scarring subsides, good results are obtained (Fig. 44.2).

PRIMARY CLOSURE OF THE LIP

Approximately one third of the lip may be sacrificed and the lip closed directly without undue changes. This rule of thumb is slightly less applicable to young patients, and there is a greater range with older patients, some of whom can have 40% of the lip removed and primary closure done (6, 7).

FLAP CLOSURE

Fan Flap

The fan flap (8) is based on the labial artery. A large superiorly based flap is constructed by through-and-through incision of the lateral portions of the upper lip and the remaining portions of the lower lip (Fig. 44.3**A**). After complete mobilization the flap is swung toward the midline of the lower lip to reconstruct the defect (Fig. 44.3**B**). As a matter of practical import, the flap is well suited for large defects but the tip of this flap has a tendency to necrose. Again, it also tends to round the commissures. Interestingly, both the fan flap and the Abbé-Estlander flap are capable of motor reinnervation (9).

Lip Switch

The lip switch is also known as the vermilion switch, Abbé flap, or Estlander flap. The basic concept involved in this approach is the borrowing of a portion of one lip for switching to the other lip. This can include something as small as vermilion and underlying muscle, which can be switched as a pedicle flap to reconstruct a vermilion defect and the pedicle severed 7–10 days later (10). In addition, it may include whole segments of lip skin in order to reconstruct large defects (11, 12; Fig. 44.4). For

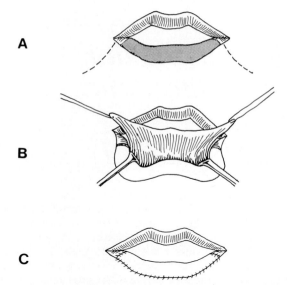

FIGURE 44.1. An artist's sketch of lip shave. **A**, Resection of mucosa and lower lip is diagrammed. **B**, Advancement of intraoral labial mucosa. **C**, Mucosa is sutured into place. Keratinization occurs with exposure.

differentiation, an Abbé flap does not include the corner of the mouth, whereas the Estlander flap does. In other respects they are basically the same. Care should be taken not to create a flap larger than one third of the donor lip because primary closure is required to repair the donor lip. Various other modifications of borrowing from one lip to another have been described and are limited only by the surgeon's imagination. However, they are based on the same principle of the labial artery being included in the wedge type of pedicle.

Nasolabial Flap

A commonly employed local flap for reconstruction of the lip is the nasolabial flap (Fig. 44.5). This is a reliable random flap that is rotated primarily without delay into rather large defects of the lips. The key is to dissect the flap down to the underlying musculature to ensure viability. In addition, the flap should be made relatively broad at its distal end in order to prevent tip necrosis and trapdooring after insetting.

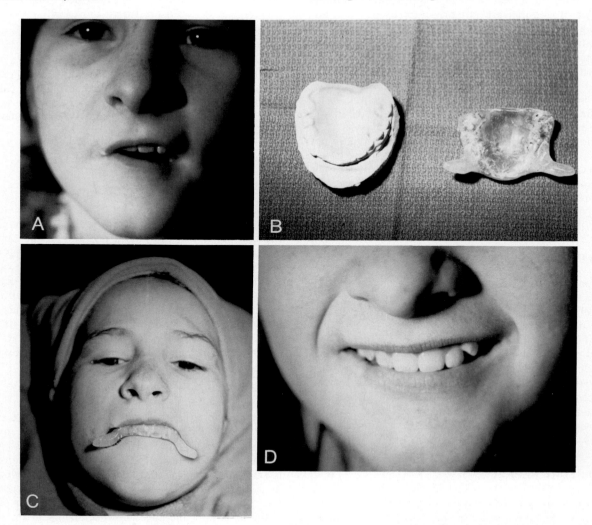

FIGURE 44.4. **A**, Infiltrating morphea-type basal cell carcinoma with vermilion retraction. **B**, Defect after Moh's chemosurgery. **C and D**, Immediate repair is performed with Abbé-Estlander flap.

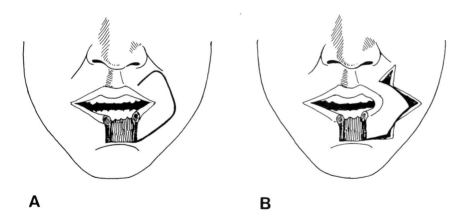

A   **B**

FIGURE 44.3. An artist's sketch of the fan flap. **A**, Construction of fan flap is performed by through-and-through incisions. **B**, The entire segment is rotated medially to close defect. Rounding of commissure occurs.

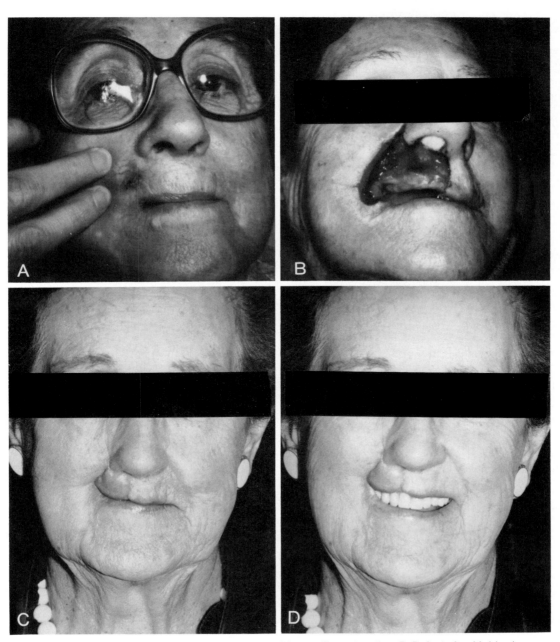

FIGURE 44.4. **A**, Infiltrating morphea-type basal cell carcinoma with vermilion retraction. **B**, Defect after Moh's chemosurgery. **C and D**, Immediate repair is performed with Abbé-Estlander flap.

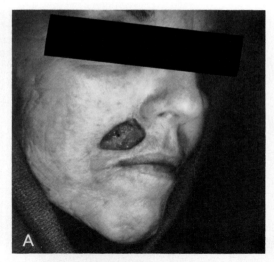

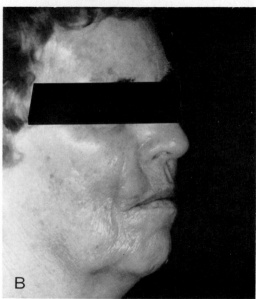

FIGURE 44.5. **A**, A defect of the cheek and lip after Moh's chemosurgery. **B**, Inset of broad nasolabial flap.

Orbicularis Oris Myocutaneous Flap (Karapandzic)

When large amounts of lower lip tissue are replaced by noninnervated, non–muscle-bearing tissue, there results a patulous lip without sphincteric action causing lack of expression and drooling. The orbicularis oris and its overlying skin may be circumferentially raised as an innervated separate myocutaneous flap to secure closure of the lip. This is done by separating it from the supporting muscles of expression while maintaining its nerve and blood supply (Fig. 44.6). Two relative shortcomings have been identified: microstomia and tightness of the lower lip (13).

TISSUE EXPANSION

Reconstruction also is possible with the use of local flaps. Although reconstruction was formerly restricted to only small defects, with the use of tissue expanders the local recruitment of tissue for areas around the face is substantial (Fig. 44.7). It is done under the same principles that govern tissue expansion in any other area of the body except that it is not as well tolerated as in some areas, with exposure not uncommon. Large amounts of skin, however, can be recruited and have substantially good blood supply (14, 15). It is a well-known fact that the area becomes highly vascular and actually makes the tissues look poor initially, with a great deal of redness and telangiectases. However, after it has been moved and sutured into place this resolves and the area achieves normal facial color again. Its inherent advantage is the recruitment of large areas of tissue similar to that of the area that requires reconstruction.

Cheek

Defects of the cheek can be repaired with small grafts, local flaps, flaps from the forehead, tissue expansion, and massive myocutaneous flaps from the area. With the advent of the musculocutaneous-type flaps surgeons

FIGURE 44.6. An artist's sketch of Karapandzic repair. **A**, Innervated and vascularized orbicularis oris myocutaneous flap is separated from the muscles of expression. **B**, Closure with some microstomia is evident.

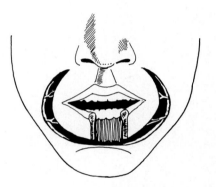

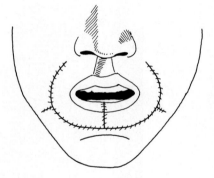

A   **B**

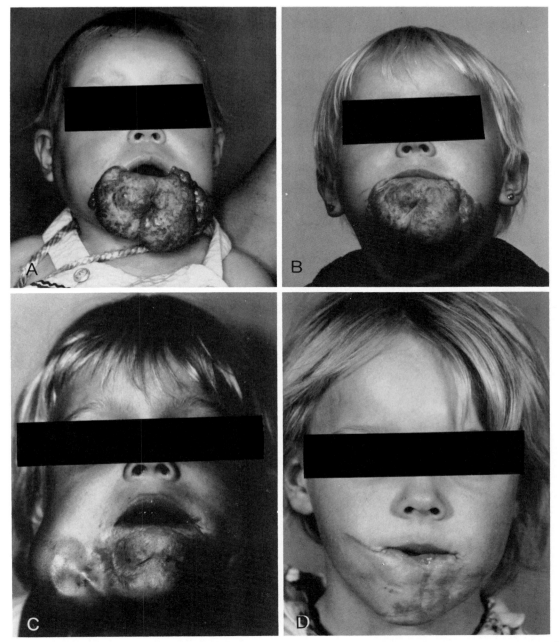

FIGURE 44.7. **A**, A massive hemangioma of the lower lip. **B**, Degree of involution after several years. **C**, Tissue expander is used in the right cheek. The expander in left cheek had ex- truded. **D**, After resection of lip and chin, expanded tissue is advanced.

achieved an enormous advantage. Previously, flaps from a distance, such as Zovickian flaps (16) and the like, were used successfully to resurface the area but at some cost to the esthetic result. In addition, a great deal of time was used in delaying flaps. In today's practice, there is good reason to use the local type of flaps, which blend very nicely with the surrounding tissues, produce a superior esthetic result, and produce an immediate result.

SKIN GRAFTS

Skin grafts either may be a temporary cover or may be used as a permanent cover. Of course, they are restricted to partial-thickness defects. A temporary cover might be employed while evaluating the area for cancer recurrence in a particularly difficult case. Later, the graft can be removed and definitive reconstruction utilized.

LOCAL FLAPS

Flaps used in cheek reconstruction are basically Mustardé-type flaps (17), which mobilize a large area to be rotated into the defect (Fig. 44.8). This can effectively cover a relatively large defect with minimal distortion and with good color match. They have a good record of survivability. Smaller types of local flaps that can be employed are Limberg-type (rhomboid) flaps, which can be used to cover medium-sized defects not through and through in nature. The fact that many of these defects are in older people with lax skin should not be forgotten, and sometimes rather large defects can be reconstructed by

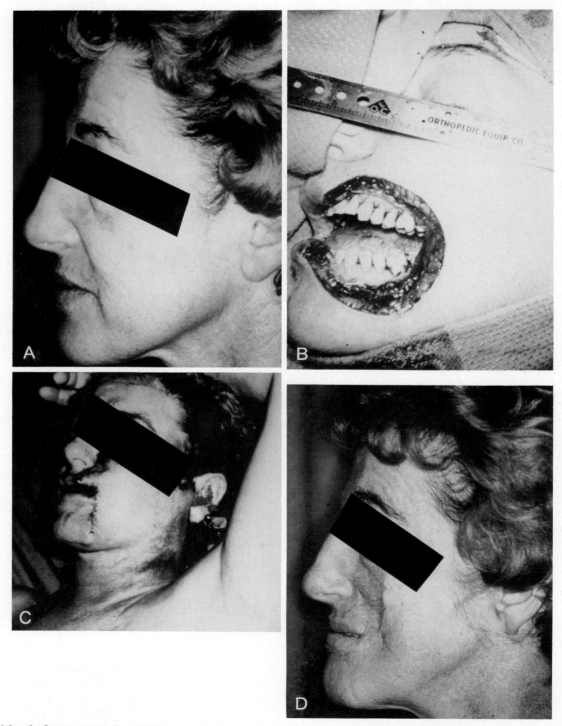

FIGURE 44.8. **A**, Squamous cell carcinoma is infiltrating the upper lip. **B**, Defect after adequate resection. **C**, Immediate repair is performed with a Mustardé-type flap. **D**, The result at 6 months.

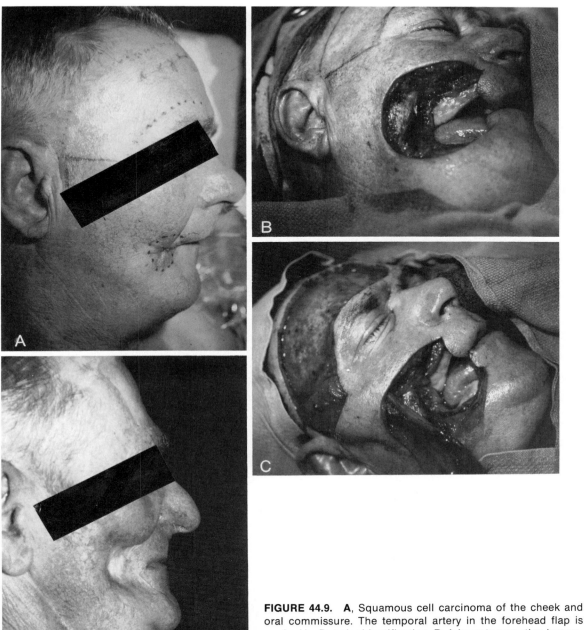

FIGURE 44.9. **A**, Squamous cell carcinoma of the cheek and oral commissure. The temporal artery in the forehead flap is marked by Doppler identification. **B**, Adequate resection is monitored by frozen section, creating a through-and-through defect. **C**, Forehead flap is passed superficial to the zygomatic arch to be inserted into the defect and covered with a graft. **D**, The final result after detaching the forehead flap and returning a portion to the forehead.

simply advancing the skin over the area with quite good esthetic results.

DISTANT FLAPS

Forehead Flap

The forehead flap (18) was formerly the most commonly used flap for the cheek area. Based on the tempo-ral artery, it is raised as a large unit taking the entire forehead and either curling it upon itself or reversing it to cover its surface with a skin graft for through-and-through defects (Fig. 44.9). The flap is relatively well hidden on the face, but the skin graft on the forehead is clearly visible, although with the passage of years it blends to an appreciable degree. There is also an indentation in the cheek as a result of the thinness of forehead compared to cheek tissue.

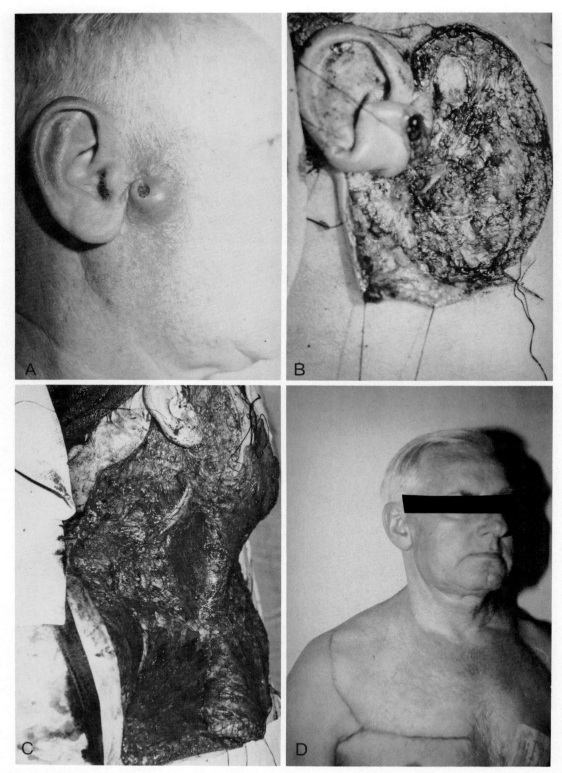

FIGURE 44.10.   **A**, Squamous cell carcinoma in cyst. **B**, The defect after adequate resection. **C**, A cervicopectoral flap is raised. **D**, The final result.

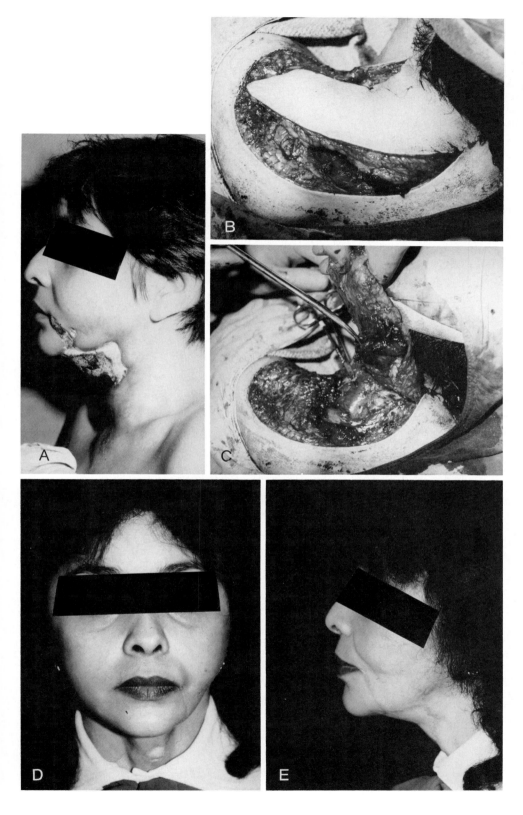

FIGURE 44.11. **A**, A tissue slough of lower cheek and upper neck. **B**, The transverse trapezius flap is raised after initial delay of distal portion. **C**, Extent of muscle incorporated into flap and preservation of spinal accessory nerve. **D and E**, The final result.

Pectoralis Major Flap

The pectoralis major myocutaneous flap is also used in reconstructing major cheek defects (19). It has supplemented the deltopectoral flap as the workhorse for head and neck reconstruction. Laterally based on the thoracoacromial artery, it can be used to cover defects as distal as the orbit. Some have believed that the flap was too bulky (20), although others have disagreed (21).

In analyzing complications of this technique in 36 patients, Mehrhof et al. (22) reported total flap necrosis in three, and partial flap necrosis in nine, with an overall complication rate of 59%. Ariyan (21) reported only partial loss of one pedicle in 20 cases. Muscle perforators from the internal mammary artery supply the muscle medially and nourish the flap when it is used as the cervicopectoral flap (Fig. 44.10). This is an excellent flap with good esthetic coverage because the tissue covering the defect is recruited from the head and neck area. The cervical portion is a random flap but needs no delay, although the platysma muscle must be incorporated within it (23).

Trapezius Flap

The trapezius myocutaneous flap provides excellent cover for the lower face. Its blood supply originates from the transverse cervical artery, which branches into ascending and descending branches. The vertical flap creates a less noticeable donor defect, but the transverse flap has an arc of rotation that makes it quite applicable to lower cheek defects. When using the transverse flap, the spinal accessory nerve can be dissected out to preserve function (Fig. 44.11). The donor defect is more apparent with the transverse flap but its skin is thinner so that it blends better with the face. Muscle is included only in the proximal portion of the flap. The distal portion of this flap is a random flap and should be delayed to ensure viability (24).

Sternocleidomastoid Flap

The sternocleidomastoid myocutaneous flap was one of the first such flaps described but was unrecognized as such at the time when first presented in 1949 (25). Its blood supply has been documented by Jabaley et al. (26). It has been used to carry up the clavicle to repair mandibular defects (27). It is not a first choice for soft tissue repair of the cheek.

Retroauricular Flap

A unique flap for reconstruction of the upper cheek has been described by Washio (28, 29). It provides for thin, nonbearing skin and an easily camouflaged donor defect. It survives on connections between the retroauricular artery and the superficial temporal artery. It is limited by the small amount of tissue available and the fact that little tailoring of the flap is possible once it is harvested. Accu-

rate preoperative planning is essential. It does provide tissue similar to that of the cheek and the donor defect is easily hidden.

Platysma Flap

The platysma flap is well described (30) and can be employed for coverage near the commissure or intraorally over the jaw. It is not a robust flap and, at least in our hands, the skin paddle can be precarious.

References

1. Spira M, Hardy SB: Vermilionectomy: Review of cases with variations in techniques. *Plast Reconstr Surg* 33:39, 1964.
2. Birt BD: The "lip shave" operation for premalignant conditions and microinvasive carcinoma of the lower lip. *J Otolaryngol* 6:407, 1977.
3. Kazanjian VH, Roopenian A: The treatment of lip deformities resulting from electric burns. *Am J Surg* 88:884, 1954.
4. Converse JM: Technique of elongation of the oral fissure and restoration of the angle of the mouth. In Kazanjian VH, Converse JM (eds): *The Surgical Treatment of Facial Injuries.* Baltimore, Williams & Wilkins Co, 1959, p 795.
5. Czerepack CS: Oral splint therapy to manage electrical burns of the mouth in children. *Clin Plast Surg* 11:685, 1984.
6. Fries R: Advantage of a basic concept in lip reconstruction after tumor resection. *J Maxillofac Surg* 1:13, 1973.
7. Madden JJ Jr, Erhardt WL Jr, Franklin JD, et al: Reconstruction of the upper and lower lip using a modified Bernard-Burow technique. *Ann Plast Surg* 5:100, 1980.
8. Gillies H, Millard DR Jr: *The Principles and Art of Plastic Surgery.* Boston, Little, Brown and Co, 1959, p 117.
9. Rea JL, Davis WE, Rittenhouse LK: Reinnervation of an Abbe-Estlander and a Gillies fan flap of the lower lip. *Arch Otolaryngol* 104:294, 1978.
10. Kawamoto HK Jr: Correction of major defects of the vermilion with a cross-lip vermilion flap. *Plast Reconstr Surg* 64:315, 1979.
11. Abbé R: A new plastic operation for the relief of deformity due to double harelip. *Med Rec* 5:477, 1898.
12. Estlander JA: Eine methode aus der einen lippe substanzverluste der anderen zu ersetzen. *Arch Klin Chir* 14:622, 1872. (Also in The Classic Reprint. Translated by Sundell B. *Plast Reconstr Surg* 42:361, 1968.)
13. Jabaley ME, Clement RL, Orcutt TW: Myocutaneous flaps in lip reconstruction; applications of the Karapandzic principle. *Plast Reconstr Surg* 59:680, 1977.
14. Sasaki GH, Pang CY: Pathophysiology of skin flaps raised on expanded pig skin. *Plast Reconstr Surg* 74:59:1984.
15. Manders EK, Schenden MJ, Furrey JA, et al: Soft tissue expansion: Concepts and complications. *Plast Reconstr Surg* 74:493, 1984.
16. Zovickian A: Pharyngeal fistulas: Repair and prevention using mastoid-occiput based shoulder flaps. *Plast Reconstr Surg* 19:355, 1957.
17. Mustardé JC: *Repair and Reconstruction in the Orbital Region. A Practical Guide.* Baltimore, Williams & Wilkins Co, 1966.
18. McGregor IA, Reid WH: The use of the temporal flap in primary repair of full-thickness defects of the cheek. *Plast Reconstr Surg* 38:1, 1966.
19. Ariyan S: The pectoralis major myocutaneous flap: A versatile flap for reconstruction in head and neck. *Plast Reconstr Surg* 63:73:1979.
20. Theogaraj SD, Merritt WH, Acharya G, et al: The pectoralis major musculocutaneous island flap in single stage reconstruction of the pharyngoesophageal region. *Plast Reconstr Surg* 65:267, 1980.
21. Ariyan S: The pectoralis major for single stage reconstruction of

the difficult wounds of the orbit and pharyngoesophagus. *Plast Reconstr Surg* 72:468, 1983.

22. Mehrhof AL Jr, Rosenstock A, Neifeld JP, et al: The pectoralis major myocutaneous flap in head and neck reconstruction. Analysis of complications. *Am J Surg* 146:478, 1983.

23. Becker DW: A cervicopectoral rotation flap for cheek coverage. *Plast Reconstr Surg* 61:868, 1978.

24. McGraw JB, Magee WP, Kalwaic H: Use of the trapezius and sternomastoid myocutaneous flaps in head and neck surgery. *Plast Reconstr Surg* 63:49, 1979.

25. Owens N: A compound neck pedicle designed for the repair of massive facial defects: Formation, development, and application. *Plast Reconstr Surg* 15:369, 1955.

26. Jabaley ME, Heckler FR, Wallace WH, et al: Sternocleidomas-

toid regional flaps; a new look at an old concept. *Br J Plast Surg* 32:106, 1979.

27. Siemssen SO, Kirby B, O'Connor TPF: Immediate reconstruction of a resected segment of the lower jaw, using a compound flap of clavicle and sternomastoid muscle. *Plast Reconstr Surg* 61:724, 1978.

28. Washio H: Retroauricular temporal flap. *Plast Reconstr Surg* 43:162, 1969.

29. Washio H: Further experiences with the retroauricular flap. *Plast Reconstr Surg* 50:160, 1972.

30. Coleman JJ III, Jurkiewicz MJ, Nahai F, et al: The platysma musculocutaneous flap: Experience with 24 cases. *Plast Reconstr Surg* 72:315, 1983.

45

Reconstruction of the Nose

Fritz E. Barton, Jr., M.D., F.A.C.S.

There is probably no better way to chronicle the development of the field of plastic surgery than to trace the series of attempts to reconstruct the human nose over the centuries. Amputation of the tip of the nose was a common form of punishment among some of the primitive Asian cultures, and it was practiced upon conquered enemies and transgressors of social laws. It is not surprising, then, that one of the earliest accounts of repair of an absent nasal part appeared in the Brahmin holy books of India, the Suśrutaś Áyurvéda (ca. 600 B.C.). Subsequent historical references are scarce until the Renaissance, when modern medicine became formalized.

The history of nasal reconstruction evolved along three basic lines: (*a*) the Indian method of midline forehead flap; (*b*) the Italian method of brachial flap; and (*c*) the French method of lateral cheek flap (1–3).

The technique of using midline forehead tissue in a pedicle flap apparently originated with early Indian cultures. With the exploration of the Indian subcontinent by the Italians and its later occupation by the British, the Indian method was carried back to Europe. The Brancas of Sicily are said to have experimented with the midline forehead flap, but documentation of its use first appeared in an article published in the *Gentleman's Magazine* of London in 1794, apparently authored by Mr. Lucas, an English surgeon residing in Madras. Joseph Carpue subsequently popularized the method in Europe as a result of his 1816 report.

The use of an arm flap for nasal reconstruction is ascribed to Gaspar Tagliacozzi in 1597, and this method still bears his name.

During the 19th century, German and French surgeons under the leadership of Dieffenbach developed several procedures involving cheek tissue to restore missing nasal parts.

Anatomy

To evaluate the various options in nasal reconstruction, one must be familiar with the component anatomy of this peculiar structure. Cottle's (4) terminology refers to the mobile lower portion of the nose as the *lobule,* and this is further divided into the *tip, alae, columella* (including the membranous septum), and *nostril sills.* The *soft triangle* consists of the area at the apex of each vestibule where the arch of the ala joins the columella (Fig. 45.1**A**).

The soft triangle is in reality a web of skin located just caudal to the dome of each alar cartilage.

To be judged "excellent," a procedure for nasal reconstruction must reproduce the normal anatomy of the nose from every perspective. The most discriminating angle is from below, the so-called worm's-eye view. For the proportions to be pleasing, the tip should be no smaller than one half of but no greater than equal to the height of the nostril as measured from the basal projection (5). The caliber and patency of the internal nasal valve must be maintained, and the thickness and stability of the alar wing must also be considered.

A cross section of the ala shows inner skin with keratinized squamous epithelium and a very thin dermal layer, perichondrium, alar cartilage, external perichondrium, a thin subcutaneous layer, and dorsal skin with a thick dermal layer and prominent sebaceous appendages. This laminar arrangement is thin enough to maintain a large intranasal caliber yet sufficiently flexible and sturdy to prevent collapse on inspiration.

The best results in nasal reconstruction often derive from combinations of several small tissue units rather than attempts to shape multiple contours from one tissue mass. Optimal placement of scar in the various tissue junctions must be kept in mind (6, 7; Fig. 45.1**B**).

Classification

When planning a nasal reconstruction, the defect must be evaluated for (*a*) its anatomical location, (*b*) surface extent, and (*c*) layers involved. Defects of similar size present vastly different reconstructive challenges when located in different anatomical regions of the nose. The surface dimension of a defect is also an important consideration because many of the reconstructive techniques are limited by the size of the available donor tissue. However, perhaps the most significant indicator of the complexity of a reconstruction is the missing layer(s).

Anatomically, the nose can be divided into the *proximal one third,* overlying the nasal bones; the *middle one third,* overlying the upper lateral cartilages; and the *distal one third,* comprising the nasal tip, alae, columella, and nostril sills. From a surgical standpoint, the nose consists of *skin cover, skeletal support,* and *lining.* Most nasal defects involve loss of external skin and various amounts of deep layers.

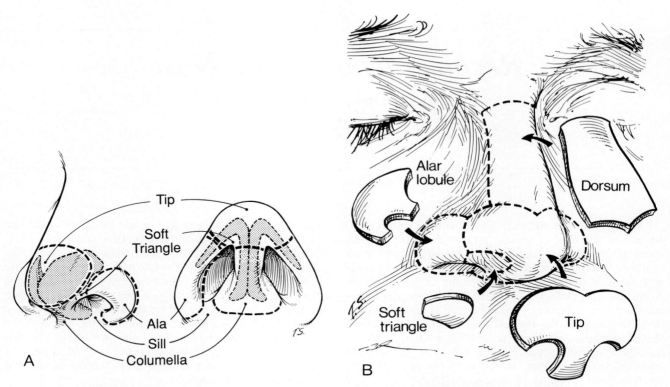

FIGURE 45.1. **A,** Anatomy of the nasal lobule. **B,** Esthetic topographical subunits of the nose.

Skin Cover

Essential considerations in choosing an appropriate cover for the missing nasal part are the color, texture, thickness, and vascularity of the skin immediately surrounding the defect. If skeletal support is needed, this will also influence the choice of coverage.

The skin of the upper two thirds of the nose is usually fine in texture, with little sebaceous gland activity and a thin dermis. The subcutaneous layer contains scant fat and acts largely as an areolar gliding plane over the periosteum. Reconstructions in the upper two thirds of the nose tend to be comparatively simple because of the abundant supply of matching skin in the adjacent nasal dorsum as well as in the postauricular and supraclavicular areas.

In contrast, the skin of the lower one third of the nose is often coarse, thick, and oily. By and large, similarly colored skin of appropriate dermal thickness and sebaceous content can only be found in the face, which limits the reconstructive options. In addition, because the skin is closely adhered to the alar cartilages, only minimal shifting of tissues is possible without risking distortion of alar shape. Esthetic repairs in the nasal lobule tend to require a measure of skeletal underpinning to preserve (or reproduce) the delicate contours of the nostril and nasal tip.

GRAFTS

Split-Thickness Skin Grafts

Split-thickness skin grafts (STSGs) invariably result in a light, shiny, and depressed patch that stands out from the surrounding nasal skin. Moreover, upon contraction, a STSG will pull and distort adjacent structures; therefore, they are reserved for use in debilitated patients with large defects to provide a healed surface on which to mount an external prosthesis.

Full-Thickness Skin Grafts

Full-thickness skin grafts (FTSGs) are useful in covering surface losses in the upper two thirds of the nose, especially if the bed is shallow and well vascularized. As the thickness of the graft dermis increases, however, so does the risk of incomplete graft take. Therefore, one should exercise caution when harvesting FTSGs from the nasolabial and posterior cervical areas. Full-thickness grafts can be a good choice of coverage for the nasal tip in certain patients, primarily women, with thin, minimally sebaceous skin. For most people, however, pedicled flaps from the nasolabial fold or forehead are safer and equally attractive options for tip coverage.

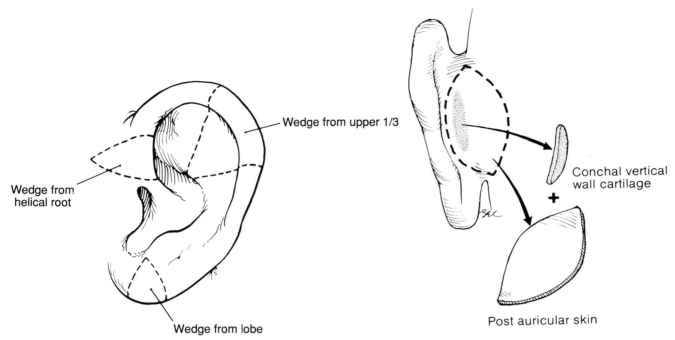

FIGURE 45.2.   Common sources of composite graft from the ear. (Figure at right from Barton FE Jr: Aesthetic aspects of partial nasal reconstruction. *Clin Plast Surg* 8:177, 1981.)

Composite Grafts

The use of composite grafts in nasal reconstruction dates to König in 1902 (8). A common source of skin-cartilage composite tissue is the ear: appropriately carved grafts from the helical root (9), helical rim (10), and concha (10) may be used to restore the alar margin, whereas composites of skin and fat from the ear lobe (11) are sometimes used to repair defects in the columella and membranous septum (Fig. 45.2).

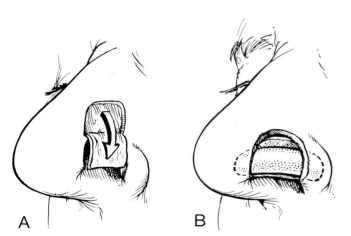

FIGURE 45.3.   A, Turn-in flap for nasal lining. **B,** Cartilage graft applied to lining flap to stabilize the alar rim.

The recipient bed of a composite graft must be carefully prepared, and no part of the graft must be more than 0.5 cm away from an adequate capillary bed if it is to survive in its entirety. All fibrotic, granulation, or scar tissue must be resected from the recipient bed before the graft is applied. Chondrocutaneous grafts to the alar margin may be combined with turn-in flaps from the edge of the wound. After the flap is opened like the pages of a book, it not only creates a good raw surface on which to seat the graft, but its skin, which now faces inward, can be used as lining (12; Fig. 45.3).

FLAPS

The usual sources of flap tissue for reconstruction of the nose are the residual nasal dorsum, adjacent cheek, forehead, and temporal scalp. Remote sites are rarely used because of the desirability of using flaps from the head and neck area that have skin with actinic exposure similar to that of the nose and that can be rotated or transposed in the simplest, most expeditious manner.

Local Nasal Flaps

A number of procedures have been designed to take advantage of the laxity of the skin in the upper two thirds of the nose. The *banner flap* is a small triangular flap based at the edge of the defect and at right angles to it

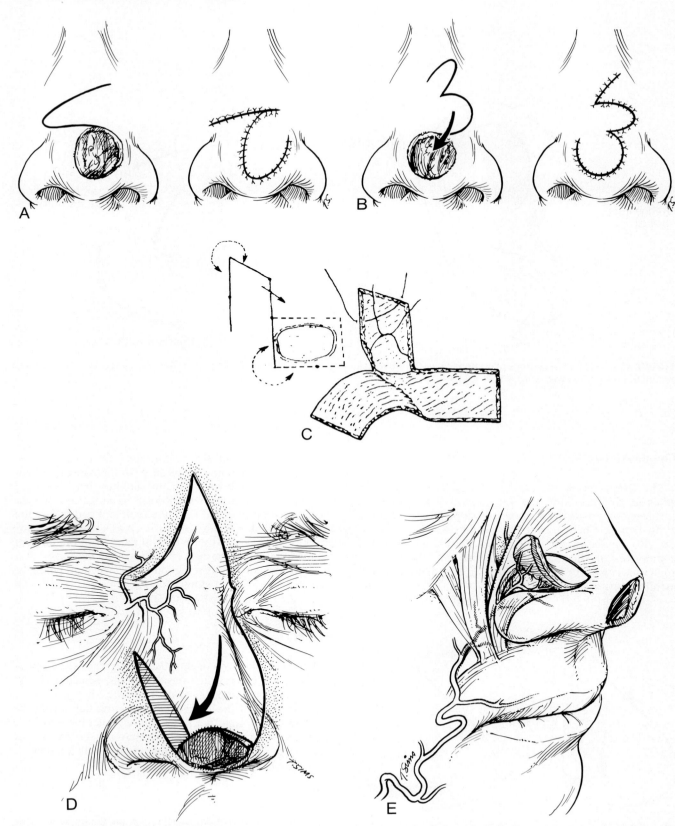

FIGURE 45.4. **A,** Banner flap. **B,** Bilobed flap. **C,** Limberg flap. **D,** Dorsal nasal flap. **E,** Nasalis sliding flap. (Figure C from Limberg AA: *The Planning of Local Plastic Operations on the Body* *Surface. Theory and Practice.* Translated by SA Wolfe. Lexington, MA, DC Heath & Co, 1984.)

(13, 14; Fig. 45.4**A**). The donor site is closed directly by undermining and advancement from the dorsum. When designed on the side of the defect, the banner flap will cover wounds up to 1.2 cm in diameter (13); based contralaterally, it serves for defects 1.5–2.0 cm (14) while causing minimal secondary asymmetry of the nasal tip.

The *bilobed flap* (15, 16; Fig. 45.4**B**) and the *geometric flaps* of Limberg and Dufourmentel (17; Fig. 45.4**C**) offer reliable alternatives in the repair of small full-thickness nasal deficits.

The *dorsal nasal flap* is based on the angular vessels at the intercanthal region and involves downward rotation of the entire nasal dorsal skin (18–21; Fig. 45.4**D**). Flap reach is increased when the flap is based contralateral to the defect.

The arc of flap rotation creates a dog-ear in the glabella, which is resected and sutured vertically to mimic one of the natural frown lines. The lower border of the flap is designed to coincide with the nostril wing–nasal sidewall depression to better hide the scar; therefore, the dorsal nasal flap will not reach over the tip and into the columella without distortion.

Small defects of the lateral lobule may be covered with sliding nasalis myocutaneous flaps from the alar crease (22; Fig. 45.4**E**).

Flaps from the Cheek

Approximately 2.5–3.0 cm of redundant skin is available from the paranasal area of the cheek for use in the nose (23). Accordingly, nasolabial flaps are a time-honored solution (24) to the problem of through-and-through losses of nasal tissue within these size limits. Nasolabial flaps may be advanced (25), transposed on a cutaneous pedicle (26, 27), or raised on a subcutaneous vascular island (28).

Nasolabial (*cheek*) *advancement* flaps are most applicable in small defects of the lateral ala. To reach the central lobule, the incision is carried along the alar crease to help camouflage the scar and to avoid taking alar skin, which is tightly bound to the alar cartilages and whose subdermal collateral supply is poor (Fig. 45.5**A**).

With the flap raised on a subcutaneous vascular pedicle, nasolabial tissue may be advanced medially to cover defects of the nostril wing or upper lateral cartilage area (28, 29). The donor site is closed in V-Y, S, or kite-like fashion (30).

Whether elevated as a direct cutaneous advancement flap or on a subcutaneous base, the sliding nasolabial technique often obliterates the natural alar groove, which must be re-created at a secondary procedure.

Nasolabial *transposition flaps* have been used in nasal reconstruction for centuries (24). They may be based inferiorly or superiorly, but the superior pedicle flap is more popular because it is more versatile. Either way, the flap may be designed to border the ala-cheek junction, thus preserving the crease and avoiding later revisions.

After transfer to the nose, the tip of a superiorly based nasolabial flap can be doubled under to serve as lining for the reconstruction (27; Fig. 45.5**B**). In these cases, a delay procedure is advised. This is an excellent option for coverage of defects of the ala and lateral lobule.

Nasolabial flaps can also be designed with the base adjacent to the alar defect, turned over so the skin of the flap faces the vestibule for lining, and rotated 90° before folding the distal flap over itself for skin cover (31). Because this method makes no provision for cartilage insertion, its primary indication is in the repair of lateral defects of the ala.

Flaps from the Forehead and Temporal Scalp

The *midline forehead flap* has been the mainstay of nasal reconstruction for centuries. As originally performed in India, the flap is elevated along a straight vertical line on the central forehead (32). However, this limits application to patients with generous foreheads; consequently, many modifications have been designed to accommodate patients with low hairlines. The flap paddle has been canted diagonally (33; Fig. 45.6**A**), angled alongside the hairline (34, 35), and given wings like a bird (36–38; Fig. 45.6**B**). Alternatively, the base of the flap can be extended caudally into the glabella (3), taking care to protect the supratrochlear vessels supplying the flap.

Adjustments in flap thickness have also been suggested to fit the method to the defect at hand (3, 35, 39). For instance, it may be necessary to resect the frontalis muscle from the undersurface of the flap and thin the subcutaneous tissue to reproduce the right degree of bulk for nostril wing. In contrast, central lobule and tip defects are best reconstructed with a full-thickness flap.

Midline forehead flaps lend themselves well to lamination with all the necessary components of a reconstruction (3, 35, 40, 41; Fig. 45.6**D**). A complete replica of the missing nasal part can be assembled on the forehead and allowed to heal in place, while blood supply and lymphatic drainage are still predictable, before flap transfer. Once the edema subsides, the pedicle is divided, and the base is replaced in the glabella.

Millard's "*seagull-shaped*" modification of the midline forehead flap combines ample skin at the tip for extensive lobular reconstruction with a pedicle no wider than 1 inch (37; Fig. 45.6**C**). The gull "wings" lie transversely on the forehead, which means they can be closed primarily and the horizontal scars can be hidden in the forehead creases. The donor site for the pedicle is sutured directly or allowed to granulate for later revision. When alar rim reconstruction is contemplated, Millard recommended applying an auricular chondrocutaneous graft to the underside of the leading edge of the appropriate "wing" (37).

To avoid a scar in the central forehead, several flaps have been designed that make use of tissue from the lateral forehead and scalp and that are supplied by the contralateral superficial temporal vessels. Foremost among these are Gillies's (42) modified *up-and-down flap*, New's (43) *sickle flap,* and Converse's (44–46) *scalping flap* (Fig. 45.7).

The original description of the *scalping flap* called for infolding the tip of the flap to create the alar rim(s). It

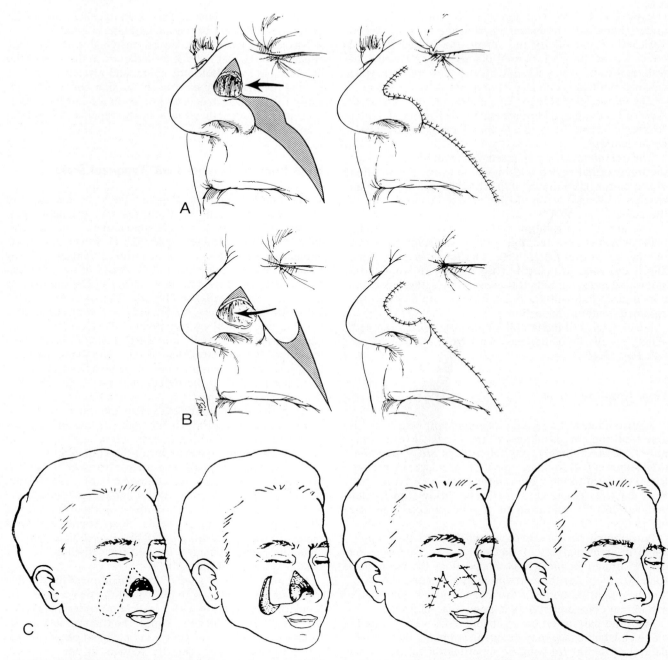

FIGURE 45.5. **A,** Nasolabial (cheek) advancement flap. **B,** Nasolabial transposition flap. **C,** The tip of a superiorly based nasolabial flap turned in for lining. (Figure C from McLaren LR: Nasolabial flap repair for alar margin defects. *Br J Plast Surg* 16:234, 1963.)

made no provision for skeletal support, and this yielded a bulky ala prone to collapse and a narrow nasal vestibule. Like the midline forehead flap, the scalping flap may be fitted with a chondrocutaneous graft while on the forehead, and the entire alar component can be prefabricated ex situ before flap transposition (40, 41). The exposed pericranium is temporarily skin grafted or kept moist with nondesiccating dressings pending return of the hair-bearing scalp after the pedicle is divided. The forehead extension of the flap is covered with a FTSG.

Retroauricular skin has also been carried to the nose based on the superficial temporal vessels (47–51). Initially described by Loeb (47), the popularity of the *auriculotemporal flap* can be traced to Washio (48) and Maillard and Montandon (51). The vascular pedicle of the flap takes advantage of the connection between the superficial temporal artery and the postauricular artery to carry the skin behind the ear without a delay procedure (Fig. 45.8). Maximum flap reach is to the midline.

A full-thickness strip of concha can be incorporated in

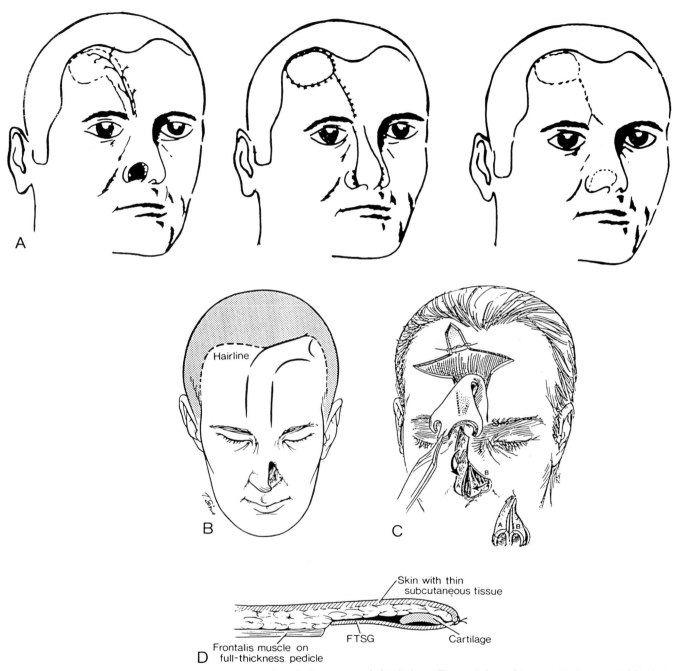

FIGURE 45.6. **A,** The slanted, off-midline forehead flap. **B,** The extended forehead flap angled along the hairline. **C,** The gullwing shaped forehead flap. **D,** The tip of the forehead flap has been laminated with cartilage for structural stability and a skin graft for lining. (Figure A from Dhawan IK, Aggarwal SB, Hariharan S: Use of an off-midline forehead flap for the repair of small nasal defects. *Plast Reconstr Surg* 53:537, 1974.)

the cutaneous paddle of the retroauricular flap to achieve nasal lining, cartilaginous flexibility, and external cover in one operation. The main drawback of the flap is that it brings postauricular rather than facial skin to the nose.

Distant Flaps

Distant flaps are a last resort in nasal reconstruction. The skin from areas other than the face tends to have different pigmentation, actinic history, texture, and hair-bearing properties. When transferred on a pedicle (52–57), the circulation of remote flaps must be protected by including a generous amount of subcutaneous tissue, which frequently results in a shapeless lump of a nose that needs multiple revisions. Transferred freely by microvascular anastomoses (58–61), distant flaps add to the complexity of the nasal reconstruction and risk considerable morbidity.

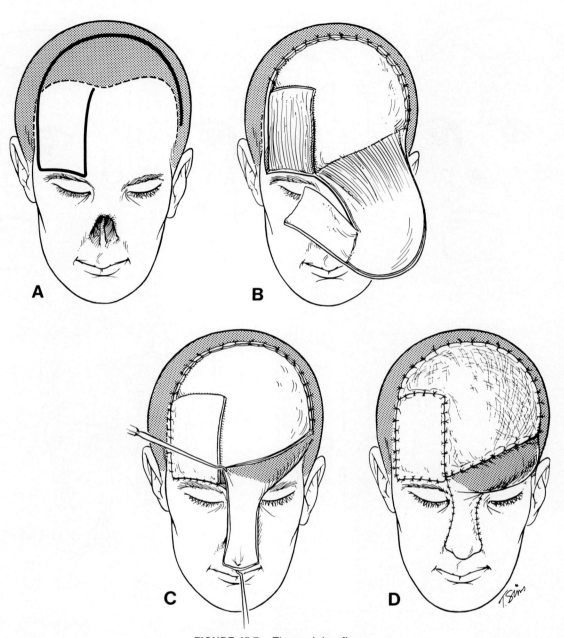

FIGURE 45.7. The scalping flap.

FIGURE 45.8. Design and transfer of the auriculotemporal flap.

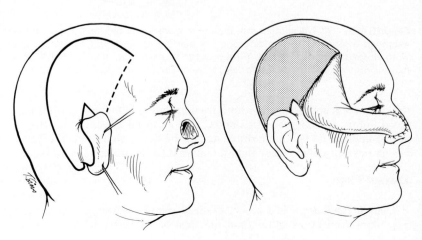

TISSUE EXPANSION

The relatively new concept of tissue expansion has been applied to traditional methods of flap transfer in nasal reconstruction in order to (a) increase the amount of skin available for coverage, or (b) facilitate closure of the flap donor site. Ortiz-Monasterio and Musolas (62) routinely expanded the forehead skin in cases of extensive defects, inserting the expander in a subgaleal plane. Kroll (63) expanded Millard's gull-wing flap slowly over several weeks, repeatedly thinning and shaping the transferred flap tissue before dividing the pedicle. All forehead flaps expanded submuscularly require considerable thinning, especially at the distal end; otherwise, there is a risk of excessive narrowing of the airway (64).

Bolton and coworkers (65) reported complete loss of nasal contour in three patients with near-total deficits as a result of flap shrinkage and accelerated resorption of the cantilever grafts used in the midline. Millard (66) opposed expansion of the flap itself because of the risk of contraction and subsequent distortion of the tissues after removal of the expander; instead, he suggested expanding the margins of the flap donor wound on the forehead to permit direct approximation.

Nasal Lining

Replacement of nasal lining is essential to the adequate function and caliber of the airway. Any raw areas left on the inside of the nose will contract with healing and distort the overlying tissues, ruining an otherwise esthetic reconstruction. The lining tissue must be thin, so as not to obstruct the lumen, yet it must be sufficiently resistant to withstand the traumatic forces associated with normal respiration.

TURNDOWN FLAPS

Turndown flaps based on the wound margin are useful in small defects of the ala, but they must be watched carefully because their blood supply crosses dense cicatricial and fibrotic tissue at the edge of the defect. In addition to providing nasal lining on their internal surface, they double externally as a vascular bed for composite grafts that may be used in reconstructing the alar rim. Meyer and Kesselring (67) based the turndown flap internally to take advantage of the existing vestibular skin/mucosa and avoid another external scar. Unfortunately, this creates another raw area farther inside the nose, which on contraction has a tendency to retract the alar margin (68).

BIPEDICLED ADVANCEMENT FLAP

When lining the lobule, Burget and Menick (69, 70) used a bipedicled advancement flap of mucosa and cartilage raised just above the defect and made to slide downward in the direction of the alar margin. The secondary lining defect is repaired with a septal hinged flap that is scored along the dorsum and bent outward to roof the nose.

EXTERNAL FLAPS

Regional flaps may be *infolded* at their tip to achieve nasal lining as well as coverage (3, 27, 39), or the undersurface of the cover flap may be *skin grafted* prior to transfer (3, 35, 40, 41, 71, 72). This adds a step to the reconstruction, but the outcome is usually better esthetically. If the graft is applied to the vestibule at the time of flap transfer, edema obscures the ultimate dimensions, and blood supply to the tissues is at its most precarious.

A popular option for lining the airway during reconstruction is to transpose a *nasolabial flap skin-side down* (38, 73, 74). As is true for external cover, this method suffers from flap bulkiness because of the thick nasofacial dermis and subcutaneous fat, which must be elevated with the flap in order to preserve its circulation.

CHONDROMUCOSAL FLAPS

Chondromucosal septal flaps are reliable, versatile, and eminently handy. Millard (36) removed the ipsilateral mucosa from the septum before swinging the flap outward, like a door hinged in the dorsal midline. The defect in the lateral nasal wall is bridged by the segment of septal cartilage with attached mucosa from the opposite nasal cavity, which becomes the new lining for the reconstruction.

When bilateral alar lining is called for, Burget and Menick (69, 70) proposed using mucoperichondrial leaves peeled from the septal pivot flap that supports the nasal dorsum. These leaves are rolled out from the midline and anchored to the medial vestibular floor on either side like a vault.

Skeletal Support

The nasal dorsum juts out from the plane of the face by virtue of a rigid cartilaginous wall, the septum. A successful reconstruction must duplicate this central longitudinal support if it is missing. This will not only ensure continued nasal projection but also resist the contraction forces of the soft tissues during healing.

When the nasal bones are intact and the anterior nasal spine is present, it may be possible to rotate the residual septal cartilage anteriorly and outward. Gillies and Millard (75) accomplished this with an *L-shaped septal flap* based superiorly near the caudal end of the nasal bones (Fig. 45.9). Burget and Menick (69, 70), in contrast, raised a huge *septal flap on an inferior base pivoting at the nasal spine* (Fig. 45.10). The flap is nourished by the septal branch of the superior labial artery.

Cantilever bone grafts offer an alternative in providing support for the nasal midline (3, 72). A strong piece of bone is anchored at the radix and follows the dorsal nasal contour to the tip, which need not be further shored up

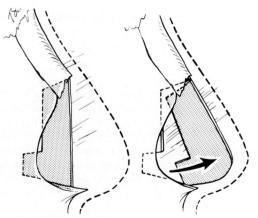

FIGURE 45.9. The L-shaped septal hinge flap.

from below (Fig. 45.11). The nasal bones are often lowered to accommodate the bone graft.

Chait and associates (76) suggested an osteochondral rib graft as cantilever, arguing that the bony portion of the graft in contact with the nasal bones solidifies in situ, while the distal cartilaginous portion maintains flexibility of the nasal tip and resists resorption. Overall, however, the long-term structural stability of cantilever grafts is remarkable (77–82).

Long pieces of cartilage fashioned as *L-struts* may also be used to span the nasal defect along the midline. The long arm of the "L" graft extends from radix to tip, where it turns a right angle downward for the short arm of the "L" to rest on the nasal spine. Gillies (83) first described the technique in 1920, and it has been widely practiced since (3, 75, 84). Once again, Chait et al. (76)

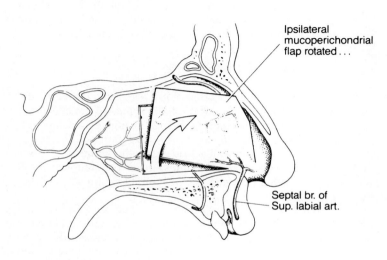

FIGURE 45.10. The septal pivot flap, based anterocaudally on the septal branch of the superior labial artery. (From Burget GC,

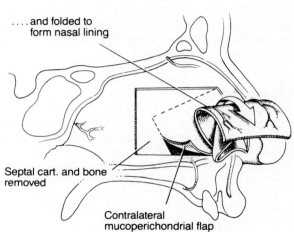

Menick FJ: Nasal support and lining: The marriage of beauty and blood supply. *Plast Reconstr Surg* 84:189, 1989.)

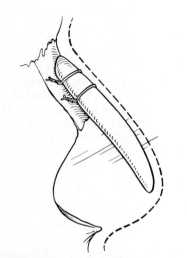

FIGURE 45.11. The cantilever bone graft.

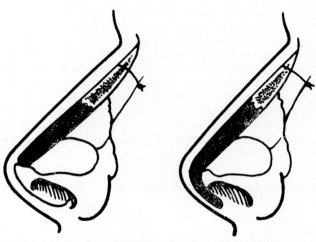

FIGURE 45.12. The osteochondral L-strut. (From Chait LA, Becker H, Cort A: The versatile costal osteochondral graft in nasal reconstruction. *Br J Plast Surg* 33:179, 1980.)

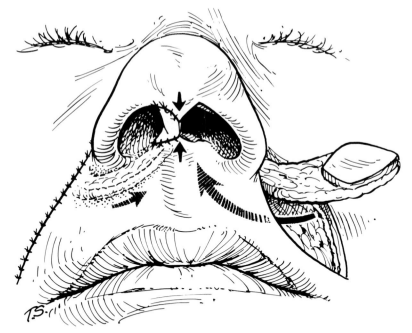

FIGURE 45.13. Bilateral nasolabial island flaps for columellar reconstruction.

preferred a combination bone-cartilage graft (Fig. 45.12) for the reasons mentioned earlier.

The importance of skeletal support in the nostril walls is unquestioned. Whether by cartilage grafts incorporated in the reconstructive flap or hinged chondromucosal flaps from the septum, skeletal elements tent the soft tissues over the airway, prevent alar collapse on inspiration, maintain flexibility of the nasal sidewalls, and obviate retraction of the alar rim.

The Columella

As an isolated defect, columellar reconstruction can be very difficult. If the vascular bed is adequate, *composite grafts of skin and fat from the earlobe* (11, 85) can be shaped to simulate a columella. Alternatively, *nasolabial flaps* may be raised unilaterally (86) or bilaterally (85), based either inferiorly (87) or superiorly (88, 89), and tunneled through the upper lip or lateral alar wall, respectively, to emerge in the midline. Here the flap tip is rolled up so as to round the projecting end (Fig. 45.13). Revision procedures for flap thinning are invariably indicated.

As part of a larger defect, the problem of a missing columella is simplified. Distal extensions of the scalping flap (46) or the gull-wing flap (37, 38) may be pinched and molded into a semblance of columella during transfer, with no additional scars on the face and the same sturdy blood supply as for the rest of the nose. Secondary defatting of these prefabricated, flap-based columellas is almost always necessary.

References

1. McDowell F, Valone JA, Brown JB: Bibliography and historical note on plastic surgery of the nose. *Plast Reconstr Surg* 10:149, 1952.
2. Ivy RH: Repair of acquired defects of the face. *JAMA* 84:181, 1925.
3. Converse JM (Ed): *Reconstructive Plastic Surgery,* ed 2. Philadelphia, WB Saunders, 1977, vol 2, chpt 29.
4. Cottle MH: *Corrective Surgery of the Nasal Septum and the External Pyramid—Study Notes and Laboratory Manual.* Chicago, American Rhinopharyngological Society, 1960.
5. Sheen JH: *Aesthetic Rhinoplasty.* St. Louis, CV Mosby, 1978.
6. Gonzalez-Ulloa M: Restoration of the face covering by means of selected skin in regional aesthetic units. *Br J Plast Surg* 9:212, 1956.
7. Millard DR Jr: Aesthetic reconstructive rhinoplasty. *Clin Plast Surg* 8:169, 1981.
8. König F: Zur Deckung von Defecten der Nasenflugel. *Berlin Klin Woch* 39:137, 1902.
9. Argamaso RV: An ideal donor site for the auricular composite graft. *Br J Plast Surg* 28:219, 1975.
10. Brown JB, Cannon B: Composite free grafts of skin and cartilage from the ear. *Surg Gynecol Obstet* 82:253, 1946.
11. Dupertuis SM: Free earlobe grafts of skin and fat. *Plast Reconstr Surg* 1:135, 1946.
12. Baker DC: Massive chondrocutaneous grafts for nasal reconstruction. Presented at the 63rd annual meeting of the American Association of Plastic Surgeons, Chicago, May 1984.
13. Elliott RA Jr: Rotation flaps of the nose. *Plast Reconstr Surg* 17:444, 1956.
14. Masson JK, Mendelson BC: The banner flap. *Am J Surg* 134:419, 1977.
15. Zimany A: The bilobed flap. *Plast Reconstr Surg* 11:424, 1953.
16. McGregor JC, Soutar DS: A critical assessment of the bilobed flap. *Br J Plast Surg* 34:197, 1981.
17. Lister GO, Gibson T: Closure of rhomboid skin defects: The flaps of Limberg and Dufourmentel. *Br J Plast Surg* 25:300, 1972.
18. Rieger RA: A local flap for repair of the nasal tip. *Plast Reconstr Surg* 40:147, 1967.
19. Lipshutz H, Penrod DS: Use of complete transverse nasal flap in repair of small defects of the nose. *Plast Reconstr Surg* 49:629, 1972.
20. Rigg BM: The dorsal nasal flap. *Plast Reconstr Surg* 52:361, 1973.
21. Marchac D, Toth B: The axial frontonasal flap revisited. *Plast Reconstr Surg* 76:686, 1985.
22. Rybka FJ: Reconstruction of the nasal tip using nasalis myocutaneous sliding flaps. *Plast Reconstr Surg* 71:40, 1983.

23. Barton FE Jr: The nasolabial flap. *Perspect Plast Surg* 3(2), 1990.
24. Dieffenbach JF: Reconstruction of the nose. In *Die operative Chirurgie*. Leipzig, 1845–48, bd 1, p 326.
25. Twyman ED: Nose defects, partial: A new modification of the "French" method of restoration with sliding flaps of adjoining tissue. *West J Surg* 48:106, 1940.
26. Hagerty RF, Smith WS: The nasolabial cheek flap. *Am Surg* 24:506, 1958.
27. McLaren LR: Nasolabial flap repair for alar margin defects. *Br J Plast Surg* 16:234, 1963.
28. Barron JN, Emmett AJJ: Subcutaneous pedicle flaps. *Br J Plast Surg* 18:51, 1965.
29. Emmett AJJ: The closure of defects by using adjacent triangular flaps with subcutaneous pedicles. *Plast Reconstr Surg* 59:45, 1977.
30. Dufourmentel C, Talaat SM: The kite flap. In *Transactions of the Fifth International Congress of Plastic and Reconstructive Surgery*. Melbourne, Butterworths, 1971, p 1223.
31. Spear SL, Kroll SS, Romm S: A new twist to the nasolabial flap for reconstruction of lateral alar defects. *Plast Reconstr Surg* 79:915, 1987.
32. Kazanjian VH: The repair of nasal defects with the median forehead flap. Primary closure of forehead wound. *Surg Gynecol Obstet* 83:37, 1946.
33. Dhawan IK, Aggarwal SB, Heriharan S: Use of an off-midline forehead flap for the repair of small nasal defects. *Plast Reconstr Surg* 53:537, 1974.
34. Sawhney CP: A longer angular midline forehead flap for the reconstruction of nasal defects. *Plast Reconstr Surg* 58:721, 1976.
35. Barton FE Jr: Aesthetic aspects of partial nasal reconstruction. *Clin Plast Surg* 8:177, 1981.
36. Millard DR Jr: Hemirhinoplasty. *Plast Reconstr Surg* 40:440, 1967.
37. Millard DR Jr: Reconstructive rhinoplasty for the lower half of a nose. *Plast Reconstr Surg* 53:133, 1974.
38. Millard Dr Jr: Reconstructive rhinoplasty for the lower two-thirds of the nose. *Plast Reconstr Surg* 57:722, 1976.
39. Blair VP: Total and subtotal restoration of the nose. *JAMA* 85:1931, 1925.
40. Barton FE Jr: Aesthetic aspects of nasal reconstruction. *Clin Plast Surg* 15:155, 1988.
41. Gillies HD: A new free graft applied to the reconstruction of the nostril. *Br J Surg* 30:305, 1943.
42. Gillies HD: The development and scope of plastic surgery. *Bull Northwest University Medical School* 35:1, 1935.
43. New GB: Sickle flap for nasal reconstruction. *Surg Gynecol Obstet* 80:497, 1945.
44. Converse JM: New forehead flap for nasal reconstruction. *Proc R Soc Med* 35:811, 1942.
45. Converse JM: Reconstruction of the nose by the scalping flap technique. *Surg Clin North Am* 39:335, 1959.
46. Converse JM: Clinical applications of the scalping flap in reconstruction of the nose. *Plast Reconstr Surg* 43:247, 1969.
47. Loeb R: Temporo-mastoid flap for reconstructions of the cheek. *Rev Lat-Am Cir Plast* 6:185, 1962.
48. Washio H: Retroauricular temporal flap. *Plast Reconstr Surg* 43:162, 1969.
49. Orticochea M: A new method for total reconstruction of the nose: The ears as donor areas. *Br J Plast Surg* 24:225, 1971.
50. Galvao MSL: A postauricular flap based on the contralateral superficial temporal vessels. *Plast Reconstr Surg* 68:891, 1981.
51. Maillard GF, Montandon D: The Washio tempororetroauricular flap: Its use in 20 patients. *Plast Reconstr Surg* 70:550, 1982.
52. Mendelson BC, Masson JK, Arnold PG, et al: Flaps used for nasal reconstruction: A perspective based on 180 cases. *Mayo Clin Proc* 54:91, 1979.
53. Young F: The repair of nasal losses. *Surgery* 20:670, 1946.
54. Gillies HD: Experiences with tubed pedicle flaps. *Surg Gynecol Obstet* 60:291, 1935.
55. Song IC, Wise AJ, Bromberg BE: Total nasal reconstruction: A further application of the deltopectoral flap. *Br J Plast Surg* 26:414, 1973.
56. Kilner TP: *Plastic Surgery in Postgraduate Surgery*, ed 3. New York, Appleton-Century-Crofts, 1937.
57. Chitrov FM: *Plastic Reconstruction of Face and Neck Defects with Filatov Tube Flaps*. Moscow, Medgiz, 1954.
58. Fujino T, Harashina T, Nakajima T: Free skin flap from the retroauricular region to the nose. *Plast Reconstr Surg* 57:338, 1976.
59. Ohmori K, Sekiguchi J, Ohmori S: Total rhinoplasty with a free osteocutaneous flap. *Plast Reconstr Surg* 63:387, 1979.
60. Shaw WW: Microvascular reconstruction of the nose. *Clin Plast Surg* 8:471, 1981.
61. Baudet J, Guimberteau JC, Nascimento E: Successful clinical transfer of two free thoraco-dorsal axillary flaps. *Plast Reconstr Surg* 58:680, 1976.
62. Ortiz-Monasterio F, Musolas A: Nasal reconstruction using forehead flaps. *Perspect Plast Surg* 3(1):71, 1989.
63. Kroll SS: Forehead flap nasal reconstruction with tissue expansion and delayed pedicle separation. *Laryngoscope* 99:448, 1989.
64. Adamson JE: Nasal reconstruction with the expanded forehead flap. *Plast Reconstr Surg* 81:12, 1988.
65. Bolton LL, Chandrasekhar B, Gottlieb ME: Forehead expansion and total nasal reconstruction. *Ann Plast Surg* 21:210, 1988.
66. Millard DR Jr: Various uses of the septum in rhinoplasty. *Plast Reconstr Surg* 81:112, 1988.
67. Meyer R, Kesselring UK: Sculpturing and reconstructive procedures in aesthetic and functional rhinoplasty. *Clin Plast Surg* 4:15, 1977.
68. Ellenbogen R: Alar rim lowering. *Plast Reconstr Surg* 79:50, 1987.
69. Burget GC, Menick FJ: Nasal reconstruction: Seeking a fourth dimension. *Plast Reconstr Surg* 78:145, 1986.
70. Burget GC, Menick FJ: Nasal support and lining: The marriage of beauty and blood supply. *Plast Reconstr Surg* 84:189, 1989.
71. Converse JM: Composite graft from the septum in nasal reconstruction. *Trans Lat Am Congr Plast Surg* 8:281, 1956.
72. Millard DR Jr: Total reconstructive rhinoplasty and a missing link. *Plast Reconstr Surg* 37:167, 1966.
73. Georgiade NG, Mladick RA, Thorne FL: The nasolabial tunnel flap. *Plast Reconstr Surg* 43:463, 1969.
74. Santos OA, Pappas JC: Repair of nostril defect with a contralateral nasolabial flap. *Plast Reconstr Surg* 57:704, 1976.
75. Gillies HD, Millard DR Jr: *The Principles and Art of Plastic Surgery*. Boston, Little Brown & Co, 1957, p 576.
76. Chait LA, Becker H, Cort A: The versatile costal osteochondral graft in nasal reconstruction. *Br J Plast Surg* 33:179, 1980.
77. Gerrie JW, Cloutier GE, Woolhouse FM: Carved cancellous bone grafts in rhinoplasty. *Plast Reconstr Surg* 6:196, 1950.
78. Wheeler ES, Kawamoto HK, Zarem HA: Bone grafts for nasal reconstruction. *Plast Reconstr Surg* 69:9, 1982.
79. Farina R, Villano JB: Follow-up of bone grafts to the nose. *Plast Reconstr Surg* 48:251, 1971.
80. Farina R: Deformity of nasal dorsum through loss of substance: Correction by bone grafting. *Ann Plast Surg* 12:466, 1984.
81. Baroudi R: An interview with Roberto Farina, M.D. *Ann Plast Surg* 12;475, 1984.
82. Jackson IT, Smith J, Mixter RC: Nasal bone grafting using split skull grafts. *Ann Plast Surg* 11:533, 1983.
83. Gillies HD: *Plastic Surgery of the Face*. London, Oxford University Press, 1920, p 224.
84. Brown JB, McDowell F: *Plastic Surgery of the Nose*. St. Louis, CV Mosby, 1951, p 320.
85. Gillies HD: The columella. *Br J Plast Surg* 2:192, 1950.
86. daSilva G: A new method of reconstructing the columella with a naso-labial flap. *Plast Reconstr Surg* 34:63, 1964.
87. Kaplan I: Reconstruction of the columella. *Br J Plast Surg* 25:37, 1972.
88. Paletta FX, van Norman RT: Total reconstruction of the columella. *Plast Reconstr Surg* 30:322, 1962.
89. Yanai A, Nagata S, Tanaka H: Reconstruction of the columella with bilateral nasolabial flaps. *Plast Reconstr Surg* 77:129, 1986.

46

Reconstruction of Eyelid Deformities

James H. Carraway, M.D., F.A.C.S. and Michael P. Vincent, M.D., F.A.C.S.

Aims of Reconstruction

The primary purpose of reconstruction of deficient eyelid tissue is to furnish cover for the sclera and cornea. The cornea is responsible for visual acuity and is very sensitive to drying and abrasion. Normal motion of the upper eyelid is responsible for wetting of the cornea as well as protecting it from threatened trauma. Tears secreted from the lacrimal gland mix with secretions from the accessory lacrimal glands of Zeis and Moll and the meibomian glands. This mixture lubricates the cornea with each blink of the upper lid. In addition to maintaining a wet cornea and sclera, the upper lid also protects the eye from wind, dust, airborne particulate matter, and other foreign bodies. During sleep, the upper lid covers and protects the cornea and sclera from drying and blocks out light. The lower lid is important in protecting the sclera as well as acting as a trough to funnel tears to the medial canthal area where the lacus lacrimalis localizes the tears, allowing drainage into the inferior punctum.

The lids are important aesthetically because the eyes are the focal point of the face. All people, young or old, need to believe that they have a normal appearance, lest they feel self-conscious. The shape of the lid can be seen from a distance across a room, whereas scars are usually visible at a conversational distance. Therefore, it is important to reconstruct the shape and motion of the lid as close to normal as possible. Lid level and the shape and placement of the medial and lateral canthi are important. The lower lid must be up and in good position without notching or ectropion. Scars should be placed in natural lines to the extent possible, and the skin used for reconstruction should be nearly the same in quality as the thin and delicate eyelid skin. Should there be excessive hollowing of the upper eyelid, bulging of the lower lid fat pad, or marked asymmetry in relation to the opposite lid, correction should be undertaken if possible.

In addition to being functional and aesthetically acceptable, the reconstructed lid must be durable. If the stiff tarsal plate is missing or the orbicularis muscle is paralyzed or absent, then the lid quickly loses its stability. These components must be incorporated into the reconstructed lid in the form of muscle continuity or fascial support for replacement of the orbicularis. Cartilage can be employed as a "stiffener" for replacement of the tarsal plate. Hair grafts intended for eyelash reconstruction often tend to lie in the wrong direction and may produce corneal irritation, but are performed occasionally, usually at the insistence of the patient. If the lid margin is unstable after serving as a donor area in a lid-sharing procedure, entropion and trichiasis may occur over a period of time. Selection of the proper donor area for grafts and flaps is important because a poor selection may result in a less than favorable color match or in skin that is thick and unpliable.

Pathology

In general, benign tumors do not present a great problem in removal and reconstruction. Often they may be "shaved," or a limited resection may be done. Primary closure after conservative excision is generally not difficult. Exceptions include hemangiomas, neurofibromas, and lymphangiomas, for which excision may be technically difficult. With hemangiomas, the most important consideration is surgical timing, especially in infants. If the visual axis is occluded, proper development of retinal functional and subsequent vision may be altered. A decision must be made on a more urgent basis if other methods of treating the hemangioma are not quickly successful (1). Neurofibromas may be difficult to manage and often involve the normal anatomical structures. Resection of the tumor without destruction of normal anatomical components and their functions is nearly impossible. Surgical excision of neurofibromas may be suboptimal with respect to the final aesthetic and functional outcome.

Malignant tumors are less common, but often present difficult challenges in reconstruction after ablation. The most important axiom in dealing with excision of malignant tumors is that adequate primary excision is imperative, particularly with regard to recurrent tumors. The amount of normal tissue margin around a tumor cannot always be measured in millimeters, but must be a matter of judgment based on the operator's experience, the type of tumor, the area of involvement, and the pathologist's findings. Primary, well-defined basal cell carcinoma may be resected with a surgical margin of 1–2 mm, whereas a basal cell carcinoma that recurs after irradiation, cautery, or inadequate surgical excision must be more widely excised. The pathologist's report is not always accurate in determining whether enough tissue has been resected, even with frozen section monitoring. Small strands of recurrent tumor may appear microscopically to resemble

FIGURE 46.1. Location of postauricular skin grafts. The *right side* demonstrates excision of entire hairless area, requiring split-thickness graft coverage.

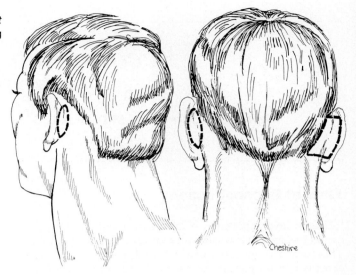

inflammatory cells or blood vessels. These small tumor nests lie dormant and give rise to recurrence even years later. Melanoma may present a problem in determining how extensive the resection must be. Judgment must be balanced between the need to conserve eyelid tissue and that of surgical excision with adequate margins. Knowledge of the level of invasion, extent of the tumor, and the patient's age are important in making a decision regarding surgical excision.

Reconstructive Techniques

GRAFTING TECHNIQUES (2)

Skin grafting of the lower lid is a common method of reconstruction, and selection of the proper donor site is important. Color match is the first consideration, with grafts above the clavicle a far better match than those from below. The most frequently selected donor sites are postauricular, upper eyelid, supraclavicular, and, occasionally, preauricular skin. The upper eyelid skin is very thin and supple and is an excellent color match, but is limited in quantity and does not have the thickness to give good support. Postauricular skin is thin and supple, provides a good color match, and also gives relatively good support where needed (2). The donor area is limited if primary closure of the donor site is desired. A larger amount of skin may be taken, including the entire hairless area (approximately 6 × 8 cm), and covered by a split-thickness graft (Fig. 46.1).

In grafting an ectropion from burn scars, overcorrection by 15–20% is preferred (3) because wound contraction may be well under way and may cause recurrent ectropion (Fig. 46.2). Where possible, unit grafting gives a better aesthetic result than a "patchy"-appearing graft. Unit grafting can be used to an even greater advantage by carrying the end of the graft in a "sling" fashion beyond the medial and lateral canthi (Fig. 46.3).

If is often somewhat more difficult to obtain a good result with grafting of the upper lid than the lower lid. Full-thickness grafts, especially if placed as a patch, tend

to wrinkle and become misshapen. The exception is a full-thickness graft from the opposite upper lid. When a large amount of scarring or a large defect is present, a split graft from the hairless medial arm is a good solution to the problem (4). Coverage of the entire upper lid as a unit is aesthetically better even though the color may be slightly lighter. The size of the defect must be measured while the lid is in the closed position, so that adequate closure may be achieved by the lid after healing. Bolus dressings are used and should be kept on at least 6–7 days, because early motion may cause some loss or increased wrinkling of the graft. During the first week, an intermarginal tarsorrhaphy suture of 6-0 Prolene (Johnson & Johnson, New Jersey) is helpful (Fig. 46.4). In the case of ectropion from scarring, or skin loss when the tarsal margin is stretched and excessive in length, a wedge tarsectomy in addition to a full-thickness graft may be performed, and the graft may be placed directly over the suture line. Tarsal resection is performed by placing a perpendicular cut in the tarsus approximately 5 mm from the lateral canthus. The two cut edges are overlapped to estimate the amount of lid resection necessary, and another perpendicular cut placed at the determined

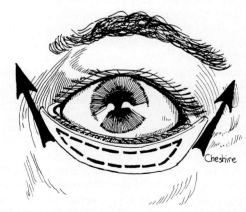

FIGURE 46.2. Graft overcorrection in the medial and lateral canthal areas shows postoperative ectropion.

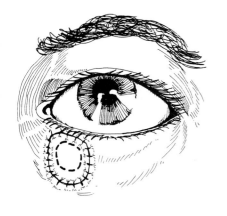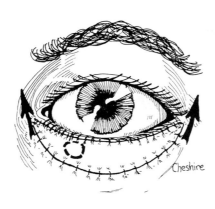

FIGURE 46.3. An incorrect patch graft (*left*) may lead to a "trap-door" appearance. *Right,* An aesthetic unit placed in a sling fashion.

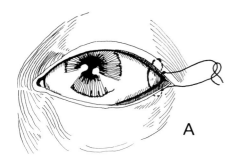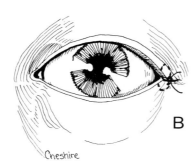

FIGURE 46.4. Temporary intermarginal tarsorrhaphy.

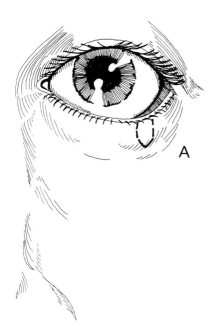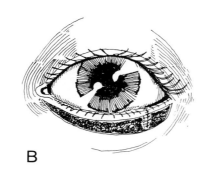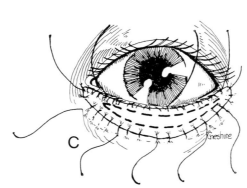

FIGURE 46.5. In cases of a cicatricial ectropion with relaxed tarsal plate, full-thickness lid excision with an overcorrected full-thickness graft provides the best result.

FIGURE 46.6. Full-thickness grafts can be utilized for coverage of medial canthal defects.

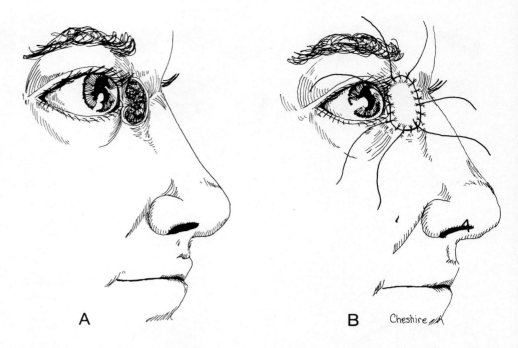

A

B

Cheshire

point of resection. Closure is performed by approximating the gray line with 6-0 silk and closing the tarsus with 6-0 chromic sutures. The muscle layer is then approximated with 6-0 chromic (Fig. 46.5).

Medial canthal defects are often closed by grafting, with upper lid or postauricular skin grafts as the donor area of choice (Fig. 46.6). After excision of the tumor, the medial canthal tendon often remains, but the graft takes well with the help of the "bridging" phenomenon. If there is bone in the base of the defect, the graft may also take, provided that no more than a few millimeters need to be covered. If there is more exposed bone, then a local

flap is probably indicated. Once the defect is closed with the graft, a bolus of cotton or Vaseline gauze is held in place with the long sutures tied over the bolus.

After enucleation, the socket must be covered with a split graft, and there is usually excellent take of this graft, even though a moderately large area of membranous bone may constitute part of the defect (Fig. 46.7). Judging the size of the defect may be more difficult than if the defect were a flat surface, but this is aided by measuring the depth of the socket and the size of the defect at the base, and adding the three sides to obtain the total. As with other grafts, sutures are left long to tie over a bolus

FIGURE 46.7. Split-thickness grafts can be utilized for socket coverage after enucleation.

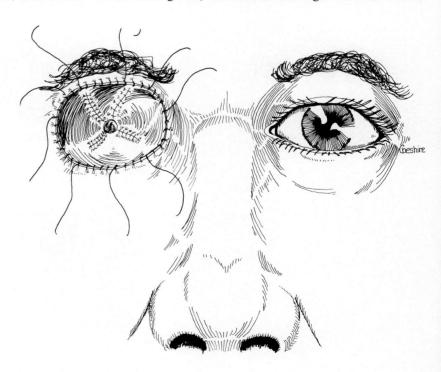

Cheshire

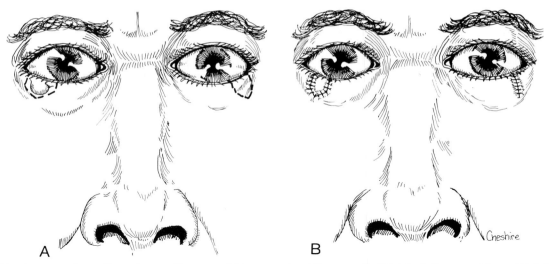

FIGURE 46.8. A composite graft may be used from one lid to reconstruct the opposite lid defect. Upper and lower lid defects may be covered by this technique.

placed in the socket over the skin graft. The bolus must be left in place about 7 days.

Composite grafts may be used for eyelid reconstruction (5). A deficit of one third of the lid margin may be managed by using a composite graft consisting of full-thickness lid (skin, tarsus, and conjunctiva) from another lid (Fig. 46.8). The take of composite grafts is quite good and may be maximized by excising all orbicularis fibers from the graft. In upper eyelid reconstruction, the superior portion of the graft should be sutured to the levator. Iced saline compresses may be useful in the postoperative period in decreasing metabolic requirements of the graft and increasing the likelihood of a successful ''take.''

LOCAL FLAPS

Nasolabial Flap

The nasolabial flap is a versatile and often used method of reconstruction of the lower lid (Fig. 46.9). The chief advantages of this flap are its rich blood supply from the superior part of the angular artery and from the supratrochlear collaterals and the good support that this thicker skin can provide to the lower lid (6). If there is a shortage of tissue in the infraorbital area, particularly in a situation in which there has been trauma, atrophy, or scarring, then subcutaneous fat may be carried with the

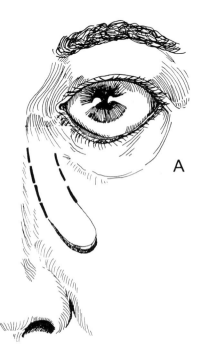
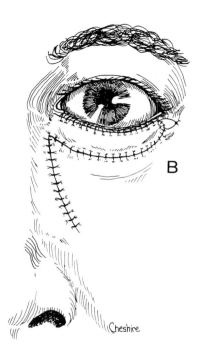

FIGURE 46.9. A nasolabial flap may be employed in cases in which full-thickness skin is needed in lower lid reconstruction.

flap. The chief disadvantage of the nasolabial flap is that the thick skin gives an abnormal appearance because it lacks the supple and delicate attributes of eyelid skin. When necessary, however, the nasolabial flap is reliable and easy to use.

The technique involves raising a flap of properly measured size, with care to maintain a relatively thick amount of tissue at the base to preserve the blood supply. The tip of the flap may be anchored into the lateral canthal tendon or the periosteum, giving added support to the lower lid. This flap will also support a cartilage-mucosa composite graft if indicated. It may be necessary in some cases to thin the flap later, which is easily accomplished.

V-Y Advancement Flap

When other flaps are not available, a V-Y advancement flap of the medial canthus and lower and upper lids may be used (7). This flap may be relatively large to replace a part of the lower lid, or small in the case of a small wound that cannot be directly closed (Fig. 46.10). The sides are cut leaving the base of the pedicle intact with subcutaneous tissue attachment. Skin hooks are used to pull the flap in the direction of the defect. Strands of subcutaneous tissue that prevent adequate mobilization are freed by blunt or sharp dissection. The flap then slides into the defect and the donor area is closed.

Lateral Cheek and Temporal Flap

In defects of the lower and upper eyelids that cannot be closed directly, use of lateral cheek or temporal skin is a sound technique. When excising full-thickness defects of the lid margin, primary closure should be attempted (Fig. 46.11). Primary closure can be used for defects of up to one third of the original lid margin, especially in older patients with greater tissue laxity. Closure is performed by placing a 6-0 silk suture at the gray line, matching up the lid edge. An absorbable suture is used to close the tarsus, which brings the conjunctival edges together. If there is excessive tension, a lateral cantholysis may provide the necessary relaxation. An incision is made horizontally from the lateral canthal angle and dissection is carried down to the periosteum of the lateral orbital rim, severing the inferior crura of the lateral canthal tendon. The skin is undermined and a determination is made as to how much cheek skin will be needed. If a small amount of relaxation is needed, then simple undermining and advancement may be done. If a larger amount of skin is needed, then a back-cut may be performed to allow better mobility. This is closed with a Z-plasty from adjacent tissue, thus filling in the defect created from the back-cut (Fig. 46.12). This approach also gives the lateral incision an upward sweep enhancing the support of the lower lid. It may be combined with a composite graft if warranted, in which case the graft is first sutured in place and the undermined cheek skin is brought over for cover (Fig. 46.13).

FIGURE 46.10. A V-Y advancement flap may be used for coverage of medial canthal defects.

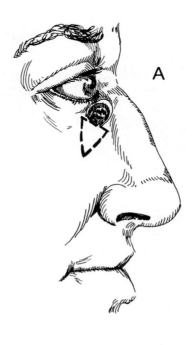

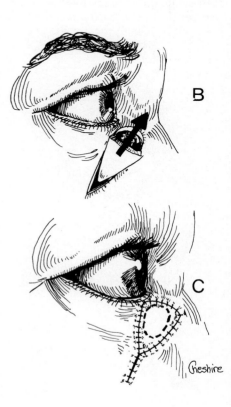

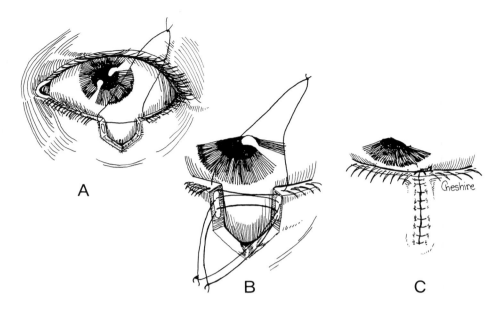

FIGURE 46.11. Primary closure can be achieved by placement of a lid margin suture initially followed by closure of the tarsus and skin. Pentagon-shaped excision gives the best closure.

Tenzel has described a semicircular flap that can be very useful for defects of the lower lid measuring one half and possibly up to two thirds of the lid (8, 9; Fig. 46.14). An incision is made at the lateral canthus in an exaggerated superior direction using a semicircle configuration. The flap does not extend beyond the point that would represent the inferior continuation of the eyebrow. The flap is undermined beneath the orbicularis muscle, and the inferior crus of the lateral canthal tendon is released to allow for flap mobility. Undermining is necessary to the point at which a tension-free closure of the defect can be accomplished. Some triangulation of the inferior aspect of the defect is usually required.

With much larger lid defects, a larger cheek flap may be indicated together with a septal chondromucosal graft. Design of the cheek flap is important, with the lateral sweeping incision rising in the temporal area in a curvilinear manner to the preauricular area as far down as the lobule. It is necessary to make a V-shaped cut to complete triangulation of the lower part of the defect to prevent a dog-ear from forming (Fig. 46.15A). It is important to make the medial incision as close to the nasomaxillary line as possible so that, when the incision is closed, the sturdier dermal attachments on the side of the nose will support the sutured cheek skin. Undermining should be done at the level of dermal subcutaneous tissue interface,

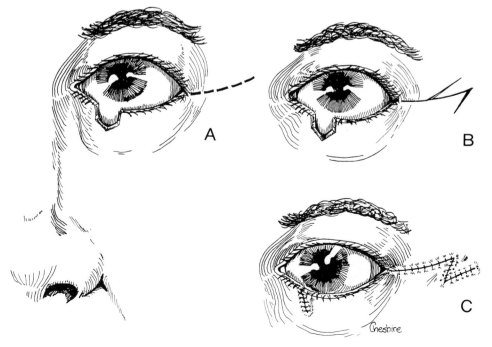

FIGURE 46.12. A lateral canthotomy with a Z-plasty closure may be used for relaxation of the lid closure for larger defects.

FIGURE 46.13. A composite chondromucosal graft (*dashed line*) may be necessary to provide lid stability.

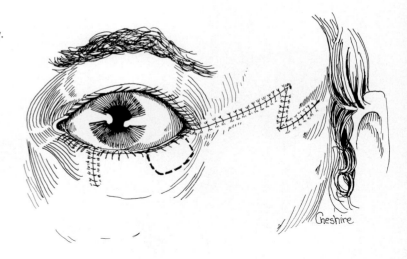

leaving about 0.5–1.0 mm of fat on the undersurface of the flap to protect the subdermal plexus. Extensive undermining is usually necessary to mobilize the flap completely without any tension in its new position. The viability of this random flap is ensured by the rich facial subdermal plexus. Once the flap is brought over into position, the upper border of the flap, at the point where it becomes the new lower lid, is sutured to the periosteum with a permanent suture to prevent ectropion postoperatively. The triangular defect is then closed with deep and superficial sutures (Fig. 46.15**B**). Before rotation and suturing of the flap, the composite chondromucosal graft is sutured in the conjunctival defect. Once the rotation oc-

curs and the flap is in place, the upper flap is sutured to a cuff of mucosa overhanging the top of the chondromucosal graft.

Advantages of the cheek flap include easy accessibility and operative technique. In the age group that presents most commonly with eyelid malignancies, there is sufficient laxity of the skin, and therefore good tissue is available to reconstruct the lower lid. Problems that can develop with this flap include hematoma, infection, or flap necrosis early in the postoperative course. Late complications include problems resulting mainly from skin tension and gravity, causing ectropion or lateral canthal distortion.

FIGURE 46.14. The semicircular flap may be useful for lower lid defects measuring up to two thirds of the lid.

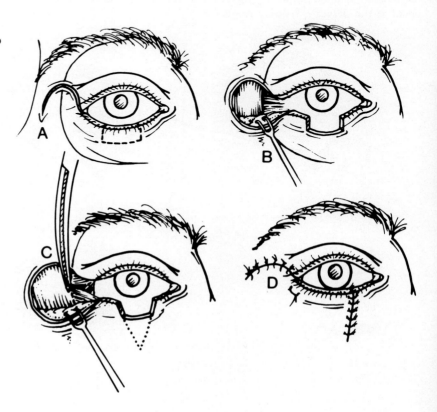

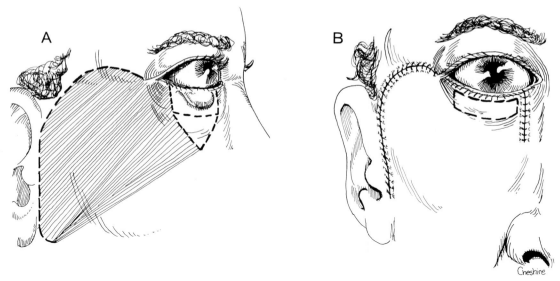

FIGURE 46.15. A Mustardé cheek flap may be used with a chondromucosal graft for reconstruction of large lid defects.

Advancement Flap

The advancement flap technique may also be used in upper lid reconstruction, and defects of greater than one half of the upper lid can be reconstructed by this technique (Fig. 46.16). The technique is basically the same as that for the lower lid, with the exception that the lateral incision is straighter and is not carried out to the preauricular area in the same manner (10). Undermining is done beneath the orbicularis muscle, with care being taken not to dissect too deep laterally because this can damage the facial nerve branches to the forehead. Before medial movement of the flap, assessment is made as to the need

for a composite cartilage-mucosa graft; if needed, it should be sutured in place to the medial and lateral edges of the defect. Very careful approximation of the cartilage graft in the medial suture line is necessary, with no visible sutures on the mucosal side after completion that could rub the cornea and cause abrasion or ulceration. After placement and suturing the graft into place, the flap is brought over the graft and sutured. The lateral cheek incision is sutured so that there is minimal tension on the vertical suture line. After completion of the procedure, a patch is placed over the eye to prevent motion for the first few postoperative days. A generous amount of antibacterial ophthalmic ointment is placed in the eye and suture

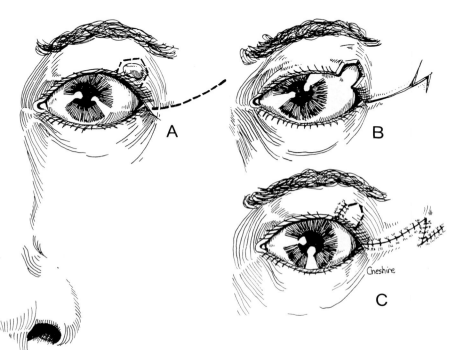

FIGURE 46.16. The upper lid may be reconstructed in a similar fashion by an advancement flap and possibly a chondromucosal graft (*dashed lines*).

FIGURE 46.17. A combination of a chondromucosal graft with a bipedicle Tripier flap can be used for lower lid reconstruction.

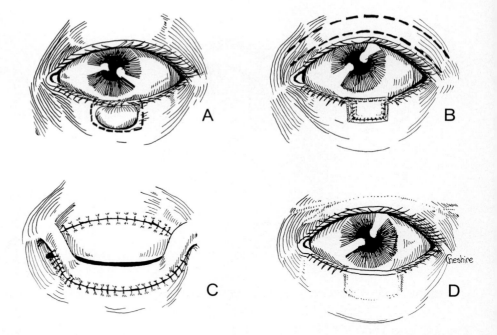

line twice daily. Reconstruction of the upper lid is much more difficult than the lower because of the need to take into consideration the continuous up and down movement.

Bipedicle "Tripier" Flap

The bipedicle Tripier flap is extremely useful for reconstruction of the horizontal defects of the lower lid. This flap is raised from the upper lid, includes skin and muscle from the area of the preseptal orbicularis muscle, and is based on medial and lateral pedicles (Fig. 46.17A). When a horizontal defect is present, the tarsus is replaced with a chondromucosal graft of the appropriate size. After the graft is sutured in place with a small flap of mucosa overlapping the upper border, the bipedicle flap is designed and elevated. The defect is directly closed by approximation of the skin only (Fig. 46.17B). The bipedicle flap is then sutured over the composite graft and the eye is treated with generous amounts of ophthalmic ointment before patching (Fig. 46.17C) for 48 hr, at which time it may be left open if desired. Clamping of both pedicles and revision of the pedicle bases may be done on about the seventh day. It is often necessary to defat the flap later (Fig. 46.17D). Although a flap from upper to lower lid is excellent, the reverse is generally not feasible.

FIGURE 46.18. **A–C,** A Mustardé cross-lid pedicle flap may be used for upper eyelid reconstruction. **D,** Detachment of the pedicle at about 10 days.

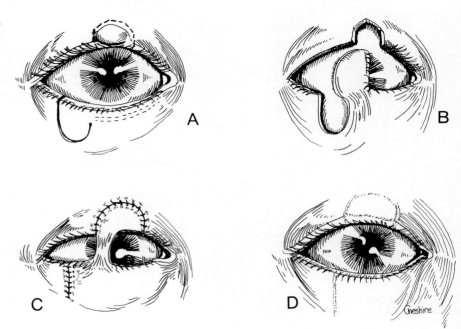

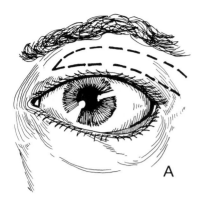 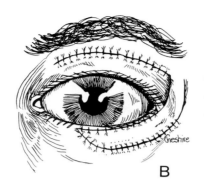

FIGURE 46.19. Single pedicle flaps may be useful for lower lid defects, medial and lateral.

Full-Thickness, Single Pedicle Flap (Cross Lid)

When a defect of the tarsal margin exists in the upper lid, it is possible to use a full-thickness lower lid flap based on the marginal arcade located between the orbicularis muscle and tarsal plate. Mustardé has used a formula for measuring the amount of replacement tissue necessary. Stated briefly, the width of the defect, minus one fourth of the width of the lid margin, is the exact width needed in the lower lid flap. Whenever possible, it should be based medially, because in closing the lower lid defect it is often necessary to mobilize cheek skin, making the vascular supply somewhat more tenuous. In addition, the flap should be oriented somewhat laterally of the defect of the upper lid to allow for rotation. Once the flap is measured and cut, the tarsal plate is completely divided, leaving the musculocutaneous pedicle intact for vascular support. The flap is rotated into place and the uppermost portion is attached to the levator aponeurosis with the tarsal margins approximated as precisely as possible. At this point the lower lid defect may be closed as described earlier (Fig. 46.18). This technique permits reconstruction of any size upper lid defect from one third to total loss. The usual outcome is a natural upper lid that functions well.

Single Pedicle Flap, Lower Lid Defect

Single pedicle flaps of the upper eyelid are easy to mobilize and generally are quite reliable. These flaps may be designed with as much as a 5:1 length ratio (Fig. 46.19). When designing the flap, a deep base should be included with muscle to enhance vascularity. These flaps may be used to cover partial-thickness loss of the lids. If a concomitant cartilage graft is needed for tarsal and conjunctival layers, the flap is usually capable of nourishing this graft.

Glabellar Flap

If the previously described techniques are not available, a glabellar flap or median forehead flap based on the supratrochlear vessels can be used to reconstruct the lids or defects in the medial canthal area (Fig. 46.20). The skin in this location is thicker than eyelid skin and should

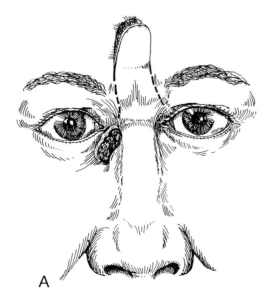 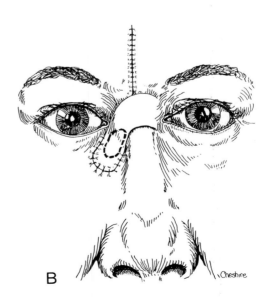

FIGURE 46.20. A glabellar flap may be used to cover larger defects of the eyelids or medial canthus. This may be essential with exposed bone.

FIGURE 46.21. A Hughes tarsoconjunctival flap with full-thickness graft coverage may be used for lower lid defects.

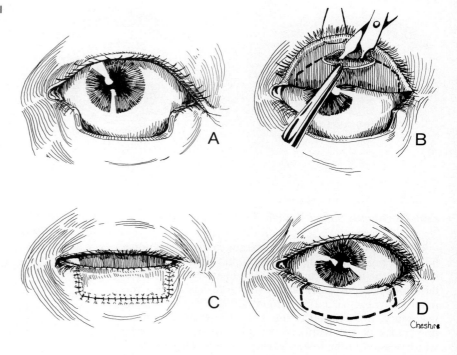

be used only if other procedures are not feasible. In general, these flaps will require subsequent thinning.

Lid-Sharing Techniques

Lid-sharing procedures can be utilized to reconstruct eyelid defects, such as the Hughes flap for horizontal defects of the lower lid (11, 12; Fig. 46.21). A tarsocon-junctival flap is rotated from the upper lid and sutured into the lower lid defect using a "tongue-in-groove" technique. This can be covered either with a full-thickness skin graft or advancement of the cheek skin. Care should be taken to leave the distal 4 mm of the tarsus intact to prevent entropion formation of the upper lid. The flap is divided about 6–8 weeks later to allow for stretching of the tarsoconjunctival flap and to ensure its vascularity. The disadvantages of this technique are that it requires

FIGURE 46.22. A Cutler-Beard flap may be advanced for upper eyelid reconstruction.

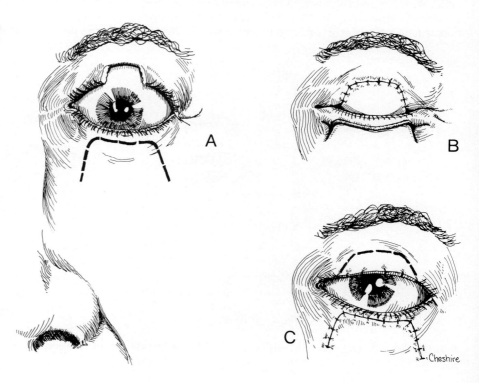

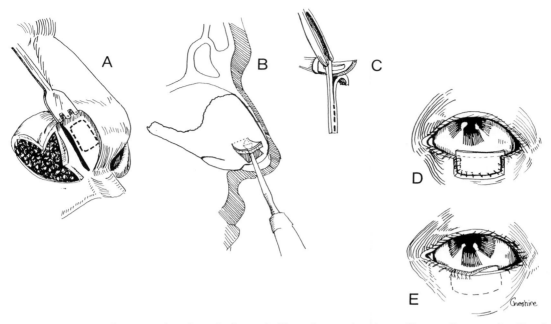

FIGURE 46.23. A thinned chondromucosal graft can be harvested from the nasal septum with a small mucosal cuff and may be used to provide lid stability in large defects.

two stages and keeps the eye covered for many weeks.

A Cutler-Beard flap may be utilized for upper lid defects (13). This involves creating a full-thickness pedicle of the lower lid just caudal to the marginal arcade and suturing it into the defect after advancement. It must be sutured to the levator to provide for upward excursion of the lid. Again, separation is carried out 8 weeks later (Fig. 46.22).

COMPOSITE CHONDROMUCOSAL GRAFTS

Composite chondromucosal septal grafts have been mentioned elsewhere in this chapter, but more must be said regarding indications and technique. These grafts should be liberally used to correct any defects of the tarsus and conjunctiva. The success of these grafts approximates 100%, and the donor area usually heals uneventfully. The largest graft that may be removed is about 2 × 3 cm, leaving the opposite septal mucosa and perichondrium to epithelialize. Once the defect is measured, a pattern is cut and laid on the nasal septum. The alar base may be incised to the caudal part of the nasal bone for more exposure. Infiltration of the septum with adrenalin solution and topical cocaine aids the dissection by encouraging hemostasis. An incision is made through the cartilage to the perichondrium of the opposite side. After undermining the mucoperichondrium, the cartilage edges are cut, either with a scalpel or sharp dissector. Once the graft is removed, cautery of some vessels posteriorly, using insulated forceps, is often necessary. If any exposed cartilage remains in the defect, it is removed so that epithelialization may occur. A piece of Gelfoam (Upjohn Co., Michigan) is cut to size, placed in the defect,

and overpacked with Vaseline gauze. The alar base incision is then closed. The cartilage is shaved on the exposed surface of the graft, which helps the graft conform to the round surface of the globe. A small (1.5-mm) cuff of mucosa is left on the upper border to suture to the covering flap. The graft is then sutured into place with either absorbable suture or a pull-out Prolene depending on the choice of the surgeon (Fig. 46.23).

When only supporting cartilage is needed without mucosal coverage, cartilage may be taken from the septum in the same manner in which a submucous resection is performed, utilizing only an anterior incision in the mucocutaneous junction. Conchal cartilage may be used in a similar manner (14). This graft is then sandwiched between the orbicularis muscle and the conjunctiva. Again, the graft is thinned to obtain the appropriate thickness and allow a subtle curvature.

LATERAL TARSAL STRIP CANTHOPLASTY

The tarsal strip canthoplasty is a very useful procedure in cases of posttraumatic, postsurgical, senile, or congenital ectropion (15, 16; Fig. 46.24). A horizontal incision is made at the lateral canthus through skin and muscle. Tenotomy scissors are then directed more vertically, and the inferior crus of the lateral canthal tendon is released. This structure may be difficult to visualize, but a distinct release can be felt. Tenotomy scissors are then placed submuscularly to release any significant cicatricial fibers. An infraciliary incision may be necessary to provide direct exposure. If the lower lid is excessively long, it can be shortened laterally. The lateral 3–4 mm are then deepithelialized, creating the lateral tarsodermal strip. This strip is then sutured to the periosteum of the superome-

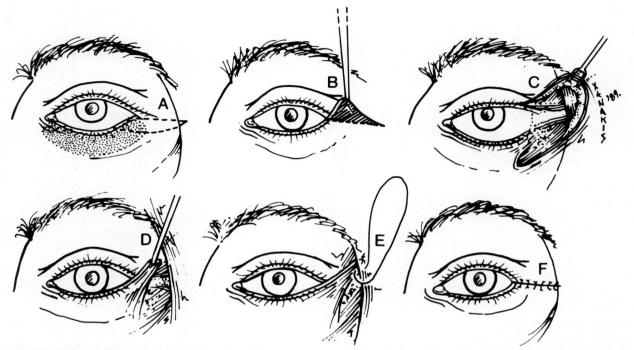

FIGURE 46.24. The lateral tarsal flap canthoplasty involves release of the inferior crura, release of any underlying adhesions, deepithelialization of a lateral tarsodermal strip, and attachment to the superomedial aspect of the lateral orbital rim.

dial aspect of the lateral orbital rim. This both raises and tightens the lower lid. A 4-0 Mersilene suture double armed on an S2 needle (Ethicon product) is a recommended suture. The lower lip should cover the inferior 2 mm of the limbus at the completion of the procedure to obtain the optimal position.

Complications

Complications may occur in eyelid reconstruction but are not frequent, owing to the precise nature of reconstruction of these small parts and the rich blood supply around the orbit.

Postoperative swelling is common, and is aggravated by inadequate hemostasis. Therefore, an absolutely dry field must be achieved in all cases. Steroids may be given postoperatively, along with head elevation and salt restriction.

A hematoma may occur and must be evacuated in order to achieve the best healing with diminished swelling and scarring. This complication can be serious if it occurs under a cheek flap and leads to partial necrosis of the flap. There is a higher incidence of necrosis in cheek flaps in patients who have had radiation therapy to this area. Loss of part or all of a flap should be treated by early débridement in most cases, and secondary coverage can be provided with a skin graft.

Corneal problems may occur, especially when a suture line is placed directly over the cornea. Examination of the deep surface of the lid to identify any suture fragments impinging on the cornea should be performed. A significant incidence of corneal problems occur after eye-

lid reconstruction, and frequent slit-lamp examinations may be indicated. Patching the eye or placing a temporary intermarginal tarsorrhaphy will help reduce the lid motion.

Notching of the lid margin at the area of closure may be excised as a secondary procedure or improved by Z-plasty technique. Irregularity of a lid margin can be reduced by opening the area over the cartilage and shaving the edge back to normal.

Asymmetry of one lid may be present, usually in the form of excess eyelid skin on the unoperated side compared to the operated side. Further revisions, including a blepharoplasty, may help in achieving symmetry of the lids.

Sagging of the lateral lid margin after reconstruction with a small or large cheek flap may be corrected by a small, laterally based flap from the upper lid. The base of this flap is superior to the lateral canthus and gives additional support to the sagging lid margin. If sagging is associated with a loose tarsal margin, removal of a tarsal wedge in addition to a small flap or graft aids in positioning the lid against the globe.

Postoperative edema caused by inadequate venous or lymphatic drainage may also be seen after cheek flap reconstruction. Although rare, these cases can be difficult to manage. Patience is critical and staged revision can be beneficial.

Lid-sharing procedures have the inherent risk of postoperative scarring in the donor lid. Some degree of lagophthalmus or retraction of the upper eyelid may occur with the Hughes or Cutler-Bear procedures. In addition, instability of the lid can be produced unless at least 3 mm of the marginal tarsal plate is preserved. Their major disadvantage, however, is that two procedures are required and the eye remains closed for many weeks.

Conclusions

Each of the reconstructive principles presented in this chapter applies equally well to defects that are congenital or result from tumor resection or trauma. Frozen section monitoring of surgical margins in tumor resection is critical. Aggressive resections are usually necessary, especially in recurrent lesions. The proper alignment of anatomical landmarks is especially important to prevent notching, asymmetry, or poor healing. The liberal use of chondromucosal grafts is recommended to facilitate lid support. Accurate attachment of any graft or flap to the levator is essential for proper upward mobility of the upper eyelid. There is a higher incidence of corneal problems in the postoperative period with upper eyelid reconstruction. All of these factors are necessary to ensure a reconstructed lid that is functional, aesthetic, and durable.

References

1. Robb RM: Refractive errors associated with hemangiomas of lids and orbit in infancy. *Am J Ophthalmol* 83:52, 1977.
2. Mustardé JC: *Repair and Reconstruction in the Orbital Region. A Practical Guide.* Edinburgh, Churchill Livingstone, 1980.
3. Grabb WC, Smith JW: *Plastic Surgery,* Boston, Little, Brown, and Co, 1979.
4. Aston SJ, Hornblass A, Meltzer MA, et al: *Third International Symposium of Plastic and Reconstructive Surgery of the Eye and Adnexa.* Baltimore, Williams & Wilkins, 1982, p 66.
5. Putterman AM: Viable composite grafting in eyelid reconstruction. *Am J Ophthalmol* 85:237, 1978.
6. Palletta FX: Lower eyelid reconstruction. *Plast Reconstr Surg* 51:653, 1973.
7. Price NM: Closure of surgical wounds using contiguous island flaps (double V to Y procedure). *Ann Plast Surg* 3:321, 1979.
8. Tenzel RR: Eyelid reconstruction by the semicircle flap technique. *Ophthalmology* 85:1164, 1978.
9. Tenzel RR: Lid reconstruction. In Della Rocca RC, Nesi FA, Lisman RD (eds): *Ophthalmic Plastic and Reconstructive Surgery.* St. Louis, CV Mosby Co, 1987, p 771.
10. McGregor IA: Eyelid reconstruction following subtotal resection of upper or lower lid. *Br J Plast Surg* 26:346, 1973.
11. Hughes WL: *Reconstructive Surgery of Eyelids.* St. Louis, CV Mosby Co, 1959.
12. McCord CD: *Oculoplastic Surgery.* New York, Raven Press, 1987.
13. Cutler NL, Beard C: Method for partial and total upper lid reconstruction. *Am J Ophthalmol* 39:1, 1955.
14. Matsuo K, Hirose T, Takahashi N, Iwasawa M, Satoh R: Lower eyelid reconstruction with a conchal cartilage graft. *Plast Reconstr Surg* 80:547, 1987.
15. Anderson RL, Gordy DD: The tarsal strip procedure. *Arch Ophthalmol* 97:2192, 1979.
16. Lisman RD, Rees T, Baker D, Smith B: Experience with tarsal suspension as a factor in lower lid blepharoplasty. *Plastic Reconstr Surg* 79:897, 1987.

47

Ear Reconstruction

David C. Leber, M.D., F.A.C.S.

Reconstruction of a deformed ear, whether of congenital or traumatic origin, presents meticulous and aesthetic challenges. Advancements in technique and alternative approaches have resulted in the achievement of favorable outcomes that are gratifying to both patient and physician. The purpose of this chapter is to present methods of ear reconstruction that have been tested and proved reliable. Emphasis is placed on the use of autologous rib cartilage, with procurement and carving for the ear framework described in detail. The coverage provided in this chapter is in no sense definitive. Appended references furnish sources with in-depth discussion of procedures that may be of assistance for particular ear reconstruction problems.

Congenital Ear Deformities

The most severe congenital deformities of the ear include anotia and microtia, in which there is complete or nearly complete absence of the external ear. Lesser deformities are those of hypoplasia of the middle third of the ear and hypoplasia of the superior third, which includes the cup ear, lop ear, cryptotia, and cockleshell ear deformities (1, 2). The least severe deformity, that of prominent ears, is discussed in Chapter 56.

TOTAL EAR RECONSTRUCTION

Historically, Gillies (3) was the first to describe total ear reconstruction with the use of carved cartilage placed under the scalp skin in 1920. The greatest advance in ear reconstruction came through the work of Tanzer in his classic description of the staged method of ear reconstruction using costocartilage as the framework (4, 5). Brent (6–8) further improved these techniques into what is now considered a state-of-the-art procedure for total ear reconstruction.

Of all other methods for total auricular reconstruction, including use of local tissues and the use of cartilage from the opposite ear, the most significant technique involves use of a silicone framework (9). This technique is discussed later.

A number of plastic surgeons suggest that reconstruction of a congenitally deformed ear be done around 6 years of age to avoid psychological trauma associated with deformity. Others, including myself, prefer to wait until about 8–10 years of age. Deferring surgery a few years allows the costocartilage to grow to sufficient size and thereby obviate fragmentary or gradual fabrication of the framework (10, 11).

The number of operations will vary depending on physical findings and patient preference regarding concha and tragus construction. At least two procedures are needed, and sometimes four or five operations can be anticipated.

Lobule formation may be done separately at an early age (4–6 years) or in combination with fabrication and insertion of the cartilage framework. The lobule can be rotated into position after insertion of the framework. When delaying framework insertion to 8 years of age or older, lobule rotation at an earlier age often reassures the patient and family that progress is being made. Recognition of an ear lobule combined with longer hair styles is psychologically rewarding to the child while awaiting the completion of reconstruction.

PREOPERATIVE PLANNING

Because it is impossible to reconstruct an ear that appears exactly like the normal ear, it is essential that the new ear be the correct size and in the proper position. Although many of the fine sculptured details are lost in a reconstructed ear because of a thicker skin cover, it is impressive how much detail will show. The anatomy of a normal ear must be well understood (Fig. 47.1). Further, characteristics of the patient's normal ear should be noted and, where possible, incorporated into the planning and carving of the framework for the new ear.

Detailed preoperative planning is essential to achieve the above goals. If the lobule is rotated as a preliminary step, its exact desired location must be determined with as much accuracy as is needed for insertion of the cartilage framework. Precise measurements of size and position of the normal ear are recorded (Fig. 47.2). The angle of inclination of the long axis of the ear usually falls between 10° and 30° in males and 2° and 20° in females (12).

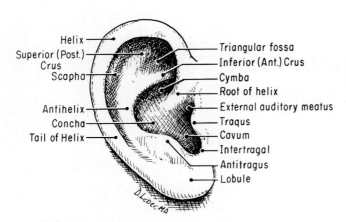

FIGURE 47.1. Anatomical landmarks of the normal ear.

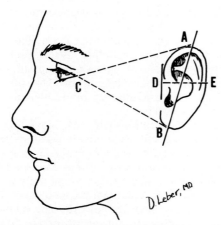

FIGURE 47.2. Measurements of normal ear: **AB** = long axis of ear; **DE** = width of ear; **AC** = distance of superior pole from lateral canthus; **BC** = distance of inferior pole from lateral canthus.

The use of clear x-ray film is helpful in determining the correct position for the reconstructed ear (Fig. 47.3). If there are problems with asymmetry of the face, as seen in hemifacial microsomia, location of the fabricated ear will need to be adjusted in proportion to the degree of hypoplasia. Patterns of the normal ear are drawn on clear x-ray film to determine the shape of the cartilage framework (Fig. 47.4). The patterns so devised are sterilized

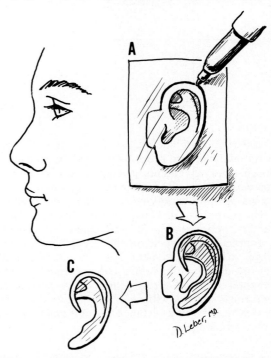

FIGURE 47.4. Patterns for a reconstructed ear. **A,** Outline the normal ear on clear x-ray film. **B,** Cut out pattern. **C,** Pattern for cartilage framework is drawn from the normal ear pattern, leaving 2 mm around outer margins for draping of skin cover.

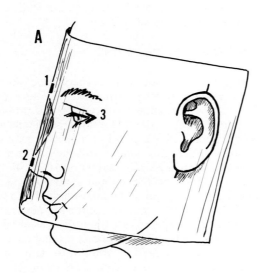

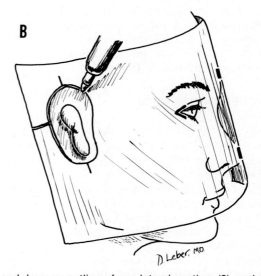

FIGURE 47.3. The method for determining the correct position of a reconstructed ear compared with the normal ear. **A,** Place ink marks on midline of forehead (**1**) and nose (**2**). Wrap a piece of clear x-ray film around the side of the face with the normal ear

and draw an outline of ear, lateral canthus (**3**), and points **1** and **2**. **B,** Cut out space within ear outline, reverse the x-ray film, line up the landmarks and draw outline where reconstructed ear should lie.

for use in the operating room during the carving process. Parallel strips of cardboard (Fig. 47.5) are helpful in checking the correct vertical position of the ear pattern (6, 8). Acrylic models of the normal ear and microtic ear as well as successive operative results provide an excellent three-dimensional record of pre- and postoperative findings. They can be used in planning proper use of the available tissue and as an aid in the operating room during carving of the framework (Fig. 47.6). These models are made from alginate molds of the ear and dental acrylic materials.

The most important preoperative aid is practice in carving an ear framework similar to the one planned for an individual patient. This helps the surgeon become familiar with the form and greatly decreases the amount of time required to carve the implant during actual surgery. If cadaver cartilage is not available for practice in carving, raw baking potatoes or balsa wood makes excellent substitute.

STAGING OF RECONSTRUCTION

Stage I: Lobule Rotation

In the classic microtia deformity, there is usually sufficient tissue to provide a lobule (Fig. 47.7) when transposed into the proper location (4, 5, 13–17). While there is vestigial cartilage in the superior portion of the ear remnant, the lower half is usually devoid of cartilage. It is best not to remove the cartilage from the upper portion at this time in order to avoid scar formation and contracture of the overlying skin, which provides excellent lining for the recess beneath the helical rim and triangular fossa area (18).

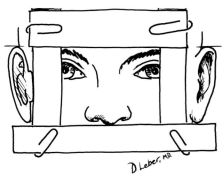

FIGURE 47.5. A guide for positioning the reconstructed ear.

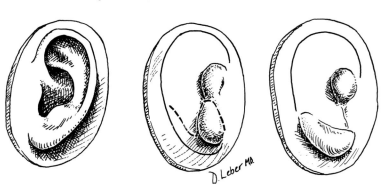

Stage II: Harvesting, Carving, and Implantation of Cartilage Framework

A method for harvesting cartilage necessary for total ear reconstruction is shown in Figure 47.8. By preserving the perichondrium, new cartilage will grow and fill the donor space, thereby precluding chest wall deformity. There is less chance of creating a pneumothorax with this technique. However, it is important to check for possible air leaks in the pleura before closing the chest wound in layers. There have been no problems with cartilage resorption after implantation in using this approach.

A step-by-step approach to rapid and accurate carving of the ear framework is demonstrated in Figures 47.9 and

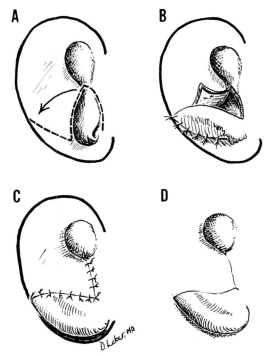

FIGURE 47.7. Lobule repositioning. **A,** Correct location of the completed ear outline must be marked so that the lobule can be accurately positioned. **B,** The lower half of microtic vestige is rotated into a new position, and posterior sutures are placed first. **C,** Anterior suture lines are completed. **D,** The well-healed lobule is ready for next stage.

FIGURE 47.6. Acrylic models showing pre- and postoperative findings.

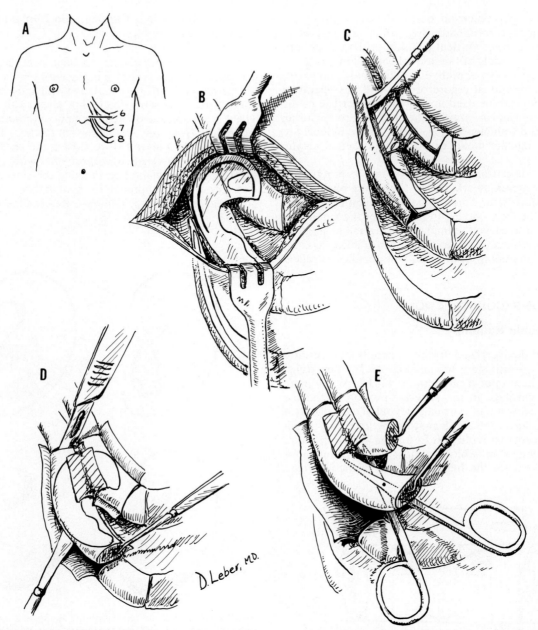

D. Leber, MD.

FIGURE 47.8. Harvesting costocartilage. **A,** Contralateral ribs 6, 7, and 8 are marked out. Transverse incision is placed in sixth interspace or inframammary fold of female patients with breast development. If skin graft is needed for conchal floor, an ellipse of full-thickness skin can be taken here. **B,** Incision transverses rectus abdominis muscle. The sixth, seventh, and eighth ribs are exposed to permit placement of framework pattern over cartilage. **C,** Superficial incisions are made through perichondrium along longitudinal axis of sixth and seventh ribs. Perichondrium is then carefully lifted up as flaps with Freer elevator. The *cross-hatched area* represents the synchondrosis of the sixth and sev-

enth ribs and is undisturbed so that continuity of the two ribs is maintained. **D,** The proximal and distal ends of the cartilage are partially cut through with a no. 15 blade and completed with a thin Freer elevator. The cartilage block is then lifted up with a hook, and the thin perichondrium is separated from the posterior surface, taking great care not to penetrate the pleural cavity. **E,** Separation of the posterior synchondrosis is completed with scissors. The eighth rib is easily removed by blunt dissection without preserving the perichondrium. A length of 10 cm is usually needed.

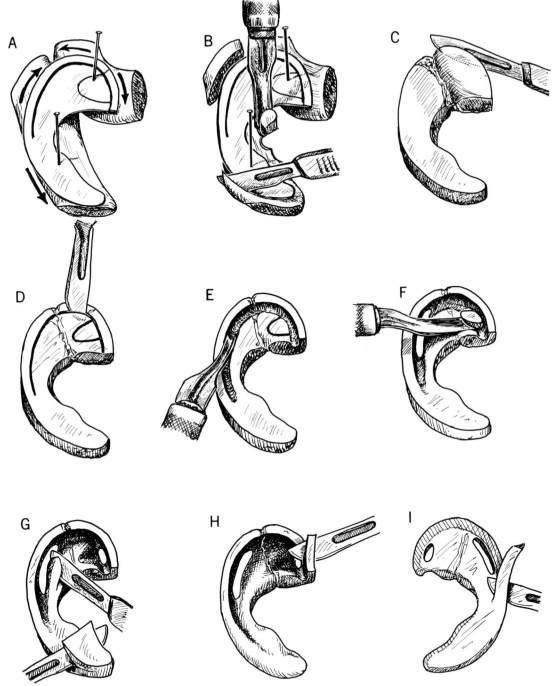

FIGURE 47.9. Carving cartilage framework. **A,** The framework pattern is fixed with two pins to cartilage. Because of grain characteristics of cartilage, knife cuts should be made with the grain in the direction of the *arrows*. There is no need to draw an outline on cartilage. **B,** The outline is cut with a no. 10 blade. The inside curve of the antihelix is quickly removed with 3/8-inch U X-ACTO_R gouge. Cuts are perpendicular to surface. **C,** The anterior surface is flattened by shaving the curved portion with a no. 10 blade (note that the synchondrosis is preserved). **D,** The inside edge of the helical rim and triangular fossa are marked out with methylene blue. A checking cut 3 mm deep is made around the helical rim; this helps prevent accidental removal of the rim in subsequent steps. **E,** Excavation of the scapha is done with a 3/32-inch U X-ACTO_R gouge. **F,** Successive cuts are made with the narrow gouge until the cartilage is removed through to the

back surface in the area of the triangular fossa and posterior scapha. Holes through the framework permit better fixation of overlying skin, thus preventing loss of detail. The triangular fossa is completed with the 3/8-inch gouge. **G,** The tail of the helical rim is thinned from the anterior surface. This allows the tail and lobular support to curve posteriorly as a result of uneven forces exerted within the cartilage (18). The antihelix is further refined with a no. 10 blade, rounding off the contours. **H,** The anterior aspect of the helical rim is reduced in height to receive the added strip of cartilage that forms the root of the helix. The edges of the lobule, antitragus, and antihelix are carefully rounded to final shape. **I,** Turning the framework over, the posterior margin of the helical rim is rounded off so that a more normal appearance is created when the ear is lifted away from the side of the head.

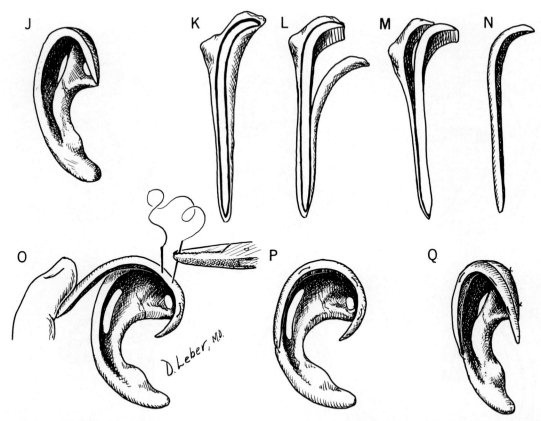

FIGURE 47.10. Carving cartilage framework (continued). **J,** Three-quarter view of completed framework base. Note undermining of helical rim. **K,** Pattern for helical rim is drawn on eighth rib (note the preformed curve in superior aspect). This will form the extension of the root of the helix. **L,** To prevent warpage, an equal amount of cartilage is removed from each side; removing the concave side first prevents accidental breakage of the narrow strip. **M,** Completion of profile cuts. **N,** The strip is also thinned on top and bottom. The outside edge is rounded while the inside edge is hollowed to increase the overhang and detail of the helical rim. **O,** The helical rim piece is easily fixed in position using 5-0 Ethilon (Ethicon, Inc.) clear monofilament nylon suture double armed with Ethicon ST-4 straight taper-point needles. The needles fix the cartilage until the suture is pulled through and tied posteriorly. When required, more flexibility of the rim can be achieved by small cuts around the outside edge. **P,** Four or five sutures complete the ear framework, which is now ready for implantation. **Q,** Three-quarter view of completed cartilage framework.

47.10. In addition to the standard surgical knife and no. 10 blade, X-ACTO$_R$ (Hunt Manufacturing Co.) gouges with a no. 6 handle are used for carving. These tools can be sterilized and are extremely sharp. When the blades become worn, they can be replaced easily. Moist 4 × 4 gauze sponges give satisfactory support while carving and prevent the cartilage from becoming dehydrated. The average time required for carving the framework and fixing the helical rim is 45 min.

The framework carved for the ear is buried under the skin of the scalp in the predetermined auricular area (Fig. 47.11**A–C**). Dissection of the scalp skin must be executed carefully in order not to interrupt the vascular supply. To hold the skin in place against the implanted framework and into the undermined helical rim, stents of loosely rolled petrolatum gauze (Fig. 47.11**E** and **F**) are sutured into position with interrupted 4-0 nylon. (Some surgeons prefer to use suction drains for this purpose, but I have found petrolatum gauze stents more reliable.) With appropriate care, there should be no concern about necrosis of the skin from excessive pressure and tension. The stents are kept in place for 3 weeks to keep the skin tightly applied to the underlying cartilage framework.

When there is insufficient skin to close the incision (Fig. 47.11**D**), a full-thickness skin graft is placed in the floor of the concha. Upon completion of the procedure, the ear is dressed with cotton, fluffed 4 × 4 gauzes, and soft pads and wrapped with a conforming gauze dressing.

Stage III: Elevation of Ear and Creation of Postauricular Sulcus

If there is sufficient height of the ear and a postauricular sulcus is not desired by the patient, this stage can be eliminated (6). However, most patients do prefer to have

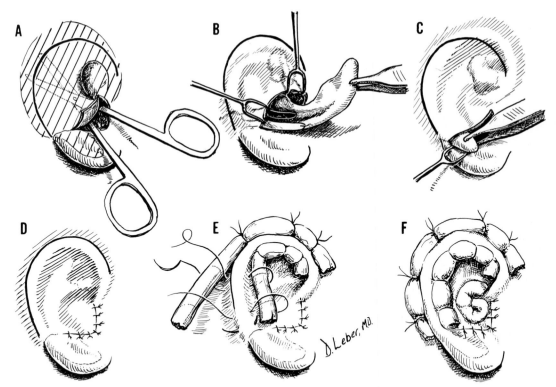

FIGURE 47.11. The cartilage framework is implanted. **A,** A subcutaneous pocket can be made through the incision of the first-stage lobule transfer. If the lobule is being transferred at the same time as the cartilage implantation, even greater exposure is available. The thin skin is carefully dissected off the rudimentary ear cartilage in the upper pole, and the deformed cartilage is removed. The pocket is dissected into the lobule to receive the tail of the helix and continued 1 cm beyond the planned ear outline. Careful hemostasis is necessary. **B,** The cartilage is inserted and rotated into position. **C,** The tail of the helix is then inserted into the lobule. **D,** The incision is closed with 5-0 nylon. If there is insufficient skin to line the conchal floor, a full-thickness skin graft can be inserted. **E,** Stents made of rolled petrolatum gauze are sutured into position with 4-0 nylon snug enough to hold the skin into the undermined helical rim but not too tight so as to cause circulatory compromise. **F,** The conchal floor is kept in place with a separate roll of gauze, which is held by a bulky soft-pressure dressing.

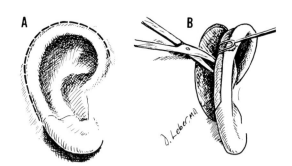

FIGURE 47.12. The auricle is elevated. **A,** A skin incision is made just outside the helical rim. **B,** The ear is lifted away from the scalp, and the sulcus is carefully dissected, avoiding exposure of the cartilage graft. **C,** The extent of the sulcus dissection is overemphasized to compensate for some contracture of the graft. The posterior scalp skin is undermined to permit advancement of the skin edge, thus reducing the size of the defect and hiding the graft behind the ear. **D,** The advanced scalp skin is sutured to underlying fascia, and the remaining defect is covered with a full-thickness skin graft. The ear is covered with a bulky pressure dressing, and a wedge of foam rubber is placed in the sulcus.

the ear elevated (Fig. 47.12). This procedure involves undermining the cartilage graft through a periauricular incision (taking care not to expose the cartilage), advancing the scalp skin (5), and covering the defect with a full-thickness skin graft. This procedure can be done 4–6 months after the cartilage is implanted. Occasionally, custom-made silicone splints are helpful in maintaining the sulcus because skin graft contracture is inevitable. A "set-back" of the normal ear may be done at the same time to provide symmetry. If cartilage and skin from the

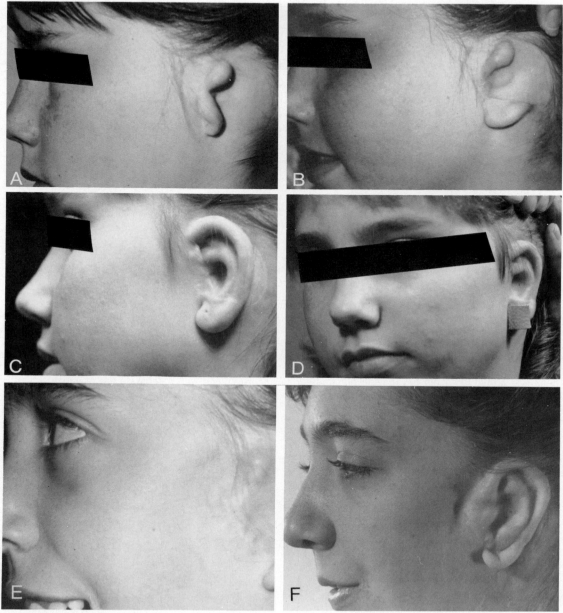

FIGURE 47.13. Results using the previously described techniques. **A,** Preoperative findings are photographed. **B,** Lobule rotation is completed. **C,** Two years after insertion of cartilage framework; no tragus has been formed at this time. **D,** Three-quarter view shows the wearing of pierced earrings. **E,** Patient with microtia and hemifacial microsomia after lobule rotation. **F,** Results after ear reconstruction and jaw advancement. **G,** Adult with normal concha and canal. **H,** After insertion of complete cartilage graft and postauricular skin graft and excision of original deformed helical rim tissue.

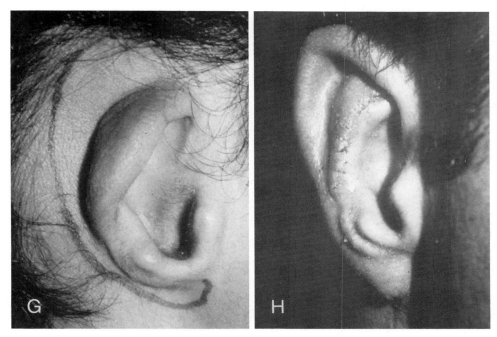

FIGURE 47.13E–H.

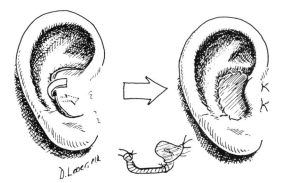

FIGURE 47.14. The concha is deepened, and the tragus is formed.

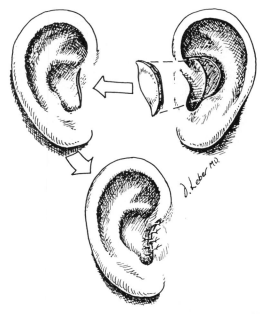

FIGURE 47.15. Tragus formation. (After Brent (8).)

normal ear are needed for tragus formation, then the set-back procedure should be deferred until a later time. Figure 47.13 shows pre- and postoperative results.

Concha and Tragus Formation

When definition of the conchal floor is lacking, the floor can be deepened. The flap of skin is advanced anteriorly to form a tragus (Fig. 47.14) and the floor is covered with a full-thickness skin graft (19). Care must be taken to avoid possible injury to the facial nerve because it may be abnormally positioned in association with the ear deformity.

When the conchal floor is sufficient, the tragus can be constructed with a composite graft of cartilage and skin from the concha of the opposite ear (Fig. 47.15). The graft is sutured in a semi-upright position to give the projection of the tragus. The donor site is closed primarily (8).

ALTERNATE METHODS OF TOTAL EAR RECONSTRUCTION

When rib cartilage is of inadequate size, an expansile framework of cartilage may be indicated (20). Problems

FIGURE 47.16. A temporalis fascia "fan flap." **A,** The temporalis fascia and periosteum are exposed and elevated. **B,** The flap is draped over the exposed implant and covered with a split-thickness skin graft while the skin flap is sutured behind the ear framework. (Redrawn from Fox JW, Edgerton MT: The fan flap: An adjunct to ear reconstruction. *Plast Reconstr Surg* 58:664, 1976.)

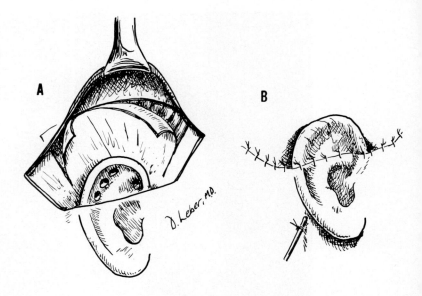

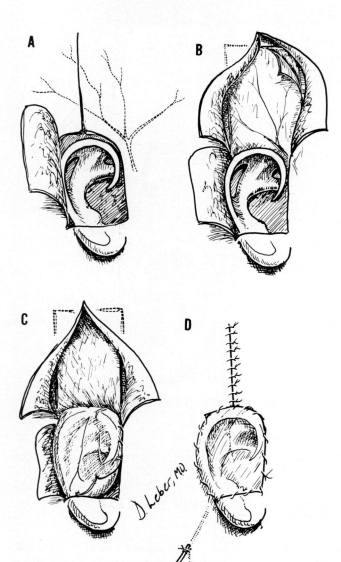

with loss of detail have been avoided by using Dacron backing on the cartilage framework (21). A method of ear reconstruction has been described that places emphasis on formation of the concha (22), using the expansile principle. With better understanding of the skin circulation, thinner flaps have been employed in a one-stage total ear reconstruction procedure (23). The advantages and disadvantages of this method should be evaluated carefully before discarding time-proven procedures. A bipedicled postauricular tubed flap has been used for less severe forms of microtia (24).

Preformed silicone frameworks are the most commonly used implants in total ear construction when cartilage is not available or used (9, 25, 26). The major disadvantage to this procedure is a high incidence of complications, such as infection and exposure of implant. However, methods are available for salvaging the exposed implant in this approach to auricular reconstruction (27).

Newer techniques of covering the silicone implants with temporal fascia "fan flaps" (28; Fig. 47.16) and temporoparietal fascia (29; Fig. 47.17), followed by skin

FIGURE 47.17. The temporoparietalis fascia flap. **A,** Skin incisions with posteriorly based flap for lining postauricular sulcus. **B,** The scalp skin is carefully elevated just below the level of the hair follicles while avoiding injury to superficial temporal vessels. The parietal fascia flap is then elevated off the underlying temporalis fascia. **C,** The fascial flap is draped over the ear implant and sutured in place with 5-0 absorbable sutures. **D,** Suction is applied through small catheter to hold the flap in place. A medium thickness skin graft from the suprascapular area is placed over the fascia flap. (Redrawn from Tegtmeier RE, Gooding RA: The use of a fascial flap in ear reconstruction. *Plast Reconstr Surg* 60:407, 1977.)

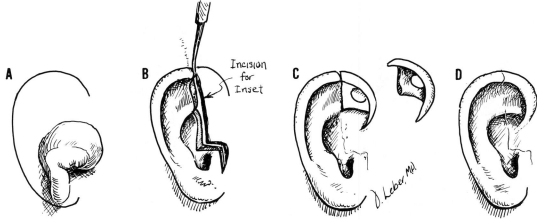

FIGURE 47.18. A cockleshell ear deformity. **A,** Typical deformity of cockleshell ear showing outline of the desired position of the ear. **B,** The anterior superior portion of the constricted ear is separated from its attachment to the side of the head and unfurled, revealing the missing anterior superior one third of the ear. Existing tissue is inserted into the scalp at this position. **C,** Several months later, a cartilage graft is carved from costocartilage and buried under the scalp skin. **D,** Three months later, the superior pole is lifted away from the head, and the sulcus is lined with a skin graft.

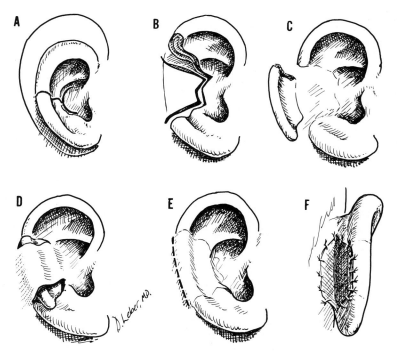

FIGURE 47.19. Reconstruction of the middle one third of the ear. **A,** Severely constricted ear showing outline for the desired size and incision for expansion. **B,** A posteriorly based scalp flap is incised. Posterior ear skin is sutured to outside margins of scalp incision. Anterior ear skin is sutured to inside flap margins. **C,** Several months later, an appropriate costocartilage graft is carved to fill the central one third of the defect. **D,** The graft is inserted into tunnel through two small incisions. **E,** After incisions have matured, the ear is lifted from the side of the head through an incision along the posterior helical margin. Care is taken not to expose the cartilage graft. **F,** A full-thickness skin graft covers the postauricular defect. (After Webster (32).)

grafting, have improved the results with less exposure of implants and good definition of auricular details. These flaps are also useful where good skin coverage is not available, such as in burn injuries (30).

PARTIAL EAR RECONSTRUCTION

Upper Third

Severe constriction and hypoplasia of the upper third of the ear is expressed in the cockleshell ear deformity (Fig. 47.18). Reconstruction is accomplished by unfurling the ear and insetting it into the scalp. After several months, a cartilage graft is carved corresponding to the defect, buried under the scalp, and then later lifted away from the side of the head (7, 31; Cramer, personal communication).

Middle Third

Hypoplasia of the middle third of the ear (Fig. 47.19) can be corrected by opening and expanding the ear in the midportion and insetting the cut edges into the scalp. An appropriately shaped cartilage graft is placed under the

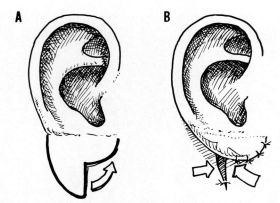

FIGURE 47.20. The lobule is reconstructed. **A,** Incisions for new lobule show that the inferior portion of the flap will be folded under the upper portion of the flap to provide double thickness. **B,** The anterior and posterior neck skin is undermined, advanced, and closed without need for a skin graft. (After Zentenio (38).)

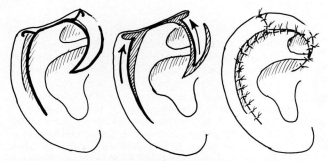

FIGURE 47.21. Small acquired defects of the superior aspect of the ear can be corrected by advancing anterior and posterior skin and cartilage flaps. Incisions are made along heavy lines, and the flaps advanced superiorly and sutured. (After Antia and Buch (47).)

mature skin. The ear is lifted away from the scalp after several months and the postauricular sulcus is covered with a skin graft (32, 33).

Lower Third or Lobule Construction

A number of methods have been suggested for lobule construction using local soft tissue flaps (32–37). A representation of one of these methods (38) is presented in Figure 47.20. Lobule reconstruction can be very disappointing if there is no internal support, such as cartilage. In the absence of support, considerable atrophy of the new lobule will occur.

Acquired Ear Deformities

Acquired ear deformities include partial and complete traumatic amputations of the ear, burns, and tumors of the ear. Accidental loss of portions or complete amputation of the external ear is not common. Methods for treating such injuries have improved considerably. Simple replantation of the entire ear or parts of the ear has been

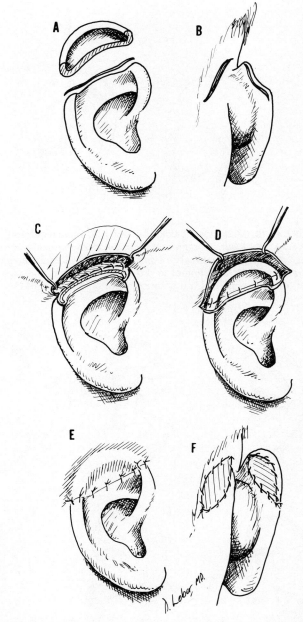

FIGURE 47.22. The upper third of the ear (tunnel procedure) is reconstructed. **A,** The size and shape of the lost ear part can be determined by placing a pattern of the normal ear over the injured ear. A cartilage framework is then carved from costal cartilage corresponding to the missing part. **B,** Incisions are made along the margin of the ear defect and over the corresponding scalp skin when the ear is pressed against the scalp. **C,** A pocket is dissected under the scalp skin. **D,** The carved cartilage framework is placed under the pocket and sutured to the margin of the remaining ear cartilage. **E,** The scalp skin is then brought over the graft and sutured to the anterior ear skin margin. The scalp skin is held against the framework either with bolsters as in Figure 47.11 or with suction. **F,** Three to 6 months later, the ear is separated from the scalp, and full-thickness skin grafts are used to cover the defects on the scalp and postauricular sulcus. (After Converse (33).)

successfully accomplished (39–42); however, the results are not dependable. Safer techniques such as the "pocket principle" (43, 44) and microsurgical anastomoses of small blood vessels (45) have improved the success rate of ear replantation.

The pocket principle requires dermabrasion of the anterior skin of the amputated part, removal of the posterior skin, fenestration of the cartilage (46), and burying the part under a scalp flap while carefully suturing the part to its original point of attachment. Two weeks later, the buried part is exteriorized and allowed to epithelialize. A graft is then used to resurface the postauricular surface.

When small portions of the ear are missing, local advancement flaps (Fig. 47.21) can be used to improve the contour (47, 48). If larger portions of the ear are absent, the "tunnel procedure" of Converse (33) is useful (Fig. 47.22).

Other adjuncts in correcting partial defects due to trauma or losses due to tumor resection include the use of small tubed pedicle flaps, skin grafts, and composite grafts from the opposite ear (49).

Full-thickness burns of the ear present a difficult challenge in reconstruction. Frameworks of cartilage are preferred (20). Skin cover seems to be best provided with either the temporalis fascia flap or the temporoparietal fascia flap covered with a skin graft (28–30; Figs. 47.16 and 47.17). A thin cervical myocutaneous flap has also been used to cover exposed ear cartilage after burn injuries (50).

In the process of repairing defects of the ear, a slightly smaller ear may be the end result. If the difference is significant, symmetry of both ears can be obtained by a reduction in size of the normal ear (51–53).

Complications

The most significant complication of ear reconstruction is exposure of the implant. The causes of exposure are usually local trauma, infection, or too much tension of the skin cover leading to necrosis of the skin. When the ear framework is of silicone, the problems are more severe and may require removal of the implant. Salvage can be accomplished at times with use of the temporal fascia flaps (28–30). Exposure of a cartilage graft can usually be treated conservatively by preventing desiccation of the exposed cartilage, trimming the edges, and allowing the skin edges to grow over the defect. Rotation flaps may be needed for larger defects (54). Prevention of exposure requires attention to many details. These include absence of tension on the skin cover, avoidance of peripheral incisions in the area of the helical rim, and great care in dissecting the pocket for implant insertion so that skin circulation is not interrupted.

References

1. Rogers B: Microtia, lop, cup and protruding ears: Four directly inheritable deformities? *Plast Reconstr Surg* 41:208, 1968.
2. Tanzer RC: The constricted (cup and lop) ear. *Plast Reconstr Surg* 55:406, 1975.
3. Gillies H: *Plastic Surgery of the Face.* London, H Frowde, Hodder and Stoughton, 1920.
4. Tanzer RC: Total reconstruction of the external ear. *Plast Reconstr Surg* 23:1, 1959.
5. Tanzer RC: Total reconstruction of the auricle. The evolution of a plan of treatment. *Plast Reconstr Surg* 47:523, 1971.
6. Brent B: The correction of microtia with autogenous cartilage grafts: I. The classic deformity. *Plast Reconstr Surg* 66:1, 980.
7. Brent B: The correction of microtia with autogenous cartilage grafts: II. Atypical and complex deformities. *Plast Reconstr Surg* 66:13, 1980.
8. Brent B: A personal approach to total auricular construction. *Clin Plast Surg* 8:211, 1981.
9. Cronin TD: Use of a Silastic frame for total and subtotal reconstruction of the external ear: Preliminary report. *Plast Reconstr Surg* 37:399, 1966.
10. Baurinka L: Congenital malformations of the auricle and their reconstruction by a new method. *Acta Chir Plast* 8:53, 1966.
11. Fukuda O, Yamada A: Reconstruction of the microtic ear with autogenous cartilage. *Clin Plast Surg* 5:351, 1978.
12. Farkas LG: Growth of normal and reconstructed auricles. In Tanzer RC, Edgerton MT (eds): *Symposium on Reconstruction of the Auricle,* St. Louis, CV Mosby Co, 1974, p 24.
13. Tanzer RC: Reconstruction of the auricle in four stages. In *Transactions of the Fifth International Congress of Plastic and Reconstructive Surgery.* Melbourne, Butterworth, 1971, p 445.
14. Tanzer RC: Correction of microtia with autogenous costal cartilage. In Tanzer RC, Edgerton MT (eds): *Symposium on Reconstruction of the Auricle.* St. Louis, CV Mosby Co, 1974, p 46.
15. Tanzer RC: Congenital deformities of the auricle. In Converse JM (ed): *Reconstructive Plastic Surgery.* Philadelphia, WB Saunders Co, 1977, p 1671.
16. Tanzer RC, Rueckert F: Reconstruction of the ear. In Grabb WC, Smith JW (eds): *Plastic Surgery, A Concise Guide to Clinical Practice,* ed 2. Boston, Little, Brown & Co, 1973, p 494.
17. Tanzer RC: Total reconstruction of the external ear. *Ann Plast Surg* 10:76, 1983.
18. Gibson T, Davis WB: The distortion of autogenous cartilage grafts: Its cause and prevention. *Br J Plast Surg* 10:257, 1958.
19. Kirkham HJD: The use of preserved cartilage in ear reconstruction. *Ann Surg* 111:896, 1940.
20. Brent B: Reconstruction of ear, eyebrow, and sideburn in the burned patient. *Plast Reconstr Surg* 55:312, 1975.
21. McGribbon B: Use of Dacron backing on the cartilage framework in the construction of ears. *Plast Reconstr Surg* 60:262, 1977.
22. Matsumoto K: A new method of reconstruction in microtia with emphasis on conchal creation. *Ann Plast Surg* 5:51, 1980.
23. Song Y, Song Y: An improved one-stage total ear reconstruction procedure. *Plast Reconstr Surg* 71:615, 1983.
24. Sarig A, Ben-Bassat M, Taube E, et al: Reconstruction of the auricle in microtia by bipedicled postauricular tubed flap. *Ann Plast Surg* 8:221, 1982.
25. Cronin TD: Reconstruction of the external ear with a Silastic frame. In *Transactions of the Fifth International Congress of Plastic and Reconstructive Surgery.* Melbourne, Butterworth, 1971, p 452.
26. Cronin TD: Use of a silastic frame for reconstruction of the auricle. In Tanzer RC, Edgerton MT (eds): *Symposium on Reconstruction of the Auricle.* St. Louis, CV Mosby Co, 1974, p 33.
27. Edgerton MT, Bacchetta C: Principles in the use and salvage of implants in ear reconstruction. In Tanzer RC, Edgerton MT (eds): *Symposium on Reconstruction of the Auricle.* St. Louis, CV Mosby Co, 1974, p 58.
28. Fox JW, Edgerton MT: The fan flap: An adjunct to ear reconstruction. *Plast Reconstr Surg* 58:663, 1976.
29. Tegtmeier RE, Gooding RA: The use of a fascial flap in ear reconstruction. *Plast Reconstr Surg* 60:406, 1977.
30. Cotlar SW: Reconstruction of the burned ear using a temporalis fascial flap. *Plast Reconstr Surg* 71:45, 1983.

31. Davis J: Repair of severe cup ear deformities. In Tanzer RC, Edgerton MT (eds): *Symposium on Reconstruction of the Auricle*. St. Louis, CV Mosby Co, 1974, p 134.
32. Webster JP: Some procedures for the correction of ear deformities. In *Transactions of the 13th Annual Meeting of the American Society for Plastic and Reconstructive Surgery*. City, Publisher, 1944, p 123.
33. Converse JM: Reconstruction of the auricle. *Plast Reconstr Surg* 22:150, 1958.
34. Davis J: Repair of traumatic defects of the auricle. In Tanzer RC, Edgerton MT (eds): *Symposium on Reconstruction of the Auricle*. St. Louis, CV Mosby Co, 1974, p 247.
35. Kazanjian VH, Converse JM: *The Surgical Treatment of Facial Injuries*. ed 2. Baltimore, Williams & Wilkins Co, 1959, p 1013.
36. Subba Rao YV, Venkatesware Rao P: A quick technique for earlobe reconstruction. *Plast Reconstr Surg* 41:13, 1968.
37. Brent B: Earlobe reconstruction with an auriculomastoid flap. *Plast Reconstr Surg* 57:389, 1976.
38. Zentenio AS: A new method for earlobe reconstruction. *Plast Reconstr Surg* 45:254, 1970.
39. McDowell F: Successful replantation of a severed half ear. *Plast Reconstr Surg* 48:281, 1971.
40. Larsen J, Pless J: Replantation of severed ear parts. *Plast Reconstr Surg* 57:176, 1976.
41. Lewis EC, Fowler JR: Two replantations of severed ear parts. *Plast Reconstr Surg* 64:703, 1979.
42. Salyapongse A, Maun LP, Suthunyarat P: Successful replantation of a totally severed ear. *Plast Reconstr Surg* 64:706, 1979.
43. Mladick RA, Horton CE, Adamson JE, et al: The pocket principle: A new technique for reattachment of severed ear part. *Plast Reconstr Surg* 48:219, 1971.
44. Mladick RA, Carraway JH: Ear reattachment by modified pocket principle. *Plast Reconstr Surg* 51:584, 1973.
45. Pennington DG, Lai MF, Pelly AD: Successful replantation of a completely avulsed ear by microvascular anastomoses. *Plast Reconstr Surg* 65:820, 1980.
46. Converse JM, Brent B: Acquired deformities of the auricle. In Converse JM (ed): *Reconstructive Plastic Surgery*, ed 2. Philadelphia, WB Saunders Co, 1977, p 1724.
47. Antia NH, Buch VI: Chondrocutaneous advancement flap for the marginal defect of the ear. *Plast Reconstr Surg* 39:472, 1967.
48. Renard A: Post auricular flap based on a dermal pedicle for ear reconstruction. *Plast Reconstr Surg* 68:159, 1981.
49. Brent B: The acquired auricular deformity: A systematic approach to its analysis and reconstruction. *Plast Reconstr Surg* 59:475, 1977.
50. McGrath MH, Ariyan S: Immediate reconstruction of full-thickness burn of the ear with an undelayed myocutaneous flap. *Plast Reconstr Surg* 62:618, 1978.
51. Peer LA, Walker JC: Total reconstruction of the ear. *J Int Coll Surg* 27:290, 1957.
52. Furnas DW: Problems in planning reconstruction in microtia. In Tanzer RC, Edgerton MT (eds): *Symposium on Reconstruction of the Auricle*. St. Louis, CV Mosby Co, 1974, p 93.
53. Tipton JB: A simple technique for reduction of the earlobe. *Plast Reconstr Surg* 66:630, 1980.
54. Tanzer RC: Reconstruction of the auricle. In Goldwyn RM (ed): *The Unfavorable Result in Plastic Surgery*. Boston, Little, Brown & Co, 1972, p 147.

48

Facial Paralysis: Principles of Treatment

Nancy Van Laeken, M.D., F.R.C.S.(C.) and Ralph T. Manktelow, M.D., F.R.C.S.(C.)

The patient with facial paralysis experiences very severe functional and cosmetic deformities related to the muscular inactivity on the affected side. The treatment goals are influenced by the aesthetic and functional deficits that are most troublesome to the patient. It is important to individualize each patient's treatment to fit the anatomical location and the degree of deformity and dysfunction. A careful history should be taken to identify clearly what it is that most bothers the patient. A detailed physical examination will then indicate the anatomical deformity that is producing the problem. From this, the surgeon can review the treatment modalities that are available for each functional and aesthetic problem and select the most appropriate procedure.

The treatment options are influenced by the age of the patient, the duration of the facial paralysis, the status of the nerve trunk, and the state of the facial musculature and soft tissues (1).

The goals of reconstruction are both functional and aesthetic. Functional recovery takes priority in the reconstruction. It is of utmost importance, in view of the possibility of corneal ulceration and blindness, to prevent eye complications in the patient with facial paralysis. Ideally, the remaining goals are to produce spontaneous facial movement and facial symmetry, both at rest and in the animated state. Animation should be spontaneous, but this is a goal that has, until recently, eluded the reconstructive surgeon. When it is clearly established that recovery will not take place spontaneously, timely reconstruction should be planned to minimize the patient's emotional stress and to take maximum benefit from the condition of the facial tissues (Fig. 48.1).

Treatment

EARLY RECONSTRUCTION (Table 48.1)

When possible, early *direct suture of divided facial nerve ends* will offer the best chance for good functional recovery (2). This should be done as soon as possible, before significant muscle degeneration occurs (preferably less than 6 months).

The nerve stumps should be realigned in fascicular groups without tension (3, 4). The repair is epineural and is performed with the aid of a microscope (5). If the nerve laceration is to a single branch and is anterior to the parotid, nerve repair is not necessary because their is overlapping function of distal branches. If multiple branches are damaged, as is usually the case, nerve repair is necessary.

To avoid tension and overcome gaps, it may be necessary to use a *nerve graft* (6). The best results are achieved using a nerve graft of appropriate cross-sectional diameter, such as a split sural nerve or the greater auricular nerve, depending on the level of nerve injury.

The results of nerve grafting are dependent upon the ability of the axons to pass through the anastomosis, the state of the muscles once the axons have reached the myoneural junction, and the appropriateness of the reinnervation (7). A major problem in the patient who obtains reinnervation through direct nerve repair, and especially through nerve grafting in the proximal portion of the facial nerve, is synkinesis. It is quite disturbing for the patient's eye to close during smiling. If the orbicularis oris contracts simultaneously with the lip elevators, the patient appears to be grimacing instead of smiling.

In situations where it is not possible to do a direct nerve repair, VIIth nerve axons may be directed to the distal end(s) of the facial nerve by *cross-facial nerve grafts* from the nonparalyzed side. Transfers from other cranial nerves, such as X, XI, and XII, to the distal nerve end(s) will provide facial muscle tone and a degree of controlled motion, and these are useful for some patients.

The technique of cross-facial nerve grafting has been described in the past by Smith, Anderl, Fisch, and Scaramella (8–12). The technique involves the utilization of a sural nerve graft to connect the functioning nerve fibers from the normal side to those on the paralyzed side. The fibers that are utilized on the normal side vary in location and number. Baker and Conley grafted the entire lower division of the nerve from the normal side onto the main trunk of the nerve on the involved side (13). Other authors, such as Anderl and Fisch, used several more pe-

Table 48.1.
Early Treatment of Facial Paralysis

Restore nerve continuity by:
  Primary nerve repair
  Nerve grafting (to overcome gaps)
  Cross-facial nerve grafting
  Nerve transfers
    Hypoglossal → facial (XII)
    Spiral accessory → facial (XI)
    Phrenic → facial (X)

Muscular and neural neurotization of paralyzed facial muscles

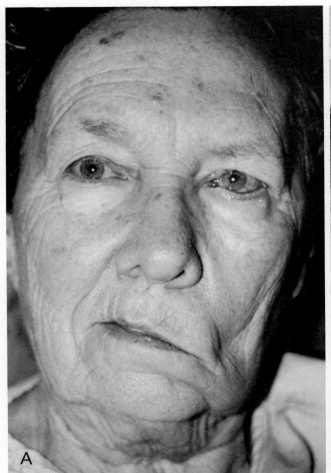
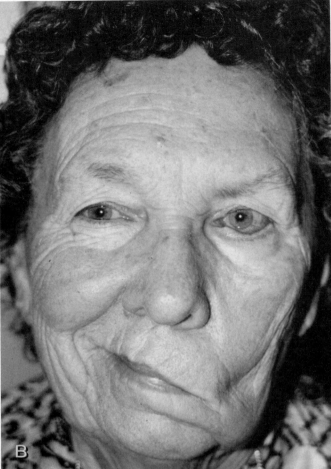

FIGURE 48.1.   A, Elderly patient with complete facial paralysis at rest. Note the marked asymmetry of the face with the paralyzed left side drooping and being drawn to the right side by the unopposed facial tone on the normal side. **B,** With smiling, the face becomes even more asymmetrical and deformed in appearance.

ripheral nerve branches in the normal side for insertion of the nerve graft (Fig. 48.2). It is possible to sacrifice approximately one half of the branches that supply any particular function without affecting function on that side. Anderl advocated a two-stage reconstruction. In the first stage, the sural nerve grafts are sutured to selected facial nerve branches on the nonparalyzed side. Four to 6 months later, when it is believed that the axons have grown through the nerve graft, the nerve graft is sutured on the paralyzed side to the corresponding branches of the facial nerve. The proposed advantages of the two-stage procedure are reduced operative time and the ability to perform the second nerve repair with axons crossing the repair shortly after its completion, rather than 6 months later.

The results of cross-facial nerve grafting have often been disappointing. These poor results are probably due to poor axonal regrowth and muscle degeneration (14–17). The present status of cross-facial nerve grafting is that it has a modest place in young patients if done within 6 months of paralysis. Tone and some spontaneous movement will occur in one half of the patients. Synkinesis can be expected. There is poor return of mouth and

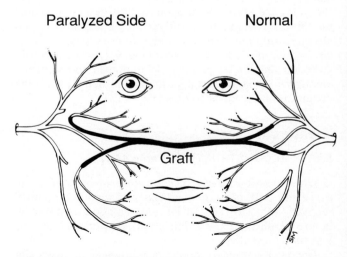

FIGURE 48.2. Cross-facial nerve graft using the sural nerve between branches of the facial nerve that supply the eye and mouth. The graft is attached to proximal branches of the face on the normal side and distal branches on the paralyzed side. Multiple grafts may be inserted, including separate grafts to the eye and separate grafts to the mouth.

eye movement. However, the spontaneity of the movement is a major advantage.

Nerve transfers have been used extensively to reinnervate the paralyzed nerve trunk. They should be done as quickly as possible after paralysis, preferably in less than 6 months. It is interesting and fortunate that patients will occasionally develop the ability to use the non-VIIth nerve transfer without being consciously aware of the process. The hypoglossal to facial nerve transfer has been used most often (18–20). The optimal result that can be expected is symmetrical resting tone with an onset at 4–6 months and maximum return at 12 months. Following transfer, the patient must learn to push the tongue against the incisors or palate in order to activate the facial muscles.

Hypoglossal transfer usually produces satisfactory orbicularis oris tone and provides adequate eye function. Another strength of the procedure is the resting muscle tone in the lower face. This produces good facial symmetry at rest for both the mouth and the eye. Further procedures will usually be required to produce a satisfactory smile. The patient rarely develops good facial movement because there is a mass firing into all of the facial nerves at once, producing synkinesis.

There are several major disadvantages of the hypoglossal transfer technique. These may include excessive resting tone, paralysis and atrophy of the ipsilateral tongue. Uncoordinated mass movement of the affected side of the face with eating, chewing, and talking occurs. Tongue paralysis results in catching of food in the vestibule on the affected side and difficulty in clear articulation and swallowing. The creation of a smile is limited by simultaneous contraction of the orbicularis oris and the lip elevators and depressors, which produces a grimace-like movement of the face.

An alternative nerve transfer has been cranial nerve XI (spinal accessory) to facial. This transfer can provide good resting tone, but the patient must elevate the shoulder to produce facial movement. A significant problem is the severe shoulder droop, which is both a cosmetic and functional deficit, if the entire nerve is used.

The phrenic nerve has also been used if both nerves XI and XII are unavailable (21). A smile can be produced while the patient is taking a deep breath. It is complicated by facial twitches and asymmetry with coughing and laughing.

An alternative to nerve transfer is *transferring functioning motor endplates* to denervated muscle via a neuromuscular pedicle graft (21). This has not been very successful in the clinical setting (22–24). Conley performed *neurotization of the denervated muscle* by placing the split surface of the masseter muscle into an area of paralyzed facial muscle (25). Axonal ingrowth into the adjacent empty neural tubules does occur and extends beyond the immediate contact surfaces (26). With this technique, Conley was able to achieve adequate physical support to the cheek and lip, as well as some voluntary movement of the lower face, including a simulated smile. It did not produce spontaneous emotional expression. Because of muscle atrophy, this technique cannot be used in cases of long-standing paralysis. An alternative

neurotization procedure is the ansa hypoglossal transfer. It is designed to produce neurotization of the paralyzed face musculature by transfer of the nerve and a small piece of musculature directly to the paralyzed facial muscle. Few surgeons have duplicated the initial successful reports.

LATE RECONSTRUCTION

In cases in which the patient is not suitable for muscle reinnervation because of long-standing paralysis and subsequent atrophy of myoneural junctions, reconstruction is achieved using static slings, dynamic slings, and free muscle transfers. Treatment is directed toward the eye, the mouth, or both.

MANAGEMENT OF THE MOUTH (Table 48.2)

There are a number of aesthetic and functional problems experienced by the patient with a facial paralysis. Asymmetry at rest and the inability to smile are the two features that most bother the patient. Other problems associated with paralysis of the oral musculature are drooling and difficulties with speech and articulation. The flaccid lip and cheek soft tissues also lead to some difficulties with chewing food, cheek biting, and depositing of

Table 48.2.
Reconstruction of the Mouth

Static slings
  Autologous materials
    Fasciae latae
    Temporalis fascia
  Synthetic materials
    Silastic rods
    Mesh
    Goretex

Dynamic transfers
  Temporalis muscle transfer
  Masseter transfer
    Split masseter transfer
    Complete masseter transfer
  Free functioning muscle transfer
    Gracilis
    Extensor digitorum brevis
    Pectoralis minor
    Serratus anterior
    Latissimus dorsi

Soft tissue procedures to improve symmetry
  Rhytidectomy
  Nasolabial fold construction
  Excision of redundant intraoral mucosa
  Z-plasty to raise corner of mouth

Procedures for drooling
  Wilkie procedure
  Submandibular gland resection with parotid duct ligation

Modification of normal side to improve symmetry
  Neurectomy
  Myectomy

---

food in the cheek pocket and buccal sulcus. The surgical solutions should be selected to solve each patient's specific problems.

Static Slings

Fascial suspension is used to achieve symmetry at rest without providing animation. It can be used alone or as an adjunct to nerve grafting or free muscle transfer to provide immediate support while awaiting muscle reinnervation (27, 28; Fig. 48.3). Autologous or synthetic material may be used (29, 30). Fascial strips harvested from the thigh (tensor fasciae latae) or temporalis muscle fascia have been used most frequently. Goretex, a substance used extensively in vascular surgery, has recently been used to provide support. Its major advantages include its soft pliable texture, ready availability, strength, and most importantly, resistance to stretching with time. The Goretex used is available in a flat sheet of 0.6-mm thickness. In our experience, the inflammatory response produced by Goretex and its susceptibility to infection detract from its usefulness.

To insert the sling, a segment of the suspensory material is cut to the appropriate length and width to span the gap from the oral commissure to the body of the zygoma and temporal fascia. It is maintained in position with multiple permanent sutures. The sutures are strategically placed in the orbicularis oris around the corner of the mouth and in the upper lip, as dictated by the patient's

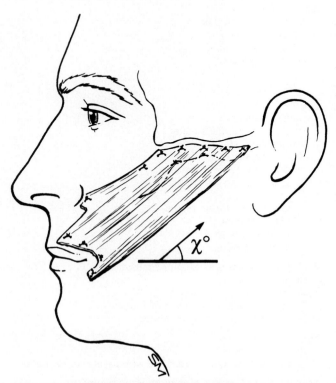

FIGURE 48.3. Static slings provide good symmetry at rest and are particularly useful in elderly patients. Fasciae latae is a reliable material.

deformity. When tension is applied, the force is distributed evenly, reproducing the resting position that is noted on the normal side. Significant overcorrection is advised to allow for some suture relaxation. The sling is attached laterally to the periosteum over the body of the zygoma and to the temporalis fascia. The position can be checked by placing the patient upright in the operating room.

Dynamic Slings

Regional muscle transfers have been used extensively for many years to achieve static support of the mouth and to produce a smile (31–36). The most frequently used muscles are the temporalis and the masseter. The digastric, platysma, and sternocleidomastoid muscles have also been used to reconstruct the depressor anguli oris (37).

Baker and Conley have described in detail the technique of transposing the masseter muscle to the skin around the mouth for oral movement (38). They advocate using the entire muscle, splitting it in its most distal portion for insertion around the mouth into the upper and lower lip. Other authors recommend separating the most anterior half of the muscle only and transposing it to the upper and lower lip. One must be cautious during the splitting dissection to avoid injury to the masseteric nerve, a branch of the trigeminal that supplies the muscle, by entering the deep surface of the muscle in its midportion.

The patient maintains voluntary control over the muscle and can activate it by clenching the teeth. Good static control of the mouth can be achieved with this technique, but the muscle does not contract with sufficient force to allow for symmetry when smiling. There is also inadequate excursion to produce a full smile, and the movement produced is too oblique for most faces. Removal of the masseter may leave a hollow above the angle of the mandible and produce a bulge in the cheek in the region of the transfer.

A more effective and versatile muscle for transfer is the temporalis (39). The temporalis muscle is harvested from its bed in the temporal fossa and turned over the zygomatic arch to extend to the oral commissure. It may be necessary to dissect the fascia off the muscle, leaving it attached superiorly to allow it to reach the oral commissure (Fig. 48.4). Baker and Conley recommended leaving a portion of the temporalis muscle anterior to the hairline to avoid an unsightly temporal hollow (38). The hollow can also be filled with a Silastic implant to improve the contour. Another aesthetic disadvantage of the temporalis transfer is the bulge of muscle that is present where the muscle passes over the arch of the zygoma. To avoid these complications, McLaughlin used an intraoral incision. By detaching the coronoid process, he was able to attach the temporalis muscle insertion into the angle of the mouth with fascial strips (40).

The temporalis provides excellent static positioning as well as voluntary activity. It is capable of producing a more vertical lift to the mouth and greater movement than the masseter transfer. The muscle is also supplied by

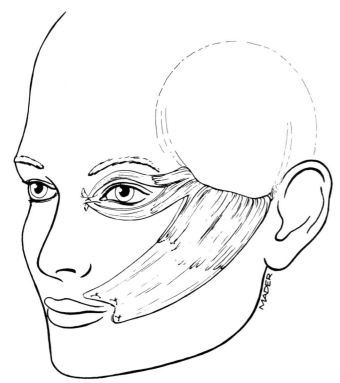

FIGURE 48.4. Temporalis transfer over the arch of the zygoma for smile reconstruction and eye closure.

the trigeminal nerve; therefore, it is activated by the voluntary action of clenching the teeth.

To achieve a proper direction of pull, the patient's smile should be analyzed. If the major direction of pull is superior and lateral, a temporalis muscle transfer would provide the most appropriate movement. If the smile is more horizontal, then a masseter transposition would be the most appropriate. Both muscles may be transferred together.

Free Muscle Transfer

The only techniques currently available to restore both spontaneous involuntary facial movement and asymmetry at rest require the use of the VIIth nerve. This nerve is most easily used with a free functioning muscle transfer.

It is not possible to restore complete symmetry of movement of all facial muscles because of the complexity and the number of facial muscles involved (41–43). There are 18 separate muscles of facial expression. At present, it is possible to transfer only one or two functioning muscles in an attempt to produce some movement. The movement that is most appropriately created is the smile because it is the deficit found to be most distressing to the patient. In addition to providing active motion, muscle transplantation can also provide a symmetrical appearance to the mouth at rest. If the facial nerve is used to reinnervate the transferred muscle, then smile and laughter will be spontaneous. When other muscle transfers are used, such as the masseteric transfer, teeth clenching is required to activate the smile.

Preoperative Planning

A vascularized, innervated muscle transfer will be successful only if various criteria are met. The basic requirement is muscle survival, and this is dependent upon patency of the microvascular anastomosis (44, 45). Muscle function then requires appropriate reinnervation. To provide adequate movement in the proper direction, the muscle size, its attachment to the origin and insertion, and its tension must be carefully calculated. Analysis of facial movement, particularly direction and type of smile, on the normal side is essential to help determine the required movement on the paralyzed side.

Muscle Selection

Various muscles have been used in the past to reanimate the paralyzed face. These include the gracilis, latissimus dorsi, serratus anterior, pectoralis minor, extensor digitorum brevis, and rectus abdominis (46). The specific muscle used is probably not as important as its placement in the face and its functional anatomy (47). A short muscle with a functional length of 4–7 cm, a contractile capability of 1.0–1.5 cm, and sufficient strength to move the facial soft tissues effectively is required. A constant vascular pedicle and nerve supply are needed to allow reliable microvascular transfer.

The muscle selected should leave no functional deficit. If two separate functions, such as eye closure and mouth movement are required, it is desirable to choose one muscle that has two separately functioning neuromuscular units, one for the mouth and one for the eye (48). The pectoralis minor, serratus anterior, and gracilis have this anatomical capability. Nevertheless, reconstruction of orbicularis oculi function has been unsatisfying to date.

Mayou et al., O'Brien et al., and Tolhurst and Bos (49–51) have reported on their experience with the use of the extensor digitorum brevis muscle transplant to reconstruct facial paralysis. This reconstruction was done in conjunction with a cross-facial nerve graft. In follow-up, they noted that the power and excursion of the muscle are inadequate to provide consistently symmetrical facial movement.

Several authors have described the use of the pectoralis minor muscle for the treatment of unilateral facial palsy (52–54). It has the advantages of easy elevation from the anterior chest wall and a good size for insertion into the face. Disadvantages include a vascular pedicle of short length and innervation by nerve branches that support both pectoralis major and minor. The location of the muscle close to the neck also makes simultaneous face and muscle dissection difficult, prolonging the procedure. Harrison described the vascular pedicle as a separate artery and vein coming directly from the axillary artery and vein (52). Terzis and Manktelow noted that the dominant pedicle is usually a branch of the thoracodorsal artery and accompanying vein (53). Harrison reported good results with this muscle; Terzis and Manktelow believe that this is a good muscle for children, but too bulky for adults.

The gracilis muscle is an excellent donor for muscle

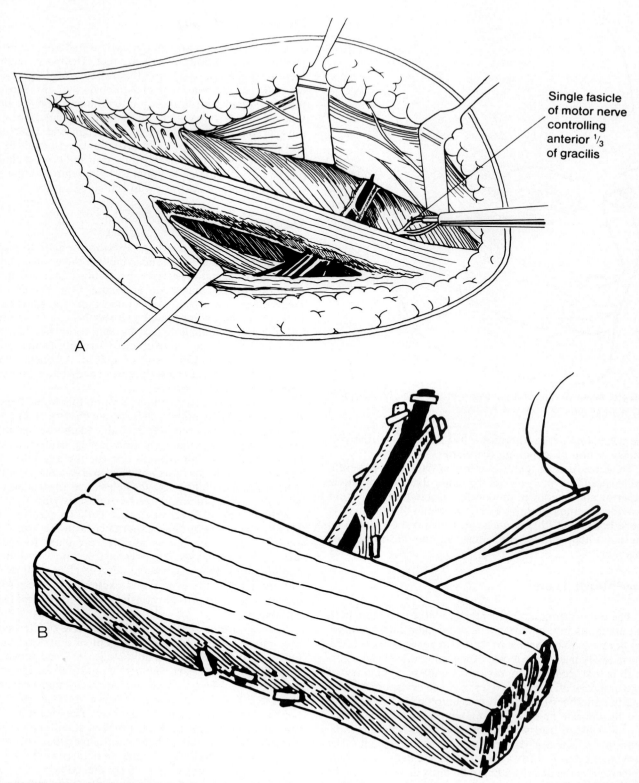

Single fasicle
of motor nerve
controlling
anterior ⅓
of gracilis

A

B

FIGURE 48.5. A portion of the gracilis muscle is transferred. **A,** The portion is based on the dominant, proximal vascular pedicle. **B,** The motor nerve may be divided into separate fascicles, and the portion of the muscle controlled by one fascicle is separated from the rest of the muscle.

transplantation (55). It leaves no functional deficit, and easy access to it is provided by a small medial thigh incision. It has a reliable vascular pedicle that is a branch of the profunda femoris artery and enters the muscle approximately 9 cm from the muscle origin. The artery is an adequate size (1.2–2.0 mm) and is accompanied by a pair of venae comitantes of size suitable for anastomosis. It is supplied by a single motor nerve, a branch of the obturator nerve, which enters the muscle obliquely just proximal to the dominant pedicle. The fascicles can be separated and individually stimulated to produce two longitudinal, separately functioning neuromuscular territories. The muscle can be cut transversely and longitudinally to produce the desired size of muscle for a transfer (Fig. 48.5).

Muscle Innervation

The choice of nerve for muscle reinnervation includes ipsilateral and contralateral facial nerve, as well as the hypoglossal, trigeminal, and accessory nerves (56). The facial nerve is the preferred source of innervation because it is the only source of nerve impulses that normally produce facial expression. It is the only means of obtaining involuntary facial movements and spontaneous expression.

If facial nerve stumps leading to the mouth are present on the paralyzed side, they are the preferred source of innervation. However, their function is usually unknown, and it is often difficult to determine which ones carry smile messages and which ones purse the lips.

If there are no suitable nerve stumps available on the paralyzed side, the preferred source of neurotization is the opposite facial nerve. A long nerve graft is placed from the normal to the paralyzed side, as originally described by Anderl and Smith. At least 50% of the normal peripheral facial nerve branches that elevate the lip are divided and attached to the cross-facial nerve graft on the normal side (Fig. 48.6). There will not be any functional deficit on the normal side.

The cross-facial nerve graft is done 9–12 months prior to muscle transplantation (Fig. 48.7). The distal end of the nerve graft is banked in front of the ear in preparation for muscle transplantation. When reinnervation of the graft has occurred, tapping over the end of the graft on the paralyzed side will elicit a Tinel's sign, which is referred to the normal side in the region of the zygoma. The Tinel's sign localizes to the musculature of the previously divided facial nerve branches. A buzzing sensation is noted as a positive Tinel's sign. This indicates that some nerve regeneration has taken place and it is time for the muscle transplantation.

In patients with bilateral facial paralysis with no VIIth nerve source for neurotization, either the hypoglossal nerve or the motor branches of the trigeminal nerve can be used. The hypoglossal nerve can be split and only one half used in order to avoid loss of tongue function (56). The motor branch to the masseter can be sacrificed with little functional deficit. The disadvantages of using these two nerves are the retraining the patients must undergo to

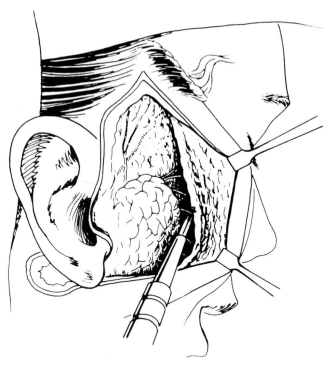

FIGURE 48.6. Staged muscle transfer for smile reconstruction is begun with a cross-facial nerve graft. This requires identification of the appropriate branches of the facial nerve that produce smile on the normal side. (From Manktelow RT: *Microvascular Reconstruction*. Heidelberg, Springer-Verlag, 1986, p 133.)

consciously smile, the likelihood that they will never develop a spontaneous smile, and the undesirable contraction of the muscle with eating.

Technique

The procedure of facial reanimation with functioning muscle transfer frequently proceeds through two stages.

If a cross-facial nerve graft is required, the sural nerve is the usual donor nerve. This nerve is harvested through a longitudinal incision with direct exposure of the nerve, or through multiple small transverse incisions and gentle avulsion of the nerve.

The nerve graft is placed through a subcutaneous tunnel from the paralyzed side to the normal side. The nerve is inserted in the normal side of the face using a face-lift incision, which allows exposure and functional evaluation of the branches of the normal facial nerve. The normal facial nerve is dissected medial to the parotid gland, and nerve stimulation is used to identify the function of the branches. For reinnervation of the nerve graft, facial nerve branches that, when stimulated, produce a smile and no other movement are selected. One half of the nerve branches that produce a smile are divided, and their proximal ends are sutured to the nerve graft using a fascicular repair with 11-0 nylon. The nerve graft is secured with a large silk suture in the preauricular area on the paralyzed side so that it can be found easily at the time of muscle transplantation.

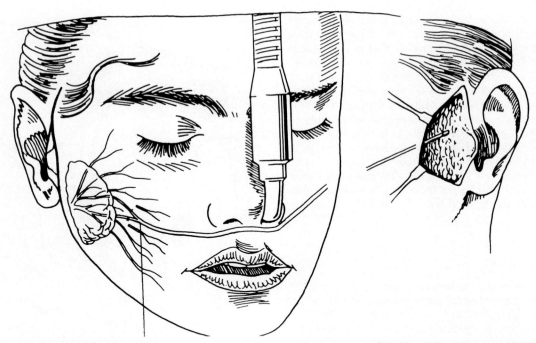

FIGURE 48.7. The cross-facial nerve graft placed across the upper lip with the end banked in front of the ear on the paralyzed side. (From Manktelow RT: *Microvascular Reconstruction.* Heidelberg, Springer-Verlag, 1986, p 134.)

The second stage is the muscle transfer, which is done 9–12 months later. Preoperative markings outline the desired location of the muscle, as determined by smile. The correct placement of the transplanted muscle is determined by analysis of the shape of the smile on the nonparalyzed side of the face. The soft tissues are assessed for skin creases at rest and while smiling. The shape of the oral commissure varies between individuals. The amount of lip eversion also varies. The direction of the upper lip and commissure movement can be measured on the patient using a goniometer. Preoperative markings are used to aid proper muscle placement and direction of pull.

Attaching the muscle to the mouth is a critical part of the procedure. It is usually inserted into the fibers of the orbicularis oris above and below the commissure and along the upper lip. The points of insertion are determined by traction on the mouth. The location and position of the traction are unchanged until the appropriate shape is achieved. The direction of movement of the commissure is determined by the origin of the muscle. It is assessed preoperatively by smile analysis. The origin is usually placed along the anterior maxilla and body and the arch of the zygoma (Figs. 48.8–48.10).

Adjunctive Procedures for Static Support

There are many additional procedures available to provide improved facial symmetry in the patient who is is not a candidate for reanimation or static slings. In certain cases, the long duration of the paralysis has produced severe facial muscle atrophy and associated skin laxity

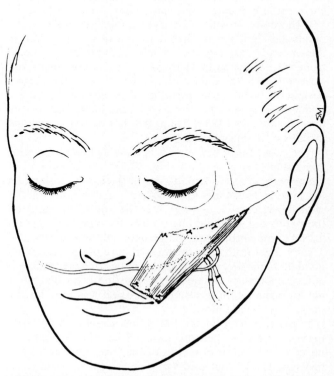

FIGURE 48.8. Attachment of the muscle to the lip, maxilla, and zygoma and appropriate repairs to the cross-facial nerve graft and facial artery and vein.

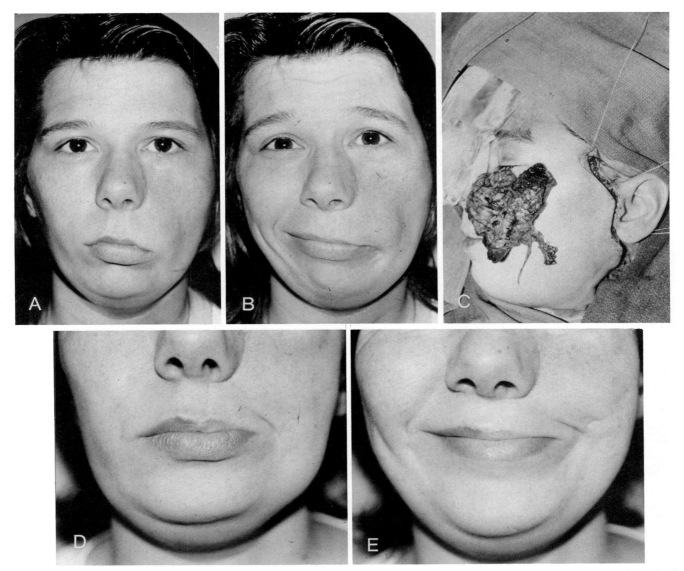

FIGURE 48.9. **A,** Patient seen 3 years after resection of an angiosarcoma with facial paralysis involving the lower portion of the left face and a significant soft tissue defect. **B,** Paralysis is observed with smiling. **C,** Patient had a lipomuscular transfer of a portion of the gracilis muscle using microneurovascular techniques. The motor nerve of the muscle is sutured to a branch of the facial nerve. **D,** Transfer provides good contour reconstruction and symmetrical position of the lips at rest. **E,** Patient has a spontaneous natural smile and good facial symmetry.

on the involved side. Procedures directed at altering the areas of skin redundancy can be of some benefit.

These procedures usually involve suspension and repositioning of the lax structures. This will include rhytidectomy, with or without SMAS plication or suspension. Improved symmetry may be obtained by direct excision of the nasolabial fold, but success with this procedure has been limited.

Treatment of Oral Incontinence

Chronic drooling can be a problem associated with facial paralysis. A lower lip ectropion secondary to paralysis of the orbicularis oris can lead to oral incontinence and drooling. There are several surgical procedures available to alleviate this problem if static and dynamic slings are not adequate.

One is redirection of the salivary flow using the Wilkie procedure. This involves creation of mucosal flaps around the orifice of the parotid duct. These flaps are tubed and then tunneled into the tonsillar fossa to divert saliva from the mouth directly into the oral pharynx. This procedure may be done in conjunction with submandibular gland resection. An alternative approach is submandibular gland resection with bilateral parotid duct ligation. Brundage et al. have recently reported great success with this procedure (57). Both procedures alleviate the

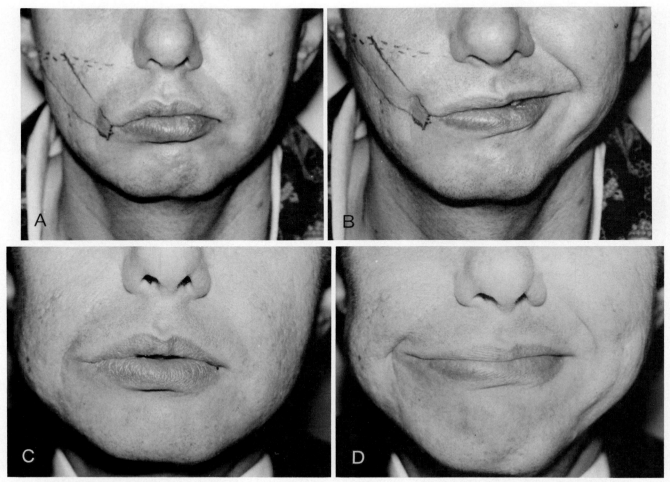

FIGURE 48.10. **A,** Patient with a near-complete congenital paralysis. Deformity is minimal at rest. **B,** Deformity is significant with smiling. Cross-facial nerve graft is dotted on cheek. Planned position of muscle is marked on cheek. It was attached by upper lip as well as commissure. **C.** Following a staged cross-facial nerve graft and microneurovascular muscle transfer, the patient has good movement of the commissure and fair movement of the upper lip. **D,** Motion is spontaneous with smiling with reasonable symmetry.

problems of drooling. Parotid duct ligation is considered to be a technically easier surgical procedure, and it has less postoperative morbidity and a reduced duration of hospitalization.

Redundant intraoral mucosa may develop following long-standing paralysis. This mucosa is prone to being bitten by the molars and can be excised to prevent constant irritation. Eversion of the paralyzed lip can be corrected by an elliptical excision of the excessive mucosa.

The Mouth: Control of Antagonistic Muscle

In a patient with a complete unilateral nerve palsy, a portion of the disfigurement occurs secondary to overactivity or unretrained activity of muscles on the normal side. With contraction, these unopposed muscles draw the paralyzed side toward the normal side, resulting in a deformity that worsens with smiling. This leads to exaggerated movement on the normal side in addition to displacement of the atonic muscle groups to that side (Fig. 48.1). One approach to this problem is to divide nerve or muscle on the normal side to decrease muscle activity (58–60).

Distortions and disfigurement result from overactivity of the levator labii superioris or inferioris, depressor anguli oris, or zygomaticus major. Attempts to improve symmetry have been made by denervation of the appropriate muscle or a reduction in muscle bulk. Myectomy of the depressor anguli oris through an intraoral approach is particularly useful. This is a beneficial procedure for the person with lower lip asymmetry resulting from hyperactivity of this muscle. A more normal appearance to the lower lip results.

Symmetry is difficult to achieve, particularly with neurotomies, because either over- or undercorrection frequently occurs.

How to Select the Appropriate Reconstruction for the Mouth

The most suitable reconstruction will depend on the surgeon's experience and the patient's requirements. It is very important to listen to each patient carefully in order to identify which aspects of the paralysis are most troublesome. If the patient is disturbed about his or her appearance at rest and is not particularly interested in smiling, a static sling may be the most suitable procedure. For the older patient with a lot of sagging of the cheek and mouth, this is a very satisfactory procedure.

A patient who wishes to be able to smile and to have better oral function will require a transfer, either a free functioning muscle transfer or a local muscle transfer such as a temporalis transfer. The advantages of the temporalis transfer are timing and reliability: the results usually occur within a few months after surgery, and most patients will get some motion and some improvement in the contour of the face at rest. A free functioning muscle transfer may be most appropriate for the person who smiles a lot and wishes to do so spontaneously without having to think of biting to produce a smile. A socially active individual who frequently eats with others may be quite upset with a temporalis transfer because of the continual cheek motion while chewing.

Free functioning muscle transfers using microneurovascular techniques are relatively new. When there is an appropriate branch of the VIIth nerve available on the side of paralysis, as may be the case following a tumor resection of the face or following facial injury, then reinnervation is more reliable, and the muscle transplantation results are obtained within a year of the procedure. If there are no branches of the facial nerve available for muscle reinnervation, a preliminary cross-facial nerve graft is required. The disadvantages of these transfers are the time that it takes until a final result is obtained, the need for reinnervation to produce movement, and the relative complexity of the procedures. However, the advantages are the spontaneity of movement of the face resulting from the fact that the muscle is governed by the VIIth nerve and the flexibility of the reconstruction technique.

It is generally recognized that reinnervation does not occur as well with older individuals. However, there is no clear definition of what is "old" in terms of muscle reinnervation. It is my practice to be cautious about doing functioning muscle transfers for individuals over 50 years of age, although there are no hard data to substantiate this. Our own results clearly show better reinnervation in the pediatric age group compared with adults. Even though this procedure is still evolving in my hands, it is quite superior to local muscle transfers for smile reconstruction.

MANAGEMENT OF THE EYE (Table 48.3)

The treatment of eye problems in a facial palsy patient is directed toward preservation of function, alleviation of

Table 48.3.
Reconstruction of the Eye

Early management
  Artificial tears
  Ophthalmic ointment
  Patching
  Moisture chambers
  Lip taping
  Forced blinking
  Contact lenses
  Lid suturing
  Tarsorrhaphy—medial/lateral

Late management
  Upper lid
    Lid weights
    Lid magnets
    Springs
  Lower lid
    Conchal cartilage
    Dermal flap
    Kuntz-Syzmonowski lid shortening procedure
    Static slings
  Both lids
    Silicon encircling band (Arion)
    Muscle transfer
      Temporalis
      Free muscle

Soft tissue procedures for improved symmetry
  Blepharoplasty
  Brow lift

symptoms, and improvement in appearance. Prevention of eye complications in a patient with facial paralysis is a primary goal of treatment. Inactivity of the orbicularis oculi combined with a relative overactivity of the levator palpebrae superioris produces a situation of chronic corneal exposure. This can lead to corneal erosions, corneal infections, and occasionally, perforation and blindness. This problem is exacerbated if there is lacrimal gland dysfunction and/or loss of corneal sensation.

Loss of the lacrimal pumping mechanism leads to inadequate drainage of tears. The tear flow mechanism is disturbed for several reasons. The orbicularis oculi muscle in a patient with a VIIth nerve palsy is not capable of producing eye closure with the upper and lower lids. It is normally the movement of the lower lid that creates a vacuum in the lacrimal system and aids in tear flow into the punctum. The lower lid paralysis also leads to lower lid laxity and ectropion, with a reduced contact between the lower lid margin, the punctum, and the globe. This eversion of the punctum also interrupts tear flow. These deficiencies lead to epiphora, which is aggravated by constant wiping, and to secondary corneal irritation, both of which then produce reflex hypersecretion of tears.

The three major functional areas of concern are, therefore, lagophthalmos with chronic corneal exposure, epiphora, and ectropion. However, patients are often greatly disturbed by the aesthetic appearance of the eye on the paralyzed side. The primary aesthetic concern is the wide-open, staring eye that is unable to show emotion. The relative overactivity of the levator palpebrae superioris and the hypotonicity of the orbicularis oris lead to an eye that appears larger than that on the normal side, with scleral show and a staring appearance.

Corneal Protection

Protection of the cornea can be provided by various ophthalmic solutions such as artificial tears, lubricants, and ophthalmic antibiotic ointments. Forced blinking, lip taping, and patching have been tried. The cornea can also be protected by the use of soft contact lenses and bubble-type moisture chambers. Temporary eye closure can be provided by lid gluing or suturing.

Lateral tarsorrhaphy has been the mainstay of treatment for lagophthalmos and lid laxity and ectropion. The McLaughlin lateral tarsorrhaphy with preservation of eyelashes for camouflage is a popular technique (61). The procedure consists of attaching the opposing surfaces of the upper and lower lid at the lateral margin. A wedge of skin, cilia, and orbicularis oculi muscle from the lower lid is excised, as well as a wedge of tarsus and conjunctiva from the upper lid. The two raw surfaces are then approximated.

By decreasing the horizontal lid length, this procedure allows for an adequate eye coverage during sleep. It may also prolong the effectiveness of the precorneal tear film. Most patients find the shorter lid aperture and the lower placement of the lateral canthus aesthetically undesirable. There is a permanent deformity of both upper and lower lids secondary to tissue loss. It is, however, the safest procedure for the patient who has a dry eye and/or an anesthetic cornea.

Lower Lid Procedures

There are many techniques available to correct lower lid laxity and ectropion. The treatment can be directed to the medial and lateral canthal area.

In medial ectropion with punctal eversion, the lower lid can be repositioned against the globe by direct excision of a tarsoconjunctival ellipse, which causes a vertical shortening of the inner aspect of the lower lid. This helps reposition the punctum against the globe. Medial canthoplasty will also support the punctum. Combinations of vertical elevation and horizontal shortening of the medial eyelid are effective in more severe cases. Propping up the lid with a full-thickness skin graft with or without a cartilage graft may also be effective.

For lateral ectropion, a horizontal lid shortening such as the modified Kuntz-Syzmanowski procedure, with or without a lateral tarsorrhaphy or canthoplasty, is an effective way to correct the lower eyelid position and maintain proper tear flow. The lateral canthoplasty can be done by mobilization of the lateral canthal tendon or by a deepithelialized dermal flap attached to the superolateral orbital margin.

Lower lid ectropion can also be supported by the insertion of a Silastic sheet or conchal cartilage in the lower eyelid (62). A piece of cartilage or Silastic is cut to the shape of the lower lid, positioned deep to the orbicularis oculi, and attached to the inferior orbital margin by sutures placed through the periosteum or bone. It sits in the lower eyelid and projects the lid upwards, advancing the lower margin of the lid.

Static support of the lower eyelid can also be supplied by a sling of fascia. The sling is placed subcutaneously in the lower lid margin from the medial canthus to the lateral orbital margin. This sling provides good elevation of the lower eyelid. The problem is obtaining adequate tension. The sling often has to be revised because it loosens in time, but when the appropriate tension is present, it is very satisfactory. This may be combined with a conchal cartilage graft and other static procedures to provide a good correction of scleral show.

The Upper Eyelid

In addition to static support for the lower eyelid, there have been many attempts to provide dynamic eye closure by modification of the upper lids. These modifications are directed to overcome the action of the levator palpebrae superioris.

Lid loading with weights is one such technique (63–65). Twenty-four carat gold is the preferred substance because of its good color match, high specific gravity, and relative nonreactivity. The appropriate weight is determined by taping or gluing a trial prosthesis to the upper lid over the tarsal plate with the patient awake. The weight is fixed in a subcutaneous position to the tarsal plate. This is a good procedure for lagophthalmos and provides good eye closure when the patient is upright or reclining. Patients may complain of the lump on the upper lid. However, this is rarely visible to the patient because it can only be seen when the eyes are closed. Complications include extrusion or a visible mass in the upper lid and are related to an inappropriate weight.

An alternative is the insertion of two small, permanently magnetized rods into the upper and lower lid (66). Mühlbauer reported good initial results in 61% of patients. This procedure is used infrequently now because of the high rate of extrusion of the magnets. Currently, he believes that, although the rods will remain permanently in some patients without extrusion, the best indication is the patient who will likely recover from the paralysis and needs a short-term solution.

Dynamic closure of the upper and lower lid may be accomplished by a number of different procedures. One technique for eyelid closure is the palpebral spring described by Morel-Fatio (67). Problems with malpositioning of the spring, spring breakage, and skin erosion, which necessitate spring removal, have prevented widespread utilization of these springs. The Arion silicon encircling band, attached at the medial canthal ligament and lateral orbital rim, has also been used. Adjustment of the proper tension allows dynamic eyelid closure. As with the other foreign materials inserted into the eyelids, the usual erosion of the Silastic band through the skin necessitates removal.

Temporalis muscle transfer with fascial strips to encircle the upper and lower eyelids has been successful in supplying dynamic eyelid closure using autologous tissue. The fascial extension of the transferred temporalis muscle is tunneled through each eyelid close to the eyelid margin. The fascia is attached to the medial canthal ligament. Laterally, the orbicularis oculi is attached to the temporalis muscle. The patient must learn to clench the teeth to produce eyelid closure.

The major problem with this technique is fascial stretching, which results in loss of effective eyelid movement, and fascial adherence, which prevents motion. With muscle contraction, the lid aperture changes from an oval to a slit shape. There may also be distortion of the palpebral aperture through lateral displacement of the eyelids, skin wrinkling over the lateral orbital margin, and a bulge at the lateral orbital margin.

Cross-facial nerve grafting with a free or pedicled muscle transfer is a newer option, but although promising in concept, it is in its infancy in development.

The Eye: Control of Antagonistic Muscles

Asymmetry and distortion can occur in the upper face as a result of apparent overactivity of muscles. Overactivity of the frontalis muscle can lead to permanent forehead wrinkling with deep furrows on the normal side. This also produces a significant discrepancy in the position of the two eyebrows. This problem can be treated by elevation of the paralyzed brow or weakening of the normal frontalis and elevation of both brows. The frontalis may be weakened by transection of the frontal branch on the normal side or resection of strips of frontalis muscle to paralyze or weaken the brow. A brow lift is useful to correct asymmetrical eyebrow positions. It can be a direct lid lift via an incision placed directly above the eyebrow, or it can be done through a coronal approach. The brow lift can be further supported by suspension from the temporalis fascia or frontal periosteum (68).

Ancillary Procedures: The Eye

Soft tissue asymmetry can be corrected in several ways. Blepharoplasty may be beneficial by the removal of lax skin from the paralyzed side in both the upper and lower lid. Extreme caution must be used in doing a lower lid blepharoplasty to avoid producing a lower lid ectropion in an already hypotonic lower lid. Lagophthalmos may be produced by excessive resection of upper lid skin.

How to Select the Appropriate Reconstruction for the Eye

Selection of the most appropriate procedures for the paralyzed eye is a difficult process. This selection depends on the patient's particular complaints and physical findings. The choice is between static and dynamic procedures. The static procedure is often adequate and gives good cosmesis. However, static procedures may not prevent epiphora, which in some patients requires a dynamic reconstruction. Reconstruction with a temporalis transfer can provide a dynamic movement; however, the transfer often becomes adherent and functions primarily as a static sling. With dynamic motion, the disadvantages are the distortion of the lateral portion of the eye and a bulge that is sometimes present over the lateral orbital margin. Free functioning muscle transfers using platysma or frontalis are still in the early stage of development, and it is not possible to predict whether these are going to have a major part to play or not. All of the variables that affect free muscle transfers for reconstruction of the mouth are present when used for the eye, and in addition, there is the requirement of a very thin slip of muscle. To date, it has been difficult to transplant a muscle without producing some increase in bulk in the eye.

Most surgeons would agree that procedures that do not employ the VIIth nerve for reanimation of either the eye or the mouth will not likely provide the final answer when the history of facial paralysis reconstruction is written. Only transfers that use the VIIth nerve have the potential for producing a spontaneous reanimation, and our reconstructive efforts should be directed toward using this nerve.

THE NOSE

The dilator alae nasi muscle plays an important role in maintaining airway patency. This is most important in the patient with unilateral facial paralysis, in which absence of dilator muscle function leads to airway collapse and malfunction of the nasal valve with each inspiration. Lack of lip and cheek elevators allows further collapse of this lateral nasal wall. Correction of airway collapse is accomplished by static support of the nasal alae with fascia or by upper lip elevation procedures. Occasionally, a septoplasty will provide an improvement in airway patency.

Summary

There are a variety of treatment modalities available for the patient with a VIIth nerve palsy. The treatment goals are directed to the functional and cosmetic deficits that are present and are individualized to suit the patient's needs. Multiple factors are considered during the decision-making process, including patient's age, duration of palsy, extent of palsy, and functional problems.

The first goal is to prevent eye complications secondary to corneal exposure. The second goal is to provide functional and cosmetic restoration of the eye, nose, and mouth. These procedures should provide static and dynamic symmetry to the face and allow the patient spontaneous facial animation.

References

1. House JW: Facial nerve grading systems. *Laryngoscope* 93:1056, 1983.
2. Sade J: Facial nerve reconstruction and its prognosis. *Ann Otolaryngol* 84:695, 1975.
3. Kempe LG: Topical organization of the distal portion of the facial nerve. *J Neurosurg* 52:671, 1980.
4. May M: Muscle of the facial nerve (spatial orientation of fibres in the temporal bone). *Laryngoscope* 83:1311, 1973.
5. Millesi H: Nerve suture and grafting to restore extratemporal facial nerve. *Clin Plast Surg* 6:333, 1979.
6. McCabe BF: Facial nerve grafting. *Plast Reconstr Surg* 45:70, 1970.
7. Gary-Bobo A, Fuentes JM: Long-term follow-up report on cross facial nerve grafting in the treatment of facial paralysis. *Br J Plast Surg* 36:48, 1983.
8. Smith JW: A new technique of facial reanimation. In Hueston JW (ed): *Transactions of the Fifth International Congress of Plastic and Reconstructive Surgery*. Melbourne, Butterworths, 1971.
9. Anderl H: Reconstruction of the face through cross face nerve transplantation in facial paralysis. *Chir Plast* 2:17, 1973.
10. Anderl H: Cross face nerve transplant. *Clin Plast Surg* 6:433, 1979.
11. Fisch U: Facial nerve grafting. *Otolaryngol Clin North Am* 7:517, 1974.
12. Scaramella L: On the repair of the injured facial nerve. *Ear Nose Throat J* 58:45, 1979.
13. Baker DC, Conley J: Facial nerve grafting: A thirty year retrospective review. *Clin Plast Surg* 6:343, 1979.
14. Salimben-Ughi G: Evaluation of results in 36 cases of facial palsy treated with nerve grafts. *Ann Plast Surg* 9:36, 1982.
15. Gary-Bobo A, Fuentes JM, Guerrier B: Cross facial nerve anastamosis in the treatment of facial paralysis: A preliminary report on 10 cases. *Br J Plast Surg* 33:195, 1980.
16. Ferreira MC: Cross facial nerve grafting. *Clin Plast Surg* 11:211, 1984.
17. Miehike A, Stennert E: New techniques for optimum reconstruction of the facial nerve in its extratemporal course. *Acta Otolaryngol* 91:497, 1981.
18. Evans DM: Hypoglossal facial anastomosis in the treatment of facial palsy. *Br J Plast Surg* 27:251, 1974.
19. Conley J, Baker DC: Hypoglossal facial nerve anastomosis for reinnervation of the paralysed face. *Plast Reconstr Surg* 63:66, 1979.
20. Bret P: Anastomosis of the spinal accessory or hypoglossal nerve to the facial nerve following cerebellopontine angle surgery. *Int J Microsurg* 2:44, 1980.
21. Tucker HM: Restoration of selective facial nerve function by the nerve muscle pedicle technique. *Clin Plast Surg* 6:293, 1979.
22. May M: Facial nerve disorders. Update 1982. *Am J Otol* 4:77, 1982.
23. Freilinger G: A new technique to correct facial paralysis. *Plast Reconstr Surg* 56:44, 1975.
24. Nicolai JP, Vingerhoets HM, Notermans SLH: Our experience with Freilinger's method for dynamic correction of facial paralysis. *Br J Plast Surg* 35:483, 1982.
25. Conley J: Mimetic neurotization from masseter muscle. *Ann Plast Surg* 10:274, 1983.
26. Frey M, Gruber H, Holle J, Freilinger G: An experimental comparison of the different kinds of muscle reinnervation: Nerve suture, nerve implantation and muscular neurotization. *Plast Reconstr Surg* 69:656, 1982.
27. Backdahl M, D'Alessio E: Experience with static reconstruction in cases of facial paralysis. *Plast Reconstr Surg* 21:211, 1958.
28. Freeman BS: An immediate combined approach for rehabilitation of the patient with facial paralysis. *Plast Reconstr Surg* 37:341, 1966.
29. Freeman BS: Review of long term results in supportive treatment of facial paralysis. *Plast Reconstr Surg* 63:214, 1979.
30. Freeman BS: Late reconstruction of the lax oral sphincter in facial paralysis. *Plast Reconstr Surg* 51:144, 1973.
31. Collier J: Reanimation in facial paralysis. *Br J Plast Surg* 5:243, 1952.
32. Battle RJV: A technique for reanimation of the face after paralysis of the seventh nerve. *Br J Plast Surg* 5:247, 1952.
33. Conway H: Muscle plastic operations for facial paralysis. *Ann Surg* 147:541, 1958.
34. Edgerton MT: Surgical correction of facial paralysis: A plea for better reconstruction. *Ann Surg* 165:986, 1967.
35. Correia PC, Zani R: Masseter muscle rotation in the treatment of inferior facial paralysis. *Plast Reconstr Surg* 52:370, 1973.
36. Ragnell A: A method for dynamic reconstruction in cases of facial paralysis. *Plast Reconstr Surg* 21:214, 1958.
37. Matthews DN: Reanimation in facial palsy. *Br J Plast Surg* 5:253, 1952.
38. Baker DC, Conley J: Regional muscle transposition for rehabilitation of the paralysed face. *Clin Plast Surg* 6:317, 1979.
39. May M: Muscle transposition for facial reanimation. *Arch Otolaryngol* 110:184, 1984.
40. McLaughlin CH: Permanent facial paralysis. *Lancet* 2:647, 1952.
41. Manktelow RT: *Microvascular Reconstruction: Anatomy, Applications and Surgical Technique*. Heidelberg, Springer-Verlag, 1986.
42. Freilinger G, Gruber H, Happak W, Pechman U: Surgical anatomy of the mimic muscle system and the facial nerve: Importance for reconstructive and aesthetic surgery. *Plast Reconstr Surg* 80:686, 1987.
43. Rubin LR: The anatomy of a smile: Its importance in the treatment of facial paralysis. *Plast Reconstr Surg* 53:384, 1974.
44. Harelius L: Transplantation of free autogenous muscle in the treatment of facial paralysis. *Scand J Plast Reconstr Surg* 8:220, 1974.
45. Terzis JK, Sweet RD, Dykes RW, Williams HB: Recovery of function in free muscle transplants using microneurovascular anastomosis. *J Hand Surg* 3:37, 1978.
46. Hamilton SGL, Terzis JK: Surgical anatomy of donor sites for free muscle transplantation to the paralysed face. *Clin Plast Surg* 11:197, 1984.
47. Frey M, Gruber H, Freilinger G: The importance of the correct resting tension in muscle transplantation: Experimental and clinical aspects. *Plast Reconstr Surg* 71:510, 1983.
48. Manktelow RT, Zuker RM: Muscle transplantation by fascicular territory. *Plast Reconstr Surg* 73:751, 1984.
49. Mayou BJ, Watson JS, Harrison DH, Parry CBW: Free microvascular and microneural transfer of the extensor digitorum brevis muscle for the treatment of unilateral facial palsy. *Br J Plast Surg* 34:362, 1981.
50. O'Brien BM, Franklin JD, Morrison WA: Cross facial nerve grafts and microneurovascular free muscle transfer for long established facial palsy. *Br J Plast Surg* 33:202, 1980.
51. Tolhurst DE, Bos KE: Free revascularized muscle grafts in facial palsy. *Plast Reconstr Surg* 69:760, 1982.
52. Harrison DH: The pectoralis minor vascularized muscle graft for the treatment of unilateral facial palsy. *Plast Reconstr Surg* 75:206, 1985.
53. Terzis JK, Manktelow RT. Pectoralis minor: A new concept in facial reanimation. *Plast Reconstr Surg Forum* 5, 1982.
54. Manktelow RT: Free muscle transplantation for facial paralysis. *Clin Plast Surg* 11:215, 1984.
55. Harii K, Ohmori Y, Torii T: Free gracilis muscle transplantation with microneurovascular anastomosis for the treatment of facial paralysis. *Plast Reconstr Surg* 57:133, 1976.
56. Zuker RM, Manktelow RT: A smile for the Moebius syndrome patient. *Ann Plast Surg* 22:188, 1989.
57. Brundage SR, Moore WD: Submandibular gland resection and bilateral parotid duct ligation as a management for chronic drooling in cerebral palsy. *Plast Reconstr Surg* 83:443, 1989.
58. Clodius L: Selective neurectomies to achieve symmetry in partial and complete facial paralysis. *Br J Plast Surg* 29:43, 1976.
59. Niklison J: Contribution to the subject of facial paralysis. *Plast Reconstr Surg* 17:276, 1956.
60. Niklison J: Facial paralysis: Moderation of non-paralysed muscles. *Br J Plast Surg* 43:397, 1965.

61. Jelks GW, Smith B, Bosniak S: The evaluation and management of the eye in facial palsy. *Clin Plast Surg* 6:397, 1979.
62. Anderl H: A simple method for correcting ectropion. *Plast Reconstr Surg* 49:156, 1972.
63. Nicolai JPA, deKoomen H, Van Leeuwen JBS, Sybrandy S: Gold weights in upper eyelids for the correction of paralytic lagophthalmos. *Eur J Plast Surg* 9:66, 1986.
64. Jobe RP: A technique for lid loading in the management of the lagophthalmos of facial palsy. *Plast Reconstr Surg* 53:29, 1974.
65. Neuman AR, Weinberg A, Sela M, Peled IJ, Wexler MR: The correction of seventh nerve palsy with gold lid load (16 years experience). *Ann Plast Surg* 22:142, 1989.
66. Mühlbauer WD, Segeth H, Viessman A: Restoration of lid function in facial palsy with permanent magnets. *Chir Plastica* 1:295, 1973.
67. Morgan LR, Rich AM: Four years experience with the Morel-Fatio palpebral spring. *Plast Reconstr Surg* 53:404, 1974.
68. Castañares S: Forehead wrinkles, glabella frown and ptosis of the eyebrows. *Plast Reconstr Surg* 34:406, 1964.

49

Cervical Masses

Gregory S. Georgiade, M.D., F.A.C.S. and Nicholas G. Georgiade, D.D.S., M.D., F.A.C.S.

Cervical masses should be evaluated by their location in relation to anatomical landmarks (i.e., the submaxillary gland, sternocleidomastoid muscle, trapezius muscle, parotid gland, trachea, hyoid bone, and thyroid gland). In order to make an adequate diagnosis, a complete history is necessary, including the initial appearance of the mass, possible systemic problems, age of the patient, and location of the mass. Visual inspection of the oral cavity and mirror laryngoscopy are of value in appraising masses in the upper cervical area.

Three classificatory groups according to area(s) of neck involvement are useful in diagnosing cervical masses: (*a*) lateral neck masses, (*b*) midcervical neck masses, and (*c*) masses that may appear any place in the neck, either as single or multiple nodules (Table 49.1). A preponderance of neck masses occur in adults, and in this group, over one half will be of malignant origin.

Lateral Neck Masses

The masses that appear most frequently in the lateral aspect of the neck are presented below.

BRANCHIAL CLEFT ANOMALIES

These developmental anomalies are the most frequently occurring masses of the lateral neck. They appear as soft, nontender, smooth, round lesions along the border of the sternocleidomastoid muscle, usually deep to the muscle. They may be located in sites extending from the region of the external auditory canal to the midclavicular area (Fig. 49.1). The tract along which they occur may extend into the lateral pharyngeal area (Rosenmuller's pouch). These lateral neck masses are usually present by 8 years of age but have also been reported in patients in the third decade of life.

Embryologically, branchial cleft anomalies and/or sinus tracts occur because of a failure of the first or second branchial arch to attain maturity. The residual remnant is trapped in the neck tissue. Anomalies may be manifest: (*a*) in the preauricular area, (*b*) posterior to the angle of the mandible, and (*c*) in the upper cervical area with extension into the bony and cartilaginous auditory canal in

close proximity to the facial nerve (Fig. 49.2). Anomalies of the second branchial arch are manifested as cysts or sinuses or fistulae found along the anterior border of the sternocleidomastoid muscle (Fig. 49.3). The cystic mass and its tract, if present, may extend through the platysma muscle and follow superiorly along the carotid sheath. In the upper neck, the tract can be located deep to the posterior belly of the digastric muscle and superficial to the

Table 49.1.
Classification of Cervical Masses by Location

Lateral neck masses
  Branchial cleft anomalies
  Cystic hygroma
  Hemangioma
  Lipoma
  Neurilemmoma
  Carotid body tumor
  Salivary gland (parotid)
    Adenoma
    Warthin's tumor
  Other
    Thyroid or parathyroid
    Adenomas
    Sebaceous cysts
    Myomas
Midline neck masses
  Aberrant thyroid tissue
  Thyroglossal duct or sinus tract cysts
  Thyroid adenomas
  Delphian node
  Dermoid cyst
Single or multiple masses in one or more locations of the
    neck
  Suppuration in neck of dental or tonsillar origin
  Metastatic tumors
  Masses of lymphatic origin
    Lymphoma
    Hodgkins
    Lymphoepithelioma
  Inflammatory masses
    Tubercular
    Actinomycotic
    Blastomycosis
    Sporotrichotic
  Teratomas (congenital)

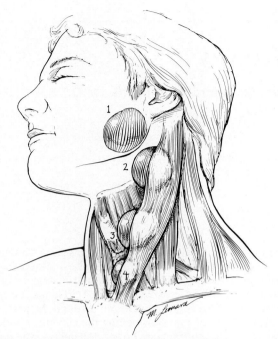

FIGURE 49.1.   Lateral neck masses may appear anywhere from the midclavicular area to the region of the external auditory canal.

hypoglossal nerve, with an opening in the base of the tonsillar fossa and lateral pharyngeal area.

Histologically, the cyst and cystic tract are typically lined with stratified squamous or low columnar epithelium. Treatment consists of surgical excision with care being taken to keep the cervical incision small. A "stepladder" approach can be executed in the crease lines, tunneling the initial tract superiorly as high as possible before the next incision is made. Anatomical landmarks (noted above) must be identified carefully because of the close proximity of the carotid vessels and the facial nerve in the superior portion of the neck.

CYSTIC HYGROMA

Cystic hygroma usually presents in a newborn or in early infancy. It appears as a soft, cystic, lobulated mass that is displaced laterally. Often, the cystic hygroma extends to the midline of the neck and beyond. The mass will transilluminate and is soft to palpation (Fig. 49.4).

A cystic hygroma is essentially a lymphangioma that arises as a developmental anomaly of the lymphatic channels. Displaced embryonic tissue results in the development of large endothelial-lined spaces from the venous system. These may be found along the branches of the jugular vein around the esophagus and larynx. The cystic hygroma interdigitates with cervical vessels, nerves, and muscle, rendering surgical removal both arduous and difficult. The size of the mass may cause respiratory difficulty. Aspiration of the yellow fluid contents may be undertaken for temporary decompression. Lymphangioma tissue may be found extending into the axillary area and inferiorly into the mediastinum. Treatment is by surgical excision, and the initial procedure should maximize removal of the tumor mass for the best long-term result.

HEMANGIOMA

The cavernous hemangioma seen in infants or children represents a vascular developmental anomaly. Histologically, it is characterized by extensive proliferation of endothelial cells with resultant large vascular spaces that fill with blood. The cavernous hemangioma appears as a soft, round, collapsible mass. A distinctive diagnostic feature is the bluish tone of the skin overlying the mass.

The management plan must include ruling out the presence of an extensive vascular abnormality. Should there be any question about the extensiveness of the tumor, further vascular studies are indicated, including a computed tomography (CT) scan and/or magnetic resonance imaging.

A single hemangiomatous mass can usually be excised surgically without difficulty. Care must be taken to main-

FIGURE 49.2.   Potential sites of branchial cleft anomalies with remnant trappings: **I,** preauricular; **II,** posterior to angle of mandible; **III,** upper cervical area.

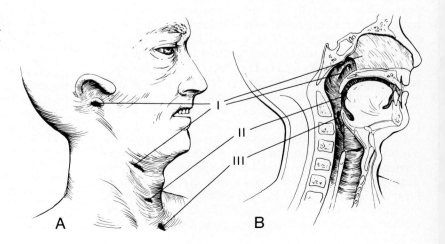

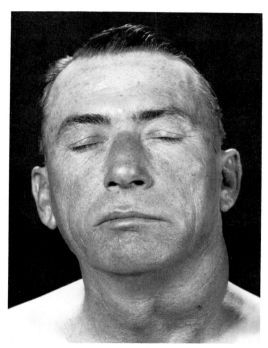

FIGURE 49.3. A patient with a branchial cyst at the anterior border of the sternocleidomastoid muscle.

tain dissection in the plane around the hemangioma to minimize bleeding from the blood-filled mass.

LIPOMA

Lipomas are often confused with branchial cleft cysts because of their relatively similar appearance, location, and softness. Treatment consists of surgical excision, which is usually accomplished easily by dissecting the lipoma free from surrounding tissue (Fig. 49.5).

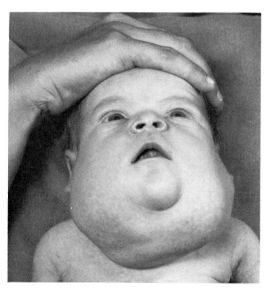

FIGURE 49.4. Cystic hygroma in an infant.

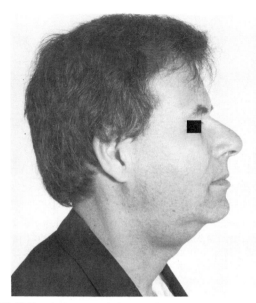

FIGURE 49.5. A lipoma of the cervical area in an adult male patient.

NEURILEMMOMA

In contrast to previously described lateral neck masses, the neurilemmoma is more solid in consistency and deeper on palpation. The clinical picture is one of a slow-growing, painless mass presenting in the mature patient. It is frequently found in association with von Reck-

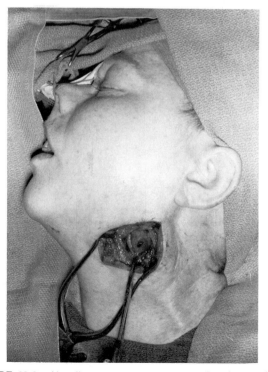

FIGURE 49.6. Neurilemmoma as an encapsulated mass in an adult female patient.

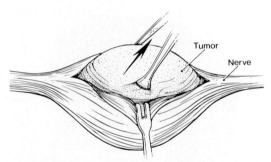

FIGURE 49.7. The typical location of a neurilemmoma encapsulated in a nerve sheath.

linghausen's disease. When the growth rate is rapid, more pain and discomfort is experienced, and the proportion of malignancies is also higher. When a neurilemmoma is involved with the sympathetic nerve chain, Horner's syndrome may occur.

Palpation of the deep-seated, encapsulated mass will allow some lateral and anterior movement. Because of the attached nerve sheath, which courses in a superior-inferior direction, no movement occurs in this vector. Treatment of the neurilemmoma consists of meticulous dissection from the encompassing nerve and usually results in no disability (Figs. 49.6 and 49.7).

CAROTID BODY TUMORS

The carotid body tumor is characterized by its slow, painless growth. It is located at the bifurcation of the carotid artery and can be removed laterally but not vertically. Carotid tumors may attain such size as to cause difficulty in swallowing, speaking, and breathing. They

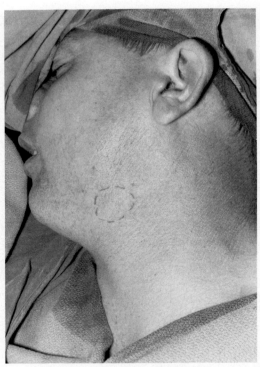

FIGURE 49.9. A patient with a submaxillary gland tumor of the parotid in the midsubmandibular area.

are usually found in patients over 50 years of age, and removal is quite hazardous. An open biopsy should be performed to rule out a malignancy, which occurs in slightly over 10% of patients. If the mass is nonmalignant and slow growing, it should probably be left in place be-

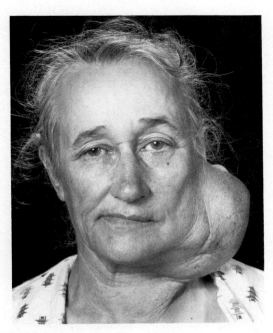

FIGURE 49.8. Warthin's tumor in the inframandibular area of the lateral neck.

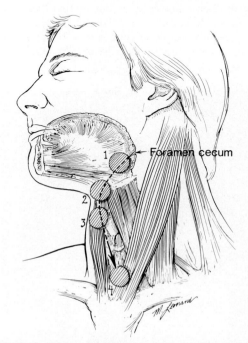

FIGURE 49.10. Thyroglossal duct cyst in midline area of neck; sinus tract cysts may occur from the region of the foramen cecum linguae to the thyroid isthmus.

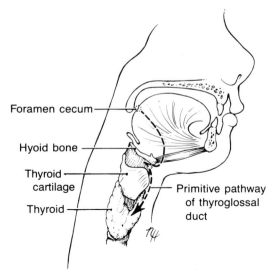

FIGURE 49.11. The primitive pathway of the thyroglossal.

cause of the hazards of excision. Morbidity accompanying removal is usually high because excision of a portion of the involved common carotid artery is included. Should surgery be the treatment of choice, extirpation of this tumor should be planned. Preoperative compression of the carotid artery against the vertebra for 15–20 min four or five times a day for a 2-week period before surgery is recommended because of the high incidence of hemiplegia after ligation of the common carotid artery.

Histologically, the carotid body tumor is composed of sheets of polyhedral and epitheloid cells with large, pale-staining nuclei and pale-staining cytoplasm. These cells occur in cords or sheets of cells with an interspersion of fibrous tissue, vessels, and large numbers of neural elements.

SALIVARY GLAND MASSES

Parotid

Occasionally, an adenoma or Warthin's tumor may present in the upper neck. Although it may be mistaken for a separate tumor mass, it is actually associated with the caudad portion of the parotid gland (Fig. 49.8). Tumors in this area are usually benign and are easily distinguished from other neck masses at the time of surgery.

Submaxillary gland tumors occur in the upper midneck and midsubmandibular area (Fig. 49.9). They will present as firm, nonmobile masses that are somewhat painful on palpation. This mass is usually a benign adenoma, or it may manifest as a large calculus in the submaxillary gland. There is associated pain and tenderness, particularly when chewing and ingesting food. Surgical extirpation of the entire gland is necessary. Diagnostic differentiation between an adenoma and salivary calculus can be made by obtaining a suitable intraoral radiograph of the floor of the mouth. Orthopan radiography of the area will often reveal the presence of a calcified mass in the submaxillary gland.

MISCELLANEOUS LATERAL MASSES

Occasionally, an aberrant *thyroid* or *parathyroid adenoma* will present in the lower lateral neck as a small, mobile mass in the region of the thyroid gland. *Sebaceous cysts* can appear in any area of the neck and are characterized by their ovoid appearance, ease of palpation, and close proximity to the skin surface. *Myomas* rarely occur in the lateral neck. When present, they are usually within the sternocleidomastoid muscle and are firm, ovoid, fixed masses that are painless.

Midline Neck Masses

Primary masses of the midcervical area include those described below.

ABERRANT THYROID TISSUE

The presence of displaced thyroid tissue, cysts, or sinus tract is a result of the epithelial lining failing to disappear. It is present during the downward progression of the thyroid tissue from the foramen cecum linguae, through the hyoid bone, to its final position in the lower midneck.

Lingual thyroid is characterized by a supralingual protruding mass in the posterior area of the tongue at the foramen cecum linguae. The aberrant thyroid tissue may be located in any position from the foramen cecum linguae to the thyroid gland proper, including the thyroid isthmus.

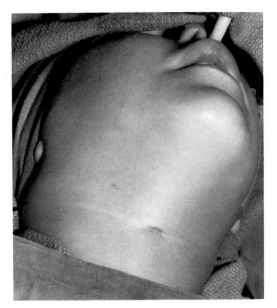

FIGURE 49.12. The thyroglossal duct sinus in an adult male patient.

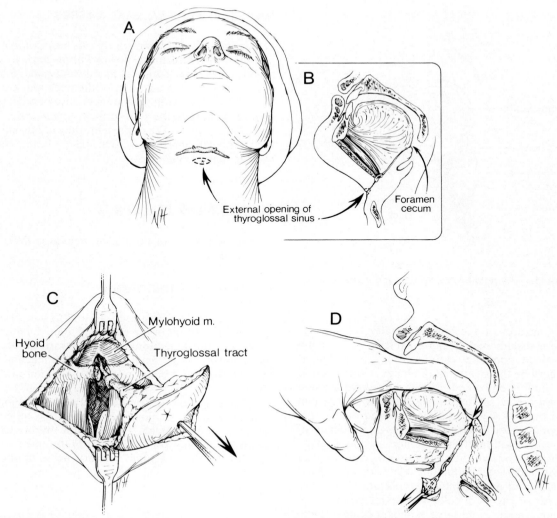

FIGURE 49.13. Horizontal excision of initial sinus tract opening. **A,** The external opening. **B,** An anteroposterior view of foramen cecum and sinus tract. **C,** The sinus tract cyst is dissected. An anterior view shows the hyoid bone combined in the surgical procedure. **D,** Intraoral digital pressure at the midline position of the foramen cecum is of assistance in identifying the superior portion of sinus tract cyst and in the dissection.

THYROGLOSSAL DUCT OR SINUS TRACT CYSTS

These masses appear at a midline site anywhere from the thyroid isthmus to the foramen cecum linguae. The sinus tract usually appears in the region of the hyoid bone and thyroid isthmus. Duct cysts occur more frequently in children (Figs. 49.10–49.12). The histopathological composition of the cyst tract is characteristically squamous cell epithelium together with some thyroid tissue. Treatment consists of horizontal excision of the initial sinus tract opening with dissection of the tract from the surrounding tissue. Traction is maintained to identify the tract better (Fig. 49.13**A** and **B**). The midportion of the hyoid bone is included in the resection (Fig. 49.13**C**). The tract is dissected superiorly to the base of the tongue. Intraoral digital pressure at the midline position of the foramen cecum linguae is beneficial in the superior dissection and in identifying the superior portion of the tract at the position of the posterior tongue (foramen cecum) (Figs. 49.13**D**, 49.14, and 49.15).

THYROID ADENOMA

This benign mass will occasionally present as an easily palpable, somewhat mobile mass.

DELPHIAN NODE

Delphian node is characterized as a firm mass that may be confused with an adenoma. It is attached to the fascia of the thyroid isthmus and may be diagnostic of a thyroid disease process or a malignancy involving the thyroid gland.

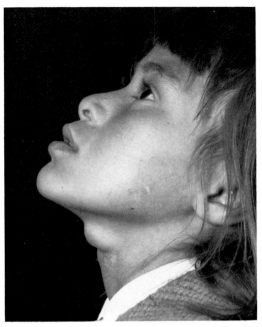

FIGURE 49.14. A sinus tract cyst shown in profile in an 8-year-old patient.

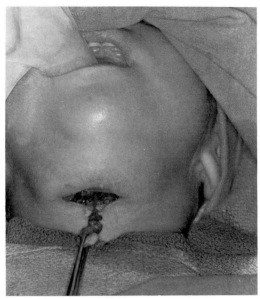

FIGURE 49.15. An anterior view of duct cyst opening in an adult patient.

DERMOID CYST

The dermoid cyst is derived from remnants of epithelial cells remaining during fusion at the midline in the embryonic stage and may contain hair follicles, sebaceous glands, and other glandular elements. The characteristic dermoid cyst appears as an intraoral mass in children, usually up to 5 years of age, and is located intraorally above the geniohyoid muscle. It may also occur in the submental area, and in this position, it is inferior to the geniohyoid muscle (Fig. 49.16). Surgery can be carried out either intraorally or through the small submental incision, depending on the location of the presenting mass.

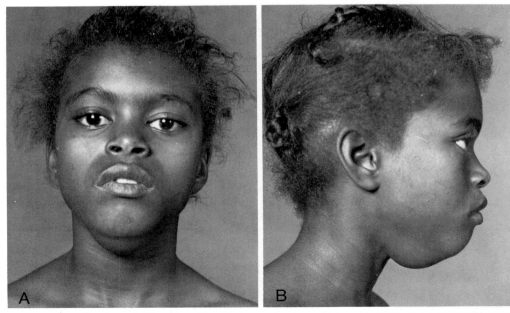

FIGURE 49.16. The frontal (**A**) and profile (**B**) views of a dermoid cyst involving the geniohyoid muscle.

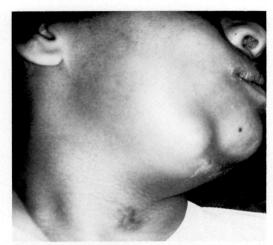

FIGURE 49.17. A patient with an infection of dental origin.

Single or Multiple Masses in One or More Neck Locations

Masses that occur in one or more locations of the neck and may appear as single or multiple nodules include those described below.

SUPPURATION IN THE NECK

An area of suppuration in the neck is most commonly of dental origin (Fig. 49.17). Infections related to the ton-

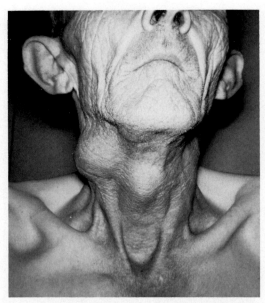

FIGURE 49.18. A metastatic tumor in the lateral neck of a patient in late maturity.

sillar area are another source. Usually, the mass is of recent origin, painful, and located at a site directly in the submandibular area. An Orthopan radiograph of the entire mandible will usually reveal the primary source as a periapical dental infection that has eroded through the cortex of the mandible into the underlying soft tissues. A

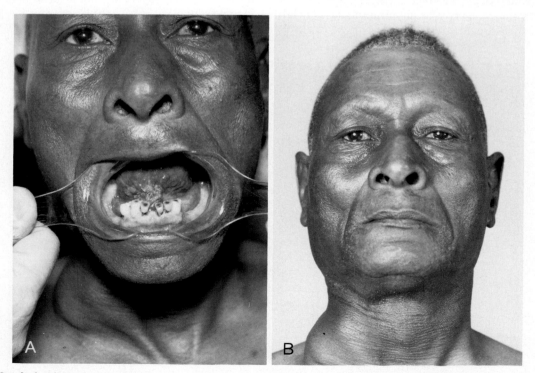

FIGURE 49.19. **A,** A primary carcinoma of the oral cavity (sublingual) in an adult male patient. **B,** Metastasis to the lateral neck is evident.

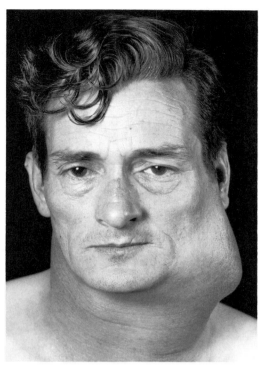

FIGURE 49.20.   Hodgkin's disease: a sizable mass in the lateral neck of an adult male patient.

neck infection of tonsillar origin will extend into the parapharyngeal space with involvement of the cervical region. Extension of the infection along the fascial space will further complicate the clinical picture. Involvement of the cervical sympathetic chain with resultant Horner's syndrome or even vagal involvement and vocal cord paralysis may occur. This condition is treated by incision and adequate drainage with removal of the offending tooth. Suitable antibiotics are prescribed.

METASTATIC TUMORS

Metastatic tumors may occur in the neck and are usually from primary carcinomas of the oral cavity, pharynx, and nasal pharynx (Figs. 49.18 and 49.19). A small group of metastatic masses occur in the lower neck and will originate from primary sites below the clavicle, including lungs, esophagus, gastrointestinal tract, or even locations such as the prostate, kidneys, or uterus.

LYMPHATIC MASSES

Neck masses of lymphatic origin, such as lymphoma, Hodgkin's disease (Fig. 49.20), and lymphoepithelioma, may appear anywhere in the neck and present as firm, mobile, painless masses, usually in clusters. Treatment, once a diagnosis is made, is usually with chemotherapy and radiation therapy.

INFLAMMATORY NECK MASSES

Inflammatory neck masses may occur occasionally as a result of tuberculosis, actinomycosis, blastomycosis, and sporotrichosis. Cat scratch fever is an inflammatory disease of viral origin usually seen in children. This disease will characteristically present as discrete neck masses that are firm and matted when palpated and are typically present for a number of weeks. A history of involvement with cats, dogs, and other animals is usual, as is intermittent low-grade fever. The disease is transmitted via a scratch, saliva, or excreta from animals (usually cats) to humans (usually children). Examination reveals moderate to tender, freely movable lymph nodes, which often may be suppurative. With exclusion of the animal, disappearance of the masses is the usual course. No antibiotics or other treatment is thought to be necessary. A skin test antigen can be used.

TERATOMAS

Teratomas of the neck can appear at any location in the cervical region, are present at birth, and may attain considerable size. A teratoma presents as a large, irregular mass that, but virtue of its size, will cause tracheal compression and respiratory difficulties as a rule. The histological appearance reveals a mixture of sebaceous squamous cell clusters and cysts containing respiratory or gastrointestinal epithelium. Teeth, neural tissues, cartilage, brain, and other tissues resulting from the presence of ectodermal, mesodermal, and entodermal germinal layers are usually present. Treatment is by surgical excision, which provides excellent long-term results if there has been careful excision of the entire mass.

Summary

Neck masses can appear at any age and in any location. About 50% occur in adults over 50 years of age. A significant number of neck masses appear in infants and children, and this dictates the need for careful evaluation and treatment. The physical examination and a complete history, including duration of symptoms, are central in determining further studies to be undertaken and subsequent management.

Suggested Readings

Cady B: Differential diagnosis of tumors of the neck. *Compr Ther* 9:33, 1983.
Chandler JR, Mitchell B: Branchial cleft cysts, sinuses, and fistulas. *Otolaryngol Clin North Am* 14:175, 1981.
Hoeprich P: *Infectious Diseases,* ed 3. Philadelphia, Harper and Row, 1983, p 1398.
Hogan D, Wilkinson RD, Williams A: Congenital anomalies of the head and neck. *Int J Dermatol* 19:479, 1980.
Karmody CS, Forston JK, Calcaterra VE: Lymphangiomas of the head and neck in adults. *Otolaryngol Head Neck Surg* 90:283, 1982.

McGoon DC: Teratomas of the neck. *Surg Clin North Am* 32:1389, 1952.

Moloy P: How to (and how not to) manage the patient with a lump in the neck. *Primary Care* 9:269, 1982.

New GB, Erich JB: Dermoid cysts of the head and neck. *Surg Gynecol Obstet* 65:48, 1937.

Padberg FT, Cady B, Persson AV: Carotid body tumor. *Am J Surg* 145:526, 1983.

Pounds LA: Neck masses of congenital origin. *Pediatr Clin North Am* 28:841, 1981.

Rood SW, Johnson J: Examination for cervical masses. *Postgrad Med* 71:189, 1982.

Sharaki MM, Talaat M, Hamam SM: Schwannoma of the neck. *Clin Otolaryngol Allied Sci* 7:245, 1982.

Simpson GT: The evaluation and management of neck masses of unknown etiology. *Otolaryngol Clin North Am* 13:489, 1980.

Watanatittan S, Othersen HB, Hughson MD: Cervical teratoma in children. *Prog Pediatr Surg* 14:225, 1981.

Weymuller EA: Problems in family practice: Evaluation of neck masses. *J Fam Pract* 11:1099, 1980.

Zitelli BJ: Neck masses in children: Adenopathy and malignant disease. *Pediatr Clin North Am* 28:813, 1981.

INDEX

Page numbers followed by t and f indicate tables and figures, respectively.

clinical aspects, 160–161
sebaceous, histopathology, 180
Epithelium, culture, 26, 250
EPM. *See* Early protected motion
Epstein-Barr virus, and carcinoma of
 nasopharynx, 457
Epulides, 455, 456f
Erich dental arch bar, 440
Erysipelas, 902
Erythema, with radiation, 1332
Erythema nuchae, 224
Erythromycin, for hand infections, 1212
Erythroplakia, oral, 457
Erythroplasia of Queyrat, 149
Escharotomy, 246f, 246–247, 249
 chest, 244, 247
 indications for, 1141
Escherichia coli, scrotal gangrene caused
 by, 958
Escherichia coli infection
 antibiotics for, 1212
 of hand, 1217
Esophageal cancer, metastases, in neck,
 605
Esophagus, cervical, reconstruction with
 jejunum, 1037, 1037f, 1038
Estane. *See* Polyurethane
Esthetic line, 323f
 in orthodontics, 321
Estlander flap, 527–528, 529f
Estrogen(s)
 effects of, and gynecomastia, 877,
 878t
 increased production of
  gynecomastia with, 877
  neoplasms with, 877–878
 and nipple discharge, 879
Estrogen-containing creams, and breast
 nodularity, 837
Ethesioneuroblastoma, midface, 512
Ethibloc, 227
Ethionamide, and gynecomastia, 878t
Ethmoid carcinoma, 512f, 513–514
Etretinate, to treat basal cell carcinoma,
 147
Eustachian tube, embryology of, 272
Ewing's sarcoma
 in hand, 1188
 mandibular involvement in, 500, 502f
Exercise(s), after replantation. *See* Early
 protected motion
Exophthalmos, 649
 in Crouzon's syndrome, 337–338
 minimal, 644
 with orbital fractures, 425, 427–428
Exorbitism, 347
 pathogenesis of, 334
 in Pfeiffer syndrome, 339
Exostoses. *See* Bony exostoses;
 Osteochondromas
Exposure osteotomy, 515
Extensor carpi radialis brachioradialis
 muscle, effects of nerve injury on,
 1138t
Extensor carpi radialis brevis muscle
 course of, 217, 217f
 effects of nerve injury on, 1138t
Extensor carpi radialis longus muscle,
 course of, 217, 217f
Extensor carpi radialis muscle, course of,
 217f
Extensor carpi ulnaris muscle, course of,
 217, 217f
Extensor carpi ulnaris tendon, course of,
 1131

Extensor communis tendons, course of,
 1131
Extensor digiti minimi tendon
 course of, 1131
 as free graft, 65
Extensor digitorum brevis muscle
 free transfer, 1018–1019
 for reanimation of paralyzed face, 585
Extensor digitorum brevis muscle flap, for
 hand coverage, 1068
Extensor digitorum communis muscle,
 course of, 217, 217f
Extensor digitorum communis tendon,
 course of, 1131, 1226
Extensor digitorum longus muscle
 course of, 217f
 as source of tendon grafts, 65
 vascular anatomy of, 42t
Extensor digitorum muscle, course of, 217f
Extensor hallucis brevis muscle, course of,
 1118f
Extensor hallucis longus muscle
 course of, 217, 217f
 leg reconstruction with, 1301, 1302f
 vascular anatomy of, 42t
Extensor indicis proprius tendon(s)
 course of, 1131
 as free grafts, 65
Extensor pollicis brevis tendon, course of,
 1131, 1226
Extensor pollicis longus tendon, course of,
 1131, 1226
Extensor tendon(s), anatomy of, 1131f,
 1131–1132, 1132f
Extensor tendon injuries, 1131
 boutonnière deformity, treatment of,
 1133
 lacerations, 1131
  boutonnière test for, 1133
  management of, 1132
 mallet finger, treatment of, 1133
 in replantation, repair of, 1077
 splinting for, 1131–1132
 tears
  severe closed, management of, 1230
  with small or medium-sized fragments,
   management of, 1230
  without bone fragment, management
   of, 1229–1230
 tenosynovitis, diagnosis of, 1165
 treatment of, 1131, 1134
  principles of, 1132–1134
External carotid artery
 course of, 206f
 ligation, for nasopharyngeal hemorrhage
  control, 410
 as recipient in microsurgical breast
  reconstruction, 873
External ear
 basal cell carcinoma of, 521–523
 squamous cell carcinoma of, 521–523
External fixation, of mandibular fractures,
 446, 446f
External genitalia. *See also* Female
 genitalia; Male genitalia
 differentiation of, 897
 embryology of, 921, 922f
 feminization of, 899–900
 masculinization of, 898–899
External jugular vein, course of, 206f
External mammary artery, course of, 823
External oblique muscle, course of, 753–
 754, 853
External oblique muscle flap, for hand
 coverage, 1068

External spermatic artery, 947f
External spermatic fascia, of scrotum, 947f
Extravasation injuries
 of foot, 1222f, 1222–1223
 of hand, 1222–1223
 prevention of, 1223
 treatment of, 1222–1223
Extremities. *See also* Lower extremity;
 Upper extremity
 embryology of, 1057–1063
 lymphedema of, 1279–1290
 position of, during development, 1061f,
 1061
 tissue expansion in, 111
Eye(s)
 bags or dark circles under, 648, 648f
 embryology of, 277
 hypofluoric acid injuries to, management
  of, 256
 management of, in facial reanimation,
  591t, 591–593
  ancillary procedures, 593
  control of antagonistic muscles, 593
  goals of, 591
  selection of appropriate procedure in,
   593
 Oriental-type, 643
 periocular pigmentation, 648
 protuberant, 644
 wrinkles around, 649
Eyebrow(s). *See also* Brow-lift
 aging-related changes in, 655, 656f
 arch, ideal, model for, 632, 646, 647f
 low, 644, 644f
  detection of, 646, 646f
 management, with facial paralysis, 593
 ptosis, 631–632, 644, 655–656, 657f
  detection of, 646, 646f
Eyebrow reconstruction, strip graft method
 for, 742, 743f
Eyelashes, loss of, after blepharoplasty, 652
Eyelash reconstruction, hair transplant for,
 551
Eyelid(s). *See also* Blepharoplasty
 aging-related changes in, 642, 655, 656f
 asymmetry
  after blepharoplasty, 652
  after eyelid reconstruction, 564
 baggy
  diagnosis of, 641
  etiology of, 641
  nomenclature for, 641
 basal cell carcinoma of, 551–552
 deformities of
  pathology of, 551–552
  reconstruction of, 551–565. *See also*
   Eyelid reconstruction
 ecchymoses. *See also* Ecchymosis,
  periorbital
  with maxillary fractures, 424
 full-thickness defects of margin, primary
  closure of, 556, 557f
 functions of, 551
 hemangioma of, 551
 injury to, treatment of, 404
 irregularities, after blepharoplasty, 652
 laxity, with facial paralysis, 592
 lower
  anatomical evaluation before
   blepharoplasty, 648–649
  anatomical variants, 648–649
  chemical peel, 666
  excess skin and orbicularis, 649
  festooning, 649, 649f
  irregularities, 649

Ganglions
  of dorsal wrist, 1167, 1167f
    differential diagnosis of, 1165
    features of, 1166
    frequency of, 1166
    pathogenesis of, 1166
  of flexor sheath (volar retinacular), 1167,
      1169f
    excision of, 1167, 1169f
  of hand, 1166–1167
    diagnosis of, 1165–1166
    differential diagnosis of, 1165
    etiology of, 1166
    frequency of, 1165
    management of, 1166–1167
    pathogenesis of, 1166
    sites for, 1166
    symptoms of, 1166
  intraosseous, symptoms of, 1166
  of volar wrist, 1167f–1168f
    with carpal arthritis, 1166
    frequency of, 1166
Gangrene, idiopathic, of scrotum, 917
Gardner's syndrome, 181, 498
Gastrocnemius muscle
  course of, 217, 217f
  vascular anatomy of, 42t
Gastrocnemius muscle flap
  lateral, leg reconstruction with, 1299,
      1300f
  medial, leg reconstruction with, 1299,
      1300f
Gastrocnemius myocutaneous flap
  lateral, leg reconstruction with, 1299–
      1300, 1301f
  medial, leg reconstruction with, 1299,
      1301f
Gastroepiploic arteries, 1033, 1034f
Gastrointestinal cancer, metastases, in
    neck, 605
Gastrointestinal tissue
  autologous transplants, vascularized, 966
  ischemia and hypoxia, metabolic
      consequences of, 968
Gender dysphoria, incidence of, 927
Gender identity, 927
Gender identity disorder, incidence of, 927
Gender identity programs, university-
    based, obstacles to formation of,
    928t
Gender reassignment surgery, 927–943
  contraindications to, 929
  female-to-male, 934–941
    ancillary procedures, 939–940
    complications of, 940–941
    phalloplasty, 935f–938f, 935–941
    surgical technique, 935–941
    urethroplasty, 935, 939, 939f–940f
  future trends in, 942–943
  male-to-female, 929–934
    body conformation and, 935f
    modified McIndoe skin graft method,
        931–932, 934f–935f
    penile flap method, 929–931, 930f–
        934f
    surgical techniques, 929–934
  patient preparation for, 929
  patient selection for, 927–929
  principles of, 929–942
  ratios of males to females requesting, 927
  results with, 941t, 941–942
Gender role, 927
Geniohyoid muscle, 435f, 436, 437f
  anatomy of, 433, 435f
  dermoid cyst involving, 603, 603f

Genioplasty, 365–369
  centering, 369
  as complementary procedure with other
      procedures, 368f–369f, 369
  jumping, 369
  lengthening, 369, 382f–384f
  reduction, 368f–369f, 369
  sliding advancement, 367
  staged serial, 369
Genital canal, 921
Genital fold, 897f
Genitalia. See also External genitalia;
      Female genitalia; Male genitalia
  embryology of, 895–900
Genital ridge, 895–896
Genital swellings, 921
Genital tract, formation of, 895
Genital tubercle, 895, 896f–897f, 898, 921
  in male, 898f
Genitofemoral nerve, 948f–949f
Gentleness, in handling of tissue, 17
Germ cells, primitive, 896
Giant cell–bearing lesions, of bone, in
      hand, 1187, 1188f
Giant cell reparative granuloma (epulides),
      499, 499f–500f, 1187
  of alveolar ridge, 455, 456f
  of bone
    recurrence rates, 1183
    treatment of, 1183
Giant cell tumor(s)
  of bone
    in hand, 1165, 1187, 1189f–1190f
      treatment of, 1187, 1189f–1190f
    recurrence rates, 1183
    treatment of, 1183
  of distal radius, 1187, 1189f–1190f
    resection of, vascularized bone transfer
        for, 1024f
    treatment of, 1187, 1189f–1190f
  of hand, frequency of, 1165
  of tendon sheath, 1177–1178
    features of, 1178, 1178f
    histology of, 1177–1178
    nerve compression with, 1178, 1179f
    recurrence of, 1178, 1180f
    treatment of, 1178, 1180f
Gigantism
  breast reduction for, 824f, 826, 827f
  hand, 1101–1102
    classification of, 1086
    partial, congenital, macrodactyly with,
        1101
Gigantomastia
  management of, 824f, 826, 827f
  unilateral, management of, 797
Girdles
  after aspirative lipoplasty, 774f, 774
  circumpress, 774f
Glabellar flap
  for dural repair, 513–514
  for eyelid reconstruction, 561f, 561–562
Glabellar frown, 656, 656f, 659, 659f
Glasgow Coma Scale, 410, 411t
Glaucoma, closed-angle, after
      blepharoplasty, 651
Glenoid fossa reconstruction, 359
Globe, evaluation of, with orbital fractures,
      427
Globulomaxillary cyst, 491–492, 492f
Glomus body, 964f
Glomus tumor
  in hand, 1193f, 1194
    treatment of, 1193f, 1194
  histopathology, 186, 186f

Glossopharyngeal nerve, course of, 276t,
      276
Glucosuria, in burn patient, 246
Gluteal thigh flap, 1005
  closure of greater trochanteric pressure
      sores with, 1269
  closure of ischial pressure sores with,
      1268, 1272f
  donor site territory, 979f
  innervated, for ischial reconstruction,
      1274
  unilateral tubed, for vaginoplasty, 923,
      924f
Gluteus gait, 58
Gluteus maximus muscle
  course of, 217, 217f
  vascular anatomy of, 41, 42t
Gluteus maximus musculocutaneous flap
  bilateral, closure of sacral pressure sores
      with, 1266f, 1268
  breast reconstruction with, 866, 868–870
  closure of ischial pressure sores with,
      1267f, 1268
  closure of sacral pressure sores with,
      1267f, 1268
  distal, closure of greater trochanteric
      pressure sores with, 1269
  inferior, closure of ischial pressure sores
      with, 1268
  inferior gluteal
    breast reconstruction with
      donor tissue selection for, 870
      flap dissection and insertion for, 870
    flap outline of, 869f
  superior gluteal
    anatomy of, 868, 869f
    breast reconstruction with, 865
      donor tissue selection for, 868
      flap dissection and insertion for, 869
    flap outline of, 869f
  total rotation, closure of sacral pressure
      sores with, 1268, 1268f
  V-Y advancement of, 42
Gluteus medius muscle, course of, 217,
      217f
Gluteus minimus muscle, course of, 217,
      217f
Glycogen-rich adenoma, of salivary gland,
      classification of, 200t
Glycosaminoglycans, 5–6
Gnathion, 324
Goldenhar syndrome, 356, 358–359
  treatment of, 358–359
Gold isotopes, for diagnosis of
      lymphedema, 1283
Gomco clamp, 901
Gonadotropins, effects of, and
      gynecomastia, 878t
Gonads
  fetal, onset of endocrine function in, 898
  primitive, 895
Gonion, 324
Goretex sling, for mouth reconstruction
      with facial paralysis, 584
Gracilis muscle
  course of, 217, 217f
  for facial reanimation, 585–587, 586f
  free transfer, nerve repair in, 1048, 1049f
  function, 1013
  innervation, 1013
  insertion, 1013
  motor nerve, 1013
  neurovascular pedicle to, 1014f
  origin, 1013
  physiology and biomechanics of, 1010

internal rigid fixation of, 392, 393f–395f
metastatic tumors involving, 502–506
miniplate systems for, 392–395
in multiple myeloma, 500, 502f
ossifying fibroma in, 504f, 506
osteogenic sarcoma of, 500, 501f
osteoid osteoma of, 498
osteomas of, 498, 498f–499f
Paget's disease in, 506
tumors of
  of bony origin, 500, 501f
  of mesodermal origin, 500, 501f
  of nonodontogenic origin, 496–500
  of odontogenic origin, 494–496
Maxillary arch bars, stabilization with
  supplementary wires, 406, 407f
Maxillary atresia, in Crouzon's syndrome,
  338
Maxillary bone graft, 321
Maxillary deformity
  with cleft lip, management of, 286–287
    orthodontics and orthopaedics for,
    286–287
  after cleft lip and palate repair, 311–313
  with lymphatic malformation, 238, 239f
Maxillary expansion devices, intraoral, for
  control of protruding premaxilla,
  290
Maxillary fracture(s). See also Le Fort
  fracture(s)
  cerebrospinal fluid rhinorrhea with, 412
  diagnosis of, 404
  reduction of, 410
  sagittal, 422–425, 423f–425f
    dental splint with, 422, 424f
    internal fixation, 422, 423f
    open reduction, 422, 423f
Maxillary growth, 372
Maxillary hypoplasia, correction of
  with bone or cartilage grafting, 312f,
  312–313
  Le Fort I advancement osteotomy for,
  312–313, 313f
Maxillary osteotomy, 385–398. See also Le
  Fort I osteotomy
  higher, requiring extraoral approaches,
  395. See also Le Fort II
  osteotomy; Le Fort III osteotomy
  Schuchardt procedure, 385
  segmental, 385, 386f–388f
  Wassmund procedure, 385, 386f–388f
Maxillary retrusion, in Pfeiffer syndrome,
  339
Maxillary sinus fracture, 418
Maxillectomy, total, reconstructive surgery
  for, 465f, 466
Maxillofacial injury. See also Midfacial
  fracture(s)
  airway obstruction with, emergency
    management of, 409–410
  aspiration with, emergency management
    of, 410
  associated injuries, evaluation for, 409
  cervical spine injury with, 410
  coma with, management of, 410–411
  early and definitive management of,
    indications for, 412
  emergency treatment of, 409–410
  evaluation of, 411–412
  hemorrhage with, emergency
    management of, 410
  and increased intracranial pressure,
    management of, 411
  preexisting facial symmetry with,
    demonstrating, 411

radiologic evaluation of, 411
soft tissue injury in, management of, 412
Maxillomandibular fixation, 440–443, 442f–
  443f
  airway control with, 450
  arch bar method, 440–441, 441f–442f
  in children, 450
  continuous loop fixation, 442–443, 443f
  with dental splints, 447
  duration of, 445
  indications for, 448–449
  with interosseous fixation of mandible,
    443
  with interosseous metal plate and screw
    method of fixation, 445
  with interosseous wire fixation of
    mandible, 443
  with Ivy loops, 441
  with Kazanjian button, 441–442, 442f
  with mandibular fractures, duration of,
    442–443
  noncontinuous loop fixation, 441–442,
    442f
  oral hygiene with, 439
  weight loss with, 439
McIndoe procedure, for Dupuytren's
  disease, 1160
McIndoe technique, of vaginal
  construction, 923, 923f
  modified, for male-to-female gender
    reassignment surgery, 931–932,
    934f–935f
McKissock pattern, for breast reduction,
  863
MCP joint. See Metacarpophalangeal joint
Measles sign, on vessel wall, 1075
Meatal stenosis
  and circumcision, 902
  with hypospadias repair, 914
Meckel's cartilage, embryology of, 273–276
Medial arm flap(s), 998, 1003
Medial canthal defect
  glabellar flap for, 561f, 561–562
  grafting technique for, 554, 554f
Median artery, embryology of, 1060
Median craniofacial dysrrhaphia, 341–342,
  342f
Median cubital vein, 981
Median forehead flap, 31t
Median nerve
  course of, 1123
  embryology of, 1060
  group fascicular repair, 1048
  partial injury, repair of, 1052f
Median nerve compression, at wrist, 1142
Median nerve division, diagnosis of, 1139
Median nerve injury
  diagnosis of, sensory area to test for,
    1139t
  effects on muscle function, 1138t
Median (naso-) palatine cyst, 492, 493f
Median raphe cyst, histopathology, 183
Median rhomboid glossitis, 456
Median vein of forearm, course of, 1119f
Mediastinitis
  major débridement for, 883
  management of
    with omental transposition flaps, 888f–
    890f, 891
    with pectoralis major muscle flaps,
    884f, 884–885
    with pectoralis major muscle rotation
    flap, 886f–887f
    with pectoralis major muscle turnover
    flap, 885, 885f–887f

by primary closure, 883–884
with rectus abdominis muscle flaps,
  886f–887f, 891
with rib grafts, 883
with skin grafts, 890f, 891
Medical-legal claims
  assisting defense attorney in, 1320–1321
  depositions for, 1321–1322
  discussion of, 1320
  expert witness testimony in, 1323–1324
  factors that cause patients to consult
    attorneys for, 1317
  interrogatories for, 1321
  investment of time in, 1320
  management of, 1319–1323
  patient planning to seek legal advice for
    identification of, 1317–1318
    management of, 1318
      advantages of, 1318
  prevention of, 1316–1319
    suggestions for, 1319
  testimony of treating physician not party
    to suit in, 1323
  trial for, 1322–1323
Medical-legal principles, 1309–1325
  damages, 1311
  duty, 1309–1310
  fraudulent concealment, 1311
  judgment, 1311
  negligence, 1310
  proximate cause, 1311
  standard of care, 1310
  statute of limitations, 1310–1311
Medical liability claims. See Medical-legal
  claims
Medical liability insurance, 1311–1312
  actions that may affect coverage, 1312
  basic policy, 1311
  claims made policy, 1312
  going bare, 1312
  irrevocable trusts, 1312
  occurrence policy, 1311–1312
  prior acts coverage, 1312
  reporting endorsement, 1312
  tail coverage, 1312
  types of coverage, 1311–1312
  umbrella policy, 1311
Medical negligence claims. See Medical-
  legal claims
Medical records
  accuracy of, 1315–1316
  altered, 1316
  correction of, 1315–1316
  dictated, accuracy of, 1315
  after the fact, 1316
  legibility of, 1316
  management of, uniform policies for,
    1319
  medical-legal significance of, 1314–
    1315
  not subject to accurate recall, 1316
  obliteration of entries in, 1316
  privileged, 1320
  promptness of, 1316
  securing and organizing, 1320
  validity of, 1316
Medpor, with orbital fractures, 428
Megalourethra, 903–904
  fusiform, 904
  scaphoid, 903
Meige's disease
  congenital anomalies associated with,
    1281
  presentation of, 1281
Meissner corpuscle, 1138t

Melanocytes, 3
  dermal, 170
  epidermal, 170
Melanocytic nevi
  clinical aspects, 172–174
  histopathology, 188–189
Melanoma, 141, 150–153
  acral lentiginous, 150, 152, 193, 194f,
        1165, 1176–1177
    histological features of, 193, 194f
    treatment of, 196
  adjuvant immunotherapy, 153
  amelanotic, 141, 150
    differential diagnosis of, 1171
  arising from giant congenital pigmented
        nevus, 171, 189
  BANS locations, 152–153
  benign juvenile, 151, 171–172
  biological behavior of, 152
  biopsy of, 151, 1176
  borderline, 151
  chemotherapy, 153, 197
  cutaneous
    biopsy, 193
    clinical presentation of, 195–196
    description of tumor invasion by
        Clark's Levels, 193, 193t
    histopathological types of, 193
    incidence of, 193
    prognostic factors, 193, 195f
    satellitosis, 193
    surgical management of, 193–198
    thickness, 193
    ulceration, 193
  desmoplastic, 150
  dysplastic nevus as precursor of, 151
  elective regional lymph node dissection,
        153
  elective versus therapeutic lymph node
        dissection with, 196–197
  epidemiology of, 150
  excision of, 1177
  of eyelids, 552
  five-year survival, 152
  follow-up, 153
  of hand
    diagnosis of, 1165
    frequency of, 1165
  histological types, 1176
  histology, 151
  immunotherapy for, 197–198
  incidence of, 150
  isolated regional perfusion, 153
  juvenile, histopathology, 190
  lentigo maligna, 144f, 150, 152, 174, 193,
        194f, 1176
    clinical presentation of, 195
    histological features of, 193, 194f
    prognosis of, 195
    treatment of, 195
  malignant
    Clark level II, of chest, 1176f
    differential diagnosis of, 151
    of hand, 1175–1177
    incidence of, 261
  versus melanocytic nevi, 188–189, 189t
  metastases, 152–153
  microscopic satellites, 144f, 152
  minimal deviation, 151
  mortality, 150
  in mucous membranes, 196
  nasal, reconstruction of, 195f, 196
  neurotropic, 150
  nevus-cell nevus, 171, 174
  nodular, 144f, 150–151, 193, 194f, 1176

histological features of, 193, 194f
  management of, 195–196
palmar, treatment of, 196
plantar, treatment of, 196, 196f
precursor lesions, 151
  surgical treatment, 153
prevalence of, 193
prognosis, 152, 1166
prognostic factors, 1176–1177
recurrent tumor, surgical removal of,
      153
resection margins, 152–153
risk factors, 1176
of salivary gland, classification of, 200t
at sites of preexisting pigmented lesions,
      151
in situ, 151
  excision, 153
of soft tissue, malignant. See Clear cell
      sarcoma
specific active immunotherapy for, 198
staging, 152
subungual, 196, 1177
and sun exposure, 150
superficial spreading, 144f, 150–152, 193,
      194f, 1176, 1176f
  histological features of, 193, 194f
  management of, 195–196
survival
  and depth, 152, 152t
  and location, 152, 152t
survival rates, 1177
treatment of, 152–153
and ultraviolet light, 260
unresectable, treatment of, 153
Melanoma in childhood. See Pigmented
      nevus, spitz
Melphalan, isolated regional perfusion
      with, for melanomas of extremity,
      153
Membranous adenoma, of salivary gland,
      classification of, 200t
Meningioma(s)
  of orbit and temporal area, 519, 521f
  of posterior cranial fossa, 524
Meningocele(s), 346
Menstrual period, breast during, 831
Mental nerve, 433, 434f
Mental retardation
  in Apert's syndrome, 338–339
  clinodactyly with, 1099
  in craniosynostosis syndromes, 337
  in Pfeiffer syndrome, 339
  in Saethre-Chotzen syndrome, 339
Menton, 323, 323f
Meperidine, side effects of, 1327
Mepivacaine (Carbocaine), drug
      interactions, 1328t, 1329
Meralgia paresthetica, 58
Merkel cell–neurite complex, 1138t
Mersilene mesh, 98
Mesh grafting, 25
Mesoderm, embryonic, 895
  proliferation of, 897f
Mesodermal skin tumors, clinical aspects,
      163–166
Mesonephric (wolffian) ducts, 896–897,
      897f, 899
Mesonephric fold, 897f
Mesonephros, 896, 896f–897f
Metabolic neuropathy, local peripheral
      nerve entrapment superimposed
      on, diagnosis of, 1139
Metacarpal bone(s)
  first (thumb)

absence of, with radial clubhand, 1087
  Matev distraction lengthening of,
      1206f, 1206–1208
head of, functional anatomy of, 1225
second, shortening of
  effects of, 1243
  management of, 1248–1249, 1249f
shaft malrotation of, management of,
      1248, 1248f
substance, loss of, management of,
      1249–1250, 1252f
third, shortening of
  effects of, 1243
  management of, 1248–1249, 1249f
Metacarpal fractures
  anatomic location of, 1244
  extra-articular, management of, 1246–
      1250
  of fifth metacarpal neck, management of,
      1246–1247
  of first (thumb) metacarpal base, intra-
      articular, 1254–1255
  frequency of, 1225
  internal fixation for, 1245–1246
  intra-articular, management of, 1250–
      1251
    options for, 1251
  management of, 1243–1246
    general concepts of, 1244–1246
    in noncompliant patients, 1257
    with minimal displacement, management
        of, 1247f, 1248
  multiple, management of, 1249, 1250f–
      1251f
  neck, management of, 1246–1248
  of second metacarpal, unstable, effects
        of, 1243
  shaft
    comminuted, management of, 1249–
        1250, 1252f
    spiral oblique, management of, 1244f,
        1245
    transverse and short oblique,
        management of, 1247f–1248f,
        1248–1249
  of third (index) metacarpal
    displaced comminuted midshaft,
        management of, 1248–1249,
        1249f
    oblique unstable, management of,
        1245, 1246f
    unstable, effects of, 1243
  of third (index) metacarpal diaphysis,
        oblique angulated displaced,
        management of, 1245f, 1245
Metacarpophalangeal joint
  arthrodesis of, indications for, 1251
  contracture, 1158
    correction of, 1158
      fasciectomy for, 1160–1161
      fasciotomy for, 1159
      wound management after, 1163
    with Dupuytren's disease, 1157
  dislocation
    with chip fracture, management of,
        1240
    complete, correction of
      longitudinal dorsal approach for, 1241
      palmar surgical approach for, 1241
      surgical approach for, 1241
    complete dorsal, of index finger,
        complications of, 1241
    dorsal
      biomechanics of, 1241
      complex, 1241

Radiation therapy—*continued*
and concurrent chemotherapy, for head and neck cancer, 469, 474–475
doses, 483. *See also* Radiation, dose
equipment for, 479–480
for head and neck cancer, 485
hyperfractionation, 483–484
and hyperthermia, 485
hypoxic cell sensitizers, 481, 484
after jejunal transplant for cervical esophagoplasty, 1038
of lymphatic malformations, 239
for malignant tumors of oral cavity, 459–460
complications of, 459
long-term effects of, 459–460
in multimodality therapy, 484–485
for neck masses, 462
for oral cavity carcinoma, aftereffects of, 1333
oxygen effect, 481
minimization of, 484
for parotid malignant tumors, 202
for pleomorphic adenoma of salivary gland, 201
postoperative, 484
preoperative, 484
for prostatic carcinoma, pelvic complications of, 1334, 1335f
radiobiological principles, 480–481
for salivary gland cancer, 208
postoperative, indications for, 206t, 208
shrinking field concept of, 483
for skin cancer, 486
skin changes induced by, 485
for soft tissue sarcoma, preoperative, with wide local excision, 216
and surgery, 484
surgery after, 485
therapeutic gain ratio, 483
of tongue tumors, 461
to treat keloid and hypertrophic scars, 11
treatment planning, 479
treatment simulator, 479
tumor regression after, 482
tumor response to, 480–481
for uterine cervical cancer, pelvic complications of, 1334, 1335f
Radiation ulcers, management of, 1333
Radical neck dissection, 462–466, 463f
Radicular cyst, 489, 490f
Radiobiology, principles of, 480–481
Radiography
Brewerton, of hand, 1250
of hand, 1166
of salivary gland tumors, 199
of soft tissue sarcoma, 211–213
Radioiodinated human serum albumin, ^{131}I-labeled, for diagnosis of lymphedema, 1283
Radioisotopes, monitoring skin flap viability with, 38
Radionecrosis, treatment of, 264
Radionuclide bone scanning, for bone tumors, 1166
Radionuclide imaging
with technetium-99 polyphosphate, of soft tissue sarcoma, 212–213, 213f
with technetium-99 stannous pyrophosphate, for diagnosis of muscle damage, 266
Radionuclide scanning, in head and neck, indications for, 459
Radiosensitivity, definition of, 480

Radiotherapy. *See* Radiation therapy
Radioulnar joint
replacement arthroplasty of, Darrach procedure for, 1148
rheumatoid arthritis in, treatment of, 1148
Radioulnar synostosis, etiology of, 1084
Radius. *See also under* Radial
absence of, with radial clubhand, 1087
as bone graft, 59
giant cell tumor of, 1187, 1189f–1190f
treatment of, 1187, 1189f–1190f
Radovan skin expander, for scalp expansion, 751
Ramus osteotomy, 363f
Ranula(s), 455, 455f
Ranula congenita, 231
Rash, from polyurethane implant, management of, 807–808
Raynaud's syndrome, ischemic ulcers in, 1295
Reading disabilities, in cleft lip/palate population, 330
Reconstructive surgery, lasers in, 124
Records. *See* Medical records
Rectum, 895, 896f
embryology of, 897
Rectus abdominis flap
elevation, 1017–1018
functional loss with removal of, 1017
incisions for, 1016f, 1017
size of, 1017
special problems with, 1018
Rectus abdominis muscle
bilateral, 887f
blood supply of, 886f
course of, 753, 853
as extended skin island musculocutaneous flap, 44, 45f
function, 1017
harvesting, 1016f
innervation, 1017
insertion, 1017
motor nerve, 1017
as muscle flap, 44, 45f
musculocutaneous perforators through, 44f
origin, 1017
sensory nerve, 1017
vascular anatomy of, 42t
vascular pedicle to, 1017f
vascular supply to, 1017
Rectus abdominis muscle flap
for hand coverage, 1068
island, thigh reconstruction with, 219f, 220
for leg reconstruction, 1305
management of mediastinitis with, 886f–887f, 891
Rectus abdominis musculocutaneous flap. *See also* Transverse rectus abdominis musculocutaneous flap
breast reconstruction with, contraindications to, 866
thigh reconstruction with, 219f, 220
Rectus abdominis myocutaneous flap, for phalloplasty, 952, 952f
Rectus abdominis myocutaneous flaps, 922
Rectus femoris muscle
course of, 217f, 870f–871f
vascular anatomy of, 42t
Red flare, correction of, 309, 309f
Reduction, definition of, 1228
Reduction mammaplasty. *See also* Breast reduction

and augmentation mammaplasty, sequence of, 797
body image distortion after, 1340
displacement of fibroglandular tissue after, 821
mammography after, 820f–821f, 821
motivation for, 1345
postoperative care for, 797
for ptosis, 829
results of, 795f
Rubin amputation procedure for, 824f
skin thickening and retraction after, 821
Reduction osteotomy, for macrodactyly, 1102
Reese drum dermatome, 22f
Reflex sympathetic dystrophy, with radial nerve laceration, 1132
Regnault incision, for abdominoplasty, 756f, 756
Reichert's cartilage, embryology of, 276
Reid thumb reconstruction, by pollicization of injured digit, 1203–1206, 1205f
Reifenstein's syndrome, gynecomastia in, 877
Renal failure, and infection, 1211
Reparative giant cell granuloma (epulides), 455, 456f, 499, 499f–500f
Replacement arthroplasty. *See specific procedure*
Replamineform, 56
Replantation, 1071–1081
after avulsion injury, 1079
bone fixation in, 1076–1077
contraindications to
absolute, 1071
relative, 1071
after crush injury, 1079
exercise(s) after. *See* Early protected motion
goal of, 1077
guidelines for, 1079–1080
history of, 1071
indications for, 1071–1072
instruments for, 1074
microsurgical, results of, 1079–1080
monitoring after, methods for, 1073
nerve grafts in, 1076
neural anastomosis in, 1077–1079
technique for, 1079
in operating room, preparation for, 1074–1075
preparation for, 1074
procedure for, 1075–1079
in psychotic self-amputee, 1071
results of, 1079–1080
revascularization for, 1075
tendon repair in, 1077, 1077f
use of leeches in, 1079
vascular anastomosis in, 1077–1079
vein grafting in, 1076
alternatives to, 1077–1078
incisions for, 1078, 1079f
sigmoid, 1079f
zig-zag, 1079f
Replant team, 1072–1073
operating room members, 1072
postoperative care members, 1072–1073
Reserpine
and gynecomastia, 878t
and nipple discharge, 879
Respiratory depression, drug-induced, reversal of, 1327
Rete testis, embryology of, 896
Retin-A, in pretreatment for chemical peel, 682

Touch perception, effect of nerve
    compression on, 1140
Tower skull. *See* Acrocephaly
Tracheostomy
    with facial injury, 399, 400f
    indications for, 409
    operative technique, 400f
Traction injury, on peripheral nerve, 1141–
    1142
    causes of, 1141
    diagnosis of, 1141
    treatment of, 1141–1142
TRAM flap. *See* Transverse rectus
    abdominis musculocutaneous flap
Transabdominal rectus myocutaneous flap,
    breast reconstruction with, 797
Transforming growth factor-beta, in wound
    healing, 10
Transsexualism, 927
    alternative (nonsurgical) treatment
        methods, 942
    diagnosis of, principles of, 928
    diagnostic criteria for, 928
    differential diagnosis, 928
    as disease, 927
    gender reassignment surgery for, 929–942
    male, gender reassignment surgery for
        and accessory feminizing operations,
            941, 942f
        postoperative complications with, 941,
            942t
    multidisciplinary approach to, 928
    nontreatment of
        follow-up and comparison to treatment
            group, 941–942
        social and personal costs of, 928
Transverse abdominal island flap. *See also*
    Transverse rectus abdominis
        musculocutaneous flap
    bilateral breast reconstruction with,
        perioperative management of, 855
    bipedicled, breast reconstruction with,
        perioperative management of, 855
    blood supply of, 853, 853f, 865
    breast reconstruction with, 851–864
        abdominal wall repair in, procedure
            for, 860–861, 860f–861f
        aesthetic management of contralateral
            breast in, 863–864
        assessment of abdominal tissue
            available for, 852
        benefits of, 865
        chest wall exposure in, 857
        complications of, 864, 864t
        contraindications to, 851–852
        flap and pedicle design for, 855–857
        flap elevation and vascular pedicle
            isolation for, 857–860, 858f–860f
        flap loss in, 864
        after Halstead radical mastectomy, 851
        indications for, relative, 851
        after modified mastectomy, 851
        operative plan for, 856, 857f
        operative procedures for, 857–863
        patient risk factor classification for,
            852t, 852
        patient selection for, 851
        perioperative management of, 855
        postoperative care for, 863
        risk factors, 851–852, 852t
        after salvage mastectomy, 851
        shaping of new breast in, 861–863,
            862f–863f
        for subcutaneous mastectomy cripple,
            851

vascular pedicle options for, 856f
    chest reconstruction with, 851, 864
    double, breast reconstruction with
        flap elevation and vascular pedicle
            isolation in, 859
        operative technique for, 857
    hemodynamics of, 855
    innervation of, 854
    muscle and fascia of, 853, 853f
    pertinent anatomy, 853–855
    single
        bilateral breast reconstruction with,
            flap elevation and vascular pedicle
            isolation, 859
        breast reconstruction with
            operative technique for, 857
            perioperative management of, 855
            vascular pedicle options for, 856f,
                856
Transverse cervical artery flap, donor site
    territory, 979f
Transverse cervical flap, 1005
Transverse perineal muscle, 946f
Transverse rectus abdominis
    musculocutaneous flap, 1010. *See
    also* Transverse abdominal island
    flap
    microvascular, breast reconstruction
        with, 865
        donor tissue selection for, 867–868
        flap dissection and insertion for, 868
Transverse retinacular ligament, course of,
    1131
Transversus abdominis muscle, course of,
    753, 853
Transvestism
    and gender reassignment surgery, 942
    versus transsexualism, 928
Trapezium, absence of, with radial
    clubhand, 1087
Trapezium replacement arthroplasty
    considerations in, 1153–1155
    postoperative care after, 1154
    for rheumatoid arthritis, results of, 1154
    with Swanson prosthesis, 1153, 1154f
Trapezius muscle
    embryology of, 1063
    vascular anatomy of, 42t
Trapezius muscle flap, for cheek
    reconstruction, 535f, 536
Trapezius myocutaneous flap, for head and
    neck, 466
Trauma, and metabolic status, 6–7
Traumatic bone cyst, of mandible and
    maxilla, 494, 494f
Traumatic cutaneous injuries, 129–133. *See
    also* Traumatic wounds
    involving soft tissue, repair of, 129–133
    repair of, 129–133
Traumatic wounds. *See also* Traumatic
    cutaneous injuries
    acute, closure of, 131
    bacterial cultures, 130
    bacterial evaluation of, 130
    clinical evaluation of patient with, 130
    contaminated
        bacterial control in, 132
        biological dressings for, 132
        closure of, 132
    contamination of, 129
        chronic, 131–132
        diagnosis of degree of, 130
    débridement of, 131
    delayed closure, 131
    dressings for, 132

evaluation of, 130
irrigation, 131
preparation for closure, 131
primary repair, 131
spontaneous closure, 131
tetanus immunoprophylaxis with, 131
tissue culture, 130
Treacher Collins–Franceschetti complex,
    352–356, 353f–356f
    alveolar bone and palate in, 354
    associated malformations, 354
    bony deficits of, 353
    buccal commissure in, 354
    cheek in, 354
    chin in, 354
    choanal atresia in, 354
    ear and facial nerve in, 354
    eyebrow in, 354
    eyes in, 353
    genetics of, 352–353
    lacrimal apparatus in, 354
    lateral canthus in, 354
    lower eyelid in, 353
    malar bone in, 354
    mandible in, 354
    maxilla and maxillary sinus in, 354
    nose in, 354
    orbit in, 354
    temporal region and muscles in, 354
    temporomandibular joint in, 354
    treatment of, 355–356, 355f–356f
    upper eyelid in, 354
Treacher Collins syndrome, 340. *See also*
    Treacher Collins–Franceschetti
    complex
    craniofacial clefts in, 345
Treatment and care, closure of, modifying
    exposure during, 1312–1314
Tretinoin, to treat basal cell carcinoma, 147
Triamcinolone, and keloid regression, 11
Triangulation technique, for microvascular
    anastomosis, 972, 972f
Triceps brachii muscle, 999f
Triceps muscle
    course of, 216, 217f, 1119f
    effects of nerve injury on, 1138t
Trichilemmal cyst, 163
Trichoadenoma, 177
Trichoepithelioma(s), 145
    clinical aspects, 160
    desmoplastic, 177
    histopathology, 177, 178f
    multiple, 177
        treatment of, 177
    solitary, 177
        treatment of, 177
Trichofolliculoma, 159
    histopathology, 177–178, 178f
Tricholemmoma
    and breast cancer, 178
    histopathology, 178
Tricyclic antidepressants, effects of, and
    gynecomastia, 878t
Trigeminal nerve, course of, 276t, 276, 302
Trigger finger, congenital, 1097
Trigger thumb, congenital, 1097
Trigonocephaly, 335, 336f
Trimetrexate, for head and neck cancer,
    471
Tripier (bipedicled) flap, for eyelid
    reconstruction, 560, 560f
Trisomy D, 921
Trisomy E, 921
Trochanteric pressure sores. *See* Greater
    trochanteric pressure sores